CONTEMPORARY ORTHODONTICS

CONTEMPORARY ORTHODONTICS

Fourth Edition

4

William R. Proffit, DDS, PhD
Kenan Professor and Chairman
Department of Orthodontics
School of Dentistry
University of North Carolina
Chapel Hill, North Carolina

Henry W. Fields, Jr., DDS, MS, MSD
Professor and Head
Section of Orthodontics
College of Dentistry
The Ohio State University
Chief, Section of Orthodontics
Department of Dentistry
Columbus Children's Hospital
Columbus, Ohio

David M. Sarver, DMD, MS
Private Practice of Orthodontics
Birmingham, Alabama
Adjunct Professor
Department of Orthodontics
School of Dentistry
University of North Carolina
Chapel Hill, North Carolina

MOSBY
ELSEVIER

Contemporary Orthodontics, 4/e
Proffit

MOSBY
An imprint of Elsevier
11830 Westline Industrial Drive
St. Louis, Missouri 63146

Original ISBN : 978-0-323-04046-4

Notice

Knowledge and best practice in this field are constantly changing. As new research and experience broaden our knowledge, changes in practice, treatment and drug therapy may become necessary or appropriate. Readers are advised to check the most current information provided (i) on procedures featured or (ii) by the manufacturer of each product to be administered, to verify the recommended dose or formula,the method and duration of administration, and contraindications. It is the responsibility of the practitioner, relying on experience and knowledge of the patient, to make diagnoses, to determine dosages and the best treatment for each individual patient, and to take all appropriate safety precautions. To the fullest extent of the law, neither the Publisher nor the Authors assume any liability for any injury and/or damage to persons or property arising out or related to any use of the material contained in this book.

THE PUBLISHER

First Printed in India 2007
Reprinted 2007

Indian Reprint ISBN : 978-81-312-0868-7

Published by Elsevier, a division of Reed Elsevier India Private Limited, Sri Pratap Udyog, 274, Captain Gaur Marg, Sriniwaspuri, New Delhi-110 065 (India).

Printed and bound at Gopsons Papers Ltd., NOIDA.

This edition is dedicated to our wives
Sara, Anne, and Valerie, respectively,
whose tolerance is best described as remarkable

PREFACE

As in previous editions, the objective of *Contemporary Orthodontics* is to provide a comprehensive overview of this subject that is accessible to students, useful for residents, and a valuable reference for practitioners. Our goal has been to put information into a perspective that facilitates clinical use in a rational way. In each section of the book, and often in individual chapters, basic background information that every dentist needs is covered first, followed by more detailed information for orthodontic residents and specialist practitioners.

This fourth edition differs from its predecessors in being more illustrated, but it follows the basic outline of previous editions. New aspects include a discussion of orthodontics as an enhancement technology (an important new way of thinking about need for treatment in all medical fields), an increased emphasis on soft tissue consideration and clinical examination in diagnosis and treatment planning, a particular focus on basing clinical decisions on data instead of on anecdote and opinion, new material on the use of implant anchorage and possible applications of distraction osteogenesis, and consideration of the changes in orthodontic technique as computer applications to appliance design become more widespread.

Literature citations in this book are of two types: the classic papers in orthodontics that are the background for current concepts, and recent contributions to the literature that not only provide current information but cite the previous publications in this particular area. These papers can open the door to a more detailed evaluation of the literature on important subjects, and are cited partly for that purpose—which reduces what would otherwise be a voluminous number of references.

For use in the dental curriculum and residency programs, the book now is also available separately in an "E-dition", which provides access to the book's own website. The E-dition provides a searchable text, which makes it easier to quickly find the answer to clinical questions. For dental students, this has proved to be a major advantage of electronic editions. In addition, the E-dition places selected illustrations from the book in a downloadable format for easier use in teaching and continuing education. The website is updated frequently to provide evaluation and commentary on current orthodontic literature.

In addition, the book is supplemented with extensive computer-based teaching materials that are compatible with delivery to students via high-speed Internet access. They are also available in CD/DVD format for both Windows and Macintosh operating systems, and have been evaluated with both dental students and advanced general dentistry residents. These programs are most useful when they serve as a major part of the background for interactive small group seminars. Suggested outlines and visuals for these seminars also are available. All of the teaching programs now include computer self-tests (for instruction, not evaluation). These self-tests not only tell students if they have correctly answered questions about the material they just studied, but also they tell them why answers are correct or incorrect and display appropriate graphics (e.g.,graphs,clinical photos) to reinforce the message.

Further information about these supplemental teaching materials, including computer teaching programs and computer self-tests, seminar outlines and visuals, and tests for evaluation, can be obtained by contacting the Department of Orthodontics, University of North Carolina School of Dentistry, Chapel Hill, NC 27599-7450, or by visiting the department's website at www.dent.unc.edu/depts/academic/ortho/.

ACKNOWLEDGMENTS

We thank Ramona Hutton-Howe for outstanding photographic support and preparation of the image files (which contain nearly 1000 new color images for this edition), and Faith Patterson for careful organization and management of the revision. Particular thanks also go to Drs. William Gierie and Dirk Weichmann for their generous sharing of clinical experience and illustrations, to Drs. Steve Dickens, Eric Bednar, and Jared Blacker for assistance during their orthodontic residency programs in locating photos and radiographs in the UNC files, and soon-to-be Drs. Kenneth Miller and Elizabeth Kelly for diligent work in scanning color slides. Orthodontic residents in the classes of 2004-2007 at Ohio State were a valuable resource in helping procure clinical illustrative material. Thanks also go to a number of individuals who have reviewed areas of the manuscript and kindly contributed illustrations; specific acknowledgment is provided at appropriate points throughout the book.

William R. Proffit
Henry W. Fields, Jr.
David M. Sarver

CONTENTS

SECTION I
THE ORTHODONTIC PROBLEM

SECTION II
THE DEVELOPMENT OF ORTHODONTIC PROBLEMS

SECTION III
DIAGNOSIS AND TREATMENT PLANNING

SECTION IV
BIOMECHANICS, MECHANICS, AND CONTEMPORARY ORTHODONTIC APPLIANCES

SECTION V
TREATMENT IN PREADOLESCENT CHILDREN

SECTION VI
COMPREHENSIVE ORTHODONTIC TREATMENT IN THE EARLY PERMANENT DENTITION

SECTION VII
TREATMENT IN ADULTS

CONTEMPORARY ORTHODONTICS

SECTION

I

THE ORTHODONTIC PROBLEM

CHAPTER 1

Malocclusion and Dentofacial Deformity in Contemporary Society

CHAPTER OUTLINE

THE CHANGING GOALS OF ORTHODONTIC TREATMENT

Crowded, irregular, and protruding teeth have been a problem for some individuals since antiquity, and attempts to correct this disorder go back at least to 1000 BC. Primitive (and surprisingly well designed) orthodontic appliances have been found in both Greek and Etruscan materials.[1] As dentistry developed in the eighteenth and nineteenth centuries, a number of devices for the "regulation" of the teeth were described by various authors and apparently used sporadically by the dentists of that era.

After 1850, the first texts that systematically described orthodontics appeared, the most notable being Norman Kingsley's *Oral Deformities*.[2] Kingsley, who had a tremendous influence on American dentistry in the latter half of the nineteenth century, was among the first to use extraoral force to correct protruding teeth. He was also a pioneer in the treatment of cleft palate and related problems.

Despite the contributions of Kingsley and his contemporaries, their emphasis in orthodontics remained the alignment of the teeth and the correction of facial proportions. Little attention was paid to bite relationships, and since it was common practice to remove teeth for many dental problems, extractions for crowding or malalignment were frequent. In an era when an intact dentition was a rarity, the details of occlusal relationships were considered unimportant.

In order to make good prosthetic replacement teeth, it was necessary to develop a concept of occlusion, and this occurred in the late 1800s. As the concepts of prosthetic occlusion developed and were refined, it was natural to extend this to the natural dentition. Edward H. Angle (Figure

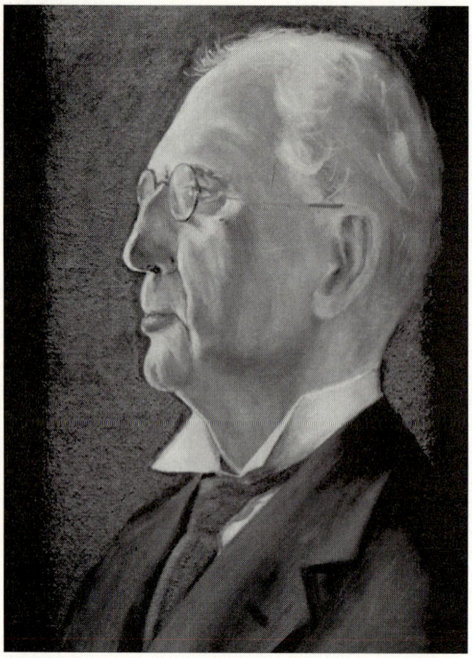

Figure 1-1 Edward H. Angle in his fifties, as the proprietor of the Angle School of Orthodontia. After establishing himself as the first dental specialist, Angle operated proprietary orthodontic schools from 1905 to 1928 in St. Louis; New London, Connecticut; and Pasadena, California, in which many of the pioneer American orthodontists were trained.

1-1), whose influence began to be felt about 1890, can be credited with much of the development of a concept of occlusion in the natural dentition. Angle's original interest was in prosthodontics, and he taught in that department in the dental schools at Pennsylvania and Minnesota in the 1880s. His increasing interest in dental occlusion and in the treatment necessary to obtain normal occlusion led directly to his development of orthodontics as a specialty, with himself as the "father of modern orthodontics."

The development of Angle's classification of malocclusion in the 1890s was an important step in the development of orthodontics because it not only subdivided major types of malocclusion but also included the first clear and simple definition of normal occlusion in the natural dentition. Angle's postulate was that the upper first molars were the key to occlusion and that the upper and lower molars should be related so that the mesiobuccal cusp of the upper molar occludes in the buccal groove of the lower molar. If the teeth were arranged on a smoothly curving line of occlusion (Figure 1-2) and this molar relationship existed (Figure 1-3), then normal occlusion would result.[3] This statement, which 100 years of experience has proved to be correct—except when there are aberrations in the size of teeth—brilliantly simplified normal occlusion.

Angle then described three classes of malocclusion, based on the occlusal relationships of the first molars:

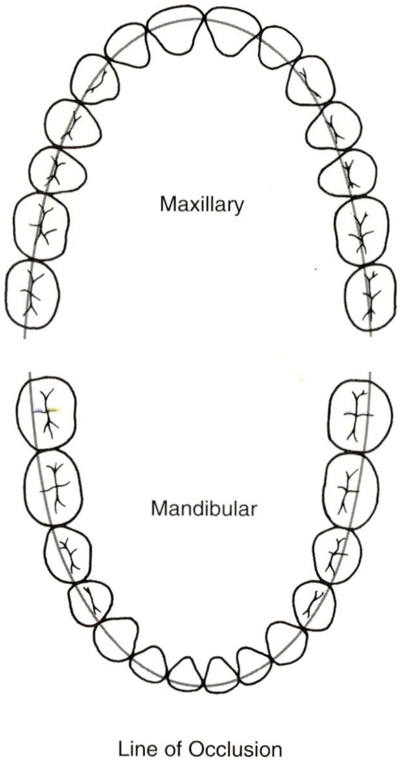

Figure 1-2 The line of occlusion is a smooth (catenary) curve passing through the central fossa of each upper molar and across the cingulum of the upper canine and incisor teeth. The same line runs along the buccal cusps and incisal edges of the lower teeth, thus specifying the occlusal as well as interarch relationships once the molar position is established.

Class I: Normal relationship of the molars, but line of occlusion incorrect because of malposed teeth, rotations, or other causes

Class II: Lower molar distally positioned relative to upper molar, line of occlusion not specified

Class III: Lower molar mesially positioned relative to upper molar, line of occlusion not specified

Note that the Angle classification has four classes: normal occlusion, Class I malocclusion, Class II malocclusion, and Class III malocclusion (see Figure 1-3). Normal occlusion and Class I malocclusion share the same molar relationship but differ in the arrangement of the teeth relative to the line of occlusion. The line of occlusion may or may not be correct in Class II and Class III.

With the establishment of a concept of normal occlusion and a classification scheme that incorporated the line of occlusion, by the early 1900s, orthodontics was no longer just the alignment of irregular teeth. Instead, it had evolved into the treatment of malocclusion, defined as any deviation from the ideal occlusal scheme described by Angle. Since precisely defined relationships required a full complement of teeth in both arches, maintaining an intact dentition became an important goal of orthodontic treatment. Angle and his

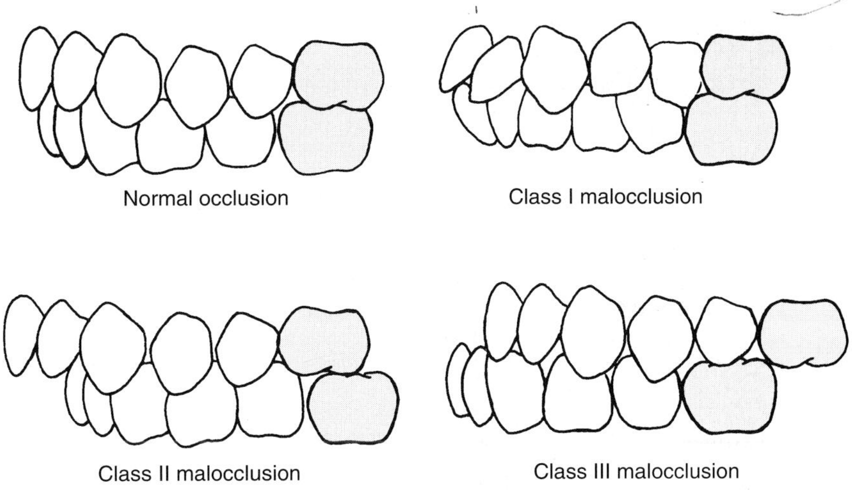

FIGURE 1-3 Normal occlusion and malocclusion classes as specified by Angle. This classification was quickly and widely adopted early in the twentieth century. It is incorporated within all contemporary descriptive and classification schemes.

followers strongly opposed extraction for orthodontic purposes. With the emphasis on dental occlusion that followed, however, less attention came to be paid to facial proportions and esthetics. Angle abandoned extra-oral force because he decided this was not necessary to achieve proper occlusal relationships.

As time passed, it became clear that even an excellent occlusion was unsatisfactory if it was achieved at the expense of proper facial proportions. Not only were there esthetic problems, it often proved impossible to maintain an occlusal relationship achieved by prolonged use of heavy elastics to pull the teeth together as Angle and his followers had suggested. Extraction of teeth was reintroduced into orthodontics in the 1930s to enhance facial esthetics and achieve better stability of the occlusal relationships.

Cephalometric radiography, which enabled orthodontists to measure the changes in tooth and jaw positions produced by growth and treatment, came into widespread use after World War II. These radiographs made it clear that many Class II and Class III malocclusions resulted from faulty jaw relationships, not just malposed teeth. By use of cephalometrics, it also was possible to see that jaw growth could be altered by orthodontic treatment. In Europe, the method of "functional jaw orthopedics" was developed to enhance growth changes, while in the United States, extraoral force came to be used for this purpose. At present, both functional and extraoral appliances are used internationally to control and modify growth and form.

In the early 21st century, orthodontics differs from what was done previously in three important ways:

1. There is more emphasis now on dental and facial appearance. This reflects a greater awareness that parents and patients seek treatment largely because of concern about facial appearance, and that psychosocial problems related to appearance can have major effects on an individual's quality of life. The advent of orthognathic surgery has made it possible to correct facial disproportions that previously were not treatable, and the development of computer imaging methods that allow the orthodontist to share facial concerns with patients in a way that was not possible until recently;
2. Patients now expect and are granted a greater degree of involvement in planning treatment. No longer is it appropriate for the paternalistic doctor to simply tell patients what treatment they should have. Now patients are given the opportunity to participate in selecting among treatment options—a process that is facilitated by computer imaging methods; and
3. Orthodontics now is offered much more frequently to older patients as part of a multidisciplinary treatment plan involving other dental and medical specialties. The goal is not necessarily the best possible dental occlusion or facial esthetics but the best chance for long-term maintenance of the dentition. This increased emphasis on treatment coordinated with other dentists has the effect of integrating orthodontics back into the mainstream of dentistry, from which Angle's teachings had tended to separate it.

All three of these recent developments are reflected in the later chapters of this book. The change in the goals of treatment represents a paradigm shift, away from an emphasis on skeletal and dental relationships and toward greater consideration of the oral and facial soft tissues. The soft tissues now are recognized as both the major limitation on orthodontic treatment and the major consideration in whether treatment can be judged to be successful.[4,5] Table 1-1 contrasts the Angle paradigm that dominated 20th century orthodontics with the soft tissue paradigm that is replacing it. The impact on diagnosis and treatment planning that the new paradigm requires is readily apparent, and is emphasized in the clinical chapters that follow.

It must be kept in mind that orthodontics is shaped by biological, psychosocial, and cultural determinants. For that reason, in defining the goals of orthodontic treatment, one has to consider not only morphologic and functional factors, but a wide range of psychosocial and bioethical issues as well.

TABLE 1-1

Angle versus Soft Tissue Paradigms: A New Way of Looking at Treatment Goals

Parameter	Angle paradigm	Soft tissue paradigm
Primary treatment goal	Ideal dental occlusion	Normal soft tissue proportions and adaptations
Secondary goal	Ideal jaw relationships	Functional occlusion
Hard/soft tissue relationships	Ideal hard tissue proportions produce ideal soft tissues	Ideal soft tissue proportions define ideal hard tissues
Diagnostic emphasis	Dental casts, cephalometric radiographs	Clinical examination of intra-oral and facial soft tissues
Treatment approach	Obtain ideal dental and skeletal relationships, assume the soft tissues will be OK	Plan ideal soft tissue relationships and then place teeth and jaws as needed to achieve this
Function emphasis	TM joint in relation to dental occlusion	Soft tissue movement in relation to display of teeth
Stability of result	Related primarily to dental occlusion	Related primarily to soft tissue pressure/equilibrium effects

These are discussed briefly in the sections of this chapter on need and demand for treatment, and in greater detail in Chapters 6-8.

The treatment sequence shown in Figures 1-4 through 1-7 demonstrates the facial as well as dental changes that can be attained through orthodontics. The focus of modern orthodontic treatment is on improving not only dental and skeletal but also soft tissue aspects of orthodontic problems, in combination with other dental treatment as needed.

THE USUAL ORTHODONTIC PROBLEMS: EPIDEMIOLOGY OF MALOCCLUSION

What Angle defined as normal occlusion more properly should be considered the ideal, especially when his criteria are applied strictly. In fact, perfectly interdigitating teeth arranged along a perfectly regular line of occlusion are quite rare. For many years, epidemiologic studies of malocclusion suffered from considerable disagreement among the investigators about how much deviation from the ideal should be accepted within the bounds of normal. As a result, between 1930 and 1965, the prevalence of malocclusion in the United States was variously estimated as 35% to 95%. These tremendous disparities were largely the result of the investigators' differing criteria for normal.

By the 1970s, a series of studies by public health or university groups in most developed countries provided a reasonably clear worldwide picture of the prevalence of various occlusal relationships or malrelationships. In the United States, two large-scale surveys carried out by the Division of Health Statistics of the U.S. Public Health Service (USPHS) covered children ages 6 to 11 between 1963 and 1965 and youths ages 12 to 17 between 1969 and 1970.[6,7] As part of a large-scale national survey of health care problems and needs in the United States in 1989-1994 (National Health and Nutrition Estimates Survey III, abbreviated as NHANES III), estimates of malocclusion again were obtained. This study of some 14,000 individuals was statistically designed to provide weighted estimates for approximately 150 million persons in the sampled racial/ethnic and age groups. The data provide current information for U.S. children and youths and include the first good data set for malocclusion in adults, with separate estimates for the major racial/ethnic groups.[8,9]

The characteristics of malocclusion evaluated in NHANES III included the irregularity index, a measure of incisor alignment (Figure 1-8), the prevalence of midline diastema >2 mm (Figure 1-9), and the prevalence of posterior crossbite (Figure 1-10). In addition, overjet (Figure 1-11) and overbite/open bite (Figure 1-12) were measured. Overjet, which reflects Angle's Class II and Class III molar relationships, can be evaluated much more precisely under epidemiologic evaluation conditions, so molar relationship was not evaluated directly.

Current data for these characteristics of malocclusion for children (age 8 to 11), youths (age 12 to 17) and adults (age 18 to 50) in the U.S. population, taken from NHANES III, are shown in Tables 1-2 and 1-3 and are displayed graphically in Figures 1-13 to 1-16.

Note that in the age 8-11 age group, just over half of U.S. children have well-aligned incisors. The rest have varying degrees of malalignment and crowding. The percent with excellent alignment decreases in the age 12-17 group as the remaining permanent teeth erupt, then remains essentially stable in the upper arch but worsens in the lower arch for adults. Only 34% of adults have well-aligned lower incisors.

Nearly 15% of adolescents and adults have severely or extremely irregular incisors, so that major arch expansion or extraction of some teeth would be necessary to align them.

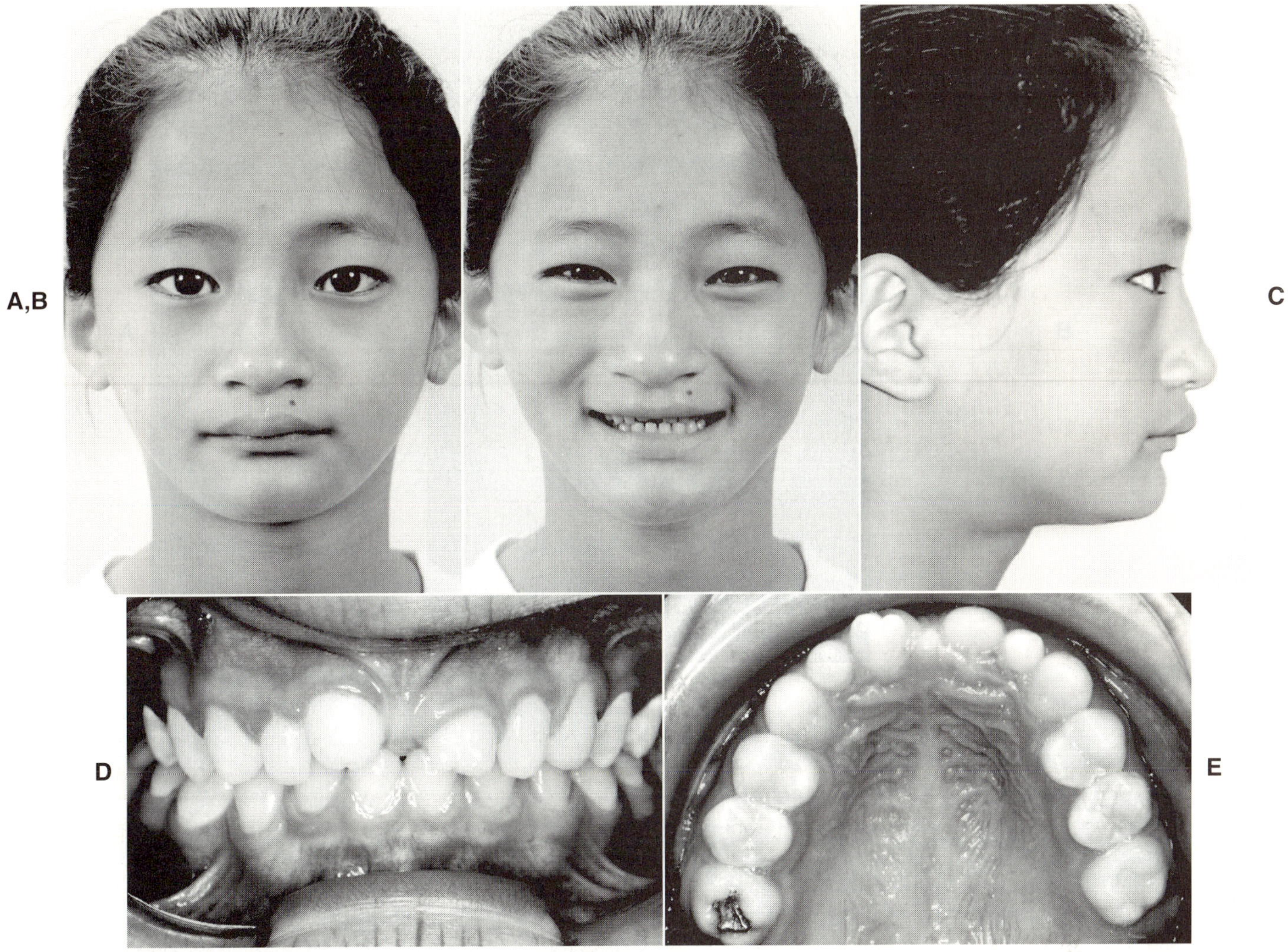

Figure 1-4 Pre-treatment facial and dental views of an 11-year-old girl. She and her parents were concerned about her facial appearance, especially the "no teeth" appearance on smile, and her difficulty in eating. **A,** On the frontal view of the face, short lower face height in proportion to facial width, a short upper lip and minimal display of the vermilion borders of the lips, and a deep labiomental fold were apparent. **B,** On smile, there was only 1 mm display of the upper incisors, which were malformed and quite small. **C,** On the profile view, an everted upper lip, short face height and incomplete development of the nose were noted. **D-E,** Intraoral examination revealed malformed maxillary incisors and short crown heights. Note the deep bite anteriorly.

A wide space between the maxillary central incisors (midline diastema) often is present in childhood (26% have >2 mm space). Although this space tends to close, over 6% of youths and adults still have a noticeable diastema that compromises the appearance of the smile. Blacks are more than twice as likely to have a midline diastema than whites or Hispanics ($p < .001$).

Posterior crossbite reflects deviations from ideal occlusion in the transverse plane of space, overjet or reverse overjet indicate antero-posterior deviations in the Class II/Class III direction, and overbite/open bite indicate vertical deviations from ideal. As Table 1-2 shows, posterior crossbite is relatively rare at all ages. Overjet of 5 mm or more, suggesting Angle's Class II malocclusion, occurs in 23% of children, 15% of youths, and 13% of adults. Reverse overjet, indicative of Class III malocclusion, is much less frequent. This affects about 1% of American children and increases slightly in youths and adults. Severe Class II and Class III problems, at the limit of orthodontic correction, occur in about 4% of the population, with severe Class II much more prevalent. Severe Class II problems are less prevalent, and severe Class III problems are more prevalent, in the Hispanic than the white or black groups.

Vertical deviations from the ideal overbite of 0-2 mm are less frequent in adults than children but occur in half the adult population, the great majority of whom have excessive overbite. Severe deep bite (overbite ≥ 5 mm) is found in nearly 20% of children and 13% of adults, while open bite

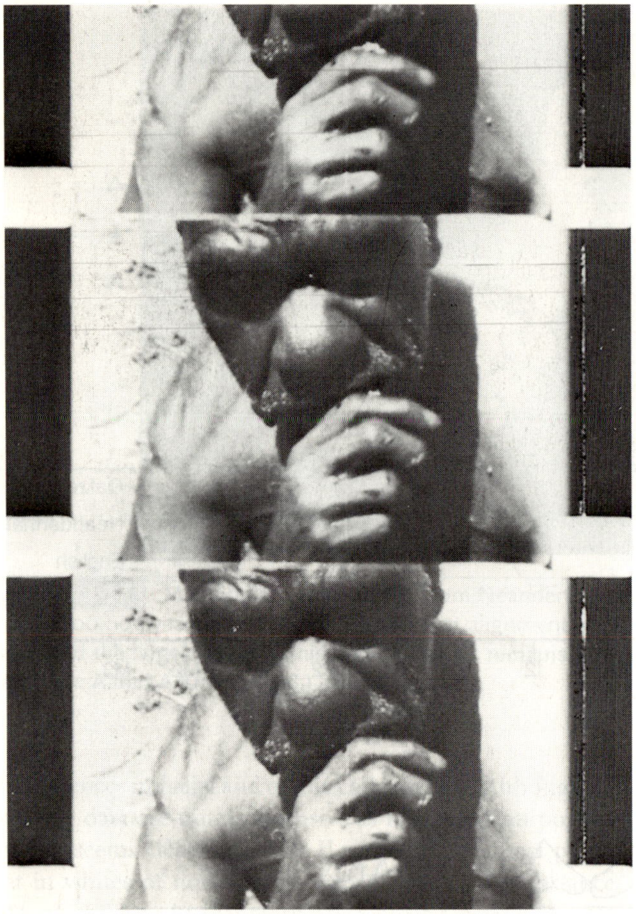

FIGURE 1-20 Sections from a 1960s movie of an Australian aboriginal man eating a kangaroo prepared in the traditional fashion. Note the activity of muscles, not only in the facial region, but throughout the neck and shoulder girdle. (Courtesy M.J. Barrett.)

but a reduction in jaw size related to disuse atrophy is hard to document, and the parallel with stress-related diseases can be carried only so far. Although it is difficult to know the precise cause of any specific malocclusion, we do know in general what the etiologic possibilities are, and these are discussed in some detail in Chapter 5.

What difference does it make if you have a malocclusion? Let us consider now the reasons for orthodontic treatment.

NEED AND DEMAND FOR ORTHODONTIC TREATMENT

Need for Orthodontic Treatment

Protruding, irregular, or maloccluded teeth can cause three types of problems for the patient: (1) discrimination because of facial appearance; (2) problems with oral function, including difficulties in jaw movement (muscle incoordination or pain), temporomandibular joint dysfunction (TMD), and problems with mastication, swallowing or speech; and (3) greater susceptibility to trauma, periodontal disease or tooth decay.

Psychosocial Problems

A number of studies in recent years have confirmed what is intuitively obvious, that severe malocclusion is likely to be a social handicap. The usual caricature of an individual who is none too bright includes protruding upper incisors. A witch not only rides a broom, she has a prominent lower jaw that would produce a Class III malocclusion. Well-aligned teeth and a pleasing smile carry positive status at all social levels and ages, whereas irregular or protruding teeth carry negative status.[15-17] Appearance can and does make a difference in teachers' expectations and therefore student progress in school, in employability, and in competition for a mate. Tests of the psychologic reactions of individuals to various dental conditions, carried out by showing photographs of various mouths to the individual whose response was being evaluated, show that cultural differences are smaller than might have been anticipated. A dental appearance pleasing to Americans was also judged pleasing in Australia and East Germany, whereas a dental appearance considered in the United States to carry with it some social handicap drew about the same response in these other cultural settings.[18] Protruding incisors are judged unattractive within populations where most individuals have prominent teeth, just as they are within less protrusive groups.[19]

There is no doubt that social responses conditioned by the appearance of the teeth can severely affect an individual's whole adaptation to life. This places the concept of "handicapping malocclusion" in a larger and more important context. If the way you interact with other individuals is affected constantly by your teeth, your dental handicap is far from trivial. It is interesting that psychic distress caused by disfiguring dental or facial conditions is not directly proportional to the anatomic severity of the problem. An individual who is grossly disfigured can anticipate a consistently negative response. An individual with an apparently less severe problem (e.g., a protruding chin or irregular incisors) is sometimes treated differently because of this but sometimes not. It seems to be easier to cope with a defect if other people's responses to it are consistent rather than if they are not. Unpredictable responses produce anxiety and can have strong deleterious effects.[20]

The impact of a physical defect on an individual also will be strongly influenced by that person's self-esteem. The result is that the same degree of anatomic abnormality can be merely a condition of no great consequence to one individual but a genuinely severe problem to another. It seems clear that the major reason people seek orthodontic treatment is to minimize psychosocial problems related to their dental and facial appearance. These problems are not "just cosmetic." They can have a major effect on the quality of life.

Oral Function

Adults with severe malocclusion routinely report difficulty in chewing, and after treatment, patients usually say that their masticatory problems are largely corrected.[21] It seems reasonable that poor dental occlusion would be a handicap to function, but there is no good test for chewing ability and no objective way to measure the extent of any functional handicap. Methods to test for jaw function would put this reason for orthodontic treatment on a more scientific basis. Scoring the efficiency of mastication from video tapes of standard tasks now offers the possibility of doing this.[22]

Severe malocclusion may make adaptive alterations in swallowing necessary. In addition, it can be difficult or impossible to produce certain sounds (see Chapter 6), and effective speech therapy may require some preliminary orthodontic treatment. Even less severe malocclusions tend to affect function, not by making it impossible but by making it difficult, so that extra effort is required to compensate for the anatomic deformity. For instance, everyone uses as many chewing strokes as it takes to reduce a food bolus to a consistency that is satisfactory for swallowing, so if chewing is less efficient in the presence of malocclusion, either the affected individual uses more effort to chew or settles for less well masticated food before swallowing it. Similarly, almost everyone can move the jaw so that proper lip relationships exist for speech, so distorted speech is rarely noted even though an individual may have to make an extraordinary effort to produce normal speech. As methods to quantify functional adaptations of this type are developed, it is likely that the effect of malocclusion on function will be appreciated more than it has been in the past.

The relationship of malocclusion and adaptive function to temporomandibular dysfunction (TMD), manifested as pain in and around the TM joint, is understood much better now than only a few years ago. The pain may result from pathologic changes within the joint, but more often is caused by muscle fatigue and spasm. Muscle pain almost always correlates with a history of clenching or grinding the teeth as a response to stressful situations, or of constantly posturing the mandible to an anterior or lateral position.

Some dentists have suggested that even minor imperfections in the occlusion serve to trigger clenching and grinding activities. If this were true, it would indicate a real need for perfecting the occlusion in everyone, to avoid the possibility of developing facial muscle pain. Because the number of people with at least moderate degrees of malocclusion (50% to 75% of the population) far exceeds the number with TMD (5% to 30%, depending on which symptoms are examined), it seems unlikely that occlusal patterns alone are enough to cause hyperactivity of the oral musculature. A reaction to stress usually is involved. Some individuals with poor occlusion have no problem with muscle pain when stressed but develop symptoms in other organ systems. Almost never does an individual have both ulcerative colitis (also a common stress-induced disease) and TMD. Some types of malocclusion (especially posterior crossbite with a shift on closure) correlate positively with TM joint problems while other types do not,[23] but even the strongest correlation coefficients are only 0.3 to 0.4. This means that for the great majority of patients, there is no association between malocclusion and TMD.

On the other hand, if a patient does respond to stress by increased oral muscle activity, improper occlusal relationships may make the problem more severe and harder to control. Therefore, malocclusion coupled with pain and spasm in the muscles of mastication may indicate a need for orthodontic treatment as an adjunct to other treatment for the muscle pain (but orthodontics as the primary treatment almost never is indicated). If the problem is a pathologic process within the joint itself, improving the dental occlusion may or may not help the patient adapt to the necessarily altered joint function (see Chapter 18).

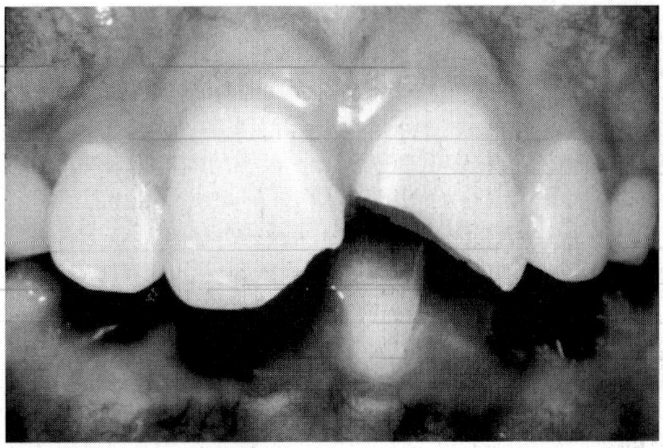

Figure 1-21 Fractured maxillary central incisors in a 10-year-old girl. There is almost one chance in three of an injury to a protruding incisor, though fortunately the damage rarely is this severe. Most of the accidents occur during normal activity, not in sports.

Relationship to Injury and Dental Disease

Malocclusion, particularly protruding maxillary incisors, can increase the likelihood of an injury to the teeth (Figure 1-21). There is about one chance in three that a child with an untreated Class II malocclusion will experience trauma to the upper incisors, but most of the time, the result is only minor chips in the enamel resulting in a fracture of the tooth and/or devitalization of the pulp. For that reason, reducing the chance of injury when incisors protrude is not a strong argument for early treatment of Class II problems (see Chapter 8). Extreme overbite, so that the lower incisors contact the palate, can cause significant tissue damage, leading to loss of the upper incisors in a few patients. Extreme wear of incisors also occurs in some patients with excessive overbite.

It seems obvious that malocclusion could contribute to both dental decay and periodontal disease, by making it harder to care for the teeth properly or by causing occlusal trauma. Current data indicate, however, that malocclusion has little if any impact on diseases of the teeth or supporting structures. An individual's willingness and motivation determine oral hygiene much more than how well the teeth are aligned, and presence or absence of dental plaque is the major determinant of the health of both the hard and soft tissues of the mouth. If individuals with malocclusion are more prone to tooth decay, the effect is small compared with hygiene status.[24] Occlusal trauma, once thought to be important in the development of periodontal disease, now is recognized to be a secondary, not a primary, etiologic factor.

Two studies carried out in the late 1970s, in which a large number of patients were carefully examined 10 to 20 years after completion of orthodontic treatment, shed some light on long-term relationships between malocclusion and oral health.[25,26] In both studies, comparison of the patients who underwent orthodontic treatment years earlier with untreated individuals in the same age group showed similar periodontal status, despite the better functional occlusions of the orthodontically treated group. There was only a tenuous link between untreated malocclusion and major periodontal disease later in life. No evidence of a beneficial effect of orthodontic treatment on future periodontal health was demonstrated, as would have been expected if untreated malocclusion had a major role in the cause of periodontal problems.

Patients with a history of orthodontic treatment appear to be more likely to seek later periodontal care than those who were not treated, and thus are over-represented among periodontal patients. Because of this, it has been suggested that previous orthodontic treatment predisposes to later periodontal disease. The long-term studies show no indication that orthodontic treatment increased the chance of later periodontal problems. The association between early orthodontic and later periodontal treatment appears to be only another manifestation of the phenomenon that one segment of the population seeks dental treatment while another avoids it. Those who have had one type of successful dental treatment, like orthodontics in childhood, are more likely to seek another like periodontal therapy in adult life.

In summary, it appears that both psychosocial and functional handicaps can produce significant need for orthodontic treatment. The evidence is less clear that orthodontic treatment reduces the development of later dental disease.

Epidemiologic Estimates of Orthodontic Treatment Need

Psychosocial and facial considerations, not just the way the teeth fit, play a role in defining orthodontic treatment need. For this reason, it is difficult to determine who needs treatment and who does not, just from an examination of dental casts or radiographs. It seems reasonable that the severity of a malocclusion correlates with need for treatment. This assumption is necessary when treatment need is estimated for population groups.

Several indices for scoring how much the teeth deviate from the normal, as indicators of orthodontic treatment need, were proposed in the 1970s. Of these, Grainger's Treatment Priority Index (TPI)[27] is the most prominent because it was used in the 1965-1970 U.S. population surveys. None of the early indices were widely accepted for screening potential patients, however.

More recently, Shaw and co-workers in the United Kingdom developed a scoring system for malocclusion, the Index of Treatment Need (IOTN),[28] that places patients in five grades from "no need for treatment" to "treatment need." The index has a dental health component derived from occlusion and alignment (Box 1-1) and an esthetic component derived from comparison of the dental appearance to standard photographs (Figure 1-22). IOTN grades seem to reflect clinical judgments better than previous methods.[29,30] There is a surprisingly good correlation between treatment need assessed by the dental health and esthetic components of IOTN (i.e., children selected as needing treatment on one of the scales are also quite likely to be selected using the other).

With some allowances for the effect of missing teeth, it is possible to calculate the percentages of U.S. children and youths who would fall into the various IOTN grades from the NHANES III data set.[9] Figure 1-23 shows the number of youths age 12-17 estimated by IOTN to have mild/moderate/severe treatment need. Although the prevalence of malocclusion is similar for the three racial/ethnic groups evaluated in NHANES III, the percentage of blacks with severe problems is higher. The TPI scores of 40 years ago placed more children toward the severe end of the malocclusion spectrum than the current IOTN grades, but it seems unlikely that there has been a major change in treatment need. To some extent, the difference may be due to the difference in the indices, but there is another factor. Many more children have orthodontic treatment now. The number of white children who receive treatment is considerably higher than blacks or Hispanics ($p < .001$). Treatment almost always produces an improvement but may not totally eliminate all the characteristics of malocclusion, so the effect is to move some individuals from the severe to the mild treatment need categories. The higher proportion of severe malocclusion among blacks, who are much less likely to receive treatment at this point than whites, probably reflects the effect of more treatment in the white group, and may not indicate the presence of more severe malocclusion in the black population.[31]

How do the IOTN scores compare with what parents and dentists think relative to orthodontic treatment need? The (rather weak) existing data suggest that in typical American neighborhoods, about 35% of adolescents are perceived by parents and peers as needing orthodontic treatment (see Figure 1-23). Note that this is larger than the number of children who would be placed in IOTN grades 4 and 5 as severe problems definitely needing treatment, but smaller than the total of grades 3, 4, and 5 for moderate and severe problems. Dentists usually judge that only about one-third of their patients have normal occlusion, and they suggest treatment for about 55% (thereby putting about 10% in a category of

Box 1-1

IOTN TREATMENT GRADES

Grade 5 (Extreme/Need Treatment)

5.i Impeded eruption of teeth (except third molars) due to crowding, displacement, the presence of supernumerary teeth, retained deciduous teeth, and any pathological cause.
5.h Extensive hypodontia with restorative implications (more than one tooth per quadrant) requiring pre-prosthetic orthodontics.
5.a Increased overjet greater than 9 mm.
5.m Reverse overjet greater than 3.5 mm with reported masticatory and speech difficulties.
5.p Defects of cleft lip and palate and other craniofacial anomalies.
5.s Submerged deciduous teeth.

Grade 4 (Severe/Need Treatment)

4.h Less extensive hypodontia requiring pre-restorative orthodontics or orthodontic space closure (one tooth per quadrant).
4.a Increased overjet greater than 6 mm but less than or equal to 9 mm.
4.b Reverse overjet greater than 3.5 mm with no masticatory or speech difficulties.
4.m Reverse overjet greater than 1 mm but less than 3.5 mm with recorded masticatory or speech difficulties.
4.c Anterior or posterior crossbites with greater than 2 mm discrepancy between retruded contact position and intercuspal position.
4.l Posterior lingual crossbite with no functional occlusal contact in one or both buccal segments.
4.d Severe contact point displacements greater than 4 mm.
4.e Extreme lateral or anterior open bits greater than 4 mm.
4.f Increased and complete overbite with gingival or palatal trauma.
4.t Partially erupted teeth, tipped, and impacted against adjacent teeth.
4.x Presence of supernumerary teeth.

Grade 3 (Moderate/Borderline Need)

3.a Increased overjet greater than 3.5 mm but less than or equal to 6 mm with incompetent lips.
3.b Reverse overjet greater than 1 mm but less than or equal to 3.5 mm.
3.c Anterior or posterior crossbites with greater than 1 mm but less than or equal to 2 mm discrepancy between retruded contact position and intercuspal position.
3.d Contact point displacements greater than 2 mm but less than or equal to 4 mm.
3.e Lateral or anterior open bite greater than 2 mm but less than or equal to 4 mm.
3.f Deep overbite complete on gingival or palatal tissues but no trauma.

Grade 2 (Mild/Little Need)

2.a Increased overjet greater than 3.5 mm but less than or equal to 6 mm with competent lips.
2.b Reverse overjet greater than 0 mm but less than or equal to 1 mm.
2.c Anterior or posterior crossbite with less than or equal to 1 mm discrepancy between retruded contact position and intercuspal position.
2.d Contact point displacements greater than 1 mm but less than or equal to 2 mm.
2.e Anterior or posterior openbite greater than 1 mm but less than or equal to 2 mm.
2.f Increased overbite greater than or equal to 3.5 mm without gingival contact.
2.g Pre-normal or post-normal occlusions with no other anomalies.

Grade 1 (No Need)

1. Extremely minor malocclusions including contact point displacements less than 1 mm.

malocclusion with little need for treatment). It appears that they would include all the children in IOTN grade 3 and some of those in grade 2 (Table 1-4) in the group who would benefit from orthodontics. Presumably, facial appearance and psychosocial considerations are used in addition to dental characteristics when parents judge treatment need or dentists decide to recommend treatment.

Demand for Orthodontic Treatment

Demand for treatment is indicated by the number of patients who actually make appointments and seek care. Not all patients with malocclusion, even those with extreme deviations from the normal, seek orthodontic treatment. Some do not recognize that they have a problem; others feel that they need treatment but cannot afford it or cannot obtain it.

Both the perceived need and demand vary with social and cultural conditions.[32] More children in urban areas are thought (by parents and peers) to need treatment than children in rural areas. Family income is a major determinant of how many children receive treatment (Figure 1-24). This appears to reflect two things, not only that higher income families can more easily afford orthodontic treatment, but also that good facial appearance and avoidance of disfiguring dental conditions are associated with more prestigious social positions and occupations. The higher the aspirations for a child, the more likely the parent is to seek orthodontic treatment for him or her. It is widely recognized

1 6

2 7

3 8

4 9

5 10

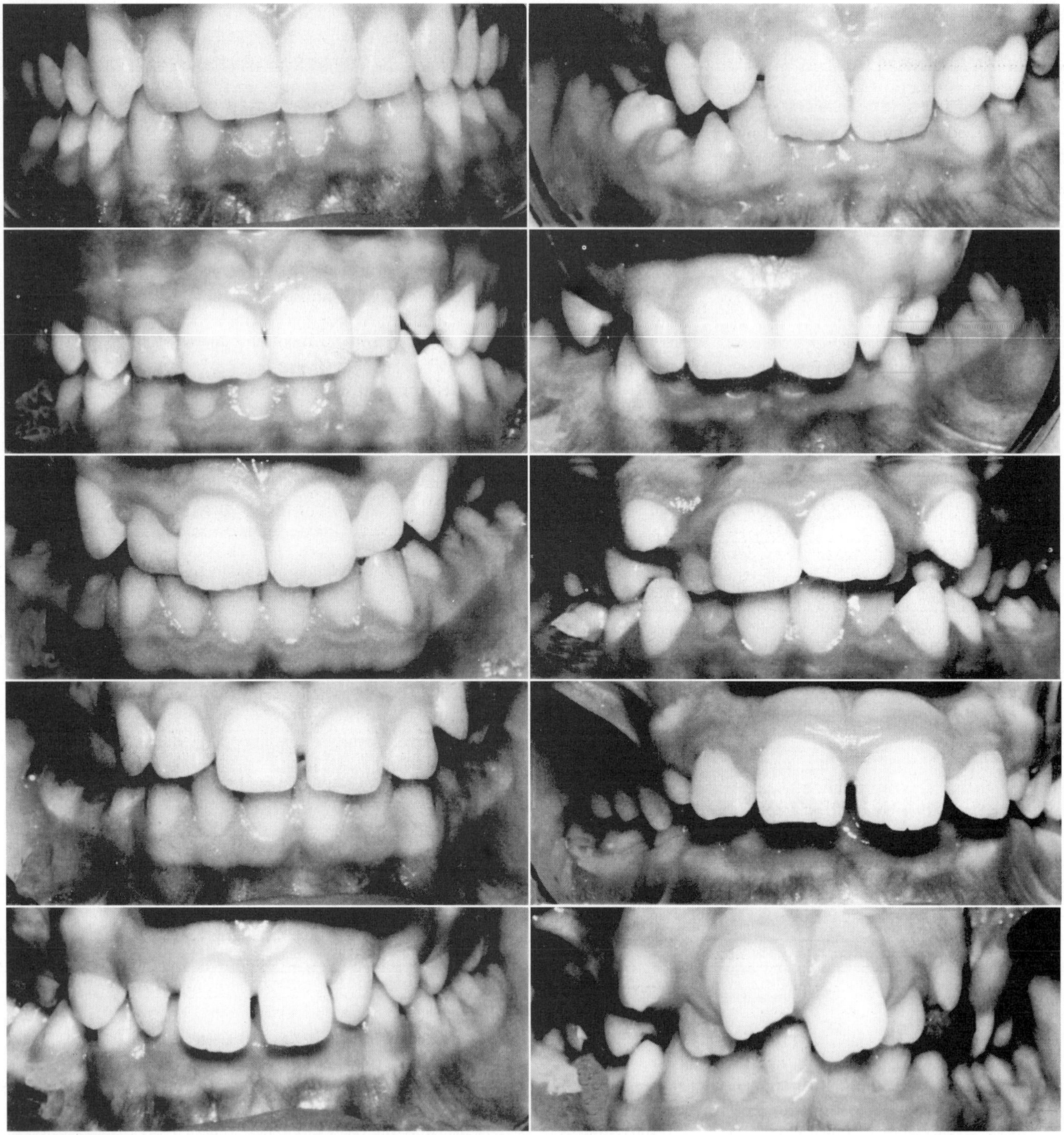

FIGURE 1-22 The stimulus photographs of the IOTN esthetic index. The score is derived from the patient's answer to "Here is a set of photographs showing a range of dental attractiveness. Number 1 is the most attractive and number 10 the least attractive arrangement. Where would you put your teeth on this scale?" Grades 8-10 indicate definite need for orthodontic treatment, 5-7 moderate/borderline need, 1-4 no/slight need.

that severe malocclusion can affect an individual's entire life adjustment, and every state now provides at least some orthodontic treatment through its Medicaid program, but Medicaid and related programs support only a tiny fraction of the population's orthodontic care. From that perspective, it is interesting that even in the lowest income group almost 5% of the youths and over 5% of adults report receiving treatment, with 10% to 15% treated at intermediate income levels. This probably reflects the importance placed on orthodontic treatment by some families as a factor in social and career progress.

The effect of financial constraints on demand can be seen most clearly by the response to third-party payment plans. When third-party copayment is available, the number of

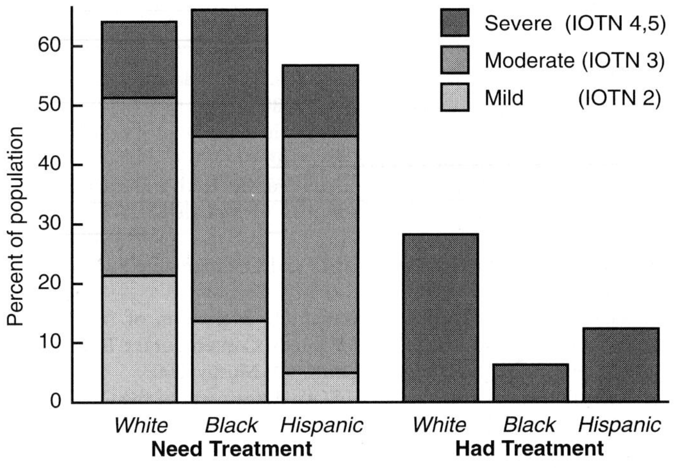

FIGURE 1-23 Orthodontic need by severity of the problem for white, black, and Mexican-American youths age 12-17 in the United States 1989-94, and the percent of each group who report receiving orthodontic treatment. The greater number of whites who receive treatment probably accounts for the smaller number of severe problems in the white population.

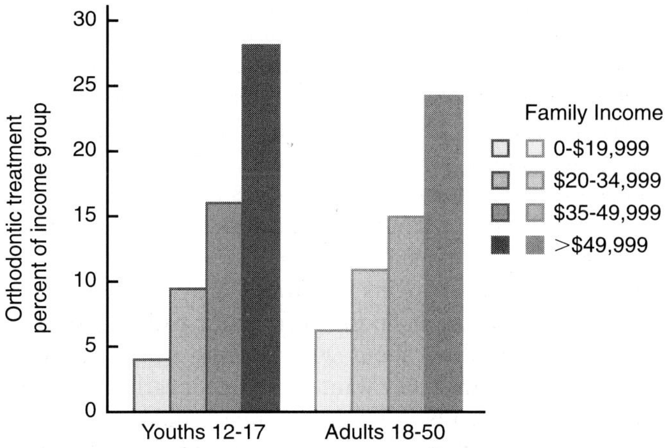

FIGURE 1-24 The percent of the U.S. population 1989-94 who received orthodontic treatment, as a function of family income. Although severe malocclusion is recognized as an important problem and all states offer at least some coverage to low-income children through their Medicaid program, this funds treatment for a very small percentage of the population. Nevertheless, nearly 5% of the lowest income group, and 10%-15% of intermediate income groups, have had some orthodontic treatment. The increasing availability of orthodontics in recent years is reflected in the larger number of youths than adults who report being treated.

TABLE 1-4

Percent of U.S. Population Estimated to Need Orthodontics, 1965-1970 versus 1989-1994

	WHITE				BLACK				HISPANIC**	
	CHILD		YOUTH		CHILD		YOUTH		CHILD	YOUTH
Age	6-11	8-11	12-17		6-11	8-11	12-17		8-11	12-17
Year	1965-70	1989-91	1965-70	1989-91	1965-70	1989-91	1965-70	1989-91	1989-91	1989-91
Index	TPI	IOTN	TPI	IOTN	TPI	IOTN	TPI	IOTN	IOTN	IOTN
No treatment need (TPI 0-1, IOTN 1)	28.7	36.5	20.0	43.7	39.7	40.4	24.3	42.2	49.4	41.5
Minimal need (TPI 2-3, IOTN 2)	33.9	16.3	25.1	16.5	28.4	8.8	27.3	9.2	11.7	8.5
Moderate need (TPI 4-6, IOTN 3)	23.7	36.4	25.7	25.3	15.0	37.1	21.0	26.0	29.9	36.8
Definite need (TPI >6, IOTN 4-5)	13.7	10.8	29.2	14.5	16.9	13.7	27.4	22.6	9.0	13.2
Had orthodontic treatment	2.5*	10.5	10.7*	27.4		3.6		6.2	1.4	11.7

Data from NHANES I and III.
*White/black combined.
**No data for 1965-1970.

CHAPTER 2

Concepts of Growth and Development

CHAPTER OUTLINE

A thorough background in craniofacial growth and development is necessary for every dentist. Even for those who never work with children, it is difficult to comprehend conditions observed in adults without understanding the developmental processes that produced these problems. For those who do interact professionally with children—and almost every dentist does so at least occasionally—it is important to distinguish normal variation from the effects of abnormal or pathologic processes. Since dentists and orthodontists are heavily involved in the development of not just the dentition but the entire dentofacial complex, a conscientious practitioner may be able to manipulate facial growth for the benefit of the patient. Obviously, it is not possible to do so without a thorough understanding of both the pattern of normal growth and the mechanisms that underlie it.

The very terms *growth* and *development* can cause difficulties in understanding. Growth and development, though closely related, are not synonymous. In conversational English, growth usually refers to an increase in size but tends to be linked more to change than anything else. Only if growth meant change, after all, could someone seriously speak of a period of economic recession as one of "negative economic growth." Since some tissues grow rapidly and then shrink or disappear, a plot of physical growth versus time may include a negative phase. On the other hand, if growth is defined solely as a process of change, the term becomes almost meaningless. As a general term, development connotes an increasing degree of organization, often with unfortunate consequences for the natural environment. In this chapter, the term *growth* usually refers to an increase in size or number. Occasionally, however, the increase will be in neither size nor number, but in complexity. More often, the term *development* will be used to refer to an increase in complexity. Development carries an overtone of increasing

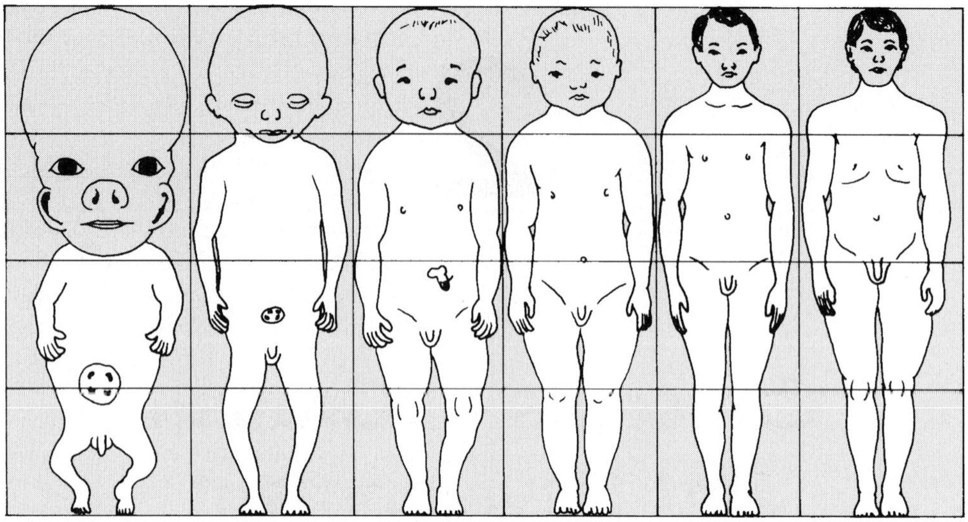

FIGURE 2-1 Schematic representation of the changes in overall body proportions during normal growth and development. After the third month of fetal life, the proportion of total body size contributed by the head and face steadily declines. (Redrawn from Robbins WJ, et al. Growth. New Haven: Yale University Press; 1928.)

specialization, so that one price of increased development is a loss of potential. Growth is largely an anatomic phenomenon, whereas development is physiologic and behavioral.

It should be kept in mind that although dentists work with the physical features of the teeth and face, a major reason for orthodontic treatment is its psychosocial effects. Furthermore, patient cooperation is necessary—eliciting it in children of different ages requires a knowledge of social and behavioral development. Both physiologic and psychosocial development are important subjects for this chapter. For convenience, not because they are innately more important, physical growth concepts are presented first, and then developmental factors are reviewed.

GROWTH: PATTERN, VARIABILITY, AND TIMING

In studies of growth and development, the concept of pattern is an important one. In a general sense, pattern (as in the pattern from which articles of clothing of different sizes are cut) reflects proportionality, usually of a complex set of proportions rather than just a single proportional relationship. Pattern in growth also represents proportionality, but in a still more complex way, because it refers not just to a set of proportional relationships at a point in time, but to the change in these proportional relationships over time. In other words, the physical arrangement of the body at any one time is a pattern of spatially proportioned parts. But there is a higher level pattern, the pattern of growth, which refers to the changes in these spatial proportions over time.

Figure 2-1 illustrates the change in overall body proportions that occurs during normal growth and development. In fetal life, at about the third month of intrauterine development, the head takes up almost 50% of the total body length. At this stage, the cranium is large relative to the face and represents more than half the total head. In contrast, the limbs are still rudimentary and the trunk is underdeveloped. By the time of birth, the trunk and limbs have grown faster than the head and face, so that the proportion of the entire body devoted to the head has decreased to about 30%. The overall pattern of growth thereafter follows this course, with a progressive reduction of the relative size of the head to about 12% of the adult. At birth, the legs represent about one third of the total body length, while in the adult, they represent about half. As Figure 2-1 illustrates, there is more growth of the lower limbs than the upper limbs during postnatal life. All of these changes, which are a part of the normal growth pattern, reflect the "cephalocaudal gradient of growth." This simply means that there is an axis of increased growth extending from the head toward the feet.

Another aspect of the normal growth pattern is that not all the tissue systems of the body grow at the same rate (Figure 2-2). Obviously, the muscular and skeletal elements grow faster than the brain and central nervous system, as reflected in the relative decrease of head size. The overall pattern of growth is a reflection of the growth of the various tissues making up the whole organism. To put it differently, one reason for gradients of growth is that different tissue systems that grow at different rates are concentrated in various parts of the body.

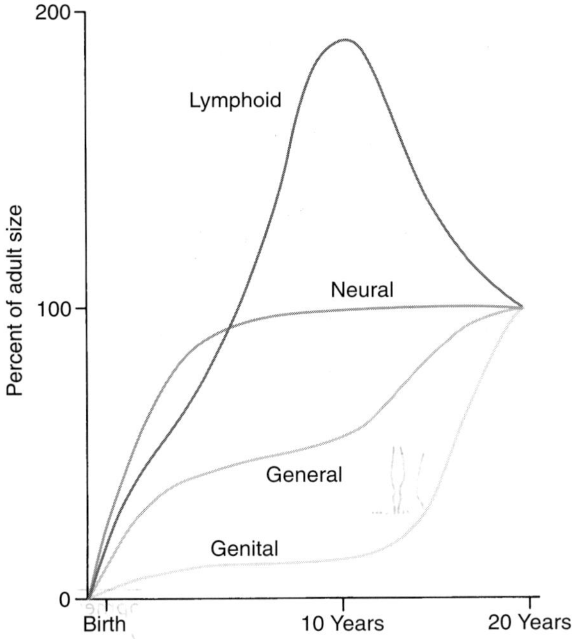

FIGURE 2-2 Scammon's curves for growth of the four major tissue systems of the body. As the graph indicates, growth of the neural tissues is nearly complete by 6 or 7 years of age. General body tissues, including muscle, bone, and viscera, show an S-shaped curve, with a definite slowing of the rate of growth during childhood and an acceleration at puberty. Lymphoid tissues proliferate far beyond the adult amount in late childhood, and then undergo involution at the same time that growth of the genital tissues accelerates rapidly. (From Scammon RD. The measurement of the body in childhood. In: Harris JA, ed. The Measurement of Man. Minneapolis: University of Minnesota Press; 1930.)

Even within the head and face, the cephalocaudal growth gradient strongly affects proportions and leads to changes in proportion with growth (Figure 2-3). When the skull of a newborn infant is compared proportionally with that of an adult, it is easy to see that the infant has a relatively much larger cranium and a much smaller face. This change in proportionality, with an emphasis on growth of the face relative to the cranium, is an important aspect of the pattern of facial growth. When the facial growth pattern is viewed against the perspective of the cephalocaudal gradient, it is not surprising that the mandible, being farther away from the brain, tends to grow more and later than the maxilla, which is closer.

An important aspect of pattern is its predictability. Patterns repeat, whether in the organization of different-colored tiles in the design of a floor or in skeletal proportions changing over time. The proportional relationships within a pattern can be specified mathematically, and the only difference between a growth pattern and a geometric one is the addition of a time dimension. Thinking about pattern in this way allows one to be more precise in defining what constitutes a change in pattern. Change, clearly, would denote an alteration in the predictable pattern of mathematical relationships. A change in growth pattern would indicate some alteration in the expected changes in body proportions.

A second important concept in the study of growth and development is variability. Obviously, everyone is not alike in the way that they grow, as in everything else. It can be difficult, but clinically very important, to decide whether an individual is merely at the extreme of the normal variation or falls outside the normal range.

Rather than categorizing people as normal or abnormal, it is more useful to think in terms of deviations from the usual pattern and to express variability quantitatively. One way to do this is to evaluate a given child relative to peers on a standard growth chart (Figure 2-4). Although charts of this

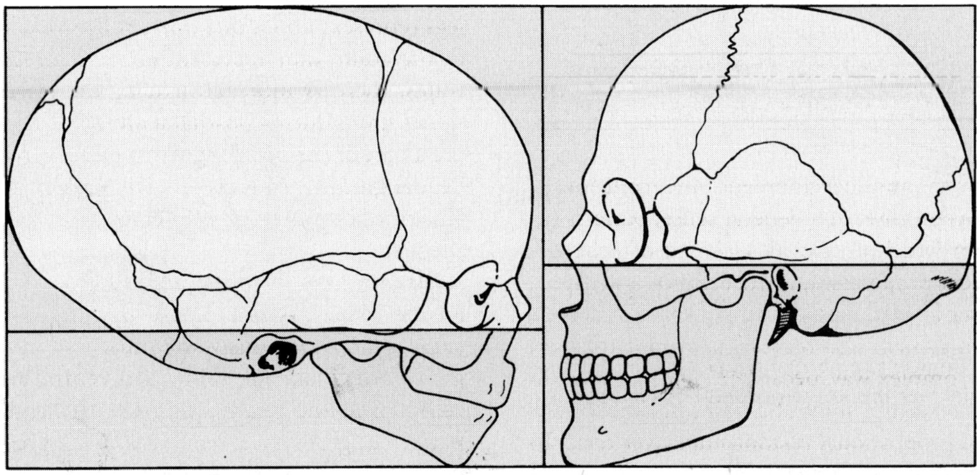

FIGURE 2-3 Changes in proportions of the head and face during growth. At birth, the face and jaws are relatively underdeveloped compared with their extent in the adult. As a result, there is much more growth of facial than cranial structures postnatally. (Redrawn from Lowery GH. Growth and Development of Children, 6th ed. Chicago: Mosby; 1973.)

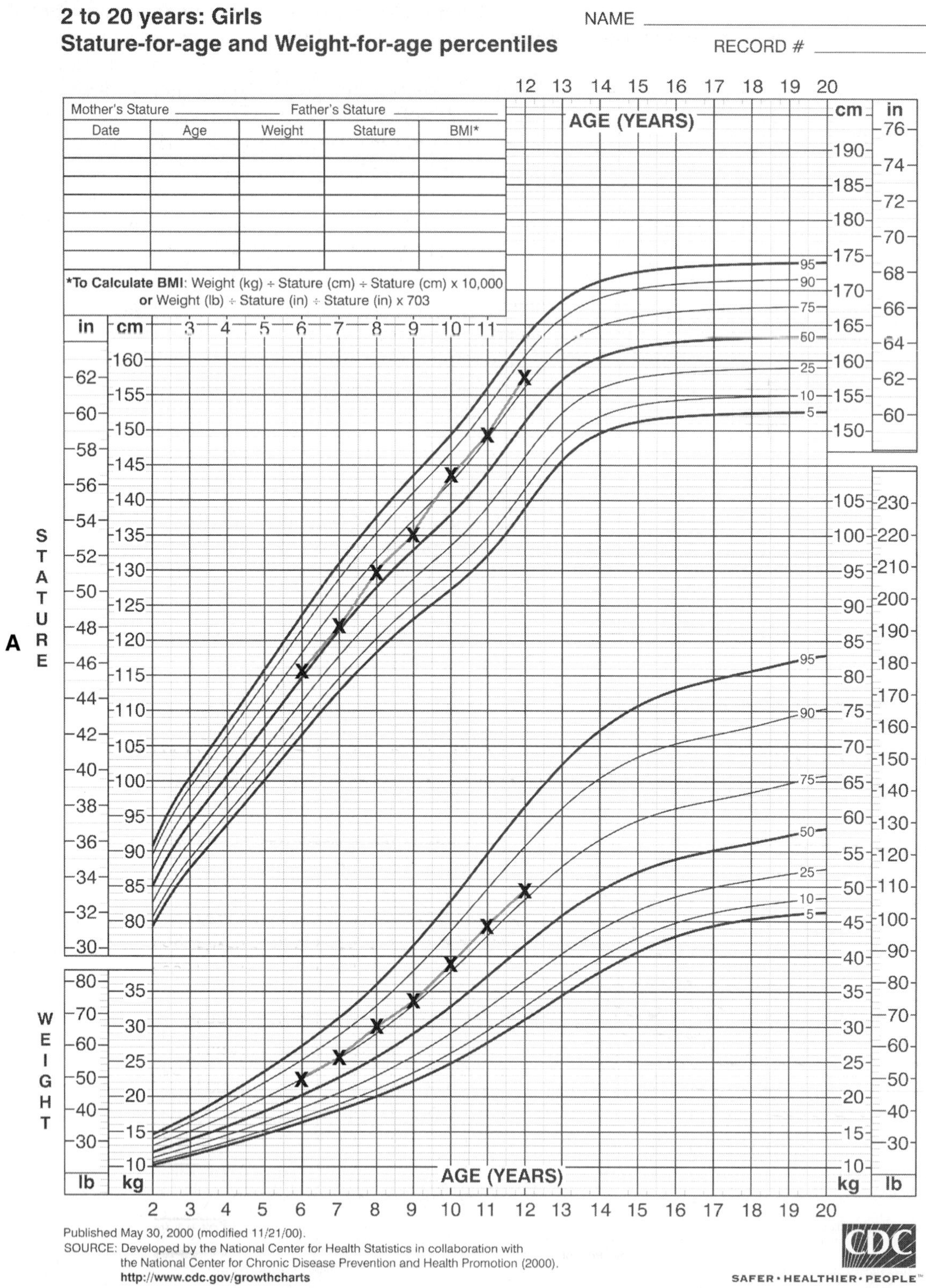

FIGURE 2-4 **A,** Growth of a normal girl plotted on the chart for females. Note that this girl remained at about the 75th percentile for height and weight over this entire period of observation.

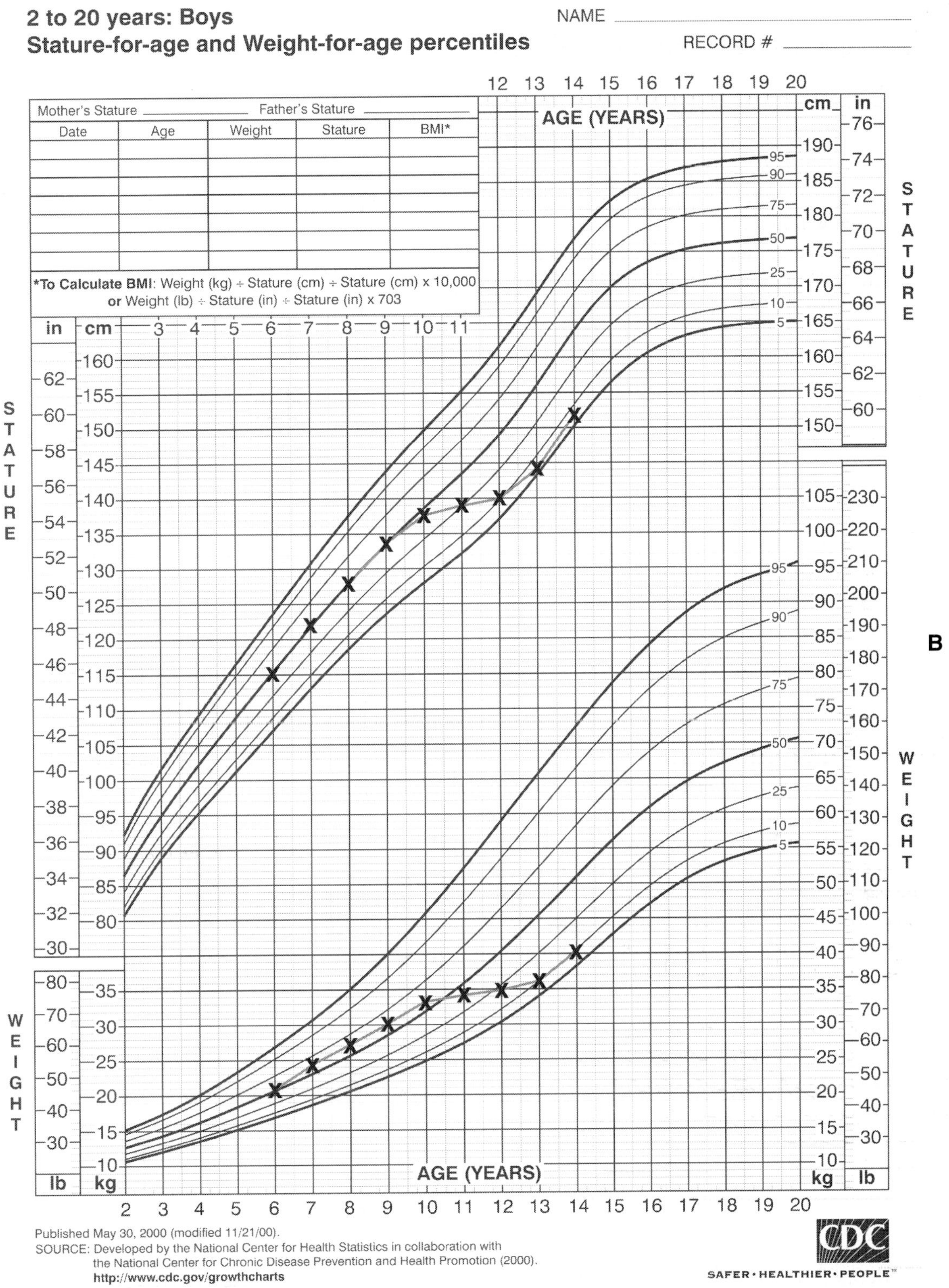

Figure 2-4 cont'd **B,** Growth of a boy who developed a medical problem that affected growth, plotted on the male chart. Note the change in pattern (crossover of lines on the chart) between ages 10 and 11. This reflects the impact of serious illness beginning at that time, with partial recovery after age 13 but a continuing effect on growth. (Data from Hamill, et al. National Center for Health Statistics, 1979; charts developed by the National Center for Health Statistics in collaboration with the National Center for Chronic Disease Prevention and Health Promotion, published May 30, 2000, revised 11/21/00.) (Charts available from http://www.ccd.gov/growth charts.)

type are commonly used for height and weight, the growth of any part of the body can be plotted in this way. The "normal variability," as derived from large-scale studies of groups of children, is shown by the solid lines on the graphs. An individual who stood exactly at the midpoint of the normal distribution would fall along the 50% line of the graph. One who was larger than 90% of the population would plot above the 90% line; one who was smaller than 90% of the population would plot below the 10% line.

These charts can be used in two ways to determine whether growth is normal or abnormal. First, the location of an individual relative to the group can be established. A general guideline is that a child who falls beyond the range of 97% of the population should receive special study before being accepted as just an extreme of the normal population. Second and perhaps more importantly, growth charts can be used to follow a child over time to evaluate whether there is an unexpected change in growth pattern. Pattern implies predictability. For the growth charts, this means that a child's growth should plot along the same percentile line at all ages. If the percentile position of an individual relative to his or her peer group changes, especially if there is a marked change (see Figure 2-4), the clinician should suspect some growth abnormality and should investigate further. Inevitably, there is a gray area at the extremes of normal variations, at which it is difficult to determine if growth is normal.

A final major concept in physical growth and development is that of timing. Variability in growth arises in several ways: from normal variation, from influences outside the normal experience (e.g., serious illness), and from timing effects. Variation in timing arises because the same event happens for different individuals at different times—or, viewed differently, the biologic clocks of different individuals are set differently.

Variations in growth and development because of timing are particularly evident in human adolescence. Some children grow rapidly and mature early, completing their growth quickly and thereby appearing on the high side of developmental charts until their growth ceases and their contemporaries begin to catch up. Others grow and develop slowly and so appear to be behind, even though, given time, they will catch up with and even surpass children who once were larger. All children undergo a spurt of growth at adolescence, which can be seen more clearly by plotting change in height or weight (Figure 2-5), but the growth spurt occurs at different times in different individuals.

Growth effects because of timing variation can be seen particularly clearly in girls, in whom the onset of menstruation, often referred to as menarche, gives an excellent indicator of the arrival of sexual maturity. Sexual maturation is accompanied by a spurt in growth. When the growth velocity curves for early-, average-, and late-maturing girls are compared in Figure 2-6, the marked differences in size between these girls during growth are apparent. At age 11, the early-maturing girl is already past the peak of her adolescent growth spurt, whereas the late-maturing girl has not

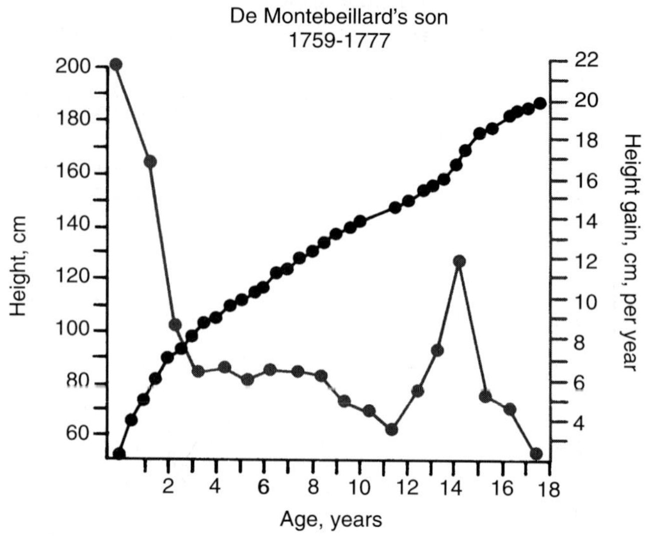

FIGURE 2-5 Growth can be plotted in either height or weight at any age (the black line here) or the amount of change in any given interval (the maroon line here, showing the same data as the black line). A curve like the black line is called a "distance curve," whereas the maroon line is a "velocity curve." Plotting velocity rather than distance makes it easier to see when accelerations and decelerations in the rate of growth occurred. These data are for the growth of one individual, the son of a French aristocrat in the late eighteenth century, whose growth followed the typical pattern. Note the acceleration of growth at adolescence, which occurred for this individual at about age 14. (Redrawn from Tanner JM. Growth at Adolescence, 2nd ed. Oxford: Blackwell Scientific Publications; 1962.)

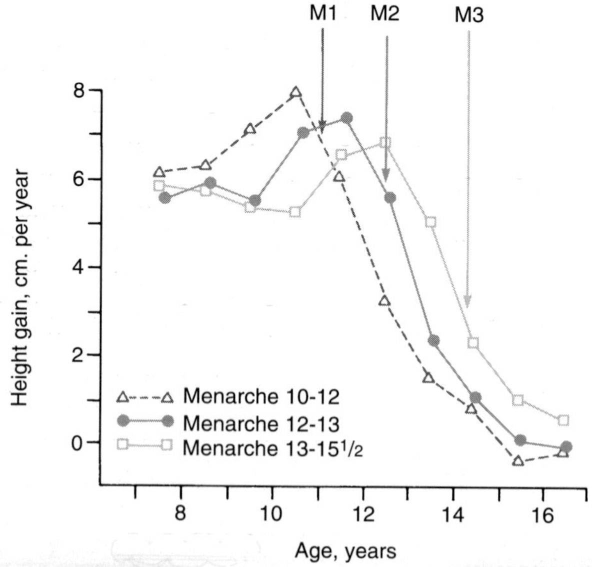

FIGURE 2-6 Growth velocity curves for early-, average-, and late-maturing girls. It is interesting to note that the earlier the adolescent growth spurt occurs, the more intense it appears to be. Obviously, at age 11 or 12, an early maturing girl would be considerably larger than one who matured late. In each case, the onset of menstruation (menarche) (M1, M2, and M3) came after the peak of growth velocity.

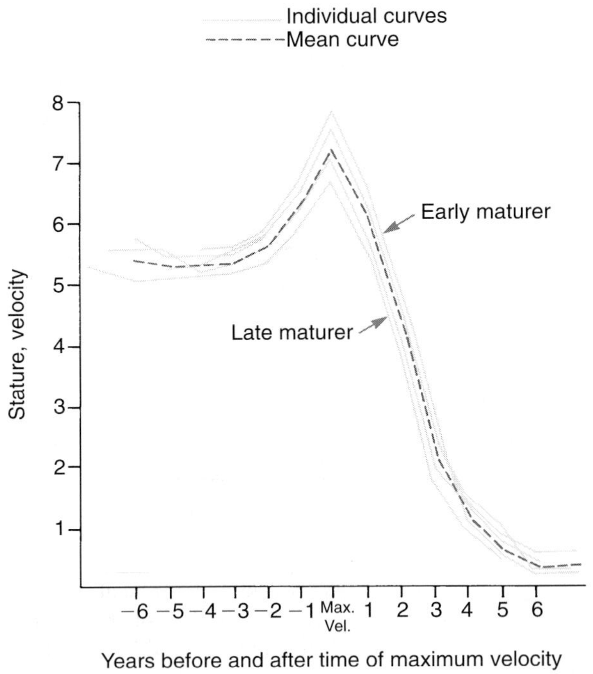

Figure 2-7 Velocity curves for four girls with quite different times of menarche, replotted using menarche as a zero time point. It is apparent that the growth pattern in each case is quite similar, with almost all of the variations resulting from timing.

even begun to grow rapidly. This sort of timing variation, which occurs in many ways other than that shown here, can be an important contributor to variability.

Although age is usually measured chronologically as the amount of time since birth or conception, it is also possible to measure age biologically, in terms of progress toward various developmental markers or stages. Timing variability can be reduced by using developmental age rather than chronologic age as an expression of an individual's growth status. For instance, if data for gain in height for girls are replotted, using menarche as a reference time point (Figure 2-7), it is apparent that girls who mature early, average, or late really follow a very similar growth pattern. This graph substitutes stage of sexual development for chronologic time to produce a biologic time scale and shows that the pattern is expressed at different times chronologically, but not at different times physiologically. The effectiveness of biologic or developmental age in reducing timing variability makes this approach useful in evaluating a child's growth status.

Methods for Studying Physical Growth

Before beginning the examination of growth data, it is important to have a reasonable idea of how the data were obtained. There are two basic approaches to studying physical growth. The first is based on techniques for measuring living animals (including humans), with the implication that the measurement itself does no harm and that the animal will be available for additional measurements at another time. The second approach uses experiments in which growth is manipulated in some way. This implies that the subject of the experiment will be available for study in some detail, and the detailed study may be destructive. For this reason, such experimental studies are largely restricted to non-human species.

Measurement Approaches

Acquiring Measurement Data

Craniometry. The first of the measurement approaches for studying growth, with which the science of physical anthropology began, is craniometry, based on measurements of skulls found among human skeletal remains. Craniometry was originally used to study the Neanderthal and Cro-Magnon peoples whose skulls were found in European caves in the eighteenth and nineteenth centuries. From such skeletal material, it has been possible to piece together a great deal of knowledge about extinct populations and to get some idea of their pattern of growth by comparing one skull with another. Craniometry has the advantage that rather precise measurements can be made on dry skulls; it has the important disadvantage for growth studies that, by necessity, all these growth data must be cross-sectional. Cross-sectional means that although different ages are represented in the population, the same individual can be measured at only one point in time.

Anthropometry. It is also possible to measure skeletal dimensions on living individuals. In this technique, called *anthropometry*, various landmarks established in studies of dry skulls are measured in living individuals simply by using soft tissue points overlying these bony landmarks. For example, it is possible to measure the length of the cranium from a point at the bridge of the nose to a point at the greatest convexity of the rear of the skull. This measurement can be made on either a dried skull or a living individual, but results would be different because of the soft tissue thickness overlying both landmarks. Although the soft tissue introduces variation, anthropometry does make it possible to follow the growth of an individual directly, making the same measurements repeatedly at different times. This produces longitudinal data: repeated measures of the same individual. In recent years, Farkas' anthropometric studies have provided valuable new data for human facial proportions and their changes over time.[1]

Cephalometric Radiology. The third measurement technique, cephalometric radiology, is of considerable importance not only in the study of growth but also in clinical evaluation of orthodontic patients. The technique depends on precisely orienting the head before making a radiograph, with equally precise control of magnification. This approach can combine the advantages of craniometry and anthropometry. It allows a direct measurement of bony

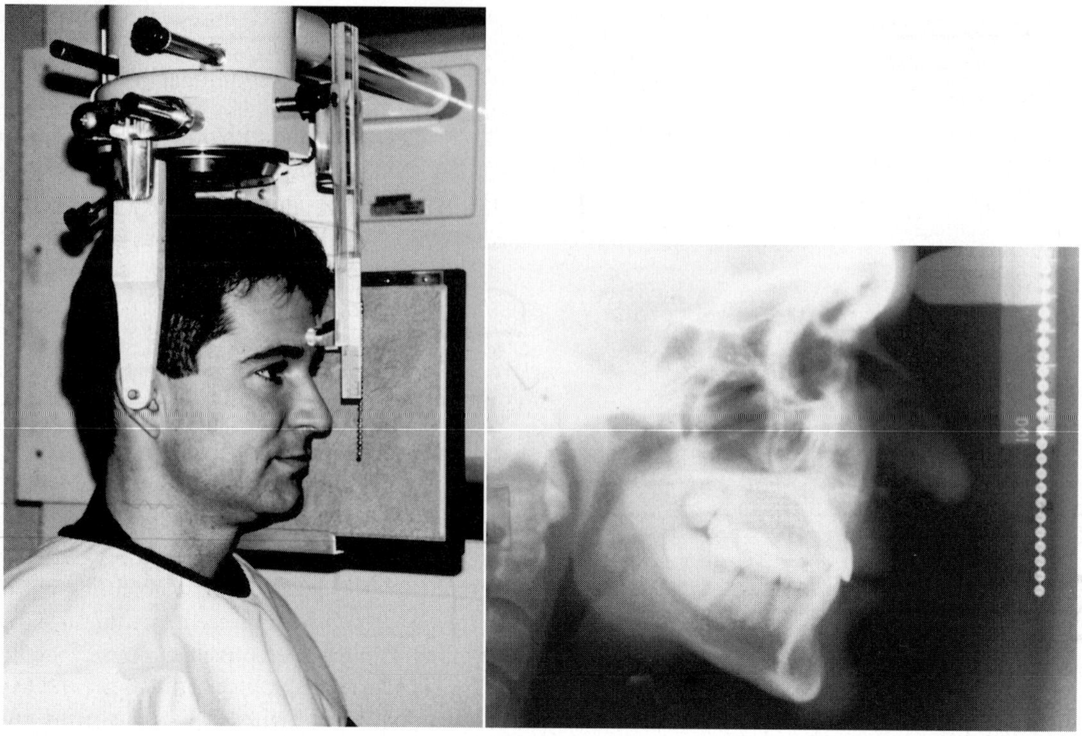
A

B

FIGURE 2-8 **A,** A cephalometric radiograph merits this name because of the use of a head positioning device to provide precise orientation of the head. This means that valid comparisons can be made between external and internal dimensions in members of the same population group, or that the same individual can be measured at two points in time, because the head orientation is reproducible. **B,** This radiograph was taken in natural head position (NHP) (see Chapter 6 for a description of this head positioning technique).

skeletal dimensions, since the bone can be seen through the soft tissue covering in a radiograph, but it also allows the same individual to be followed over time. Growth studies are done by superimposing a tracing or digital model of a later cephalogram on an earlier one, so that the changes can be measured. Both the locations and amounts of growth can be observed in this way (Figure 2-8). Cephalometric superimposition techniques are described in detail in Chapter 6.

The disadvantage of a standard cephalometric radiograph is that it produces a two-dimensional representation of a three-dimensional structure, and so, even with precise head positioning, not all measurements are possible. To some extent, this can be overcome by making more than one radiograph at different orientations and using triangulation to calculate oblique distances. The general pattern of craniofacial growth was known from craniometric and anthropometric studies before cephalometric radiography was invented, but much of the current picture of craniofacial growth is based on cephalometric studies.

Three-Dimensional Imaging. New information now is being obtained with the application of three-dimensional imaging techniques. Computed axial tomography (CAT or just CT) allows 3-D reconstructions of the cranium and face, and this method has been applied for several years to plan surgical treatment for patients with facial deformities (Figure 2-9). Recently, cone beam rather than spiral CT has been applied to facial scans, significantly reducing the radiation dose and allowing scans of patients with radiation exposure that is much closer to the dose from cephalograms. Superimposition of 3-D images is much more difficult than the superimpositions used with 2-D cephalometric radiographs, but methods developed recently are overcoming this difficulty (Figure 2-10).[2] Magnetic resonance imaging (MRI) also provides 3-D images that can be useful in studies of growth, with the advantage that there is no radiation exposure with this technique. This method already has been applied to analysis of the growth changes produced by functional appliances.[3] A more detailed examination of 3-D changes in growing patients almost surely will add to current knowledge of growth patterns in the near future.

Analysis of Measurement Data

Both anthropometric and cephalometric data can be expressed cross-sectionally rather than longitudinally. Obviously, it would be much easier and quicker to do a cross-sectional study, gathering data once for any individual and including subjects of different ages, rather than spending many years on a study in which the same individuals are measured repeatedly. For this reason, most studies are cross-sectional. When this approach is used, however, variability

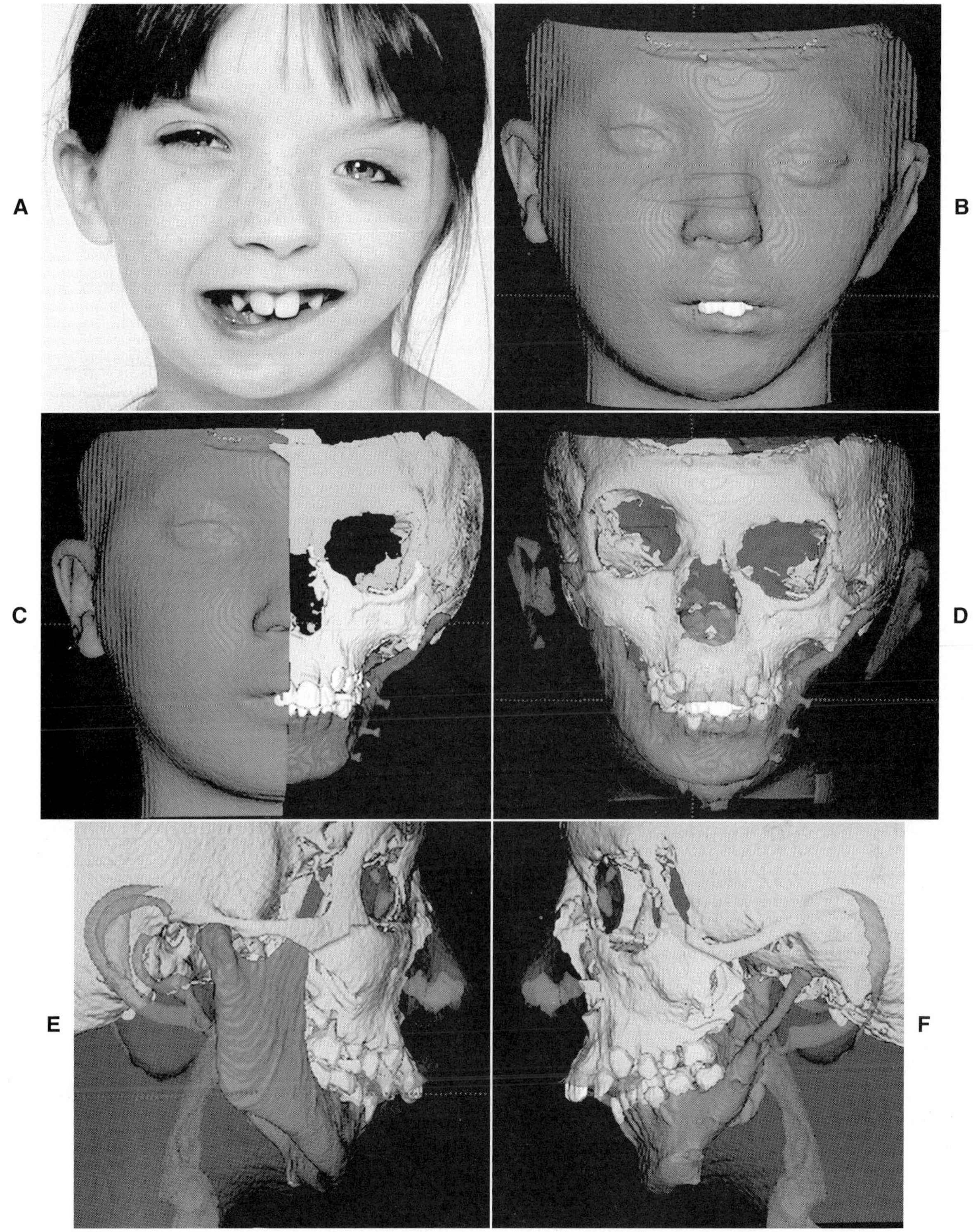

Figure 2-9 Computed tomography (CT) scans are the best way to determine the details of skeletal deformities. These views of a 9-year-old girl with severe hemifacial microsomia (and previous surgical treatment to build up the affected side of the mandible) illustrate that CT scans can show both skin contours and bony relationships from any aspect. Color can be added to different structures to make it easier to visualize them, and surface layers can be made transparent (as in **C–F**) to reveal the skeletal structures beneath. Views of this type greatly facilitate surgical treatment planning.

A

B

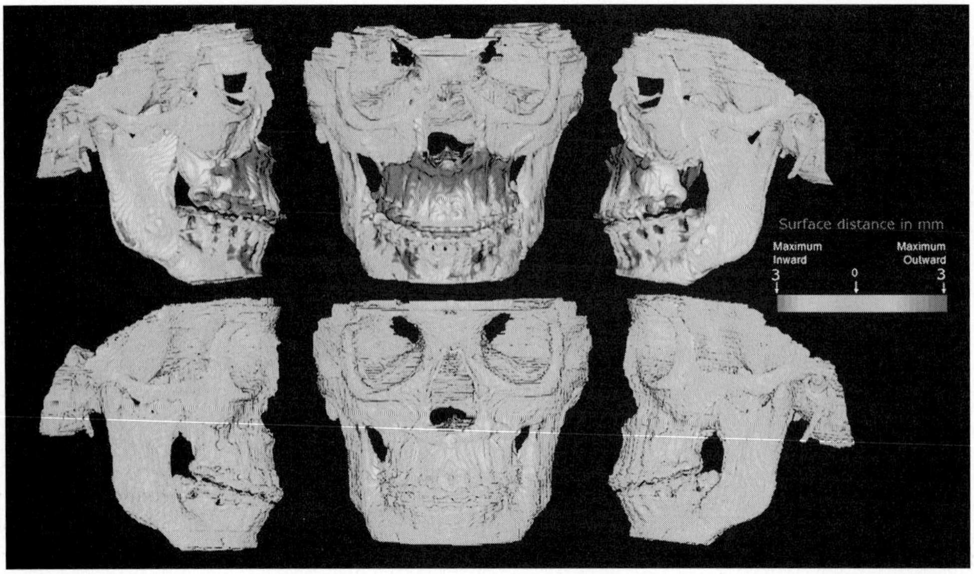

FIGURE 2-10 Superimposition of CT images is much more difficult than superimposition of cephalometric tracings but is necessary to detect the amount of change and can be used to see changes in exquisite detail. These images are based on a superimposition of a surface map of the cranial base. They show the amount of change in various areas in a patient who had both maxillary and mandibular surgery to correct a skeletal Class III problem (in three views for each time period) **(A)** from pre- to post-surgery, and **(B)** from immediately post-surgery to 1 year afterward. Note that areas in green had little or no change; areas in red moved outward; and areas in blue moved inward. It is apparent that the maxilla was rotated down in front as it was advanced (red at the superior areas, green below) and that the mandibular ramus was slightly rotated transversely more on the right side than the left (medial surface of coronoid process shades toward yellow, distal surface of ramus shades toward blue). There were minimal changes in the first post-surgical year, but some remodeling of the upper part of the advanced maxilla (shading toward blue) can be detected. Growth changes could be observed in the same way.

within the sample can conceal details of the growth pattern, particularly when there is no correction for timing variation (Figure 2-11). Fluctuations in the growth curve that may occur for nearly every individual would be seen in a cross-sectional study only if they occurred at the same time for each person, which is unlikely. Longitudinal studies are efficient in the sense that a great deal of information can be gained from a relatively small number of subjects, fewer than would be needed in a cross-sectional study. In addition, the longitudinal data highlight individual variations, particularly variations caused by timing effects.

Measurement data can be presented graphically in a number of different ways, and frequently, it is possible to clarify growth changes by varying the method of display. For example, we have already seen that growth data can be presented by plotting the size attained as a function of age, which is called a "distance" curve, or as a "velocity" curve, showing not the total length but the increment added each year (see Figure 2-5). Changes in the rate of growth are much more easily seen in the velocity curve than the distance curve.

Various other mathematical transformations can be used with growth data to make them easier to understand. For instance, the growth in weight of any embryo at an early stage follows a logarithmic or exponential curve, because the growth is based on division of cells; the more cells there are, the more cell divisions can occur. If the same data are plotted using the logarithm of the weight, a straight-line plot is attained (Figure 2-12). This demonstrates that the rate of multiplication for cells in the embryo is remaining more or less constant.

More complex mathematical transformations were used many years ago by D'Arcy Thompson[4] to reveal similarities in proportions and growth changes that had not previously been suspected (Figure 2-13). To correctly interpret data after mathematical transformation, it is important to understand how the data were transformed, but the approach is a powerful one in clarifying growth concepts. Thompson's classic presentation remains stimulating reading.

Experimental Approaches

Vital Staining

Much has been learned about skeletal growth using the technique called *vital staining,* in which dyes that stain mineralizing tissues (or occasionally, soft tissues) are injected into an animal. These dyes remain in the bones and teeth and can be detected later after sacrifice of the animal. This method was originated by the great English anatomist John Hunter in the eighteenth century. Hunter observed that the bones of pigs that occasionally were fed textile waste were often stained in an interesting way. He discovered that the active

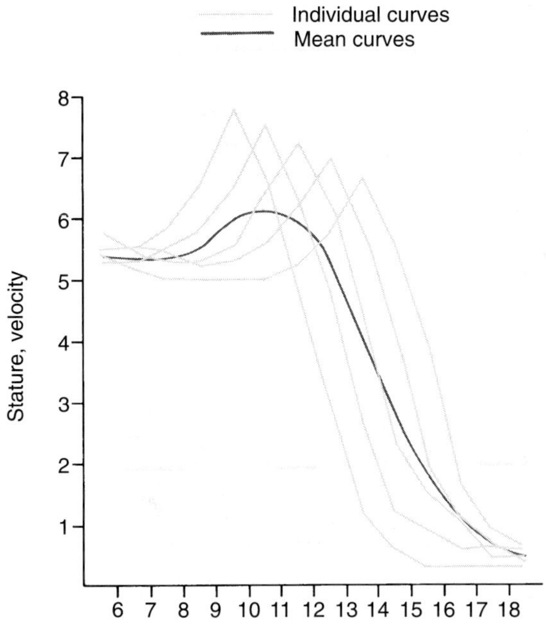

FIGURE 2-11 If growth velocity data for a group of individuals with a different timing of the adolescent growth spurt are plotted on a chronologic scale, it is apparent that the average curve is not an accurate representation of the pattern of growth for any particular individual. This smoothing of individual variation is a characteristic of cross-sectional data and a major limitation in use of the cross-sectional method for studies of growth. Only by following individuals through time in a longitudinal study is it possible to see the details of growth patterns.

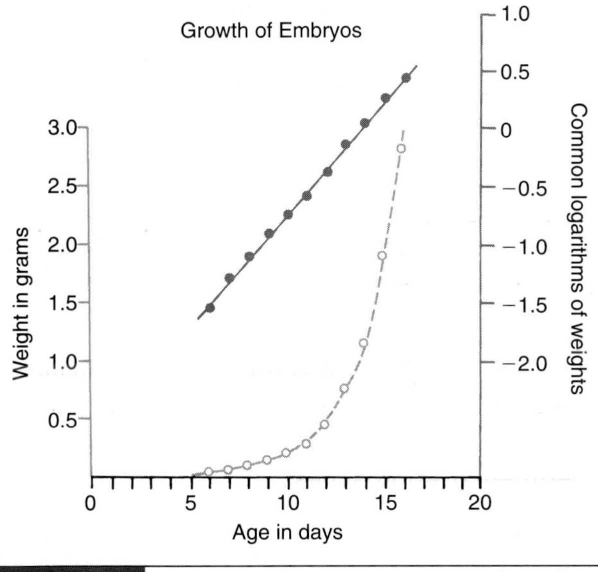

FIGURE 2-12 Data for the increase in weight of early embryos, with the raw data plotted in green and the same data plotted after logarithmic transformation in blue. At this stage, the weight of the embryo increases dramatically, but, as shown by the straight line after transformation, the rate of multiplication of individual cells remains fairly constant. When more cells are present, more divisions can occur, the weight increases faster. (From Lowery GH. Growth and Development of Children, 8th ed. Chicago: Mosby; 1986.)

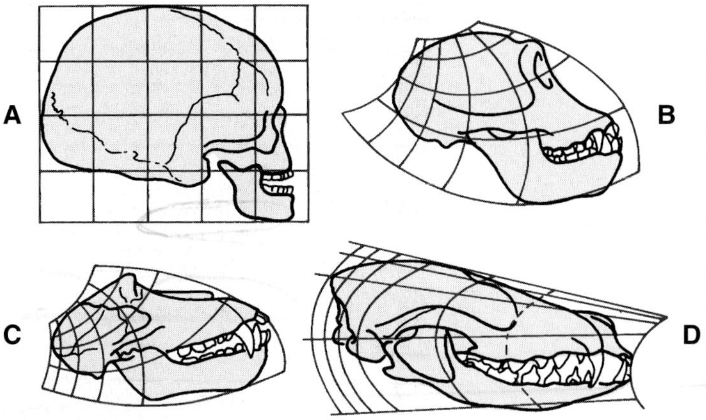

FIGURE 2-13 In the early 1900s, D'Arcy Thompson showed that mathematical transformation of a grid could account for the changes in the shape of the face from man **(A)** to chimpanzee **(B)**, monkey **(C)**, dog **(D)**, or other animals. Application of this method revealed previously unsuspected similarities among various species. (Redrawn from Thompson JT. On Growth and Form. Cambridge, Mass: Cambridge University Press; 1971.)

agent was a dye called alizarin, which still is used for vital staining studies (Figure 2-14). Alizarin reacts strongly with calcium at sites where bone calcification is occurring. Since these are the sites of active skeletal growth, the dye marks the locations at which active growth was occurring when it was injected. Bone remodels rapidly, and areas from which bone is being removed also can be identified by the fact that vital stained material has been removed from these locations. Highly detailed vital staining studies of bony changes in craniofacial development in experimental animals now are available.[5]

Although studies using vital stains are not possible in humans, vital staining can occur. Many children born in the late 1950s and early 1960s were treated for recurrent infections with the antibiotic tetracycline. It was discovered too late that tetracycline is an excellent vital stain that binds to calcium at growth sites in the same way as alizarin. The discoloration of incisor teeth that results from tetracycline given when the teeth are mineralizing has been an esthetic disaster for some individuals (Figure 2-15).

With the development of radioactive tracers, it has become possible to use almost any radioactively labeled metabolite that becomes incorporated into the tissues as a sort of vital stain. The location is detected by the weak radioactivity given off at the site where the material was incorporated. The gamma-emitting isotope ^{99m}Tc can be used to detect areas of rapid bone growth in humans, but these images are more useful in diagnosis of localized growth problems (see Chapter 19) than for studies of growth patterns. For most studies of growth, radioactively labeled materials in the tissues of experimental animals are detected by the technique of autoradiography, in which a film emulsion is placed over a thin section of tissue containing the

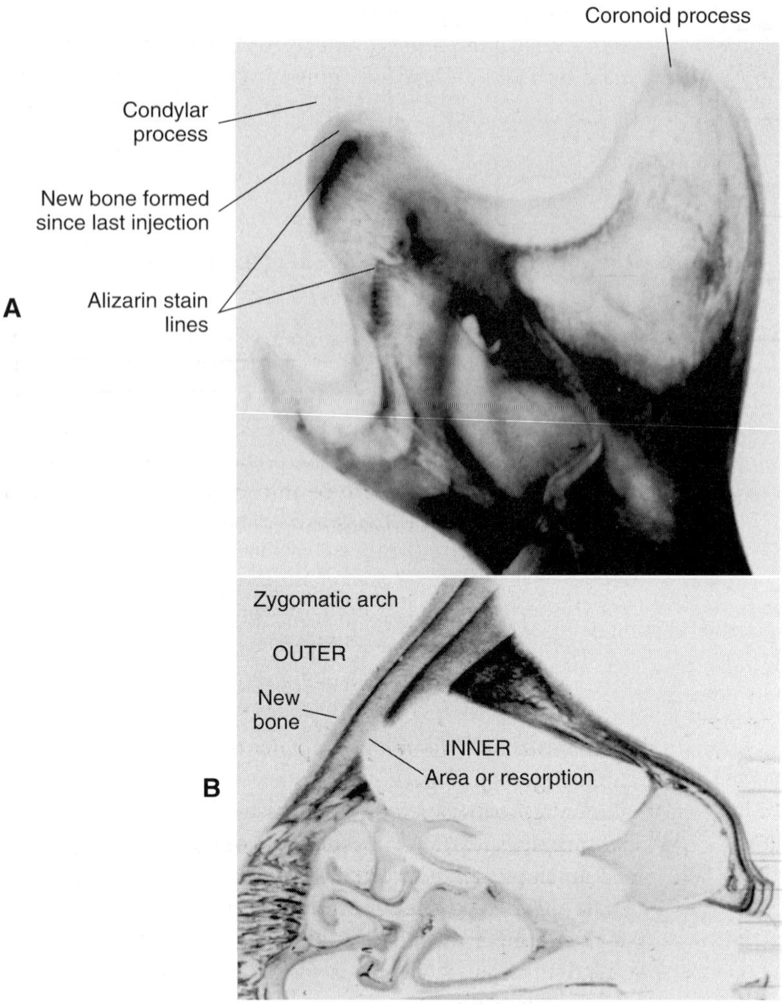

FIGURE 2-14 **A,** The mandible of a growing rat that received four injections of alizarin (red-blue-red-blue) at 2-week intervals and was sacrificed 2 weeks after the last injection (so the bone formed since then is white). Remodeling of the bone as it grows blurs some of the lines of intensely colored bone created by each injection, but the red-blue sequential lines in the condylar process can be seen clearly. **B,** Section through the zygomatic arch, from the same animal. The zygomatic arch grows outward by apposition of bone on the outer surface and removal from the inner surface. The interruptions in the staining lines on the inner surface clearly show the areas where bone is being removed. What was the outer surface of the zygomatic arch at one point becomes the inner surface a relatively short time later, and then is removed.

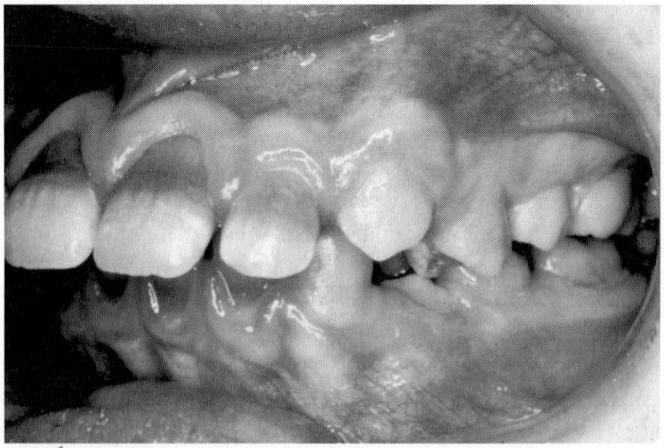

FIGURE 2-15 Tetracycline staining in the teeth of a boy who received large doses of tetracycline because of repeated upper respiratory infections in early childhood. From the location of the staining, it is apparent that tetracycline was not administered in infancy but was given in large doses beginning when the crowns of the central incisors were about half formed, or at approximately 30 months.

isotope and then is exposed in the dark by the radiation. After the film is developed, the location of the radiation that indicates where growth is occurring can be observed by looking at the tissue section through the film (Figure 2-16).

Implant Radiography

Another experimental method applicable to studies of humans is implant radiography. In this technique, inert metal pins are placed in bones anywhere in the skeleton, including the face and jaws. These metal pins are well tolerated by the skeleton and become permanently incorporated into the bone without causing any problems (Figure 2-17). If metallic implants are placed in the jaws, a considerable increase in the accuracy of a longitudinal cephalometric analysis of growth pattern can be achieved. This method of study, developed by Professor Arne Bjork and coworkers at the Royal Dental College in Copenhagen, Denmark,[6] and used extensively by workers there (see Chapter 4), provided important new information about the growth pattern of the jaws. The metal pins stay where they were placed within the bones in the absence of infection or inflammation, which is

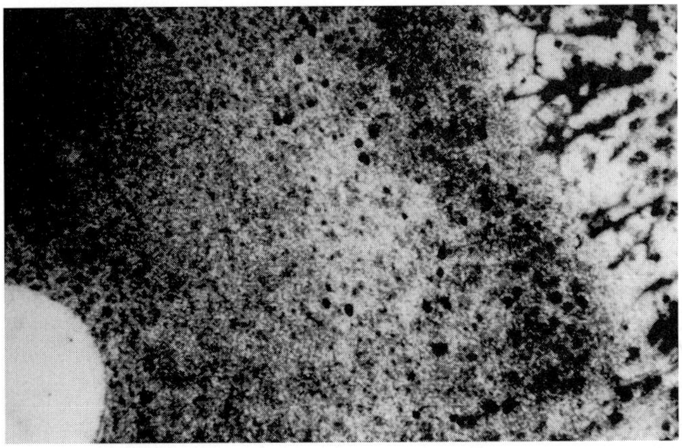

Figure 2-16 Autoradiograph of fetal rat bones growing in organ culture, with ^{14}C-proline and ^{3}H-thymidine incorporated in the culture medium. Thymidine is incorporated into DNA, which is replicated when a cell divides, so labeled nuclei are those of cells that underwent mitosis in culture. Because proline is a major constituent of collagen, cytoplasmic labeling indicates areas where proline was incorporated, primarily into extracellularly secreted collagen.

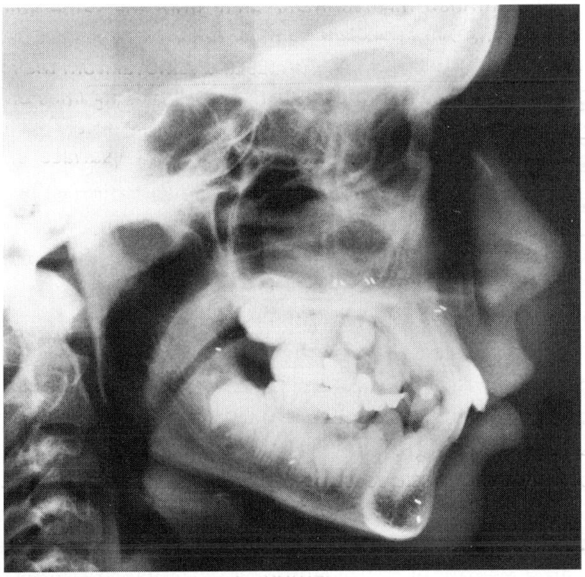

Figure 2-17 Lateral cephalometric radiograph from the archives of Bjork's implant studies, showing a subject with six maxillary and five mandibular tantalum implants. (Courtesy Dept. of Orthodontics, University of Copenhagen, Denmark.)

rarely a problem. Superimposing cephalometric radiographs on the implanted pins allows precise observation of both changes in the position of one bone relative to another and changes in the external contours of individual bones. Before radiographic studies using implants, the extent of remodeling changes in the contours of the jaw bones was underestimated, and the rotational pattern of jaw growth described in Chapter 4 was not appreciated.

At this point, precise evaluation of dentofacial growth in humans using implant cephalograms has largely been superseded by 3-dimensional imaging via computed tomography or MRI, but it still can be helpful to use implants to provide landmarks for superimposition.

Genetic Influences on Growth

Rapid advances in molecular genetics are providing new information about growth and its control. For example, the importance of homeobox genes in the establishment of body plan, pattern formation and morphogenesis is well recognized,[7] and the whole family of transforming growth factor-beta genes now is known to be important in regulating cell growth and organ development.[8] The proper functioning of families of growth factors and their cognate receptors remains indispensable in regulating embryonic processes of cell growth and organ development, as well as a myriad of postnatal processes that include growth, wound healing, bone remodeling and homeostasis. The proper growth of the mandible, for instance, requires epithelial–mesenchymal interactions and the temporospatial orchestration of thousands of gene products.

Interaction between different tissues within the craniofacial complex creates yet another level of regulation of growth and development. One example of this is the convergence of the development of the muscles that attach to the mandible and the bony areas to which they attach. While there are a number of genes involved in determining mandibular size,[9] genetic alterations in muscle development and function translate into changes in the forces on areas of bone where muscles attach, and this leads to modification of skeletal areas like the coronoid process and gonial angle area of the mandible; genetic alterations that affect muscle also would affect these skeletal areas. To understand this, it is necessary both to identify specific genes involved and to deduce how their activity is modified, but already it is apparent that gene expression can be up- or down-regulated by mechanical stresses.[10,11]

An exciting prospect is a better understanding of how patients with orthodontic problems that are known to have a genetic component (Class III malocclusion being the best example) will respond to treatment. It is clear that there are multiple sub-types of Class III, and a necessary first step is better characterization of these phenotypes. Establishing phenotypic markers (distinct clinical characteristics) makes it possible to establish definitive correlations with modes of inheritance and is necessary for linkage studies that will clarify the genetic basis for the problem. It is likely that in the future, genetic screening of blood or other tissue samples will be used to identify patients with orthodontic problems who are likely to respond well or poorly to specific treatment modalities, in the same way that the likely response to drug therapies already is being determined.

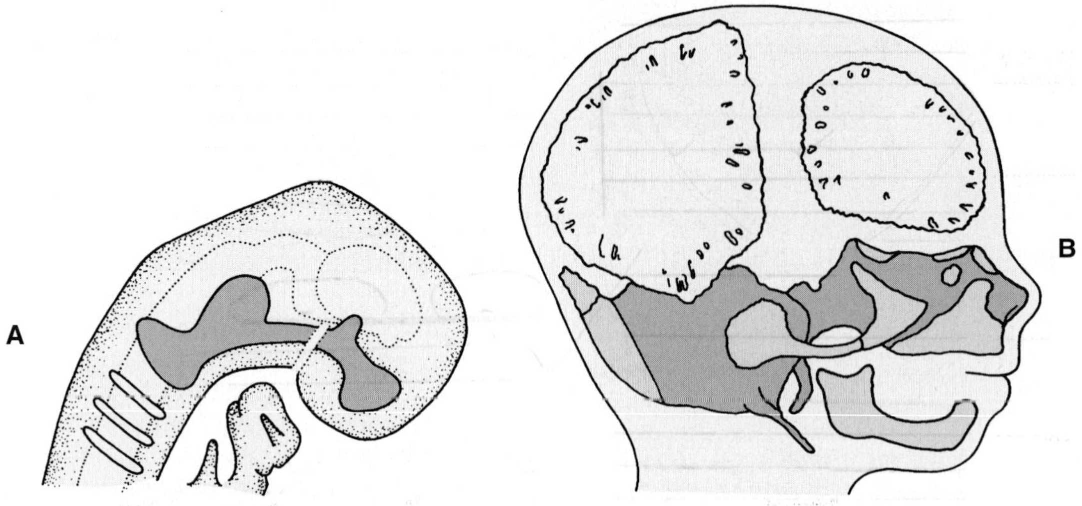

FIGURE 2-18 Development and maturation of the chondrocranium (cartilage: light blue; bone: stippled dark blue). **A,** Diagrammatic representation at about 8 weeks. Note that an essentially solid bar of cartilage extends from the nasal capsule anteriorly to the occipital area posteriorly. **B,** Skeletal development at 12 weeks. Ossification centers have appeared in the midline cartilage structures, and, in addition, intramembranous bone formation of the jaws and brain case has begun. From this point on, bone replaces cartilage of the original chondrocranium rapidly, so that only the small cartilaginous synchondroses connecting the bones of the cranial base remain.

Experiments that clarify how growth is controlled at the cellular level offer exciting prospects for better control of growth in the future. It is estimated that about two-thirds of the 25,000 human genes play a role in craniofacial development, so complex patterns of genetic activity obviously are involved, and complex interactions exist with external influences on growth. It is unlikely that genetic analysis will ever be applicable to planning treatment for the majority of orthodontic problems, but it could yield valuable information about the best approach to some of the most difficult skeletal malocclusions.

THE NATURE OF SKELETAL GROWTH

At the cellular level, there are only three possibilities for growth. The first is an increase in the size of individual cells, which is referred to as *hypertrophy.* The second possibility is an increase in the number of the cells, which is called *hyperplasia.* The third is for the cells to *secrete extracellular material,* thus contributing to an increase in size independent of the number or size of the cells themselves.

In fact, all three of these processes occur in skeletal growth. Hyperplasia is a prominent feature of all forms of growth. Hypertrophy occurs in a number of special circumstances but is a less important mechanism than hyperplasia in most instances. Although tissues throughout the body secrete extracellular material, this phenomenon is particularly important in the growth of the skeletal system, where extracellular material later mineralizes.

The fact that the extracellular material of the skeleton becomes mineralized leads to an important distinction between growth of the soft or nonmineralized tissues of the body and the hard or calcified tissues. Hard tissues are bones, teeth, and sometimes cartilages. Soft tissues are everything else. In most instances, cartilage, particularly the cartilage significantly involved in growth, behaves like soft tissue and should be thought of in that group, rather than as hard tissue.

Growth of soft tissues occurs by a combination of hyperplasia and hypertrophy. These processes go on everywhere within the tissues, and the result is what is called *interstitial growth,* which simply means that it occurs at all points within the tissue. Secretion of extracellular material can also accompany interstitial growth, but hyperplasia primarily and hypertrophy secondarily are its characteristics. Interstitial growth is characteristic of nearly all soft tissues and of uncalcified cartilage within the skeletal system.

In contrast, when mineralization takes place so that hard tissue is formed, interstitial growth becomes impossible. Hyperplasia, hypertrophy, and secretion of extracellular material all are still possible, but in mineralized tissues, these processes can occur only on the surface, not within the mineralized mass. Direct addition of new bone to the surface of existing bone can and does occur through the activity of cells in the periosteum—the soft tissue membrane that covers bone. Formation of new cells occurs in the periosteum, and extracellular material secreted there is mineralized and becomes new bone. This process is called *direct* or *surface apposition* of bone. Interstitial growth is a prominent aspect of overall skeletal growth because a major portion of the skeletal system is originally modeled in cartilage. This includes the basal part of the skull as well as the trunk and limbs.

Figure 2-18 shows the cartilaginous or chondrocranium at 8 and 12 weeks of intrauterine development. The height

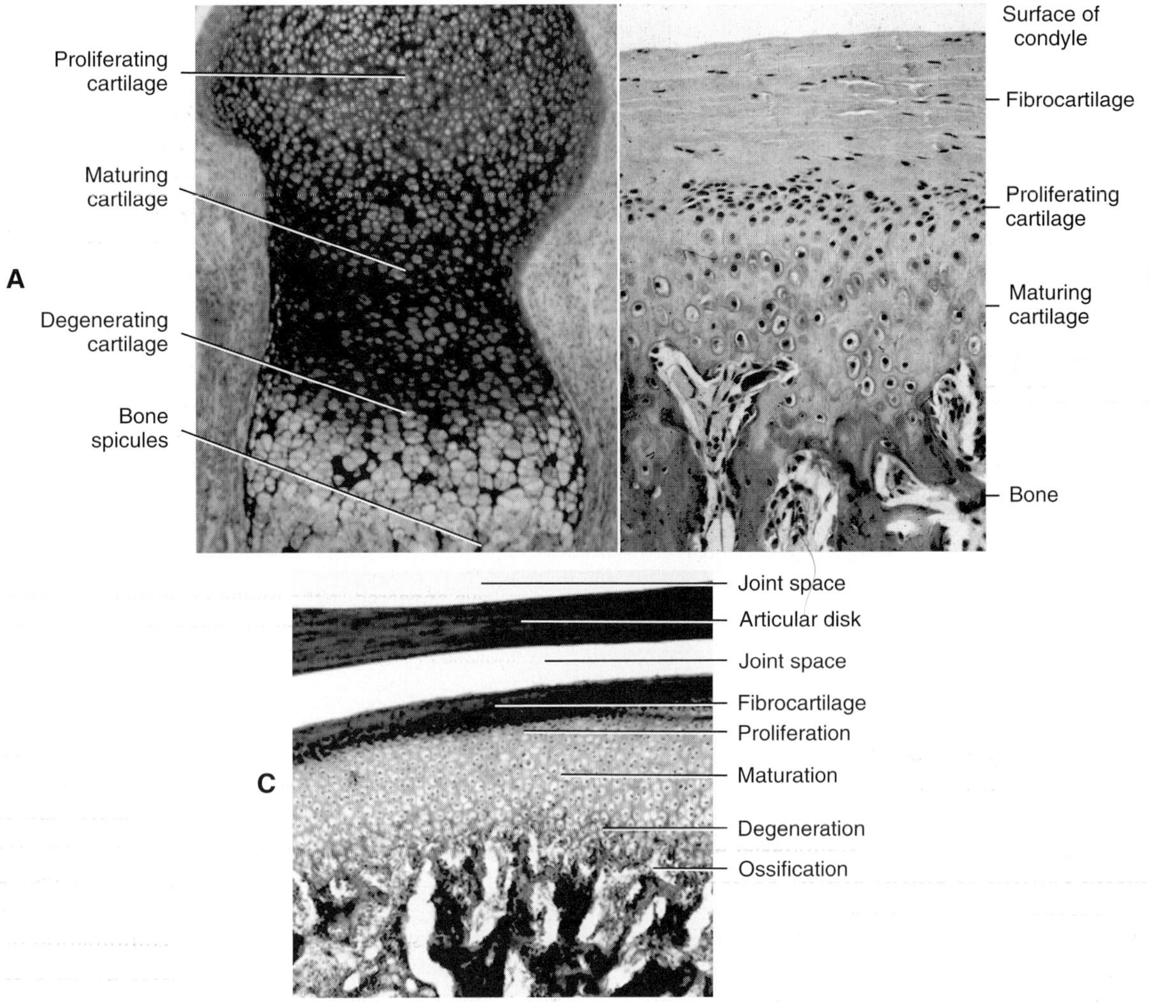

FIGURE 2-19 **A,** Endochondral ossification at an epiphyseal plate. Growth occurs by proliferation of cartilage, occurring here at the top. Maturing cartilage cells are displaced away from the area of proliferation, undergo hypertrophy, degenerate, and are replaced by spicules of bone, as seen in the bottom. **B** and **C,** Endochondral ossification in the head of the condyle. A layer of fibrocartilage lies on the surface, with proliferating cells just beneath. Maturing and degenerating cartilage cells can be seen toward the area of ossification.

of cartilaginous skeletal development occurs during the third month of intrauterine life. A continuous plate of cartilage extends from the nasal capsule posteriorly all the way to the foramen magnum at the base of the skull. It must be kept in mind that cartilage is a nearly avascular tissue whose internal cells are supplied by diffusion through the outer layers. This means, of course, that the cartilage must be thin. At early stages in development, the extremely small size of the embryo makes a chondroskeleton feasible, but with further growth, such an arrangement is no longer possible without an internal blood supply.

During the fourth month in utero, there is an ingrowth of blood vascular elements into various points of the chondrocranium (and the other parts of the early cartilaginous skeleton). These areas become centers of ossification, at which cartilage is transformed into bone, and islands of bone appear in the sea of surrounding cartilage (see Figure 2-18, *B*). The cartilage continues to grow rapidly but is replaced by bone with equal rapidity. The result is that the amount of bone increases rapidly and the relative (but not the absolute) amount of cartilage decreases. Eventually, the old chondrocranium is represented only by small areas of cartilage interposed between large sections of bone, which assume the characteristic form of the ethmoid, sphenoid, and basioccipital bones. Growth at these cartilaginous connections between the skeletal bones is similar to growth in the limbs.

In the long bones of the extremities, areas of ossification appear in the center of the bones and at the ends, ultimately producing a central shaft called the *diaphysis* and a bony cap on each end called the *epiphysis.* Between the epiphysis and diaphysis is a remaining area of uncalcified cartilage called the *epiphyseal plate* (Figure 2-19). The epiphyseal plate cartilage of the long bones is a major center for their growth, and in fact, this cartilage is responsible for almost all growth

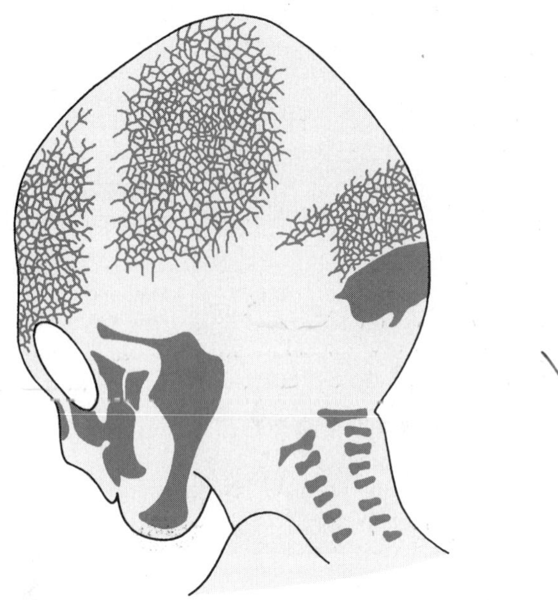

FIGURE 2-20 The bones of the skull of a 12-week-old fetus, drawn from a cleared alizarin-stained specimen. (Redrawn from Sadler TW, Langman J. Langman's Medical Embryology, 9th ed. Philadelphia: Lippincott Williams & Wilkins; 2003.)

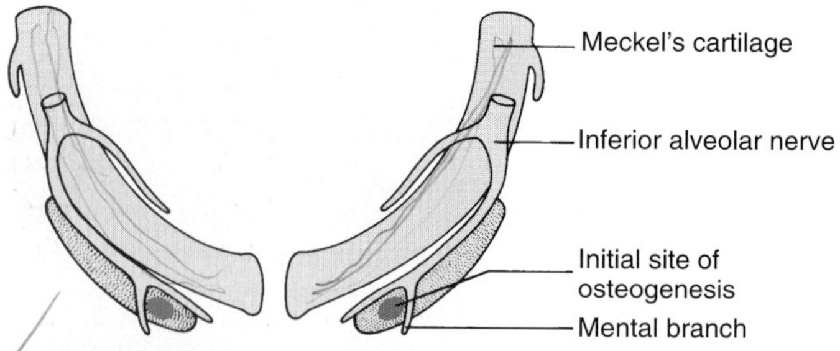

FIGURE 2-21 Diagrammatic representation of the relation of initial bone formation in the mandible to Meckel's cartilage and the inferior alveolar nerve. Bone formation begins just lateral to Meckel's cartilage and spreads posteriorly along it without any direct replacement of the cartilage by the newly forming bone of the mandible. (Redrawn from Ten Cate AR. Oral Histology: Development, Structure and Function, 5th ed. St. Louis: Mosby; 1998.)

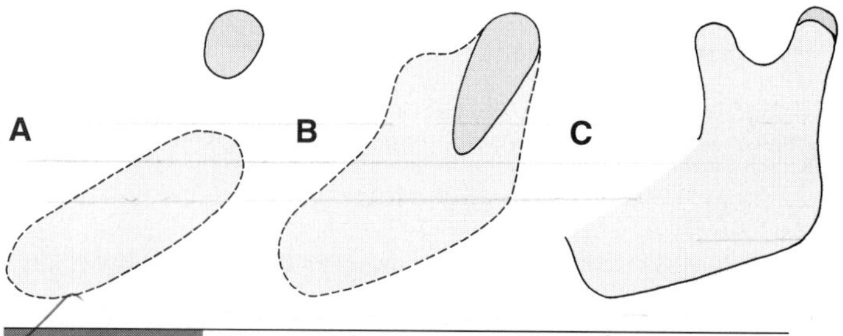

FIGURE 2-22 The condylar cartilage (*blue*) develops initially as a separate area of condensation from that of the body of the mandible, and only later is incorporated within it. **A,** Separate areas of mesenchymal condensation, at 8 weeks. **B,** Fusion of the cartilage with the mandibular body, at 4 months. **C,** Situation at birth (reduced to scale).

in length of these bones. The periosteum on the surfaces of the bones also plays an important role in adding to thickness and in reshaping the external contours.

Near the outer end of each epiphyseal plate is a zone of actively dividing cartilage cells. Some of these, pushed toward the diaphysis by proliferative activity beneath, undergo hypertrophy, secrete an extracellular matrix, and eventually degenerate as the matrix begins to mineralize and then is rapidly replaced by bone (see Figure 2-19). As long as the rate at which cartilage cells proliferate is equal to or greater than the rate at which they mature, growth will continue. Eventually, however, toward the end of the normal growth period, the rate of maturation exceeds the rate of proliferation, the last of the cartilage is replaced by bone, and the epiphyseal plate disappears. At that point, the growth of the bone is complete, except for surface changes in thickness, which can be produced by the periosteum.

Not all bones of the adult skeleton were represented in the embryonic cartilaginous model, and it is possible for bone to form by secretion of bone matrix directly within connective tissues, without any intermediate formation of cartilage. Bone formation of this type is called *intramembranous bone formation.* This type of ossification occurs in the cranial vault and both jaws (Figure 2-20).

Early in embryonic life, the mandible of higher animals develops in the same area as the cartilage of the first pharyngeal arch—Meckel's cartilage. It would seem that the mandible should be a bony replacement for this cartilage in the same way that the sphenoid bone beneath the brain replaces the cartilage in that area. In fact, development of the mandible begins as a condensation of mesenchyme just lateral to Meckel's cartilage and proceeds entirely as an intramembranous bone formation (Figure 2-21). Meckel's cartilage disintegrates and largely disappears as the bony mandible develops. Remnants of this cartilage are transformed into a portion of two of the small bones that form the conductive ossicles of the middle ear but not into a significant part of the mandible. Its perichondrium persists as the sphenomandibular ligament. The condylar cartilage develops initially as an independent secondary cartilage, which is separated by a considerable gap from the body of the mandible (Figure 2-22). Early in fetal life, it fuses with the developing mandibular ramus.

The maxilla forms initially from a center of mesenchymal condensation in the maxillary process. This area is located on the lateral surface of the nasal capsule, the most anterior part of the chondrocranium, but although the growth cartilage contributes to lengthening of the head and anterior displacement of the maxilla, it does not contribute directly to formation of the maxillary bone. An accessory cartilage, the

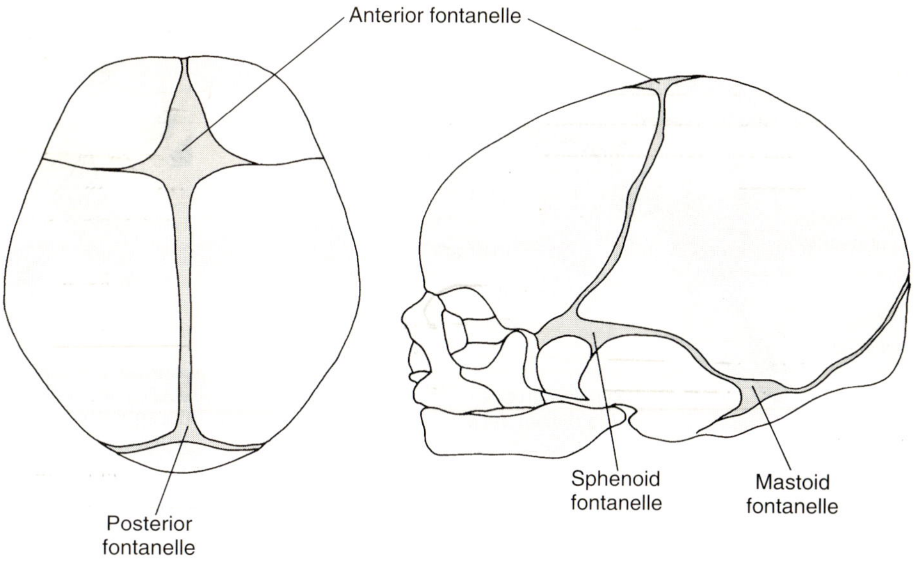

Figure 2-23 The fontanelles of the newborn skull (*blue*).

zygomatic or malar cartilage, which forms in the developing malar process, disappears and is totally replaced by bone well before birth, unlike the mandibular condylar cartilage, which persists.

Whatever the location for intramembranous bone formation, interstitial growth within the mineralized mass is impossible, and the bone must be formed entirely by apposition of new bone to free surfaces. Its shape can be changed through removal (resorption) of bone in one area and addition (apposition) of bone in another (see Figure 2-14). This balance of apposition and resorption, with new bone being formed in some areas while old bone is removed in others, is an essential component of the growth process. *Remodeling* of this type is seen at the surfaces of bones that are growing primarily by endochondral replacement, as well as in bones that formed directly within a connective tissue membrane.

Sites and Types of Growth in the Craniofacial Complex

To understand growth in any area of the body, it is necessary to understand: (1) the sites or location of growth, (2) the type of growth occurring at that location, and (3) the determinant or controlling factors in that growth.

For the following discussion of sites and types of growth, it is convenient to divide the craniofacial complex into four areas that grow rather differently: (1) the cranial vault, the bones that cover the upper and outer surface of the brain; (2) the cranial base, the bony floor under the brain, which also is the dividing line between the cranium and the face; (3) the nasomaxillary complex, made up of the nose, maxilla, and associated small bones; and (4) the mandible. Determinants or controlling factors, as they are viewed from the perspective of current theories of growth control, are discussed in the following section.

Cranial Vault

The cranial vault is made up of a number of flat bones that are formed directly by intramembranous bone formation, without cartilaginous precursors. From the time that ossification begins at a number of centers that foreshadow the eventual anatomic bony units, the growth process is entirely the result of periosteal activity at the surfaces of the bones. Remodeling and growth occur primarily at the periosteum-lined contact areas between adjacent skull bones, the *cranial sutures,* but periosteal activity also changes both the inner and outer surfaces of these platelike bones.

At birth, the flat bones of the skull are rather widely separated by relatively loose connective tissues (Figure 2-23). These open spaces, the fontanelles, allow a considerable amount of deformation of the skull at birth. This is important in allowing the relatively large head to pass through the birth canal (see Chapter 3 for more detail). After birth, apposition of bone along the edges of the fontanelles eliminates these open spaces fairly quickly, but the bones remain separated by a thin, periosteum-lined suture for many years, eventually fusing in adult life.

Despite their small size, apposition of new bone at these sutures is the major mechanism for growth of the cranial vault. Although the majority of growth in the cranial vault occurs at the sutures, there is a tendency for bone to be removed from the inner surface of the cranial vault, while at the same time, new bone is added on the exterior surface. This remodeling of the inner and outer surfaces allows for changes in contour during growth.

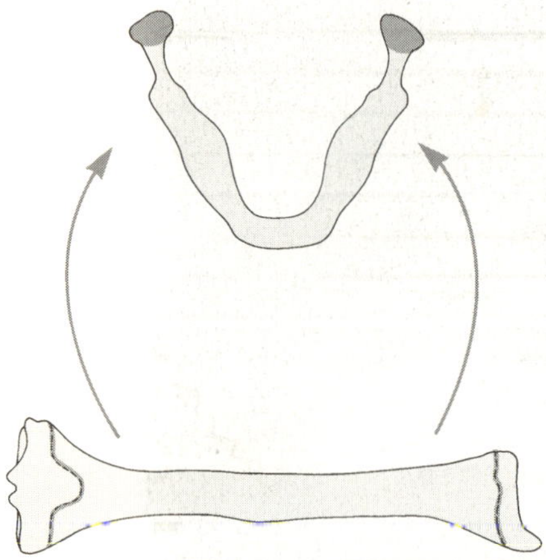

FIGURE 2-36 The mandible was once viewed conceptually as being analogous to a long bone that had been modified by (1) removal of the epiphysis, leaving the epiphyseal plates exposed, and (2) bending of the shaft into a horseshoe shape. If this analogy were correct, of course, the cartilage at the mandibular condyles should behave like true growth cartilage. Modern experiments indicate that, although the analogy is attractive, it is incorrect.

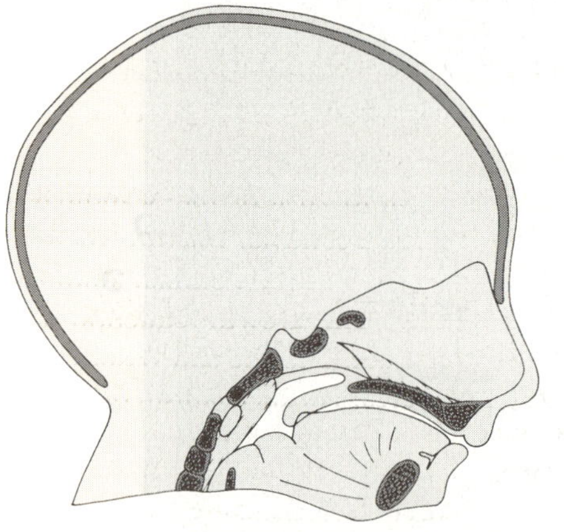

FIGURE 2-37 Diagrammatic representation of the chondrocranium at an early stage of development, showing the large amount of cartilage in the anterior region that eventually becomes the cartilaginous nasal septum.

Two kinds of experiments have been carried out to test the idea that cartilage can serve as a true growth center. These involve an analysis of the results of transplanting cartilage and an evaluation of the effect on growth of removing cartilage at an early age.

Transplantation experiments demonstrate that not all skeletal cartilage acts the same when transplanted. If a piece of the epiphyseal plate of a long bone is transplanted, it will continue to grow in a new location or in culture, indicating that these cartilages do have innate growth potential. Cartilage from the spheno-occipital synchondrosis of the cranial base also grows when transplanted, but not as well. It is difficult to obtain cartilage from the cranial base to transplant, particularly at an early age, when the cartilage is actively growing under normal conditions; perhaps this explains why it does not grow in vitro as much as epiphyseal plate cartilage. In early experiments, transplanting cartilage from the nasal septum gave equivocal results: sometimes it grew, sometimes it did not. In more precise recent experiments, however, nasal septal cartilage was found to grow nearly as well in culture as epiphyseal plate cartilage.[13] Little or no growth was observed when the mandibular condyle was transplanted, and cartilage from the mandibular condyle showed significantly less growth in culture than the other cartilages.[14] From these experiments, the other cartilages appear capable of acting as growth centers, but the mandibular condylar cartilage does not.

Experiments to test the effect of removing cartilages are also informative. The basic idea is that if removing a cartilaginous area stops or diminishes growth, perhaps it really was an important center for growth. In rodents, removing a segment of the cartilaginous nasal septum causes a considerable deficit in growth of the midface. It does not necessarily follow, however, that the entire effect on growth in such experiments results from loss of the cartilage. It can be argued that the surgery itself and the accompanying interference with blood supply to the area, not the loss of the cartilage, cause the growth changes.

There are few reported cases of early loss of the cartilaginous nasal septum in humans. One individual in whom the entire septum was removed at age 8 after an injury is shown in Figure 2-38. It is apparent that a midface deficiency developed, but one cannot confidently attribute this to the loss of the cartilage. Nevertheless, the loss of growth in experimental animals when this cartilage is removed is great enough to lead most observers to conclude that the septal cartilage does have some innate growth potential, whose loss makes a difference in maxillary growth, and the rare human cases support this view.

The neck of the mandibular condyle is a relatively fragile area. When the side of the jaw is struck sharply, the mandible often fractures just below the opposite condyle. When this happens, the condyle fragment is usually retracted well away from its previous location by the pull of the lateral pterygoid muscle (Figure 2-39). The condyle literally has been removed when this occurs, and it resorbs over a period of time. Condylar fractures occur relatively frequently in children. If the condyle was an important growth center, one would expect to see severe growth impairment after such an injury at an early age. If so, surgical intervention to locate the condylar segment and put it back into position would be the logical treatment.

Two excellent studies carried out in Scandinavia disproved this concept. Both Gilhuus-Moe[15] and Lund[16] demonstrated that after fracture of the mandibular condyle in a child, there was an excellent chance that the condylar process would regenerate to approximately its original size

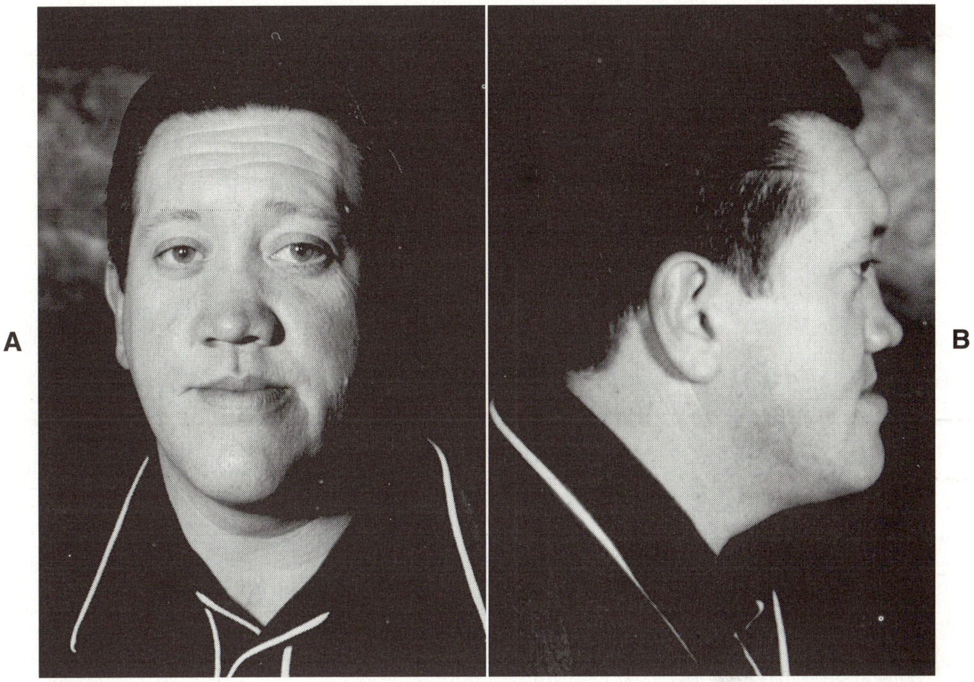

Figure 2-38 Profile view of a man whose cartilaginous nasal septum was removed at age 8, after an injury. The obvious midface deficiency developed after the septum was removed.

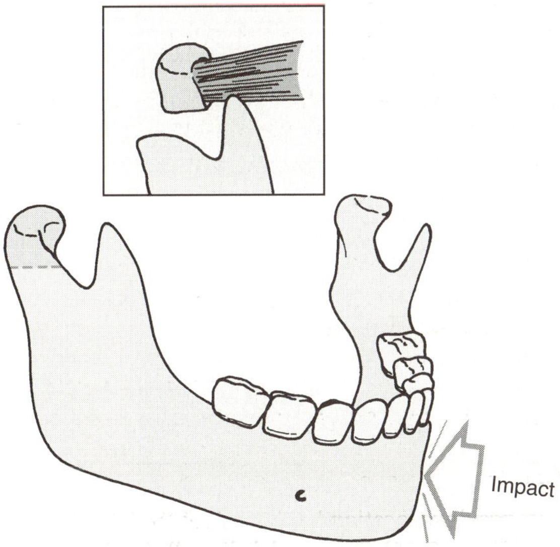

Figure 2-39 A blow to one side of the mandible may fracture the condylar process on the opposite side. When this happens, the pull of the lateral pterygoid muscle distracts the condylar fragment, including all the cartilage, and it subsequently resorbs.

and a small chance that it would overgrow after the injury. In experimental animals and in children, after a fracture, all of the original bone and cartilage resorb, and a new condyle regenerates directly from periosteum at the fracture site (Figure 2-40). Eventually, at least in experimental animals, a new layer of cartilage forms at the condylar surface. Although there is no direct evidence that the cartilage layer itself regenerates in children after condylar fractures, it is likely that this occurs in humans also.

However, in 15% to 20% of the Scandinavian children studied who suffered a condylar fracture, there was a reduction in growth after the injury. Similar findings have been reported elsewhere.[17] This growth reduction seems to relate to the amount of trauma to the soft tissues and the resultant scarring in the area. The mechanism by which this occurs is discussed in the following section.

In summary, it appears that epiphyseal cartilages and (probably) the cranial base synchondroses can and do act as independently growing centers, as can the nasal septum (perhaps to a lesser extent). Transplantation experiments and experiments in which the condyle is removed lend no support to the idea that the cartilage of the mandibular condyle is an important center. Neither do studies of the cartilage itself in comparison to primary growth cartilage. It appears that the growth at the mandibular condyles is much more analogous to growth at the sutures of the maxilla—entirely reactive—than to growth at an epiphyseal plate.

Functional Matrix Theory of Growth

If neither bone nor cartilage was the determinant for growth of the craniofacial skeleton, it would appear that the control would have to lie in the adjacent soft tissues. This point of view was put formally in the 1960s by Moss, in his "functional matrix theory" of growth, and was reviewed and updated by him in the 1990s.[18] While granting the innate

A

B

C

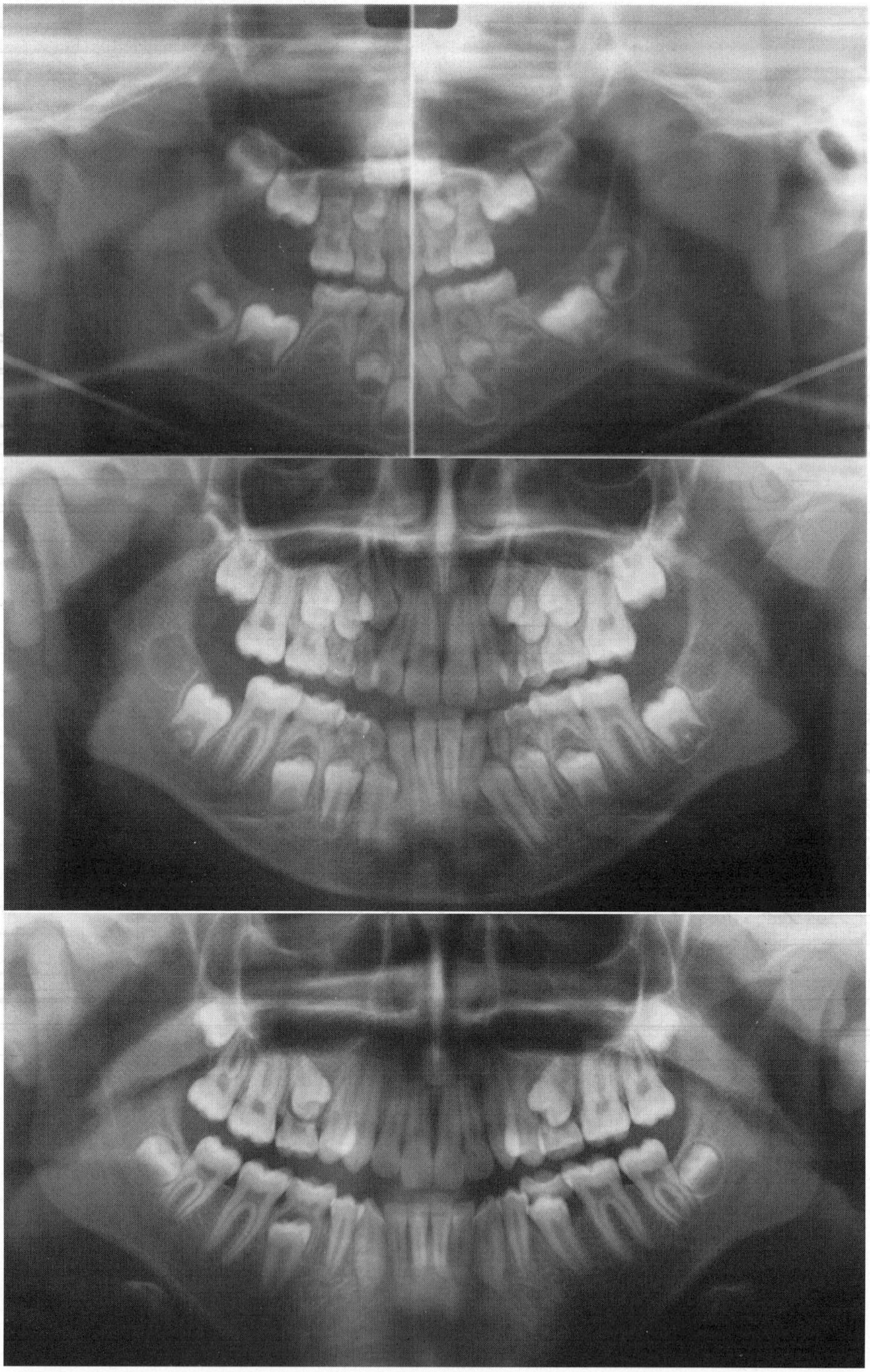

Figure 2-40 After a condylar fracture and resorption of the condyle, regeneration of a new condyle is quite possible in humans. Whether it occurs is a function of the severity of the soft tissue injury that accompanied the fracture. **A,** Age 5, at the time mandibular asymmetry was noticed on a routine dental visit. Note that the left condylar process is missing. The history included a fall at age 2 with a blow to the chin that created a condylar fracture, with no regeneration up to that time. **B,** Age 8, after treatment with an asymmetric functional appliance that led to growth on the affected side and a reduction in the asymmetry. **C,** Age 14, at the end of the adolescent growth spurt. Regeneration of a condyle on the affected side is apparent in **(B)** and **(C).**

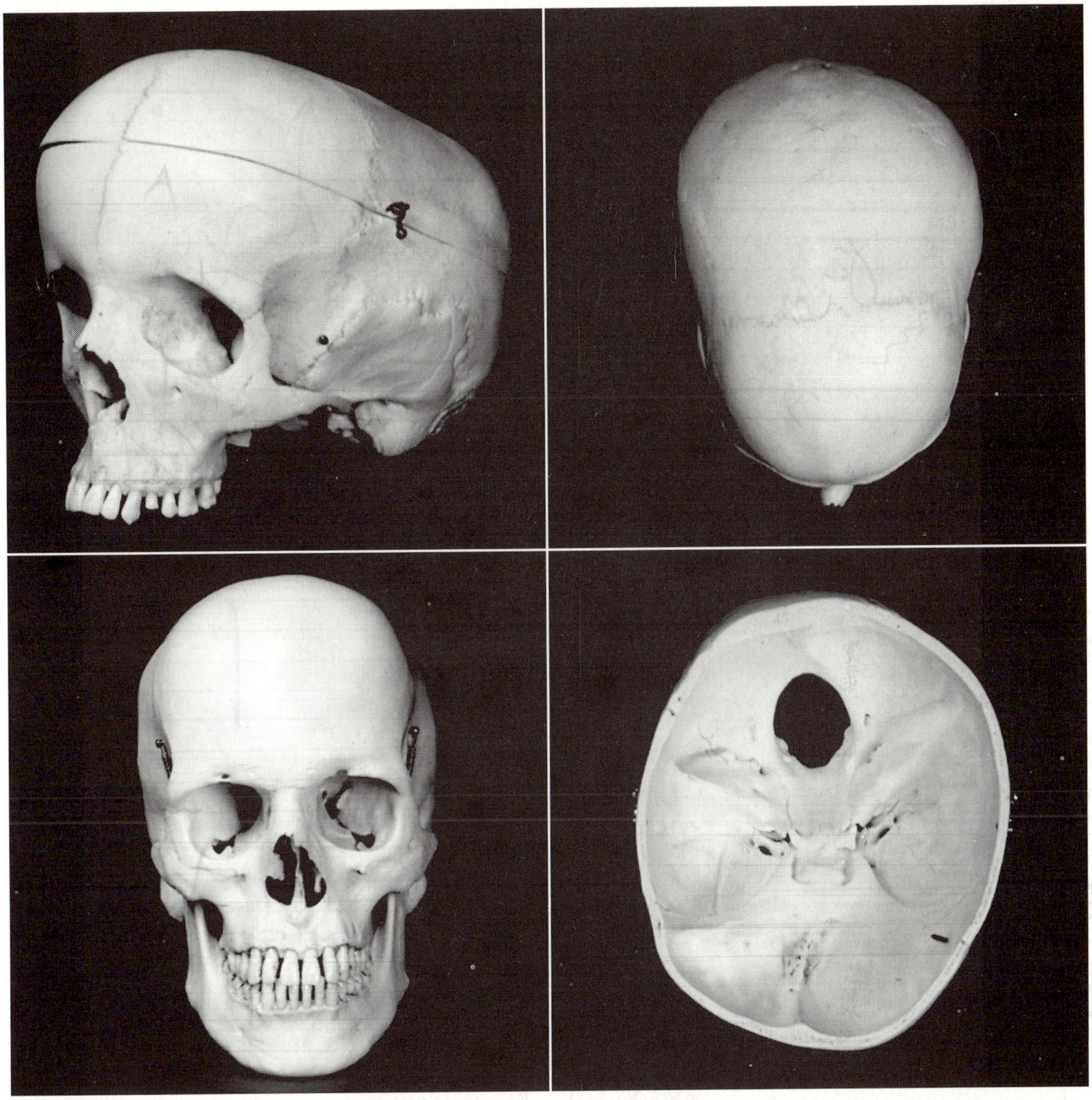

Figure 2-41 **A,** The skull of a young child who had hydrocephaly. Note the tremendous enlargement of the brain case in response to the increased intracranial pressure. **B** and **C,** Superior and front views of the skull of an individual with scaphocephaly, in which the midsagittal suture fuses prematurely. Note the absence of the midsagittal suture and the extremely narrow width of the cranium. In compensation for its inability to grow laterally, the brain and brain case have become abnormally long posteriorly. **D,** Cranial base of an individual with premature fusion of sutures on the right side, leading to a marked asymmetry that affected both the cranium and cranial base.

growth potential of cartilages of the long bones, his theory holds that neither the cartilage of the mandibular condyle nor the nasal septum cartilage is a determinant of jaw growth. Instead, he theorizes that growth of the face occurs as a response to functional needs and neurotrophic influences and is mediated by the soft tissue in which the jaws are embedded. In this conceptual view, the soft tissues grow, and both bone and cartilage react.

The growth of the cranium illustrates this view of skeletal growth very well. There can be little question that the growth of the cranial vault is a direct response to the growth of the brain. Pressure exerted by the growing brain separates the cranial bones at the sutures, and new bone passively fills in at these sites so that the brain case fits the brain.

This phenomenon can be seen readily in humans in two experiments of nature (Figure 2-41). First, when the brain is very small, the cranium is also very small, and the condition of microcephaly results. In this case, the size of the head is an accurate representation of the size of the brain. A second natural experiment is the condition called hydrocephaly. In this case, reabsorption of cerebrospinal fluid is impeded, the fluid accumulates, and intracranial pressure builds up. The

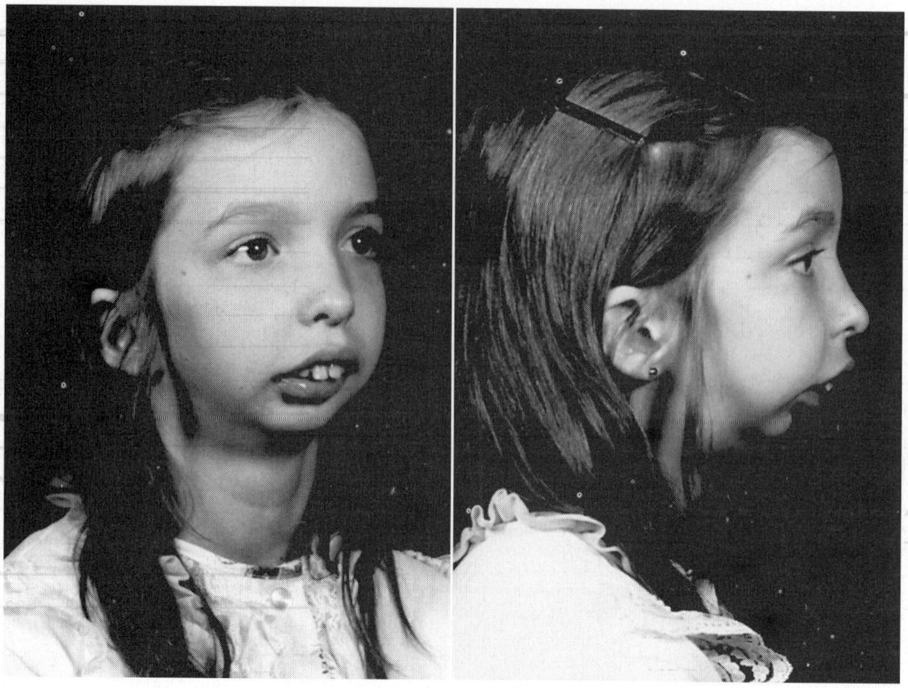

FIGURE 2-42 Oblique **(A)** and profile **(B)** views of a girl in whom a severe infection of the mastoid air cells involved the temporomandibular joint and led to ankylosis of the mandible. The resulting restriction of mandibular growth is apparent.

increased intracranial pressure impedes development of the brain, so the hydrocephalic may have a small brain and be mentally retarded; but this condition also leads to an enormous growth of the cranial vault. Uncontrolled hydrocephaly may lead to a cranium two or three times its normal size, with enormously enlarged frontal, parietal, and occipital bones. This is perhaps the clearest example of a "functional matrix" in operation. Another excellent example is the relationship between the size of the eye and the size of the orbit. An enlarged eye or a small eye will cause a corresponding change in the size of the orbital cavity. In this instance, the eye is the functional matrix.

Moss theorizes that the major determinant of growth of the maxilla and mandible is the enlargement of the nasal and oral cavities, which grow in response to functional needs. The theory does not make it clear how functional needs are transmitted to the tissues around the mouth and nose, but it does predict that the cartilages of the nasal septum and mandibular condyles are not important determinants of growth, and that their loss would have little effect on growth if proper function could be obtained. From the view of this theory, however, absence of normal function would have wide-ranging effects.

We have already noted that in 75% to 80% of human children who suffer a condylar fracture, the resulting loss of the condyle does not impede mandibular growth. The condyle regenerates very nicely. What about the 20% to 25% of children in whom a growth deficit occurs after condylar fracture?[19] Could some interference with function be the reason for the growth deficiency?

The answer seems to be a clear *yes*. It has been known for many years that mandibular growth is greatly impaired by an ankylosis (see Figure 2-39), defined as a fusion across the joint so that motion is prevented or extremely limited. Mandibular ankylosis can develop in a number of ways. For instance, one possible cause is a severe infection in the area of the temporomandibular joint, leading to destruction of tissues and ultimate scarring (Figure 2-42). Another cause, of course, is trauma, which can result in a growth deficiency if there is enough soft tissue injury to lead to severe scarring as the injury heals. It appears that the mechanical restriction caused by scar tissue in the vicinity of the temporomandibular joint impedes translation of the mandible as the adjacent soft tissues grow, and that this is the reason for growth deficiency in some children after condylar fractures.

It is interesting, and potentially quite significant clinically, that under some circumstances, bone can be induced to grow at surgically created sites by the method called *distraction osteogenesis* (Figure 2-43). The Russian surgeon Alizarov discovered in the 1950s that if cuts were made through the cortex of a long bone of the limbs, the arm or leg then could be lengthened by tension to separate the bony segments. Current research shows that the best results are obtained if this type of distraction starts after a few days of initial healing and callus formation, and if the segments are separated at a rate of a 0.5-1.5 millimeters per day. Surprisingly, large amounts of new bone can form at the surgical site, lengthening the arm or leg by several centimeters in some cases. Distraction osteogenesis now is widely used to correct

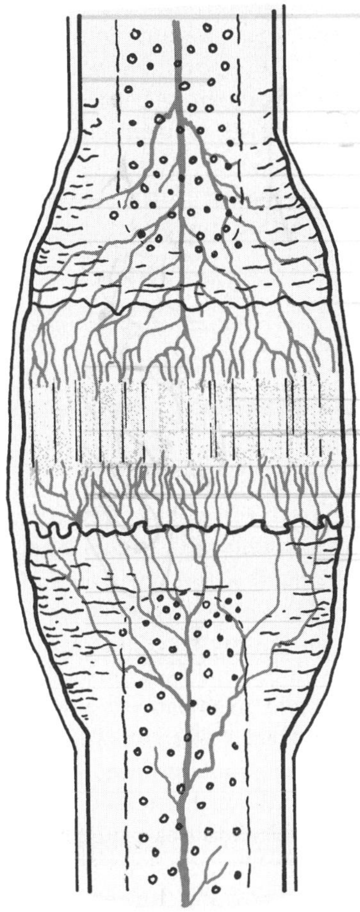

Figure 2-43 Diagrammatic representation of distraction osteogenesis in a long bone. The drawing represents the situation after bone cuts through the cortex, initial healing, and then a few weeks of distraction. In the center, a fibrous radiolucent interzone with longitudinally oriented collagen bundles in the area where lengthening of the bone is occurring. Proliferating fibroblasts and undifferentiated mesenchymal cells are found throughout this area. Osteoblasts appear at the edge of the interzone. On both sides of the interzone, a rich blood supply is present in a zone of mineralization. Beneath that, a zone of remodeling exists. This sequence of formation of a stretched collagen matrix, mineralization, and remodeling is typical of distraction osteogenesis. (Redrawn from Samchukov, et al. In: McNamara J, Trotman C, eds. Distraction Osteogenesis and Tissue Engineering. Ann Arbor, Mich: The University of Michigan Center for Human Growth and Development; 1998.)

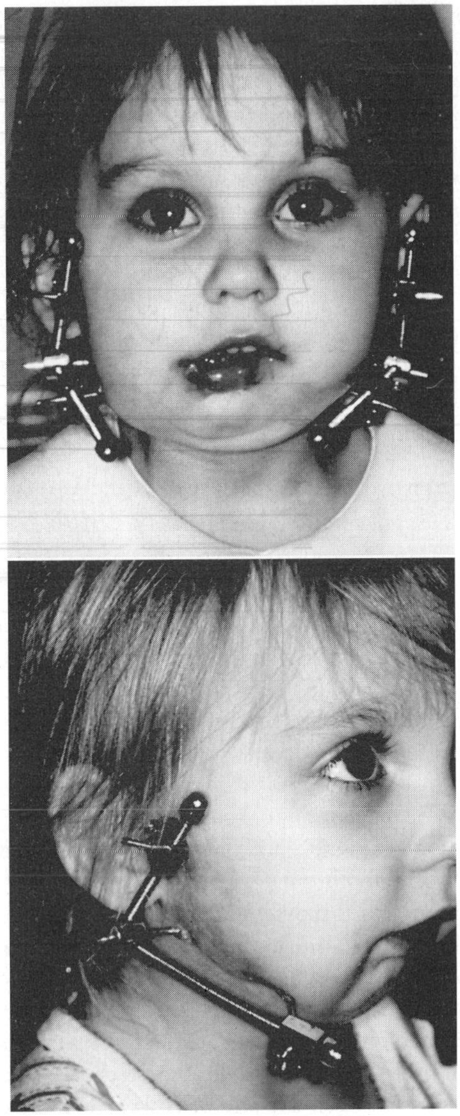

Figure 2-44 External fixation for lengthening the mandible by distraction osteogenesis in a child with severe asymmetric mandibular deficiency secondary to injury at an early age.

limb deformities, especially after injury but also in patients with congenital problems.

The bone of the mandible is quite similar in its internal structure to the bone of the limbs, even though its developmental course is rather different. Lengthening the mandible via distraction osteogenesis clearly is possible (Figure 2-44), and major changes in mandibular length (a centimeter or more) are managed best in this way. Precise positioning of the jaw is not possible, however, so conventional orthognathic surgery remains the preferred way to treat mandibular deficiency. In a sense, inducing maxillary growth by separating cranial and facial bones at their sutures is a distraction method. Manipulating maxillary growth by influencing growth at the sutures has been a major part of orthodontic treatment for many years, and this can be done at later ages with surgical assistance. The current status of distraction osteogenesis as a method to correct deficient growth in the face and jaws is reviewed in some detail in Chapter 19.

In summary, it appears that growth of the cranium occurs almost entirely in response to growth of the brain. Growth of the cranial base is primarily the result of endochondral growth and bony replacement at the synchondroses, which have independent growth potential but perhaps are influenced by the growth of the brain. Growth of the maxilla and its associated structures occurs from a combination of growth at sutures and direct remodeling of the surfaces of the bone. The maxilla is translated downward and forward as the face grows, and new bone fills in at the sutures. The extent to which growth of cartilage of the nasal septum leads to translation of the maxilla remains unknown, but both the surrounding soft tissues and this cartilage probably contribute to the forward repositioning of the maxilla. Growth of the mandible occurs by both endochondral proliferation at the condyle and apposition and resorption of bone at surfaces. It seems clear that the mandible is translated in space by the growth of muscles and other adjacent soft tissues, and that addition of new bone at the condyle is in response to the soft tissue changes.

Social and Behavioral Development

F.T. McIver and W.R. Proffit

Physical growth can be considered the outcome of an interaction between genetically controlled cell proliferation and environmental influences that modify the genetic program. Similarly, behavior can be viewed as the result of an interaction between innate or instinctual behavioral patterns and behaviors learned after birth. In animals, it appears that the majority of behaviors are instinctive, although even lower animals are capable of a degree of learned behavior. In humans, on the other hand, it is generally conceded that the great majority of behaviors are learned.

For this reason, it is less easy to construct stages of behavioral development in humans than stages of physical development. The higher proportion of learned behavior means that what might be considered environmental effects can greatly modify behavior. On the other hand, there are human instinctual behaviors (e.g., the sex drive), and, in a sense, the outcome of behavior hinges on how the instinctual behavioral urges have been modified by learning. As a general rule, the older the individual, the more complex the behavioral pattern and the more important the learned overlay of behavior will be.

In this section, a brief overview of social, cognitive and behavioral development is presented, greatly simplifying a complex subject and emphasizing the evaluation and management of children who will be receiving dental and orthodontic treatment. First, the process by which behavior can be learned is presented. Second, the structural substrate of behavior, which appears to relate both to the organization of the nervous system at various stages and to emotional components underlying the expression of behavior, will be reviewed. The relevance of the theoretical concepts to the day-to-day treatment of patients is emphasized.

Learning and the Development of Behavior

The basic mechanisms of learning appear to be essentially the same at all ages. As learning proceeds, more complex skills and behaviors appear, but it is difficult to define the process in distinct stages—a continuous flow model appears more appropriate. It is important to remember that this discussion is of the development of behavioral patterns, not the acquisition of knowledge or intellectual skills in the academic sense.

At present, psychologists generally consider that there are three distinct mechanisms by which behavioral responses are learned: (1) classical conditioning, (2) operant conditioning, and (3) observational learning.

Classical Conditioning

Classical conditioning was first described by the Russian physiologist Ivan Pavlov, who discovered in the nineteenth century during his studies of reflexes that apparently unassociated stimuli could produce reflexive behavior. Pavlov's classic experiments involved the presentation of food to a hungry animal, along with some other stimulus, for example, the ringing of a bell. The sight and sound of food normally elicit salivation by a reflex mechanism. If a bell is rung each time food is presented, the auditory stimulus of the ringing bell will become associated with the food presentation stimulus, and, in a relatively short time, the ringing of a bell by itself will elicit salivation. Classical conditioning, then, operates by the simple process of association of one stimulus with another. For that reason, this mode of learning is sometimes referred to as learning by association.

Classical conditioning occurs readily with young children and can have a considerable impact on a young child's behavior on the first visit to a dental office. By the time a child is brought for the first visit to a dentist, even if that visit is at an early age, it is highly likely that he or she will have had many experiences with pediatricians and medical personnel. When a child experiences pain, the reflex reaction is crying and withdrawal. In Pavlovian terms, the infliction of pain is an unconditioned stimulus, but a number of aspects of the setting in which the pain occurs can come to be associated with this unconditioned stimulus.

For instance, it is unusual for a child to encounter people who are dressed entirely in white uniforms or long white coats. If the unconditioned stimulus of painful treatment comes to be associated with the conditioned stimulus of white coats (Figure 2-45), a child may cry and withdraw immediately at the first sight of a white-coated dentist or dental assistant. In this case, the child has learned to associate the conditioned stimulus of pain and the unconditioned stimulus of a white-coated adult, and the mere sight of the white coat is enough to produce the reflex behavior initially associated with pain.

Associations of this type tend to become generalized. Painful and unpleasant experiences associated with medical treatment can become generalized to the atmosphere of a physician's office, so that the whole atmosphere of a waiting room, receptionist, and other waiting children may produce crying and withdrawal after several experiences in the physician's office, even if there is no sign of a white coat.

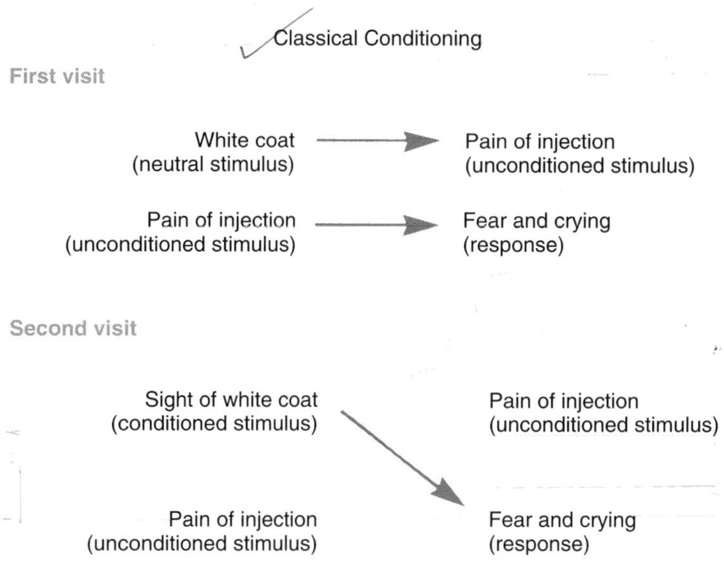

FIGURE 2-45 Classical conditioning causes an originally neutral stimulus to become associated with one that leads to a specific reaction. If individuals in white coats are the ones who give painful injections that cause crying, the sight of an individual in a white coat soon may provoke an outburst of crying.

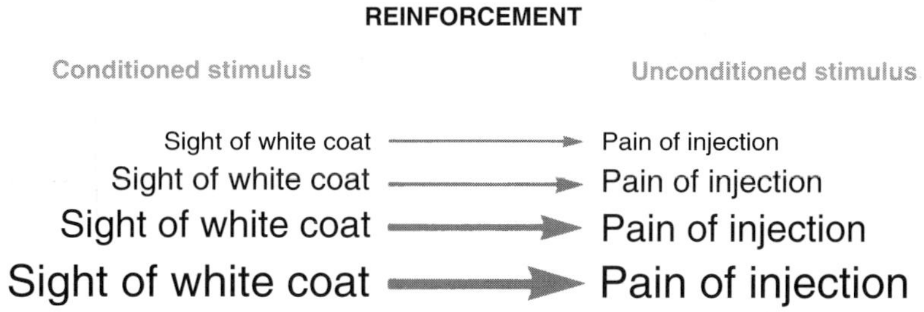

FIGURE 2-46 Every time they occur, the association between a conditioned and unconditioned stimulus is strengthened. This process is called reinforcement.

Because of this association, behavior management in the dentist's office is easier if the dental office looks as little like the typical pediatrician's office or hospital clinic as possible. In practices where the dentist and auxiliaries work with young children, they have found it helps in reducing children's anxiety if their appearance is different from that associated with the physician. It also helps if they can make the child's first visit as different as possible from the previous visits to the physician. Treatment that might produce pain should be avoided if at all possible on the first visit to the dental office.

The association between a conditioned and an unconditioned stimulus is strengthened or reinforced every time they occur together (Figure 2-46). Every time a child is taken to a hospital clinic where something painful is done, the association between pain and the general atmosphere of that clinic becomes stronger, as the child becomes more sure of his conclusion that bad things happen in such a place. Conversely, if the association between a conditioned and an unconditioned stimulus is not reinforced, the association between them will become less strong, and eventually, the conditioned response will no longer occur. This phenomenon is referred to as *extinction of the conditioned behavior*. Once a conditioned response has been established, it is necessary to reinforce it only occasionally to maintain it. If the conditioned association of pain with the doctor's office is strong, it can take many visits without unpleasant experiences and pain to extinguish the associated crying and avoidance.

The opposite of generalization of a conditioned stimulus is discrimination. The conditioned association of white coats with pain can easily be generalized to any office setting. If a child is taken into other office settings that are somewhat different from the one where painful things happen, a dental office, for instance, where painful injections are not necessary, a discrimination between the two types of offices soon will develop, and the generalized response to any office as a place where painful things occur will be extinguished.

Operant Conditioning

Operant conditioning, which can be viewed conceptually as a significant extension of classical conditioning, was emphasized by the preeminent behavioral theorist of recent years, B. F. Skinner. Skinner contended that the most complex human behaviors can be explained by operant conditioning. His theories, which downplay the role of the individual's conscious determination in favor of unconscious determined behavior, have met with much resistance but have been remarkably successful in explaining many aspects of social behavior far too complicated to be understood from the perspective of classical conditioning.

Since the theory of operant conditioning explains—or attempts to explain—complex behavior, it is not surprising that the theory itself is more complex. Although it is not possible here to explore operant conditioning in any detail, a brief overview is presented as an aid in understanding the acquisition of behavior that older children are likely to demonstrate in the dentist's or orthodontist's office.

The basic principle of operant conditioning is that the consequence of a behavior is in itself a stimulus that can affect future behavior (Figure 2-47). In other words, the consequence that follows a response will alter the probability of that response occurring again in a similar situation. In classical conditioning, a stimulus leads to a response; in operant conditioning, a response becomes a further stimulus. The general rule is that if the consequence of a certain response is pleasant or desirable, that response is more likely to be used again in the future; but if a particular response produces an unpleasant consequence, the probability of that response being used in the future is diminished.

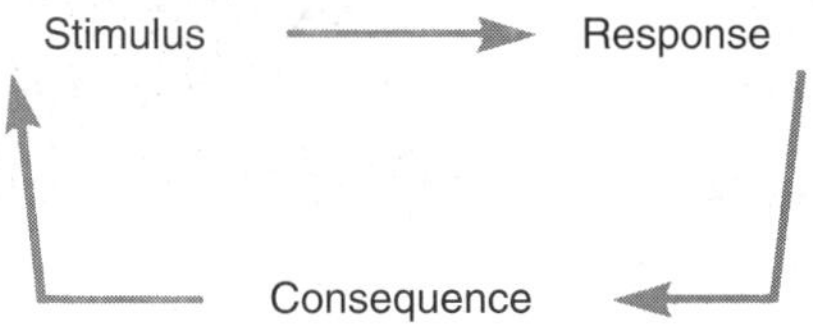

FIGURE 2-47 Operant conditioning differs from classical conditioning in that the consequence of a behavior is considered a stimulus for future behavior. This means that the consequence of any particular response will affect the probability of that response occurring again in a similar situation.

Skinner described four basic types of operant conditioning, distinguished by the nature of the consequence (Figure 2-48). The first of these is *positive reinforcement*. If a pleasant consequence follows a response, the response has been positively reinforced, and the behavior that led to this pleasant consequence becomes more likely in the future. For example, if a child is given a reward such as a toy for behaving well during her first dental visit, she is more likely to behave well during future dental visits; her behavior was positively reinforced.

A second type of operant conditioning, called *negative reinforcement*, involves the withdrawal of an unpleasant stimulus after a response. Like positive reinforcement, negative reinforcement increases the likelihood of a response in the future. In this context, the word *negative* is somewhat misleading. It merely refers to the fact that the response that is reinforced is a response that leads to the removal of an undesirable stimulus. Note that negative reinforcement is not a synonym for *punishment*, another type of operant conditioning.

As an example, a child who views a visit to the hospital clinic as an unpleasant experience may throw a temper tantrum at the prospect of having to go there. If this behavior (response) succeeds in allowing the child to escape the visit to the clinic, the behavior has been negatively reinforced and is more likely to occur the next time a visit to the clinic is proposed. The same can be true, of course, in the dentist's office. If behavior considered unacceptable by the dentist and his staff nevertheless succeeds in allowing the child to escape from dental treatment, that behavior has been negatively reinforced and is more likely to occur the next time the child is in the dental office. In dental practice, it is important to reinforce only desired behavior, and it is equally important to avoid reinforcing behavior that is not desired.[20]

The other two types of operant conditioning decrease the likelihood of a response. The third type, *omission* (also called time-out), involves removal of a pleasant stimulus after a

	Probability of Response Increases	Probability of Response Decreases
Pleasant stimulus (S_1)	I S_1 Presented Positive reinforcement or reward	III S_1 Withdrawn Omission or time-out
Unpleasant stimulus (S_2)	II S_2 Withdrawn Negative reinforcement or escape	IV S_2 Presented Punishment

FIGURE 2-48 The four basic types of operant conditioning.

particular response. For example, if a child who throws a temper tantrum has his favorite toy taken away for a short time as a consequence of this behavior, the probability of similar misbehavior is decreased. Because children are likely to regard attention by others as a very pleasant stimulus, withholding attention following undesirable behavior is a use of omission that is likely to reduce the unwanted behavior.

The fourth type of operant conditioning, *punishment*, occurs when an unpleasant stimulus is presented after a response. This also decreases the probability that the behavior that prompted punishment will occur in the future. Punishment, like the other forms of operant conditioning, is effective at all ages, not just with children. For example, if the dentist with her new sports car receives a ticket for driving 50 miles per hour down a street marked for 35 miles per hour, she is likely to drive more slowly down that particular street in the future, particularly if she thinks that the same radar speed trap is still operating. Punishment, of course, has traditionally been used as a method of behavior modification in children, more so in some societies than others.

In general, positive and negative reinforcement are the most suitable types of operant conditioning for use in the dental office, particularly for motivating orthodontic patients who must cooperate at home even more than in the dental office. Both types of reinforcement increase the likelihood of a particular behavior recurring, rather than attempting to suppress a behavior as punishment and omission do. Simply praising a child for desirable behavior produces positive reinforcement, and additional positive reinforcement can be achieved by presenting some tangible reward.

Older children are just as susceptible to positive reinforcement as younger ones. Adolescents in the orthodontic treatment age, for instance, can obtain positive reinforcement from a simple pin saying, "World's Greatest Orthodontic Patient," or something similar. A reward system, perhaps providing a T-shirt with some slogan as a prize for three consecutive appointments with good hygiene, is another simple example of positive reinforcement (Figure 2-49).

Negative reinforcement, which also accentuates the probability of any given behavior, is more difficult to utilize as a behavioral management tool in the dental office, but it can be used effectively if the circumstances permit. If a child is concerned about a treatment procedure but behaves well and understands that the procedure has been shortened because of his good behavior, the desired behavior has been negatively reinforced. In orthodontic treatment, long bonding and banding appointments may go more efficiently and smoothly if the child understands that his helpful behavior has shortened the procedure and reduced the possibility that the procedure will need to be redone.

The other two types of operant conditioning, omission and punishment, should be used sparingly and with caution in the dental office. Since a positive stimulus is removed in omission, the child may react with anger or frustration. When punishment is used, both fear and anger sometimes result. In fact, punishment can lead to a classically conditioned fear response. Obviously, it is a good idea for the dentist and staff to avoid creating fear and anger in a child (or adult) patient, and thus these two types of operant conditioning should be used cautiously.

One mild form of punishment that can be used with children is called "voice control." Voice control involves speaking to the child in a firm voice to gain his (or her) attention, telling him that his present behavior is unacceptable, and directing him as to how he (or she) should behave. This technique should be used with care, and the child should be immediately rewarded for an improvement in his behavior. It is most effective when a warm, caring relationship has been established between the dental team and the patient.[31]

A

B

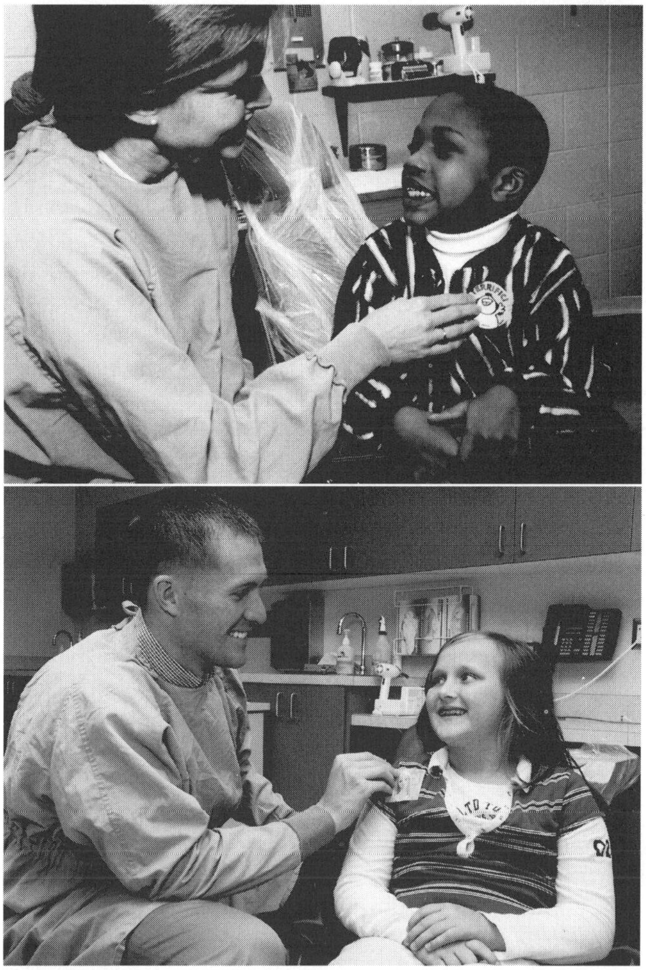

FIGURE 2-49 **A,** This 8-year-old boy is being positively reinforced by receiving a "terrific patient" button after his visit to the dentist. **B,** The same methods work well for older orthodontic patients, who enjoy receiving a reward like a "great patient" sticker to put on a shirt or a T-shirt with a message related to orthodontic treatment (for example, "Braces are *Cool*").

There is no doubt that operant conditioning can be used to modify behavior in individuals of any age, and that it forms the basis for many of the behavior patterns of life. Behavioral theorists believe that operant conditioning forms the pattern of essentially all behavior, not just the relatively superficial ones. Whether or not this is true, operant conditioning is a powerful tool for learning of behavior and an important influence throughout life.

Concepts of reinforcement as opposed to extinction, and generalization as opposed to discrimination, apply to operant conditioning as well as to classical conditioning. In operant conditioning, of course, the concepts apply to the situation in which a response leads to a particular consequence, not to the conditioned stimulus that directly controls the conditioned response. Positive or negative reinforcement becomes even more effective if repeated, although it is not necessary to provide a reward at every visit to the dental office to obtain positive reinforcement. Similarly, conditioning obtained through positive reinforcement can be extinguished if the desired behavior is now followed by omission, punishment, or simply a lack of further positive reinforcement.

Operant conditioning that occurs in one situation can also be generalized to similar situations. For example, a child who has been positively reinforced for good behavior in the pediatrician's office is likely to behave well on the first visit to a dentist's office because he or she will anticipate a reward at the dentist's also, based on the similarity of the situation. A child who continues to be rewarded for good behavior in the pediatrician's office but does not receive similar rewards in the dentist's office, however, will learn to discriminate between the two situations and may eventually behave better for the pediatrician than for the dentist.

Observational Learning (Modeling)

Another potent way that behavior is acquired is through imitation of behavior observed in a social context. This type of learning appears to be distinct from learning by either classical or operant conditioning. Acquisition of behavior through imitation of the behavior of others, of course, is entirely compatible with both classical and operant conditioning. Some theorists emphasize the importance of learning by imitation in a social context,[22] whereas others, especially Skinner and his followers, argue that conditioning is more important, although recognizing that learning by imitation can occur. It certainly seems that much of a child's behavior in a dental office can be learned from observing siblings, other children, or even parents.

There are two distinct stages in observational learning: *acquisition* of the behavior by observing it, and the actual *performance* of that behavior (Figure 2-50). A child can observe many behaviors and thereby acquire the potential to perform them, without immediately demonstrating or performing that behavior. Children are capable of acquiring almost any behavior that they observe closely and that is not too complex for them to perform at their level of physical development. A child is exposed to a tremendous range of possible behaviors, most of which he acquires even though the behavior may not be expressed immediately or ever.

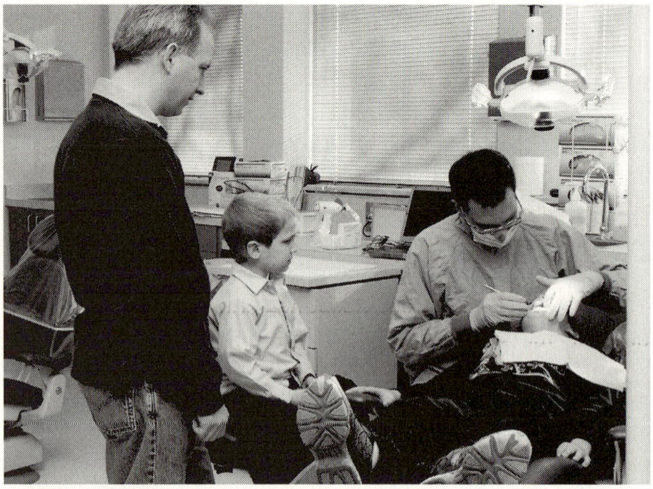

FIGURE 2-50 Observational learning: a child acquires a behavior by first observing it and then actually performing it. For that reason, allowing a younger child to observe an older one calmly receiving dental treatment (in this case, an orthodontic examination that will include impressions of the teeth) greatly increases the chance that he will behave in the same calm way when it is his turn to be examined.

Whether a child will actually perform an acquired behavior depends on several factors. Important among these are the characteristics of the role model. If the model is liked or respected, the child is more likely to imitate him or her. For this reason, a parent or older sibling is often the object of imitation by the child. For children in the elementary and junior high school age groups, peers within their own age group, or individuals slightly older, are increasingly important role models, while the influence of parents and older siblings decreases. For adolescents, the peer group is the major source of role models.

Another important influence on whether a behavior is performed is the expected consequences of the behavior. If a child observes an older sibling refuse to obey his father's command and then sees punishment follow this refusal, he is less likely to defy the father on a future occasion, but he probably still has acquired the behavior, and if he should become defiant, is likely to stage it in a similar way.

Observational learning can be an important tool in management of dental treatment. If a young child observes an older sibling undergoing dental treatment without complaint or uncooperative behavior, he or she is likely to imitate this behavior. If the older sibling is observed being rewarded, the younger child will also expect a reward for behaving well. Because the parent is an important role model for a young child, the mother's attitude toward dental treatment is likely to influence the child's approach.

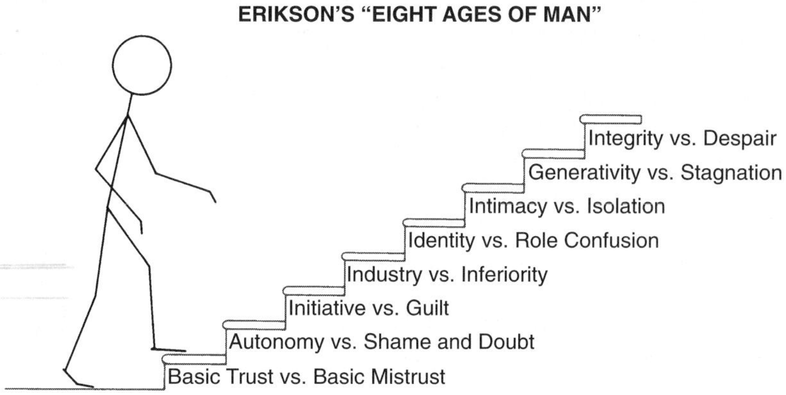

FIGURE 2-51 Erikson's stages of emotional development: the sequence is more fixed than the time when each stage is reached. Some adults never reach the final steps on the developmental staircase.

Research has demonstrated that one of the best predictors of how anxious a child will be during dental treatment is how anxious the mother is. A mother who is calm and relaxed about the prospect of dental treatment teaches the child by observation that this is the appropriate approach to being treated, whereas an anxious and alarmed mother tends to elicit the same set of responses in her child.[23]

Observational learning can be used to advantage in the design of treatment areas. At one time, it was routine for dentists to provide small private cubicles in which all patients, children and adults, were treated. The modern trend, particularly in treatment of children and adolescents but to some extent with adults also, is to carry out dental treatment in open areas with several treatment stations.

Sitting in one dental chair watching the dentist work with someone else in an adjacent chair can provide a great deal of observational learning about what the experience will be like. Direct communication among patients, answering questions about exactly what happened, can add even further learning. Both children and adolescents do better, it appears, if they are treated in open clinics rather than in private cubicles, and observational learning plays an important part in this. The dentist hopes, of course, that the patient waiting for treatment observes appropriate behavior and responses on the part of the patient who is being treated, which will be the case in a well-managed clinical setting.

Stages of Emotional and Cognitive Development

Emotional Development

In contrast to continuous learning by conditioning and observation, both emotional or personality development and cognitive or intellectual development seem to pass through relatively discrete stages. The contemporary description of emotional development is based on Sigmund Freud's psychoanalytic theory of personality development but was greatly extended by Erik Erikson.[24] Erikson's work, although connected to Freud's, represents a great departure from psychosexual stages as proposed by Freud. His "eight ages of man" illustrate a progression through a series of personality development stages. In Erikson's view, "psychosocial development proceeds by critical steps—'critical' being a characteristic of turning points, of moments of decision between progress and regression, integration and retardation." In this view, each developmental stage represents a "psychosocial crisis" in which individuals are influenced by their social environment to develop more or less toward one extreme of the conflicting personality qualities dominant at that stage.

Although chronologic ages are associated with Erikson's developmental stages, the chronologic age varies among individuals but the sequence of the developmental stages is constant. This, of course, is similar to what also happens in physical development. Rather differently from physical development, it is possible and indeed probable that qualities associated with earlier stages may be evident in later stages because of incomplete resolution of the earlier stages.

Erikson's stages of emotional development are as follows (Figure 2-51):

1. Development of Basic Trust (Birth to 18 Months). In this initial stage of emotional development a basic trust—or lack of trust—in the environment is developed. Successful development of trust depends on a caring and consistent mother or mother substitute, who meets both the physiologic and emotional needs of the infant. There are strongly held theories but no clear answers to exactly what constitutes proper mothering, but it is important that a strong bond develop between parent and child. This bond must be maintained to allow the child to develop basic trust in the world. In fact, physical growth can be significantly retarded unless the child's emotional needs are met by appropriate mothering.

The syndrome of "maternal deprivation," in which a child receives inadequate maternal support, is well recognized though fortunately rare. Such infants fail to gain weight and are retarded in their physical as well as emotional growth. The maternal deprivation must be extreme to produce a deficit in physical growth. Unstable mothering that produces no apparent physical effects can result in a lack of sense of basic trust. This may occur in children from broken families or who have lived in a series of foster homes.

The tight bond between parent and child at this early stage of emotional development is reflected in a strong sense of "separation anxiety" in the child when separated from the parent. If it is necessary to provide dental treatment at an early age, it usually is preferable to do so with the parent present and, if possible, while the child is being held by one of the parents. At later ages, a child who never developed a sense of basic trust will have difficulty entering into situations that require trust and confidence in another person. Such an individual is likely to be an extremely frightened and uncooperative patient who needs special effort to establish rapport and trust with the dentist and staff.

2. Development of Autonomy (18 Months to 3 Years). Children around the age of 2 often are said to be undergoing the "terrible two's" because of their uncooperative and frequently obnoxious behavior. At this stage of emotional development, the child is moving away from the mother and developing a sense of individual identity or autonomy. Typically, the child struggles to exercise free choice in his or her life. He or she varies between being a little devil who says no to every wish of the parents and insists on having his own way, and being a little angel who retreats to the parents in moments of dependence. The parents and other adults with whom the child reacts at this stage must protect him against the consequences of dangerous and unacceptable behavior, while providing opportunities to develop independent behavior. Consistently enforced limits on behavior at this time allow the child to further develop trust in a predictable environment (Figure 2-52).

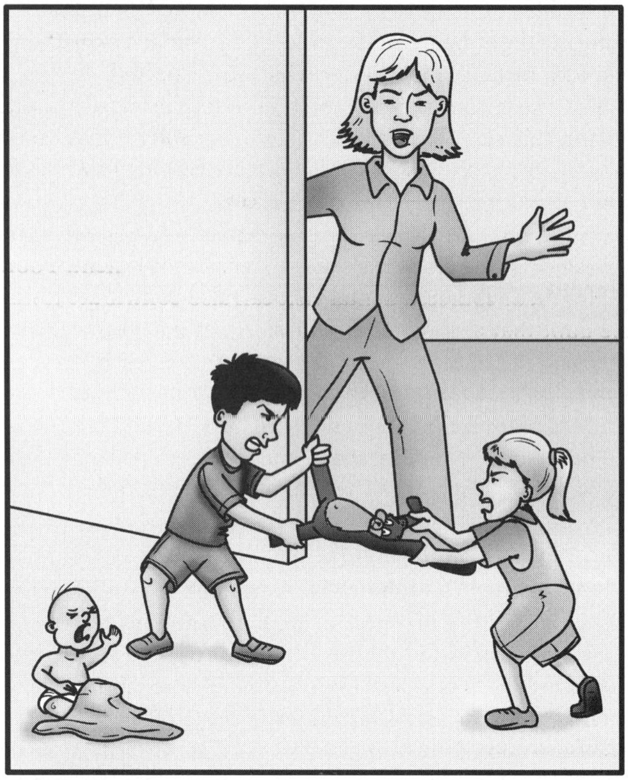

Figure 2-52 During the period in which children are developing autonomy, conflicts with siblings, peers and parents can seem never-ending. Consistently enforced limits on behavior during this stage, often called the "terrible two's," are needed to allow the child to develop trust in a predictable environment.

Failure to develop a proper sense of autonomy results in the development of doubts in the child's mind about his ability to stand alone, and this in turn produces doubts about others. Erikson defines the resulting state as one of shame, a feeling of having all one's shortcomings exposed. Autonomy in control of bodily functions is an important part of this stage, as the young child is toilet trained and taken out of diapers. At this stage (and later!), wetting one's pants produces a feeling of shame. This stage is considered decisive in producing the personality characteristics of love as opposed to hate, cooperation as opposed to selfishness, and freedom of expression as opposed to self-consciousness. To quote Erikson, "From a sense of self-control without a loss of self-esteem comes a lasting sense of good will and pride; from a sense of loss of self-control and foreign over-control come a lasting propensity for doubt and shame."[24]

A key toward obtaining cooperation with treatment from a child at this stage is to have the child think that whatever the dentist wants was his or her own choice, not something required by another person. For a 2-year-old seeking autonomy, it is all right to open your mouth if you want to, but almost psychologically unacceptable to do it if someone tells you to. One way around this is to offer the child reasonable choices whenever possible, for instance, either a green or a yellow napkin for the neck.

A child at this stage who finds the situation threatening is likely to retreat to Mother and be unwilling to separate from her. Allowing the parent to be present during treatment may be needed for even the simplest procedures. Complex dental treatment of children at this age is quite challenging and may require extraordinary behavior management procedures such as sedation or general anesthesia.

3. Development of Initiative (3 to 6 Years). In this stage, the child continues to develop greater autonomy, but now adds to it planning and vigorous pursuit of various activities. The initiative is shown by physical activity and motion, extreme curiosity and questioning, and aggressive talking. A major task for parents and teachers at this stage is to channel the activity into manageable tasks, arranging things so that the child is able to succeed, and preventing him or her from undertaking tasks where success is not possible. At this stage, a child is inherently teachable. One part of initiative is the eager modeling of behavior of those whom he respects.

The opposite of initiative is guilt resulting from goals that are contemplated but not attained, from acts initiated but not completed, or from faults or acts rebuked by persons the child respects. In Erikson's view, the child's ultimate ability to initiate new ideas or activities depends on how well he or she is able at this stage to express new thoughts and do new things without being made to feel guilty about expressing a bad idea or failing to achieve what was expected.

For most children, the first visit to the dentist comes during this stage of initiative. Going to the dentist can be constructed as a new and challenging adventure in which the child can experience success. Success in coping with the anxiety of visiting the dentist can help develop greater independence and produce a sense of accomplishment. Poorly managed, of course, a dental visit can also contribute toward the guilt that accompanies failure. A child at this stage will be intensely curious about the dentist's office and eager to learn about the things found there. An exploratory visit with the mother present and with little treatment accomplished usually is important in getting the dental experience off to a good start. After the initial experience, a child at this stage can usually tolerate being separated from the mother for treatment and is likely to behave better in this arrangement, so that independence rather than dependence is reinforced.

4. Mastery of Skills (Age 7 to 11 Years). At this stage, the child is working to acquire the academic and social skills that will allow him or her to compete in an environment where significant recognition is given to those who produce. At the same time, the child is learning the rules by which that world is organized. In Erikson's terms, the child acquires industriousness and begins the preparation for entrance into a competitive and working world. Competition with others within a reward system becomes a reality; at the same time, it becomes clear that some tasks can be accomplished only by cooperating with others. The influence of parents as role models decreases and the influence of the peer group increases.

The negative side of emotional and personality development at this stage can be the acquisition of a sense of inferiority. A child who begins to compete academically, socially, and physically is certain to find that others do some things better, and that whatever he or she does best, someone does it better. Somebody else gets put in the advanced section, is selected as leader of the group, or is chosen first for the team. It is necessary to learn to accept this, but failure to measure up to the peer group on a broad scale predisposes toward personality characteristics of inadequacy, inferiority and uselessness. Again, it is important for responsible adults to attempt to structure an environment that provides challenges that have a reasonable chance of being met, rather than guarantee failure.

By this stage, a child should already have experienced the first visit to the dentist, although a significant number will not have done so. Orthodontic treatment often begins during this stage of development. Children at this age are trying to learn the skills and rules that define success in any situation, and that includes the dental office. A key to behavioral guidance is setting attainable intermediate goals, clearly outlining for the child how to achieve those goals and positively reinforcing success in achieving these goals. Because of the child's drive for a sense of industry and accomplishment, cooperation with treatment can be obtained.

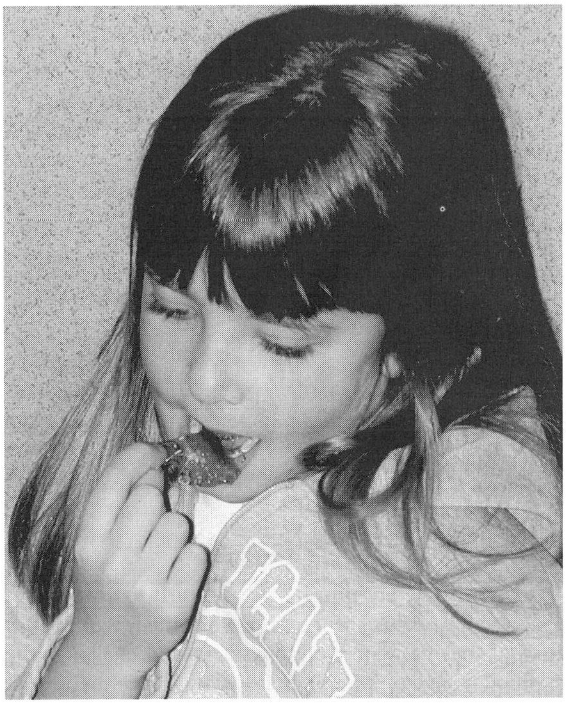

Figure 2-53 Instructions for a young child who will be wearing a removable orthodontic appliance must be explicit and concrete. Children at this stage cannot be motivated by abstract concepts but are influenced by improved acceptance or status from the peer group.

Orthodontic treatment in this age group is likely to involve the faithful wearing of removable appliances (Figure 2-53). Whether a child will do so is determined in large part by whether he or she understands what is needed to please the dentist and parents, whether the peer group is supportive, and whether the desired behavior is reinforced by the dentist.

Children at this stage still are not likely to be motivated by abstract concepts such as, "If you wear this appliance, your bite will be better." They can be motivated, however, by improved acceptance or status from the peer group. This means that emphasizing how the teeth will look better as the child cooperates is more likely to be a motivating factor than emphasizing a better dental occlusion, which the peer group is not likely to notice.

5. Development of Personal Identity (Age 12 to 17 Years). Adolescence, a period of intense physical development, is also the stage in psychosocial development in which a unique personal identity is acquired. This sense of identity includes both a feeling of belonging to a larger group and a realization that one can exist outside the family. It is an extremely complex stage because of the many new opportunities that arise. Emerging sexuality complicates relationships with others. At the same time, physical ability changes, tional child, however, the word "coat" is initially associated with only the one he or she wears, and the garment that Daddy wears would require another word.

A particularly prominent feature of thought processes of children at this age is the concrete nature of the process and hence, the concrete or literal nature of their language. In this sense, concrete is the opposite of abstract. Children in the preoperational period understand the world in the way they sense it through the five primary senses. Concepts that cannot be seen, heard, smelled, tasted, or felt—for example, time and health—are very difficult for preoperational children to grasp. At this age, children use and understand language in a literal sense and thus understand words only as they have learned them. They are not able to comprehend more than the literal meaning of idioms, and sarcastic or ironic statements are likely to be misinterpreted.

A general feature of thought processes and language during the preoperational period is *egocentrism,* meaning that the child is incapable of assuming another person's point of view. At this stage, his own perspective is all that he can manage—assuming another's view is simply beyond his mental capabilities.

Still another characteristic of thought processes at this stage is *animism,* investing inanimate objects with life. Essentially everything is seen as being alive by a young child, and so stories that invest the most improbable objects with life are quite acceptable to children of this age. Animism can be used to the dental team's advantage by giving dental instruments and equipment lifelike names and qualities. For example, the handpiece can be called "Whistling Willie" who is happy while he works at polishing the child's teeth.

At this stage, capabilities for logical reasoning are limited, and the child's thought processes are dominated by immediate sensory impressions. This characteristic can be illustrated by asking the child to solve a liquid conservation problem. The child is first shown two equal-size glasses with water in them. The child agrees that both contain the same amount of water. Then the contents of one glass are poured into a taller, narrower glass while the child watches. Now when asked which container has more water, the child will usually say that the tall one does. Her impressions are dominated by the greater height of the water in the tall glass.

For this reason, the dental staff should use immediate sensations rather than abstract reasoning in discussing concepts like prevention of dental problems with a child at this stage. Excellent oral hygiene is very important when an orthodontic appliance is present (a lingual arch to prevent drift of teeth, for instance). A preoperational child will have trouble understanding a chain of reasoning like the following: "Brushing and flossing remove food particles, which in turn prevents bacteria from forming acids, which cause tooth decay." He or she is much more likely to understand: "Brushing makes your teeth feel clean and smooth," and, "Toothpaste makes your mouth taste good," because these statements rely on things the child can taste or feel immediately.

A knowledge of these thought processes obviously can be used to improve communication with children of this age.[26] A further example would be talking to a 4-year-old about how desirable it would be to stop thumb sucking. The dentist might have little problem in getting the child to accept the idea that "Mr. Thumb" was the problem, and that the dentist and the child should form a partnership to control Mr. Thumb, who wishes to get into the child's mouth. Animism, in other words, can apply even to parts of the child's own body, which seem to take on a life of their own in this view.

On the other hand, it would not be useful to point out to the child how proud his father would be if he stopped sucking his thumb, since the child would think his father's attitude was the same as the child's (egocentrism). Since the child's view of time is centered around the present, and he or she is dominated by how things look, feel, taste, and sound now, there also is no point in talking to the 4-year-old about how much better his teeth will look in the future if he stops sucking his thumb. Telling him that the teeth will feel better now or talking about how bad his thumb tastes, however, may make an impact, since he can relate to that.

3. Period of Concrete Operations. As a child moves into this stage, typically after a year or so of preschool and first grade activity, an improved ability to reason emerges. He or she can use a limited number of logical processes, especially those involving objects that can be handled and manipulated (i.e., concrete objects). Thus an 8-year-old could watch the water being poured from one glass to another, imagine the reverse of that process, and conclude that the amount of water remains the same no matter what size the container is. If a child in this stage is given a similar problem, however, stated only in words with no concrete objects to illustrate it, the child may fail to solve it. The child's thinking is still strongly tied to concrete situations, and the ability to reason on an abstract level is limited.

By this stage, the ability to see another point of view develops, while animism declines. Children in this period are much more like adults in the way they view the world, but they are still cognitively different from adults. Presenting ideas as abstract concepts rather than illustrating them with concrete objects can be a major barrier to communication. Instructions must be illustrated with concrete objects. "Now, wear your retainer every night and be sure to keep it clean," is too abstract. More concrete directions would be: "This is your retainer. Put it in your mouth like this, and take it out like that. Put it in every evening right after dinner before you go to bed, and take it out before breakfast every morning. Brush it like this with an old toothbrush to keep it clean."

4. Period of Formal Operations. For most children, the ability to deal with abstract concepts and abstract reasoning develops by about age 11. At this stage, the child's thought process has become similar to that of an adult, and the child is capable of understanding concepts like health, disease, and preventive treatment. At this stage, intellectually, the child can and should be treated as an adult. It is as great a mistake to talk down to a child who has developed the ability to deal with abstract concepts, using the concrete approach needed with an 8-year-old, as it is to assume that the 8-year-old can handle abstract ideas. Successful communication, in other words, requires a feel for the child's stage of intellectual development.

In addition to the ability to deal with abstractions, teenagers have developed cognitively to the point where they can think about thinking. They are now aware that others think, but usually, in a new expression of egocentrism, presume that they and others are thinking about the same thing. Because young adolescents are experiencing tremendous biologic changes in growth and sexual development, they are preoccupied with these events. When an adolescent considers what others are thinking about, he assumes that others are thinking about the same thing he is thinking about, namely, himself. Adolescents assume that others are as concerned with their bodies, actions, and feelings as they themselves are. They feel as though they are constantly "on stage," being observed and criticized by those around them. This phenomenon has been called the "imaginary audience" by Elkind.[27]

The imaginary audience is a powerful influence on young adolescents, making them quite self-conscious and particularly susceptible to peer influence. They are very worried about what peers will think about their appearance and actions, not realizing that others are too busy with themselves to be paying attention to much other than themselves.

The reaction of the imaginary audience to braces on the teeth, of course, is an important consideration to a teenage patient. As orthodontic treatment has become more common, adolescents have less concern about being singled out because they have braces on their teeth, but they are very susceptible to suggestions from their peers about how the braces should look. In some settings, this has led to pleas for tooth-colored plastic or ceramic brackets (to make them less visible); at other times, brightly colored ligatures and elastics have been popular (because everybody is wearing them).

The notion that "others really care about my appearance and feelings as much as I do" leads adolescents to think they are quite unique, special individuals. If this were not so, why would others be so interested in them? As a result of this thought, a second phenomenon emerges, which Elkind called the "personal fable." This concept holds that "because I am unique, I am not subject to the consequences others will experience." The personal fable is a powerful motivator that allows us to cope in a dangerous world. It permits us to do things such as travel on airplanes while knowing that "occasionally they crash, but the one I'm on will arrive safely."

While both the imaginary audience and the personal fable have useful functions in helping us develop a social awareness and allowing us to cope in a dangerous environment, they may also lead to dysfunctional behavior and even foolhardy risk-taking. The adolescent may drive too fast, thinking, "I am unique. I'm especially skilled at driving. Other less skillful drivers may have wrecks, but not I." These phenomena are likely to have significant influence on orthodontic treatment. The imaginary audience, depending on what the adolescent believes, may influence him to accept or reject treatment, and to wear or not wear appliances. The personal fable may make a patient ignore threats to health, such as decalcification of teeth from poor oral hygiene during orthodontic therapy. The thought, of course, is, "Others may have to worry about that, but I don't."

The challenge for the dentist is not to try to impose change on reality as perceived by adolescents, but rather to help them more clearly see the actual reality that surrounds them. A teenage patient may protest to his orthodontist that he does not want to wear a particular appliance because others will think it makes him "look goofy." In this situation, telling the patient that he should not be concerned because many of his peers also are wearing this appliance does little to encourage him to wear it. A more useful approach, one does not deny the point of view of the patient, is to agree with him that he may be right in what others will think, but ask him to give it a try for a specified time. If his peers do respond as the teenager predicts, then a different, but less desirable, treatment technique can be discussed. This test of the teenager's perceived reality usually demonstrates that the audience does not respond negatively to the appliance, or that the patient can successfully cope with the peer response. Wearing interarch elastics while in public often falls into this category. Encouraging a reluctant teenager to try it and judge his peers' response is much more likely to get him to wear the elastics than telling him everybody else does it so he should too (Figure 2-56).

Sometimes, teenage patients have experience with the imaginary audience regarding a particular appliance but have incorrectly measured the response of the audience. They may require guidance to help them accurately assess the view of the audience. Experience with 13-year-old Beth illustrates this point. Following the loss of a maxillary central incisor in an accident, treatment for Beth included a removable partial denture to replace the tooth. She and her parents had been told on several occasions that it would be necessary to wear the removable appliance until enough healing and growth had occurred to permit treatment with a fixed bridge. At a routine recall appointment, Beth asked if the bridge could be placed now. Realizing that this must be a significant concern for Beth, the dentist commented "Beth, wearing this partial must be a problem. Tell me more about it." Beth replied, "It's embarrassing." Inquiring further, the dentist asked, "When is it embarrassing?" Beth said, "When I spend the night at other girls' homes and have to take it out to brush my teeth." "Well, what is the response of the girls when they see you remove your tooth?" Beth replied, "They think it's neat." Nothing more was said about the tooth and the conversation moved to the vacation that Beth's family was planning.

This illustration indicates how it is possible to provide guidance toward a more accurate evaluation of the attitude

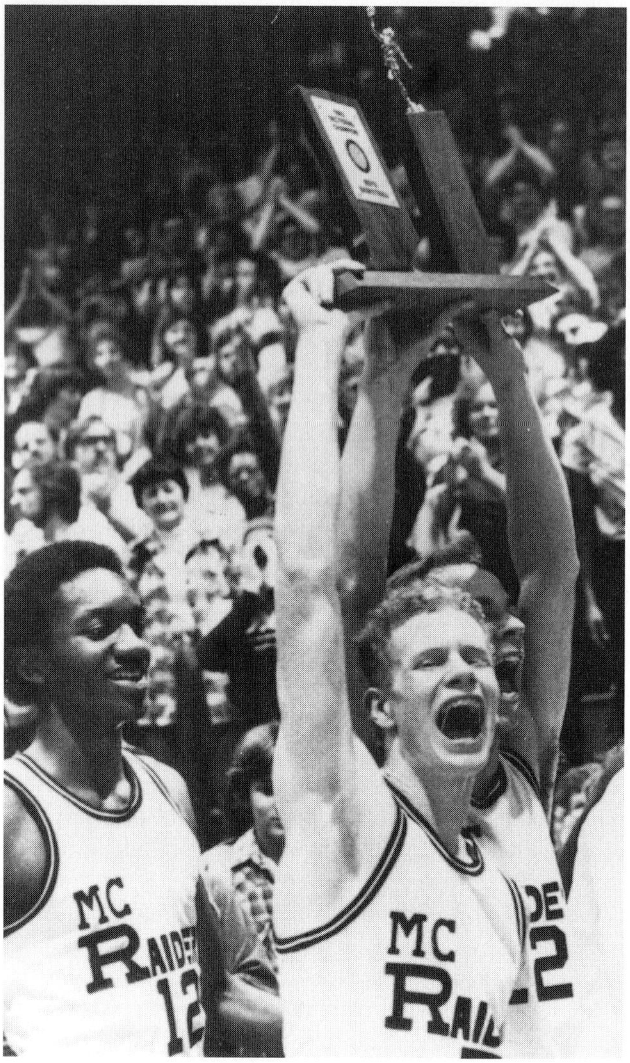

FIGURE 2-56 Wearing your orthodontic elastics during the championship high school basketball game, as this newspaper photo shows he obviously was doing, is acceptable to your peers—but the orthodontist is more likely to convince a teenager of that by encouraging him to try it and test their response, than by telling him that he should do it because everybody else does. (Courtesy T.P. Laboratories.)

of the audience and thus allow teenagers to solve their own problems. This approach on the part of the dentist neither argues with the teenager's reality nor uncritically accepts it. One role of an effective dental professional is to help teenagers test the reality that actually surrounds them.

To be received, the dentist's message must be presented in terms that correspond to the stage of cognitive and psychosocial development that a particular child has reached. It is the job of the dentist to carefully evaluate the development of the child, and to adapt his or her language so that concepts are presented in a way that the patient can understand them. The adage "different strokes for different folks" applies strongly to children, whose variations in intellectual and psychosocial development affect the way they receive orthodontic treatment, just as their differing stages of physical development do.

REFERENCES

1. Farkas LG. Anthropometry of the Head and Face. New York: Raven Press; 1994.
2. Cevidanes LHS, Bailey LJ, Tucker SF, et al. Superimposition of 3D cone-beam CT models of orthognathic surgery patients. Dentomaxillofacial Radiol 34:369-375, 2005.
3. Cevidanes LHS, Franco AA, Gerig G, et al. Comparison of relative mandibular growth vectors with high-resolution 3-dimensional imaging. Am J Orthod Dentofac Orthop, 128:27-34, 2005.
4. Thompson DT. On Growth and Form. Cambridge, Mass: Cambridge University Press; 1971.
5. Baer MJ, Bosma JF, Ackerman JL. The Postnatal Development of the Rat Skull. Ann Arbor, Mich: The University of Michigan Press; 1983.
6. Bjork A. The use of metallic implants in the study of facial growth in children: Method and application. Am J Phys Anthropol 29:243-250, 1968.
7. Allapat S, Zhang ZY, Chen YP. Msx homeobox gene family and craniofacial development. Cell Res 13:429-442, 2003.
8. Dixon D, Hoyte D, Running O. Fundamentals of Craniofacial Growth. Boca Raton, Fla: CRC Press; 1997.
9. Klingenberg CP, Leamy LJ, Cheverud JM. Integration and modularity of quantitative locus effects on geometric shape of the mouse mandible. Genetics 166:1909-1921, 2004.
10. Rabie AB, She TT, Harley VR. Forward mandibular positioning upregulates SOX9 and type II collagen expression in the glenoid fossa. J Dent Res 82:725-730, 2003.
11. Tang GH, Rabie AB. Runx2 regulates endochondral ossification in condyle during mandibular advancement. J Dent Res 84:166-171, 2005.
12. Enlow DH, Hans MG. Essentials of Facial Growth. Philadelphia: WB Saunders; 1996.
13. Copray JC. Growth of the nasal septal cartilage of the rat in vitro. J Anat 144:99-111, 1986.
14. Delatte M, Von den Hoff JW, van Rheden RE, Kuijpers-Jagtman AM. Primary and secondary cartilages of the neonatal rat: The femoral head and the mandibular condyle. Eur J Oral Sci 112:156-162, 2004.
15. Gilhuus-Moe O. Fractures of the Mandibular Condyle in the Growth Period. Stockholm: Scandinavian University Books, Universitatsforlaget; 1969.
16. Lund K. Mandibular growth and remodelling process after mandibular fractures. Acta Odontol Scand 32:(suppl 64), 1974.
17. Sahm G, Witt E. Long-term results after childhood condylar fracture: A CT study. Eur J Orthod 11:154-160, 1990.
18. Moss ML. The functional matrix hypothesis revisited. Am J Orthod Dentofac Orthop 112:8-11, 221-226, 338-342, 410-417, 1997.
19. Proffit WR, Vig KWL, Turvey TA. Early fracture of the mandibular condyles: Frequently an unsuspected cause of growth disturbances. Am J Orthod 78:1-24, 1980.
20. Feigal RJ. Guiding and managing the child dental patient. J Dent Ed 65:1369-1377, 2001.
21. Greenbaum PE, Turner C, Cook EW III, Melamed BG. Dentists' voice control: Effects on children's disruptive and affective behavior. Health Psychol 9:546-558, 1990.
22. Miltenberger RG. Behavior Modification: Principles and Procedures. 3rd ed. Pacific Grove, Calif: Brooks/Cole; 2004.

23. Baghadi ZD. Principles and application of learning theory in child patient management. Quintessence International 32:135-141, 2001.
24. Erikson EH. A way of looking at things—selected papers from 1930 to 1980 (S. Schlein, editor). New York: WW Norton & Co; 1987.
25. Wadsworth BJ. Piaget's Theory of Cognitive and Affective Development. New York: Longman; 1989.
26. Delitala G. Incorporating Piaget's theories into behavior management techniques for the child dental patient. Gen Dent 48:74-76, 2000.
27. Elkind D. The teenager's reality. Pediatr Dent 9:337-341, 1987.

CHAPTER 3

Early Stages of Development

CHAPTER OUTLINE

PRENATAL INFLUENCES ON FACIAL DEVELOPMENT

A general understanding of the formation of the face, as presented in the standard embryology texts, is presumed in the discussion that follows. The focus here is on the events in prenatal development that are particularly pertinent to orthodontic problems later in life.

Embryologic Development

In broad overview, nearly all the tissues of the face and neck originate from ectoderm. This includes the muscular and skeletal elements that elsewhere in the body are derived from mesoderm. Most of these tissues develop from neural crest cells that migrate downward beside the neural tube and laterally under the surface ectoderm.[1] After the crest cells have completed their migration, facial growth is dominated by regional growth centers as the organ systems are formed and the final differentiation of tissues occurs.

There are five principal stages in craniofacial development (Table 3-1): (1) germ layer formation and initial organization of craniofacial structures; (2) neural tube formation and initial formation of the oropharynx; (3) origins, migrations and interactions of cell populations, especially neural crest cells; (4) formation of organ systems, especially the pharyngeal arches and the primary and secondary palates; and (5) final differentiation of tissues (skeletal, muscular, and nervous elements).[2] Some specific abnormalities in facial form and jaw relationships can be traced to the very early first and second stages. For example, the characteristic facies of fetal alcohol syndrome (FAS) (Figure 3-1) is due to deficiencies of midline tissue of the neural plate very early

TABLE 3-1

Stages of Embryonic Craniofacial Development

Stage	Time (humans) (post-fertilization)	Related syndromes
Germ layer formation and initial organization of structures	Day 17	Fetal alcohol syndrome (FAS)
Neural tube formation	Days 18-23	Anencephaly
Origin, migration, and interaction of cell populations	Days 19-28	Hemifacial microsomia Mandibulofacial dysostosis (Treacher Collins syndrome) Limb abnormalities
Formation of organ systems		
Primary palate	Days 28-38	Cleft lip and/or palate, other facial clefts
Secondary palate	Days 42-55	Cleft palate
Final differentiation of tissues	Day 50-birth	Achondroplasia Synostosis syndromes (Crouzon's, Apert's, etc.)

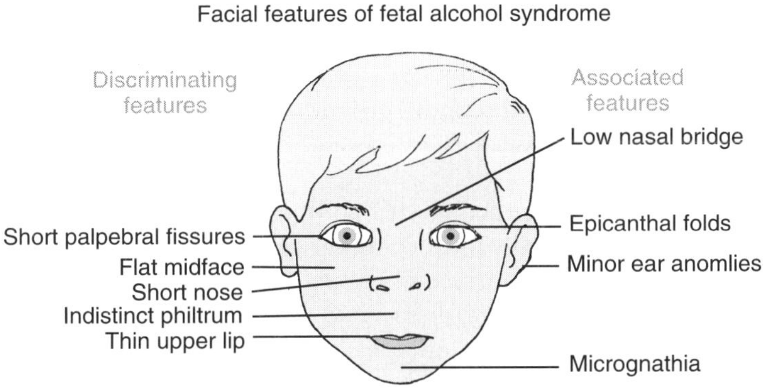

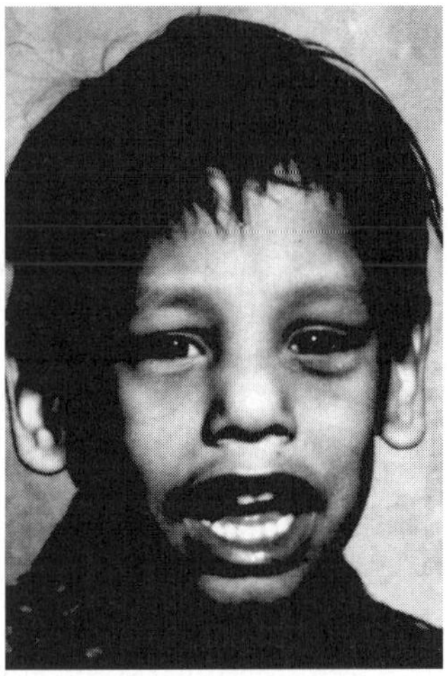

FIGURE 3-1 The characteristic facial appearance of fetal alcohol syndrome (FAS), caused by exposure to very high blood alcohol levels during the first trimester of pregnancy.

in embryonic development, caused by exposure to very high levels of ethanol. Although such blood levels can be reached only in extreme intoxication in chronic alcoholics, the resulting facial deformity occurs frequently enough to be implicated in many cases of midface deficiency.[3]

Neural Crest Cell Problems

Many of the problems that result in craniofacial anomalies arise in the third stage of development, neural crest cell origin and migration. Since most structures of the face are ultimately derived from migrating neural crest cells (Figure 3-2), it is not surprising that interferences with this migration produce facial deformities. At the completion of the migration of the neural crest cells in the fourth week of human embryonic life, they form practically all of the loose mesenchymal tissue in the facial region that lies between the surface ectoderm and the underlying forebrain and eye and most of the mesenchyme in the mandibular arch. Most of the neural crest cells in the facial area later differentiate into skeletal and connective tissues, including the bones of the jaw and the teeth.

The importance of neural crest migration and the possibility of drug-induced impairment has been demonstrated clearly by unfortunate experience. In the 1960s and 70s, exposure to thalidomide caused major congenital defects including facial anomalies in thousands of children. In the 1980s, severe facial malformations related to the anti-acne drug isotretinoin (Accutane) were reported. The similarities

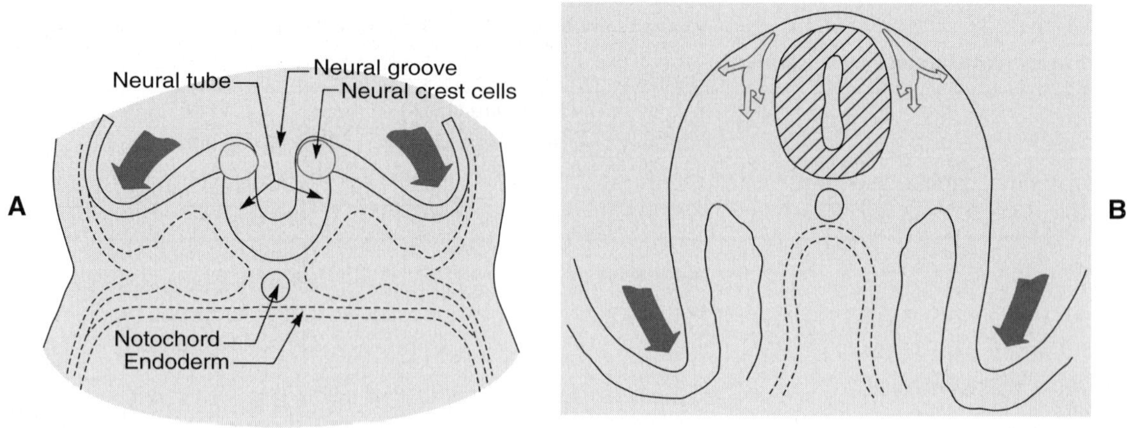

FIGURE 3-2 Diagrammatic lateral sections of embryos at 20 and 24 days, showing formation of the neural folds, neural groove and neural crest. **A,** At 20 days, neural crest cells can be identified at the lips of the deepening neural groove, forerunner of the central nervous system. **B,** At 24 days, the neural crest cells *(pink)* have separated from the neural tube and are beginning their extensive migration beneath the surface ectoderm. The migration is so extensive, and the role of these neural crest cells so important in formation of structures of the head and face, that they can almost be considered a fourth primary germ layer.

in the defects make it likely that both these drugs affect the formation and/or migration of neural crest cells.

Altered neural crest development also has been implicated in mandibulofacial dysostosis (Treacher Collins syndrome) and hemifacial microsomia. In Treacher Collins syndrome, both the maxilla and mandible are underdeveloped as a result of a generalized lack of mesenchymal tissue (Figure 3-3). The best evidence suggests that the problem arises because of excessive cell death (cause unknown) in the trigeminal ganglion, which secondarily affects neural crest–derived cells.[4]

Hemifacial microsomia, as the name suggests, is primarily a unilateral and always an asymmetrical problem. It is characterized by a lack of tissue on the affected side of the face (Figure 3-4). Typically, the external ear is deformed and both the ramus of the mandible and associated soft tissues (muscle, fascia) are deficient or missing (see Figure 3-4). An early explanation of the condition was that it was due to hemorrhage from the stapedial artery at the time, about 6 weeks after conception, when the maxillary artery takes over the blood supply to the affected area. More recent work suggests that, although hemorrhage at the critical time may be involved, hemifacial microsomia arises primarily from early loss of neural crest cells.[2] Neural crest cells with the longest migration path, those taking a circuitous route to the lateral and lower areas of the face, are most affected, whereas those going to the central face tend to complete their migratory movement. This explains why midline facial defects including clefts rarely are part of the syndrome. Some degree of asymmetry may be present, but both sides are affected. Neural crest cells migrating to lower regions are important in the formation of the great vessels (aorta, pulmonary artery, aortic arch), and they also are likely to be affected. For this reason defects in the great vessels (as in the tetralogy of Fallot) are common in children with hemifacial microsomia. The spectrum of deformities induced by thalidomide and isotretinoin includes conditions similar to both mandibulofacial dysostosis and hemifacial microsomia.

Facial Cleft Problems

The most common congenital defect involving the face and jaws, second only to clubfoot in the entire spectrum of congenital deformities, is clefting of the lip, palate, or, less commonly, other facial structures. Clefts arise during the fourth developmental stage. Exactly where they appear is determined by the locations at which fusion of the various facial processes failed to occur (Figures 3-5 and 3-6), and this in turn is influenced by the time in embryologic life when some interference with development occurred.

Clefting of the lip occurs because of a failure of fusion between the median and lateral nasal processes and the maxillary prominence, which normally occurs in humans during the sixth week of development. At least theoretically a midline cleft of the upper lip could develop because of a split within the median nasal process, but this almost never occurs. Instead, clefts of the lip occur lateral to the midline on either or both sides (Figure 3-7). Since the fusion of these processes during primary palate formation creates not only the lip but the area of the alveolar ridge containing the central and lateral incisors, it is likely that a notch in the alveolar process will accompany a cleft lip even if there is no cleft of the secondary palate.

Closure of the secondary palate by elevation of the palatal shelves (Figures 3-8 and 3-9) follows that of the primary palate by nearly 2 weeks, which means that an interference with lip closure that still is present can also affect the palate.

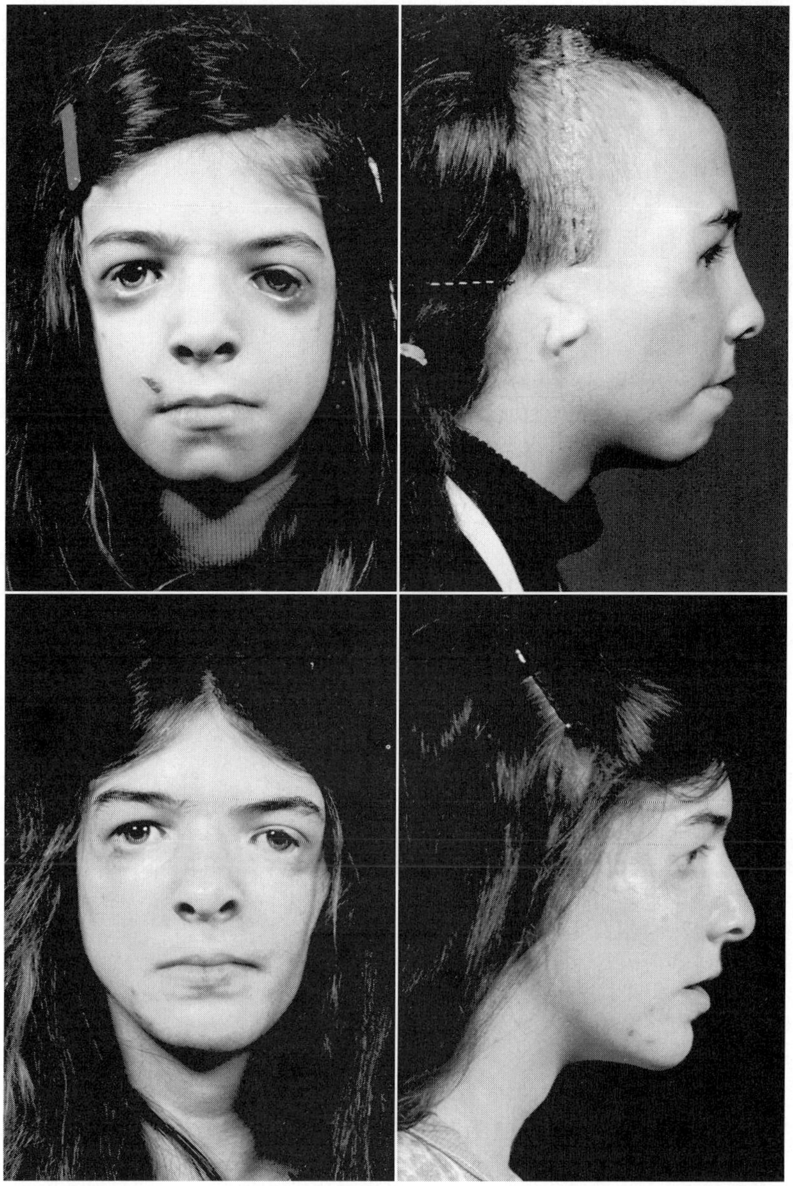

Figure 3-3 In the Treacher Collins syndrome (also called mandibulofacial dysostosis), a generalized lack of mesenchymal tissue in the lateral part of the face is the major cause of the characteristic facial appearance. Note the underdevelopment of the lateral orbital and zygomatic areas. The ears also may be affected. **A,** Patient at age 12 before and, **B,** immediately after surgical treatment to advance the mid-face. **C,D,** Age 16. Note the change in the lateral orbital margins.

About 60% of individuals with a cleft lip also have a palatal cleft (Figure 3-10). An isolated cleft of the secondary palate is the result of a problem that arose after lip closure was completed. Incomplete fusion of the secondary palate, which produces a notch in its posterior extent (sometimes only a bifid uvula), indicates a very late-appearing interference with fusion.

The width of the mouth is determined by fusion of the maxillary and mandibular processes at their lateral extent, and so a failure of fusion in this area could produce an exceptionally wide mouth, or macrostomia. Failure of fusion between the maxillary and lateral processes could produce an obliquely directed cleft of the face. Other patterns of facial clefts are possible, based on the details of fusion.[5] Fortunately, these conditions are rare.

Morphogenetic movements of the tissues are a prominent part of the fourth stage of facial development. As these have become better understood, the way in which clefts of the lip and palate develop has been clarified. For example, it is known now that cigarette smoking by the mother is an etiologic factor in the development of cleft lip and palate.[6] An important initial step in development of the primary palate is a forward movement of the lateral nasal process, which positions it so that contact with the median nasal process is possible. The hypoxia associated with smoking probably interferes with this movement.

Synostosis Problems

Another major group of craniofacial malformations arise considerably later than the ones discussed so far, during the final stage of facial development and in the fetal rather than the embryologic period of prenatal life. These are the craniosynostosis syndromes, which result from early closure of the sutures between the cranial and facial bones. In fetal life, normal cranial and facial development is dependent on growth adjustments at the sutures in response to growth of the brain and facial soft tissues. Early closure of a suture, called *synostosis,* leads to characteristic distortions depending on the location of the early fusion.[7]

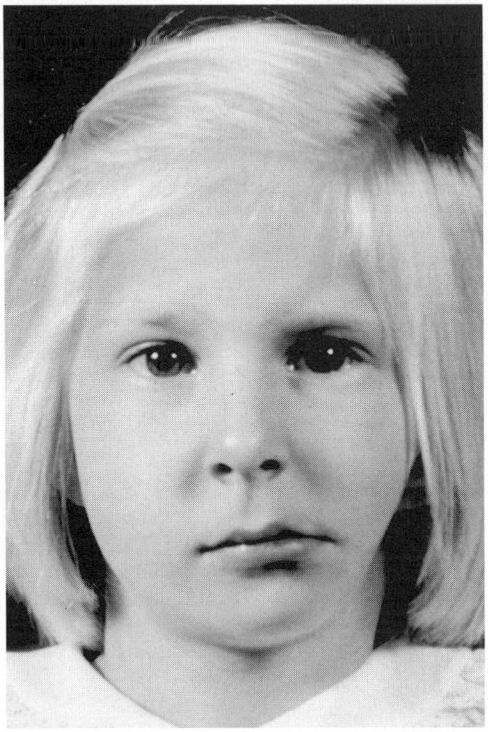

FIGURE 3-4 In hemifacial microsomia, both the external ear and the mandibular ramus are deficient or absent on the affected side. (From Proffit WR, White RP, Sarver DM. Contemporary Treatment of Dentofacial Deformity. St. Louis: Mosby; 2003.)

Crouzon's syndrome is the most frequently occurring member of this group. It is characterized by underdevelopment of the midface and eyes that seem to bulge from their sockets (Figure 3-11). Crouzon's syndrome arises because of prenatal fusion of the superior and posterior sutures of the maxilla, along the wall of the orbit. The premature fusion frequently extends posteriorly into the cranium, producing distortions of the cranial vault as well. If fusion in the orbital area prevents the maxilla from translating downward and forward, the result must be severe underdevelopment of the middle third of the face. The characteristic protrusion of the eyes is largely an illusion—the eyes appear to bulge outward because the area beneath them is underdeveloped. There may be a component of true extrusion of the eyes, however, because when cranial sutures become synostosed, intracranial pressure increases.

Although the characteristic deformity is recognized at birth, the situation worsens as growth disturbances caused by the fused sutures continue postnatally. Surgery to release the sutures is necessary at an early age.

Late Fetal Development and Birth

By the third trimester of intrauterine life, the human fetus weighs approximately 1000 grams and though far from ready for life outside the protective intrauterine environment, can often survive premature birth. During the last 3 months of intrauterine life, continued rapid growth results in a tripling of body mass to about 3000 grams. Dental development, which begins in the third month, proceeds rapidly thereafter (Table 3-2). Development of all primary teeth and the permanent first molars starts well before birth.

Although the proportion of the total body mass represented by the head decreases from the fourth month of intrauterine life onward, at birth the head is still nearly half the total body mass and represents the largest impediment to passage of the infant through the birth canal. Making the head longer and narrower obviously would facilitate birth,

TABLE 3-2

Chronology of Tooth Development, Primary Dentition

	CALCIFICATION BEGINS		CROWN COMPLETED		ERUPTION		ROOT COMPLETED	
Tooth	*Max.*	*Mand.*	*Max.*	*Mand.*	*Max.*	*Mand.*	*Max.*	*Mand.*
Central	14 wk. in utero	14 wk. in utero	1½ mo.	2½ mo	10 mo.	8 mo.	1½ yr.	1½ yr.
Lateral	16 wk. in utero	16 wk. in utero	2½ mo.	3 mo.	11 mo.	13 mo.	2 yr.	1½ yr.
Canine	17 wk. in utero	17 wk. in utero	9 mo.	9 mo.	19 mo.	20 mo.	3¼ yr.	3¼ yr.
1st Molar	15 wk. in utero	15 wk. in utero	6 mo.	5½ mo.	16 mo.	16 mo.	2½ yr.	2¼ yr.
2nd Molar	19 wk. in utero	18 wk. in utero	11 mo.	10 mo.	29 mo.	27 mo.	3 yr.	3 yr.

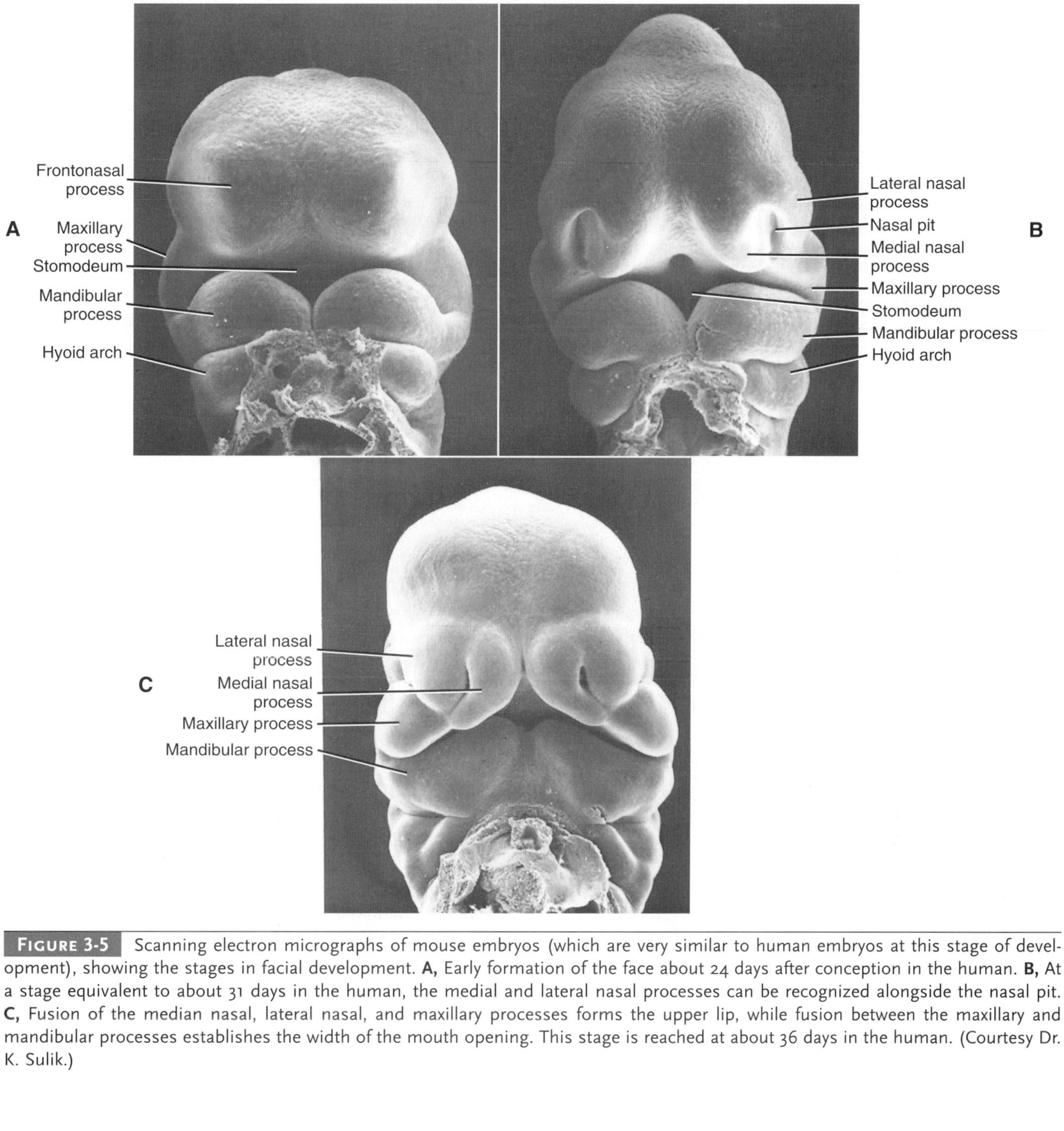

FIGURE 3-5 Scanning electron micrographs of mouse embryos (which are very similar to human embryos at this stage of development), showing the stages in facial development. **A,** Early formation of the face about 24 days after conception in the human. **B,** At a stage equivalent to about 31 days in the human, the medial and lateral nasal processes can be recognized alongside the nasal pit. **C,** Fusion of the median nasal, lateral nasal, and maxillary processes forms the upper lip, while fusion between the maxillary and mandibular processes establishes the width of the mouth opening. This stage is reached at about 36 days in the human. (Courtesy Dr. K. Sulik.)

and this is accomplished by a literal distortion of its shape (Figure 3-12). The change of shape is possible because at birth, relatively large uncalcified fontanelles persist between the flat bones of the brain case. As the head is compressed within the birth canal, the brain case (calvarium) can increase in length and decrease in width, assuming the desired tubular form and easing passage through the birth canal.

The relative lack of growth of the lower jaw prenatally also makes birth easier, since a prominent bony chin at the time of birth would be a considerable problem in passage through the birth canal. Many a young dentist, acutely aware of the orthodontic problems that can arise later because of skeletal mandibular deficiency, has been shocked to discover how incredibly mandibular deficient his or her own newborn is, and has required reassurance that this is a perfectly normal and indeed desirable phenomenon. Postnatally, the mandible grows more than the other facial structures and gradually catches up, producing the eventual adult proportions.

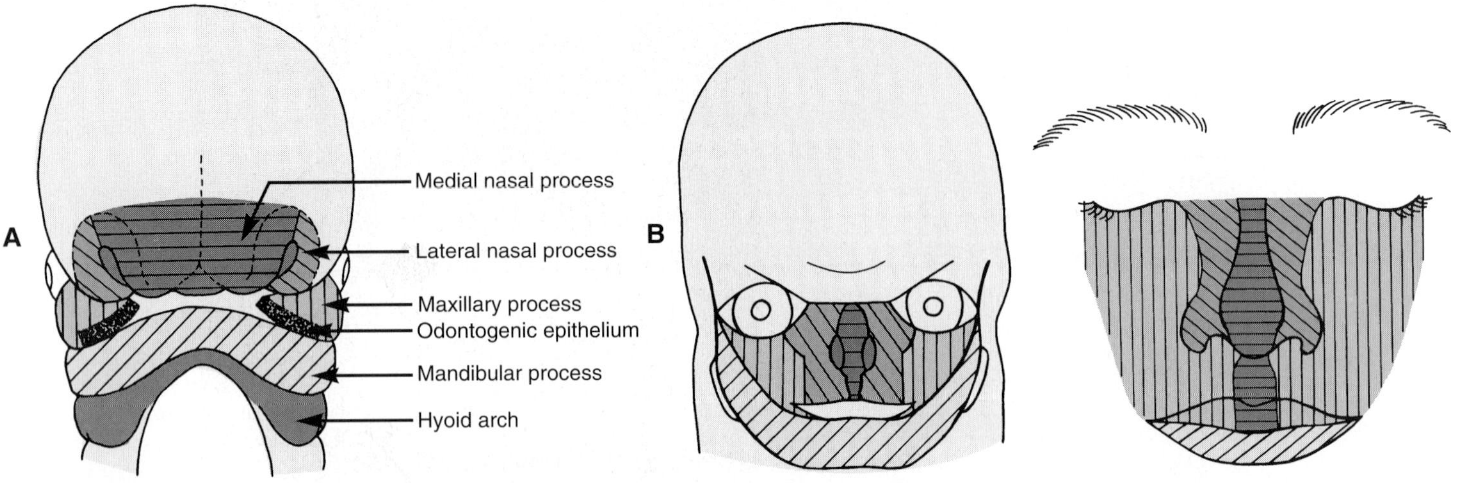

FIGURE 3-6 Schematic representations of fusion of the facial processes. **A,** Diagrammatic representation of structures at 31 days, when fusion is just beginning. **B,** Relationships at 35 days, when the fusion process is well-advanced. **C,** Schematic representation of the contribution of the embryonic facial processes to the structures of the adult face. The medial nasal process contributes the central part of the nose and the philtrum of the lip. The lateral nasal process forms the outer parts of the nose, and the maxillary process forms the bulk of the upper lip and the cheeks. (**B,** Redrawn from Ten Cate AR. Oral Histology, ed 3. St Louis: Mosby; 1989; **C,** redrawn from Sulik KK, Johnston MC. Scan Elect Microsc 1:309-322, 1982.)

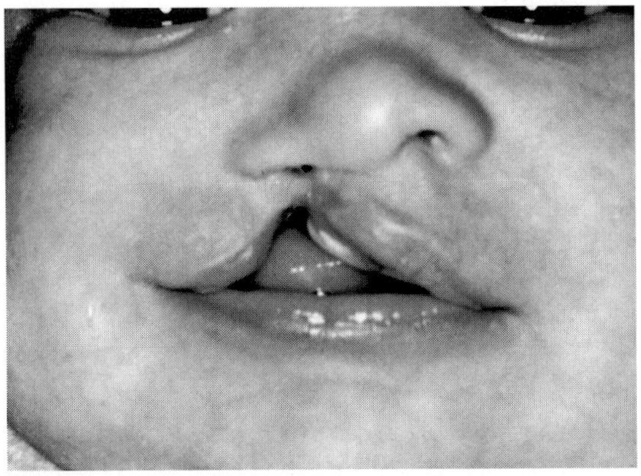

FIGURE 3-7 Unilateral cleft lip in an infant. Note that the cleft is not in the midline, but lateral to the midline.

Despite the physical adaptations that facilitate it, birth is a traumatic process. In the best of circumstances, being thrust into the world requires a dramatic set of physiologic adaptations. For a short period, growth ceases and often there is a small decrease in weight during the first 7 to 10 days of life. Such an interruption in growth produces a physical effect in skeletal tissues that are forming at the time, because the orderly sequence of calcification is disturbed. The result is a noticeable line across both bones and teeth that are forming at the time. However, bones are not visible and are remodeled to such an extent that any lines caused by the growth arrest at birth would soon be covered over at any rate.

Teeth, on the other hand, are quite visible, and the extent of any growth disturbance related to birth can be seen in the enamel, which is not remodeled. Almost every child has a "neonatal line" across the surface of the primary teeth, its location varying from tooth to tooth depending on the stage of development at birth (Figure 3-13). Under normal circumstances, the line is so slight that it can be seen only if the tooth surface is magnified, but if the neonatal period was stormy, a prominent area of stained, distorted, or poorly calcified enamel can be the result.[8]

Birth is not the only circumstance that can have this effect. As a general rule, it can be anticipated that growth disturbances lasting 1 to 2 weeks or more, such as the one that accompanies birth or a growth cessation caused by a febrile illness later, will leave a visible record in the enamel of teeth forming at the time. Permanent as well as primary teeth can be affected by illnesses during infancy and early childhood.

INFANCY AND EARLY CHILDHOOD: THE PRIMARY DENTITION YEARS

Physical Development in the Preschool Years

The general pattern of physical development after birth is a continuation of the pattern of the late fetal period: rapid

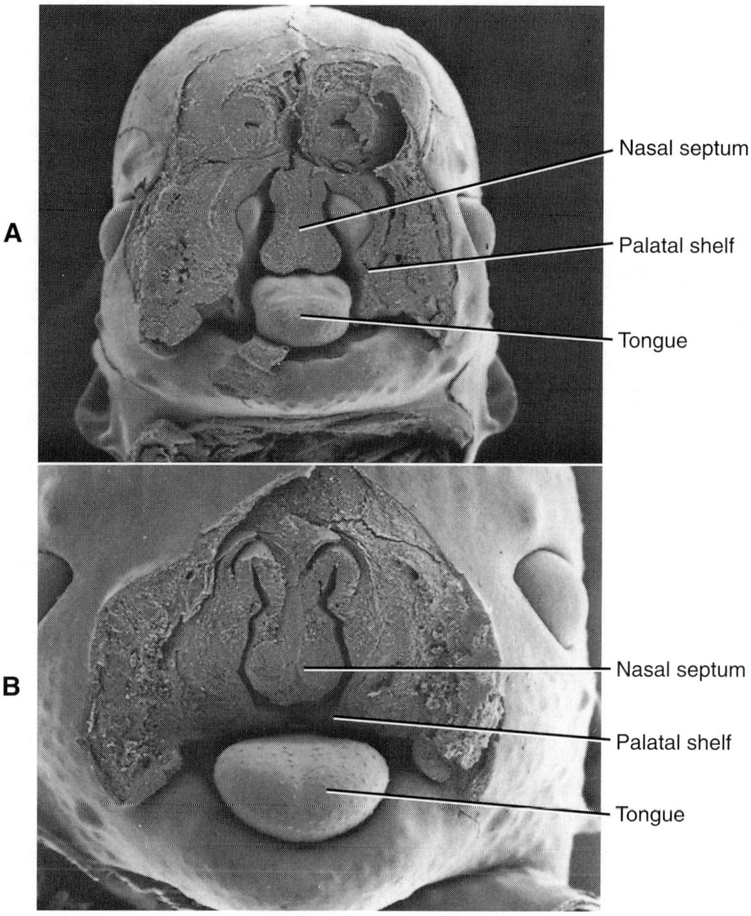

FIGURE 3-8 Scanning electron micrographs of mouse embryos sectioned in the frontal plane. **A,** Before elevation of the palatal shelves. **B,** Immediately after depression of the tongue and elevation of the shelves. (Courtesy Dr. K. Sulik.)

growth continues, with a relatively steady increase in height and weight, although the rate of growth declines as a percentage of the previous body size (Figure 3-14).

Three circumstances merit special attention:

1. Premature birth (low birth weight). Infants weighing less than 2500 gm at birth are at greater risk of problems in the immediate postnatal period. Since low birth weight is a reflection of premature birth, it is reasonable to establish the prognosis in terms of birth weight rather than estimated gestational age. Until recent years, children with birth weights below 1500 gm often did not survive. Even with the best current specialized neonatal services, the chances of survival for extremely low birth weight infants (less than 1000 gm) are not good, though some now are saved.

If a premature infant survives the neonatal period, however, there is every reason to expect that growth will follow the normal pattern and that the child will gradually overcome the initial handicap (Figure 3-15). Premature infants can be expected to be small throughout the first and into the second years of life. In many instances, by the third year of life premature and normal-term infants are indistinguishable in attainment of developmental milestones.[9]

2. Chronic illness. Skeletal growth is a process that can occur only when the other requirements of the individual have been met. A certain amount of energy is necessary to maintain life. An additional amount is needed for activity, and a further increment is necessary for growth. For a normal child, perhaps 90% of the available energy must be "taken off the top" to meet the requirements for survival and activity, leaving 10% for growth.

Chronic illness alters this balance, leaving relatively less of the total energy available to support growth. Chronically ill children typically fall behind their healthier peers, and if the illness persists, the growth deficit is cumulative. An episode of acute illness leads to a temporary cessation of growth, but if the growth interruption is relatively brief, there will be no long-term effect. The more chronic the illness, the greater the cumulative impact. Obviously, the more severe the illness, the greater the impact at any given time. Children with congenital hormone deficiencies provide an excellent example. If the hormone is replaced, a dramatic improvement in growth and recovery toward normal height and weight often occurs (Figure 3-16). A congenital heart defect can have a similar effect on growth, and similarly dramatic effects on growth can accompany repair of the defect.[10]

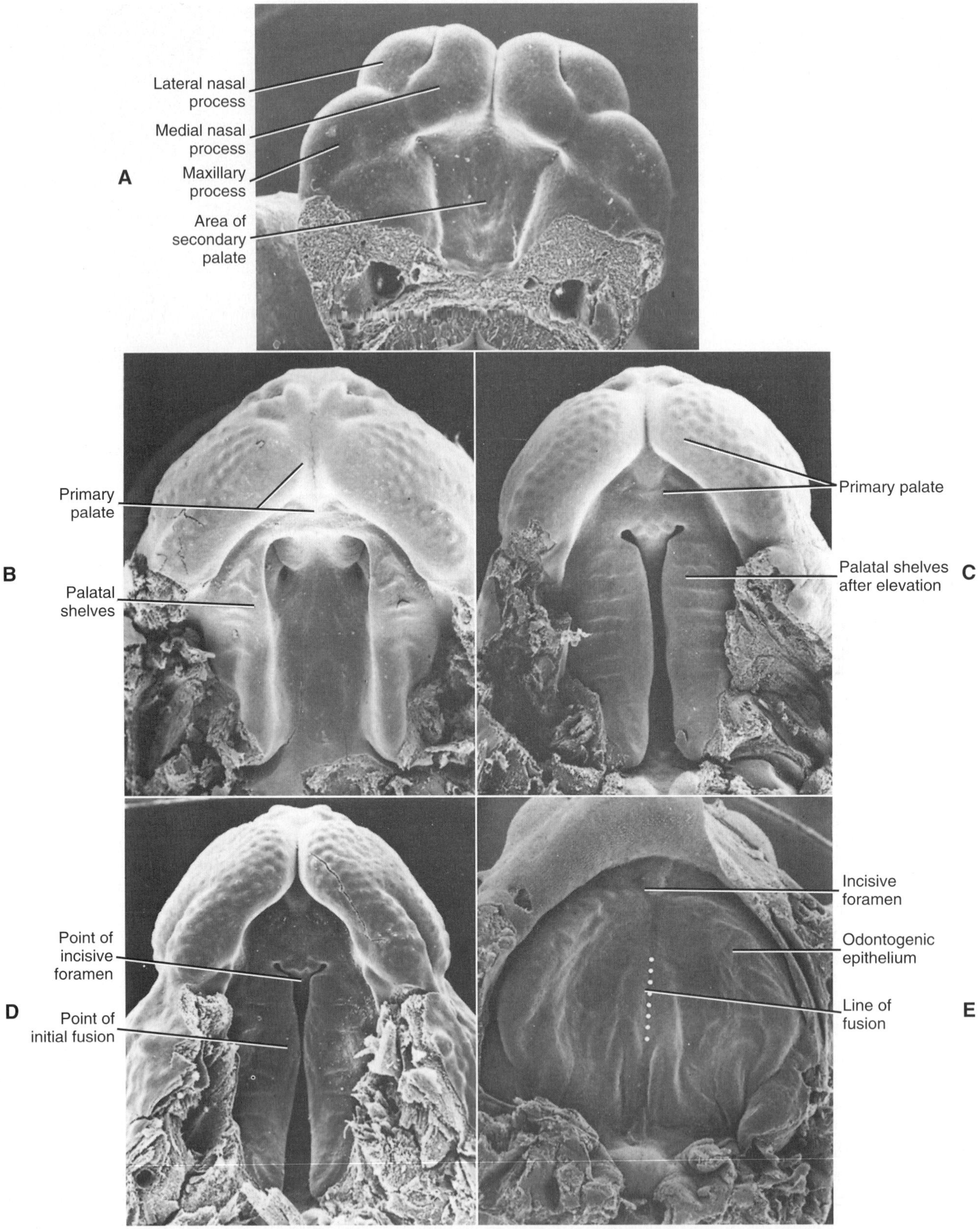

FIGURE 3-9 Scanning electron micrographs of the stages in palate closure (mouse embryos sectioned so that the lower jaw has been removed), analogous to the same stages in human embryos. **A,** At the completion of primary palate formation. **B,** Before elevation of the palatal shelves, equivalent to Figure 3-8, *A*; **C,** Shelves during elevation. **D,** Initial fusion of the shelves at a point about one third of the way back along their length. **E,** Secondary palate immediately after fusion. (Courtesy Dr. K. Sulik.)

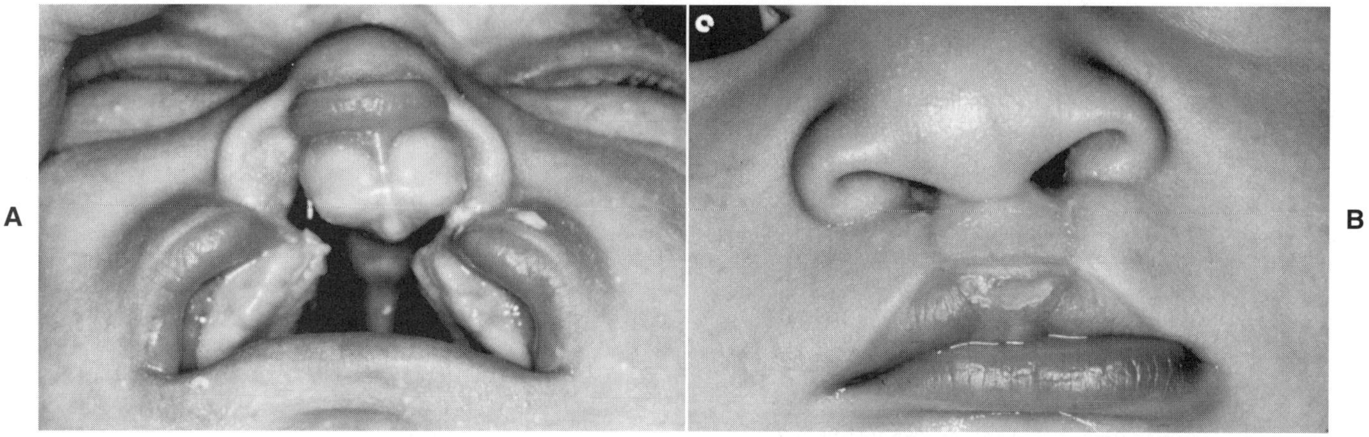

FIGURE 3-10 **A,** Bilateral cleft lip and palate in an infant. The separation of the premaxilla from the remainder of the maxilla is shown clearly. **B,** Same child after lip repair.

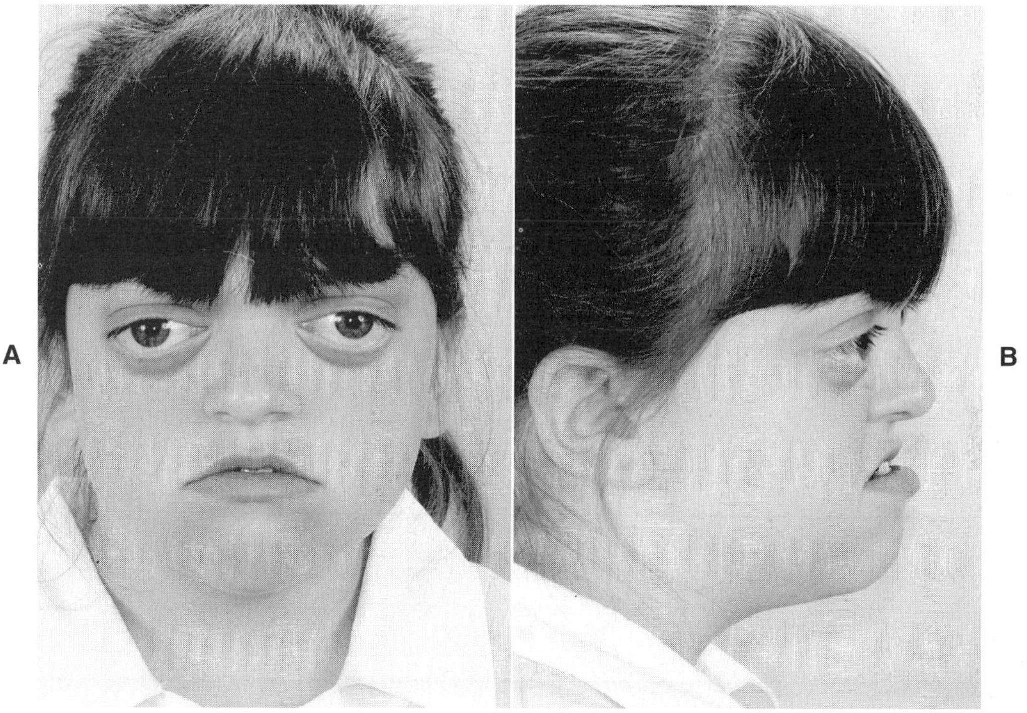

FIGURE 3-11 Facial appearance in Crouzon's syndrome of moderate severity, at age 8 years 8 months. Note the wide separation of the eyes (hypertelorism) and deficiency of the midfacial structures, both of which are characteristic of this syndrome. Because of premature suture fusion, forward development of the midface is retarded, which produces the apparent protrusion of the eyes.

Psychologic and emotional stress in extreme cases can affect physical growth in somewhat the same way as chronic illness (Figure 3-17).

3. Nutritional status. For growth to occur, there must be a nutritional supply in excess of the amount necessary for mere survival. Chronically inadequate nutrition, therefore, has an effect similar to chronic illness. On the other hand, once a level of nutritional adequacy has been achieved, additional nutritional intake is not a stimulus to more rapid growth. Adequate nutrition, like reasonable overall health, is a necessary condition for normal growth but is not a stimulus to it.

An interesting phenomenon of the last 300 or 400 years, particularly the twentieth century, has been a generalized increase in size of most individuals. There has also been a lowering in the age of sexual maturation, so that children

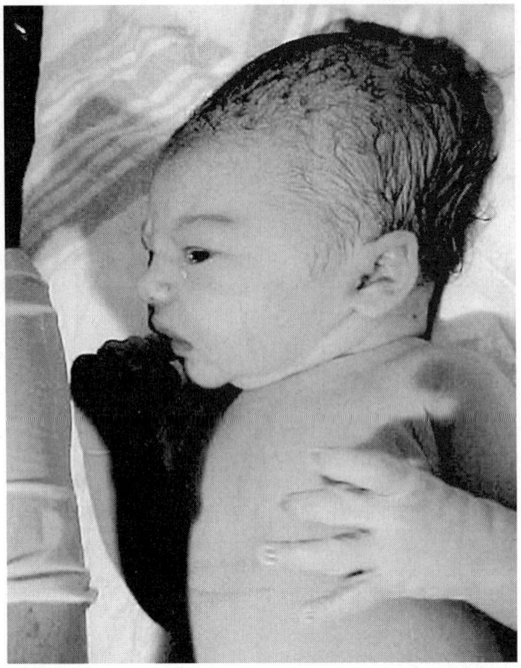

FIGURE 3-12 This photograph of a newborn infant clearly shows the head distortion that accompanies (and facilitates) passage through the birth canal. Note that the head has been squeezed into a more elliptical or tubular "cone-head" shape, a distortion made possible by the presence of the relatively large fontanelles.

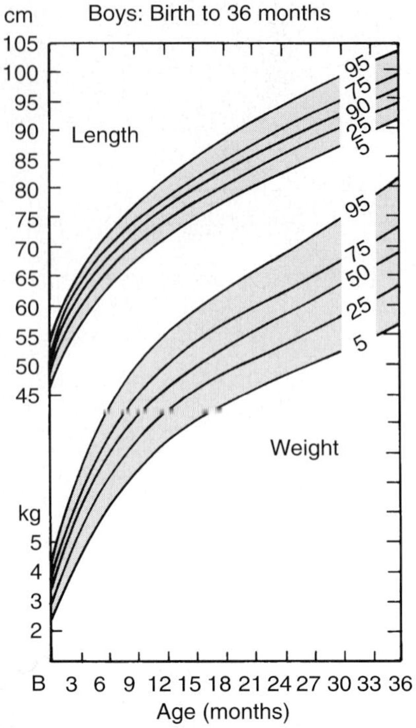

FIGURE 3-14 Graphs of growth in length and weight in infancy for boys (the curves for girls are almost identical at these ages). Note the extremely rapid growth in early infancy, with a progressive slowing after the first 6 months. (Based on data from the National Center for Health Statistics.)

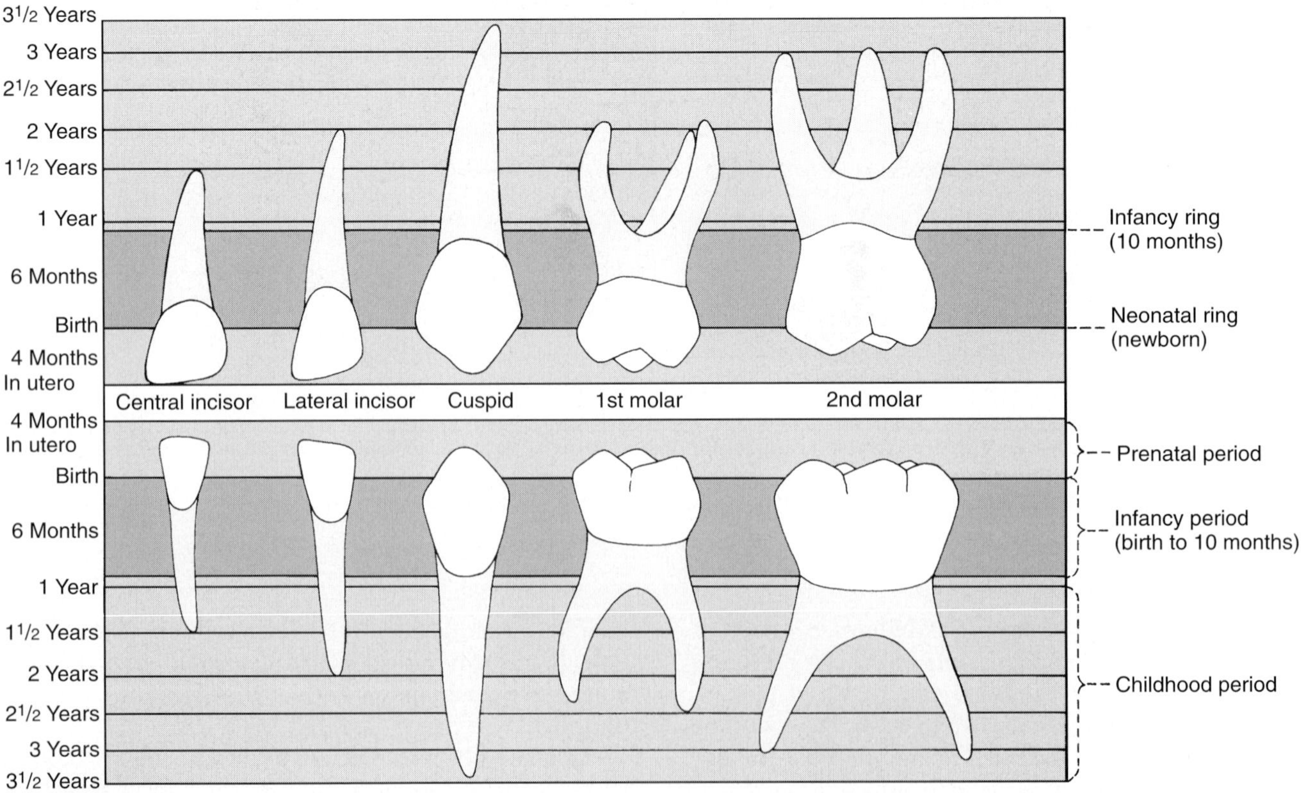

FIGURE 3-13 Primary teeth shown on a developmental scale that indicates the expected location of the neonatal line. From a chart of this type, the timing of illness or traumatic events that led to disturbances of enamel formation can be deduced from the location of enamel lines on various teeth.

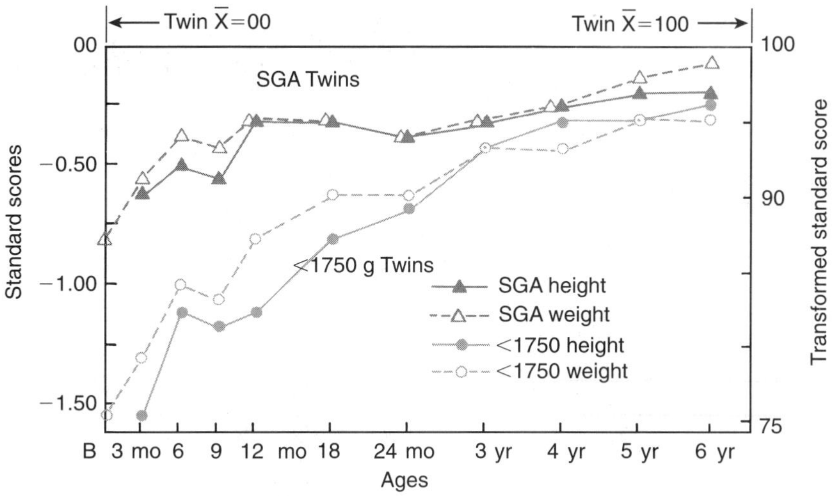

FIGURE 3-15 Growth curves for two groups of at-risk groups of infants: small-for-gestational age (SGA) twins and twins of less than 1750 grams birth weight (premature birth). In this graph, 100 is the expected height and weight for normal, full-term infants. Note the recovery of the low birth weight infants over time. (Redrawn from Lowery GH. Growth and Development of Children, ed 8. Chicago: Mosby; 1986.)

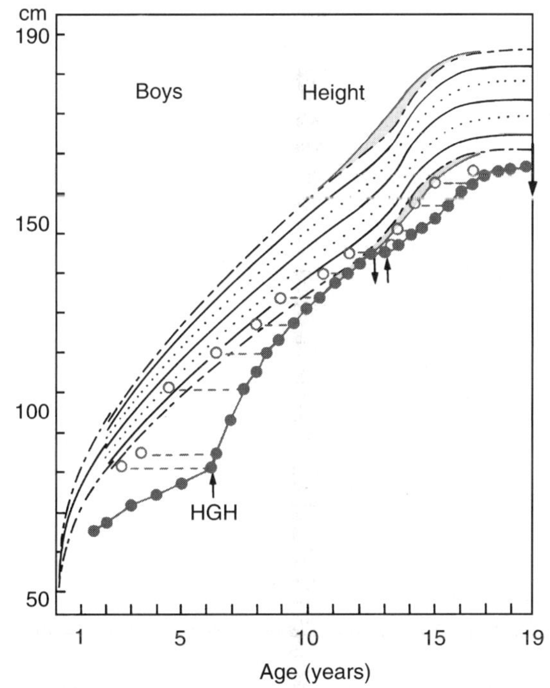

FIGURE 3-16 The curve for growth in height for a boy with isolated growth hormone deficiency. No treatment was possible until he was 6.2 years of age. At that point, human growth hormone (HGH) became available, and it was administered regularly from then until age 19, except for 6 months between 12.5 and 13 years. The beginning and end of HGH administration are indicated by the arrows. The open circles represent height plotted against bone age, thus delay in bone age is represented by the length of each horizontal dashed line. It is 3.5 years at the beginning of treatment, and 0.8 years at 11 to 12 years, when catch-up was essentially complete. Note the very high growth rate immediately after treatment started, equal to the average rate of a 1-year old infant. (Redrawn from Tanner JM, Whitehouse RH. Atlas of Children's Growth. London: Academic Press; 1982.)

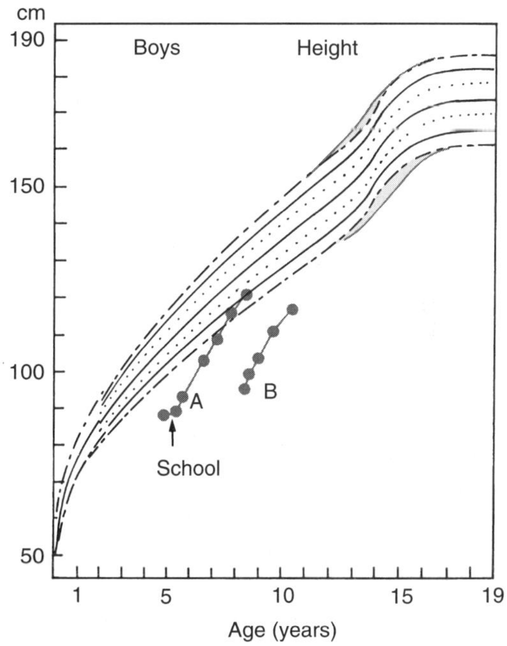

FIGURE 3-17 The effect of a change in social environment on growth of two children who had an obviously disturbed home environment, but no identifiable organic cause for the growth problem. When both children were placed in a special boarding school where presumably their psychosocial stress was lessened, both responded with above-average growth though the more severely affected child was still outside the normal range 4 years later. The mechanism by which psychosocial stress can affect growth so markedly is thought to be induction of a reversible growth hormone deficiency, accompanied by disturbance of the nearby appetite center. (Redrawn from Tanner JM, Whitehouse RH. Atlas of Children's Growth. London: Academic Press; 1982.)

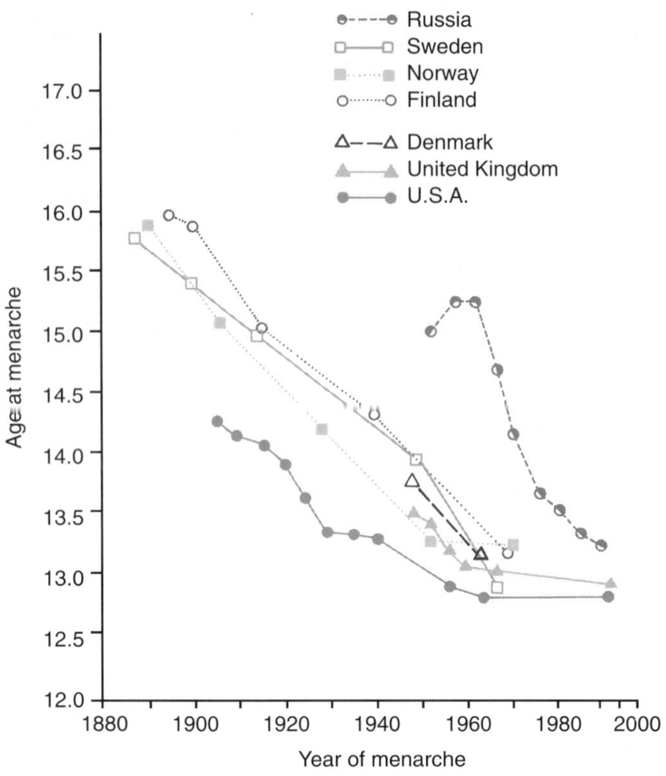

FIGURE 3-18 Age at menarche declined in both the United States and northern European countries in the first half of the 20th century. On the average, children are now larger at any given age than in the early 1900s, and they also mature more quickly. This secular trend seems to have leveled off recently. (Redrawn from Tanner JM. Foetus Into Man. Cambridge, Mass: Harvard University Press; 1978; 1995 U.S. data from Herman-Giddens, et al. Pediatrics 99:597-598, 1997; 1995 English data from Cooper C, et al. Br J Obstet Gynecol 103:814-817, 1996; Russian data from Dubrova YE, et al. Hum Biol 67:755-767, 1995.)

recently have grown faster and matured earlier than they did previously. Since 1900, in the United States the average height has increased 2 to 3 inches, and the average age of girls at first menstruation, the most reliable sign of sexual maturity, has decreased by more than 1 year (Figure 3-18). This "secular trend" toward more rapid growth and earlier maturation has continued until very recently and may still be occurring. Recent data suggest that signs of sexual maturation now appear in many girls much earlier than the previously-accepted standard dates.[11]

The trend undoubtedly is related to better nutrition, which allows the faster weight gain that by itself can trigger earlier maturation. Because a secular trend also has been observed in populations whose nutritional status does not seem to have improved significantly, nutrition may not be the entire explanation. Exposure to environmental chemicals that have estrogenic effects (like some pesticides, for instance) may be contributing to earlier sexual maturation. On the other hand, a deficiency in one or two essential nutritional components can serve to limit the rate of growth, even if the diet is generally adequate. Physical growth requires the formation of new protein, and it is likely that the amount of protein may have been a limiting factor for many populations in the past. A generally adequate diet that was low in trace minerals, vitamins, or other minor but important components may have limited the rate of growth in the past, so that even a small change to supply previously deficient items may in some instances have allowed a considerable increase in growth.

Secular changes in body proportions, which presumably reflect environmental influences, also have been observed. It is interesting that skull proportions have changed during the last century, with the head and face becoming taller and narrower.[12] Some anthropologists feel that such changes are related to the trend toward a softer diet and less functional loading of the facial skeleton (see Chapter 5), but firm evidence does not exist.

Maturation of Oral Function

The principal physiologic functions of the oral cavity are respiration, swallowing, mastication and speech. Although it may seem odd to list respiration as an oral function, since the major portal for respiration is the nose, respiratory needs are a primary determinant of posture of the mandible and tongue.

At birth, if the newborn infant is to survive, an airway must be established within a very few minutes and must be maintained thereafter. As Bosma demonstrated with a classic radiographic study of newborn infants,[13] to open the airway, the mandible must be positioned downward and the tongue moved downward and forward away from the posterior pharyngeal wall. This allows air to be moved through the nose and across the pharynx into the lungs. Newborn infants are obligatory nasal breathers and may not survive if the nasal passage is blocked at birth. Later, breathing through the mouth becomes physiologically possible. At all times during life, respiratory needs can alter the postural basis from which oral activities begin.

Respiratory movements are "practiced" in utero, although of course the lungs do not inflate at that time. Swallowing also occurs during the last months of fetal life, and it appears that swallowed amniotic fluid may be an important stimulus to activation of the infant's immune system.

Once an airway has been established, the newborn infant's next physiologic priority is to obtain milk and transfer it into the gastrointestinal system. This is accomplished by two maneuvers: suckling (not sucking, with which it is frequently confused) and swallowing.

The milk ducts of lactating mammals are surrounded by smooth muscle, which contracts to force out the milk. To obtain milk, the infant does not have to suck it from the mother's breast and probably could not do so. Instead, the infant's role is to stimulate the smooth muscle to contract and squirt milk into his mouth. This is done by suckling,

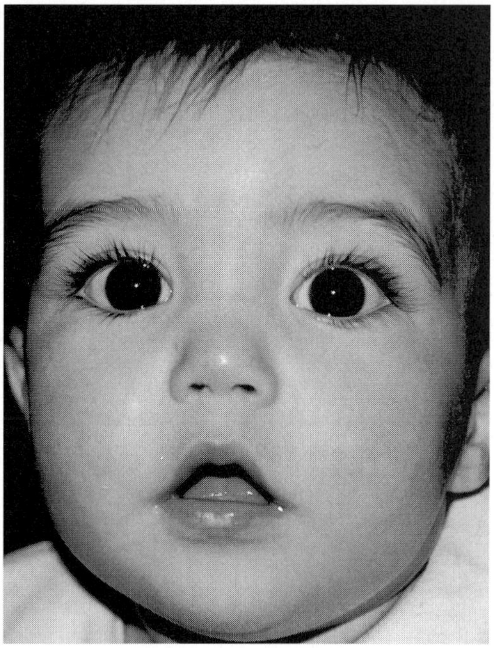

Figure 3-19 Characteristic placement of the tongue against the lower lip in an infant of a few months of age. At this stage of development, tongue contact with the lip is maintained most of the time.

consisting of small nibbling movements of the lips, a reflex action in infants. When the milk is squirted into the mouth, it is only necessary for the infant to groove the tongue and allow the milk to flow posteriorly into the pharynx and esophagus. The tongue, however, must be placed anteriorly in contact with the lower lip, so that milk is in fact deposited on the tongue.

This sequence of events defines an infantile swallow, which is characterized by active contractions of the musculature of the lips, a tongue tip brought forward into contact with the lower lip, and little activity of the posterior tongue or pharyngeal musculature. Tongue-to-lower lip apposition is so common in infants that this posture is usually adopted at rest, and it is frequently possible to gently move the infant's lip and note that the tongue tip moves with it, almost as if the two were glued together (Figure 3-19). The suckling reflex and the infantile swallow normally disappear during the first year of life.

As the infant matures, there is increasing activation of the elevator muscles of the mandible as the child swallows. As semisolid and eventually solid foods are added to the diet, it is necessary for the child to use the tongue in a more complex way to gather up a bolus, position it along the middle of the tongue, and transport it posteriorly. The chewing movements of a young child typically involve moving the mandible laterally as it opens, then bringing it back toward the midline and closing to bring the teeth into contact with the food. By the time the primary molars begin to erupt, this sort of juvenile chewing pattern is well established. By this time also, the more complex movements of the posterior part of the tongue have produced a definite transition beyond the infantile swallow.

Maturation of oral function can be characterized in general as following a gradient from anterior to posterior. At birth, the lips are relatively mature and capable of vigorous suckling activity, whereas more posterior structures are quite immature. As time passes, greater activity by the posterior parts of the tongue and more complex motions of the pharyngeal structures are required.

This principle of front-to-back maturation is particularly well illustrated by the acquisition of speech. The first speech sounds are the bilabial sounds /m/, /p/, and /b/—which is why an infant's first word is likely to be "mama" or "papa." Somewhat later, the tongue tip consonants like /t/ and /d/ appear. The sibilant /s/ and /z/ sounds, which require that the tongue tip be placed close to but not against the palate, come later still, and the last speech sound, /r/, which requires precise positioning of the posterior tongue, often is not acquired until age 4 or 5.

Nearly all modern infants engage in some sort of habitual non-nutritive sucking—sucking a thumb, finger, or a similarly shaped object. Some fetuses have been reported to suck their thumbs in utero, and the vast majority of infants do so during the period from 6 months to 2 years or later. This practice is culturally determined to some extent, since children in primitive groups who are allowed ready access to the mother's breast for a long period rarely suck any other object.[14]

After the eruption of the primary molars during the second year, drinking from a cup replaces drinking from a bottle or continued nursing at the mother's breast, and the number of children who engage in non-nutritive sucking diminishes. When sucking activity stops, a continued transition in the pattern of swallow leads to the acquisition of an adult pattern. This type of swallow is characterized by a cessation of lip activity (i.e., lips relaxed, the placement of the tongue tip against the alveolar process behind the upper incisors, and the posterior teeth brought into occlusion during swallowing). As long as sucking habits persist, however, there will not be a total transition to the adult swallow.

Surveys of American children indicate that at age 8, about 60% have achieved an adult swallow, while the remaining 40% are still somewhere in the transition.[15] After sucking habits are extinguished, a complete transition to the adult swallow may require some months. This is complicated, however, by the fact that an anterior open bite, which may well be present if a sucking habit has persisted for a long time, can delay the transition even further because of the physiologic need to seal the anterior space. The relationship of tongue position and the pattern of swallowing to malocclusion is discussed further in Chapter 5.

The chewing pattern of the adult is quite different from that of a typical child: an adult typically opens straight down, then moves the jaw laterally and brings the teeth into contact, whereas a child moves the jaw laterally on opening

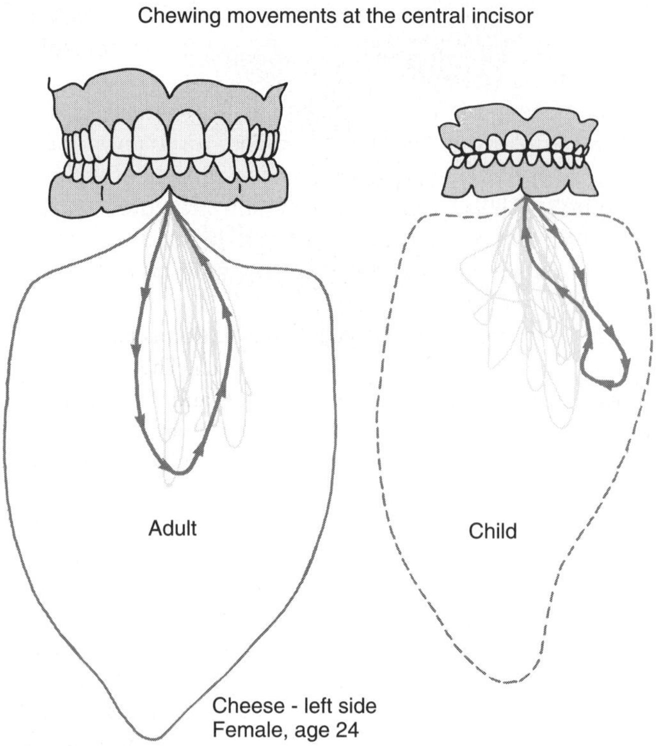

FIGURE 3-20 Chewing movements of an adult contrasted to a child. Children move the jaw laterally on opening, while adults open straight down, then move the jaw laterally. (Redrawn from Lundeen HC, Gibbs CH. Advances in Occlusion. Boston, Mass: John Wright's PSG; 1982.)

(Figure 3-20). The transition from the juvenile to adult chewing pattern appears to develop in conjunction with eruption of the permanent canines, at about age 12. Interestingly, adults who do not achieve normal function of the canine teeth because of a severe anterior open bite retain the juvenile chewing pattern.[16]

Eruption of the Primary Teeth

At birth, neither the maxillary nor the mandibular alveolar process is well developed. Occasionally, a "natal tooth" is present, although the first primary teeth normally do not erupt until approximately 6 months of age. The natal tooth may be a supernumerary one, formed by an aberration in the development of the dental lamina, but usually is merely a very early but otherwise normal central incisor. Because of the possibility that it is perfectly normal, such a natal tooth should not be extracted casually.

The timing and sequence of eruption of the primary teeth are shown in Table 3-2. The dates of eruption are relatively variable; up to 6 months of acceleration or delay is within the normal range. The eruption sequence, however, is usually preserved. One can expect that the mandibular central incisors will erupt first, closely followed by the other incisors. After a 3-to-4 month interval, the mandibular and maxillary

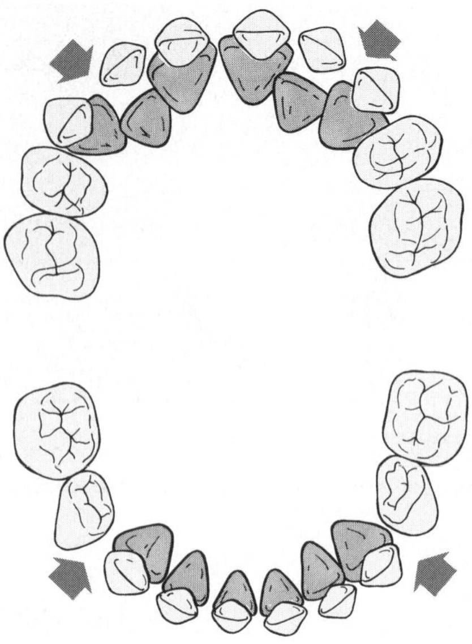

FIGURE 3-21 The crowns of the permanent incisors *(gray)* lie lingual to the crowns of the primary incisors *(yellow)*, particularly in the case of the maxillary laterals. Arrows point to the primate spaces.

first molars erupt, followed in another 3 or 4 months by the maxillary and mandibular canines, which nearly fill the space between the lateral incisor and first molar. The primary dentition is usually completed at 24 to 30 months as the mandibular, then the maxillary second molars erupt.

Spacing is normal throughout the anterior part of the primary dentition but is most noticeable in two locations, called the primate spaces. (Most subhuman primates have these spaces throughout life, thus the name.) In the maxillary arch, the primate space is located between the lateral incisors and canines, whereas in the mandibular arch, the space is between the canines and first molars (Figure 3-21). The primate spaces are normally present from the time the teeth erupt. Developmental spaces between the incisors are often present from the beginning, but become somewhat larger as the child grows and the alveolar processes expand. Generalized spacing of the primary teeth is a requirement for proper alignment of the permanent incisors.

LATE CHILDHOOD: THE MIXED DENTITION YEARS

Physical Development in Late Childhood

Late childhood, from age 5 or 6 to the onset of puberty, is characterized by important social and behavioral changes (see Chapter 2) but the physical development pattern of the previous period continues. The normally different rates of growth for different tissue systems, however, must be kept in mind. The maximum disparity in the development of

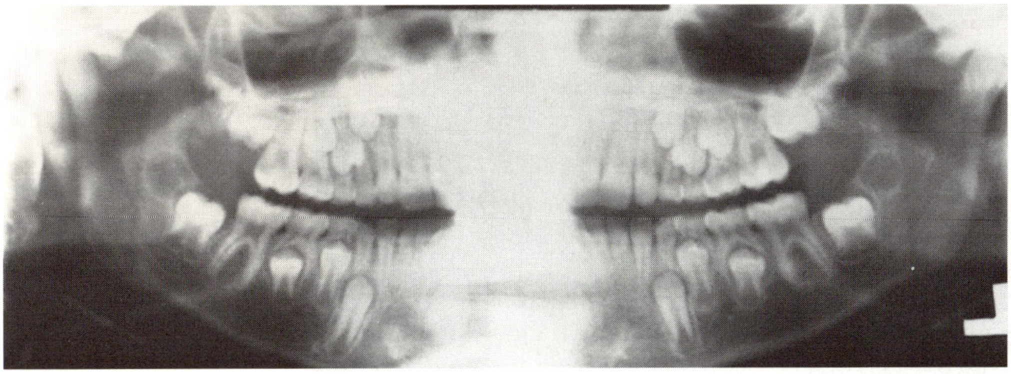

Figure 3-22 Panoramic radiograph of normal eruption in a 10-year-old boy. Note that the permanent teeth erupt as resorption of overlying primary teeth and bone occurs. Resorption must occur to make eruption possible.

different tissue systems occurs in late childhood (see Figure 2-2).

By age 7, a child has essentially completed his or her neural growth. The brain and the brain case are as large as they will ever be, and it is never necessary to buy a child a larger baseball cap because of growth (unless, of course, the growth is of uncut hair). Lymphoid tissue throughout the body has proliferated beyond the usual adult levels, and large tonsils and adenoids are common. In contrast, growth of the sex organs has hardly begun and general body growth is only modestly advanced. During early childhood the rate of general body growth declines from the rapid pace of infancy, then stabilizes at a moderate lower level during late childhood. Both nutrition and general health can affect the level at which stabilization occurs.

Eruption of the Permanent Teeth

The eruption of any tooth can be divided into several stages. This includes the primary teeth: the physiologic principles underlying eruption that are discussed in this section are not different for the primary teeth, despite the root resorption that eventually causes their loss. The nature of eruption and its control before the emergence of the tooth into the mouth are somewhat different from eruption after emergence, and we will consider these major stages separately.

Preemergent Eruption

During the period when the crown of a tooth is being formed, there is a very slow labial or buccal drift of the tooth follicle within the bone, but this follicular drift is not attributed to the eruption mechanism itself. In fact, the amount of change in the position of the tooth follicle is extremely small, observable only with vital staining experiments and so small that a follicle can be used as a natural marker in radiographic studies of growth. Eruptive movement begins soon after the root begins to form. This supports the idea that metabolic activity within the periodontal ligament is necessary for eruption.

Two processes are necessary for preemergent eruption. First, there must be resorption of bone and primary tooth roots overlying the crown of the erupting tooth; second, the eruption mechanism itself then must move the tooth in the direction where the path has been cleared (Figure 3-22). Although the two mechanisms normally operate in concert, in some circumstances they do not. Investigations of the results of a failure of bone resorption, or alternately, of a failure of the eruption mechanism when bone resorption is normal, have yielded considerable insight into the control of preemergent eruption.

Defective bone resorption occurs in a mutant species of mice, appropriately labeled *Ia,* for Incisors absent. In these animals, the deficient bone resorption means that the incisor teeth cannot erupt, and they never appear in the mouth. Failure of teeth to erupt because of a failure of bone resorption also occurs in humans, as for instance in the syndrome of cleidocranial dysplasia (Figure 3-23). In children with this condition, not only is resorption of primary teeth and bone deficient, but heavy fibrous gingiva and multiple supernumerary teeth also impede normal eruption. All of these serve to mechanically block the succedaneous teeth (those replacing primary teeth) from erupting. If the interferences are removed, the teeth often erupt and can be brought into occlusion.[17]

It has been demonstrated experimentally in animals that the rate of bone resorption and the rate of tooth eruption are not controlled physiologically by the same mechanism. For instance, if the tooth bud of a dog premolar is wired to the lower border of the mandible, the tooth can no longer erupt because of this mechanical obstruction, but resorption of overlying bone proceeds at the usual rate, resulting in a large cystic cavity overlying the ligated tooth bud.[18]

On at least two occasions, the same experiment has inadvertently been done to a child, in whom an unerupted permanent tooth was inadvertently wired to the lower border of the mandible when a mandibular fracture was repaired (Figure 3-24). The result was the same as in the animal premolars are still in the stage of crown completion or just at the beginning of root formation.

Dental age 8 (Figure 3-31) is characterized by the eruption of the maxillary lateral incisors. After these teeth come into the arch, there is a delay of 2 to 3 years before any further permanent teeth appear.

Since no teeth are erupting at that time, dental ages 9 and 10 must be distinguished by the extent of resorption of the primary canines and premolars and the extent of root development of their permanent successors. At dental age 9, the primary canines, first molars, and second molars are present. Approximately one third of the root of the mandibular canine and the mandibular first premolar is completed. Root development is just beginning, if it has started at all, on the mandibular second premolar (Figure 3-32). In the maxillary arch, root development has begun on the first premolar but is just beginning, if it is present at all, on both the canine and the second premolar.

Dental age 10 is characterized by a greater amount of both root resorption of the primary canines and molars, and root development of their permanent successors. At dental age 10, approximately one half of the roots of the mandibular canine and mandibular first premolar have been completed; nearly half the root of the upper first premolar is complete; and there is significant root development of the mandibular second premolar, maxillary canine, and maxillary second premolar.

Teeth usually emerge when three fourths of their roots are completed.[24] Thus a signal that a tooth should be appearing in the mouth is root development approaching this level. It takes 2 to 3 years for roots to be completed after a tooth has erupted into occlusion.

TABLE 3-3

Chronology of Tooth Development, Permanent Dentition

	CALCIFICATION BEGINS		CROWN COMPLETED		ERUPTION		ROOT COMPLETED	
Tooth	*Max.*	*Mand.*	*Max.*	*Mand.*	*Max.*	*Mand.*	*Max.*	*Mand.*
Central	3 mo.	3 mo.	4½ yr.	3½ yr.	7¼ yr.	6¼ yr.	10½ yr.	9½ yr.
Lateral	11 mo.	3 mo.	5½ yr.	4 yr.	8¼ yr.	7½ yr.	11 yr.	10 yr.
Canine	4 mo.	4 mo.	6 yr.	5¾ yr.	11½ yr.	10½ yr.	13½ yr	12¾ yr.
1st Premolar	20 mo.	22 mo.	7 yr.	6¾ yr.	10¼ yr.	10½ yr.	13½ yr.	13½ yr.
2nd Premolar	27 mo.	28 mo.	7¾ yr.	7½ yr.	11 yr.	11¼ yr.	14½ yr.	15 yr.
1st Molar	32 wk. in utero	32 wk. in utero	4¼ yr.	3¾ yr.	6¼ yr.	6 yr.	10½ yr.	10½ yr.
2nd Molar	27 mo.	27 mo.	7¾ yr.	7½ yr.	12½ yr.	12 yr.	15¾ yr.	16 yr.
3rd Molar	8 yr.	9 yr.	14 yr.	14 yr.	20 yr.	20 yr.	22 yr.	22 yr.

A

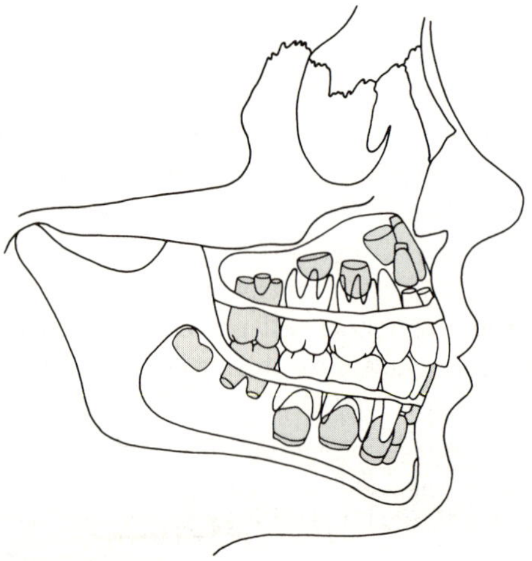

B

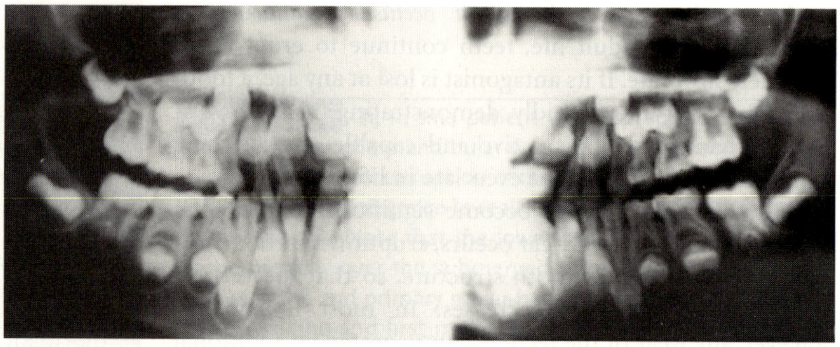

FIGURE 3-30 The first stage of eruption of the permanent teeth, at age 6, is characterized by the near-simultaneous eruption of the mandibular central incisors, the mandibular first molars, and the maxillary first molars. **A,** Drawing of right side. **B,** Panoramic radiograph.

Another indicator of dental age 10, therefore, would be completion of the roots of the mandibular incisor teeth and near completion of the roots of the maxillary laterals. By dental age 11, the roots of all incisors and first permanent molars should be well completed.

Dental age 11 (Figure 3-33) is characterized by the eruption of another group of teeth: the mandibular canine, mandibular first premolar, and maxillary first premolar, which all erupt more or less simultaneously. In the mandibular arch, the mandibular canine most often appears just ahead of the first premolar, but the similarity in the time of eruption, not the most frequent sequence, is the important point. In the maxillary arch, on the other hand, the first premolar usually erupts well ahead of the canine. At dental age 11, the only remaining primary teeth are the maxillary canine and second molar, and the mandibular second molar.

At dental age 12 (Figure 3-34), the remaining succedaneous permanent teeth erupt. *Succedaneous* refers to permanent teeth that replace primary predecessors; thus a canine is a succedaneous tooth, whereas a first molar is not. In addition, at age 12 the second permanent molars in both arches are nearing eruption. The succedaneous teeth complete their eruption before the emergence of the second molars in most but by no means all normal children. Although

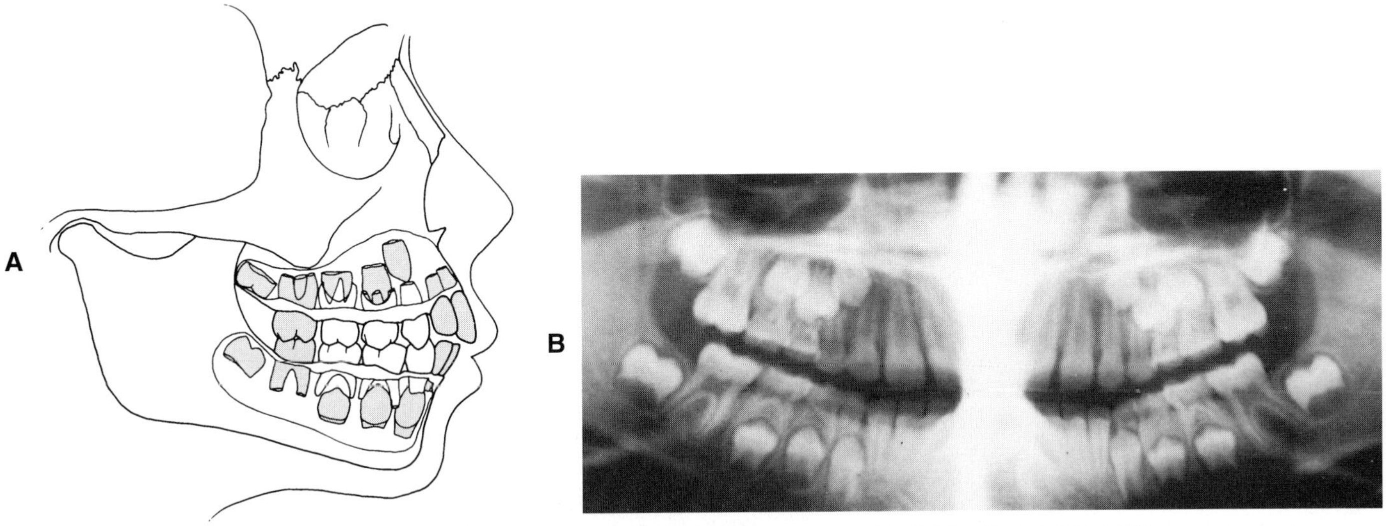

FIGURE 3-31 Dental age 8 is characterized by eruption of the maxillary lateral incisors.

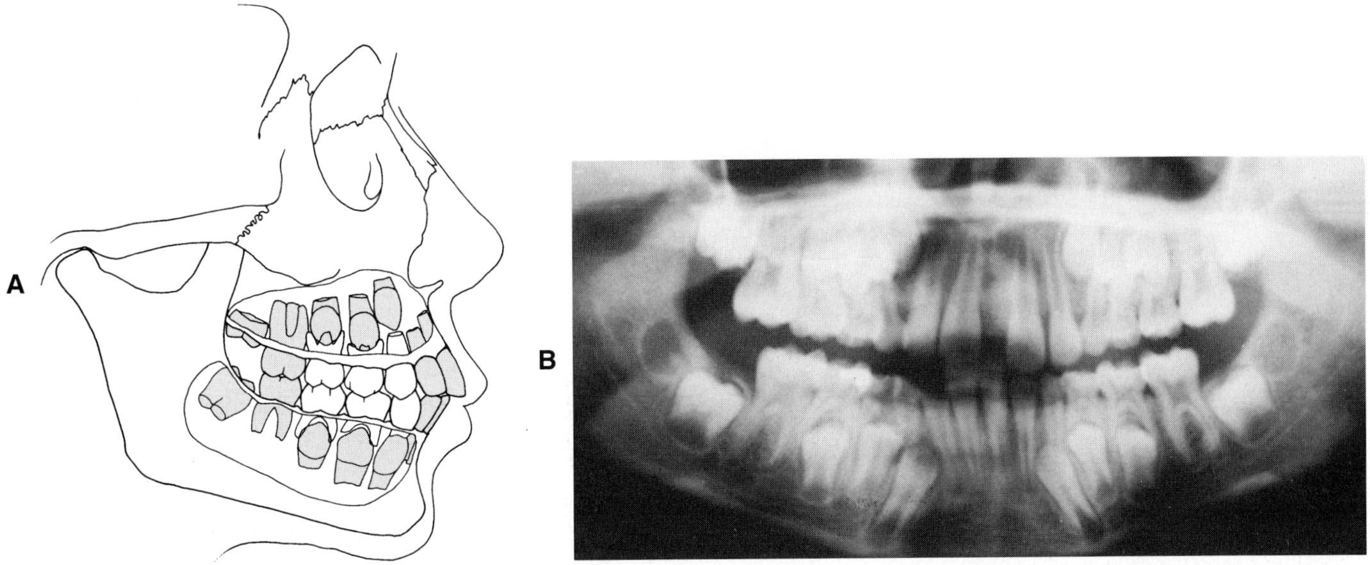

FIGURE 3-32 At dental age 9, the maxillary lateral incisors have been in place for 1 year, and root formation on other incisors and first molars is nearly complete. Root development of the maxillary canines and all second premolars is just beginning, while about one third of the root of the mandibular canines and all of the first premolars have been completed.

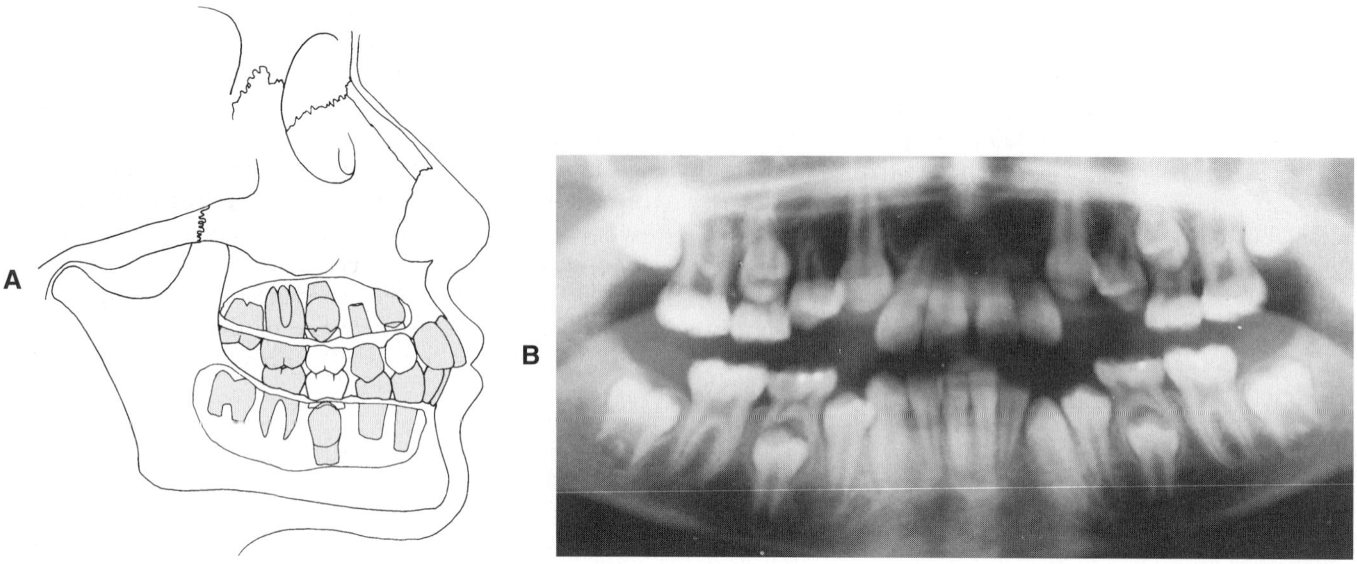

FIGURE 3-33 Dental age 11 is characterized by the more or less simultaneous eruption of the mandibular canines, mandibular first premolars, and maxillary first premolars.

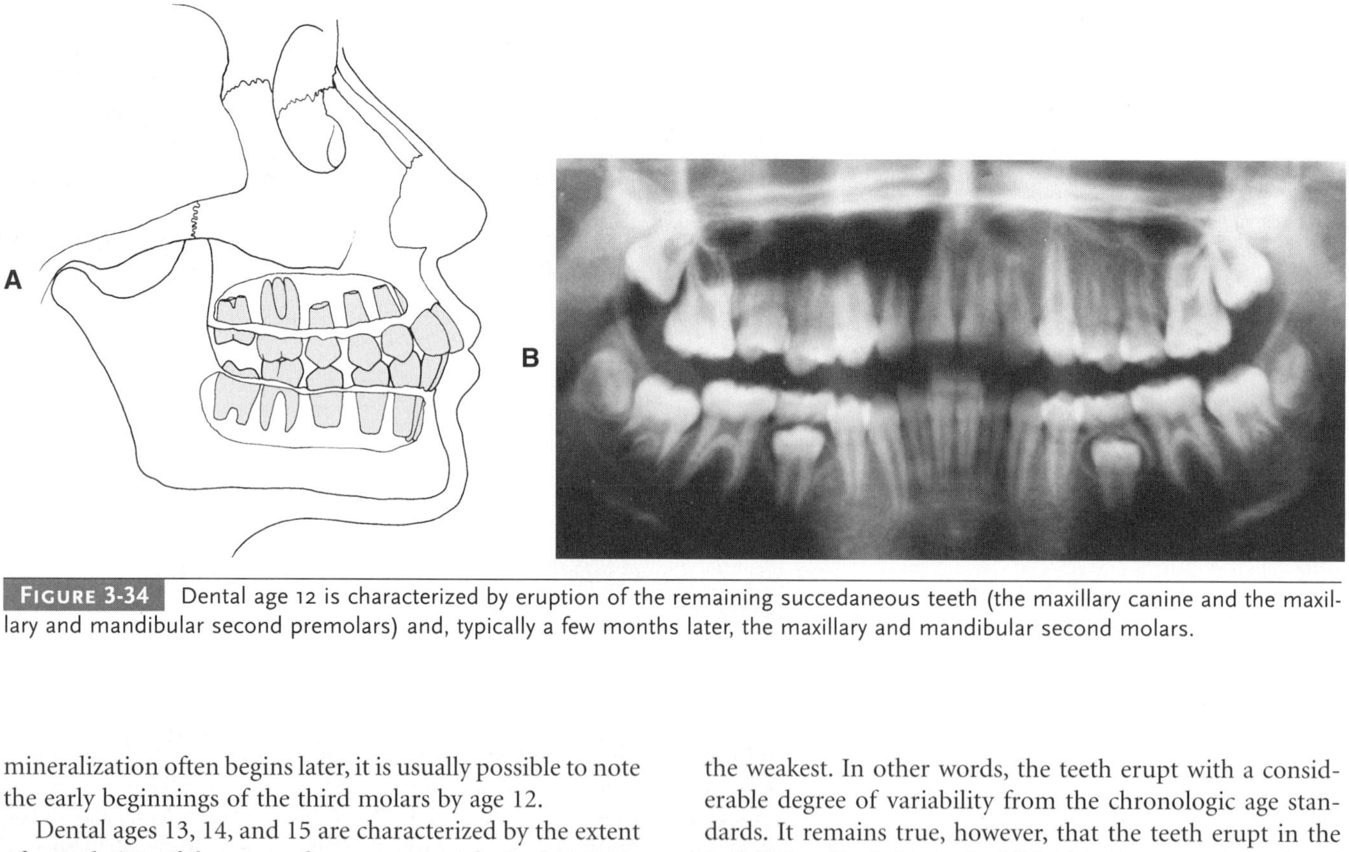

FIGURE 3-34 Dental age 12 is characterized by eruption of the remaining succedaneous teeth (the maxillary canine and the maxillary and mandibular second premolars) and, typically a few months later, the maxillary and mandibular second molars.

mineralization often begins later, it is usually possible to note the early beginnings of the third molars by age 12.

Dental ages 13, 14, and 15 are characterized by the extent of completion of the roots of permanent teeth. By dental age 15 (Figure 3-35), if a third molar is going to form, it should be apparent on the radiographs, and the roots of all other permanent teeth should be complete.

Like all other developmental ages (discussed in more detail in paragraphs following), dental age correlates with chronologic age—but the correlation for dental age is one of the weakest. In other words, the teeth erupt with a considerable degree of variability from the chronologic age standards. It remains true, however, that the teeth erupt in the stages described above. A child who has precocious dental development might have the mandibular central incisors and first molars erupt at age 5 and could reach dental age 12 by chronologic age 10. A child with slow dental development might not reach dental age 12 until chronologic age 14.

A change in the sequence of eruption is a much more reliable sign of a disturbance in normal development than a

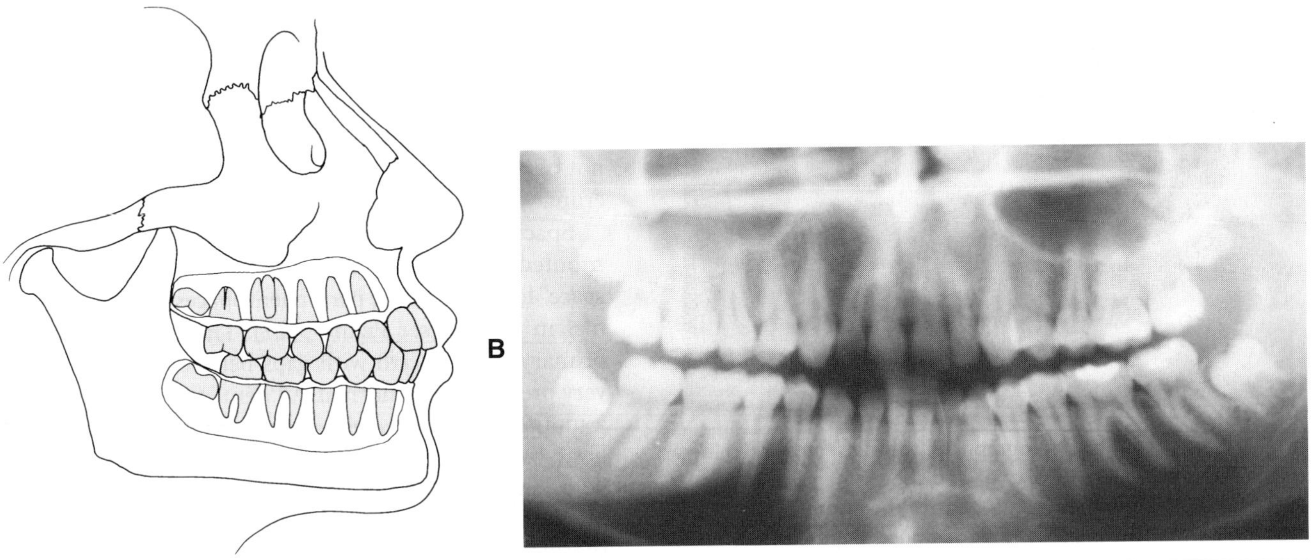

A

B

FIGURE 3-35 By dental age 15, the roots of all permanent teeth except the third molars are complete, and crown formation of third molars often has been completed.

generalized delay or acceleration. The more a tooth deviates from its expected position in the sequence, the greater the likelihood of some sort of problem. For example, a delay in eruption of maxillary canines to age 14 is within normal variation if the second premolars are also delayed, but if the second premolars have erupted at age 12 and the canines have not, something is probably wrong.

Several reasonably normal variations in eruption sequence have clinical significance and should be recognized. These are: (1) eruption of second molars ahead of premolars in the mandibular arch, (2) eruption of canines ahead of premolars in the maxillary arch, and (3) asymmetries in eruption between the right and left sides.

Early eruption of the mandibular second molars can be unfortunate in a dental arch where room to accommodate the teeth is marginal. The eruption of the second molar before the second premolar tends to decrease the space for the second premolar and may lead to its being partially blocked out of the arch. Some dental intervention may be needed to get the second premolar into the arch when the mandibular second molar erupts early.

If a maxillary canine erupts at about the same time as the maxillary first premolar (remember that this is the normal eruption sequence of the lower arch but is abnormal in the upper), the canine probably will be forced labially. Labial positioning of maxillary canines often occurs when there is an overall lack of space in the arch, because this tooth is the last to erupt normally; but displacement of the canine also can be an unfortunate consequence of an eruption sequence abnormality.

An asymmetry in the rate of eruption on the two sides of the dental arch is a frequent enough variation to approach the bounds of normal. A striking illustration of genetic influences on eruption timing is seen in identical twins, who frequently have mirror-image asymmetries in the dentition at the various stages of eruption. For example, if the premolars erupt a little earlier on the left in one of the twins, they will erupt a little earlier on the right in the other. The normal variation is only a few months, however. As a general rule, if a permanent tooth on one side erupts but its counterpart on the other does not within 6 months, a radiograph should be taken to investigate the cause of the problem. Although small variations from one side to the other are normal, large ones often indicate a problem.

Space Relationships in Replacement of the Incisors

If a dissected skull is examined, it can be seen that in both the maxillary and mandibular arches, the permanent incisor tooth buds lie lingual as well as apical to the primary incisors (Figure 3-36; also see Figure 3-21). The result is a tendency for the mandibular permanent incisors to erupt somewhat lingually and in a slightly irregular position, even in children who have normal dental arches and normal spacing within the arches. In the maxillary arch, the lateral incisor is likely to be lingually positioned at the time of its emergence and to remain in that position if there is any crowding in the arch. The permanent canines are positioned to lie more nearly in line with the primary canines. If there are problems in eruption, these teeth can be displaced either lingually or labially, but usually they are displaced labially if there is not enough room for them.

The permanent incisor teeth are considerably larger than the primary incisors that they replace. For instance, the mandibular permanent central incisor is about 5.5 mm in

19. Proffit WR, Vig KWL. Primary failure of eruption: a possible cause of posterior open bite. Am J Orthod 80:173-190, 1981.
20. Frazier-Bowers S, Koehler K, Ackerman JL, Proffit WR. Primary failure of eruption: further characterization of a rare eruption disorder. Am J Orthod Dentofac Orthop, in press.
21. Craddock HL, Youngson CC. Eruptive tooth movement—the current state of knowledge. Br Dent J 197:385-391, 2004.
22. Risinger RK, Proffit WR. Continuous overnight observation of human premolar eruption. Arch Oral Biol 41:779-789, 1996.
23. Trentini CJ, Proffit WR. High resolution observations of human premolar eruption. Arch Oral Biol 41:63-68, 1996.
24. Cheek CC, Paterson RL, Proffit WR. Response of erupting human second premolars to blood flow changes. Arch Oral Biol 47:851-858, 2002.
25. Moorrees CFA, Chadha JM. Available space for the incisors during dental development—a growth study based on physiologic age. Angle Orthod 35:12-22, 1965.
26. Edwards JG. The diastema, the frenum, the frenectomy. Am J Orthod 71:489-508, 1977.
27. Tanner JM. Assessment of Skeletal Maturity and Prediction of Adult Height. New York: WB Saunders; 2001.
28. Baccetti T, Franchi L, McNamara JA Jr. The cervical vertebral maturation (CVM) method for the assessment of optimal treatment timing in dentofacial orthopedics. Sem Orthod 11:119-129, 2005.

CHAPTER

4

Later Stages of Development

CHAPTER OUTLINE

ADOLESCENCE: THE EARLY PERMANENT DENTITION YEARS

Adolescence is a sexual phenomenon, the period of life when sexual maturity is attained. More specifically, it is the transitional period between the juvenile stage and adulthood, during which secondary sexual characteristics appear, the adolescent growth spurt takes place, fertility is attained, and profound physiologic changes occur. All these developments are associated with the maturation of the sex organs and the accompanying surge in secretion of sex hormones.

This period is particularly important in dental and orthodontic treatment, because the physical changes at adolescence significantly affect the face and dentition. Major events in dentofacial development that occur during adolescence include the exchange from the mixed to the permanent dentition, an acceleration in the overall rate of facial growth, and differential growth of the jaws.

Initiation of Adolescence

The first events of puberty occur in the brain, and although considerable research progress has been made in this area, the precise stimulus for their unfolding remains unknown. For whatever reason, apparently influenced both by an internal clock and external stimuli, brain cells in the hypothalamus begin to secrete substances called releasing factors. Both the cells and their method of action are somewhat unusual. These neuroendocrine cells look like typical neurons, but they secrete materials in the cell body, which are carried by cytoplasmic transport down the axon toward a richly vascular area at the base of the hypothalamus near the pituitary gland (Figure 4-1). The substances secreted by the nerve cells

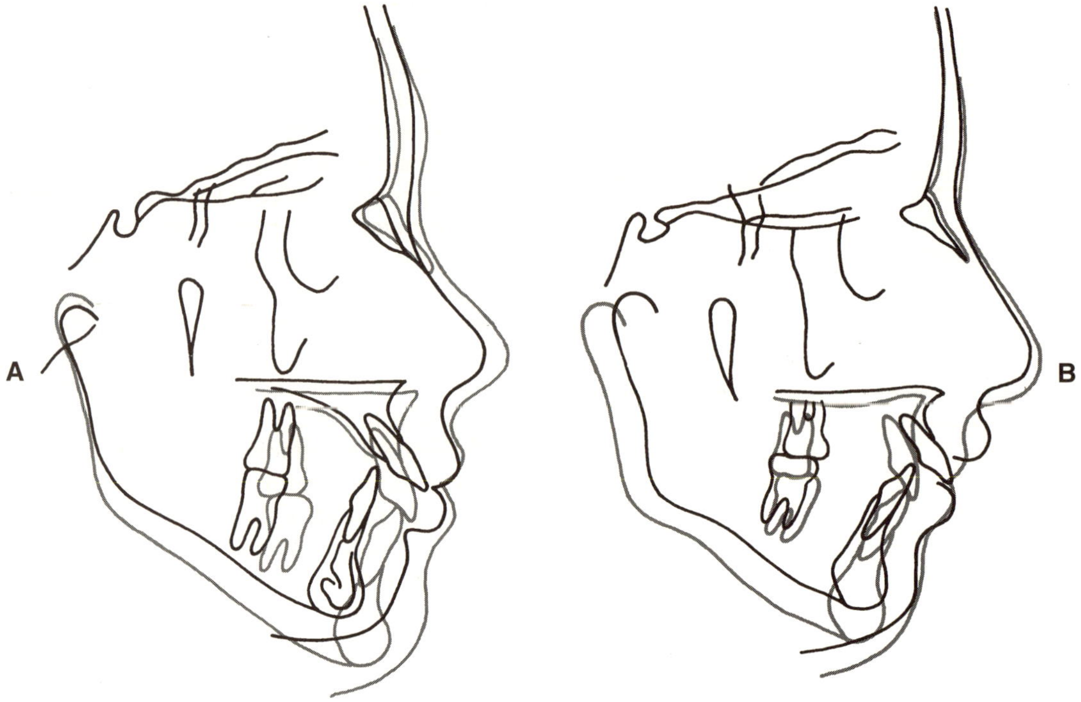

FIGURE 4-9 Cephalometric tracings showing growth in two patients during the orthodontic correction of moderate Class II malocclusion (superimposed on sphenoethmoid triad in cranial base). **A,** Changes from age 11 years 10 months to age 14 years 11 months. In this patient, approximately 7 mm of mandibular growth was expressed entirely as forward movement of the chin, while the area of the temporomandibular (TM) joint remained in the same anteroposterior position relative to the cranial base. **B,** Changes from age 11 years 8 months to age 15 years 0 months. This patient also had approximately 7 mm of mandibular growth, but the TM joint area moved downward and backward relative to the cranial base, so that much of the growth was not expressed as forward movement of the chin. (Courtesy Dr. V. Kokich.)

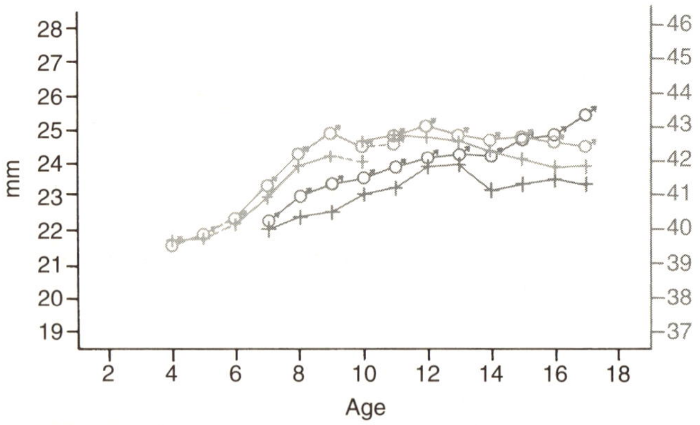

FIGURE 4-10 Average changes in mandibular canine and molar widths in both sexes during growth. Molar widths are shown in blue, canine widths in green. (From Moyers RE, et al. Standards of Human Occlusal Development. Ann Arbor, Mich: University of Michigan Center for Human Growth and Development; 1976.)

does not occur until the early twenties in boys, somewhat earlier in girls.

Rotation of Jaws During Growth

Implant Studies of Jaw Rotation

Until longitudinal studies of growth using metallic implants in the jaws were carried out in the 1960s (see Chapter 2), primarily by Bjork and coworkers in Copenhagen, the extent to which both the maxilla and mandible rotate during growth was not appreciated. The reason is that the rotation that occurs in the core of each jaw, called *internal rotation,* tends to be masked by surface changes and alterations in the rate of tooth eruption. The surface changes produce *external rotation.* Obviously, the overall change in the orientation of each jaw, as judged by the palatal plane and mandibular plane, results from a combination of internal and external rotation.

The terminology for describing these rotational changes is itself confusing. The descriptive terms used here, in an effort to simplify and clarify a complex and difficult subject, are not those Bjork used in the original papers on this

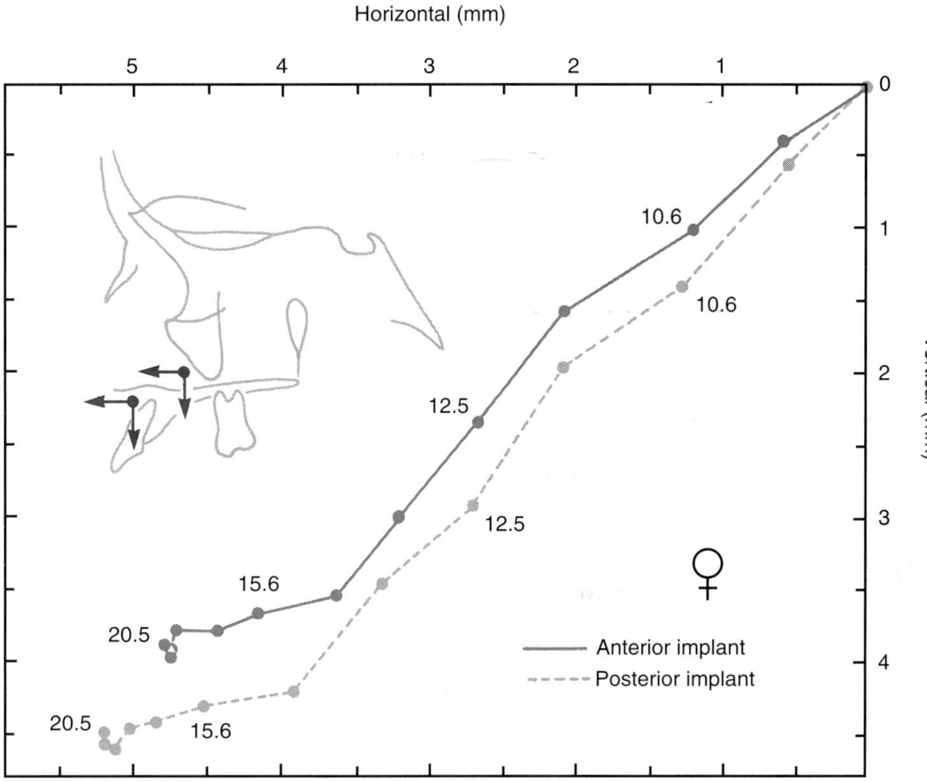

FIGURE 4-11 Mean growth tracks of anterior and posterior maxillary implants relative to the cranial base and its perpendicular, in a group of Danish girls. The two tracks are shown with their origins superimposed to facilitate comparison. Note that the posterior implant moves down and forward more than the anterior one, with growth continuing into the late teens at a slow rate. (Courtesy Dr. B. Solow.)

TABLE 4-4

Terminology, Rotational Changes of the Jaws

Condition	Bjork	Shudy	
Anterior growth greater than posterior	Forward rotation	Clockwise rotation	
Posterior growth greater than anterior	Backward rotation	Counterclockwise rotation	
	Bjork	**Solow, Houston**	**Proffit**
Rotation of mandibular core relative to cranial base	Total rotation	True rotation	Internal rotation
Rotation of mandibular plane relative to cranial base	Matrix rotation	Apparent rotation	Total rotation
Rotation of mandibular plane relative to core of mandible	Intramatrix rotation	Angular remodeling of lower border	External rotation

Proffit: Total rotation = internal rotation − external rotation
Bjork: Matrix rotation = total rotation − intramatrix rotation
Solow: Apparent rotation = true rotation − angular remodeling of lower border

subject, or exactly the same as suggested in some previous papers.[8,9] See Table 4-4 for a comparison of terms.

It is easier to visualize the internal and external rotation of the jaws by considering the mandible first. The core of the mandible is the bone that surrounds the inferior alveolar nerve. The rest of the mandible consists of its several functional processes (Figure 4-12). These are the alveolar process (bone supporting the teeth and providing for mastication), the muscular processes (the bone to which the muscles of mastication attach), and the condylar process, the function in this case being the articulation of the jaw with the skull. If implants are placed in areas of stable bone away from the functional processes, it can be observed that in most individuals, the core of the mandible rotates during growth in a way that would tend to decrease the mandibular plane angle (i.e., up anteriorly and down posteriorly).

Bjork and Skieller[10] distinguished two contributions to internal rotation (which they called total rotation) of the

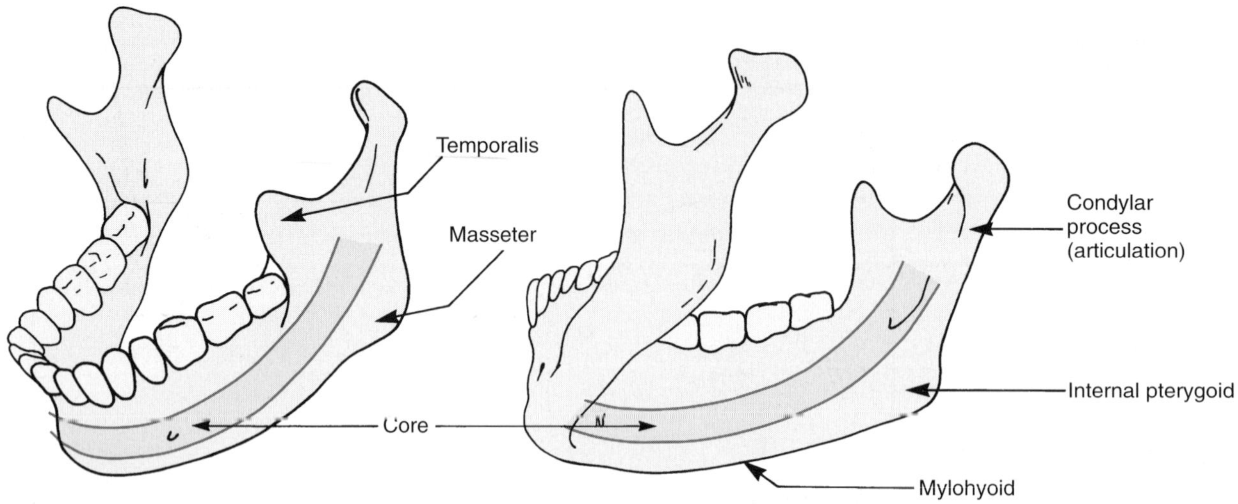

FIGURE 4-12 The mandible can be visualized as consisting of a core of bone surrounding the inferior alveolar neurovascular bundle and a series of functional processes: the alveolar process, serving the function of mastication; the muscular processes, serving for muscle attachments; and the condylar process, serving to articulate the bone with the rest of the skull.

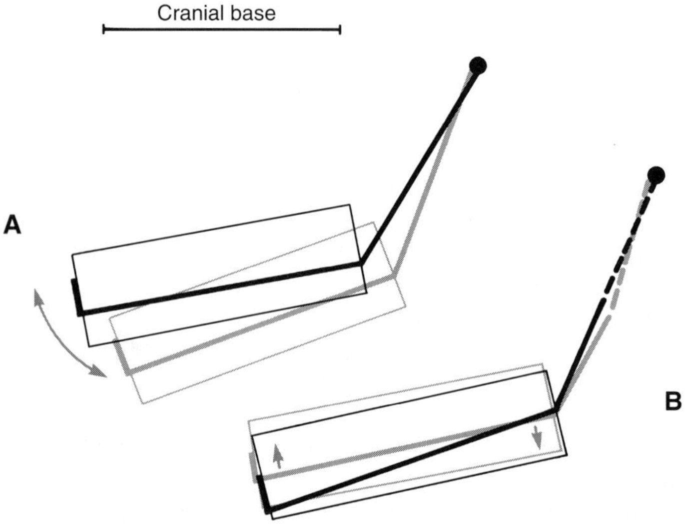

FIGURE 4-13 Internal rotation of the mandible (i.e., rotation of the core relative to the cranial base) has two components: **A,** Rotation around the condyle, or matrix rotation. **B,** Rotations centered within the body of the mandible, or intramatrix rotation. (Redrawn from Bjork A, Skieller V. Eur J Orthod 5:1-46, 1983.)

mandible: (1) matrix rotation, or rotation around the condyle; and (2) intramatrix rotation, or rotation centered within the body of the mandible (Figure 4-13). By convention, the rotation of either jaw is considered "forward" and given a negative sign if there is more growth posteriorly than anteriorly. The rotation is "backward" and given a positive direction if it lengthens anterior dimensions more than posterior ones, bringing the chin downward and backward.

One of the features of internal rotation of the mandible is the variation between individuals, ranging up to 10 to 15 degrees. The pattern of vertical facial development, discussed in more detail later, is strongly related to the rotation of both jaws. For an average individual with normal vertical facial proportions, however, there is about a −15 degree internal rotation from age 4 to adult life. Of this, about 25% results from matrix rotation and 75% results from intramatrix rotation.

During the time that the core of the mandible rotates forward an average of 15 degrees, the mandibular plane angle, representing the orientation of the jaw to an outside observer, decreases only 2 to 4 degrees on the average. The reason that the internal rotation is not expressed in jaw orientation, of course, is that surface changes (external rotation) tend to compensate. This means that the posterior part of the lower border of the mandible must be an area of resorption, while the anterior aspect of the lower border is unchanged or undergoes slight apposition. Studies of surface changes reveal exactly this as the usual pattern of apposition and resorption (Figure 4-14). On the average, then, there is about 15 degrees of internal, forward rotation and 11 to 12 degrees of external, backward rotation producing the 3 to 4 degree decrease in mandibular plane angle observed in the average individual during childhood and adolescence.

It is less easy to divide the maxilla into a core of bone and a series of functional processes. The alveolar process is certainly a functional process in the classic sense, but there are no areas of muscle attachment analogous to those of the mandible. The parts of the bone surrounding the air passages serve the function of respiration, and the form–function relationships involved are poorly understood. If implants are placed above the maxillary alveolar process, however, one can observe a core of the maxilla that undergoes a small and variable degree of rotation, forward or backward (Figure 4-15).[8,11] This internal rotation is analogous to the intramatrix rotation of the mandible. Matrix

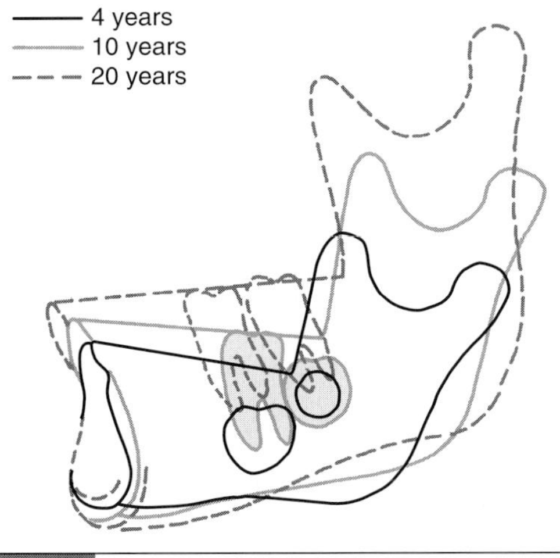

FIGURE 4-14 Superimposition on implants for an individual with a normal pattern of growth, showing surface changes in the mandible from ages 4 to 20 years. For this patient there was −19 degrees internal rotation but only −3 degrees change in the mandibular plane angle. Note how the dramatic remodeling (external rotation) compensates for and conceals the extent of the internal rotation. (From Bjork A, Skieller V. Eur J Orthod 5:1-46, 1983.)

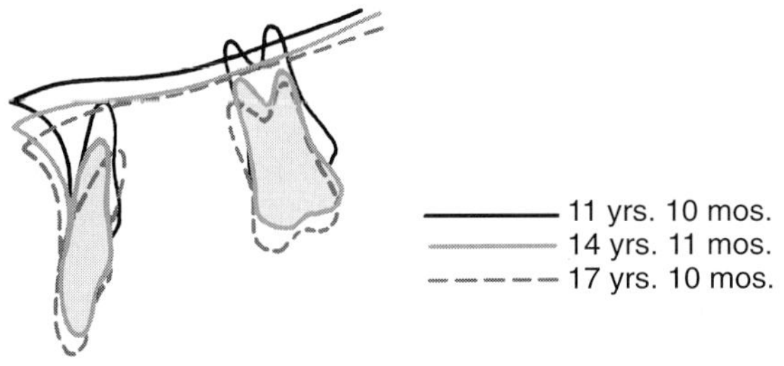

FIGURE 4-15 Superimposition on implants in the maxilla reveals that this patient experienced a small amount of backward internal rotation of the maxilla (i.e., down anteriorly). A small amount of forward rotation is the more usual pattern, but backward rotation occurs frequently. (From Bjork A, Skieller V. Am J Orthod 62:357, 1972.)

rotation, as defined for the mandible, is not possible for the maxilla.

At the same time that internal rotation of the maxilla is occurring, there also are varying degrees of resorption of bone on the nasal side and apposition of bone on the palatal side in the anterior and posterior parts of the palate. Similar variations in the amount of eruption of the incisors and molars occur. These changes amount, of course, to an external rotation. For most patients, the external rotation is opposite in direction and equal in magnitude to the internal rotation, so that the two rotations cancel and the net change in jaw orientation (as evaluated by the palatal plane) is zero (see Figure 3-27). Until the implant studies were done, rotation of the maxilla during normal growth had not been suspected.

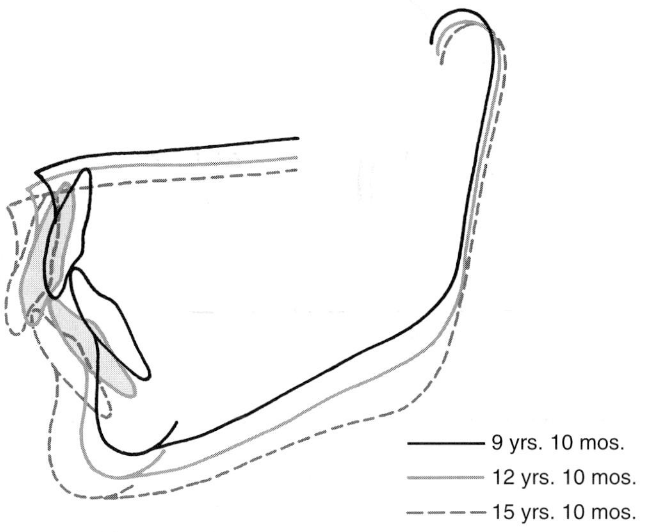

FIGURE 4-16 Cranial base superimposition shows the characteristic pattern of forward mandibular rotation in an individual developing in the "short face" pattern. The forward rotation flattens the mandibular plane and tends to increase overbite. (From Bjork A, Skieller V. Am J Orthod 62:344, 1972.)

Although both internal and external rotation occur in everybody, variations from the average pattern are common. Greater or lesser degrees of both internal and external rotation often occur, altering the extent to which external changes compensate for the internal rotation.[12] The result is moderate variation in jaw orientation, even in individuals with normal facial proportions. In addition, the rotational patterns of growth are quite different for individuals who have what are called the short face and long face types of vertical facial development.[13]

Individuals of the short face type, who are characterized by short anterior lower face height, have excessive forward rotation of the mandible during growth, resulting from both an increase in the normal internal rotation and a decrease in external compensation. The result is a nearly horizontal palatal plane and mandibular morphology of the "square jaw" type, with a low mandibular plane angle and a square gonial angle (Figure 4-16). A deep bite malocclusion and crowded incisors usually accompany this type of rotation (see following sections).

In long face individuals, who have excessive lower anterior face height, the palatal plane rotates down posteriorly, often creating a negative rather than the normal positive inclination to the true horizontal. The mandible shows an opposite, backward rotation, with an increase in the mandibular plane angle (Figure 4-17). The mandibular changes result primarily from a lack of the normal forward internal rotation or even a backward internal rotation. The internal rotation, in turn, is primarily matrix rotation (centered at the condyle), not intramatrix rotation. This type of rotation is associated with anterior open bite malocclusion and mandibular deficiency (because the chin rotates back as

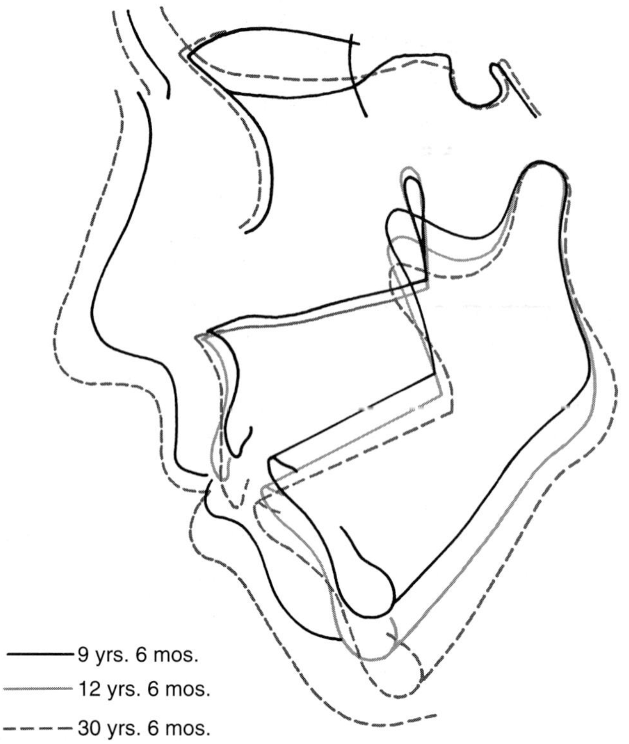

Figure 4-17 The pattern of jaw rotation in an individual with the "long face" pattern of growth (cranial base superimposition). As the mandible rotates backward, anterior face height increases, there is a tendency toward anterior open bite, and the incisors are thrust forward relative to the mandible. (From Bjork A, Skieller V. Eur J Orthod 5:29, 1983.)

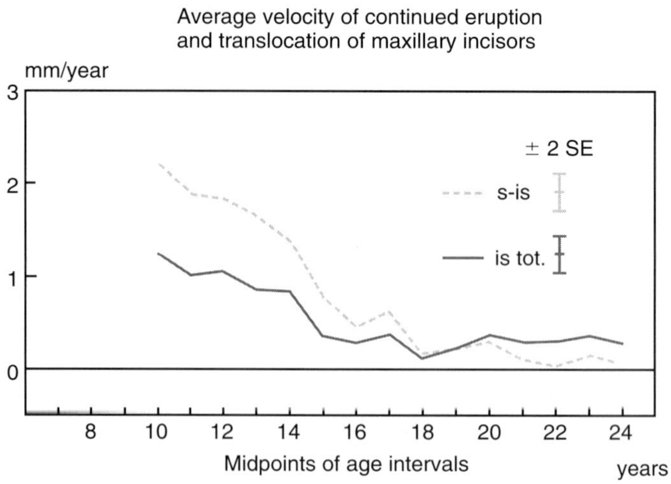

Figure 4-18 The average velocity of continued eruption (movement of the incisors relative to implants in the maxilla) and translocation (movement away from the cranial base) of maxillary incisors in Danish girls, from a mixed longitudinal sample. (Redrawn from Solow and Haluk. In: Davidovitch S, Norton L, eds. Biological Mechanisms of Tooth Movement and Craniofacial Adaptation. Boston, Mass: Harvard Society for Advancement of Orthodontics; 1996.)

well as down). As one would expect, changes in face height correlate better with changes in the mandibular plane angle (which reflects total rotation) than with changes in the corpus axis (which reflects internal rotation). This is another reflection of the fact that the total change is determined by the interaction between internal and external changes. Backward rotation of the mandible also occurs in patients with abnormalities or pathologic changes affecting the temporomandibular joints. In these individuals, growth at the condyle is restricted. The interesting result in three cases documented by Bjork and Skieller[13] was an intramatrix rotation centered in the body of the mandible, rather than the backward rotation at the condyle that dominated in individuals of the classic long face type. Jaw orientation changes in both the backward-rotating types, however, are similar, and the same types of malocclusions develop.

Interaction Between Jaw Rotation and Tooth Eruption

As we have discussed, growth of the mandible away from the maxilla creates a space into which the teeth erupt. The rotational pattern of jaw growth obviously influences the magnitude of tooth eruption. To a surprising extent, it can also influence the direction of eruption and the ultimate anteroposterior position of the incisor teeth.

The path of eruption of the maxillary teeth is downward and somewhat forward (see Figure 4-11). In normal growth, the maxilla usually rotates a few degrees forward but frequently rotates slightly backward. Forward rotation would tend to tip the incisors forward, increasing their prominence, while backward rotation directs the anterior teeth more posteriorly than would have been the case without the rotation, relatively uprighting them and decreasing their prominence. Movement of the teeth relative to the cranial base obviously could be produced by a combination of *translocation* as the tooth moved along with the jaw in which it was embedded, and true *eruption,* movement of the tooth within its jaw. As Figure 4-18 shows, translocation contributes about half the total maxillary tooth movement during adolescent growth.

The eruption path of mandibular teeth is upward and somewhat forward. The normal internal rotation of the mandible carries the jaw upward in front. This rotation alters the eruption path of the incisors, tending to direct them more posteriorly than would otherwise have been the case (Figure 4-19). Because the internal jaw rotation tends to upright the incisors, the molars migrate further mesially during growth than do the incisors, and this migration is reflected in the decrease in arch length that normally occurs (Figure 4-20). Since the forward internal rotation of the mandible is greater than that of the maxilla, it is not surprising that the normal decrease in mandibular arch length is somewhat greater than the decrease in maxillary arch length.

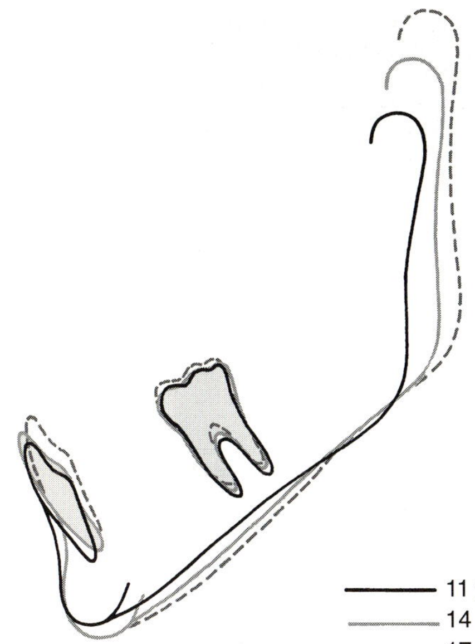

Figure 4-19 Superimposition on mandibular implants shows the lingual positioning of the mandibular incisors relative to the mandible that often accompanies forward rotation during growth. (From Bjork A, Skieller V. Am J Orthod 62:357, 1972.)

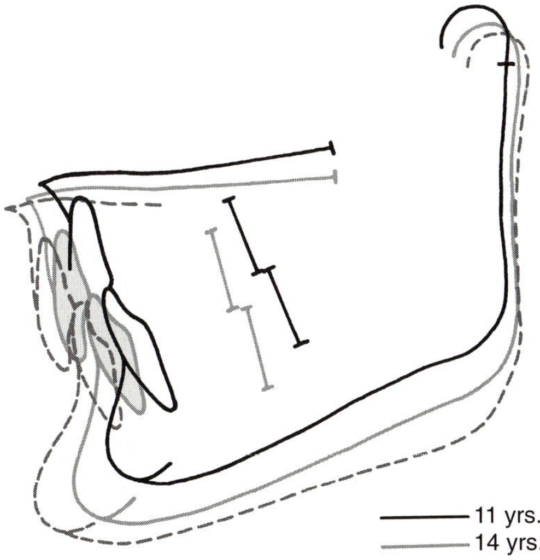

Figure 4-20 Cranial base superimposition for a patient with the short face pattern of growth. As the mandible rotates upward and forward, the vertical overlap of the teeth tends to increase, creating a deep bite malocclusion. In addition, even though both the upper and lower teeth do move forward relative to cranial base, lingual displacement of incisors relative to the maxilla and mandible increases the tendency toward crowding. (From Bjork A, Skieller V. Am J Orthod 62:355, 1972.)

Note that this explanation for the decrease in arch length that normally occurs in both jaws is different from the traditional interpretation that emphasizes forward migration of the molar teeth. The modern view places relatively greater importance on lingual movement of the incisors and relatively less importance on the forward movement of molars. In fact, the same implant studies that revealed the internal jaw rotation also confirmed that changes in anteroposterior position of the incisor teeth are a major influence on arch length changes.

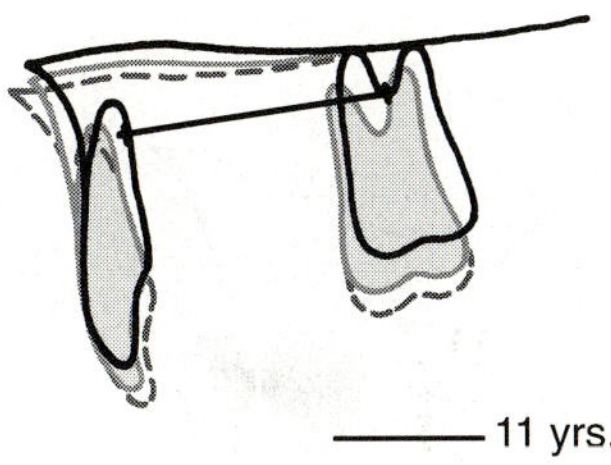

Figure 4-21 Superimposition on the maxilla reveals uprighting of the maxillary incisors in the short face growth pattern (same patient as Figure 4-20). This decreases arch length and contributes to progressive crowding. (From Bjork A, Skieller V. Am J Orthod 62:355, 1972.)

Given this relationship between jaw rotation and incisor position, it is not surprising that both the vertical and anteroposterior positions of the incisors are affected in short face and long face individuals. When excessive rotation occurs in the short face type of development, the incisors tend to be carried into an overlapping position even if they erupt very little; hence the tendency for deep bite malocclusion in short face individuals (Figure 4-21). The rotation also progressively uprights the incisors, displacing them lingually and causing a tendency toward crowding. In the long face growth pattern, on the other hand, an anterior open bite will develop as anterior face height increases unless the incisors erupt for an extreme distance. The rotation of the jaws also carries the incisors forward, creating dental protrusion.

The interaction between tooth eruption and jaw rotation explains a number of previously puzzling aspects of tooth positioning in patients who have vertical facial disproportions. This topic is discussed from an etiologic perspective in Chapter 5 and is reviewed from the point of view of treatment planning in Chapter 8.

Maturational and Aging Changes

Maturational changes affect both the soft and hard tissues of the face and jaws, with greater long-term changes in the soft tissues. There are important effects on the teeth, their supporting structures and the dental occlusion itself, as well as changes in jaw relationships as slow growth continues in adult life.

Changes in Facial Soft Tissues

An important concept is that changes in facial soft tissues not only continue with aging, they are much larger in

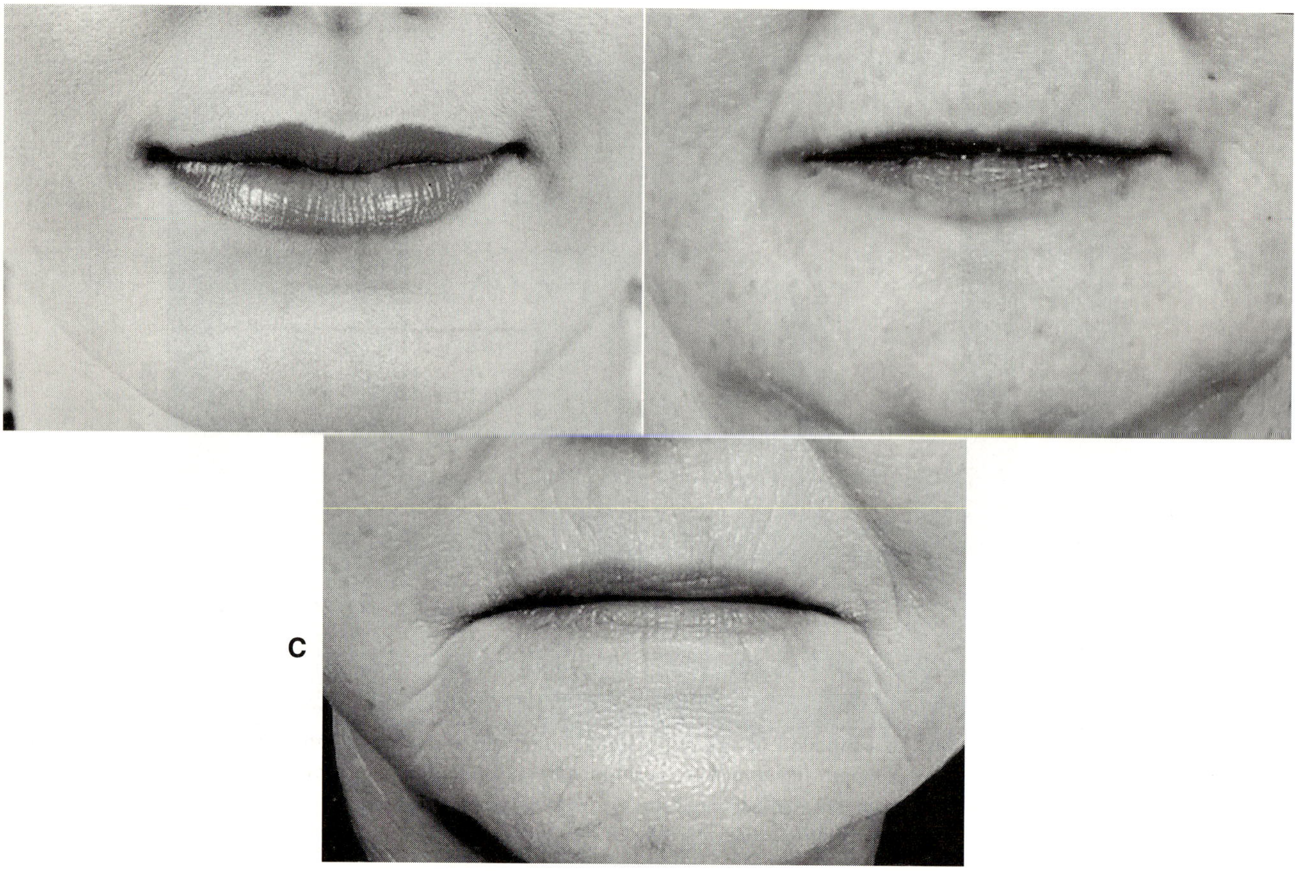

Figure 4-25 A decrease in the fullness of the lips is an obvious sign of aging. **A,** Age 20. **B,** Age 40. **C,** Age 70.

the accompanying eruption of the teeth, than from downward migration of the gingival attachment. As we have noted previously, vertical growth of the jaws and an increase in face height continue after transverse and anteroposterior growth have been completed. By the time the jaws all but stop growing vertically in the late teens, the gingival attachment is usually near the cementoenamel junction. In the absence of inflammation, mechanical abrasion, or pathologic changes, the gingival attachment should remain at about the same level almost indefinitely. In fact, however, most individuals experience some pathology of the gingiva or periodontium as they age, and so further recession of the gingiva is common.

At one time, it was thought that "passive eruption" occurred, defined as an actual gingival migration of the attachment without any eruption of the tooth. It now appears that as long as the gingival tissues are entirely healthy, this sort of downward migration of the soft tissue attachment does not occur. What was once thought to be apical migration of the gingiva during the teens is really active eruption, compensating for the vertical jaw growth still occurring at that time (Figure 4-27).

Both occlusal and interproximal wear, often to a severe degree, occurred in primitive people eating an extremely coarse diet. The elimination of most coarse particles from modern diets has also largely eliminated wear of this type. With few exceptions (tobacco chewing is one), wear facets on the teeth now indicate bruxism, not what the individual has been eating.

Changes in Alignment and Occlusion

Individuals in primitive societies who experienced wear of the teeth lost tooth substance interproximally as well as from the occlusal surfaces. The alveolar bone bends during heavy mastication, allowing the teeth to move relative to each other (see Chapter 9 for more details). On a coarse diet, this movement causes both interproximal and occlusal wear. The result in many primitive populations was a reduction in arch circumference of 10 mm or more after completion of the permanent dentition at adolescence.

When this type of interproximal wear occurs, spaces do not open up between the posterior teeth, although some spacing may develop anteriorly. Instead, the permanent molars migrate mesially, keeping the contacts reasonably tight even as the contact points are worn off and the mesiodistal width of each tooth decreases.

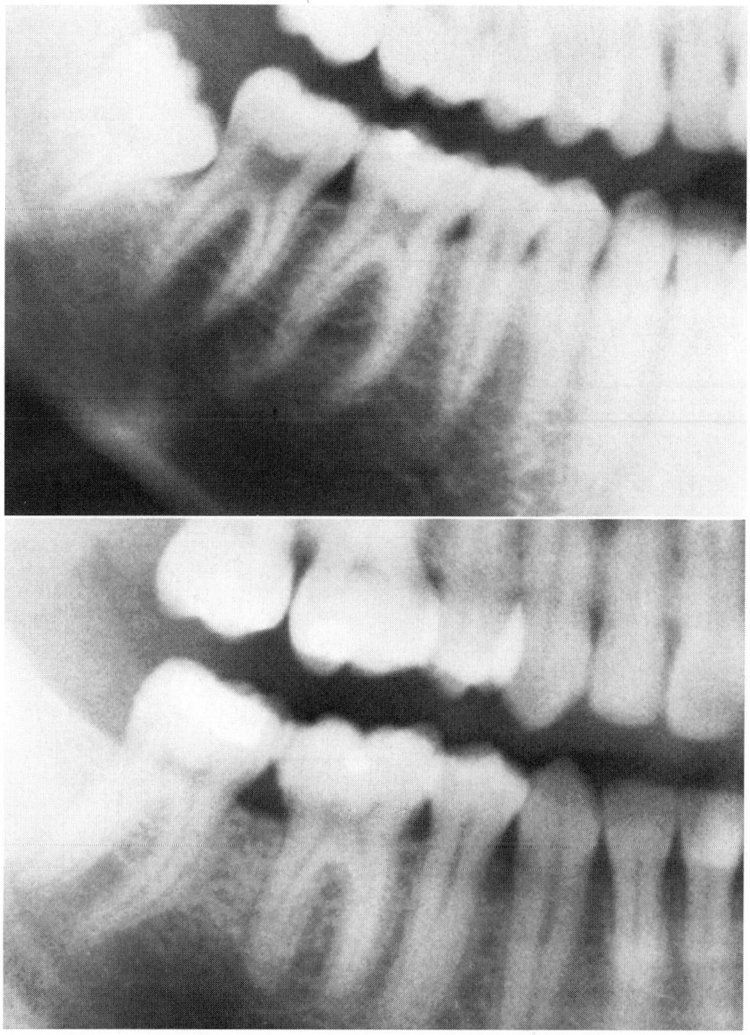

Figure 4-26 The size of the pulp chambers of permanent teeth decreases during adolescence then continues to fill in more slowly for the rest of adult life. **A,** Age 16. **B,** Age 26.

In modern populations, there is a strong tendency for crowding of the mandibular incisor teeth to develop in the late teens and early twenties, no matter how well aligned the teeth were initially. Mild crowding of the lower incisors tends to develop if the teeth were initially well aligned, or initially mild crowding becomes worse (Figure 4-28). These changes appear as early as age 17 to 18 in some individuals and as late as the mid-twenties in others. Three major theories to account for this crowding have been proposed:

1. Lack of "normal attrition" in the modern diet. As noted in Chapter 1, primitive populations tend to have a much smaller prevalence of malocclusion than do contemporary populations in developed countries. If a shortening of arch length and a mesial migration of the permanent molars is a natural phenomenon, it would seem reasonable that crowding would develop unless the amount of tooth structure was reduced during the final stages of growth. Raymond Begg, a pioneer Australian orthodontist, noted in his studies of the Australian aborigines[14] that malocclusion is uncommon but large amounts of interproximal and occlusal attrition occurred (Figure 4-29). He concluded that in modern populations the teeth became crowded when attrition did not occur with soft diets, and advocated widespread extraction of premolar teeth to provide the equivalent of the attrition he saw in aborigines. More recent observations have shown that when Australian aborigines change to a modern diet, as happened in most of this group by the late 20th century, occlusal and interproximal wear all but disappears. Late crowding rarely develops,[15] although periodontal disease does become a major problem. It has been observed in other population groups that late crowding may develop even after premolars are extracted and arch length is reduced by modern orthodontic treatment. Thus the Begg theory, though superficially attractive, does not explain late crowding.

2. Pressure from third molars. Late crowding develops at about the time the third molars should erupt. In most individuals, these teeth are hopelessly impacted because the jaw

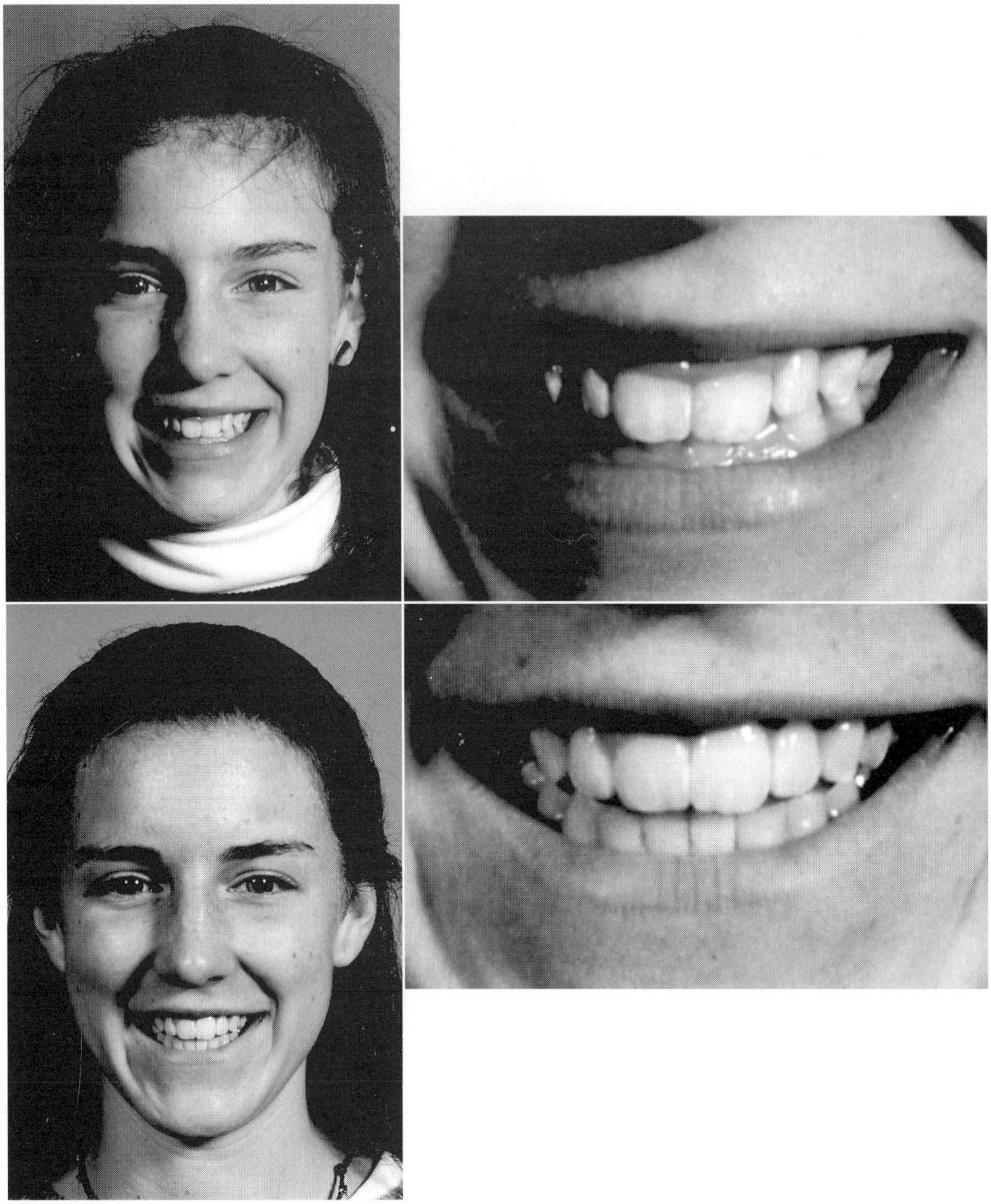

Figure 4-27 The increasing crown height of permanent teeth during adolescence was once thought to result from a downward migration of the gingival attachment but now is recognized to occur mostly from tooth eruption in response to vertical growth. **A,** Age 10. **B,** Age 16.

length did not increase enough to accommodate them via backward remodeling of the ramus (Figure 4-30). It has seemed entirely logical to dentists and patients that pressure from third molars with no room to erupt is the cause of late incisor crowding. It is difficult to detect such a force, however, even with modern instrumentation that should have found it if it exists.[16] In fact, late crowding of lower incisors can and often does develop in individuals whose lower third molars are congenitally missing. There is some evidence that incisor crowding may be lessened by early removal of second molars, which presumably would relieve pressure from third molars, but pressure from third molars clearly is not the total explanation either.[17]

3. Late mandibular growth. As a result of the cephalocaudal gradient of growth discussed in Chapter 2, the mandible can and does undergo more growth in the late

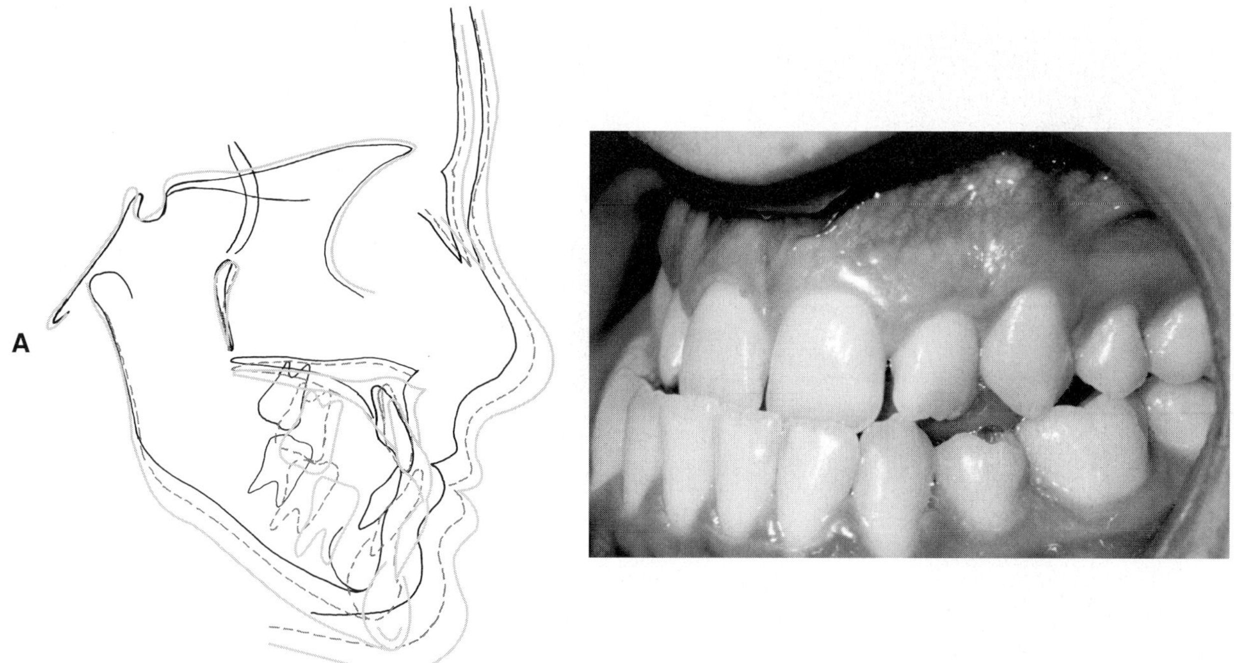

FIGURE 4-28 In this patient with a prolonged pattern of excessive mandibular growth **(A)**, the lower incisors were increasingly tipped lingually as the mandible grew forward and were noticeably retroclined **(B)** by the end of adolescent growth. This is a more obvious demonstration of what often happens under normal circumstances, when a small amount of late mandibular growth occurs in the late teens after maxillary growth stops. Late mandibular growth is a major cause of the mandibular incisor crowding that frequently develops at that time.

teens than the maxilla. Is it possible that late mandibular growth somehow causes late mandibular incisor crowding? If so, how? Bjork's implant studies have provided an understanding of why late crowding occurs and how it indeed relates to the growth pattern of the jaw.

The position of the dentition relative to the maxilla and mandible is influenced by the pattern of growth of the jaws, a concept explored in some detail in previous sections. When the mandible grows forward relative to the maxilla, as it usually does in the late teens as well as earlier, the mandibular incisor teeth tend to be displaced lingually (see Figure 4-19), particularly if any excessive rotation is also present.

In patients with a tight anterior occlusion before late mandibular growth occurs, the contact relationship of the lower incisors with the upper incisors must change if the mandible grows forward. In that circumstance, one of three events must occur: (1) the mandible is displaced distally, accompanied by a distortion of temporomandibular joint function and displacement of the articular disc; (2) the upper incisors flare forward, opening space between these teeth; or (3) the lower incisors displace distally and become crowded.

All three of these phenomena have been reported. The second response, flaring and spacing of the maxillary incisors, is the least common. Posterior displacement of a "trapped mandible" can happen and may occasionally be related to myofascial pain and dysfunction, but despite the claims of some occlusion theorists, this too seems to be quite rare. Distal displacement of the lower incisors, with concomitant crowding and a decrease in the lower intercanine distance, is the most likely response.

It is not even necessary for the incisors to be in occlusal contact for late crowding to develop. This also occurs commonly in individuals who have an anterior open bite and backward, not forward, rotation of the mandible (see Figure 4-20). In this situation, the rotation of the mandible carries the dentition forward, thrusting the incisors against the lip. This creates light but lasting pressure by the lip, which tends to reposition the protruding incisors somewhat lingually, reducing arch length and causing crowding.

The current concept is that late incisor crowding almost always develops as the mandibular incisors, and perhaps the entire mandibular dentition, move distally relative to the body of the mandible late in mandibular growth. This also sheds some light on the possible role of the third molars in determining whether crowding will occur, and how severe it will be. If space were available at the distal end of the mandibular arch, it might be possible for all the mandibular teeth to shift slightly distally, allowing the lower incisors to upright without becoming crowded. On the other hand, impacted third molars at the distal end of the lower arch would prevent the posterior teeth from shifting distally, and

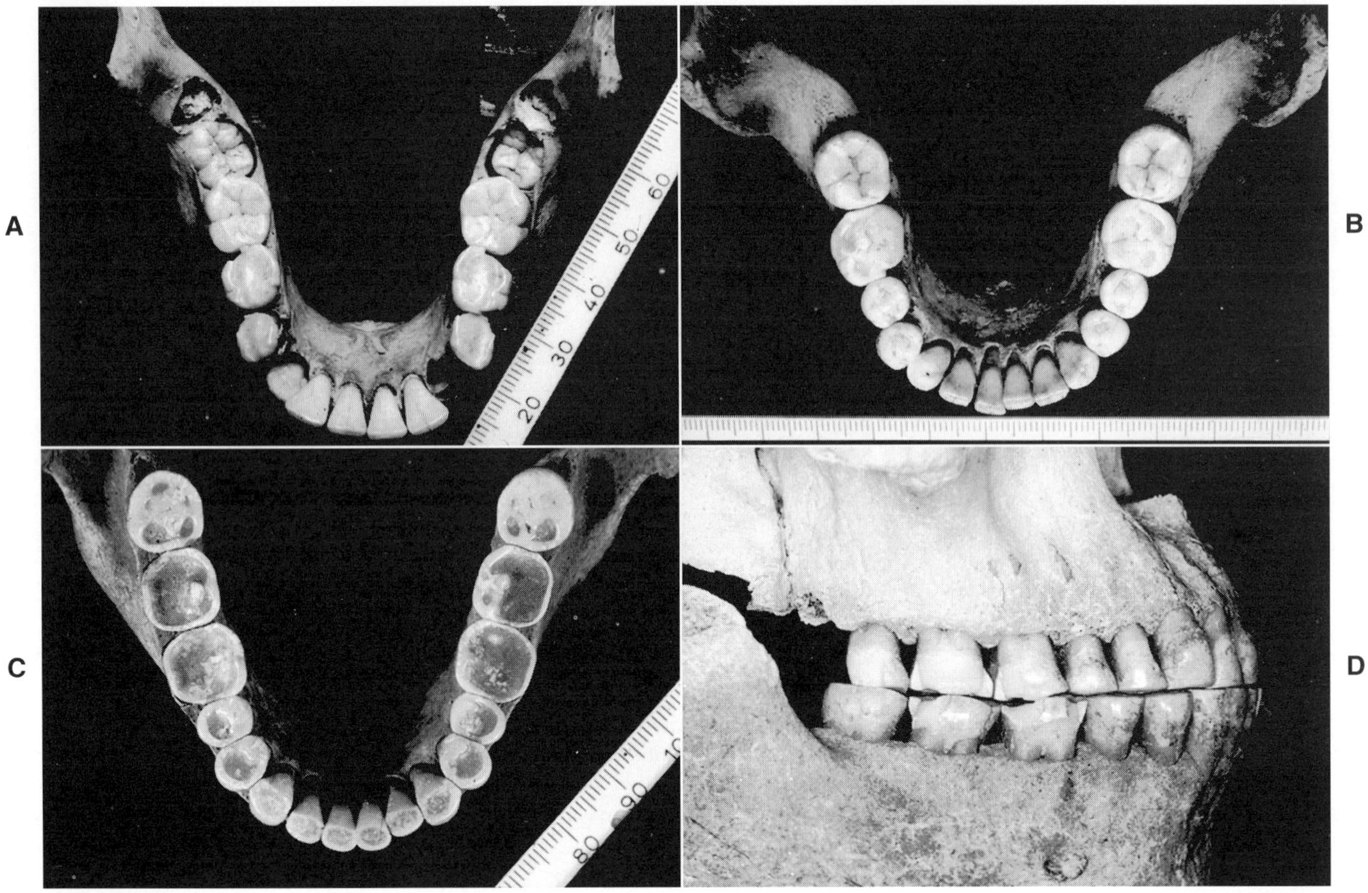

FIGURE 4-29 Australian aboriginal mandibles for **(A)** a child approximately at dental age 8, **(B)** an adolescent at approximately dental age 14, and **(C, D)** an adult of indeterminate age. Note the increasing attrition of the teeth in the younger specimens and the severe attrition of the adult's teeth, with interproximal as well as occlusal wear. Arch length in this population shortened by 1 cm or more after adolescence because of the extensive interproximal wear. (Specimens from the Begg Collection, University of Adelaide; Courtesy Prof. W. Sampson.)

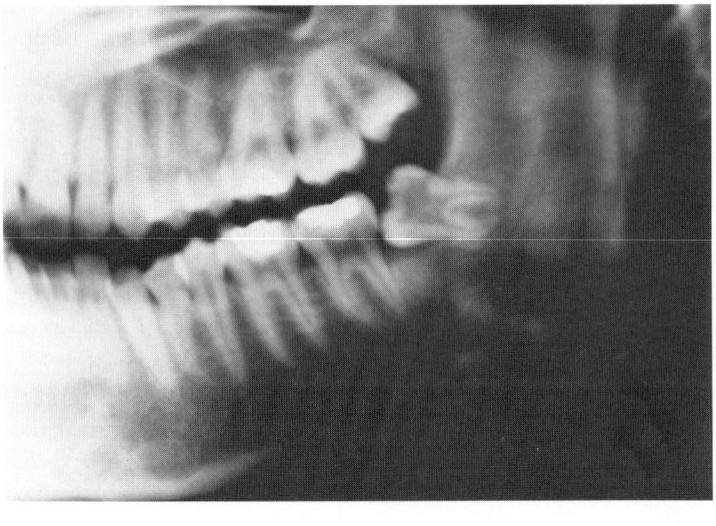

FIGURE 4-30 It seems reasonable that a horizontally impacted third molar would provide pressure against the dental arch, but it is highly unlikely that there is enough pressure from this source to cause the crowding of mandibular incisors that often develops in the late teens.

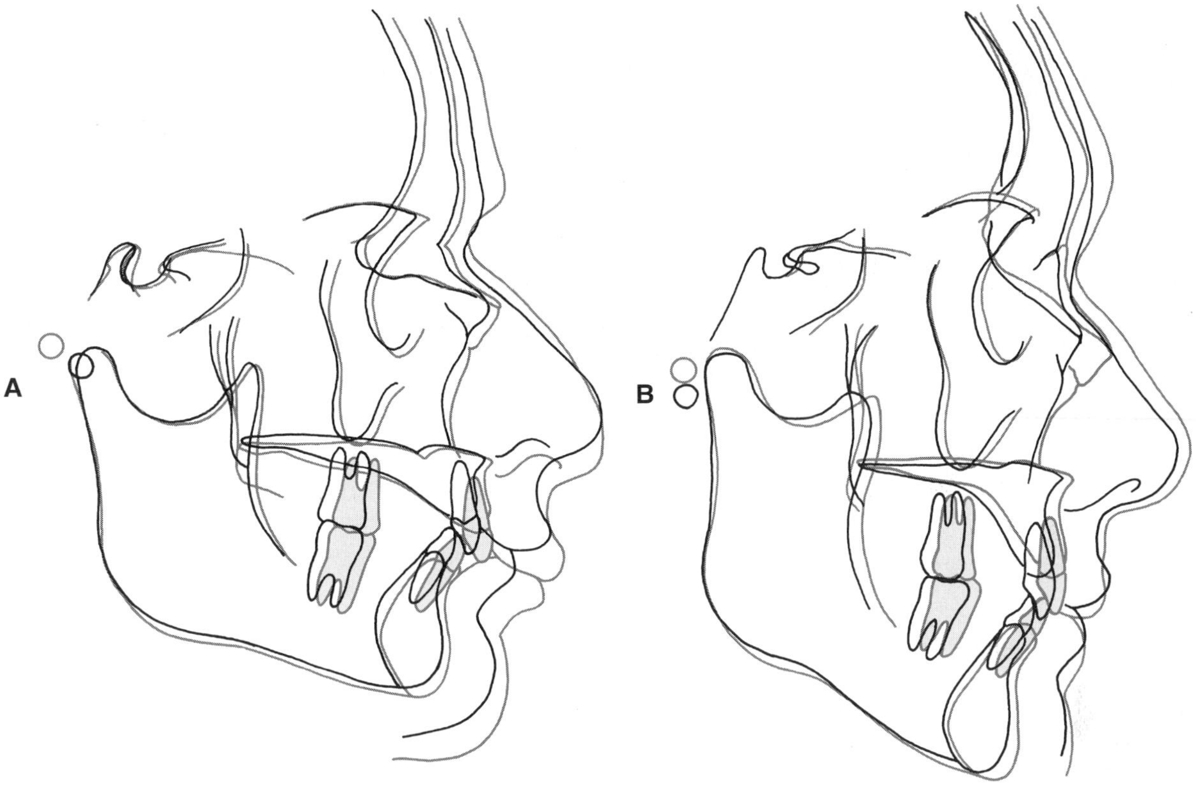

FIGURE 4-31 Growth changes in adults. **A,** Changes in a male from age 37 (*black*) to age 77 (*red*). Note that both the maxilla and mandible grew forward, and the nose grew considerably. **B,** Growth changes in a woman between age 34 (*black*) and 83 (*red*). Note that both jaws grew forward and somewhat downward, and that the nasal structures enlarged. (From Behrents RG. A Treatise on the Continuum of Growth in the Aging Craniofacial Skeleton. Ann Arbor, Mich: University of Michigan Center for Human Growth and Development; 1984.)

if differential mandibular growth occurred, their presence might guarantee that crowding would develop. In this case, the lower third molars could be the "last straw" in a chain of events that led to late incisor crowding. As noted previously, however, late incisor crowding occurs in individuals with no third molars at all, and so the presence of these teeth is not the critical variable. The extent of late mandibular growth is. The more your mandible grows after other growth has essentially stopped, the greater the chance your lower incisors will become crowded.

Facial Growth in Adults

Until recently, although some anthropologists in the 1930s had reported small amounts of growth continuing into middle age, it was generally assumed that growth of the facial skeleton ceased in the late teens or early twenties. In the early 1980s, Behrents[18] succeeded in recalling over 100 individuals who had participated in the Bolton growth study in Cleveland in the 1930s and late 1940s, more than 40 years previously. Most had never had orthodontic treatment; a few did. While they were participants in the study, the growth of these individuals had been carefully evaluated and recorded, by both measurements and serial cephalometric films. The magnification in the radiographs was known precisely, and it was possible to obtain new radiographs more than 4 decades later with known magnification, so that precise measurements of facial dimensions could be made.

The results were surprising but unequivocal: facial growth had continued during adult life (Figure 4-31). There was an increase in essentially all of the facial dimensions, but both size and shape of the craniofacial complex altered with time. Vertical changes in adult life were more prominent than anteroposterior changes, whereas width changes were least evident, and so the alterations observed in the adult facial skeleton seem to be a continuation of the pattern seen during maturation. In a point of particular interest, an apparent deceleration of growth in females in the late teens was followed by a resumption of growth during the twenties. It appears that a woman's first pregnancy often produces some growth of her jaws. Although the magnitude of the adult growth changes, assessed on a millimeters per year basis, was quite small, the cumulative effect over decades was surprisingly large (Figure 4-32).

The data also revealed that rotation of both jaws continued into adult life, in concert with the vertical changes

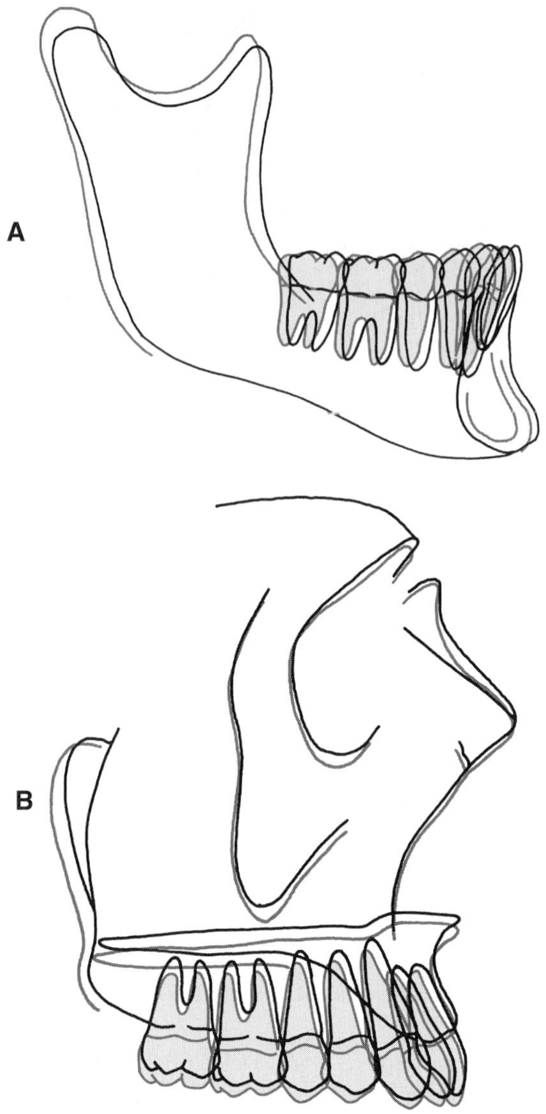

Figure 4-32 Growth changes in adults. **A,** Mean dimensional changes in the mandible for males in adult life. It is apparent that the pattern of juvenile and adolescent growth continues at a slower but ultimately significant rate. **B,** The mean positional changes in the maxilla during adult life, for both sexes combined. Note that the maxilla moves forward and slightly downward, continuing the previous pattern of growth. (From Behrents RG. A Treatise on the Continuum of Growth in the Aging Craniofacial Skeleton. Ann Arbor, Mich: University of Michigan Center for Human Growth and Development; 1984.)

and eruption of teeth. Because implants were not used in these patients, it was not possible to precisely differentiate internal from external rotation, but it seems likely that both internal rotation and surface changes did continue. In general, males showed a net rotation of the jaws in a forward direction, slightly decreasing the mandibular plane angle, whereas females had a tendency toward backward rotation, with an increase in the mandibular plane angle. In both groups, compensatory changes were noted in the dentition, so that occlusal relationships largely were maintained.

Both a history of orthodontic treatment and loss of multiple teeth had an impact on facial morphology in these adults and on the pattern of change. In the smaller group of patients who had orthodontic treatment many years previously, Behrents noted that the pattern of growth associated with the original malocclusion continued to express itself even in adult life. This finding is consistent with previous observations of growth in the late teens but also indicates how a gradual worsening of occlusal relationships could occur in some patients long after the completion of orthodontic treatment.

As expected, changes in the facial soft tissue profile were greater than changes in the facial skeleton. The soft tissue changes involved an elongation of the nose (which often became significantly longer during adult life), flattening of the lips, and an augmentation of the chin. A knowledge of soft tissue changes during aging is important in planning modern orthodontic treatment, and this is reviewed in detail in Chapter 6.

In the light of Behrents' findings, it seems clear that the view of facial growth as a process that ends in the late teens or early twenties must be revised. It is correct, however, to view the growth process as one that declines to a basal level after the attainment of sexual maturity, that continues to show a cephalocaudal gradient (i.e., more mandibular than maxillary changes in adult life), and that affects the three planes of space differently. Growth in width is not only the first to drop to adult levels, usually reaching essential completion by the onset of puberty, but the basal or adult level observed thereafter is quite low.[19] Anteroposterior growth continues at a noticeable rate for a longer period, declining to basal levels only after puberty, with small but noticeable changes continuing throughout adult life. Vertical growth, which had previously been observed to continue well after puberty in both males and females, continues at a modest level far into adult life. The existing data are not adequate to answer the question of whether growth rates are greater in early than late adult life, but even if they are, skeletal growth comes much closer to being a process that continues throughout life than most observers had previously suspected.

References

1. Marshall WA, Tanner JM. Puberty. In: Falkner F, Tanner JM, eds. Human Growth, vol 2, ed 2. New York: Plenum Publishing; 1986.
2. Anderson DL, Thompson GW, Popovich F. Interrelationship of dental maturity, skeletal maturity, height and weight from age 4 to 14 years. Growth 39:453-462, 1975.
3. Sisk CL, Foster DL. The neural basis of puberty and adolescence. Nature Neurosci 7:1040-1047, 2004.
4. Enlow DH, Hans MG. Essentials of Facial Growth. Philadelphia: WB Saunders; 1996.
5. Agronin KJ, Kokich VG. Displacement of the glenoid fossa: A cephalometric evaluation of growth during treatment. Am J Orthod Dentofacial Orthop 91:42-48, 1987.

6. Bishara SE, Jakobsen JR, Treder J, Nowak A. Arch width changes from 6 weeks to 45 years of age. Am J Orthod Dentofac Orthop 111:401-409, 1997.
7. Solow B, Iseri H. Maxillary growth revisited: an update based on recent implant studies. In: Davidovitch Z, Norton LA, eds. Biological Mechanisms of Tooth Movement and Craniofacial Adaptation. Boston, Mass: Harvard Society for Advancement of Orthodontics; 1996.
8. Bjork A. The use of metallic implants in the study of facial growth in children: Method and application. Am J Phys Anthropol 29:243-254, 1968.
9. Solow B, Houston WJ. Mandibular rotations: Concept and terminology. Eur J Orthod 10:177-179, 1988.
10. Bjork A, Skieller V. Normal and abnormal growth of the mandible: A synthesis of longitudinal cephalometric implant studies over a period of 25 years. Eur J Orthod 5:1-46, 1983.
11. Bjork A, Skieller V. Postnatal growth and development of the maxillary complex. In: McNamara JA, ed. Factors Affecting Growth of the Midface. Ann Arbor, Mich: University of Michigan Center for Human Growth and Development; 1976.
12. Houston WJ. Mandibular growth rotations—their mechanisms and importance. Eur J Orthod 10:369-373, 1988.
13. Bjork A, Skieller V. Contrasting mandibular growth and facial development in long face syndrome, juvenile rheumatoid arthritis and mandibulofacial dysostosis. J Craniofac Genet Dev Biol 1(suppl):127-138, 1985.
14. Begg PR. Stone age man's dentition. Am J Orthod 40:298-312, 373-383, 462-475, 517-531, 1954.
15. Corruccini RS. Australian aboriginal tooth succession, interproximal attrition and Begg's theory. Am J Orthod Dentofacial Orthop 97:349-357, 1990.
16. Southard TE, Southard KA, Weeda LW. Mesial force from unerupted third molars. Am J Orthod Dentofacial Orthop 99:220-225, 1991.
17. Richardson ME. The etiology of late lower arch crowding alternative to mesially directed forces: A review. Am J Orthod Dentofac Orthop 105:592-597, 1994.
18. Behrents RG. A Treatise on the Continuum of Growth in the Aging Craniofacial Skeleton. Ann Arbor, Mich: University of Michigan Center for Human Growth and Development; 1984.
19. Harris EF. A longitudinal study of arch size and form in untreated adults. Am J Orthod Dentofac Orthop 111:419-427, 1997.

CHAPTER

5

The Etiology of Orthodontic Problems

CHAPTER OUTLINE

Malocclusion is a developmental condition. In most instances, malocclusion and dentofacial deformity are caused, not by some pathologic process, but by moderate distortions of normal development. Occasionally a single specific cause is apparent, as for example, mandibular deficiency secondary to a childhood fracture of the jaw or the characteristic malocclusion that accompanies some genetic syndromes. More often these problems result from a complex interaction among multiple factors that influence growth and development, and it is impossible to describe a specific etiologic factor (Figure 5-1).

Although it is difficult to know the precise cause of most malocclusions, we do know in general what the possibilities are, and these must be considered when treatment is considered. In this chapter, we examine etiologic factors for malocclusion under three major headings: specific causes, hereditary influences, and environmental influences. The chapter concludes with a perspective on the interaction of hereditary and environmental influences in the development of the major types of malocclusion.

SPECIFIC CAUSES OF MALOCCLUSION

Disturbances in Embryologic Development

Defects in embryologic development usually result in death of the embryo. As many as 20% of early pregnancies terminate because of lethal embryologic defects, often so early that the mother is not even aware of conception. Only a relatively small number of recognizable conditions that produce orthodontic problems are compatible with long-term survival. The more common of these conditions and their embryologic origins are discussed briefly and illustrated in

Chapter 3. Further details are provided in current texts on facial syndromes[1] and dentofacial deformity.[2]

A variety of causes exist for embryologic defects, ranging from genetic disturbances to specific environmental insults. Chemical and other agents capable of producing embryologic defects if given at the critical time are called *teratogens.* Most drugs do not interfere with normal development or, at high doses, kill the embryo without producing defects, and therefore are not teratogenic. Teratogens typically cause specific defects if present at low levels but if given in higher doses, do have lethal effects. Teratogens known to produce orthodontic problems are listed in Table 5-1.

Problems that can be traced to embryologic defects, though devastating to the affected individual, fortunately are relatively rare. The best estimate is that fewer than 1% of children who need orthodontics had a disturbance in embryologic development as a major contributing cause.

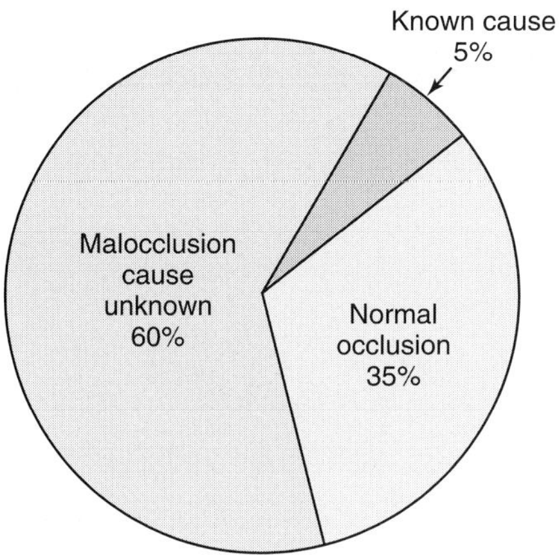

FIGURE 5-1 From a broad perspective, only about one third of the U.S. population has normal occlusion, while two thirds have some degree of malocclusion. In the malocclusion group, a small minority have problems attributable in a specific known cause; the remainder are the result of a complex and poorly-understood combination of inherited and environmental influences.

Skeletal Growth Disturbances

Fetal Molding and Birth Injuries

Injuries apparent at birth fall into two major categories: (1) intrauterine molding and (2) trauma to the mandible during the birth process, particularly from the use of forceps in delivery.

Intrauterine Molding. Pressure against the developing face prenatally can lead to distortion of rapidly growing areas. Strictly speaking, this is not a birth injury, but because the effects are noted at birth, it is considered in that category. On rare occasions an arm is pressed across the face in utero, resulting in severe maxillary deficiency at birth (Figure 5-2). Occasionally a fetus' head is flexed tightly against the chest in utero, preventing the mandible from growing forward normally. This is related to a decreased volume of amniotic fluid, which can occur for any of several reasons. The result is an extremely small mandible at birth, usually accompanied by a cleft palate because the restriction on displacement of the mandible forces the tongue upward and prevents normal closure of the palatal shelves.

This extreme mandibular deficiency at birth is termed the Pierre Robin anomalad or sequence. It is not a syndrome that

TABLE 5-1

Teratogens Affecting Dentofacial Development

Teratogens	Effect
Aminopterin	Anencephaly
Aspirin	Cleft lip and palate
Cigarette smoke (hypoxia)	Cleft lip and palate
Cytomegalovirus	Microcephaly, hydrocephaly, microphthalmia
Dilantin	Cleft lip and palate
Ethyl alcohol	Central mid-face deficiency
6-Mercaptopurine	Cleft palate
13-cis Retinoic acid (Accutane)	Retinoic acid syndrome: malformations virtually same as hemifacial microsomia, Treacher Collins syndrome
Rubella virus	Microphthalmia, cataracts, deafness
Thalidomide	Malformations similar to hemifacial microsomia, Treacher Collins syndrome
Toxoplasma	Microcephaly, hydrocephaly, microphthalmia
X-radiation	Microcephaly
Valium	Cleft lip and palate
Vitamin D excess	Premature suture closure

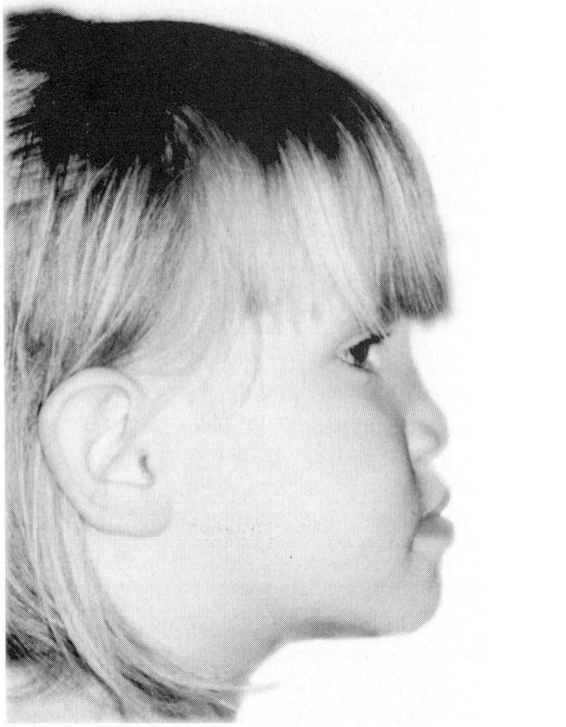

FIGURE 5-2 Midface deficiency in a 3-year-old, still apparent though much improved from the severe deficiency that was present at birth because of intrauterine molding. Prior to birth, one arm was pressed across the face. (From Proffit WR, White RP, Sarver DM. Contemporary Treatment of Dentofacial Deformity. St. Louis: Mosby; 2003.)

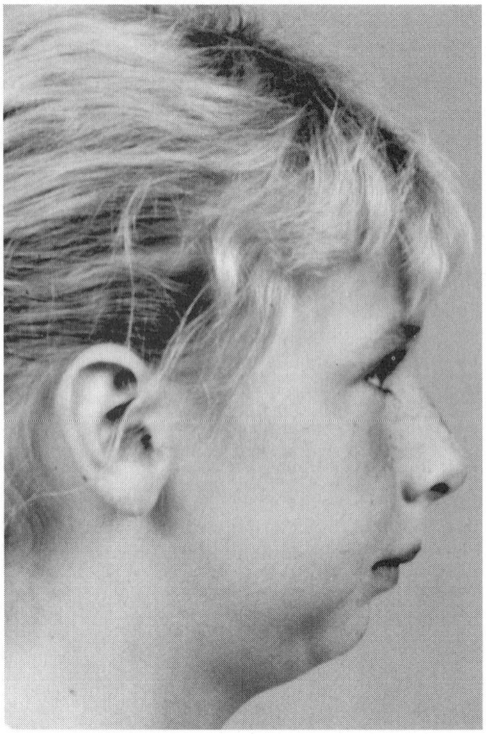

FIGURE 5-3 This girl was diagnosed at birth as having the Pierre Robin anomalad, consisting of a very small mandible, airway obstruction and cleft palate. Some children with this condition have enough postnatal mandibular growth to largely correct the jaw deficiency, but the majority do not. At age 9, her mandibular deficiency persists but the initial airway problems do not. (From Proffit WR, White RP, Sarver DM. Contemporary Treatment of Dentofacial Deformity. St. Louis: Mosby; 2003.)

has a defined cause; instead, multiple causes can lead to the same sequence of events that produce the deformity. The reduced volume of the oral cavity can lead to respiratory difficulty at birth, and it may be necessary to perform a tracheostomy so the infant can breathe.[3] Early mandibular advancement via distraction osteogenesis has been used recently in these severely affected infants to provide more space for an airway so that the tracheostomy can be closed.[4]

Because the pressure against the face that caused the growth problem would not be present after birth, there is the possibility of normal growth thereafter and perhaps eventually a complete recovery. Some children with Pierre Robin sequence at birth do have favorable mandibular growth thereafter. Others never make up the deficit (Figure 5-3) and surgical intervention is needed. It has been estimated that about one-third of the Pierre Robin patients have a defect in cartilage formation and can be said to have Stickler syndrome. Not surprisingly, this group have limited growth potential. Catch-up growth is most likely when the original problem was mechanical growth restriction that no longer existed after birth.

Birth Trauma to the Mandible. Many deformity patterns now known to result from other causes once were blamed on injuries during birth. Many parents, despite explanations from their doctors, will refer to their child's facial deformity as being caused by a birth injury even if a congenital syndrome pattern is evident. No matter what the parents say later, Treacher Collins syndrome or Crouzon's syndrome (see Chapter 3) obviously did not arise because of birth trauma.

In some difficult births, however, the use of forceps to the head to assist in delivery might damage either or both the temporomandibular joints. At least in theory, heavy pressure in the area of the temporomandibular joints could cause internal hemorrhage, loss of tissue, and a subsequent underdevelopment of the mandible. At one time this was a common explanation for mandibular deficiency. If the cartilage of the mandibular condyle were an important growth center, of course, the risk from damage to a presumably critical area would seem much greater. In light of the contemporary understanding that the condylar cartilage is not critical for proper growth of the mandible, it is not as easy to blame underdevelopment of the mandible on birth injuries.

It is interesting to note that although the use of forceps in deliveries has decreased considerably over the last 50 years, the prevalence of Class II malocclusion due to mandibular deficiency has not decreased. In short, injury to the mandible during a traumatic delivery appears to be a rare and unusual cause of facial deformity. Children with deformities involving the mandible are much more likely to have a congenital syndrome.

Childhood Fractures of the Jaw

The falls and impacts of childhood can fracture jaws just like other parts of the body. The condylar neck of the mandible is particularly vulnerable, and fractures of this area in childhood are relatively common. Fortunately, the condylar process tends to regenerate well after early fractures. The best human data suggest that about 75% of children with early fractures of the mandibular condylar process have normal mandibular growth, and therefore do not develop malocclusions that they would not have had in the absence of such trauma (see Chapter 2). Interestingly, the prognosis is better the earlier the condylar fracture occurs, perhaps because the growth potential is greater early in life. From the number of children with later growth problems whose original fracture was not diagnosed, it appears that many early fractures of the condylar process go completely unnoticed. It seems to be relatively common for a child to crash the bicycle, chip a tooth and fracture a condyle, cry a bit, and then continue to develop normally, complete with total regeneration of the condyle.

When a problem does arise following condylar fracture, it usually is asymmetric growth, with the previously injured side lagging behind (Figure 5-4). A survey of patients seen in the Dentofacial Clinic at the University of North Carolina indicates that only about 5% of patients referred for evaluation of severe mandibular deficiency have clinical and/or historical evidence of an early fracture of the jaw.[5] This suggests that childhood jaw fractures, though potentially a cause of severe orthodontic problems, do not make a large contribution to the total pool of patients with malocclusion.

It is important to understand the mechanism by which trauma can produce a distortion in subsequent growth. The maxilla normally grows downward and forward because of a combination of push from behind by the lengthening cranial base (which is largely complete at an early age) and pull from in front by anteriorly positioned tissue elements (probably including but not limited to the cartilaginous nasal septum). The mandible seems to be almost entirely pulled forward by the soft tissue matrix in which it is embedded. After an injury, growth problems arise when there is enough scarring in the area to restrict the normal growth movements, so that the maxilla or, more frequently, the mandible cannot be pulled forward along with the rest of the growing face. If there is more scarring and restriction on one side, subsequent growth will be asymmetric.

This concept is highly relevant to the management of condylar fractures in children. It suggests, and clinical experience confirms, that there would be little if any advantage from surgical open reduction of a condylar fracture in a child. The additional scarring produced by surgery could make things worse. The best therapy therefore is conservative management at the time of injury and early mobilization of the jaw to minimize any restriction on movement.

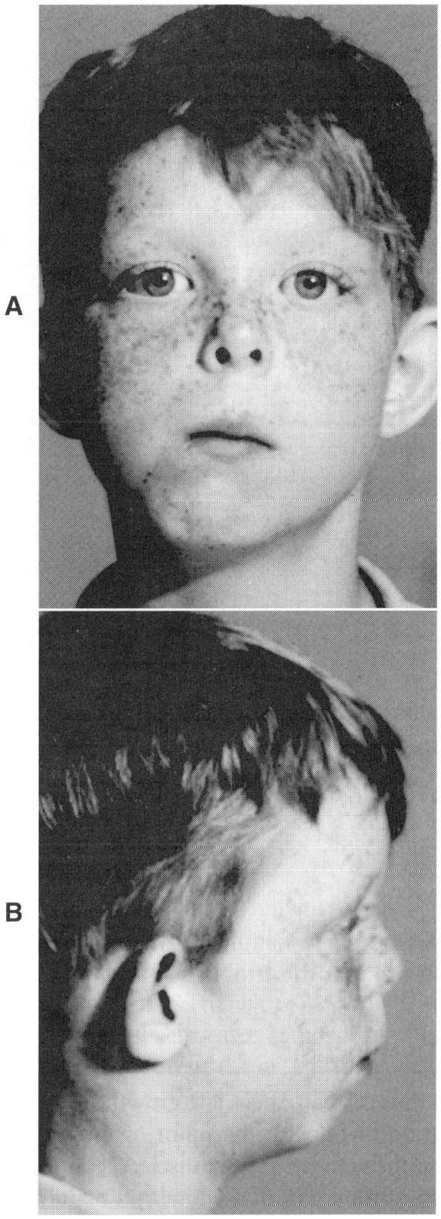

FIGURE 5-4 Mandibular asymmetry in an 8-year-old boy, due to deficient growth on the affected side after fracture of the left condylar process, probably at age 2. For this patient, growth was normal despite the complete loss of the mandibular condyle until age 6, when an attachment of the condylar process to the underside of the zygomatic arch on the injured side began to restrict growth; then facial asymmetry developed rapidly. (From Proffit WR, White RP, Sarver DM. Contemporary Treatment of Dentofacial Deformity. St. Louis: Mosby; 2003.)

An old condylar fracture is the most likely cause of asymmetric mandibular deficiency in a child, but other destructive processes that involve the temporomandibular joint such as rheumatoid arthritis (Figure 5-5), or a congenital

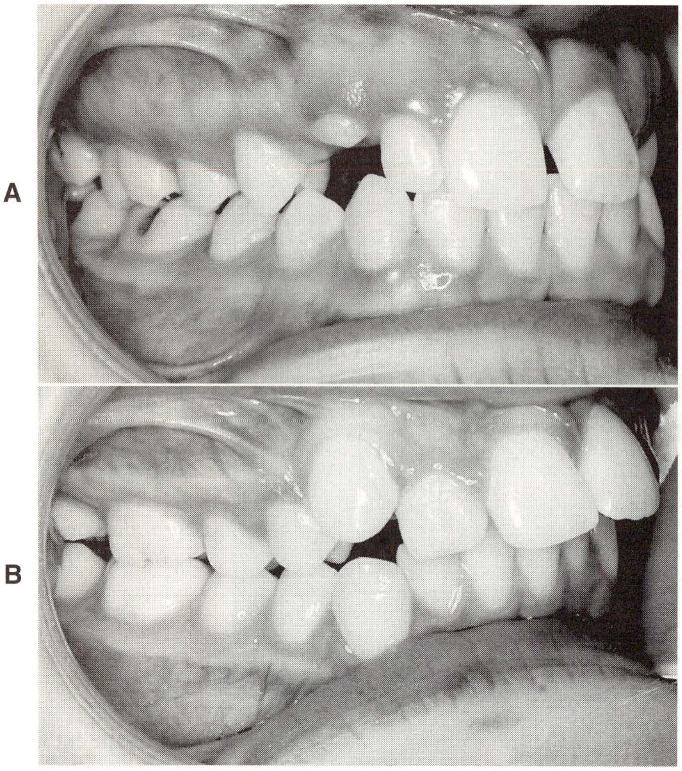

Figure 5-12 Disproportionately small **(A)** or large **(B)** maxillary lateral incisors are relatively common. This creates a tooth-size discrepancy that makes normal alignment and occlusion almost impossible. It is easier to build up small laterals than reduce the size of large ones, because dentin is likely to be exposed interproximally after more than 1-2 mm in width reduction.

Malformed and Supernumerary Teeth

Abnormalities in tooth size and shape result from disturbances during the morphodifferentiation stage of development, perhaps with some carryover from the histodifferentiation stage. The most common abnormality is a variation in size, particularly of maxillary lateral incisors (Figure 5-12) and second premolars. About 5% of the total population have a significant "tooth size discrepancy" because of disproportionate sizes of the upper and lower teeth. Unless the teeth are matched for size, normal occlusion is impossible. As might be expected, the most variable teeth, the maxillary lateral incisors, are the major culprits. The diagnosis of tooth size discrepancy, discussed in Chapter 6, is based on comparison of the widths of teeth to published tables of expected tooth sizes.

Occasionally, tooth buds may fuse or geminate (partially split) during their development. Fusion results in teeth with separate pulp chambers joined at the dentin, whereas gemination results in teeth with a common pulp chamber. The differentiation between gemination and fusion can be difficult and is usually confirmed by counting the number of teeth in an area. If the other central and both lateral incisors are present, a bifurcated central incisor is the result of either gemination or, less probably, fusion with a supernumerary incisor. On the other hand, if the lateral incisor on the affected side is missing, the problem probably is fusion of the central and lateral incisor buds. Normal occlusion, of course, is all but impossible in the presence of geminated, fused or otherwise malformed teeth.

Supernumerary or extra teeth also result from disturbances during the initiation and proliferation stages of dental development. The most common supernumerary tooth appears in the maxillary midline and is called a *mesiodens.* Supernumerary lateral incisors also occur; extra premolars occasionally appear; a few patients have fourth as well as third molars. The presence of an extra tooth obviously has great potential to disrupt normal occlusal development (Figure 5-13), and early intervention to remove it is usually required to obtain reasonable alignment and occlusal relationships. Multiple supernumerary teeth are most often seen in the congenital syndrome of cleidocranial dysplasia (see Figure 3-23), which is characterized by missing clavicles (collar bones), many supernumerary and unerupted teeth, and failure of the succedaneous teeth to erupt (see further discussion following).

Interference With Eruption

For a permanent tooth to erupt, the overlying bone as well as the primary tooth roots must resorb, and the tooth must make its way through the gingiva. Supernumerary teeth, sclerotic bone, and heavy fibrous gingiva can obstruct eruption.

All of these interferences are present in cleidocranial dysplasia. The multiple supernumerary teeth contribute an element of mechanical interference. More seriously, children with this condition have a defect in bone resorption, and the gingiva is quite heavy and fibrous.[11] If the eruption path can be cleared, the permanent teeth will erupt (see Figure 3-23). To accomplish this, it is necessary not only to extract any supernumerary teeth that may be in the way but also to remove the bone overlying the permanent teeth and reflect the gingiva so that the teeth can break through into the mouth.

In patients with less severe interferences with eruption, delayed eruption of some permanent teeth contributes to malocclusion only when other teeth drift to improper positions in the arch. In 5% to 10% of U.S. children, at least one primary molar becomes ankylosed (fused to the bone) before it finally resorbs and exfoliates. Although this delays eruption of its permanent successor, there is usually no lasting effect, but a primary molar that becomes ankylosed at a young age can become totally submerged. In that case, the primary molar is unlikely to exfoliate, the permanent premolar is severely delayed, and drift of other permanent teeth into the space of the delayed tooth can create a significant malocclusion.

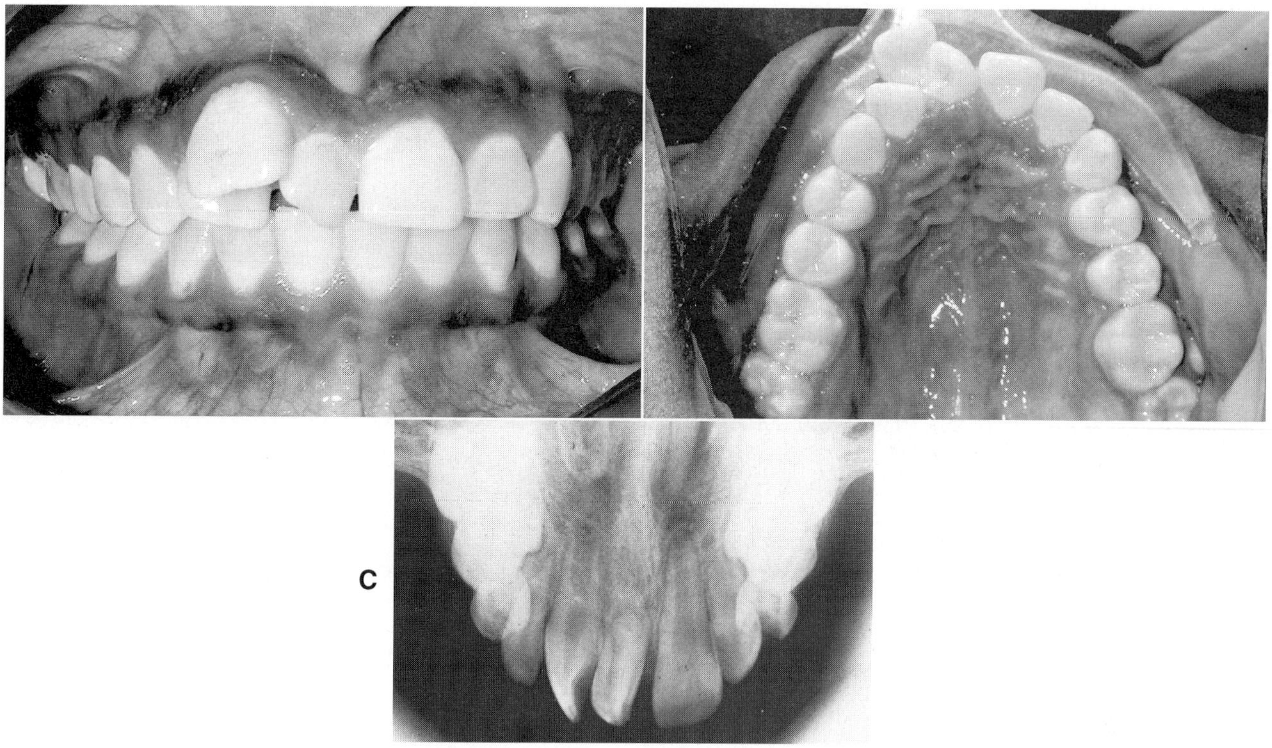

Figure 5-13 The maxillary midline is the most common location for a supernumerary tooth, which can be of almost any shape. The supernumerary may block the eruption of one or both the central incisors, or as in this girl, may separate them widely and also displace the lateral incisors.

Ectopic Eruption

Occasionally, malposition of a permanent tooth bud can lead to eruption in the wrong place. This condition is called *ectopic eruption* and is most likely to occur in the eruption of maxillary first molars. If the eruption path of the maxillary first molar carries it too far mesially at an early stage, the permanent molar is unable to erupt, and the root of the second primary molar may be damaged (Figure 5-14). The mesial position of the permanent molar means that the arch will be crowded unless the child receives treatment.

Ectopic eruption of other teeth is rare but can result in transposition of teeth or bizarre eruption positions. Mandibular second premolars sometimes erupt distally, and can end up beneath the permanent molars or even in the ramus (Figure 5-15).[12] A poor eruption direction of other teeth, especially maxillary canines, usually is due to the eruption path being altered by a lack of space.

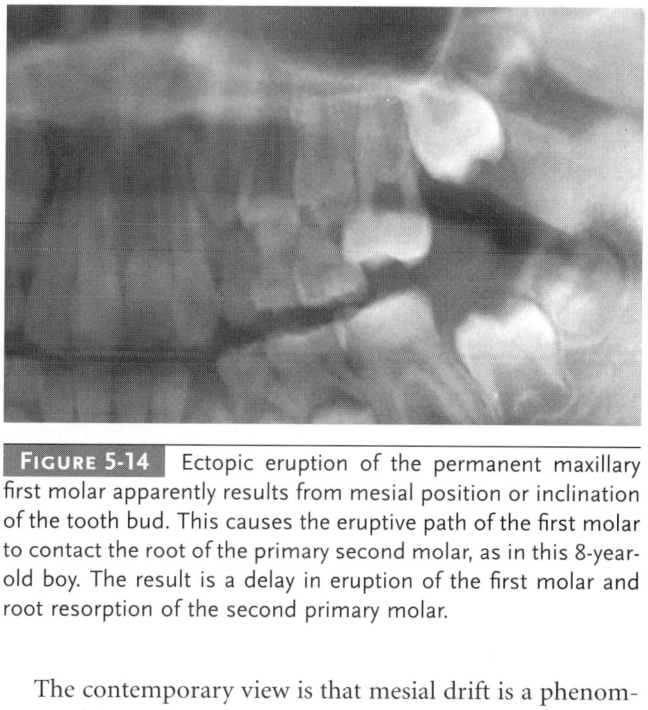

Figure 5-14 Ectopic eruption of the permanent maxillary first molar apparently results from mesial position or inclination of the tooth bud. This causes the eruptive path of the first molar to contact the root of the primary second molar, as in this 8-year-old boy. The result is a delay in eruption of the first molar and root resorption of the second primary molar.

Early Loss of Primary Teeth

When a unit within the dental arch is lost, the arch tends to contract and the space to close. At one time, this space closure was attributed entirely to mesial drift of posterior teeth, which in turn was confidently ascribed to forces from occlusion. Although a mesially-directed force when posterior teeth are brought together,[13] it probably is not a major factor in closure of spaces within the dental arches.

The contemporary view is that mesial drift is a phenomenon of the permanent molars only. The major reason these teeth move mesially when a space opens up is their mesial inclination, so that they erupt mesially as well as occlusally. Experimental data suggest that, rather than causing mesial

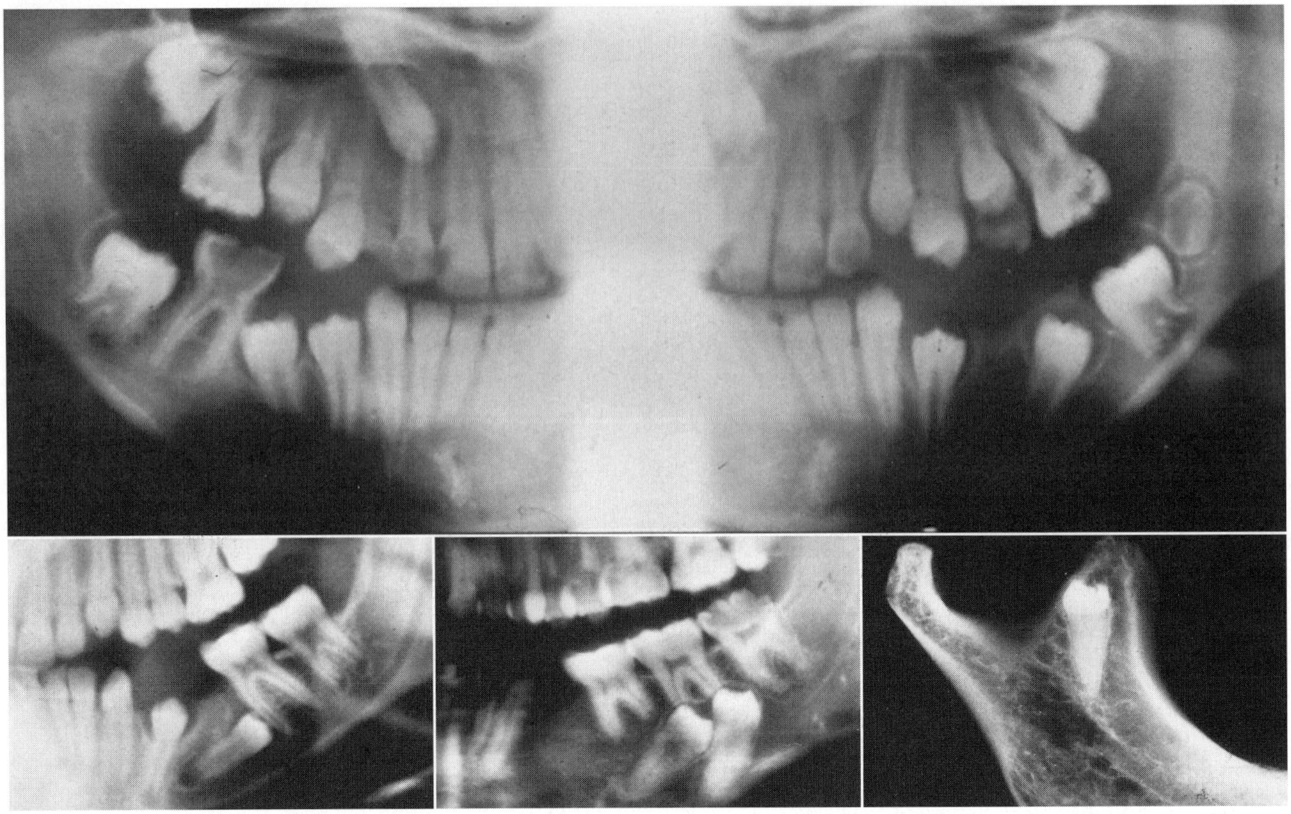

FIGURE 5-15 **A,** Mandibular second premolars tend to erupt tipped distally, and are prone to horizontal impaction, especially if the first molar is lost prematurely, but orthodontic correction is possible. **B,** If the first molar is lost prematurely and the unerupted second premolars are tipped distally, the second premolar can migrate back against the second molar, and may erupt in tight contact with it. **C,** Rarely, the premolars migrate distally beneath the permanent molars, and D, extreme migration into the mandibular ramus, even to the point that a premolar is found at the top of the coronoid process, is possible. (**D,** Courtesy Dr. K. Mitchell.)

drift, forces from occlusion actually retard it.[14] In other words, a permanent molar is likely to drift mesially more rapidly in the absence of occlusal contacts than if they are present.

Mesial drift of the permanent first molar after a primary second molar is lost prematurely (Figure 5-16) can significantly contribute to the development of crowding in the posterior part of the dental arch. This has been a significant cause of crowding and malalignment of premolars in the past. For this reason, maintenance of the space after a primary second molar has been lost is indicated (see Chapter 11).

When a primary first molar or canine is lost prematurely, there is also a tendency for the space to close. This occurs primarily by distal drift of incisors, not by mesial drift of posterior teeth (Figure 5-16, *B*). The impetus for distal drift appears to have two sources: force from active contraction of transseptal fibers in the gingiva, and pressures from the lips and cheeks.[15] The pull from transseptal fibers probably is the more consistent contributor to this space closure tendency, whereas lip pressure adds a variable component (see the following section on equilibrium). If a primary canine or first molar is lost prematurely on only one side, the permanent teeth drift distally only on that side, leading to an asymmetry in the occlusion as well as a tendency toward crowding.

From this description, it is apparent that early loss of primary teeth can cause crowding and malalignment within the dental arches. Is this a major cause of Class I crowding problems? The impact of fluoridation and other caries-preventive treatment on the prevalence of malocclusion indicates that it is not. Although fluoridation greatly reduced caries and early loss of primary teeth in typical U.S. communities, there was little or no impact on the prevalence of malocclusion. Even without fluoridation, in other words, most crowding problems are not caused by early loss of primary teeth.

Traumatic Displacement of Teeth

Almost all children fall and hit their teeth during their formative years. Occasionally, the impact is intense enough to knock out or severely displace a primary or permanent tooth. Dental trauma can lead to the development of malocclusion in three ways: (1) damage to permanent tooth buds from an injury to primary teeth, (2) drift of permanent teeth after premature loss of primary teeth, and (3) direct injury to permanent teeth.

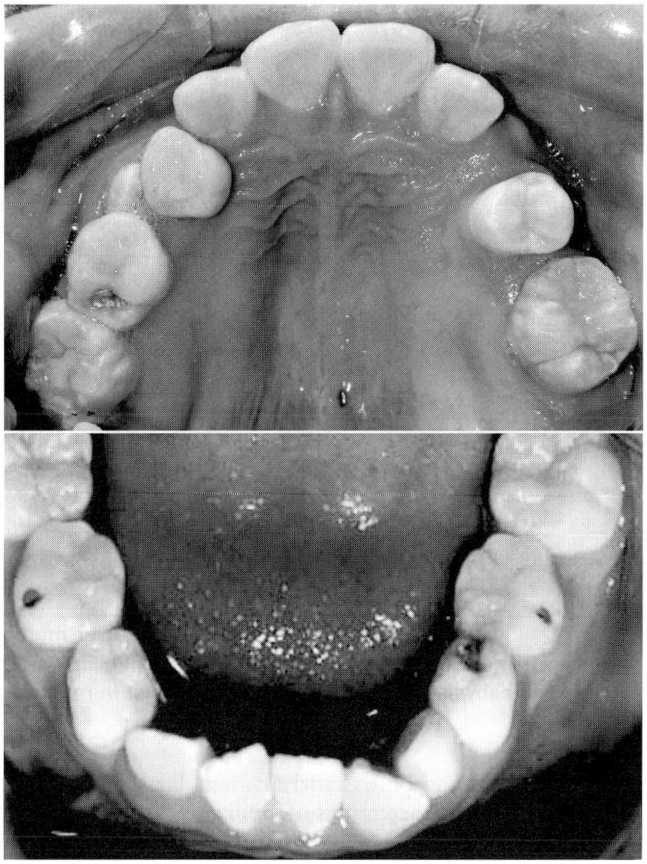

Figure 5-16 **A,** In this child's maxillary arch, early loss of the left second primary molar led to marked mesial drift of the permanent first molar. Note the space closure on the patient's left side (the right side of this mirror image photo), where almost no room for the second premolar remains. **B,** In this child's mandibular arch, early loss of the left primary canine led to a shift of the permanent incisors lingually and to the left.

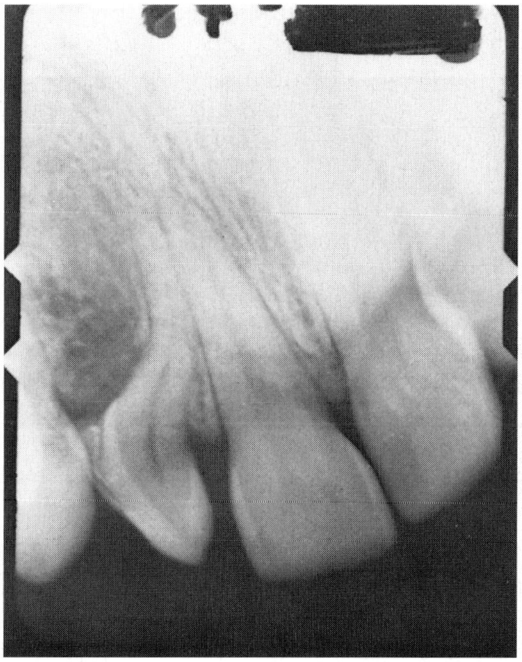

Figure 5-17 Distortion of the root (termed dilaceration) of this lateral incisor resulted from trauma at an earlier age that displaced the crown relative to the forming root.

Trauma to a primary tooth can displace the permanent tooth bud underlying it. There are two possible results. First, if the trauma occurs while the crown of the permanent tooth is forming, enamel formation will be disturbed and there will be a defect in the crown of the permanent tooth.

Second, if the trauma occurs after the crown is complete, the crown may be displaced relative to the root. Root formation may stop, leaving a permanently shortened root. More frequently, root formation continues, but the remaining portion of the root then forms at an angle to the traumatically displaced crown (Figure 5-17). This distortion of root form is called *dilaceration,* defined as a distorted root form. Dilaceration may result from mechanical interference with eruption (as from an ankylosed primary tooth that does not resorb), but its usual cause, particularly in permanent incisor teeth, is trauma to primary teeth that also displaced the permanent buds.

If distortion of root position is severe enough, it is almost impossible for the crown to assume its proper position—that might require the root to extend out through the alveolar bone. For this reason, it may be necessary to extract a severely dilacerated tooth. Traumatically displaced permanent teeth in children should be repositioned as early as possible (see Chapter 12). Immediately after the accident, an intact tooth usually can be moved back to its original position rapidly and easily. After healing (which takes 2 to 3 weeks), it is difficult to reposition the tooth, and ankylosis may develop that makes it impossible.

Genetic Influences

A strong influence of heredity on facial features is obvious at a glance—it is easy to recognize familial tendencies in the tilt of the nose, the shape of the jaw, and the look of the smile. Certain types of malocclusion run in families. The Hapsburg jaw, the prognathic mandible of this European royal family, is the best known example (Figure 5-18), but dentists routinely see repeated instances of similar malocclusions in parents and their offspring. The pertinent question for the etiology of malocclusion is not whether there are inherited influences on the jaws and teeth, because obviously there are, but whether different types of malocclusion can be directly caused by inherited characteristics.

For much of the 20th century, thoughts about how malocclusion could be produced by inherited characteristics focused on two major possibilities. The first would be an inherited disproportion between the size of the teeth and the pressures from lips, cheeks, and tongue at rest are maintained most of the time, one would expect these pressures to affect tooth position.

It is easy to demonstrate that this is indeed the case. For example, if an injury to the soft tissue of the lip results in scarring and contracture, the incisors in this vicinity will be moved lingually as the lip tightens against them (Figure 5-21). On the other hand, if restraining pressure by the lip or cheek is removed, the teeth move outward in response to unopposed pressure from the tongue (Figure 5-22, *A*). Pressure from the tongue, whether from an enlargement of the tongue from a tumor or other source or because its posture has changed, will result in labial displacement of the teeth even though the lips and cheeks are intact, because the equilibrium is altered (Figure 5-22, *B*).

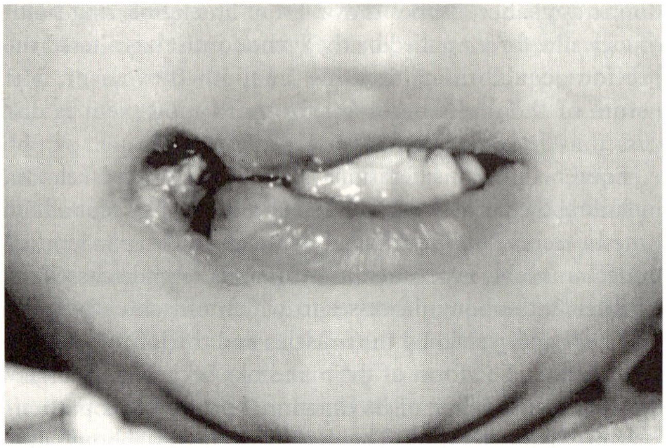

Figure 5-21 Scarring of the corner of the mouth in this child will occur as the burn from biting an electrical cord heals. From equilibrium theory, one would expect a distortion in the form of the dental arch in the region of the contracting scar, and exactly this occurs after an injury of this type.

These observations make it plain that, in contrast to forces from mastication, light sustained pressures from lips, cheeks, and tongue at rest are important determinants of tooth position. It seems unlikely, however, that the intermittent short-duration pressures created when the tongue and lips contact the teeth during swallowing or speaking would have any significant impact on tooth position. As with masticatory forces, the pressure magnitudes would be great enough to move a tooth, but the duration is inadequate (Table 5-2).

Another possible contributor to the equilibrium could be pressures from external sources, of which various habits and orthodontic appliances would be most prominent. As an example, an orthodontic appliance that created light pressure on the inside of the dental arch might be used to expand the teeth laterally and anteriorly, creating enough space to bring all teeth into alignment. After a certain amount of arch expansion, cheek and lip pressure begins to increase. One

A

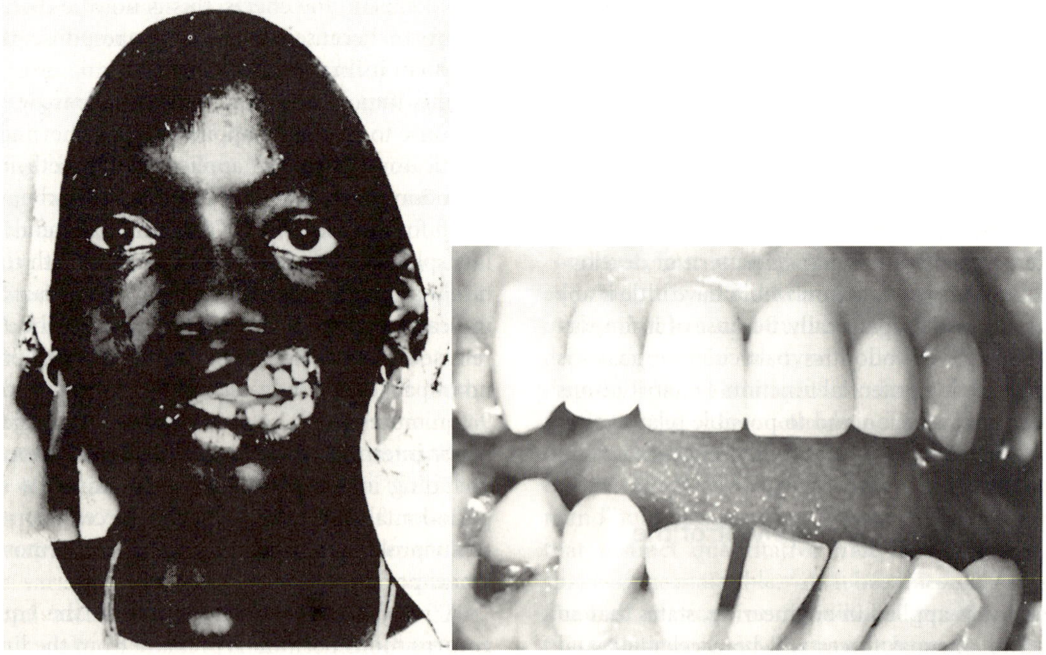

B

Figure 5-22 The effect of a change in lip/tongue force on the dentition. Constant light pressure from soft tissues can move teeth. The key is not so much the pressure magnitude as its duration. **A,** In this unfortunate individual, a large portion of the cheek was lost because of a tropical infection. Note the outward splaying of the teeth when the restraining force of the check was lost. (Courtesy Prof. J.P. Moss). **B,** After a paralytic stroke, this patient's tongue rested against the mandibular posterior teeth. Before the stroke, the occlusion was normal. In this patient, an outward splaying of the teeth occurred on the affected side because of the increase in resting tongue pressure. (Courtesy Dr. T. Wallen.)

Table 5-2

Possible Equilibrium Influences: Magnitude and Duration of Force Against the Teeth During Function

Possible equilibrium influence	Force magnitude	Force duration
Tooth contacts		
Mastication	Very heavy	Very short
Swallowing	Light	Very short
Soft tissue pressures of lip, cheek, and tongue		
Swallowing	Moderate	Short
Speaking	Light	Very short
Resting	Very light	Long
External pressures		
Habits	Moderate	Variable
Orthodontics	Moderate	Variable
Intrinsic pressures		
PDL fibers	Light	Long
Gingival fibers	Variable	Long

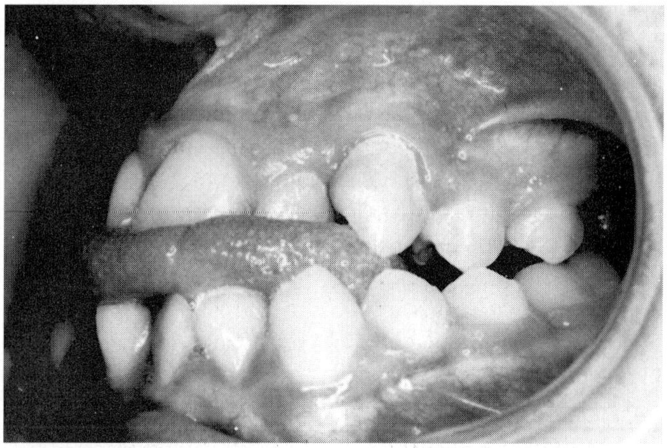

Figure 5-23 A large tongue, as in this patient with a history of thyroid deficiency from infancy onward, may contribute to the development of mandibular prognathism by causing the mandible to be positioned forward at all times.

could expect that as long as the appliance remained in place, even though it no longer exerted any active force, it would serve as a retainer to counter these increased forces. When the appliance was removed, however, the equilibrium would again be unbalanced, and the teeth would collapse lingually until a new position of balance was reached.

Whether a habit can serve in the same way as an orthodontic appliance to change the position of the teeth has been the subject of controversy since at least the first century AD, when Celsus recommended that a child with a crooked tooth be instructed to apply finger pressure against it to move it to its proper position. From our present understanding of equilibrium, we would expect that this might work, *if* the child kept the finger pressure against the tooth for 6 hours or more per day.

The same reasoning can be applied to other habits: if a habit like thumbsucking created pressure against the teeth for more than the threshold duration (6 hours or more per day), it certainly could move teeth and might affect the direction of jaw growth (Figure 5-23). On the other hand, if the habit had a shorter duration little or no effect would be expected, no matter how heavy the pressure. Whether a behavior pattern is essential or nonessential, innate or learned, its effect on the position of the teeth is determined not by the force that it applies to the teeth but by how long that force is sustained.

This concept also makes it easier to understand how playing a musical instrument might relate to the development of a malocclusion. In the past, many clinicians have suspected that playing a wind instrument might affect the position of the anterior teeth, and some have prescribed instruments as part of orthodontic therapy. Playing a clarinet, for instance, might lead to increased overjet because of the way the reeds are placed between the incisors, and this instrument could be considered both a potential cause of a Class II malocclusion and a therapeutic device for treatment of Class III. String instruments like the violin and viola require a specific head and jaw posture that affects tongue vs lip/cheek pressures and could produce asymmetries in arch form. Although the expected types of displacement of teeth are seen in professional musicians,[28] even in this group the effects are not dramatic, and little or no effect is observed in most children.[29] It seems quite likely that the duration of tongue and lip pressures associated with playing the instrument is too short to make any difference, except in the most devoted musician.

Another possible contributor to the dental equilibrium is the periodontal fiber system, both in the gingival tissues and within the periodontal ligament. We have already noted that if a tooth is lost, the space tends to close, in part because of force created by the transseptal fibers in the gingiva. The importance of this force has been demonstrated experimentally in monkeys by extracting a tooth and then making repeated incisions in the gingiva so that the transseptal fiber network is disrupted and cannot reestablish continuity. Space closure is almost completely abolished under these circumstances.[30]

The same gingival fiber network stretches elastically during orthodontic treatment and tends to pull the teeth back toward their original position. Clinical experience has shown that after orthodontic treatment, it is often wise to eliminate this force by making gingival incisions that sever the stretched transseptal fibers, thereby allowing them to heal with the teeth properly aligned (see Chapter 17). In the absence of a space created by extraction or orthodontic tooth movement, however, the gingival fiber network apparently has minimal effects on the dental equilibrium.

The periodontal ligament itself can contribute to the forces that make up the dental equilibrium. Exactly how the eruption mechanism works is still not completely understood, but it seems clear now that the eruptive force is generated within the periodontal ligament. This force is large enough and sustained enough to move a tooth. It seems likely that the same metabolic activity can and does produce forces that serve as a part of "active stabilization" for teeth, directly contributing to the equilibrium. The extent to which this occurs in teeth that are not erupting is not known. It is known, however, that the eruption mechanism remains at least potentially active throughout life, since a tooth can begin to erupt again many years after eruptive movements have apparently ceased, if its antagonist is extracted. Thus there is at least the potential for metabolic activity in the periodontal ligament to affect equilibrium.

Consideration of eruptive forces leads to a final aspect of the dental equilibrium: the effect of forces against the teeth must be considered, not only in the anteroposterior and transverse planes of space that relate to the position of a tooth within the arch, but also vertically in relation to how much or how little a tooth erupts. The vertical position of any tooth, of course, is determined by the equilibrium between the forces that produce eruption and those that oppose it. Forces from mastication are the primary ones opposing eruption, but lighter, more sustained forces from soft tissues such as the tongue interposed between the teeth probably are more important, just as they are for the horizontal equilibrium.

Equilibrium Effects on Jaw Size and Shape

The jaws, particularly the mandible, can be thought of as consisting of a core of bone to which functional processes are attached (see Figure 4-12). The functional processes of bones will be altered if the function is lost or changed. For example, the bone of the alveolar process exists only to support the teeth. If a tooth fails to erupt, alveolar bone never forms in the area it would have occupied, and if a tooth is extracted, the alveolus in that region resorbs until finally it completely atrophies. When one of a pair of opposing teeth is extracted, the other usually begins to erupt again, and even as bone is resorbing in one jaw where the tooth was lost, new alveolar bone forms in the other as the erupting tooth brings bone with it. The position of the tooth, not the functional load on it, determines the shape of the alveolar ridge.

The same is true for the muscular processes: the location of the muscle attachments is more important in determining bone shape than mechanical loading or degree of activity. Growth of the muscle, however, determines the position of the attachment, and so muscle growth can produce a change in shape of the jaw, particularly at the coronoid process and angle of the mandible.

If the condylar processes of the mandible can be considered functional processes serving to articulate the mandible with the rest of the facial skeleton, as apparently they can, the intriguing possibility is raised that altering the position of the mandible might alter mandibular growth. The idea that holding the mandible forward or pressing it backward would change its growth has been accepted, rejected, and partially accepted again during the past century. Obviously, this theory has important implications for the etiology of malocclusion. For example, if a child positions his mandible forward on closure because of incisor interferences or because his tongue is large, will this stimulate the mandible to grow larger and ultimately produce a Class III malocclusion? Would allowing a young child to sleep on his stomach, so that the weight of the head rested on the chin, cause underdevelopment of the mandible and a Class II malocclusion?

The effect of force duration is not as clear for equilibrium effects on the jaws as for the teeth. It appears, however, that the same principle applies: the magnitude of force is less important than its duration. Positioning the jaw forward only when the teeth are brought into occlusion means that most of the time, when the mandible is in its rest position, there is no protrusion. We would expect no effects on a functional process from repeated intermittent force because of the short total duration, and the condylar process seems to respond in accordance with this principle. Neither experimental nor clinical evidence suggests that mandibular growth is any different because of occlusal interferences (though it should be kept in mind that tooth eruption, and thereby the final position of the teeth, can be altered).

If the mandible were protruded at all times, as might well be the case if the tongue were unusually large, the duration threshold could be surpassed, and growth effects might be observed. On clinical examination, individuals who appear to have a large tongue almost always have a well-developed mandible, but it is very difficult to establish tongue size. Only in extreme cases, as with a patient with early-onset thyroid deficiency, is it possible to be reasonably sure that an enlarged tongue contributed to excessive growth of the mandible (Figure 5-24). This is unlikely to be a major cause of mandibular prognathism.[31]

It was widely believed in Edward Angle's era that pressures against the mandible from various habits, particularly sleeping on the stomach, interfered with growth and caused Class II malocclusion. Little or no evidence supports this contention. Growth of the soft tissue matrix that moves the mandible forward and creates a space between the condyle and the temporal fossa is the normal mechanism by which growth occurs. Inhibition of mandibular growth by pressure is not a feature of normal development and is much harder to achieve, if indeed it is possible at all.

From the perspective of equilibrium theory, then, we can conclude that intermittent pressures or forces have little if any effect on either the position of the teeth or the size and shape of the jaws. Density of bone in the alveolar process and

A,B 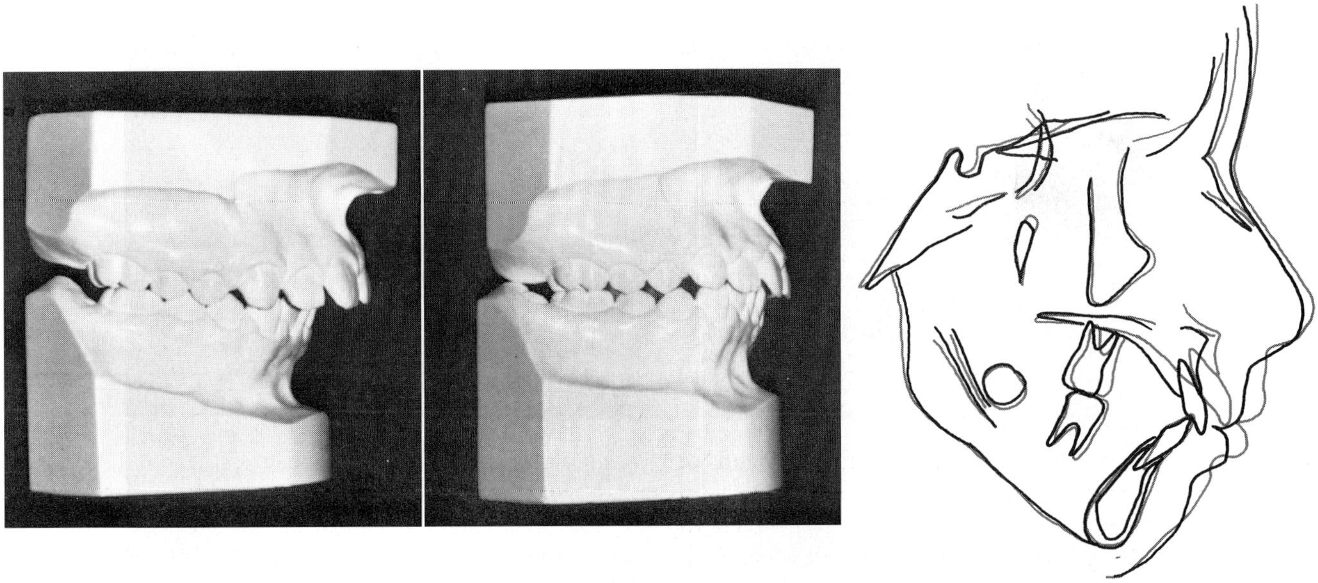 C

FIGURE 5-24 In this pair of identical twins, one sucked her thumb up to the time of orthodontic records at age 11 while the other did not. **A,** Occlusal relationships in the non-thumbsucking and **(B)** the thumbsucking girl. Note the increased overjet and forward displacement of the maxillary dentition in the thumbsucker. **C,** Cephalometric tracings of the two girls superimposed on the cranial base for the two girls. As one would expect with identical twins, the cranial base morphology is nearly identical. Note the forward displacement of not only the maxillary dentition but also the maxilla itself. (Courtesy Dr. T. Wallen.)

throughout the basal areas of the jaws should differ as a function of masticatory forces, but shape should not. Neither masticatory forces nor soft tissue pressures during swallowing and speaking should have any major influence on tooth position.

Major equilibrium influences for the teeth should be the light but long-lasting pressures from tongue, lips, and cheeks at rest. In addition, significant equilibrium effects should be expected from the elasticity of gingival fibers and from metabolic activity within the periodontal ligament (see Table 5-2). These equilibrium influences would affect the vertical as well as horizontal position of the teeth and could have a profound effect on how much tooth eruption occurred as well as where a tooth was positioned within the dental arch. The major equilibrium influences on the jaws should be positional changes affecting the functional processes, including the condylar process.

In the remainder of this section, functional patterns and habits that might produce malocclusion are examined as potential etiologic agents from the perspective of equilibrium theory.

Functional Influences on Dentofacial Development

Masticatory Function

The pressures generated by chewing activity potentially could affect dentofacial development in two ways: (1) greater use of the jaws, with higher and/or more prolonged biting force, could increase the dimensions of the jaws and dental arches. Less use of the jaws might then lead to underdeveloped dental arches, and to crowded and irregular teeth; (2) decreased biting force could affect how much the teeth erupt, thereby affecting lower face height and overbite/open bite relationships. Let us now examine both possibilities in more detail.

Function and Dental Arch Size. Equilibrium theory, as reviewed earlier, suggests that the size and shape of the muscular processes of the jaws should reflect muscle size and activity. Enlargement of the mandibular gonial angles can be seen in humans with hypertrophy of the mandibular elevator muscles (Figure 5-25), and changes in the form of the coronoid processes occur in children when temporalis muscle function is altered after injuries, so there is no doubt that the muscular processes of the jaws are affected by muscle function in humans. Equilibrium theory also suggests that heavy intermittent forces produced during mastication should have little direct effect on tooth positions, and therefore that size of the dental arches would be affected by function only if their bony base were widened. Does the extent of masticatory activity affect the width of the base of the dental arches?

It seems likely that differences between human racial groups, to some extent, reflect dietary differences and the accompanying masticatory effort. The characteristic craniofacial morphology of Eskimos, which includes broad dental arches, is best explained as an adaptation to the extreme stress they place on jaws and teeth, and changes in craniofa-

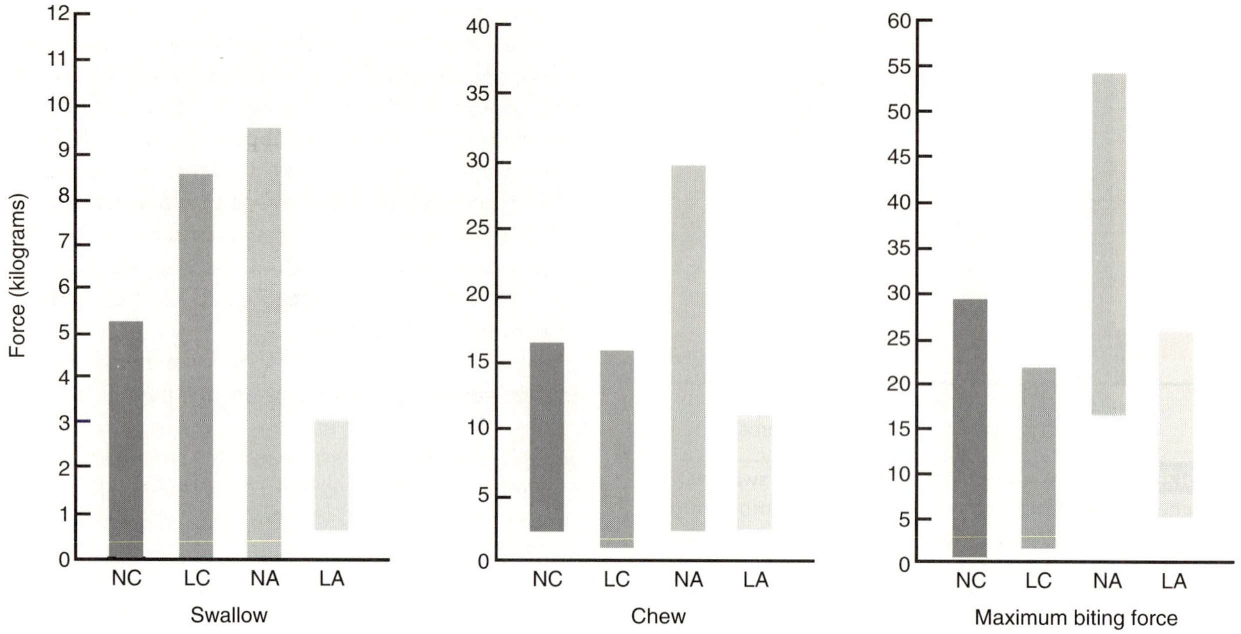

FIGURE 5-27 Comparison of occlusal forces in normal-face children (*NC*, blue), long-face children (*LC*, aqua), normal-face adults (*NA*, green), and long-face adults (*LA*, light green). Values for both groups of children and the long-face adults are similar; values for normal adults are significantly higher than any of the other three groups. The implication is that the differences in occlusal force in adults result from failure of the long-face group to gain strength during adolescence, not to the long condition itself. (From Proffit WR, Fields HW. Occlusal forces in normal and long face children. J Dent Res 62:571-574, 1983.)

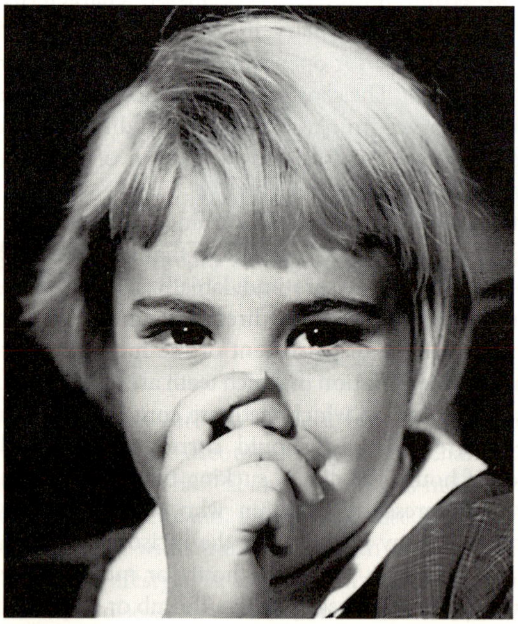

FIGURE 5-28 A child sucking his thumb usually places it against the roof of the mouth, causing pressure that pushes the lower incisors lingually and the upper incisors labially. In addition, the jaw is positioned downward, providing additional opportunity for posterior teeth to erupt, and cheek pressure is increased while the tongue is lowered vertically away from the maxillary posterior teeth, altering the equilibrium that controls width dimensions. If the thumb is placed on one side instead of in the midline, the symmetry of the arch may be affected.

there is more eruption of posterior teeth than might otherwise have occurred. Because of the geometry of the jaws, 1 mm of elongation posteriorly opens the bite about 2 mm anteriorly, so this can be a powerful contributor to the development of anterior open bite (Figure 5-29).

Although negative pressure is created within the mouth during sucking, there is no reason to believe that this is responsible for the constriction of the maxillary arch that usually accompanies sucking habits. Instead, arch form is affected by an alteration in the balance between cheek and tongue pressures. If the thumb is placed between the teeth, the tongue must be lowered, which decreases pressure by the tongue against the lingual of upper posterior teeth. At the same time, cheek pressure against these teeth is increased as the buccinator muscle contracts during sucking (Figure 5-30). Cheek pressures are greatest at the corners of the mouth, and this probably explains why the maxillary arch tends to become V-shaped, with more constriction across the canines than the molars. A child who sucks vigorously is more likely to have a narrow upper arch than one who just places the thumb between the teeth.

Although sucking habits can be a powerful contributor to malocclusion, sucking by itself does not create a severe malocclusion unless the habit persists well into the mixed dentition years. Mild displacement of the primary incisor teeth is often noted in a 3- or 4-year-old thumbsucker, but if sucking stops at this stage, normal lip and cheek pressures soon restore the teeth to their usual positions. If the habit

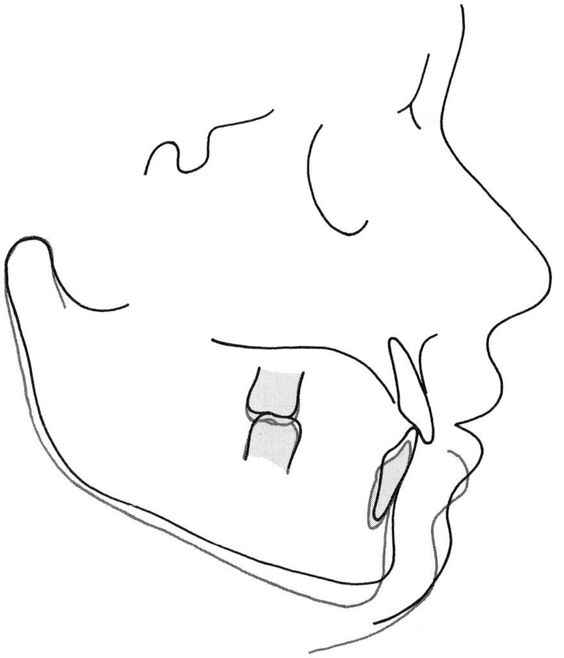

Figure 5-29 Cephalometric tracing showing the effects of posterior eruption on the extent of anterior opening. The only difference between the red and black tracings is that the first molars have been elongated 2 mm in the red tracing. Note that the result is 4 mm of separation of the incisors, because of the geometry of the jaw.

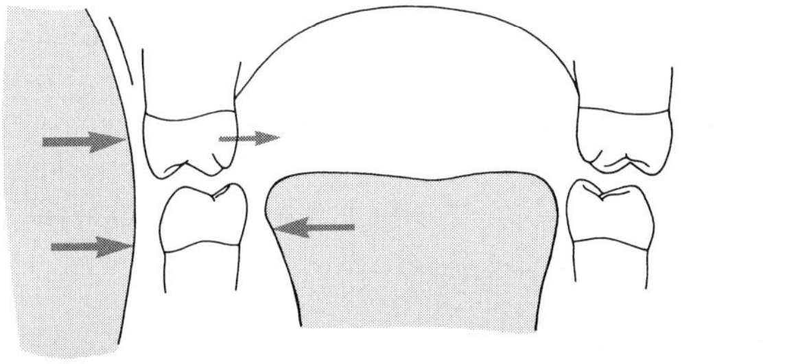

Figure 5-30 Diagrammatic representation of soft tissue pressures in the molar region in a child with a sucking habit. As the tongue is lowered and the cheeks contract during sucking, the pressure balance against the upper teeth is altered, and the upper but not the lower molars are displaced lingually.

persists after the permanent incisors begin to erupt, orthodontic treatment may be necessary to overcome the resulting tooth displacements. The constricted maxillary arch is the aspect of the malocclusion least likely to correct spontaneously. In many children, if the maxillary arch is expanded transversely, both the incisor protrusion and anterior open bite will improve spontaneously (see Chapter 12). There is no point in beginning orthodontic therapy, of course, until the habit has stopped.

Many other habits have been indicted as causes of malocclusion. As noted previously, a "sleeping habit" in which the weight of the head rested on the chin once was thought to be a major cause of Class II malocclusion. Facial asymmetries have been attributed to always sleeping on one side of the face or even to "leaning habits," as when an inattentive child leans the side of his face against one hand to doze without falling out of the classroom chair.

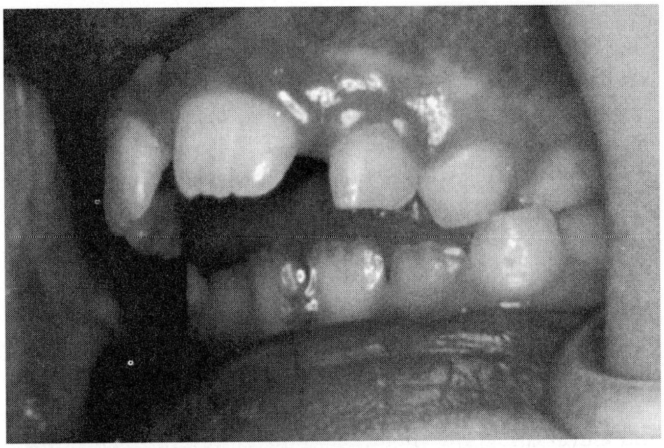

Figure 5-31 The typical appearance of a "tongue thrust swallow" with the lip pulled back. Note the tongue tip between the incisors protruding forward toward contact with the elevated lower lip.

It is not nearly as easy to distort the facial skeleton as these views implied. Sucking habits often exceed the time threshold necessary to produce an effect on the teeth, but even prolonged sucking has little impact on the underlying form of the jaws. On close analysis most other habits have such a short duration that dental effects, much less skeletal effects, are unlikely.

Tongue Thrusting

Much attention has been paid at various times to the tongue and tongue habits as possible etiologic factors in malocclusion. The possible deleterious effects of "tongue thrust swallowing" (Figure 5-31), defined as placement of the tongue tip forward between the incisors during swallowing, received particular emphasis in the 1950s and 1960s.

Laboratory studies indicate that individuals who place the tongue tip forward when they swallow usually do not have more tongue force against the teeth than those who keep the tongue tip back; in fact, tongue pressure may be lower.[38] The term *tongue thrust* is therefore something of a misnomer, since it implies that the tongue is forcefully thrust forward. Swallowing is not a learned behavior, but is integrated and controlled physiologically at subconscious levels, so whatever the pattern of swallow, it cannot be considered a habit in the usual sense. It is true, however, that individuals with an anterior open bite malocclusion place the tongue between the anterior teeth when they swallow while those who have a normal incisor relationship usually do not, and it is tempting to blame the open bite on this pattern of tongue activity.

Maturation of oral activities, including swallowing, has been discussed in some detail in Chapter 2. The mature or adult swallow pattern appears in some normal children as early as age 3, but is not present in the majority until about age 6 and is never achieved in 10% to 15% of a typical population. Tongue thrust swallowing in older patients superficially resembles the infantile swallow (described in Chapter 3), and sometimes children or adults who place the tongue between the anterior teeth are spoken of as having a retained infantile swallow. This is clearly incorrect. Only brain damaged children retain a truly infantile swallow in which the posterior part of the tongue has little or no role.

Since coordinated movements of the posterior tongue and elevation of the mandible tend to develop before protrusion of the tongue tip between the incisor teeth disappears, what is called "tongue thrusting" in young children is often a normal transitional stage in swallowing. During the transition from an infantile to a mature swallow, a child can be expected to pass through a stage in which the swallow is characterized by muscular activity to bring the lips together, separation of the posterior teeth, and forward protrusion of the tongue between the teeth. This is also a description of the classic tongue thrust swallow. A delay in the normal swallow transition can be expected when a child has a sucking habit.

When there is an anterior open bite and/or upper incisor protrusion, as often occurs from sucking habits, it is more difficult to seal off the front of the mouth during swallowing to prevent food or liquids from escaping. Bringing the lips together and placing the tongue between the separated anterior teeth is a successful maneuver to close off the front of the mouth and form an anterior seal. In other words, a tongue thrust swallow is a useful physiologic adaptation if you have an open bite, which is why an individual with an open bite also has a tongue thrust swallow. The reverse is not true—a tongue thrust swallow is often present in children with good anterior occlusion. After a sucking habit stops, the anterior open bite tends to close spontaneously, but the position of the tongue between the anterior teeth persists for a while as the open bite closes. Until the open bite disappears, an anterior seal by the tongue tip remains necessary.

The modern viewpoint is, in short, that tongue thrust swallowing is seen primarily in two circumstances: in younger children with reasonably normal occlusion, in whom it represents only a transitional stage in normal physiologic maturation; and in individuals of any age with displaced incisors, in whom it is an adaptation to the space between the teeth. The presence of overjet (often) and anterior open bite (nearly always) conditions a child or adult to place the tongue between the anterior teeth. A tongue thrust swallow therefore should be considered the result of displaced incisors, not the cause. It follows, of course, that correcting the tooth position should cause a change in swallow pattern, and this usually happens. It is neither necessary nor desirable to try to teach the patient to swallow differently before beginning orthodontic treatment.

This is not to say that the tongue has no etiologic role in the development of open bite malocclusion. From equilibrium theory, light but sustained pressure by the tongue against the teeth would be expected to have significant effects. Tongue thrust swallowing simply has too short a duration to have an impact on tooth position. Pressure by the tongue against the teeth during a typical swallow lasts for approximately 1 second. A typical individual swallows about 800 times per day while awake but has only a few swallows per hour while asleep. The total per day therefore is usually under 1000. One thousand seconds of pressure, of course, totals only a few minutes, not nearly enough to affect the equilibrium.

On the other hand, if a patient has a forward resting posture of the tongue, the duration of this pressure, even if very light, could affect tooth position, vertically or horizontally. Tongue tip protrusion during swallowing is sometimes associated with a forward tongue posture. If the position from which tongue movements start is different from normal, so that the pattern of resting pressures is different, there is likely to be an effect on the teeth, whereas if the postural position is normal, the tongue thrust swallow has no clinical significance.

Perhaps this point can best be put in perspective by comparing the number of children who have an anterior open bite malocclusion with the number of children of the same age reported to have a tongue thrust swallow. As Figure 5-32 shows, at every age above 6, the number of children reported to have a tongue thrust swallow is about 10 times greater than the number reported to have an anterior open bite. Thus there is no reason to believe that a tongue thrust swallow always implies an altered rest position and will lead to malocclusion. The odds are approximately 10 to 1 that this is not the case for any given child. In a child who has an open bite, tongue posture may be a factor, but the swallow itself is not.

Respiratory Pattern

Respiratory needs are the primary determinant of the posture of the jaws and tongue (and of the head itself, to a lesser extent). Therefore it seems entirely reasonable that an altered respiratory pattern, such as breathing through the mouth rather than the nose, could change the posture of the head, jaw, and tongue. This in turn could alter the equilibrium of pressures on the jaws and teeth and affect both jaw growth and tooth position. In order to breathe through the mouth, it is necessary to lower the mandible and tongue, and extend (tip back) the head. If these postural changes were maintained, face height would increase, and posterior teeth would super-erupt; unless there was unusual vertical growth of the ramus, the mandible would rotate down and back, opening the bite anteriorly and increasing overjet; and increased pressure from the stretched cheeks might cause a narrower maxillary dental arch.

Exactly this type of malocclusion often is associated with mouth breathing (note its similarity to the pattern also

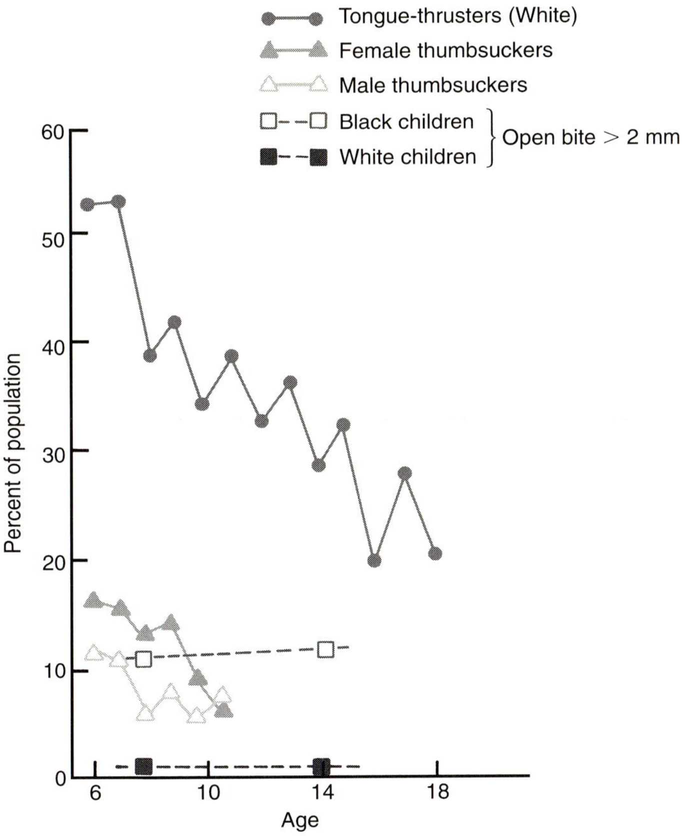

FIGURE 5-32 Prevalence of anterior open bite, thumbsucking, and tongue thrust swallowing as a function of age. Open bite occurs much more frequently in blacks than in whites. Note that the prevalence of anterior open bite at any age is only a small fraction of the prevalence of tongue thrust swallowing and is also less than the prevalence of thumbsucking. (Data from Fletcher SG, et al. J Speech Hear Disord 26:201-208, 1961; Kelly JE, et al. DHEW Pub No [HRA] 77-144, 1977.)

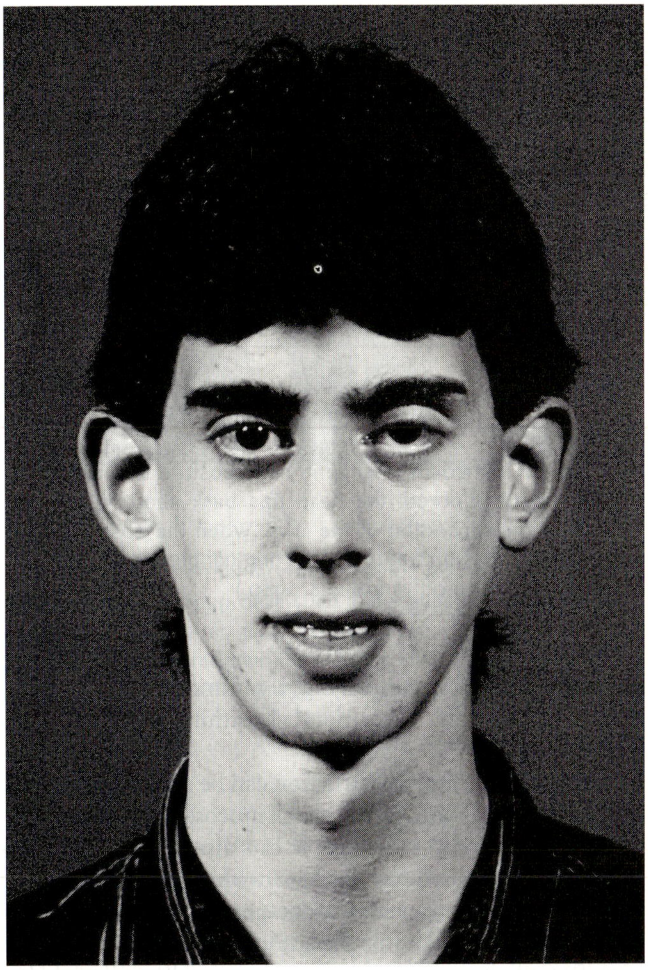

FIGURE 5-33 The classic "adenoid facies," characterized by narrow width dimensions, protruding teeth and lips separated at rest, has often been attributed to mouth breathing. Since it is perfectly possible to breathe through the nose with the lips separated, simply by creating an oral seal posteriorly with the soft palate, the facial appearance is not diagnostic of the respiratory mode. On careful study, many of these patients are found not to be obligatory mouth breathers.

blamed on sucking habits and tongue thrust swallow). The association has been noted for many years: the descriptive term *adenoid facies* has appeared in the English literature for at least a century, probably longer (Figure 5-33). Unfortunately, the relationship between mouth breathing, altered posture, and the development of malocclusion is not so clear-cut as the theoretical outcome of shifting to oral respiration might appear at first glance.[39] Recent experimental studies have only partially clarified the situation.

In analyzing this, it is important to understand first that although humans are primarily nasal breathers, everyone breathes partially through the mouth under certain physiologic conditions, the most prominent being an increased need for air during exercise. For the average individual, there is a transition to partial oral breathing when ventilatory exchange rates above 40 to 45 L/min are reached. At maximum effort, 80 or more L/min of air are needed, about half of which is obtained through the mouth. At rest, minimum airflow is 20 to 25 L/min, but heavy mental concentration or even normal conversation lead to increased airflow and a transition to partial mouth breathing.

During resting conditions, greater effort is required to breathe through the nose than through the mouth—the tortuous nasal passages introduce an element of resistance to airflow as they perform their function of warming and humidifying the inspired air. The increased work for nasal respiration is physiologically acceptable up to a point, and indeed respiration is most efficient with modest resistance present in the system. If the nose is partially obstructed, the work associated with nasal breathing increases, and at a certain level of resistance to nasal airflow, the individual switches to partial mouth breathing. This crossover point varies among individuals, but is usually reached at resistance levels of about 3.5 to 4 cm H-2-O/L/min.[40] The swelling of

MEDICAL HISTORY
(Child/Adolescent)

PATIENT NAME: ______________________________ DATE: ____________________
BIRTH DATE: __________
Name of your child's physician: ____________________ Office Phone: ______________
Address of your child's physician: ____________________ Date of last exam: __________

1. Is your child in good health? .... Yes No Don't know
2. Does your child have a health problem? .... Yes No Don't know
   If yes, explain: ____
3. Has your child ever been hospitalized, had general anesthesia, or emergency room visits? .... Yes No Don't know
   If yes, explain: ____
4. Are your child's immunizations up to date? .... Yes No Don't know
5. Does your child have allergies to medications (drugs), medical products (latex), or the environment (dust, mites, pollen, mold)? .... Yes No Don't know
   If yes, please list: ____
6. List past medications taken by child: ______________________________________
7. List daily medications child is now taking: __________________________________
8. Has your child ever had or been treated by a physician for:

Check one for each condition

Yes	No	?			Yes	No	?	
			a. Problems at birth					p. Cancer
			b. Heart murmur					q. Cerebral palsy
			c. Heart disease					r. Seizures
			d. Rheumatic fever					s. Asthma
			e. Anemia					t. Cleft lip/palate
			f. Sickle cell anemia					u. Speech or hearing problems
			g. Bleeding/hemophilia					v. Eye problems/contact lenses
			h. Blood transfusion					w. Skin problems
			i. Hepatitis					x. Tonsil/adenoid/sinus problems
			j. AIDS or HIV+					y. Sleep problems
			k. Tuberculosis					z. Emotional/behavior problems
			l. Liver disease					aa. Radiation therapy
			m. Kidney disease					bb. Growth problems
			n. Diabetes					cc. Attention deficit disorders
			o. Arthritis					

9. Has your child had any recent rapid growth? ________ If so, how much? ______________
10. Parents: (Father) Ht: _____ Wt: _____ (Mother) Ht: _____ Wt: _____
11. Older brothers and sisters: (1) Ht: ____ Wt: ____ (2) Ht: ____ Wt: ____ (3) Ht: _____ Wt: _____
12. Females: Has menstruation begun? _______ If yes, when? ____________ Pregnant? _______
    Using birth control pills? ____________
13. If yes to any above, please explain this or any other problem: ______________________
    ____
14. Child's grade in school: ____________ Child's school: ______________________________
15. Do you consider your child to be (check one): Advanced in learning ___ Progressing normally ___
    Slow learner ___

Figure 6-2 Form for obtaining medical/dental history for young orthodontic patients. A separate but similar form is needed for adult patients. Annotated comments, explaining why some of the questions are asked, are placed immediately below the form and are keyed by number to the question to which they refer.

DENTAL HISTORY

16. What is your main concern about your child's dental condition? ______________________

17. Has your child been to a dentist before? No Yes If yes, date of last visit: ______________

18. Regular dentist's name: ____

19. Check one for each condition:

Yes	No	?	
			a. Has your child ever had dental x-rays? Date of last x-rays? __________
			b. Will your child be uncooperative? If yes, explain: __________
			c. Has your child experienced any complications following dental treatment? If yes, explain: __________
			d. Has your child had cavities and / or toothaches?
			e. Are your child's teeth sensitive to temperature or food?
			f. Did you or your child ever get instructions in brushing?
			g. Do your child's gums bleed when brushed?
			h. Does your child use fluoride products: rinses, drops, tabs?
			i. Does or has your child had any clicking or pain in the jaw joint?
			j. Does or has your child had any problems opening or closing their mouth?
			k. Has your child inherited any family facial or dental characteristics? If yes, explain: __________
			l. Has your child ever injured his/her teeth?
			m. Has your child ever injured his/her jaws or face?
			n. Does or did your child use a pacifier?
			o. Does or did your child suck his/her fingers or thumb?

20. Does your child have any other dental problems we should know about? ______ Please explain: ___

____

21. Whom may we thank for referring you to our office? ______________________

22. PERSON COMPLETING THIS FORM: Signature ______________________

Relationship to patient: ______________________

ANNOTATIONS ON SELECTED QUESTIONS

2. This helps establish the patient's social-emotional status.
3. This helps establish a history of trauma.
4. In the instance of oral-facial trauma the DPT status is critical. Soft tissue injury is increased with appliances in place.
5. This helps identify allergies to all types of allergens. One must also consider latex used in dental treatment gloves and elastics. This sensitivity is increasing rapidly in the population.

8b,c,d,f: These patients need antibiotic coverage during banding and debanding procedures.
8g,h,i,j,k. With modern infection control procedures, these patients can be treated, but the treatment may need to be modified.
8o. This may relate to mandibular growth and development.
8p. This will help determine treatments using radiation or chemotherapy that can alter dental development, jaw growth, or somatic growth, depending on the site of the lesion and the treatment.
8x. This can help with evaluation of respiratory problems and tooth sensitivity.
8aa. Radiation therapy to the jaws can greatly alter local dental and skeletal development. The risks of osteoradioecrosis is also a risk in these patients depending on the radiation dosage and the type of treatment under consideration.
8bb. Some children with growth problems may be treated with growth hormones, which can have implications for growth modification treatment timing. In some cancer patients, growth hormones can be part of the post-radiation treatment regime. This, too, can affect treatment timing.
8cc. Attention Deficit Disorders can be treated with numerous drugs. The affect on growth of some of these medications is unclear.
9-12. These questions help establish growth status and timing. Birth control pills can be rendered ineffective by antibiotics used for SBE prevention and oral infections. Patients should be alerted to this problem.
16. The chief complaint is critical to determine why the patient is seeking care. This must be considered carefully in the planning of the treatment.
19a. Reduction in unnecessary radiation is critical to the highest quality care. Many practitioners will request films as part of the examination procedures. Patients seeking second opinions often have already had some records obtained.
19g. Orthodontic treatment in the face of periodontal disease, either acute or chronic, is contraindicated until the disease stage is either controlled or reversed.
19i. A previous history of TMJ problems or treatment merits pretreatment investigation.
19j. Limitations or problems with opening or closing can indicate TMJ problems.
19k. Familial tendency is indicated in some skeletal patterns, and missing teeth have a documented genetic component.
19l. Dental trauma may have implications during tooth movement due to the increased possibility of root resorption.
19n,o. Habits may explain some aspects of the malocclusion.
22. This helps establish the authenticity of the historian.

FIGURE 6-2 cont'd

A

B

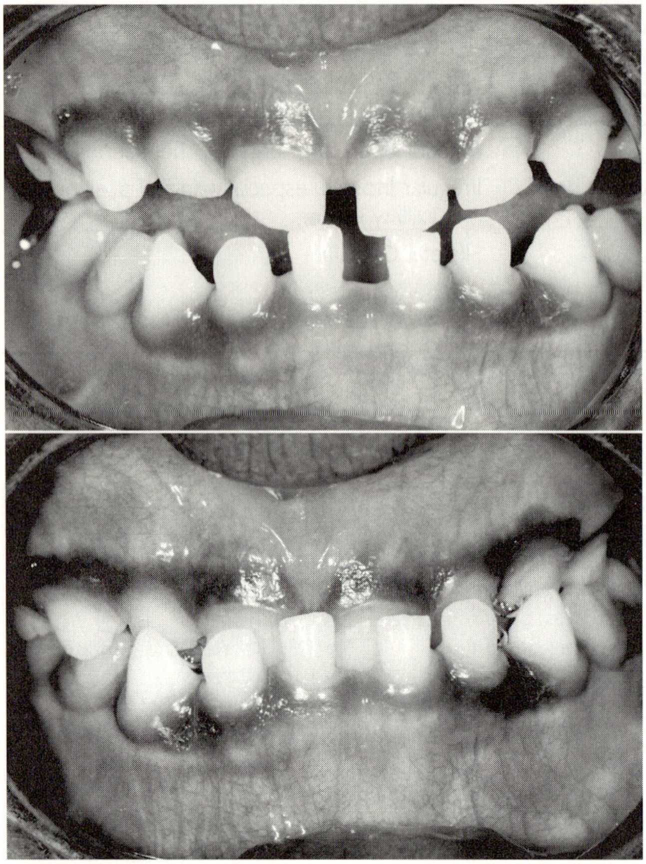

Figure 6-7 The anterior crossbite in this 5-year-old child results largely from an anterior shift of the mandible because of incisor interferences: **A,** Initial contact. **B,** Forward and lateral shift into occlusion. This shift into anterior crossbite is often referred to as a pseudo–Class III relationship because it frequently is not a reflection of a true Class III jaw relationship.

when the occlusal changes produced by orthodontic treatment are nearing completion.

Evaluation of Facial and Dental Appearance

A systematic examination of facial and dental appearance should be done in three steps:

1. The face in all three planes of space (macro-esthetics). Examples of problems that would be noted in that first step would be asymmetry, excessive or deficient face height, mandibular deficiency or excess, etc.
2. The smile framework (mini-esthetics). The smile framework is bordered by the upper and lower lips on smile animation and includes such assessments as excessive gingival display on smile, inadequate anterior tooth display, inappropriate gingival heights, and excessive buccal corridors.
3. The teeth (micro-esthetics). This includes assessment of tooth proportions in height and width, gingival shape and contour, connectors and embrasures, black triangular holes, and tooth shade.

Facial Proportions: Macro-Esthetics

The first step in evaluating facial proportions is to take a good look at the patient, examining him or her for developmental characteristics and a general impression. With faces as with everything else, looking too quickly at the details carries the risk of missing the big picture.

Assessment of Developmental Age. In a step particularly important for children around the age of puberty when most orthodontic treatment is carried out, the patient's developmental age should be assessed. Everyone becomes a more or less accurate judge of other people's ages—we expect to come within a year or two simply by observing the other person's facial appearance. Occasionally, we are fooled, as when we say that a 12-year-old girl looks 15, or a 15-year-old boy looks 12. With adolescents, the judgment is of physical maturity.

The attainment of recognizable secondary sexual characteristics for girls and boys and the correlation between stages of sexual maturation and facial growth are discussed in Chapter 4, and are summarized in Table 6-2. The degree of physical development is much more important than chronologic age in determining how much growth remains.

Facial Esthetics versus Facial Proportions. Because a major reason for orthodontic treatment is to overcome psychosocial difficulties relating to facial and dental appearance and enhance the quality of life in doing so, evaluating dental and facial esthetics is an important part of the clinical examination. Whether a face is considered beautiful is greatly affected by cultural and ethnic factors, but whatever the culture, a disproportionate face becomes a psychosocial problem. For that reason, it helps to recast the purpose of this part of the clinical evaluation as an evaluation of facial proportions, not esthetics per se. Distorted and asymmetric facial features are a major contributor to facial esthetic problems, whereas proportionate features are acceptable if not always beautiful. An appropriate goal for the facial examination therefore is to detect disproportions.

Frontal Examination. The first step in analyzing facial proportions is to examine the face in frontal view. Low set ears, or eyes that are unusually far apart (hypertelorism) may indicate either the presence of a syndrome or a microform of a craniofacial anomaly. If a syndrome is suspected, the patient's hands should be examined for syndactyly, since there are a number of dental-digital syndromes. In the frontal view, one looks for bilateral symmetry in the fifths of the face and for proportionality of the widths of the eyes/nose/mouth (Figure 6-8).

A small degree of bilateral facial asymmetry exists in essentially all normal individuals. This can be revealed most readily by comparing the real full face photograph with composites consisting of two right or two left sides (Figure 6-9). This "normal asymmetry," which usually results from a small size difference between the two sides, should be distinguished from a chin or nose that deviates to one side, which can produce severe disproportion and esthetic problems (see Figure 6-3).

Table 6-2

Adolescent Growth Stages versus Secondary Sexual Characteristics

	Girls **Total duration of adolescent growth: 3½ years**
Stage 1	
Beginning of adolescent growth	Appearance of breast buds, initial pubic hair
Stage 2 (about 12 months later)	
Peak velocity in height	Noticeable breast development, axillary hair, darker/more abundant pubic hair
Stage 3 (12-18 months later)	
Growth spurt ending	Menses, broadening of hips with adult fat distribution, breasts completed
	Boys **Total duration of adolescent growth: 5 years**
Stage 1	
Beginning of adolescent growth	"Fat spurt" weight gain, feminine fat distribution
Stage 2 (about 12 months later)	
Height spurt beginning	Redistribution/reduction in fat, pubic hair, growth of penis
Stage 3 (8-12 months later)	
Peak velocity in height	Facial hair appears on upper lip only, axillary hair, muscular growth with harder/more angular body form
Stage 4 (15-24 months later)	
Growth spurt ending	Facial hair on chin and lip, adult distribution/color of pubic and axillary hair, adult body form

Prior to the advent of cephalometric radiography, dentists and orthodontists often used anthropometric measurements (i.e., measurements made directly during the clinical examination) to help establish facial proportions (Figure 6-10). Although for orthodontists, this method was largely replaced by cephalometric analysis for many years, the recent emphasis on soft tissue proportions has brought soft tissue evaluation back into prominence. Farkas' modern studies of Canadians of northern European origin provided the data for Tables 6-3 and 6-4.[5]

Note that some of the measurements in Table 6-3 could be made on a cephalometric radiograph, but many could not. When there are questions about facial proportions, it is better to make the measurements clinically rather than waiting for the cephalometric analysis, because soft-tissue proportions, as seen clinically, determine facial appearance.

The proportional relationship of facial height to width (the facial index), more than the absolute value of either, establishes the overall facial type and the basic proportions of the face. It is important to remember that face height cannot be evaluated unless face width is known—and face width often is not taken into account when a cephalometric radiograph is analyzed.

The normal values for the facial index and other proportions that may be clinically useful are shown in Table 6-4. Differences in facial types and body types obviously must be taken into account when facial proportions are assessed, and variations from the average ratios can be compatible with good facial esthetics. An important point, however, is to avoid treatment that would change the ratios in the wrong direction—for example, treatment with interarch elastics that could rotate the mandible downward in a patient whose face already is too long for its width.

Finally, the face in frontal view should be examined from the perspective of the vertical facial thirds. The artists of the Renaissance period, primarily da Vinci and Durer, established the proportions that should be used in drawing anatomically correct human faces (Figure 6-11). They concluded that the distance from the hairline to the base of the nose, base of nose to bottom of nose, and nose to chin should be the same. Farkas' studies show that in modern Caucasians of European descent, the lower third is very slightly longer. The artists also saw that the lower third has a proportion of $^1/_3$ to $^2/_3$, and the Farkas data show that this is still true.

It is important to note the cause of vertical problems such as excessive display of the maxillary gingiva, which is done

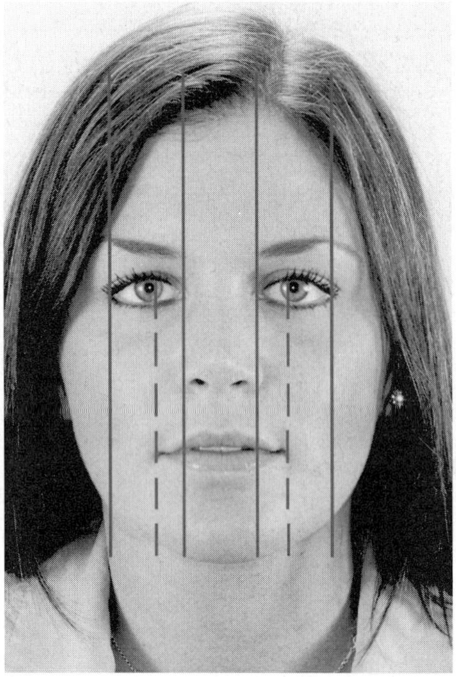

Figure 6-8 Facial proportions and symmetry in the frontal plane. An ideally proportional face can be divided into central, medial, and lateral equal fifths. The separation of the eyes and the width of the eyes, which should be equal, determine the central and medial fifths. The nose and chin should be centered within the central fifth, with the width of the nose the same as or slightly wider than the central fifth. The inter-pupillary distance *(dotted line)* should equal the width of the mouth.

Table 6-3

Facial Anthropometric Measurements (Young Adults)

Parameter	Male	Female
1. Zygomatic width (zy-zy) (mm)	137 (4.3)	130 (5.3)
2. Gonial width (go-go)	97 (5.8)	91 (5.9)
3. Intercanthal distance	33 (2.7)	32 (2.4)
4. Pupil-midfacial distance	33 (2.0)	31 (1.8)
5. Nasal base width	35 (2.6)	31 (1.9)
6. Mouth width	53 (3.3)	50 (3.2)
7. Face height (N-gn)	121 (6.8)	112 (5.2)
8. Lower face height (subnasale-gn)	72 (6.0)	66 (4.5)
9. Upper lip vermilion	8.9 (1.5)	8.4 (1.3)
10. Lower lip vermilion	10.4 (1.9)	9.7 (1.6)
11. Nasolabial angle (degrees)	99 (8.0)	99 (8.7)
12. Nasofrontal angle (degrees)	131 (8.1)	134 (1.8)

Data from Farkas LG: *Anthropometry of the head and face in medicine*, New York, 1981, Elsevier Science Publishing Co.
Measurements are illustrated in Figure 6-10.
Standard deviation is in parenthesis.

A,B

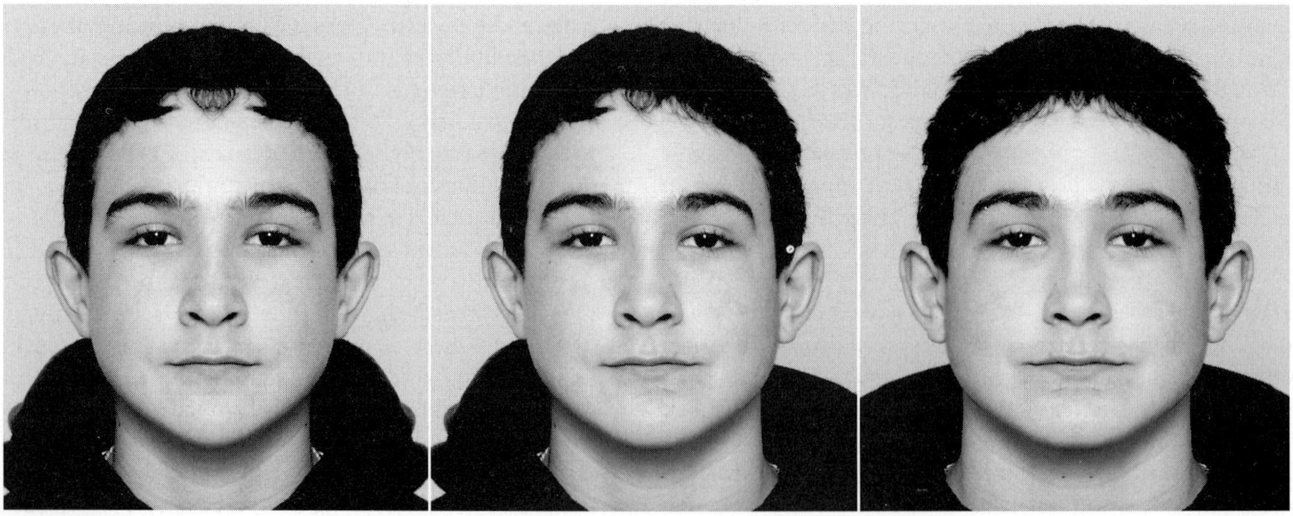

C

Figure 6-9 Composite photographs are the best way to indicate normal facial asymmetry. For this boy, whose mild asymmetry rarely would be noticed and is not a problem, the true photograph is in the center. On the right is a composite of the two right sides, while on the left is a composite of the two left sides. This technique dramatically illustrates the difference in the two sides. Although the normal asymmetry usually is less than in this boy, mild asymmetry is the rule rather than the exception. Usually, the right side of the face is a little larger than the left, rather than the reverse as in this individual.

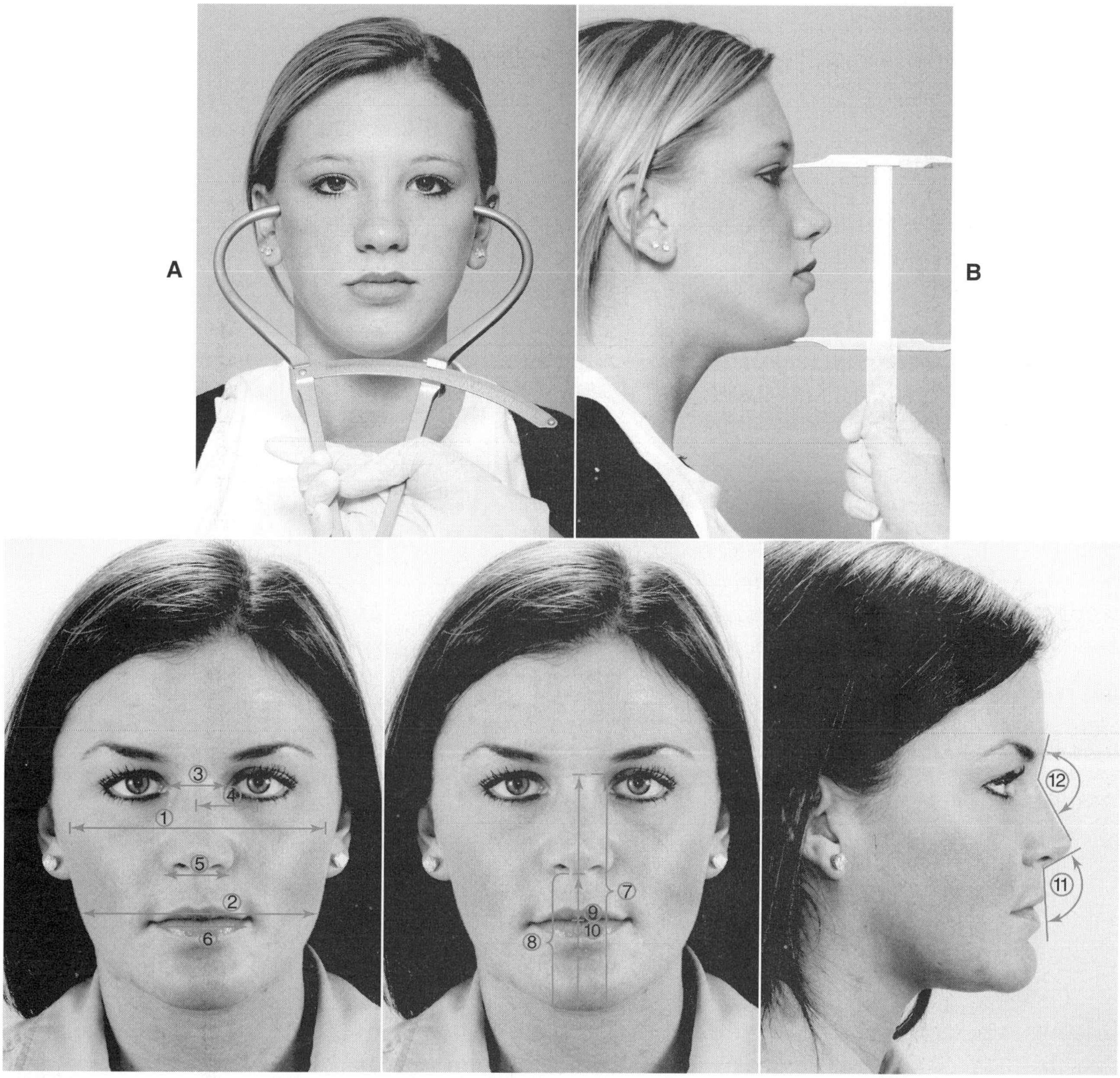

FIGURE 6-10 Facial measurements for anthropometric analysis are made with either bow calipers **(A)** or straight calipers **(B)**. **C** to **E**, Frequently-used facial anthropometric measurements (numbers are keyed to Table 6-3).

best by examining the position of lips and teeth relative to the vertical thirds of the face (Figure 6-12).

Dental-facial characteristics that should be noted as part of the facial examination are shown in Box 6-2. This checklist is just that: a list of things that should be noted systematically during the clinical examination. As in many other things, if you don't look for it, you won't see it. Precise measurements are not necessary, but deviations from the normal should be taken into account when the problem list is developed. Current computer programs already make it possible for an assistant to quickly enter positive findings as the doctor reviews them, and have them "flow through" to the preliminary problem list.

Profile Analysis. A careful examination of the facial profile yields the same information, though in less detail for the underlying skeletal relationships, as that obtained from analysis of lateral cephalometric radiographs. For diagnostic purposes, particularly to identify patients with severe disproportions, careful clinical evaluation is adequate. For this reason, the technique of facial profile analysis has sometimes been called the "poor man's cephalometric analysis." This is a vital diagnostic technique for all dentists. It must be

TABLE 6-4

Facial Indices (Young Adults)

Index	Measurements	Male	Female
Facial	n-gn/zy-zy	88.5 (5.1)	86.2 (4.6)
Mandible-face width	go-go/zy-zy	70.8 (3.8)	70.1 (4.2)
Upper face	n-sto-/zy-zy	54.0 (3.1)	52.4 (3.1)
Mandibular width—face height	go-go/n-gn	80.3 (6.8)	81.7 (6.0)
Mandibular	sto-gn/go-go	51.8 (6.2)	49.8 (4.8)
Mouth-face with	ch-ch × 100/zy-zy	38.9 (2.5)	38.4 (2.5)
Lower face—face height	sn-gn/n-gn	59.2 (2.7)	58.6 (2.9)
Mandible-face height	sto-gn/n-gn	41.2 (2.3)	40.4 (2.1)
Mandible-upper face height	sto-ng/n-sto	67.7 (5.3)	66.5 (4.5)
Mandible-lower face height	sto-ng/sn-gn	69.6 (2.7)	69.1 (2.8)
Chin-face height	sl-gn × 100/sn-gn	25.0 (2.4)	25.4 (1.9)

From Farkas LG, Munro JR: *Anthropometric facial proportions in medicine*, Spring field, III, 1987, Charles C Thomas.
Standard deviation is in parenthesis.

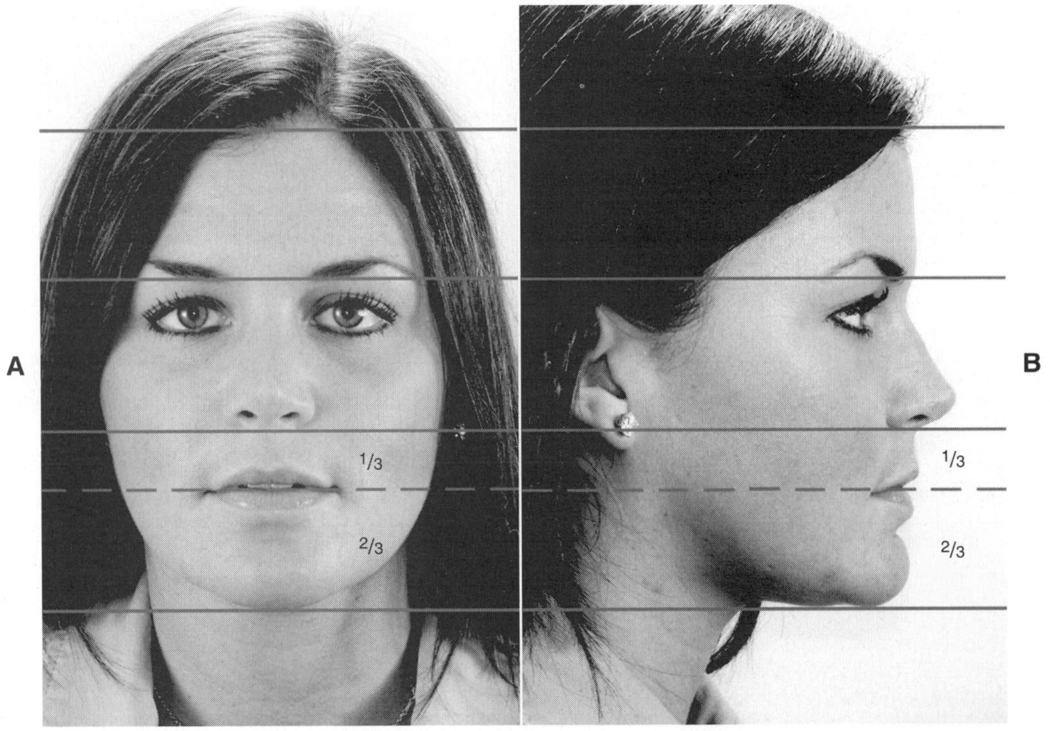

FIGURE 6-11 Vertical facial proportions in the frontal and lateral views are best evaluated in the context of the facial thirds, which the Renaissance artists noted were equal in height in well-proportioned faces. In modern Caucasians, the lower facial third often is slightly longer than the central third. The lower third has thirds: the mouth should be one-third of the way between the base of the nose and the chin.

A

B

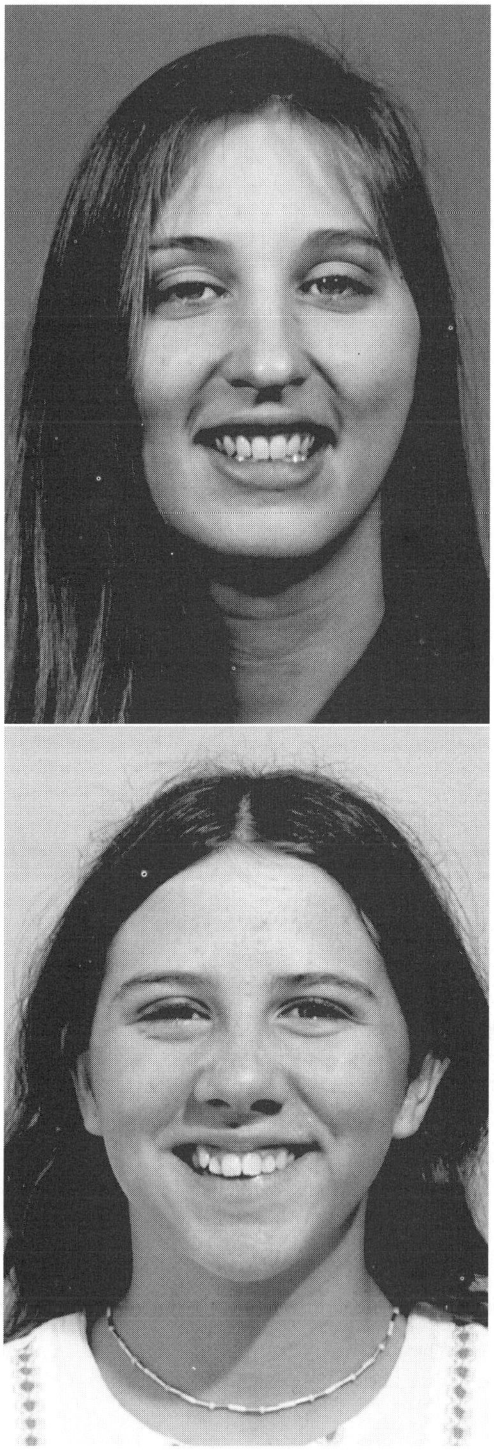

FIGURE 6-12 There are two possible causes of excessive display of maxillary gingiva. The usual cause **(A)** is a long face due to excessive downward growth of the maxilla, which results in a disproportionately long lower third of the face. This should not be confused with **(B)** a short upper lip, which can result in excessive gingival display in a patient with normal facial thirds.

mastered by all those who will see patients for primary care in dentistry, not just by orthodontists.

There are three goals of facial profile analysis, approached in three clear and distinct steps. These are:

1. Establishing whether the jaws are proportionately positioned in the anteroposterior plane of space. This step requires placing the patient in the physiologic natural head position, the head position the individual adopts in the absence of other cues. This can be done with the patient either sitting upright or standing, but not reclining in a dental chair, and looking at the horizon or a distant object. With the head in this position, note the relationship between two lines, one dropped from the bridge of the nose to the base of the upper lip, and a second one extending from that point downward to the chin (Figure 6-13). These line segments should form a nearly straight line. An angle between them indicates either profile convexity (upper jaw prominent relative to chin) or profile concavity (upper jaw behind chin). A convex profile therefore indicates a skeletal Class II jaw relationship, whereas a concave profile indicates a skeletal Class III jaw relationship.

If the profile is approximately straight, it does not matter whether it slopes either anteriorly (anterior divergence) or posteriorly (posterior divergence) (Figure 6-14). Divergence of the face (the term was coined by the eminent orthodontist-anthropologist Milo Hellman[6]) is influenced by the patient's racial and ethnic background. American Indians and Asians, for example, tend to have anteriorly divergent faces, whereas whites of northern European ancestry are likely to be posteriorly divergent. A straight profile line, regardless of whether the face is divergent, does not indicate a problem. Convexity or concavity does.

2. Evaluation of lip posture and incisor prominence. Detecting excessive incisor protrusion (which is relatively common) or retrusion (which is rare) is important because of the effect on space within the dental arches. If the incisors protrude, they align themselves on the arc of a larger circle as they lean forward, whereas if the incisors are upright or retrusive, less space is available (Figure 6-15). In the extreme case, incisor protrusion can produce ideal alignment of the teeth instead of severely crowded incisors, at the expense of lips that protrude and are difficult to bring into function over the protruding teeth. This is *bimaxillary dentoalveolar protrusion,* meaning simply that in both jaws the teeth protrude (Figure 6-16). Dentists often refer to the condition as just *bimaxillary protrusion,* a simpler term but a misnomer since it is not the jaws but the teeth that protrude. (Physical anthropologists use bimaxillary protrusion to describe faces in which both jaws are prominent relative to the cranium. Such a face would have an anteriorly divergent profile if jaw sizes were proportional.)

Determining how much incisor prominence is too much can be difficult but is simplified by understanding the relationship between lip posture and the position of the incisors. The teeth protrude excessively if (and only if) two conditions are met: (1) the lips are prominent and everted, and (2) the

Box 6-2

CHECKLIST OF FACIAL DIMENSIONS TO EVALUATE DURING CLINICAL EXAMINATION

Frontal at Rest

To mid-sagittal plane
- Nasal tip
- Maxillary dental mid-line
- Mandibular dental mid-line
- Chin (mid-symphysis)

Vertical
- Lip separation (lips relaxed)
- Lip vermilion display
- Maxillary incisor display (lips relaxed)
- Lower face height
- Philtrum length
- Commissure height
- Chin height

Frontal Smile
- Maxillary incisor display
- Maxillary incisor crown height
- Gingival display
- Smile arc
- Occlusal plane cant?

Frontal Widths
- Alar base
- Nasal tip
- Buccal corridor

Profile

Lower face
- Maxillary projection
- Mandibular projection
- Chin projection
- Lower face height

Nose
- Nasal radix
- Nasal dorsum contour
- Nasal tip projection

Lips
- Lip fullness
- Labiomental sulcus

Throat form
- Chin–throat angle
- Throat length
- Submental contour (fat pad)

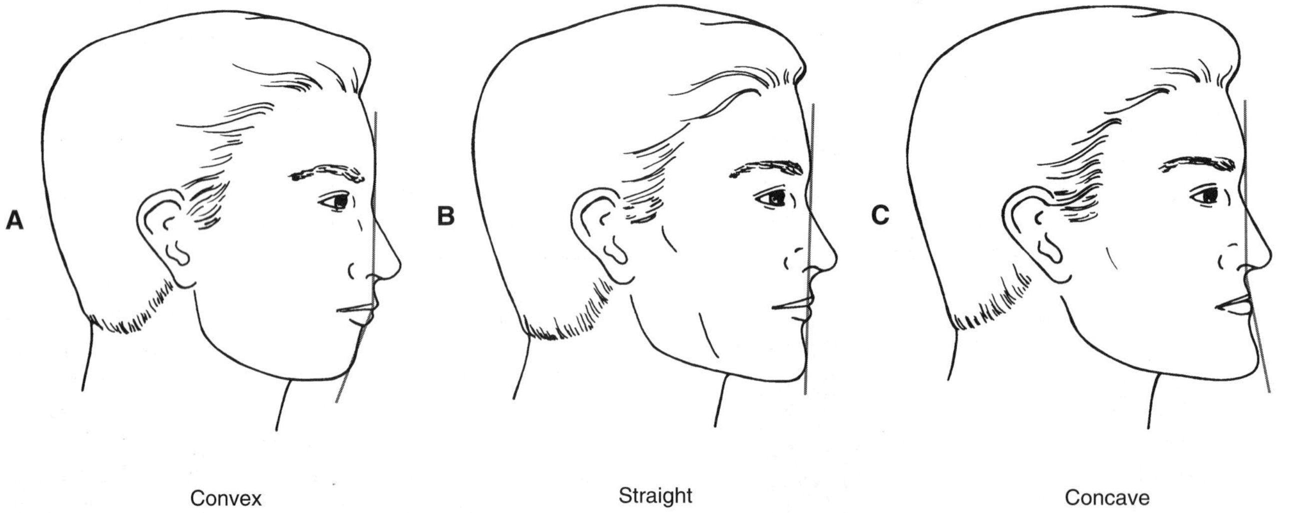

Figure 6-13 Profile convexity or concavity results from a disproportion in the size of the jaws, but does not by itself indicate which jaw is at fault. A convex facial profile **(A)** indicates a Class II jaw relationship, which can result from either a maxilla that projects too far forward or a mandible too far back. A concave profile **(C)** indicates a Class III relationship, which can result from either a maxilla that is too far back or a mandible that protrudes forward.

lips are separated at rest by more than 3 to 4 mm (which is sometimes termed *lip incompetence*). In other words, excessive protrusion of the incisors is revealed by prominent lips that are separated when they are relaxed, so that the patient must strain to bring the lips together over the protruding teeth (see Figure 6-16). For such a patient, retracting the teeth tends to improve both lip function and facial esthetics. On the other hand, if the lips are prominent but close over the teeth without strain, the lip posture is largely independent of tooth position. For that individual, retracting the incisor teeth would have little effect on lip function or prominence.

Like facial divergence, lip prominence is strongly influenced by racial and ethnic characteristics. Whites of northern European backgrounds often have relatively thin lips, with minimal lip and incisor prominence. Whites of southern European and middle eastern origin normally have more lip and incisor prominence than their northern cousins.

A,B 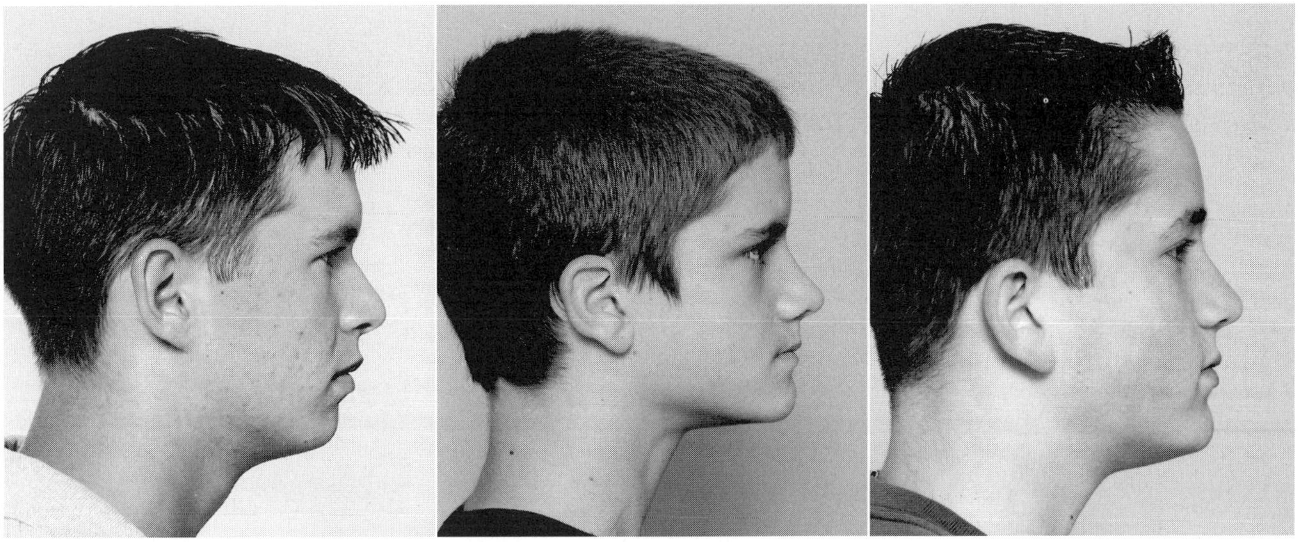 C

Figure 6-14 Divergence of the face is defined as an anterior or posterior inclination of the lower face relative to the forehead. Divergence of a straight profile line does not indicate facial or dental disproportions: all the individuals pictured here have normal dental occlusion and an acceptable dental and facial appearance. To some extent, facial divergence is a racial and ethnic characteristic. It must be distinguished from the profile convexity or concavity that does indicate disproportions. **A,** Despite this boy's posteriorly divergent profile, he has only minimal overjet and no complaints about facial esthetics. This facial pattern is particularly likely in northern Europeans. **B,** A straight profile produces a strong chin and a more masculine appearance. It is seen more frequently in whites of eastern and southern European descent, and is the usual finding in those of Asian and African descent. **C,** An anteriorly divergent profile is uncommon in whites but often is seen in those of Asian and African descent. It is quite compatible with normal dental occlusion.

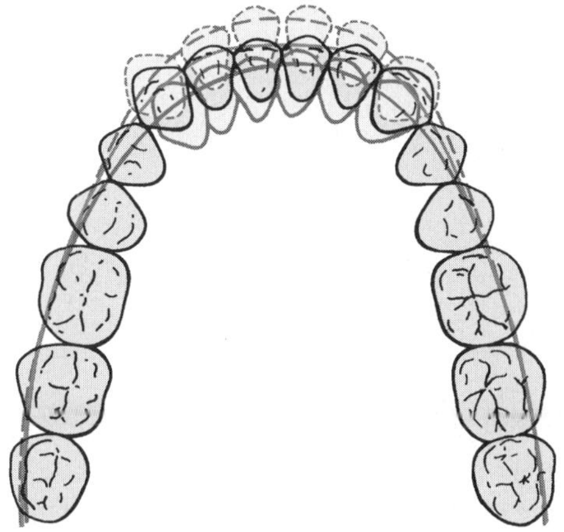

Figure 6-15 If the incisors flare forward, they can align themselves along the arc of a larger circle, which provides more space to accommodate the teeth and alleviates crowding. Conversely, if the incisors move lingually, there is less space, and crowding becomes worse. For this reason, crowding and protrusion of incisors must be considered two aspects of the same thing: how crowded and irregular the incisors are reflects both how much room is available and where the incisors are positioned relative to supporting bone.

Greater degrees of lip and incisor prominence normally occur in individuals of Asians and African descent, so a lip and tooth position normal for Asians or blacks would be excessively protrusive for most whites.

Lip posture and incisor prominence should be evaluated by viewing the profile with the patient's lips relaxed. This is done by relating the upper lip to a true vertical line passing through the concavity at the base of the upper lip (soft tissue point A) and by relating the lower lip to a similar true vertical line through the concavity between the lower lip and chin (soft tissue point B) (Figure 6-17). If the lip is significantly forward from this line, it can be judged to be prominent; if the lip falls behind the line, it is retrusive. If the lips are both prominent and incompetent (separated by more than 3 to 4 mm), the anterior teeth are excessively protrusive.

In evaluating lip protrusion, it is important to keep in mind that everything is relative, and in this case the relationships that count are the lip relationships with the nose and chin. The larger the nose, the more prominent the chin must be to balance it, and the greater the amount of lip prominence that will be esthetically acceptable (Figure 6-18). Vertical facial and dental relationships also play a role here. Some patients with short lower face height have everted and protrusive lips because they are over-closed and the upper lip presses against the lower lip, not because the teeth protrude.

A,B 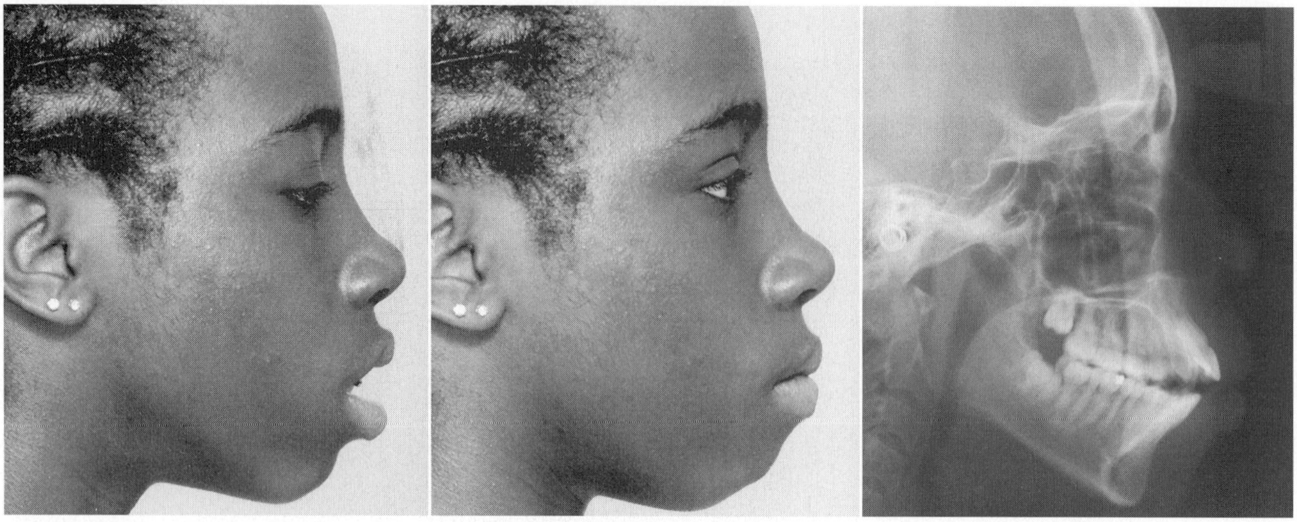 C

FIGURE 6-16 Bimaxillary dentoalveolar protrusion is seen in the facial appearance in three ways: **A,** Excessive separation of the lips at rest (lip incompetence). The general guideline (which holds for all racial groups) is that lip separation at rest should be not more than 4 mm. **B,** Excessive effort to bring the lips into closure (lip strain): and prominence of lips in the profile view (as in both **A** and **B**). Remember that all three soft tissue characteristics must be present to make the diagnosis of dental protrusion, not just protruding teeth as seen in a cephalometric radiograph (**C,** the ceph for the same girl). Different racial groups, and individuals within those groups, have different degrees of lip prominence that are independent of tooth position. As a result, excessive dental protrusion must be a clinical diagnosis. It cannot be made accurately from cephalometric radiographs.

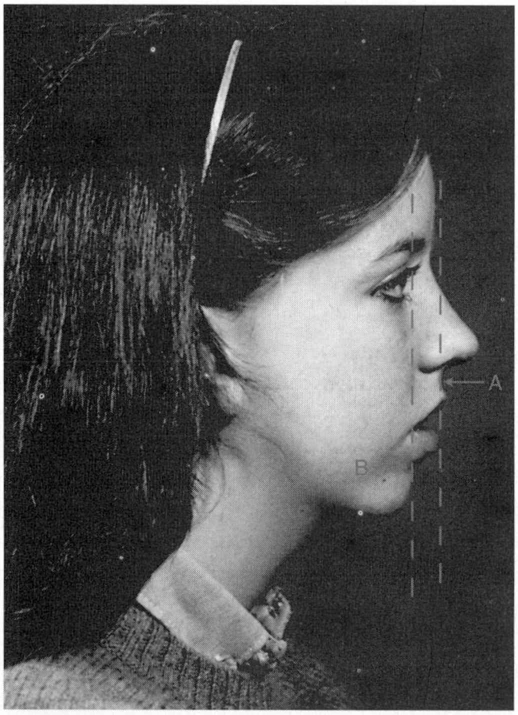

FIGURE 6-17 Lip prominence is evaluated by observing the distance that each lip projects forward from a true vertical line through the depth of the concavity at its base (soft tissue points A and B) (i.e., a different reference line is used for each lip, as shown here). Lip prominence of more than 2 to 3 mm in the presence of lip incompetence (excessive separation of the lips at rest, as in this girl), indicates dentoalveolar protrusion.

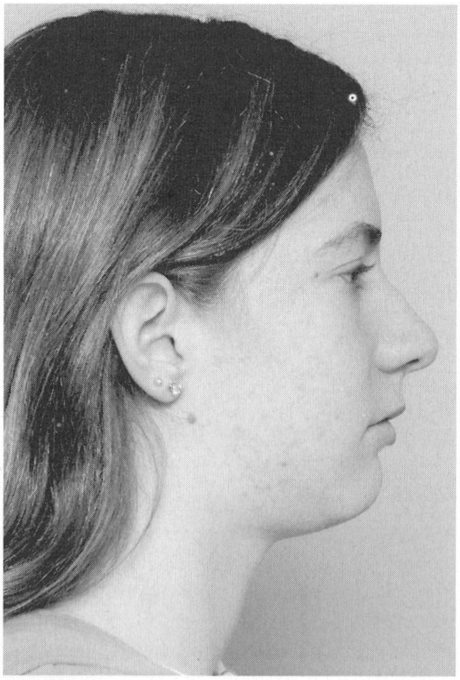

FIGURE 6-18 For this girl with Class II malocclusion, retraction of the maxillary incisors would damage facial appearance by making the relatively large nose look even bigger. The size of the nose must be considered when the position of the incisors and amount of lip support are evaluated.

A 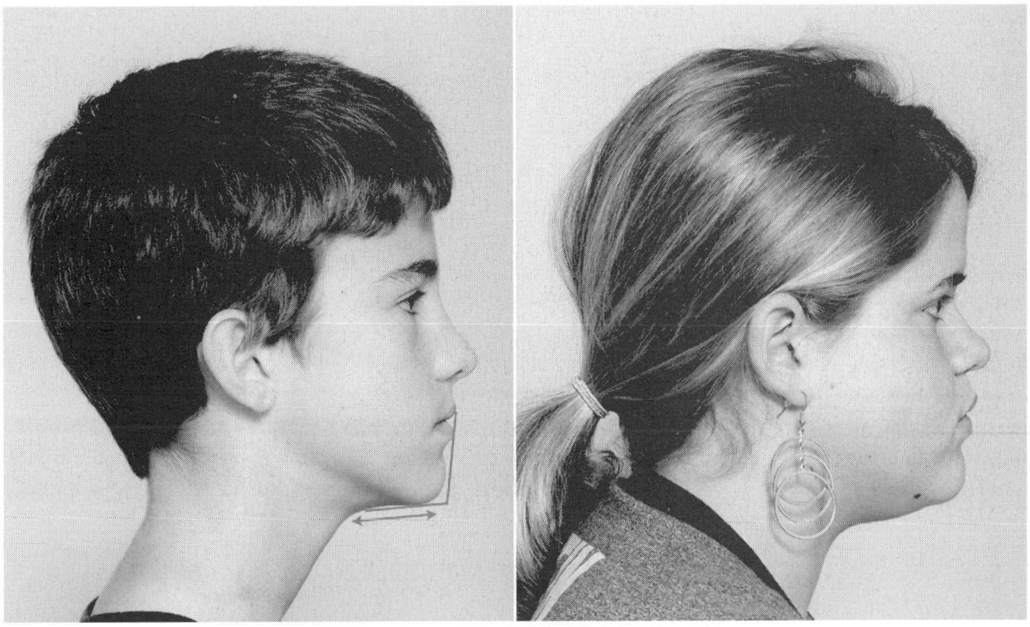 B

Figure 6-19 Throat form is evaluated in terms of the contour of the submental tissues (straight is better), chin-throat angle (which ideally should be close to 90°) and throat length (longer is better, up to a point). Both submental fat deposition and a low tongue posture contribute to a stepped throat contour, which becomes a "double chin" when extreme. **A,** For this boy whose Class II malocclusion has a component of mandibular deficiency, throat contour and the chin–throat angle are good but throat length is short (as usually is the case when the mandible is short). **B,** For this girl with a similar Class II malocclusion but better jaw proportions, throat contour is affected by submental fat and the chin-throat angle is somewhat obtuse, but throat length is good.

Not only the prominence of the chin, but also the submental soft tissue contours, should be evaluated. Throat form is an important factor in establishing optimal facial esthetics, and poor throat form is a major contributor to esthetic impairment in patients with mandibular deficiency (Figure 6-19).

3. Re-evaluation of vertical facial proportions, and evaluation of mandibular plane angle. Vertical proportions can be observed during the full face examination (see above) but sometimes can be seen more clearly in profile. In the clinical examination, the inclination of the mandibular plane to the true horizontal should be noted. The mandibular plane is visualized readily by placing a finger or mirror handle along the lower border (Figure 6-20). This is important because a steep mandibular plane angle usually indicates long anterior facial vertical dimensions and a skeletal open bite tendency, while a flat mandibular plane angle often correlates with short anterior facial height and deep bite malocclusion.

Facial form analysis carried out this way takes only a couple of minutes but provides information that simply is not present from dental radiographs and casts. Such an evaluation by the primary care practitioner is an essential part of the evaluation of every prospective orthodontic patient.

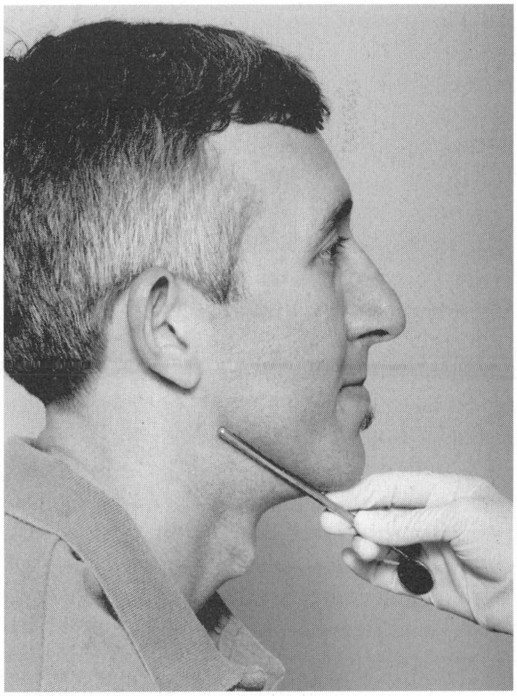

Figure 6-20 The mandibular plane angle can be visualized clinically by placing a mirror handle or other instrument along the border of the mandible. For this patient the mandibular plane angle is normal, neither too steep nor too flat.

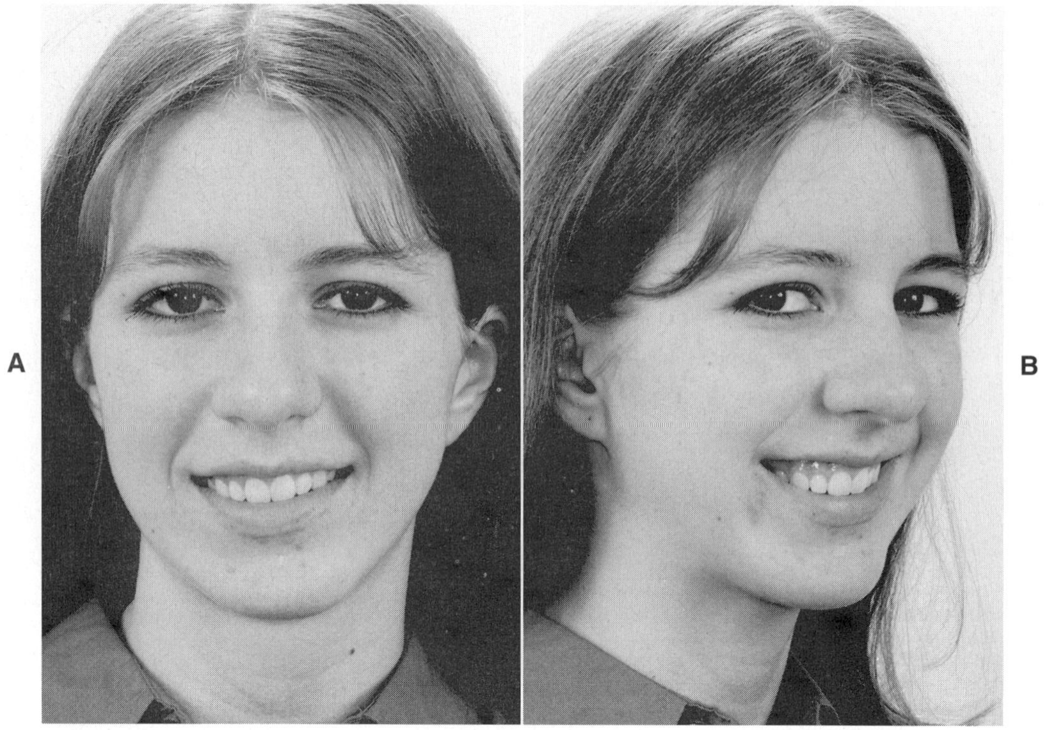

FIGURE 6-21 A cant to the occlusal plane can be seen in both frontal **(A)** and oblique **(B)** views. It becomes an esthetic problem if it is noticeable, and lay observers do notice a cant of this degree of severity.

Tooth–Lip Relationships: Mini-Esthetics

Tooth–Lip Relationships. It is important to evaluate not only the characteristics of the face, but the relationship of the dentition to the face (see Box 6-2). This can begin with an examination of symmetry, in which it is particularly important to note the relationship of the dental midline of each arch to the skeletal midline of that jaw (i.e., the lower incisor midline related to the midline of the mandible, and the upper incisor midline related to the midline of the maxilla). Dental casts, even if mounted on an articulator, will show the relationship of the midlines to each other but provide no information about the dental-skeletal midlines. This must be recorded during the clinical examination.

A second aspect of dental to soft tissue relationships is the vertical relationship of the teeth to the lips, at rest and on smile. At a minimum, the amount of incisor display should be noted. For patients with excessive incisor display, the usual cause is a long lower third of the face, but of course that is not the only possibility—a short upper lip could produce the same thing (see Figure 6-12). Recording lip height at the philtrum and the commissures can clarify the source of the problem.

A third important relationship to note is whether an up-down transverse rotation of the dentition is revealed when the patient smiles or the lips are separated at rest (Figure 6-21). This often is called a transverse cant of the occlusal plane, but is better described as a transverse roll of the esthetic line of the dentition (see the section of this chapter below on classification by dentofacial traits). Neither dental casts nor a photograph with lip retractors will reveal this. Dentists detect a transverse roll at 1mm from side to side, where laypersons are more forgiving and see it only at 3mm—but at that point, it is a problem.[7]

Smile Analysis. Facial attractiveness is defined more by the smile than by soft tissue relationships at rest. For this reason, it is important to analyze the characteristics of the smile, and to think about how the dentition relates to the facial soft tissues dynamically as well as statically. There are two types of smiles: the posed or social smile, and the emotional smile. The social smile is reproducible, and is the one that is presented to the world routinely. The emotional smile varies with the emotion being displayed (for instance, the smile when you're introduced to a new colleague differs from the smile when your team just won in the year's biggest upset). The social smile is the focus of orthodontic diagnosis.

In smile analysis, the oblique ($^3/_4$) view as well as the frontal and profile views are important. Three things need to be considered:

Amount of Incisor and Gingival Display. The guideline is that elevation of the upper lip on smile should stop at or near the gingival margin, so that all of the upper incisor is seen. Some display of gingiva is acceptable, and can be both esthetic and youthful appearing. Lip elevation that does not

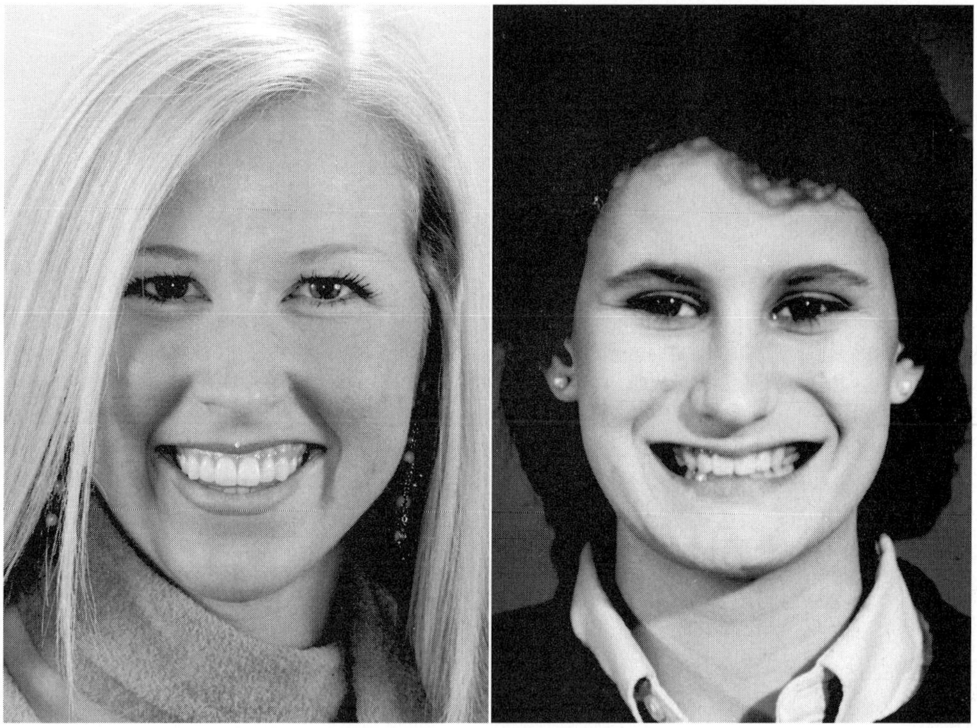
A B

Figure 6-22 **A,** Display of all the incisors and some maxillary gingiva on smiling is a youthful and appealing characteristic. **B,** Less display is less attractive although it is not considered objectionable by lay observers.

reach 100% display of the incisor crowns is less attractive (Figure 6-22). Although lay observers usually rate a smile as acceptable if there is 2 mm or more display of the maxillary incisors,[7] display of 75% of the crowns is about the minimum for excellent esthetics, and it is better to display some gingiva than too little of the incisor crowns.

It also is important to remember that the vertical relationship of the lip to the incisors will change over time, with the amount of incisor exposure decreasing (see Chapter 4). This makes it even more important to note the vertical tooth-lip relationships during the diagnostic evaluation, and to keep it in mind during treatment.

Transverse Dimensions of the Smile Relative to the Upper Arch. Depending on the facial index, i.e., the width of the face relative to its height, a broad smile may be more attractive than a narrow one—but what does that mean exactly? A dimension of interest to prosthodontists, and more recently to orthodontists, is the amount of buccal corridor that is displayed on smile, that is, the distance between the maxillary posterior teeth (especially the premolars) and the inside of the cheek (Figure 6-23). Prosthodontists consider that excessively wide buccal corridors (sometimes called "negative space") are unesthetic, and orthodontists have noted that widening the maxillary arch can improve the appearance of the smile if cheek drape is significantly wider than the dental arch. Early studies of smile esthetics in the natural dentition did not suggest that buccal corridor width was an important consideration.[8] Recent studies have indicated, however, that lay persons can detect differences in buccal corridor width, and that they tend to prefer wider dental arches and narrower buccal corridors even though wide corridors often are judged acceptable.[9,10]

It should be kept in mind, however, that arch expansion like anything else, can be overdone. Too broad a smile, so that there is no buccal corridor, is unesthetic and can be characterized as making the natural dentition look like a cheap denture. The transverse width of the dental arches, therefore, can and should be related to the width of the face (Figure 6-24). The relationship of the cheeks to the posterior teeth on smile is just another way of evaluating this relationship.

The Smile Arc. The smile arc is defined as the contour of the incisal edges of the maxillary anterior teeth relative to the curvature of the lower lip during a social smile (Figure 6-25). For best appearance, the contour of these teeth should match that of the lower lip. If the lip and dental contours match, they are said to be consonant.

Good evidence exists now that a consonant (ideal) smile arc is an important aspect of smile esthetics. Lay observers significantly prefer an ideal smile arc, and a flattened smile arc decreases the attractiveness of a male or female smile.[9] A flattened smile arc can pose either or both of two problems: It is less attractive, and it tends to make the patient look older (because older individuals often have wear of the incisors that tends to flatten the arc of the teeth). The characteristics of the smile arc must be monitored during orthodontic

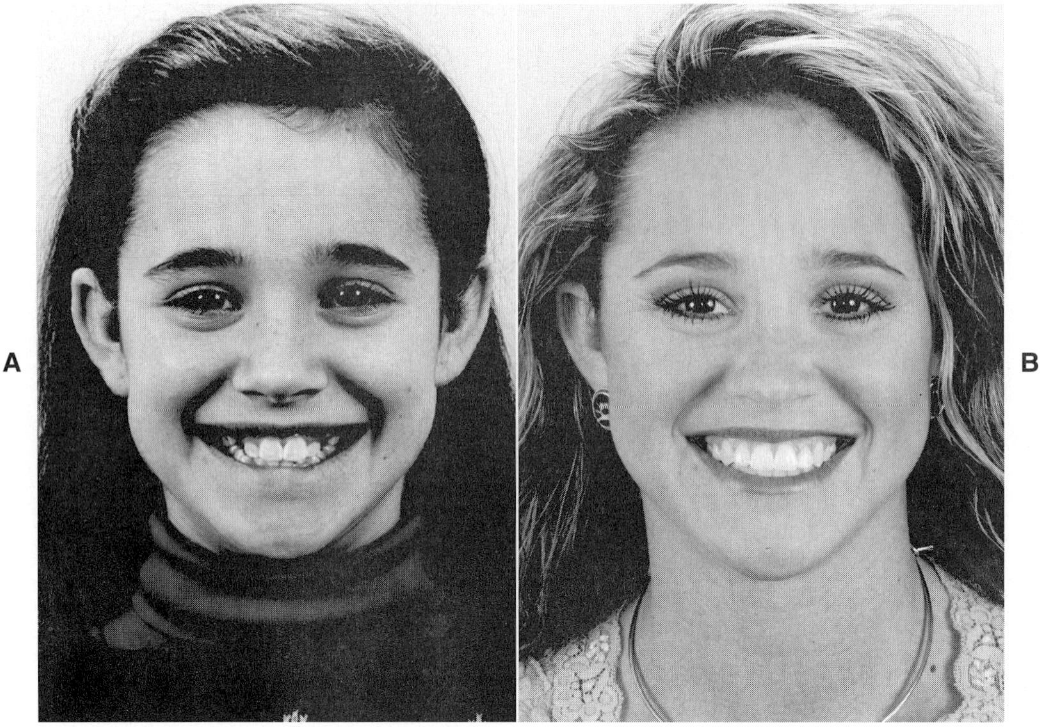

Figure 6-23 **A,** Prior to treatment, this girl had a narrow maxillary arch with wide buccal corridors. She was treated with arch expansion. **B,** On 5-year recall, the broader smile (with narrow but not obliterated buccal corridors) is part of the esthetic improvement created by orthodontic treatment.

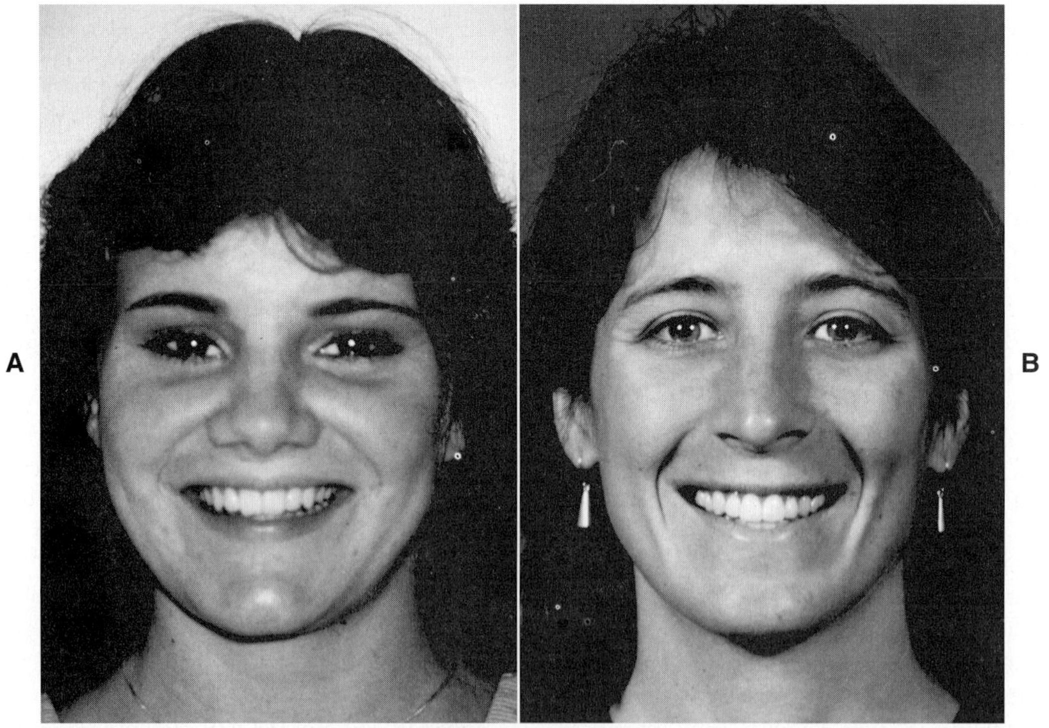

Figure 6-24 The width of the maxillary dental arch, as seen on smile, should be proportional to the width of the mid-face. **A,** A broad smile is appropriate for a face with relatively large width across the zygomatic arches, while **(B)** a narrower smile is preferred when the face width is narrow. The patient in **B** was appropriately treated with maxillary premolar extraction to prevent over-expansion during treatment.

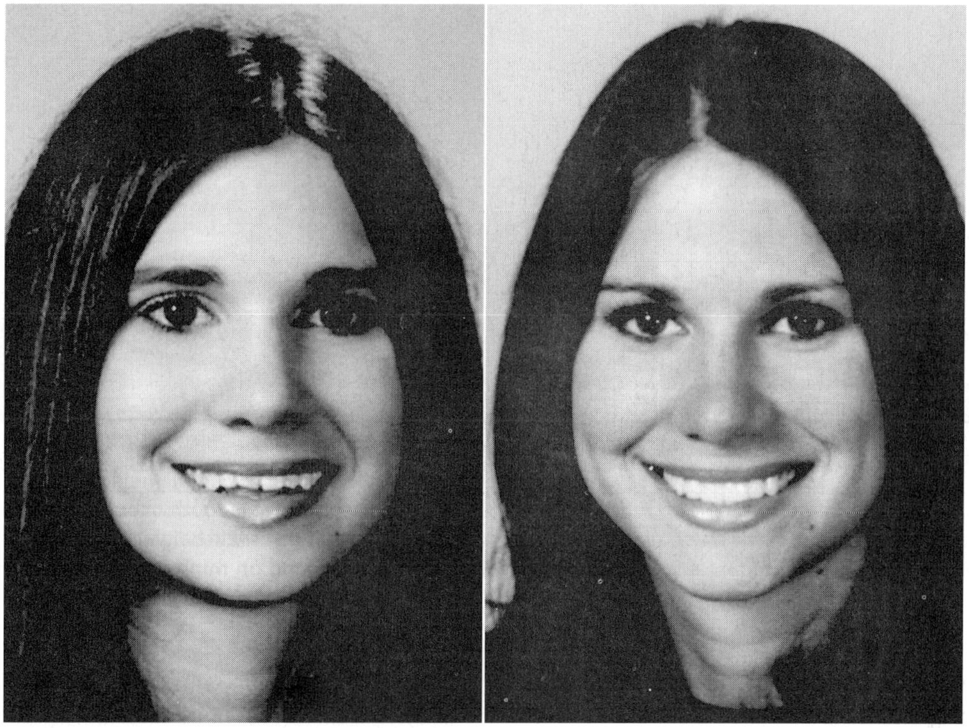

FIGURE 6-25 The smile arc is the relationship of the curvature of the lower lip to the curvature of the maxillary incisors. The appearance of the smile is best when the curvatures match. **A,** A flattened smile arc is less attractive in both males and females. **B,** The improvement in this girl's smile was created solely by lengthening her maxillary incisors—in her case, with dental laminates rather than orthodontics.

treatment because it is surprisingly easy to flatten it in the pursuit of other treatment objectives. The data indicate that this is much more important as a factor in smile esthetics than buccal corridor width.

Dental Appearance: Micro-Esthetics

Subtleties in the proportions and shape of the teeth and associated gingival contours have been emphasized in the burgeoning literature on "cosmetic dentistry" in recent years. A similar evaluation is necessary in the development of an orthodontic problem list if an optimal esthetic result is to be obtained. Treatment planning to correct problems of this type is discussed in Chapter 8.

Tooth Proportions. The smile, of course, reveals the maxillary anterior teeth, and two aspects of proportional relationships are important components of their appearance: the tooth widths in relation to each other, and the height/width proportions of the individual teeth.

Width Relationships and the "Golden Proportion." The apparent widths of the maxillary anterior teeth on smile, and their actual mesio-distal width, differ because of the curvature of the dental arch. Particularly, only a portion of the canine crown can be seen in a frontal view. For best appearance, the apparent width of the lateral incisor (as one would perceive it from a direct frontal examination) should be 62% of the width of the central incisor, the apparent width of the canine should be 62% of that of the lateral incisor, and the apparent width of the first premolar should be 62% of that of the canine (Figure 6-26). This ratio of recurring 62% proportions appears in a number of other relationships in human anatomy, and sometimes is referred to as the "golden proportion." Whether or not it has any mystic significance,

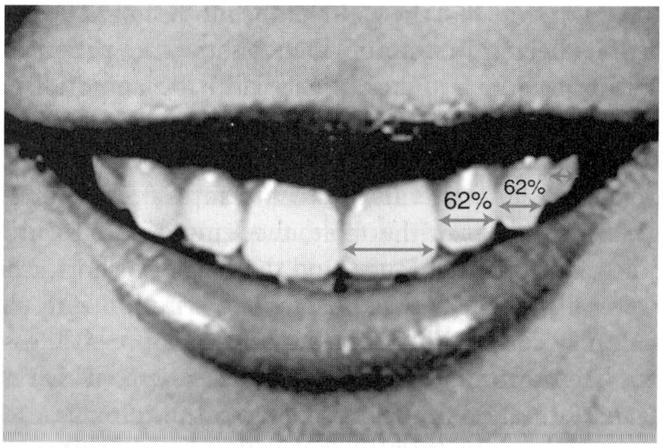

FIGURE 6-26 Ideal tooth width proportions when viewed from the front are one of many illustrations of the "golden proportion," 1.0 : 0.62 : 0.38 : 0.24, etc. In this close-up view of attractive teeth on smile, it can be seen that the width of the lateral incisor is 62% of the width of the central incisor; the (apparent) width of the canine is 62% of the width of the lateral incisor; and the (apparent) width of the first premolar is 62% of the width of the canine.

TABLE 6-6

Moyers Prediction Values (75% level)

Total mandibular-incisor width		19.5	20.0	20.5	21.0	21.5	22.0	22.5	23.0
Predicted width of canine and premolars	Maxilla	20.6	20.9	21.2	21.3	21.8	22.0	22.3	22.6
	Mandible	20.1	20.4	20.7	21.0	21.3	21.6	21.9	22.2

From Moyers RE: Handbook of orthodontics, ed 3, Chicago, 1973, Mosby.

A

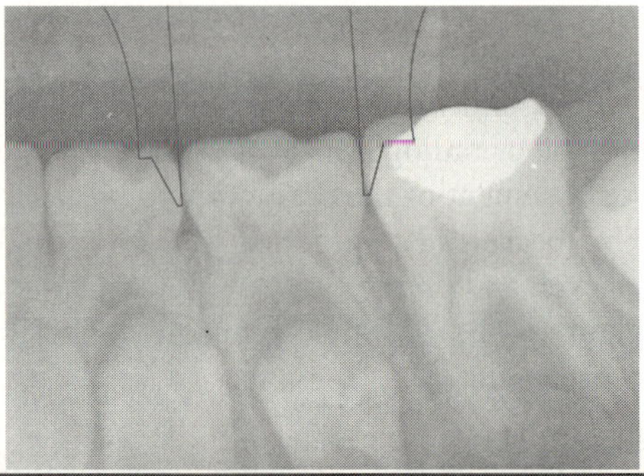

B

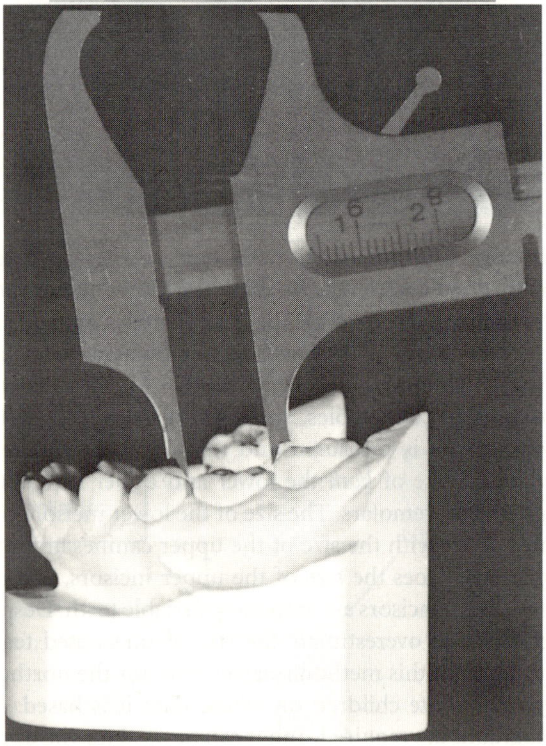

FIGURE 6-35 To correct for magnification in films, the same object is measured on the cast **(B)** and on the film **(A)**, which will yield the percentage of magnification. This ratio is used to correct for magnification on unerupted teeth.

both arches and under-estimate the space required in the lower arch for African-American males.[19]

Most computer algorithms for space analysis are based on correlations of tooth sizes, and should be used with caution if the radiographs show anything unusual (unless the computer program allows for introduction of radiographic information).

3. Combination of radiographic and prediction table methods. Since the major problem with using radiographic images comes in evaluating the canine teeth, it would seem reasonable to use the size of permanent incisors measured from the dental casts and the size of unerupted premolars measured from the radiographs to predict the size of unerupted canines. A graph developed by Staley and Kerber from Iowa growth data (Figure 6-36) allows canine width to be read directly from the sum of incisor and premolar widths. This method can be used only for the mandibular arch and, of course, requires periapical radiographs. For children of European ancestry, it is quite accurate.

Which of these methods is best for an individual patient depends on the circumstances. The prediction tables work surprisingly well when applied to the population group from which they were developed. The Moyers, Tanaka-Johnston, and Staley-Kerber predictions are all based on data from white school children of northern European descent. If the patient fits this population group, the Staley-Kerber method will give the best prediction, followed by the Tanaka-Johnston and Moyers approaches that are the basis of most computer algorithms. These methods are superior to measurement from radiographs. On balance, the Tanaka-Johnston method probably is most practical for manual calculation because no radiographs are required and the simple ratio can be printed right on the space analysis form, so that no reference tables must be consulted.

On the other hand, if the patient does not fit the population group, as an African or Asian child would not, direct measurement from the radiographs is the best approach and

Box 6-3

TANAKA AND JOHNSTON PREDICTION VALUES

One half of the mesiodistal width of the four lower incisors	+10.5 m =	estimated width of mandibular canine and premolars in one quadrant
	+11.0 mm =	estimated width of maxillary canine and premolars in one quadrant

From Tanaka MM, Johnston LE: *J Am Dent Assoc* 88:798, 1974.

23.5	24.0	24.5	25.0	25.5	26.0	26.5	27.0	27.5	28.0	28.5	29.0
22.9	23.1	23.4	23.7	24.0	24.2	24.5	24.8	25.0	25.3	25.6	25.9
22.5	22.8	23.1	23.4	23.7	24.0	24.3	24.6	24.8	25.1	25.4	25.7

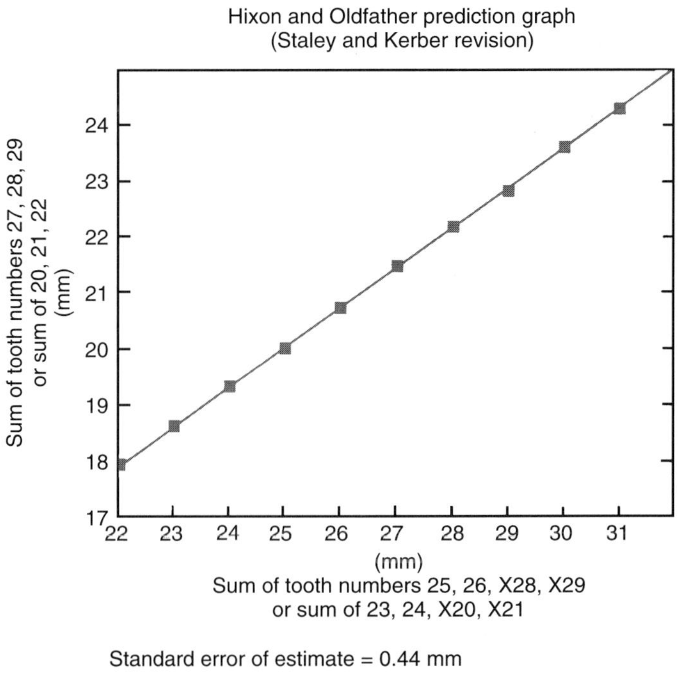

FIGURE 6-36 Graph showing relationship between size of lower incisors measured from cast plus lower first and second premolars measured from radiographs *(x-axis)* and size of canine plus premolars *(y-axis)*. (Redrawn from Staley RN, Kerber RE. Am J Orthod 78:296-302, 1980.)

TABLE 6-7

Tooth Size Relationships

Maxillary anterior sum of 3-3	Mandibular anterior sum of 3-3	Maxillary total sum of 6-6	Mandibular total sum of 6-6
40	30.9	86	78.5
41	31.7	88	80.3
42	32.4	90	82.1
43	33.2	92	84.0
44	34.0	94	85.8
45	34.7	96	87.6
46	35.5	98	89.5
47	36.3	100	91.3
48	37.1	102	93.1
49	37.8	104	95.0
50	38.6	106	96.8
51	39.4	108	98.6
52	40.1	110	100.4
53	40.9		
54	41.7		
55	42.5		

computer analysis should be avoided unless a modified equation from Tanaka-Johnston is available for that particular group. In addition, if obvious anomalies in tooth size or form are seen in the radiographs, the correlation methods (which assume normal tooth size relationships) should not be used.

A contemporary form for mixed dentition space analysis is shown in Figure 6-37. Note that: (1) a correction for mesial movement of the lower molars following the exchange of the dentition is included, (2) the Tanaka-Johnston method for predicting the size of unerupted canines and premolars is used, and (3) the result from facial form analysis is requested to check for appropriateness of the entire method and for interpretation of the results. A screen capture from computer analysis is shown in Figure 6-38. Computer analysis is faster and easier, but its accuracy will depend on how well the patient meets the assumptions that underlie its approach.

Tooth Size Analysis

For good occlusion, the teeth must be proportional in size. If large upper teeth are combined with small lower teeth, as in a denture setup with mismatched sizes, there is no way to achieve ideal occlusion. Although the natural teeth match very well in most individuals, approximately 5% of the population have some degree of disproportion among the sizes of individual teeth. This is defined as *tooth size discrepancy.* An anomaly in the size of the upper lateral incisors is the most common cause, but variation in premolars or other teeth may be present. Occasionally, all the upper teeth will be too large or too small to fit properly with the lower teeth.

Tooth size analysis, sometimes called Bolton analysis after its developer,[20] is carried out by measuring the mesiodistal width of each permanent tooth. A standard table (Table 6-7) is then used to compare the summed widths of the

UNIVERSITY OF NORTH CAROLINA AT CHAPEL HILL
SCHOOL OF DENTISTRY

SPACE ANALYSIS FORM

Patient's Name: ______________________ Date: __________

SECTION 1
AVAILABLE MANDIBULAR SPACE

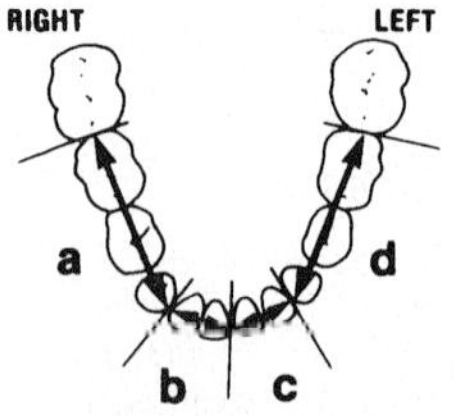

Arch Segment Lengths

a: _____mm
b: _____mm
c: _____mm
d: _____mm
TOTAL: _____mm

SECTION 2
MANDIBULAR INCISOR WIDTH

#23: _____mm
#24: _____mm
#25: _____mm
#26: _____mm
TOTAL: _____mm

SECTION 3
AVAILABLE MAXILLARY SPACE

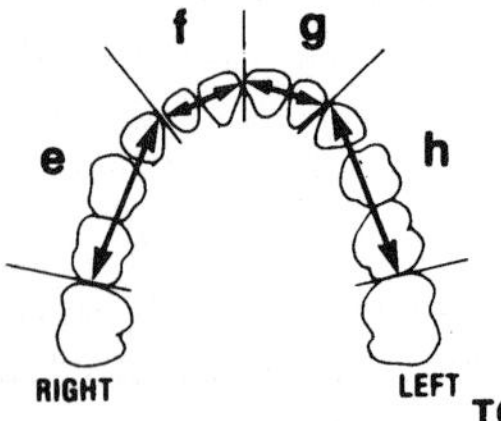

Arch Segment Lengths

e: _____mm
f: _____mm
g: _____mm
h: _____mm
TOTAL: _____mm

SECTION 4
MAXILLARY INCISOR WIDTH

#7: _____mm
#8: _____mm
#9: _____mm
#10: _____mm
TOTAL: _____mm

SECTION 5
MANDIBULAR SPACE ANALYSIS

a. TOTAL SPACE AVAILABLE *(from Section 1)* _____
b. SUM OF MAND. INCISOR WIDTHS *(from Section 2)* _____
c. SUM OF LEFT CANINE & PREMOLARS *(estimated below from mand. incisors)* _____
d. SUM OF RIGHT CANINE & PREMOLARS *(estimated below from mand. incisors)* _____
e. TOTAL SPACE REQUIRED *(b + c + d)* _____
f. DISCREPANCY *(a – e)* _____

SECTION 6
MAXILLARY SPACE ANALYSIS

a. TOTAL SPACE AVAILABLE *(from Section 3)* _____
b. SUM OF MAX. INCISOR WIDTHS *(from Section 4)* _____
c. SUM OF RIGHT CANINE & PREMOLARS *(estimated below from mand. incisors)* _____
d. SUM OF LEFT CANINE & PREMOLARS *(estimated below from mand. incisors)* _____
e. TOTAL SPACE REQUIRED *(b + c + d)* _____
f. DISCREPANCY *(a – e)* _____

SECTION 7
SKELETAL JAW RELATIONSHIP
(from Facial Profile Analysis)

( ) CLASS I; ( ) CLASS II; ( ) CLASS III

SECTION 8
OCCLUSION OF PERMANENT FIRST MOLARS

RIGHT SIDE		LEFT SIDE
( )	ANGLE CLASS I	( )
( )	END-TO-END	( )
( )	ANGLE CLASS II	( )
( )	ANGLE CLASS III	( )

SECTION 9
MOLAR SHIFT *(From end-to-end to Class I)*
For Skeletal Class I only

RIGHT SIDE + LEFT SIDE = TOTAL SHIFT
___mm + ___mm = ___mm TOTAL

SECTION 10
LIP POSTURE *(from Facial Profile Analysis)*
( ) ACCEPTABLE; ( ) PROTRUSIVE; ( ) RETRUSIVE

MANDIBULAR INCISOR POSITION
(from Facial Profile Analysis and casts)
( ) ACCEPTABLE; ( ) PROTRUSIVE; ( ) RETRUSIVE

INTERPRETATION OF NUMERICAL RESULTS *(based on observations in Sections 7 — 10)*

To estimate the size of the unerupted canine and premolars in each quadrant [method of Tanaka and Johnston, J Am Dent Assn 88:798, 1974]:

Mandibular quadrant: ½ the sum of the widths of the mandibular incisors, plus 10.5 mm. _____ [ENTER ON LINE 5c and 5d ABOVE]

Maxillary quadrant: ½ the sum of the widths of the mandibular incisors, plus 11.0 mm. _____ [ENTER ON LINE 6c and 6d ABOVE]

FIGURE 6-37 Space analysis form.

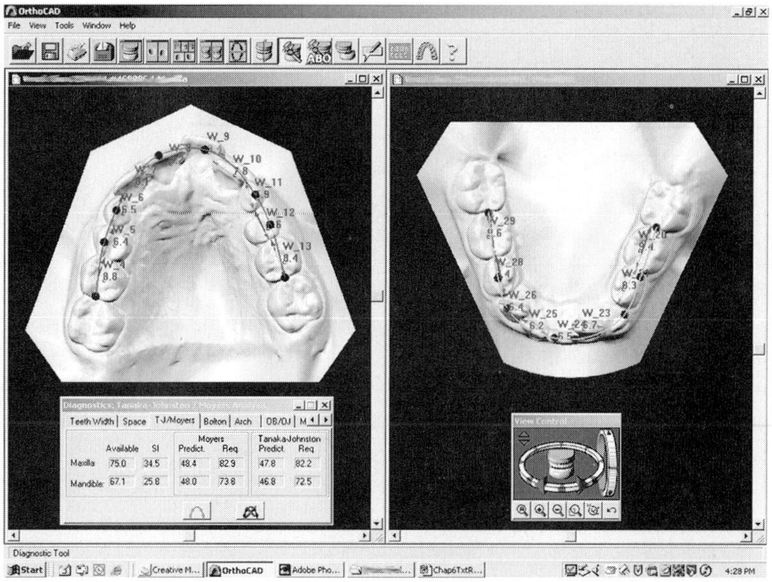

Figure 6-38 Space analysis now can be accomplished by a computer algorithm. The data for arch dimensions and tooth widths can be entered into a template on the computer screen so that the computer does the calculations, but if laser scans have created digital casts, the information already is present and space analysis based on correlations in tooth sizes becomes just a matter of requesting it.

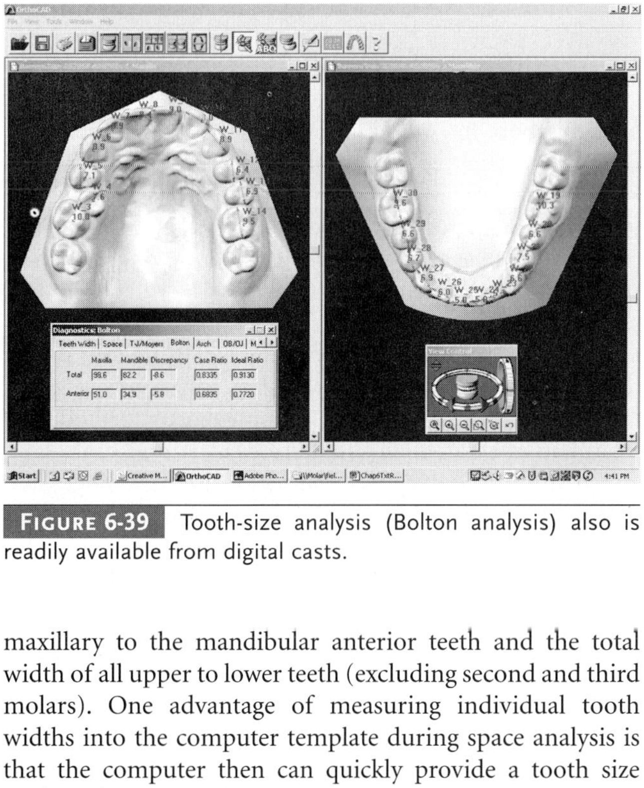

Figure 6-39 Tooth-size analysis (Bolton analysis) also is readily available from digital casts.

maxillary to the mandibular anterior teeth and the total width of all upper to lower teeth (excluding second and third molars). One advantage of measuring individual tooth widths into the computer template during space analysis is that the computer then can quickly provide a tooth size analysis (Figure 6-39).

A quick check for anterior tooth size discrepancy can be done by comparing the size of upper and lower lateral incisors. Unless the upper laterals are wider, a discrepancy almost surely exists. A quick check for posterior tooth size discrepancy is to compare the size of upper and lower second premolars, which should be about equal size. A tooth size discrepancy of less than 1.5 mm is rarely significant, but larger discrepancies create treatment problems and must be included in the orthodontic problem list.

Cephalometric Analysis

The introduction of radiographic cephalometrics in 1934 by Hofrath in Germany and Broadbent in the United States provided both a research and a clinical tool for the study of malocclusion and underlying skeletal disproportions (Figure 6-40). The original purpose of cephalometrics was research on growth patterns in the craniofacial complex. The concepts of normal development presented in Chapters 2 and 3 were largely derived from such cephalometric studies.

It soon became clear, however, that cephalometric radiographs could be used to evaluate dentofacial proportions and clarify the anatomic basis for a malocclusion. The orthodontist needs to know how the major functional components of the face (cranial base, jaws, teeth) are related to each other (Figure 6-41). Any malocclusion is the result of an interaction between jaw position and the position the teeth assume as they erupt, which is affected by the jaw relationships (see Chapter 4 for a discussion of dental compensation or adaptation). For this reason, apparently similar malocclusions as evaluated from the dental occlusions may turn out to be quite different when evaluated more completely (Figure 6-42). Although careful observation of the face can provide this information, cephalometric analysis allows greater precision.

Cephalometric radiographs are not taken as a screen for pathology, but the possibility of observing pathologic changes on these radiographs should not be overlooked. Occasionally, previously-unsuspected anomalies in the cervical spine (Figure 6-43) or degenerative changes in the vertebrae are revealed in a cephalometric radiograph, and sometimes other pathologic changes in the skull, jaws or cranial base can be observed.[21]

Perhaps the most important clinical use of radiographic cephalometrics is in recognizing and evaluating changes

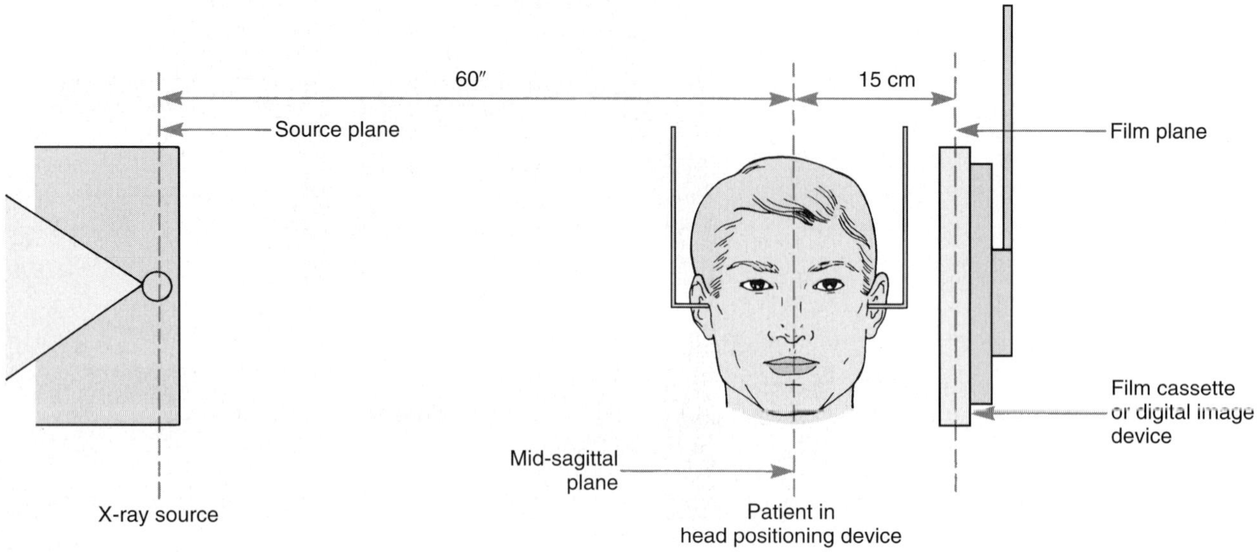

FIGURE 6-40 Diagrammatic representation of the American standard cephalometric arrangement. By convention, the distance from the x-ray source to the subject's midsagittal plane is 5 feet. The distance from the midsagittal plane to the cassette can vary in many machines but must be the same for each patient every time.

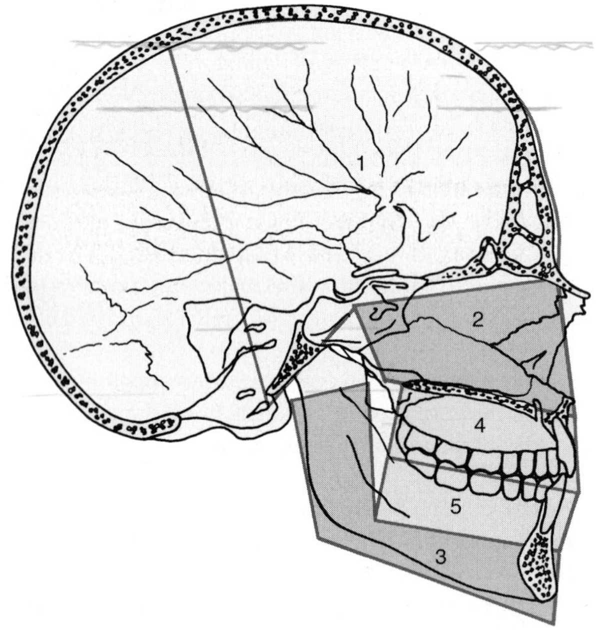

FIGURE 6-41 The structural components of the face, shown superimposed on the anatomic drawing. The cranium and cranial base *(1)*, the skeletal maxilla and nasomaxillary complex *(2)*, and the skeletal mandible *(3)* are parts of the face that exist whether or not there is a dentition. The maxillary teeth and alveolar process *(4)* and the mandibular teeth and alveolar process *(5)* are independent functional units, which can be displaced relative to the supporting bone of the maxilla and mandible, respectively. The goal of cephalometric analysis is to establish the relationship of these components in both the anteroposterior and vertical planes of space.

brought about by orthodontic treatment. Superimpositions taken from serial cephalometric radiographs before, during, and after treatment can be superimposed to study changes in jaw and tooth positions retrospectively (Figure 6-44). The observed changes result from a combination of growth and treatment (except in nongrowing adults). It is all but impossible to know what is really occurring during treatment of a growing patient without reviewing cephalometric superimpositions, which is the reason that cephalometric radiographs are required for comprehensive orthodontic treatment of children and adolescents.

For diagnostic purposes, the major use of radiographic cephalometrics is in characterizing the patient's dental and skeletal relationships. In this section, we focus on the use of cephalometric analysis to compare a patient to his or her peers, using population standards. The use of cephalometric predictions to estimate orthodontic and surgical treatment effects is covered in Chapter 8.

Development of Cephalometric Analysis

Cephalometric analysis is commonly carried out, not on the radiograph itself, but on a tracing or digital model that emphasizes the relationship of selected points. In essence, the tracing or model is used to reduce the amount of information on the radiograph to a manageable level. The common cephalometric landmarks and a typical tracing are shown in Figures 6-45 and 6-46.

Cephalometric landmarks can be represented as a series of points, which are usually defined as locations on a physical structure (for example, the most anterior point on the bony chin), or occasionally as constructed points such as the

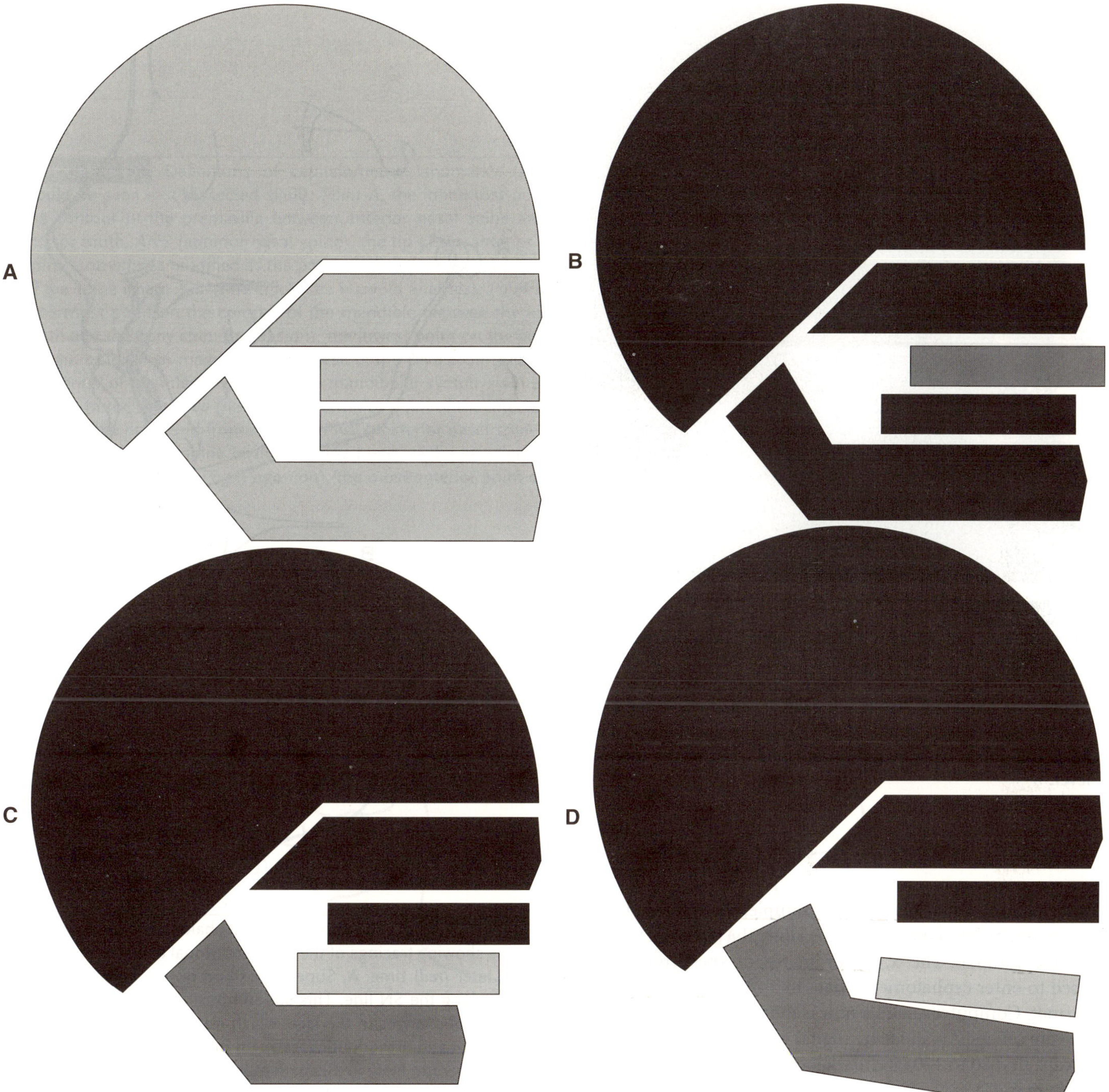

Figure 6-42 The ideal relationships of the facial and dental components can be represented as shown in **A.** Cephalometric analysis can distinguish and clarify the differing dental and skeletal contributions to malocclusions that present identical dental relationships. A Class II division 1 malocclusion, for example, could be produced by **(B)** protrusion of the maxillary teeth although the jaw relationship was normal, **(C)** mandibular deficiency with the teeth of both arches normally related to the jaw, **(D)** downward-backward rotation of the mandible produced by excessive vertical growth of the maxilla, or a number of other possibilities. The objective of cephalometric analysis is to visualize the contribution of skeletal and dental relationships to the malocclusion in this way, not to generate a table of numbers that are estimators of relationships. Measurements and other analytic procedures are a means to the end of understanding dental and skeletal relationships for an individual patient, not ends in themselves.

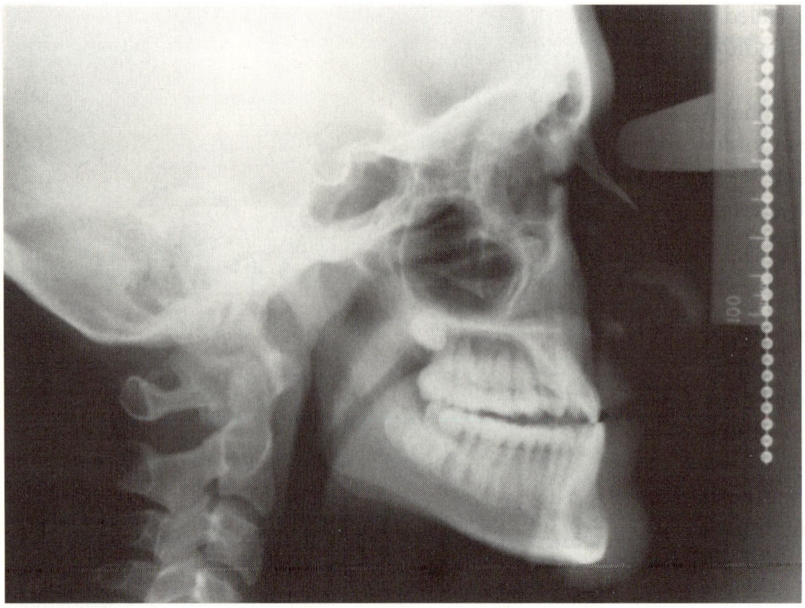

Figure 6-49 If the cephalometric film is taken with the patient in natural head position (NHP), a line perpendicular to the true vertical (shown by the image of the freely-suspended chain that is seen on the edge of the film) is the true (physiologic) horizontal line. NHP is preferred in modern cephalometrics to anatomic head positioning.

and incline their heads up and down in increasingly smaller movements until they feel comfortably positioned. The natural head position can be reproduced within 1 or 2 degrees.[28]

In contemporary usage, cephalometric radiographs should be taken in the natural head position (NHP), so that the physiologic true horizontal plane is established (Figure 6-49). Although NHP is not as precisely reproducible as orienting the head to the Frankfort plane, the potential errors from lower reproducibility are smaller than those from inaccurate head orientation.[29] The inclination of SN to the true horizontal plane (or to the Frankfort plane if true horizontal plane is not known) should always be noted, and if the inclination of SN differs significantly from 6 degrees, any measurements based on SN should be corrected by this difference.

Steiner Analysis. The Steiner analysis, developed and promoted by Cecil Steiner in the 1950s, can be considered the first of the modern cephalometric analyses for two reasons: it displayed measurements in a way that emphasized not just the individual measurements but their interrelationship into a pattern, and it offered specific guides for use of cephalometric measurements in treatment planning. Elements of it remain useful today.

In the Steiner analysis, the first measurement is the angle SNA, which is designed to evaluate the anteroposterior position of the maxilla relative to the anterior cranial base (Figure 6-50). The "norm" for SNA is 82 ± 2 degrees. Thus if a patient's SNA were greater than 84 degrees, this would be interpreted as maxillary protrusion, while SNA values of less than 80 degrees would be interpreted as maxillary retrusion. Similarly, the angle SNB is used to evaluate the anteroposterior position of the mandible, for which the norm is 78 ± 2 degrees. This interpretation is valid only if the SN

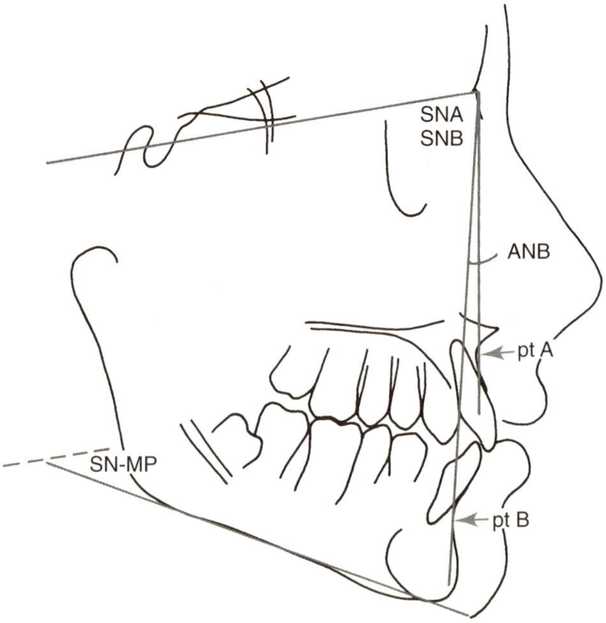

Figure 6-50 In the Steiner analysis, the angles *SNA* and *SNB* are used to establish the relationship of the maxilla and mandible to the cranial base, while the *SN-MP* (mandibular plane) angle is used to establish the vertical position of the mandible.

plane is normally inclined to the true horizontal (or if the value is corrected as described above) and the position of N is normal.

The difference between SNA and SNB—the ANB angle—indicates the magnitude of the skeletal jaw discrepancy, and this to Steiner was the measurement of real interest. One can argue, as he did, that which jaw is at fault is of mostly theo-

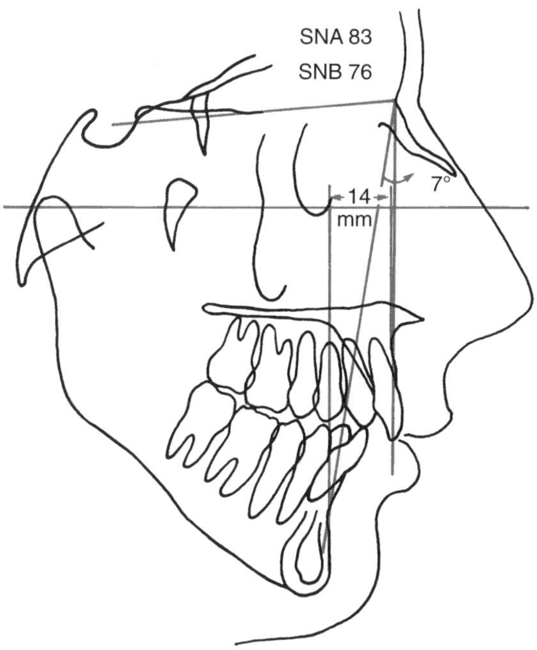

Figure 6-51 The *ANB* angle can be misleading when nasion is displaced anteriorly, as in this individual. Note that the *ANB* angle is only 7 degrees, but the *A-B* difference projected to the true horizontal is 14 mm. *ANB,* at best, is an indirect measurement of the *A-B* difference, and must be used with full awareness of its limitations.

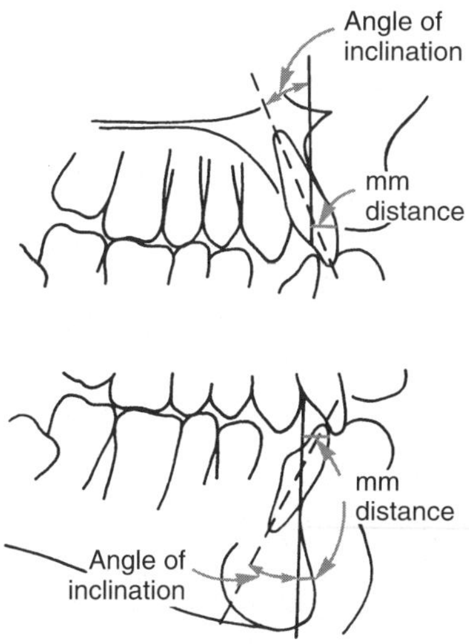

Figure 6-52 In the Steiner analysis, the relationship of the upper incisor to the NA line is used to establish the position of the maxillary dentition relative to the maxilla. Both the millimeter distance that the labial surface of the incisor is in front of the line and the inclination of the long axis of the incisor to the line are measured. The position of the lower incisor relative to the mandible is established by similar measurements to the line NB. In addition, the prominence of the chin is established by measuring the millimeter distance from the NB line to pogonion, the most prominent point on the bony chin.

retical interest: what really matters is the magnitude of the discrepancy between the jaws that must be overcome in treatment, and this is what the ANB angle measures.

The magnitude of the ANB angle, however, is influenced by two factors other than the anteroposterior difference in jaw position. One is the vertical height of the face. As the vertical distance between nasion and points A and B increases, the ANB angle will decrease. The second is that if the anteroposterior position of nasion is abnormal, the size of the angle will be affected (Figure 6-51). In addition, as SNA and SNB become larger and the jaws are more protrusive, even if their horizontal relationship is unchanged, it will be registered as a larger ANB angle. The validity of these criticisms has led to use of different indicators of jaw discrepancy in the later analyses presented in the following sections.

The next step in the Steiner analysis is to evaluate the relationship of the upper incisor to the NA line and both the lower incisor and the chin to the NB line, thus establishing the relative protrusion of the dentition (Figure 6-52). Tweed had earlier suggested that the lower incisor should be positioned at 65 degrees to the Frankfort plane, thus compensating in the incisor position for the steepness of the mandibular plane. In the Steiner analysis, both the angular inclination of each incisor and the millimeter distance of the incisal edge from the vertical line are measured. The millimeter distance establishes how prominent the incisor is relative to its supporting bone, while the inclination indicates whether the tooth has been tipped to its position or has moved there bodily. The prominence of the chin (pogonion) compared with the prominence of the lower incisor establishes the balance between them: the more prominent the chin, the more prominent the incisor can be, and vice versa. This important relationship is often referred to as the *Holdaway ratio.* The final measurement included in the Steiner analysis is the inclination of the mandibular plane to SN, its only indicator of the vertical proportions of the face (see Figure 6-50). Tabulated standard values for five racial groups are given in Table 6-8.

The various measurements incorporated in the Steiner analysis from the beginning were represented graphically as “Steiner sticks” or “chevrons,” a convenient shorthand for presenting the measurements. Steiner calculated what compromises in incisor positions would be necessary to achieve normal occlusion when the ANB angle was not ideal. This was a major step in applying cephalometrics to routine treatment planning. The Steiner compromises, and the method for establishing them for any given patient, are illustrated in Figure 6-53. These figures can be helpful in establishing how much tooth movement is needed to correct any malocclusion.

However, it should not be overlooked that relying on tooth movement alone to correct skeletal malocclusion,

TABLE 6-8

Cephalometric Values for Selected Groups (All Values in Degrees Except As Indicated)

	American white	American black	Israeli	Chinese (Taiwan)	Japanese
SNA	82	85	82	82	81
SNB	80	81	78	79	77
ANB	2	4	4	3	4
$\underline{1}$-NA	4 mm 22	7 mm 23	5 mm 24	5 mm 24	6 mm 24
$\overline{1}$-NB	4 mm 25	10 mm 34	6 mm 29	6 mm 27	8 mm 31
$\underline{1}$ to $\overline{1}$	131	119	124	126	120
GoGn-SN	32	32	35	32	34
$\overline{1}$-MnPl	93	100	93	93	96
$\overline{1}$-FH	62	51	57	57	57
Y axis	61	63	61	61	62

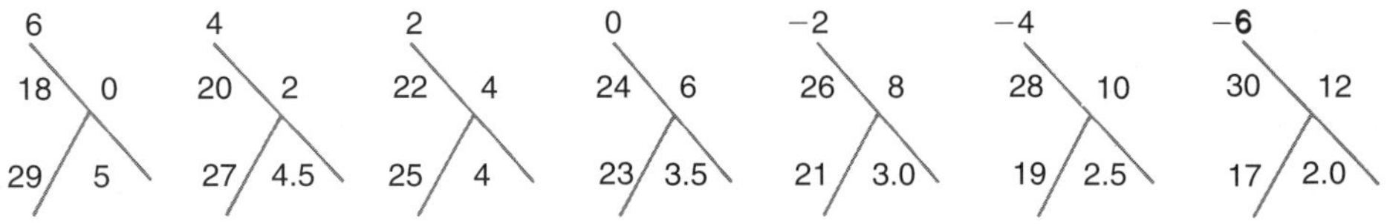

FIGURE 6-53 In the Steiner analysis, the ideal relationship of the incisors is expected when the ANB angle is 2 degrees, as indicated in the third diagram from the left. The inclination of the upper incisor to the NA line in degrees and its prominence in millimeters are shown on the second vertical line (22 degrees and 4 mm for an ANB of 2 degrees). The inclination of the lower incisor to the NB line and its prominence in millimeters are shown on the third line (25 degrees and 4 mm for an ANB of 2 degrees). If the ANB angle is different from 2 degrees, the different positioning of the incisors given by the inclination and protrusion figures will produce a dental compromise that leads to correct occlusion despite the jaw discrepancy. The fact that this degree of compensation in tooth position for jaw discrepancy can be produced by orthodontic treatment does not, of course, indicate that these compromises are necessarily the best possible treatment results.

particularly as the skeletal discrepancies become large, is not necessarily the best approach to orthodontic treatment. It is usually better to correct skeletal discrepancies at their source than to attempt only to achieve a dental compromise or camouflage (see Chapter 8 for further discussion of this important point). It is fair to say that the Steiner compromises reflect the prevailing attitude of Steiner's era, that the effects of orthodontic treatment are almost entirely limited to the alveolar process.

Sassouni Analysis. The Sassouni analysis was the first cephalometric method to emphasize vertical as well as horizontal relationships and the interaction between vertical and horizontal proportions. Sassouni pointed out that the horizontal anatomic planes—the inclination of the anterior cranial base, Frankfort plane, palatal plane, occlusal plane, and mandibular plane—tend to converge toward a single point in well-proportioned faces. The inclination of these planes to each other reflects the vertical proportionality of the face (Figure 6-54).

If the planes intersect relatively close to the face and diverge quickly as they pass anteriorly, the facial proportions are long anteriorly and short posteriorly, which predisposes the individual to an open bite malocclusion. Sassouni coined the term *skeletal open bite* for this anatomic relationship. If the planes are nearly parallel, so that they converge far behind the face and diverge only slowly as they pass anteriorly, there is a skeletal predisposition toward anterior deep bite, and the condition is termed *skeletal deep bite.*

In addition, an unusual inclination of one of the planes stands out because it misses the general area of intersection. Rotation of the maxilla down in back and up in front may contribute to skeletal open bite, for instance. The tipped palatal plane reveals this clearly (Figure 6-55).

Sassouni evaluated the anteroposterior position of the face and dentition by noting the relationship of various points to arcs drawn from the area of intersection of the planes. In a well-proportioned face, the anterior nasal spine (representing the anterior extent of the maxilla), the maxil-

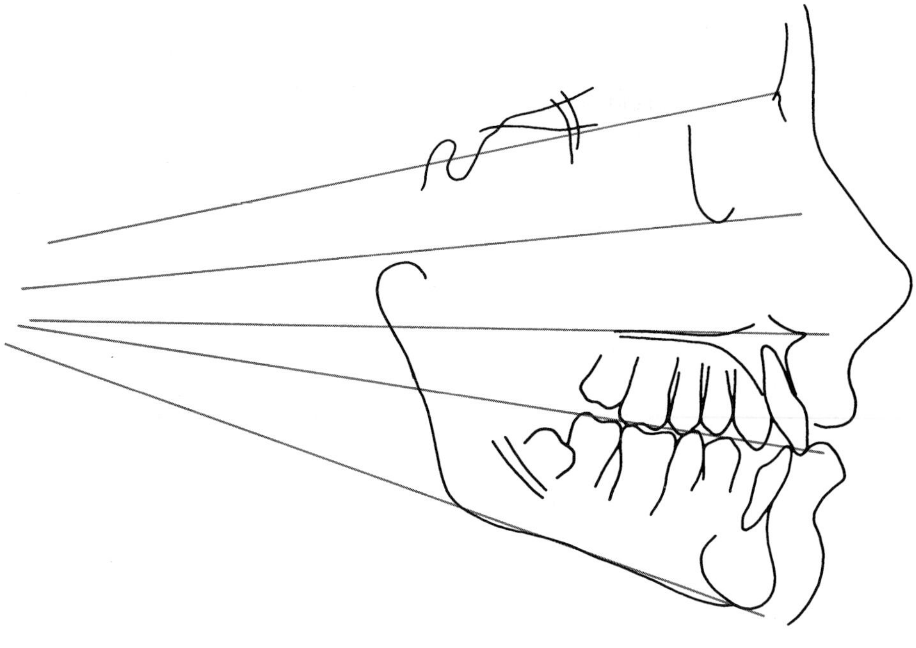

FIGURE 6-54 Sassouni[23] contributed the idea that if a series of horizontal planes are drawn from the SN line at the top to the mandibular plane below they will project toward a common meeting point in a well-proportioned face.

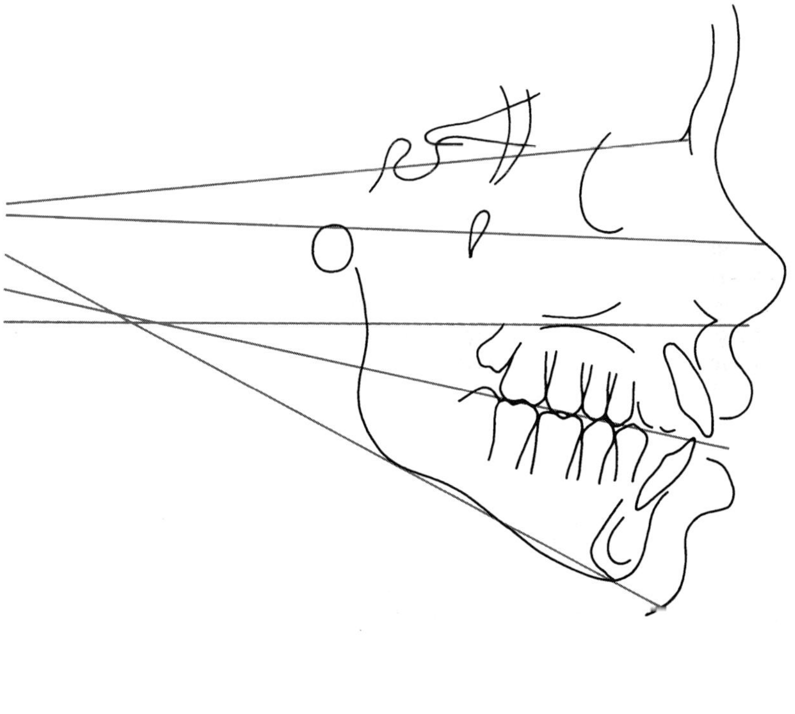

FIGURE 6-55 Inspection of the horizontal planes for this patient makes it clear that the maxilla is rotated downward posteriorly and the mandible rotated downward anteriorly. These rotations of the jaws contribute to an open bite tendency, so the skeletal pattern revealed here is often referred to as "skeletal open bite."

lary incisor, and the bony chin should be located along the same arc. As with vertical proportions, it could be seen visually if a single point deviated from the expected position, and in what direction. Unfortunately, as a face becomes more disproportionate, it is more and more difficult to establish the center for the arc, and the anteroposterior evaluation becomes more and more arbitrary.

Although the total arcial analysis described by Sassouni is no longer widely used, his analysis of vertical facial proportions has become an integral part of the overall analysis of a patient. In addition to any other measurements that might be made, it is valuable in any patient to analyze the divergence of the horizontal planes and to examine whether one of the planes is clearly disproportionate to the others.

Harvold Analysis, Wits Analysis. Both the Harvold and Wits analyses are aimed solely at describing the severity or degree of jaw disharmony. Harvold, using data derived from the Burlington growth study, developed standards for the "unit length" of the maxilla and mandible. The maxillary unit length is measured from the posterior border of the mandibular condyle to the anterior nasal spine, while the mandibular unit length is measured from the same point to the anterior point of the chin (Figure 6-56). The difference between these numbers provides an indication of the size discrepancy between the jaws. In analyzing the difference between maxillary and mandibular unit lengths, it must be kept in mind that the shorter the vertical distance between the maxilla and mandible, the more anteriorly the chin will be placed for any given unit difference, and vice versa. Harvold did quantify the lower face height to account for this factor. The position of the teeth has no influence on the Harvold figures (Table 6-9).

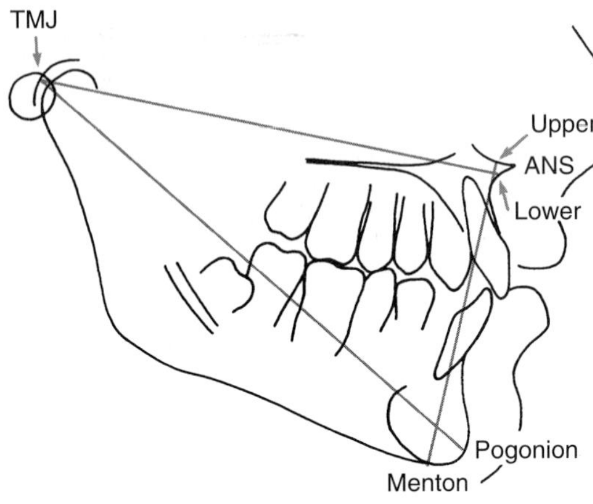

FIGURE 6-56 Measurements used in the Harvold analysis. Maxillary length is measured from *TMJ*, the posterior wall of the glenoid fossa, to lower *ANS*, defined as the point on the lower shadow of the anterior nasal spine where the projecting spine is 3 mm thick. Mandibular length is measured from *TMJ* to prognathion, the point on the bony chin contour giving the maximum length from the temporomandibular joint (close to *pogonion*), while lower face height is measured from *upper ANS*, the similar point on the upper contour of the spine where it is 3 mm thick, to *menton*.

The Wits analysis was conceived primarily as a way to overcome the limitations of ANB as an indicator of jaw discrepancy. It is based on a projection of points A and B to the occlusal plane, along which the linear difference between these points is measured. If the anteroposterior position of the jaws is normal, the projections from points A and B will intersect the occlusal plane at very nearly the same point. The magnitude of a discrepancy in the Class II direction can be estimated by how many millimeters the point A projection is in front of the point B projection, and vice versa for Class III.

The Wits analysis, in contrast to the Harvold analysis, is influenced by the teeth both horizontally and vertically—horizontally because points A and B are somewhat influenced by the dentition and vertically because the occlusal plane is determined by the vertical position of the teeth. It is important for Wits analysis that the *functional occlusal plane*, drawn along the maximum intercuspation of the posterior teeth, be used rather than an occlusal plane influenced by the vertical position of the incisors. Even so, this approach fails to distinguish skeletal discrepancies from problems caused by displacement of the dentition or specify which jaw is at fault if there is a skeletal problem, and if the Wits analysis is used, these limitations must be kept in mind.

The cephalometric approach developed by Ricketts in the 1960s was used in the original computer cephalometric system, and was widely employed at one time. Its greatest weakness was that the normative data for many of the measurements were based on unspecified samples collected by Ricketts, and the method therefore had limited scientific validity.

TABLE 6-9

Harvold Standard Values (mm)

		MALE		FEMALE	
	Age	Mean value	Standard deviation	Mean value	Standard deviation
Maxillary length (temporomandibular point to ANS) (see Figure 6-40)	6	82	3.2	80	3.0
	9	87	3.4	85	3.4
	12	92	3.7	90	4.1
	14	96	4.5	92	3.7
	16	100	4.2	93	3.5
Mandibular length (temporomandibular point to prognathion)	6	99	3.9	97	3.6
	9	107	4.4	105	3.9
	12	114	4.9	113	5.2
	14	121	6.1	117	3.6
	16	127	5.3	119	4.4
Lower face height (ANS-Me)	6	59	3.6	57	3.2
	9	62	4.3	60	3.6
	12	64	4.6	62	4.4
	14	68	5.2	64	4.4
	16	71	5.7	65	4.7

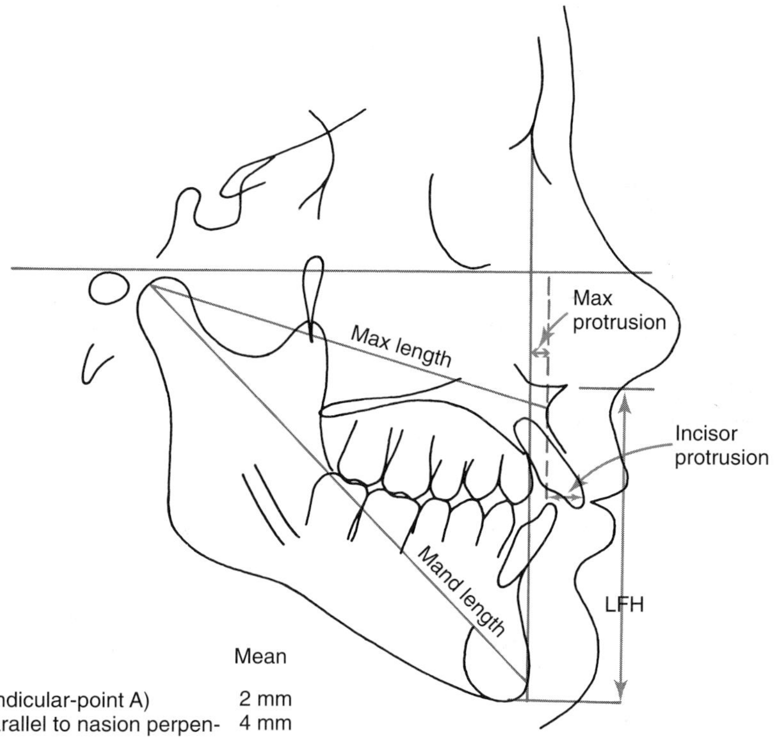

Measurements	Mean
Maxillary protrusion (mm distance from nasion perpendicular-point A)	2 mm
Maxillary incisor protrusion (mm distance from line parallel to nasion perpendicular to labial surface of incisor)	4 mm
Maxillary length	As in Harvold analysis
Mandibular length	As in Harvold analysis
Lower face height (LFH)	As in Harvold analysis

Figure 6-57 Measurements used in the McNamara analysis: Maxillary protrusion (mm distance from nasion perpendicular-point A), mean is 2 mm; maxillary incisor protrusion (mm distance from line parallel to nasion perpendicular to labial surface of incisor), mean is 4 mm; maxillary length, mandibular length, and lower face height (LFH) as in Harvold analysis.

McNamara Analysis. The McNamara analysis, originally published in 1983,[30] combines elements of previous approaches (Ricketts and Harvold) with original measurements to attempt a more precise definition of jaw and tooth positions. In this method, both the anatomic Frankfort plane and the basion–nasion line are used as reference planes. The anteroposterior position of the maxilla is evaluated with regard to its position relative to the "nasion perpendicular," a vertical line extending downward from nasion perpendicular to the Frankfort plane (Figure 6-57). The maxilla should be on or slightly ahead of this line. The second step in the procedure is a comparison of maxillary and mandibular length, using Harvold's approach. The mandible is positioned in space utilizing the lower anterior face height (ANS-menton). The upper incisor is related to the maxilla using a line through point A perpendicular to the Frankfort plane, similar to but slightly different from Steiner's relationship of the incisor to the NA line. The lower incisor is related as in the Ricketts analysis, primarily using the A-pogonion line (Figure 6-58).

The McNamara analysis has two major strengths:

1. It relates the jaws via the nasion perpendicular, in essence projecting the difference in anteroposterior position of the jaws to an approximation of the true vertical line. (Using a true vertical line, perpendicular to the true horizontal rather than anatomic Frankfort, would be better yet; the major reason for not doing so in constructing the analysis is that the cephalometric radiographs from which the normative data were derived were not taken in NHP.) This means that anteroposterior differences in jaw relationships are measured along the dimension (nearly true horizontal) in which they are visualized by both the patient and the diagnostician.
2. The normative data are based on the well-defined Bolton sample, which is also available in template form, meaning that the McNamara measurements are highly compatible with preliminary analysis by comparison with the Bolton templates.

Counterpart Analysis. A major problem with any analysis based on individual measurements is that any one measurement is affected by others within the same face. Not only are the measurements not independent, it is quite possible for a deviation in one relationship to be compensated wholly or partially by changes in other relationships. This applies to both skeletal and dental relationships. Compensatory changes in the dentition to make the teeth fit in spite of the

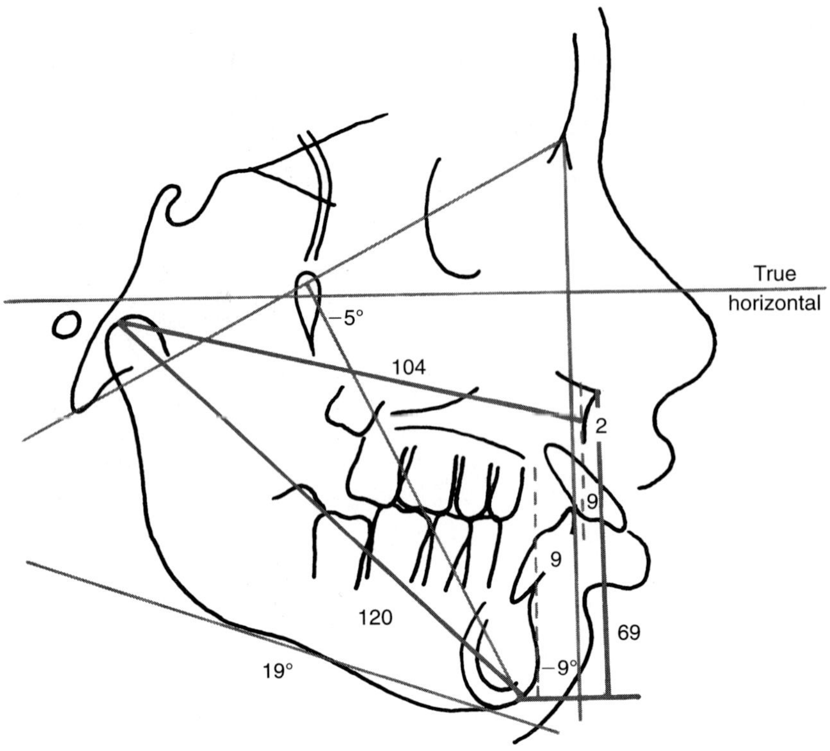

FIGURE 6-58 Analysis of a 12-year-old male, using the McNamara approach.

fact that the jaws do not are well known, and often are the goal of orthodontic treatment. Compensatory changes in skeletal components of the face are less well known, but occur frequently, and can lead to incorrect conclusions from measurements if not recognized.

The basic idea of interrelated dimensions leading to an ultimately balanced or unbalanced facial pattern was expressed well by Enlow in the 1960s, in his "counterpart analysis."[31] As Enlow et al pointed out, both the dimensions and alignment of craniofacial components are important in determining the overall facial balance. Consider dimensions first (Figure 6-59). If anterior face height is long, facial balance and proper proportion are preserved if posterior face height and mandibular ramus height also are relatively large. On the other hand, short posterior face height can lead to a skeletal open bite tendency even if anterior face height is normal, because the proportionality is disturbed. The same is true for anteroposterior dimensions. If both maxillary and mandibular lengths are normal but the cranial base is long, the maxilla will be carried forward relative to the mandible and maxillary protrusion will result. By the same token, a short maxilla could compensate perfectly for a long cranial base. Alignment would affect both the vertical and a-p position of the various skeletal units and could compensate for or worsen a tendency toward imbalance. For example, if the maxilla were rotated down posteriorly, a long ramus and acute gonial angle would compensate and allow normal facial proportions and normal occlusion, but even a slightly short ramus would produce downward-backward mandibular rotation and a long face-open bite tendency.

One way to bring the insights of counterpart analysis into clinical practice is from examination of the patient's proportions versus those of a "normal" template (see Figure 6-60). Another, increasingly popular in the last few years, is the use of "floating point" norms for measurements.[31] The idea is to use standards derived from the individual's facial type rather than relating individual cephalometric values to population means, taking advantage of the correlations between the individual values. Rather than judging normality or abnormality based on individual values, the judgment then would be based on how the values were related to each other—some combinations would be acceptable as normal even if the individual measurements were outside the normal range. Other combinations could be judged as reflecting an abnormal pattern even though the individual measurements were within the normal range. Assessing skeletal relationships in this way is particularly valuable for patients who are candidates for growth modification therapy or orthognathic surgery.

In the half-century that cephalometrics has been used clinically, dozens if not hundreds of other patterns of measurements have been published as named analyses.[26,27] In some of these methods, it is apparent what relationship the measurements are supposed to estimate, and it is clear where the normative data came from. In others, both the measurements and the norms take on almost mystical properties.

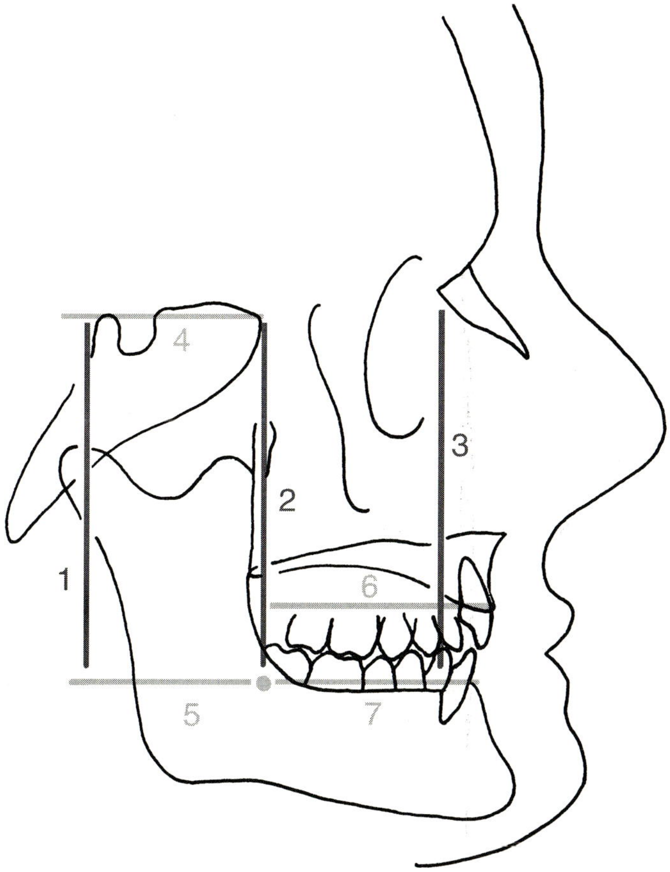

Figure 6-59 Enlow's counterpart analysis emphasizes the way changes in proportions in one part of the head and face can either add to increase a jaw discrepancy or compensate so that the jaws fit correctly even though there are skeletal discrepancies. For example, if the maxilla is long (measurement 6), there is no problem if the mandible (7) also is long, but malocclusion will result if the mandibular body length is merely normal. The same would be true for anterior versus posterior vertical dimensions (1-3). If these dimensions match each other, there is no problem, but if they do not, whether short or long, malocclusion will result.

Unless one is careful, it is easy to lose sight of the goal of cephalometric analysis: to estimate the relationships, vertically and horizontally, of the jaws to the cranial base and to each other, and the relationships of the teeth to their supporting bone. Unfortunately, analyses based on a limited set of standard measurements often differ in their assessment of both skeletal and dental relationships, even when there are significant dentofacial deviations. This occurs because of differences among the samples from which the analysis was derived, and especially because often there was no control for vertical face height, which has a distinct influence on anteroposterior relationships.

An approach that addresses this problem is available now for patients with a northern European (Caucasian) ancestry. First, determine from facial analysis whether the patient has normal vertical facial proportions. If so, an anteroposterior evaluation can be made using one of the common cephalometric methods and norms (Table 6-10) that were derived by ROC curve evaluation for 10-18 year old Caucasian subjects who had facial and dental relationships that were compatible (i.e., Class I faces with Class I dentitions, Class II faces with Class II dentitions, etc.) and normal face height. The ROC method evaluates the diagnostic ability of a test and is an objective way to detect the trade-offs between sensitivity and specificity for the cephalometric measures. It was used to determine a "cut point" (the cephalometric value) which distinguished between Class I and Class II or Class III skeletal relationships. This is the value with the maximum statistical probability for the point where one skeletal classification changes to another (e.g., Class I changes to Class II). These norms were derived and validated on independent samples and have proven to be less discordant (conflicting) when applied to individual Caucasian patients.[33] The benefit from using these standards is that one set of values can be used for each measurement regardless of the age or gender of the patient, and the performance will be equal to or better than using traditional values.

Table 6-10

Anteroposterior Cephalometric Values for Caucasian Males and Females Ages 10-18 With Normal Vertical Proportions

Measure	Classification	Range
ANB°	Class I	0.1 to 3.6°
	Class II	>3.6°
	Class III	<0.1°
McNamara (A–Pog horizontal distance)	Class I	−3.3 to 2.8 mm
	Class II	>2.8 mm
	Class III	<−3.3 mm
WITS (A-B difference)	Class I	−4 to 2.1 mm
	Class II	>2.1 mm
	Class III	<−4 mm
APDI	Class I	97.9 to 83.6
	Class II	<83.6
	Class III	>97.9
Unit mm Difference	Class I	26.9 to 32.7
	Class II	<26.9 mm
	Class III	>32.7 mm

Template Analysis

In the early years of cephalometric analysis, it was recognized that representing the norm in graphic form might make it easier to recognize a pattern of relationships. The "Moorrees mesh," which was developed in the 1960s and updated more recently, presents the patient's disproportions as the distortion of a grid.[33,34] In recent years, direct comparison of patients with templates derived from the various growth

Summary of Contemporary Cephalometric Methodology

In its early years, cephalometric analysis was correctly criticized as being just a "numbers game," leading to orthodontic treatment aimed at producing certain numbers on a cephalometric radiograph. That might or might not represent the best treatment result for that patient. Totally accepting the Steiner compromises and setting treatment goals solely in terms of producing these numbers could certainly be criticized on that basis. At present, competent clinicians use cephalometric analysis to better understand the underlying basis for a malocclusion. To do this, they look not just at individual measurements compared with a norm but at the pattern of relationships, including soft tissue relationships. Any measurements are a means to this end, not the end in itself.

Whatever the later steps (measurement or template superimposition), the place to begin cephalometric analysis is by drawing the Sassouni horizontal planes and examining their interrelationships. This simple step highlights rotations of the jaws (remember that both the maxilla and mandible can be rotated) and makes vertical proportions more apparent.

At that point, the analysis should turn to the anteroposterior relationships of the jaws and the dentition of each jaw. Superimposition of Bolton (or other) templates is one way to do that. The same information can be obtained by using a true vertical line across the front of the face as a reference, as in McNamara analysis, which is a straightforward way to establish skeletal relationships without having the measurements affected by tooth position. Moving the true vertical line so that it passes through point A, and then through point B, reveals the amount of dental protrusion or retrusion of the maxillary and mandibular teeth respectively.

Finally, any other measurements needed to clarify relationships that are not clear should be made. Often this includes measurements of face height, maxillary and mandibular unit lengths or other components of the various analyses that have been discussed. The goal of modern cephalometrics is to evaluate the relationship of the functional units shown in Figure 6-40 and to do whatever is necessary to establish the position, horizontally and vertically, of each of those units. Because what is required amounts to pattern analysis, almost never can any single measurement be viewed in isolation. Instead, the interrelationship among various measurements and observed relationships must be taken into account. In a measurement analysis system, the appropriate floating norms always should be employed.

ORTHODONTIC CLASSIFICATION

Classification has traditionally been an important tool in the diagnosis-treatment planning procedure. An ideal classification would summarize the diagnostic data and imply the treatment plan. In our concept of diagnosis, classification can be viewed as the (orderly) reduction of the database to a list of the patient's problems (Figure 6-63).

Development of Classification Systems

The first useful orthodontic classification, still important now, was Angle's classification of malocclusion into Classes I, II, and III (see Chapter 1). The basis of the Angle classification was the relationship of the first molar teeth and the alignment (or lack of it) of the teeth relative to the line of occlusion. Angle's classification thus created four groups:

Normal occlusion	Normal (Class I) molar relationship, teeth on line of occlusion
Class I malocclusion	Normal (Class I) molar relationship, teeth crowded, rotated, etc.
Class II malocclusion	Lower molar distal to upper molar, relationship of other teeth to line of occlusion not specified
Class III malocclusion	Lower molar mesial to upper molar, relationship of other teeth to line of occlusion not specified

The Angle system was a tremendous step forward, not only because it provided an orderly way to classify maloc-

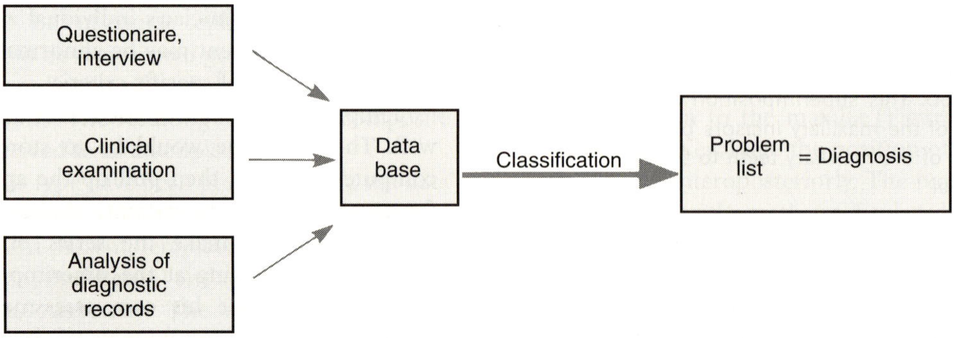

FIGURE 6-63 Conceptually, classification can be viewed as an orderly way to derive a list of the patient's problems from the database.

clusion but also because for the first time it provided a simple definition of normal occlusion, and thereby a way to distinguish normal occlusion from malocclusion.

Almost immediately, it was recognized that the Angle classification was not complete, because it did not include important characteristics of the patient's problem. The deficiencies in the original Angle system led to a series of informal additions at an early stage. A series of subdivisions of Class I were proposed by Martin Dewey, initially Angle's protégé but later his rival. Gradually Angle's classification numbers were extended to refer to four distinct but related characteristics: the classification of malocclusion, as in the original plan; the molar relationship; the skeletal jaw relationship; and the pattern of growth (Figure 6-64). Thus a Class II jaw relationship meant the mandible was positioned distally relative to the maxilla. This was usually found in connection with a Class II molar relationship but occasionally could be present despite a Class I molar relationship. Similarly, a Class II growth pattern was defined as a downward and backward growth direction of the mandible, which would tend to create and maintain Class II jaw and molar relationships. Class I and Class III growth patterns show balanced and disproportionate forward mandibular growth, respectively.

In the 1960s, Ackerman and Proffit formalized the system of informal additions to the Angle method by identifying five major characteristics of malocclusion to be considered and systematically described in classification (Figure 6-65). The approach overcame the major weaknesses of the Angle scheme. Specifically, it (1) incorporated an evaluation of crowding and asymmetry within the dental arches and included an evaluation of incisor protrusion, (2) recognized the relationship between protrusion and crowding, (3) included the transverse and vertical as well as the anteroposterior planes of space, and (4) incorporated information about skeletal jaw proportions at the appropriate point, that is, in the description of relationships in each of the planes of space. Experience has confirmed that a minimum of five characteristics must be considered in a complete diagnostic evaluation.

Although the elements of the Ackerman-Proffit scheme are often not combined exactly as originally proposed, classification by five major characteristics is now widely used. Like other aspects of orthodontic diagnosis, classification is affected by the major changes that have occurred recently, such as the development of three-dimensional imaging and other advances in orthodontic technology. The most important change, however, is the greater emphasis now on evaluating facial soft tissue proportions and the relationship of the dentition to the lips and cheeks, on smile as well as at rest.

Recent revision of the classification scheme has focused on broadening it to incorporate these new aspects of orthodontic diagnosis.[36] Forty years ago, most orthodontists viewed their role as correcting malocclusion by straightening teeth. At present, the goal of treatment takes into account facial and dental appearance as well as the relationships of the teeth. Today, evaluation of dentofacial appearance includes full-face evaluation, consideration of anterior tooth display at rest and during smile, and assessment of soft tissues in oblique ($^3/_4$) as well as frontal and profile views. Little has changed regarding the description of crowding or spacing within the dental arches, but a clearer understanding of the line of occlusion in relationship to the goals of treatment now is required. The goal of treatment no longer is to just correct malocclusion, but to correct it while also bringing the dentition and facial skeleton into normal

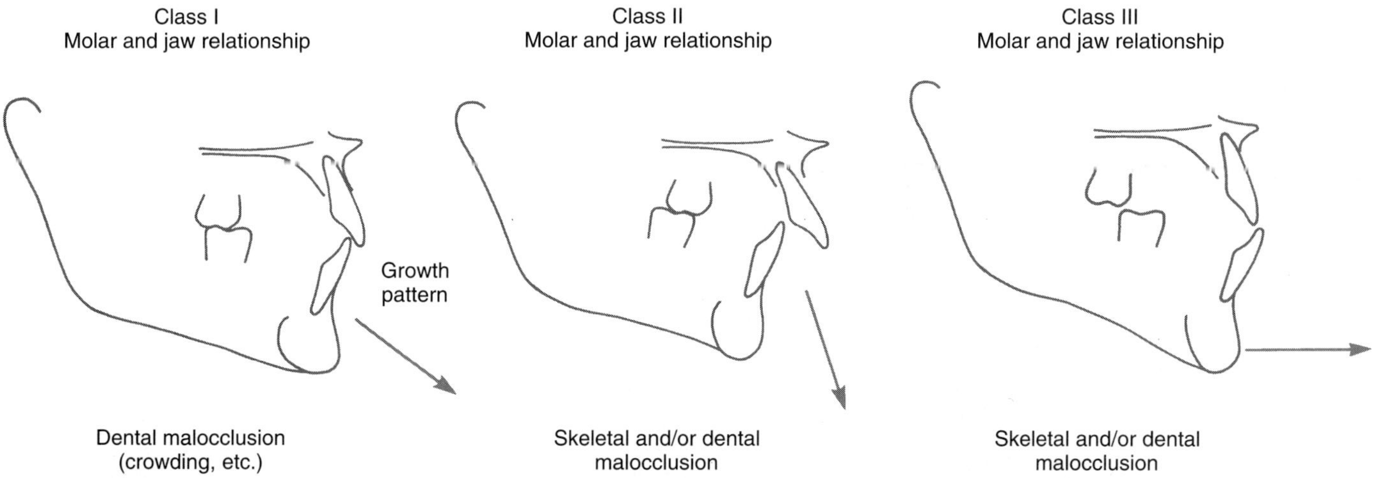

Figure 6-64 The Angle classification has come to describe four different characteristics: the type of malocclusion, the molar relationship, the jaw relationship, and the pattern of growth, as shown here diagrammatically. Although the jaw relationship and growth pattern correlate with the molar relationship, the correlations are far from perfect. It is not unusual to observe a Class I molar relationship in a patient with a Class II jaw relationship or to find that an individual with a Class I molar and jaw relationship grows in a Class III pattern, which ultimately will produce a Class III malocclusion.

relationships with the facial and intra-oral soft tissues—which means that a more thorough analysis of dentofacial traits is required.

Additions to the Five-Characteristics Classification System

Two things particularly help this more thorough analysis: (1) evaluating the orientation of the *esthetic line of the dentition,* which is related to but different from Angle's functional line of occlusion, and (2) supplementing the traditional three-dimensional description of facial and dental relationships with rotational characteristics around each plane of space. Considering these in turn:

1. *Esthetic line of the dentition.* For over a century, Angle's line of occlusion has been used to characterize the positions of the teeth within the dental arch and as a reference for assessing arch form and arch symmetry. Angle's concept was that if the buccal occlusal line of the mandibular dental arch was coincident with the central fossae line of the maxillary dental arch and the teeth were well-aligned, ideal occlusion would result. The line of occlusion is hidden from view when the maxillary and mandibular teeth are in contact.

   In modern analysis, another curved line characterizing the appearance of the dentition is important, the one that is seen when evaluating anterior tooth display (Figure 6-66). This line, the esthetic line of the dentition, follows the facial edges of the maxillary anterior and posterior teeth. The orientation of this line, like the orientation of the head and jaws, is best described when the rotational axes of pitch, roll and yaw are considered in addition to transverse, anteroposterior and vertical planes of space.

2. *Pitch, roll, and yaw in systematic description.* A key aspect of our previous classification system was its incorporation of systematic analysis of skeletal and dental relationships in all three planes of space, so that deviations in any direction would be incorporated into the patient's problem list. A complete description, however, requires consideration of both translation (forward/backward, up/down, right left) in three-dimensional space and rotation about three perpendicular axes (pitch, roll and yaw) (Figure 6-67). This is exactly analogous to what would be necessary to describe the position of an airplane in space. The introduction of rotational axes into systematic description of dentofacial traits significantly improves the precision of the description, and thereby facilitates development of the problem list.

   Pitch, roll and yaw of the esthetic line of the dentition is a particularly useful way to evaluate the relationship of the teeth to the soft tissues that frame their display. From this perspective, an excessive upward/downward rotation of the

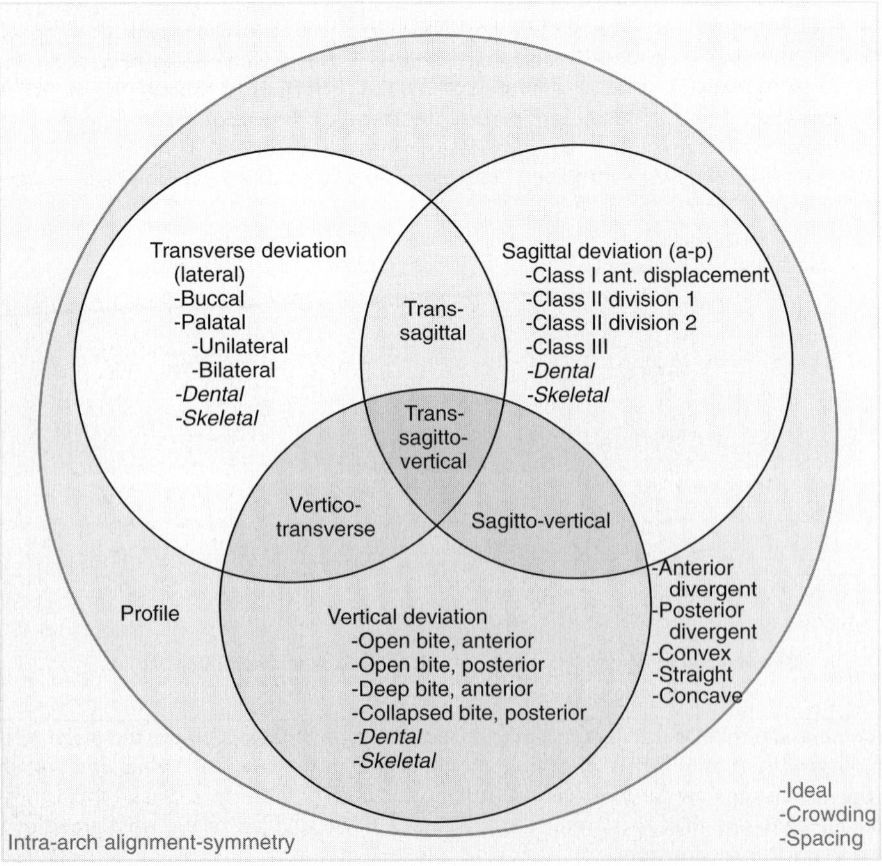

FIGURE 6-65 Ackerman and Proffit represented the five major characteristics of malocclusion via a Venn diagram. The sequential description of the major characteristics, not their graphic representation, is the key to this classification system; but the interaction of the tooth and jaw relationships with facial appearance must be kept in mind.

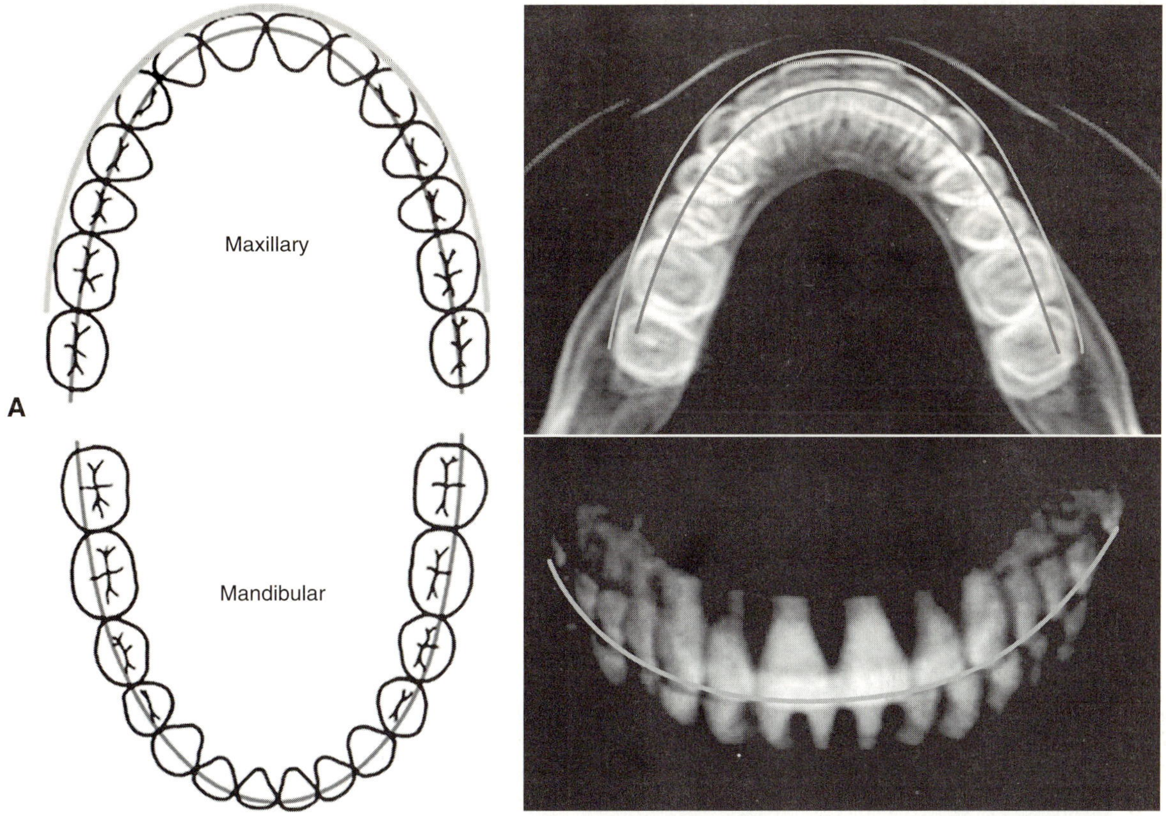

Figure 6-66 **A,** The relationship of the teeth to Angle's line of occlusion *(red)* has long been the basis for analysis of dental arch symmetry and crowding. A curved *(green)* line along the incisal edges and cusp tips of the maxillary teeth, the esthetic line of the dentition, now is used to incorporate tooth-lip relationships into the diagnostic evaluation of tooth positions. **B,** In vivo submental-vertex cone-beam computed tomographic (CBCT) view of an individual with normal occlusion, showing the maxillary dentition superimposed on the mandibular dentition as it is in life. For this individual, the teeth are aligned and positioned so that the line of occlusion is almost ideally placed for both arches. If a patient has an asymmetry characterized by rotation of the maxilla, mandible, dentition (or any or all of the above) around the vertical axis it can be detected in this radiographic projection. The esthetic line of the dentition *(green)* also can be seen in this projection, drawn as it was in **A. C,** A cross-sectional "block" of a CBCT image can be manipulated on the computer screen around all three rotational axes. This is simply a different perspective of the image shown in **B,** on which the esthetic line of the dentition is shown in its relationship to the incisal edges and cusp tips of the upper teeth.

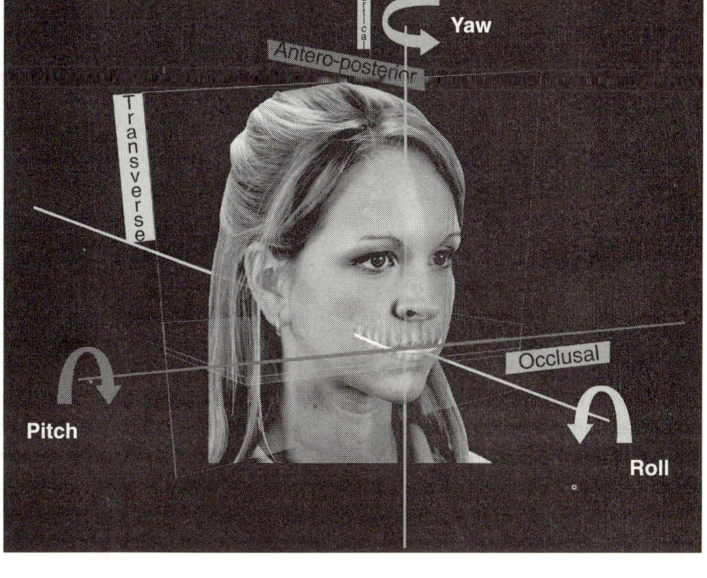

Figure 6-67 In addition to relationships in the transverse, antero-posterior, and vertical planes of space used in traditional 3-dimensional analysis, rotations around axes perpendicular to these planes also must be evaluated. These rotations are pitch, viewed as up-down deviations around the antero-posterior axis; roll, viewed as up-down deviations around the transverse axis; and yaw, viewed as left-right deviations around the vertical axis. The rotations should be evaluated for the jaws and for the esthetic line of the dentition.

Table 6-11

Arch Width Measurements*

AGE	MALE			FEMALE		
	MAXILLARY ARCH					
	Canine	First premolar	First molar	Canine	First premolar	First molar
6	27.5†	32.3†	41.9	26.9†	31.7†	41.3
8	29.7†	33.7†	43.1	29.1†	33.0†	42.4
10	30.5†	34.4†	44.5	29.8†	33.6†	43.5
12	32.5	35.7	45.3	31.5	35.1	44.6
14	32.5	36.0	45.9	31.3	34.9	44.3
16	32.3	36.6	46.6	31.4	35.2	45.0
18	32.3	36.7	46.7	31.2	34.6	43.9
	MANDIBULAR ARCH					
6	23.3†	28.7†	40.2	22.2†	28.4†	40.0
8	24.3†	29.7†	40.9	24.0†	29.5†	40.3
10	24.6†	30.2†	41.5	24.1†	29.7†	41.0
12	25.1	32.5	42.1	24.8	31.6	41.8
14	24.8	32.3	42.1	24.4	31.0	41.1
16	24.7	32.3	42.8	23.9	31.0	41.5
18	24.8	32.8	43.0	23.1	30.8	41.7

Data from Moyers RE et al: *Standards of human occlusal development,* Monograph 5, Craniofacial Growth Series. Ann Arbor, Mich., 1976, University of Michigan, Center for Human Growth and Development.
*mm distance between centers of teeth.
†Primary predecessor.

crossbite and measurements across the arch show that the mandible is wide while the maxillary arch is normal, a skeletal mandibular discrepancy probably is present.

Step 4: Evaluation of Skeletal and Dental Relationships in the Anteroposterior Plane of Space.

Examining the dental casts in occlusion will reveal any anteroposterior problems in the buccal occlusion or in the anterior relationships. The Angle classification, in its extended form, describes this well.

It is important to ask whether an end-to-end, Class II or Class III buccal segment relationship, or excessive overjet or reverse overjet of the incisors, is caused by a jaw (skeletal) discrepancy, displaced teeth on well-proportioned jaws (dental Class II or III), or a combination of skeletal and dental displacement. Deficient or excessive jaw growth almost always produces an occlusal discrepancy as well, but if the jaw discrepancy is the cause, the problem should be described as a *skeletal* Class II or Class III. The terminology simply means that the skeletal or jaw relationship is the cause of the Class II dental occlusion. The distinction between dental and skeletal is important, because the treatment for a skeletal Class II relationship in a child or adult will be different from treatment for a dental Class II problem. Cephalometric analysis is needed to be precise about the nature of the problem. The object is to accurately evaluate the underlying anatomic basis of the malocclusion (Figure 6-72).

Occasionally the molar occlusion is Class II on one side, and Class I on the other. Angle called this a Class II subdivision right or left, depending on which was the Class II side. In modern classification the subdivision label rarely is useful because it does not describe the real problem. The asymmetric molar relationship reflects either an asymmetry within one or both the dental arches (typically due to loss of space when one primary second molar was lost prematurely), or a yaw discrepancy of the jaw or dentition. These must be distinguished and should already have been addressed in the first or second steps in the classification procedure.

Step 5: Evaluation of Skeletal and Dental Relationships in the Vertical Plane of Space.

With the casts in occlusion, vertical problems can be described as anterior open bite (failure of the incisor teeth to overlap), anterior deep bite (excessive overlap of the anterior teeth), or posterior open bite (failure of the posterior teeth to occlude, unilaterally or bilaterally). As with all

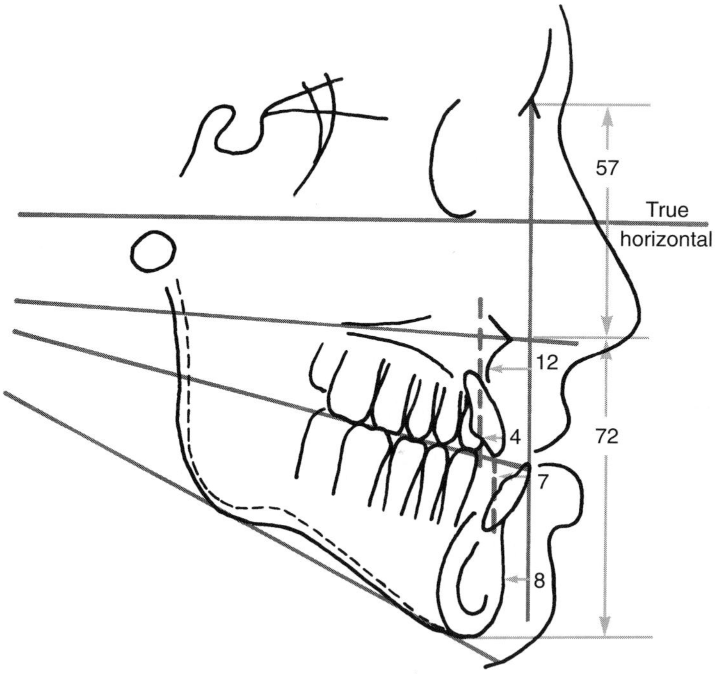

Figure 6-72 Cephalometric analysis combining elements of the measurement approaches presented earlier. A description in words of this patient's problems would be that the maxilla is quite deficient relative to the mandible and the cranial base, but the maxillary teeth are reasonably well related to the maxilla. The mandible is fairly well related in the anteroposterior plane of space to the cranial base, but the mandibular teeth protrude relative to the mandible. Vertical proportions are good.

aspects of malocclusion, it is important to ask, "Why does the open bite (or other problem) exist?" Since vertical problems, particularly anterior open bite, can result from environmental causes or habits, the "why" in this instance has two important components: at what anatomic location is the discrepancy, and can a cause be identified?

It is obvious that if the posterior teeth erupt a normal amount but the anterior teeth do not, there will be a pitch discrepancy of the line of occlusion and the esthetic line of the dentition. This would result in two related problems: an anterior open bite and less than the normal display of the maxillary anterior teeth. Upward pitch anteriorly of the maxillary dentition is possible but rarely is the major reason for an anterior open bite. Instead, anterior open bite patients usually have at least some excessive eruption of maxillary posterior teeth. If the anterior teeth erupt a normal amount but the posterior teeth erupt too much, anterior open bite is inevitable. In this case, the relationship of the anterior teeth to the lips would be normal, and there would be excessive display of the posterior teeth. The line of occlusion and the esthetic line of the dentition then would be pitched down posteriorly (see Figure 6-67).

This leads to an important but sometimes difficult concept: a patient with a *skeletal* open bite will usually have an anterior bite malocclusion that is characterized by excessive eruption of posterior teeth, downward rotation of the mandible and maxilla, and normal (or even excessive) eruption of anterior teeth (Figure 6-73). This facial and dental pattern is sometimes called the "long face syndrome." The reverse is true in a short face, skeletal deep bite relationship (Figure 6-74). In that circumstance, one would expect to see a normal amount of eruption of incisor teeth but rotation of both jaws in the opposite direction and insufficient eruption of the posterior teeth. The skeletal component is revealed by the rotation of the jaws, reflected in the palatal and mandibular plane angles. If the angle between the mandibular and palatal planes is low, there is a skeletal deep bite tendency (i.e., a jaw relationship that predisposes to an anterior deep bite, regardless of whether one is present). Similarly, if the mandibular-palatal angle is high, there is a skeletal open bite tendency.

It is important to remember that if the mandibular plane angle is unusually flat or steep, correcting an accompanying deep bite or open bite may require an alteration in the vertical position of posterior teeth so that the mandible can rotate to a more normal inclination. Cephalometric analysis is required for evaluation of patients with skeletal vertical problems, again with the goal of accurately describing skeletal and dental relationships. As the tracings in this chapter illustrate, most published analyses do a much better job of identifying anteroposterior than vertical problems. Adequate analysis of long- or short-face patients requires additional measurements to meet the needs of the specific case, or careful superimposition of templates and inspection of the relationships.

A careful clinical evaluation of the relationship of the dentition to the soft tissues also is critically important. Open bites and deep bites can result from almost any combination

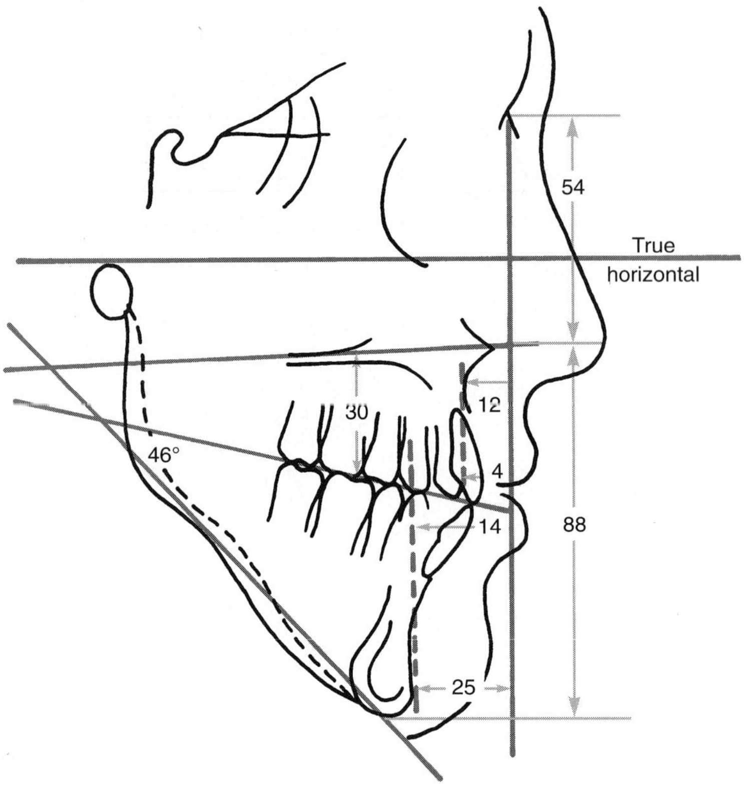

FIGURE 6-73 Cephalometric analysis for a patient with severe vertical problems. Note that the Sassouni lines clearly indicate the skeletal open bite pattern and that the measurements confirm both long anterior facial dimensions and severe mandibular deficiency related to downward and backward rotation of the mandible. Measurements of the distance from the upper first molar mesial cusp to the palatal plane confirms that excessive eruption of the upper molar has occurred.

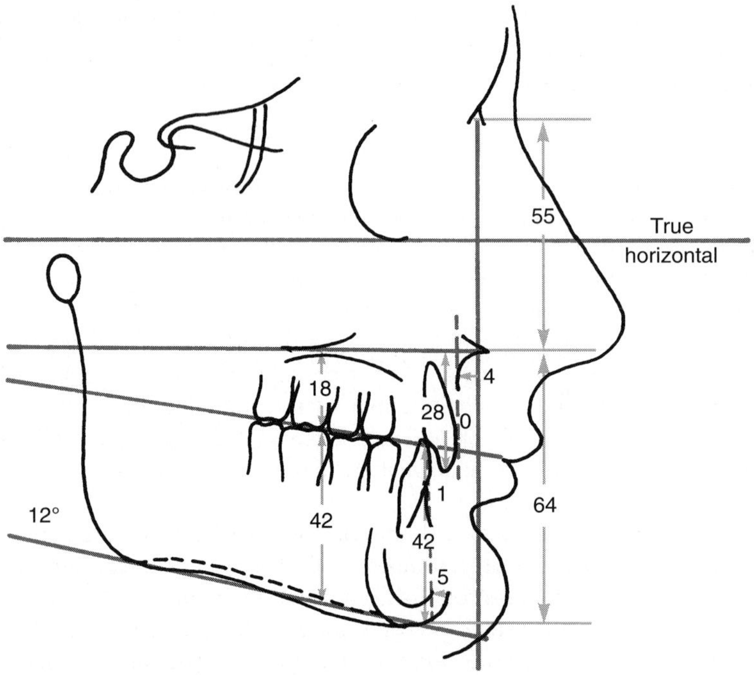

FIGURE 6-74 Cephalometric analysis of a patient with short anterior vertical dimensions. The measurements show excessive eruption of the lower molar compared with the upper molar and document the distal displacement of the lower incisor relative to the mandible. Note that the Sassouni planes are almost parallel, confirming the skeletal deep bite tendency.

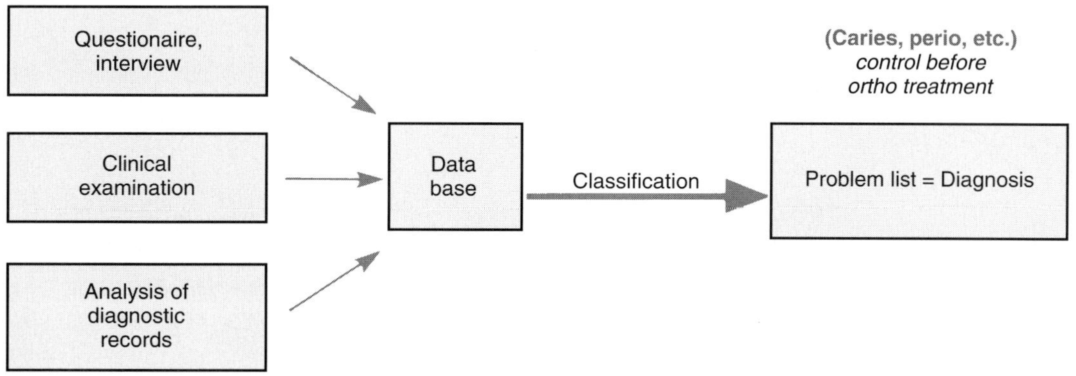

FIGURE 6-75 As a final step in diagnosis, the patient's problems related to pathology should be separated from the developmental problems, so that the pathology can be treated first.

of skeletal and dental components, and the problem is likely to include improper tooth–lip relationships. Careful analysis is required if the approach to treatment is to be esthetic and stable.

DEVELOPMENT OF A PROBLEM LIST

If positive findings from a systematic description of the patient are recorded (i.e., if the procedure described above is used), the automatic and important result is a list of the patient's problems. The step-by-step procedure is designed to ensure that the important distinctions have been made and that nothing has been overlooked.

The problem list often includes two types of problems: (1) those relating to disease or pathologic processes and (2) those relating to disturbances of development that have created the patient's malocclusion (Figure 6-75). The set of developmental abnormalities related to malocclusion is the orthodontic problem list. A developmental problem is just that (e.g., mandibular deficiency), not the findings that indicate its presence (e.g., posterior divergence, increased facial convexity, and increased ANB angle all are findings, not problems).

For efficient clinical application of the method, it is important to group different aspects of the same thing into a single major problem area related to the Ackerman-Proffit classification. This means that it would be impossible for a patient to have more than five major developmental problems, though several sub-problems within a major category would be quite possible. For instance, lingual position of the lateral incisors, labial position of the canines, and rotation of the central incisors all are problems, but they can and should be lumped under the general problem of incisor crowding/malalignment. Similarly, anterior open bite, rotation of the maxilla down posteriorly and rotation of the mandible down anteriorly, and extreme lip incompetence are all aspects of skeletal open bite. Where possible, the problems should be indicated quantitatively, or at least classified as mild, moderate, or severe (i.e., 5 mm mandibular incisor crowding, severe mandibular deficiency, etc.).

The initial diagnostic records for a patient with moderately severe orthodontic problems, whose primary reason for treatment was improvement of her dental and facial appearance, are shown in Figures 6-76 to 6-79 and the steps in developing a problem list are illustrated in Boxes 6-5 to 6-8. Similar diagnostic work-ups for patients with more severe problems are briefly reviewed in Chapters 18 and 19.

With the completion of a problem list, the diagnostic phase of diagnosis and treatment planning is completed, and

Box 6-5

PATIENT F.P: INTERVIEW DATA

Chief Complaint

"I don't like the way my teeth stick out and look ugly."

Medical, Dental, Social History

- Hemangioma removed from leg at age 4
- No chronic medications
- Regular dental care, no restorations
- Lives with both parents, good progress in school, seems well adjusted without any major social problems

Motivation

- Largely external, mother wants treatment for a problem that she perceives as important
- Patient agrees that she needs treatment, will have to be convinced that this requires her cooperation

Expectation

- General improvement in appearance, seems realistic

Other Pertinent Information

- Older brother treated successfully previously; mother very supportive of orthodontic treatment, father much less so

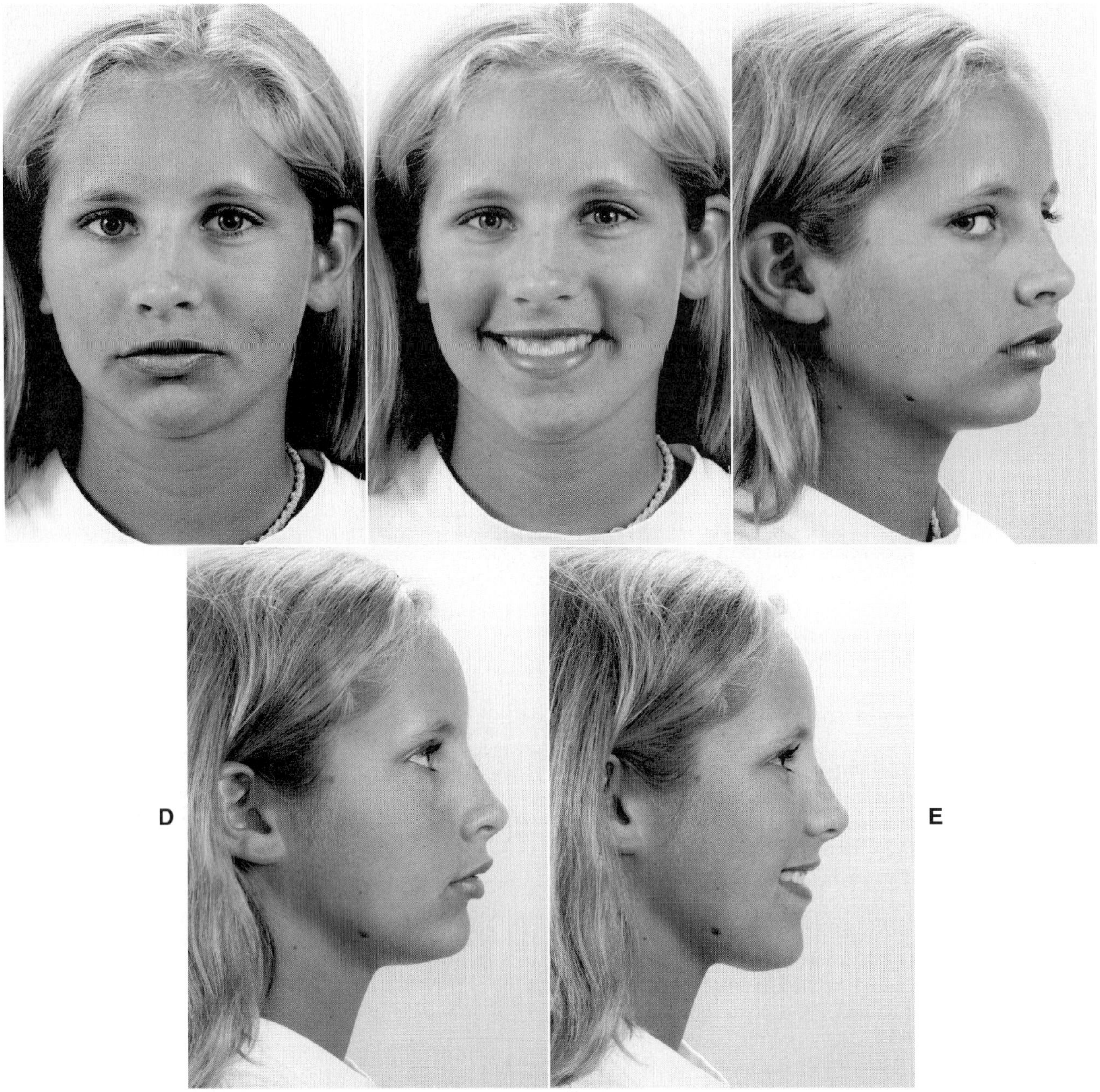

Figure 6-76 Patient F.P., age 12-3, facial views prior to treatment. Note the mildly short anterior face height, lack of mandibular projection, and the appearance of the maxillary incisors on smile (very upright with short clinical crowns but minimal gingival display).

A,B C D E

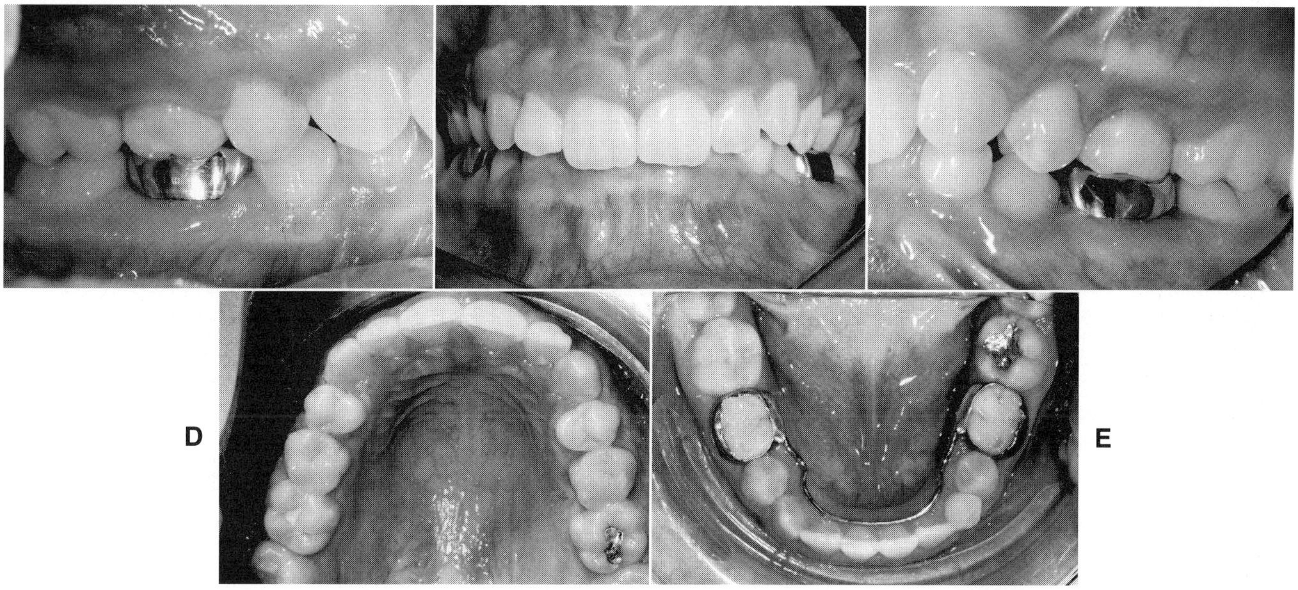

Figure 6-77 Patient F.P., age 12-3, intraoral views prior to treatment. There is moderate maxillary incisor crowding, with the midline off due to displacement of the maxillary incisors. The maxillary incisors are tipped lingually, there is minimal overjet despite Class II buccal segments, and overbite is excessive. A pediatric dentist had placed a lingual arch to maintain alignment of the lower incisors.

Box 6-6

PATIENT F.P: CLINICAL EXAMINATION DATA

Dentofacial Proportions

- Mildly short lower third of face
- Moderate mandibular deficiency
- Inadequate display of maxillary incisors
- Maxillary incisors as wide as they are tall: short maxillary incisor crowns
- Moderate facial and dental asymmetry: mild roll down on right and yaw to left are not severe enough to be noticed as a problem

Health of Hard and Soft Tissues

- Hypoplastic area, upper left first premolar
- Mild gingivitis
- Moderate overgrowth of gingiva, anterior maxilla

Jaw Function

- Maximum opening 45 mm
- Normal range of motion
- No joint sounds
- No pain on palpation

Box 6-7

PATIENT F.P: ANALYSIS OF DIAGNOSTIC RECORDS

(using the Ackerman-Proffit classification to generate the initial problem list)

1. **Facial Proportions and Esthetics**
   - Deficient chin projection, mandibular deficiency
   - Mildly short lower third of face
   - Maxillary incisors tipped lingually, short crowns
2. **Dental Alignment/Symmetry**
   - Moderate maxillary incisor crowding
   - Dental midline off, maxillary incisor displaced
3. **Transverse Relationships**
   - Normal arch widths, no crossbite
4. **Anteroposterior Relationships**
   - Moderate mandibular deficiency
   - Class II buccal segments, minimal overjet
5. **Vertical Relationships**
   - Deep bite, excessive eruption of lower incisors
   - Mildly short face

A

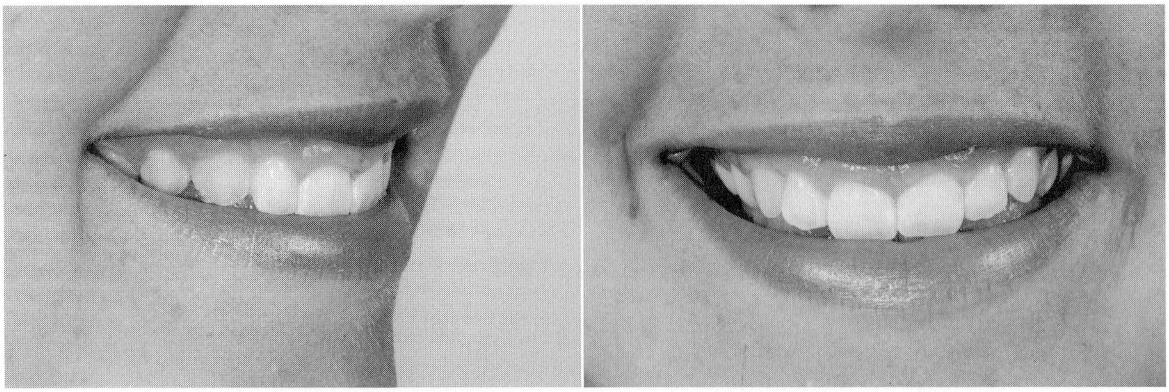

B

FIGURE 6-78 Patient F.P. age 12-3. Close-up views of the smile can be a valuable part of the diagnostic records when dental and facial appearance is an important consideration in developing a treatment plan. For this patient, the short clinical crowns coupled with almost no display of the gingiva should be noted in the problem list. Note that the oblique smile view allows an excellent view of these characteristics.

A

B

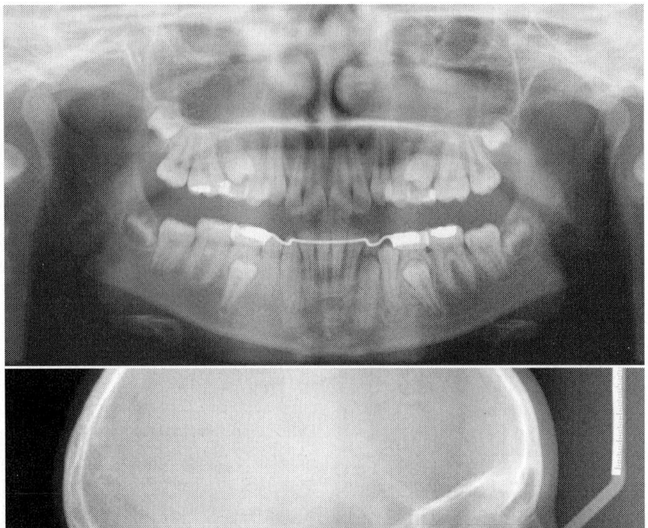

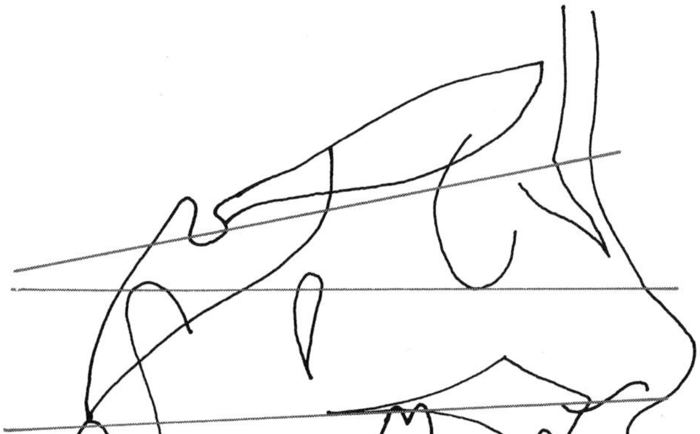

C

FIGURE 6-79 Patient F.P. age 12-3, panoramic **(A)** and cephalometric **(B)** radiographs prior to treatment. **C,** Cephalometric tracing prior to treatment. To assist in visualization of skeletal and dental relationships, drawing this set of horizontal and vertical reference lines and evaluating relationships relative to the true horizontal line and perpendiculars to it is recommended. Note that mandibular deficiency is the major contributor to her Class II malocclusion, and that the deep overbite is primarily due to excessive eruption of the lower incisors. The maxillary incisors are tipped lingually, which is the reason that overjet is not excessive despite the skeletal Class II relationship and the Class II molar relationship.

Box 6-8

PATIENT F.P.: PROBLEM LIST (DIAGNOSIS)

(in the order they appeared in the evaluation sequence)

- Mild gingivitis, mild gingival overgrowth
- Hypoplastic area maxillary left premolar
- Mandibular deficiency
- Maxillary incisors tipped lingually, short crowns
- Moderate maxillary incisor crowding
- Class II buccal segments, minimal overjet
- Deep bite, excessive eruption mandibular incisors

the more subjective process of treatment planning begins. Thorough diagnostic evaluation means that all problems have been identified and characterized at this stage, omitting nothing of significance. The steps in treatment planning and the outcome of treatment for the patient above are presented at the end of Chapter 7, Boxes 7-1 to 7-7, and Figures 7-25 to 7-28.

References

1. Kenealy P, Frude N, Shaw W. An evaluation of the psychological and social effects of malocclusion: Some implications for dental policy making, Social Sci Med 28:583-591, 1989.
2. Tanner JM. Assessment of Skeletal Maturity in Prediction of Adult Height. Philadelphia: WB Saunders; 2001.
3. Deicke M, Pancherz H. Is radius-union an indicator for completed facial growth? Angle Orthod 75:295-299, 2005.
4. Okeson JP. Management of Temporomandibular Disorders and Occlusion, ed 5. St. Louis: Mosby; 2002.
5. Farkas LG. Anthropometry of the Head and Face in Medicine, ed 2. New York: Raven Press; 1994.
6. Hellman M. Variations in occlusion. Dental Cosmos 63:608-619, 1921.
7. Kokich VO Jr, Kiyak HA, Shapiro PA. Comparing the perception of dentists and lay people to altered dental esthetics. J Esthet Dent 11:311-324, 1999.
8. Hulsey CM. An esthetic evaluation of lip-teeth relationships present in the smile. Am J Orthod 57:132-144, 1970.
9. Parekh J, Fields HW, Beck FM, Rosenstiel S. Attractiveness of variations in the smile arc and buccal corridor space as judged by orthodontists and laymen, Angle Orthod 76:557-563, 2005.
10. Moore T, Southard KA, Casko JS, Qian F, Southard TE. Buccal corridors and smile esthetics. Am J Orthod Dentofac Orthop 127:208-213, 2005.
11. Atchison KA, Luke LS, White SC. An algorithm for ordering pretreatment orthodontic radiographs. Am J Orthod Dentofac Orthop 102:29-44, 1992.
12. Web site for new radiographic guidelines, January 2005. Available at: www.ada.org/prof/resources/topics/radiography.asp
13. Jacobs SG. Localization of the unerupted maxillary canine: How to and when to. Am J Orthod Dentofac Orthop 115:314-322, 1999.
14. Armstrong C, Johnston C, Burden D, Stevenson M. Localizing ectopic maxillary canines—horizontal or vertical parallax? Eur J Orthod 25:585-589, 2003.
15. Herring JT. Localization of impacted maxillary canines: the effectiveness of orthodontists and oral radiologists using cone-beam CT and parallax methods. Univ of North Carolina School of Dentistry, MS Thesis, 2006.
16. Brooks SA, Brand JW, Gibbs SJ, et al. Imaging of the temporomandibular joint—a position paper of the American Academy of Oral and Maxillofacial Radiology. Oral Surg Oral Med Oral Pathol 83:609-618, 1997.
17. Tripodakis AP, Smulow JB, Mehta NR, Clark RE. Clinical study of location and reproducibility of three mandibular positions in relation to body posture and muscle function. J Pros Dent 73:190-198, 1995.
18. Trpkova B, Prasad NG, Lam EW, et al. Assessment of facial asymmetries from posteroanterior cephalograms: Validity of reference lines. Am J Orthod Dentofac Orthop 123:512-520, 2003.
19. Altherr ER, Koroluk LA, Phillips C. The influence of gender and ethnic tooth-size differences on mixed dentition space analysis. Am J Orthod Dentofac Orthop, in press.
20. Bolton WA. The clinical application of a tooth-size analysis. Am J Orthod 48:504-529, 1962.
21. Kantor ML, Norton LA. Normal radiographic anatomy and common anomalies seen in cephalometric films. Am J Orthod Dentofacial Orthop 91:414-426, 1987.
22. Downs WB. Variations in facial relationships: Their significance in treatment and prognosis. Am J Orthod 34:812, 1948.
23. Riolo ML, et al. An Atlas of Craniofacial Growth, Monograph 2, Craniofacial Growth Series. Ann Arbor, Mich: University of Michigan, Center for Human Growth and Development; 1974.
24. Popovich F, Thompson GW. Craniofacial templates for orthodontic case analysis. Am J Orthod 71:406-420, 1977.
25. Broadbent BH Sr, Broadbent BH Jr, Golden WH. Bolton Standards of Dentofacial Developmental Growth. St. Louis: Mosby; 1975.
26. Jacobson A. Radiographic Cephalometry: From Basics to Videoimaging. Chicago: Quintessence; 1995.
27. Athanasiou AE. Orthodontic Cephalometry. Chicago: Mosby; 1995.
28. Cooke MS. Five-year reproducibility of natural head posture: A longitudinal study. Am J Orthod Dentofacial Orthop 97:487-494, 1990.
29. Lundstrom A, Lundstrom F, Lebret LM, Moorrees CF. Natural head position and natural head orientation: Basic considerations in cephalometric analysis. Eur J Orthod 17:111-120, 1995.
30. McNamara JA Jr. A method of cephalometric analysis. In: Clinical Alteration of the Growing Face, Monograph 12, Craniofacial Growth Series. Ann Arbor, Mich: University of Michigan, Center for Human Growth and Development; 1983.
31. Enlow DH, Moyers RE, Hunter WS, McNamara JA. A procedure for the analysis of intrinsic facial form and growth. Am J Orthod 56:6-14, 1969.
32. Franchi L, Baccetti T, McNamara JA. Cephalometric floating norms for North American adults. Angle Orthod 68:497-502, 1998.
33. Anderson G, Fields HW, Beck FM, Chacon G, Vig KWL. Development of cephalometric norms using a unified facial and dental approach. Angle Orthod, 76:612-618, 2006
34. Faustini MM, Hale C, Cisneros GJ. Mesh diagram analysis: Developing a norm for African Americans. Angle Orthod 67:121-128, 1997.
35. Evanko AM, Freeman K, Cisneros GJ. Mesh diagram analysis: Developing a norm for Puerto Rican Americans. Angle Orthod 67:381-388, 1997.
36. Ackerman JL, Proffit WR, Sarver DM, Ackerman MB, Kean MR. Systematic analysis of dentofacial traits: An update on classification. Am J Orthod Dentofac Orthop, in press.
37. Severt TR, Proffit WR. The prevalence of facial asymmetry in the dentofacial deformities population at the University of North Carolina. Int J Adult Orthod Orthogn Surg 12:171-176, 1997.

CHAPTER 7

Orthodontic Treatment Planning: From Problem List to Specific Plan

CHAPTER OUTLINE

TREATMENT PLANNING CONCEPTS AND GOALS

Orthodontic diagnosis is complete when a comprehensive list of the patient's problems has been developed and pathologic and developmental problems have been separated. At that point, the objective in treatment planning is to design the strategy that a wise and prudent clinician, using his or her best judgment, would employ to address the problems while maximizing benefit to the patient and minimizing cost and risk.

It is important to view the goal of treatment in that way. Otherwise, an inappropriate emphasis on some aspect of the case is likely, whether the proposed treatment is medical, dental, or just orthodontics. For example, consider a patient who seeks dental care because she is concerned about the status of old restorations. For that individual, controlling periodontal disease might be more beneficial than replacing old amalgams, and this should be emphasized when a treatment plan is discussed with the patient, even though he or she initially sought only restorative treatment. The same principle applies when orthodontic treatment is planned. The orthodontic treatment plan should be developed, in collaboration with the patient, to do what, on balance, would be best for that individual.

When a group of dentists and dental specialists meet to plan treatment for a patient with complex problems, important orthodontic questions often asked are, "Could you retract the incisors enough to correct the overjet?" or "Could you develop incisal guidance for this patient?" To a question phrased as, "Could you . . .?" the answer often is yes, given an unlimited commitment to treatment. The more appropriate question is not "Could you . . .?" but "Should you . . .?"

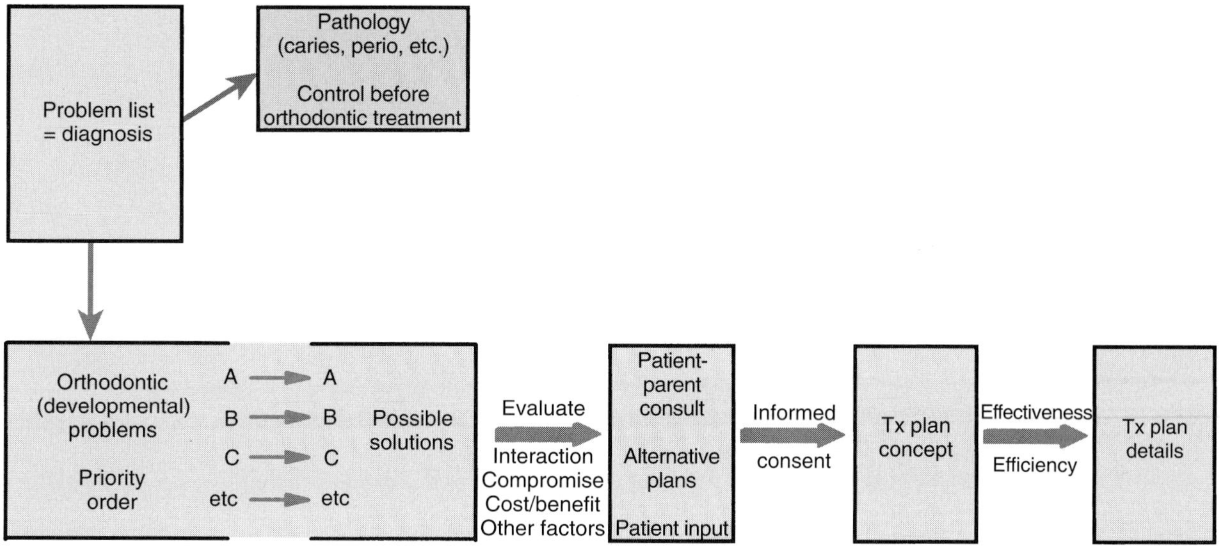

FIGURE 7-1 The treatment planning sequence. In treatment planning, the goal is wisdom, not scientific truth—judgment is required. Interaction with the patient and parent, so that they are involved in the decisions that lead to the final plan, is the key to informed consent.

or "Would it be best for the patient to . . .?" Cost-benefit and risk-benefit analyses are introduced appropriately when the question is rephrased.

A treatment plan in orthodontics, as in any other field, may be less than optimal if it does not take full advantage of the possibilities or if it is too ambitious. There is always a temptation to jump to conclusions and proceed with a superficially obvious plan without considering all the pertinent factors. The treatment planning approach advocated here is specifically designed to avoid both missed opportunities (the false negative or undertreatment side of treatment planning) and excessive treatment (the false positive or overtreatment side), while appropriately involving the patient in the planning process (Figure 7-1).

For the patient whose diagnostic work-up is illustrated at the end of Chapter 6, the development of a treatment plan and the treatment outcome are shown below in the section on comprehensive treatment (see Figures 7-22, 7-25 to 7-28). At this point, let us examine some important concepts that underlie treatment planning more generally.

Need for Treatment

Indications for Orthodontic Treatment

In broad terms, there are six reasons for orthodontic treatment, in the approximate order of their frequency as the reason that patients seek treatment: to (1) remove, or at least alleviate, the social handicap created by an unacceptable dental and/or facial appearance; (2) enhance dental and facial appearance in individuals who already are socially acceptable but wish to improve their quality of life; (3) maintain as normal a developmental process as possible; (4) improve jaw function and correct problems related to functional impairment; (5) reduce the impact on the dentition of trauma or disease, and (6) facilitate other dental treatment, as an adjunct to restorative, prosthodontic or periodontal therapy. These are discussed in Chapter 1, and references to the appropriate literature are provided there. The goal here is to summarize what is known about need for orthodontic treatment.

Psychosocial Indications. Research has documented the effect of an unfortunate facial appearance on both social interactions and self-perception, and orthodontic treatment is justifiable on this basis when the appearance of the face and/or teeth creates a psychosocial problem for the patient. Although the severity of the malocclusion correlates with its psychosocial effect, measuring how much the teeth protrude or how irregular they are is not sufficient to determine individual treatment need. This is case- and patient-specific. A malocclusion that is not a problem for one individual can be a significant problem for another. The major reason patients seek treatment is their concern about appearance and its impact on their life adjustment.

Developmental Indications. Problems related to the development of the dentition occur relatively frequently, and often orthodontic treatment is needed to maintain dental health and continue normal development. For example, it is much better to extract maxillary primary canines early to improve the chance that the permanent canine will erupt in that area than to correct it after the tooth becomes impacted or erupts far from its normal position (Figure 7-2). Treatment to control the attrition of tooth structure that can occur when a tooth is out of position, or to control loss of space if a tooth is missing or lost, also is easily justified. Problems of dental development almost always should be corrected when noticed.

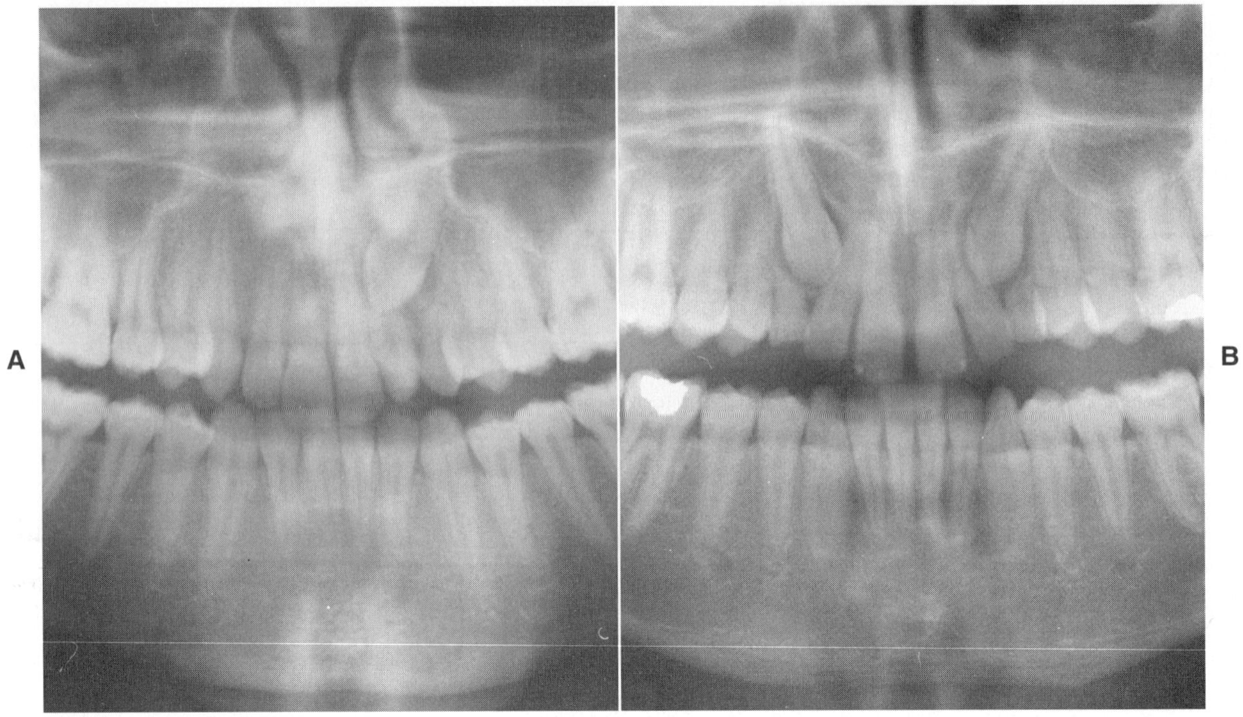

Figure 7-2 Unilateral **(A)** and bilateral **(B)** impacted maxillary canines in young adults. The permanent canines moved mesial to the primary canines rather than replacing them. Extraction of the primary canines at the time the mesial position of the permanent canines was just developing probably could have prevented impaction.

Functional Indications. Severe malocclusion affects function, usually not by making it impossible, but by making it more difficult for the affected individual to breathe, incise, chew, swallow and speak normally (see Chapter 5). The reverse also is true: alterations or adaptations in function can be etiologic factors for malocclusion, by influencing the pattern of growth and development. The extent to which improved function justifies orthodontic treatment remains poorly defined. Current thinking can be summarized as follows:

- Respiration—There seem to be numerous weak relationships between respiratory mode and malocclusion, but the more refined and rigorous the investigations, the more questionable specific links become. The evidence does not support orthodontic referrals of children for surgery to open the nasal airway (by removing adenoids, turbinates, or other presumed obstacles to nasal airflow), because the effect on the future facial growth pattern is unpredictable. For the same reason, expanding the maxillary dental arch by opening the midpalatal suture, which also widens the nasal passages, cannot be supported as an effective way of changing the respiratory pattern toward nasal breathing and away from mouth breathing.
- Chewing, jaw function, and temporomandibular joint dysfunction (TMD)—It seems obvious that chewing should be easier and more efficient with good dental occlusion, but individuals expend the effort necessary to accomplish important tasks like chewing, and there is little evidence to support any impact of malocclusion on nutritional status. Except for the most extreme malocclusions, the effect appears to be increased work to prepare a satisfactory bolus for swallowing. Masticatory effort is difficult to measure accurately, so there are no good data for how much difference it makes to have mild, moderate, or severe malocclusion.

It is possible that functional problems related to malocclusion would appear as temporomandibular dysfunction. Little or no data support the idea that orthodontic treatment is needed at any age to prevent the development of TMD. A recent population-based study in Germany, with a sample of 7008 individuals from a population of 212,157, found essentially no link between malocclusion or functional occlusion and TMD.[1] Some studies have found correlations between some types of malocclusion and TMD, but they are not strong enough to explain even a small fraction of TMD problems.

- Swallowing/speech—Both the pattern of activity in swallowing and tongue-lip function during speech are affected by the presence of the teeth. The most effective way to eliminate a "tongue thrust swallow" is to retract protruding incisors and close an open bite, so orthodontics can have an effect on swallowing, but rarely is this a reason for treatment. Normal speech is possible in the presence of extreme anatomic deviations. Certain types of malocclusion are related to difficulty with specific sounds (see Chapter 6, Table 6-1), and occasionally a reason for orthodontic treatment is that it would facilitate speech therapy. Usually, however, speech problems are not a reason for orthodontics.

Trauma/Disease Control Indications. At one time it was thought that malocclusion contributed to the development of periodontal disease, but this link is so tenuous that almost never is it a reason for orthodontic treatment. In older patients, orthodontics as an adjunct to periodontal therapy may be indicated. In children and adolescents, orthodontics cannot be justified for disease control. Contact of the lower incisors with the palatal mucosa or the upper incisors with the mandibular anterior gingiva, which often occurs in deep overbite, can lead to loss of soft tissue and periodontal defects. Correcting tissue impingement by the teeth, therefore, can be a benefit from orthodontic treatment at any age—but better data are needed to clarify the amount of benefit. Although there is ample evidence that protruding incisors are more likely to be damaged, the severity of the injury varies greatly, and often is trivial. Only in the most accident-prone child is this a valid reason for reducing overjet.

Adjunctive Treatment Indications. Especially in adults who need extensive restorations or replacement of missing teeth, conventional dental treatment often is destined to fall short of an optimal result because of tooth positions that can be improved by limited orthodontic treatment. For example, redistributing space within the dental arches makes better restorations possible, periodontal conditions or therapy can be altered by moving teeth adjacent to bony defects, and traumatically displaced teeth can be repositioned to improve their prognosis and provide better endodontic access.

The bottom line: orthodontic treatment almost always is elective, but it can produce significant benefits in psychosocial well-being, normal development, jaw function, dental/oral health and improved outcomes in the treatment of dental disease. Orthodontics is needed if it would produce these benefits—and not needed if it would not.

Type of Treatment: Evidence-Based Selection

If treatment is needed, how do you decide what sort of treatment to use? The present trend in health care is strongly toward evidence-based treatment, that is, treatment procedures should be chosen on the basis of clear evidence that the selected method is the most successful approach to that particular patient's problem(s).[2] The better the evidence, of course, the easier the decision.

The problem-oriented approach to diagnosis and treatment planning is built around identifying the patient's problems, then considering and evaluating the possible solutions to those specific problems. The best way to evaluate alternative treatment methods is with a randomized clinical trial, in which great care is taken to control variables that might affect the outcomes, so that differences attributable to the treatment procedures become apparent. A second acceptable way to replace opinion with evidence is from careful study of treatment outcomes under well-defined conditions. Clinical trial data are just becoming available in orthodontics, and not all decisions about alternative treatment possibilities can be based on good evidence of any type. In Chapter 8, the quality of clinical evidence relative for current orthodontic procedures is examined in detail. In this and the subsequent chapters, recommendations for treatment are based insofar as possible on solid clinical evidence. Where this is not available, the authors' current opinions are provided and labeled as such.

Treatment Goals: The Soft Tissue Paradigm

A paradigm can be defined as *"a set of shared beliefs and assumptions that represent the conceptual foundation of an area of science or clinical practice."* The re-orientation of orthodontics from the Angle paradigm that dominated the 20th century toward the soft tissue paradigm was reviewed briefly in Chapter 1, and the differences between the Angle and soft tissue paradigms are tabulated there (see Table 1-1). As clinicians increasingly now accept the new paradigm, which states that both the goals and limitations of orthodontic treatment are established more by soft tissue considerations than skeletal/dental relationships, treatment planning inevitably is affected.

What difference does the soft tissue paradigm make in planning treatment? There are several major effects.

The primary goal of treatment becomes soft tissue relationships and adaptations, not Angle's ideal occlusion. The broader goal is not incompatible with Angle's ideal occlusion, but it acknowledges that in order to provide maximum benefit for the patient, ideal occlusion cannot always be the major focus of a treatment plan. Soft tissue relationships, both the proportions of the soft tissue integument of the face and the relationship of the dentition to the lips and face, are the major determinants of facial appearance. Soft tissue adaptations to the position of the teeth (or lack thereof) determine whether or not the orthodontic result will be stable. Keeping this in mind while planning treatment is critically important.

The secondary goal of treatment becomes *functional* occlusion. What does that have to do with soft tissues? Temporomandibular dysfunction, to the extent that it relates to the dental occlusion, is best thought of as due to injury to the patient from clenching and grinding the teeth. Given that, an important goal of treatment is to arrange the occlusion to minimize the chance of injury. In this also, Angle's ideal occlusion is not incompatible with the broader goal—but deviations from the Angle ideal may provide greater benefit for some patients, and should be considered when treatment is planned.

The thought process that goes into "solving the patient's problems" is reversed. In the past, the clinician's focus was on dental and skeletal relationships, with the tacit assumption that if these were correct, the soft tissue relationships would take care of themselves. With the broader focus on facial and oral soft tissues, the thought process is to establish what these soft tissue relationships should be, and then determine how the teeth and jaws would have to be arranged to meet the soft tissue goals.

This approach is entirely compatible with problem-oriented diagnosis and treatment planning. The problem list will reflect soft tissue considerations in a way that it might not have previously, and this has been emphasized in the previous chapter. The goal of treatment is exactly the same: to solve those problems in a way that maximizes benefit to the patient, with benefit defined from the broader perspective.

Major Issues in Planning Treatment

Once a patient's orthodontic problems have been identified and prioritized, three issues must be faced as treatment planning begins: (1) the complexity of the treatment that would be required, (2) the predictability of success with a given treatment approach, and (3) the patient's (and parents') goals and desires. Considering these briefly in turn:

Complexity of Treatment

The complexity of the treatment that would be required affects treatment planning especially in the context of who should do the treatment. In orthodontics as in all areas of dentistry, it makes sense that the less complex cases would be selected for treatment in general or family practice, while the more complex cases would be referred to a specialist. In family practice, an important issue is how you rationally select patients for treatment or referral. A formal scheme is presented below for separating patients most appropriate for orthodontic treatment in family practice from those more likely to require complex treatment.

Predictability of Treatment

If alternative methods of treatment are available—as usually is the case—which one should be chosen? Data gradually are accumulating to allow choices to be based on evidence of outcomes rather than anecdotal reports and the claims of advocates of particular approaches. The quality of evidence for clinical decisions, and how to evaluate the data as evaluations of treatment become available, are emphasized in Chapter 8.

Patient Input

Finally but most important, treatment planning must be an interactive process. No longer can the doctor decide, in a paternalistic way, what is best for a patient. Both ethically and practically, patients must be involved in the decision-making process. Ethically, patients have the right to control what happens to them in treatment—treatment is something done for them, not to them. Practically, the patient's compliance is likely to be a critical issue in success or failure, and there is little reason to select a mode of treatment that the patient would not support. Informed consent, in its modern form, requires the involvement of the patient in the treatment planning process. This is emphasized in the procedure for presenting treatment recommendations that is presented below.

Orthodontic Triage: Distinguishing Moderate From Complex Treatment Problems

For a patient with malocclusion, the first question is whether orthodontic treatment is needed. If the answer is yes, the second question, typically faced by the family dentist seeing a child who needs orthodontic intervention now, is who should do the treatment. Does this patient warrant referral to a specialist?

In military and emergency medicine, triage is the process used to separate casualties by the severity of their injuries. Its purpose is twofold: to separate patients who can be treated at the scene of the injury from those who need transportation to specialized facilities, and to develop a sequence for handling patients so that those most likely to benefit from immediate treatment will be treated first. Since orthodontic problems almost never are an emergency, the process of sorting orthodontic problems by their severity is analogous to triage in only one sense of the word. On the other hand, it is very important for the primary care dentist to be able to distinguish moderate from complex problems, because this process determines which patients are appropriately treated within family practice and which are most appropriately referred to a specialist.

As with all components of dental practice, a generalist's decision of whether to include orthodontic treatment as a component of his or her services is an individual one, best based on experience and ability. The principle that the less severe problems are handled within the context of general practice and the more severe problems are referred should remain the same, however, regardless of the practitioner's interest in orthodontics. Only the cutoff points for treating a patient in the general practice or referral should change.

This section presents a logical scheme for orthodontic triage for children, to select children for referral on the basis of the severity of their malocclusion and the likely complexity of their evaluation and treatment. It is based on the diagnostic approach developed in Chapter 6 and incorporates the principles of determining treatment need that are discussed above. An adequate database and a thorough problem list, of course, are necessary to carry out the triage process. A cephalometric radiograph is not required, but appropriate dental radiographs are needed (usually, a panoramic film; occasionally, bitewings supplemented with anterior occlusal radiographs). A flow chart illustrating the steps in the triage sequence accompanies this section.

Step 1: Syndromes and Developmental Abnormalities

The first step in the triage process is to separate out patients with facial syndromes and similarly complex problems (Figure 7-3). From physical appearance, the medical and

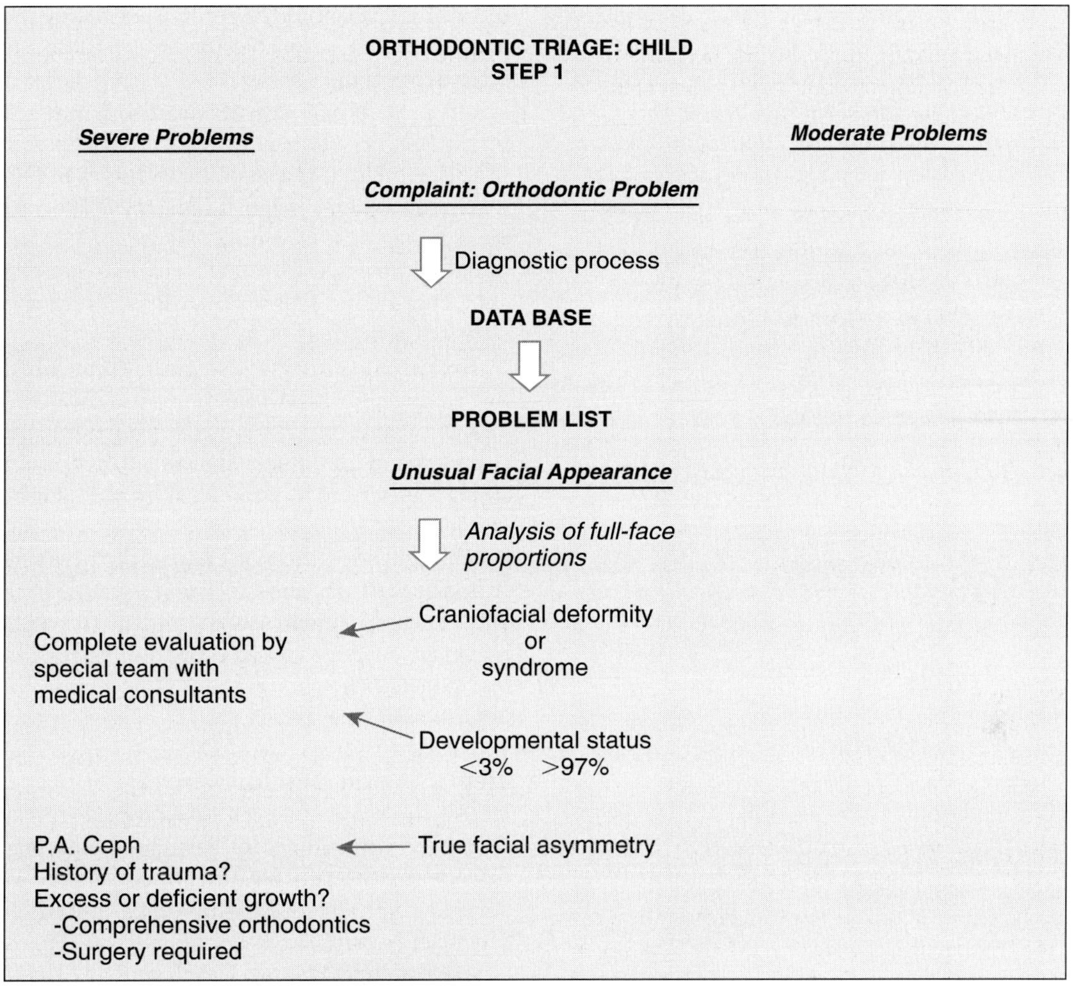

FIGURE 7-3 Orthodontic triage, Step 1.

dental histories, and an evaluation of developmental status, nearly all such patients are easily recognized. Examples of these disorders are cleft lip or palate, Treacher-Collins' syndrome, hemifacial microsomia, and Crouzon's syndrome (see Chapter 3). The multidisciplinary treatment approach now considered as the standard of care for these patients should lead to their referral to a craniofacial team of specialists at a regional medical center for evaluation and treatment. The American Cleft Palate Association publishes a directory of these teams,[3] who now cover the whole spectrum of craniofacial problems, not just cleft palate.

A similar route of referral and medical evaluation is recommended for patients who appear to be developing either above the 97th or below the third percentiles on standard growth charts. Growth disorders may demand that any orthodontic treatment be carried out in conjunction with endocrine, nutritional, or psychological therapy. For these patients and those with diseases that affect growth, such as juvenile rheumatoid arthritis, the proper orthodontic therapy must be combined with identification and control of the disease process.

Patients with significant skeletal asymmetry (not necessarily those whose asymmetry results from only a functional shift of the mandible) always fall into the severe problem category (Figure 7-4). These patients could have a developmental problem or the growth anomaly could be the result of injury. They require evaluation including posteroanterior and lateral cephalometric radiographs. Treatment is likely to involve surgery in addition to comprehensive orthodontics. Timing of intervention is affected by whether the cause of the asymmetry is deficient or excessive growth (see Chapter 8), but early comprehensive evaluation is indicated even if treatment ultimately is deferred.

Step 2: Facial Profile Analysis

(Figure 7-5)

Anteroposterior and Vertical Problems. Skeletal Class II and Class III problems and vertical deformities of the long face and short face types, regardless of their cause, require thorough cephalometric evaluation to plan appropriate treatment and must be considered complex problems (Figure 7-6). As with asymmetry, early evaluation is indicated even if treatment would be deferred, so early referral is appropriate. Issues in treatment planning for growth modification are discussed in Chapter 8, and the appropriate treatment techniques are described in Chapter 13.

Excessive Dental Protrusion or Retrusion. Severe dental protrusion or retrusion, which also is a complex treatment problem, should be recognized during the facial profile analysis. Excessive protrusion or retrusion of incisor teeth often accompanies skeletal jaw discrepancies, and if protrusion is present in a patient who also has a skeletal problem, this should be subordinated to the skeletal problem in planning treatment. It is also possible, however, for an individual with good skeletal proportions to have protrusion of incisor teeth rather than crowding (Figure 7-7). When this occurs, the space analysis will show a small or nonexistent discrepancy, because the incisor protrusion has compensated for the potential crowding.

Excessive protrusion of incisors (bimaxillary protrusion, not excessive overjet) usually is an indication for premolar extraction and retraction of the protruding incisors. This is complex and prolonged treatment. Because of the profile changes produced by adolescent growth, it is better for most children to defer extraction to correct protrusion until late in the mixed dentition or early in the permanent dentition. It is definitely an error to begin extraction early and then allow the permanent molars to drift forward, because this will make effective incisor retraction impossible. Techniques for controlling the amount of incisor retraction are described in Chapter 15.

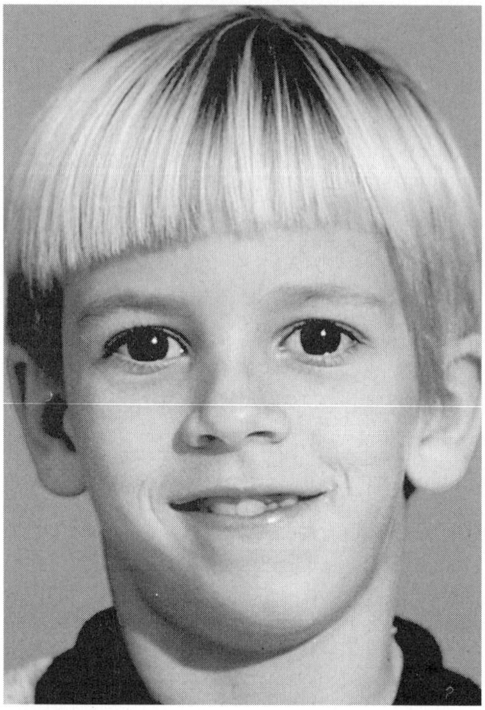

FIGURE 7-4 At age 8, this boy has a noticeable mandibular asymmetry, with the chin several millimeters off to the left. A problem of this type is likely to become progressively worse, and is an indication for referral for comprehensive evaluation by a facial deformities team. (From Proffit WR, White RP, Sarver DM. Contemporary Treatment of Dentofacial Deformity. St. Louis: Mosby; 2003.)

Step 3: Dental Development

Unlike the more complex skeletal problems and problems related to protruding incisors, problems involving dental development usually need treatment as soon as they are discovered, typically during the early mixed dentition, and often can be handled in family practice (Figure 7-8).

Asymmetric Dental Development. Treatment for an abnormal sequence of dental development should be planned only after a careful determination of the underlying cause. Asymmetric eruption (one side ahead of the other) is significant if the difference is 6 months or more. Appropriate treatment involves careful monitoring of the situation, and in the absence of outright pathology, often requires

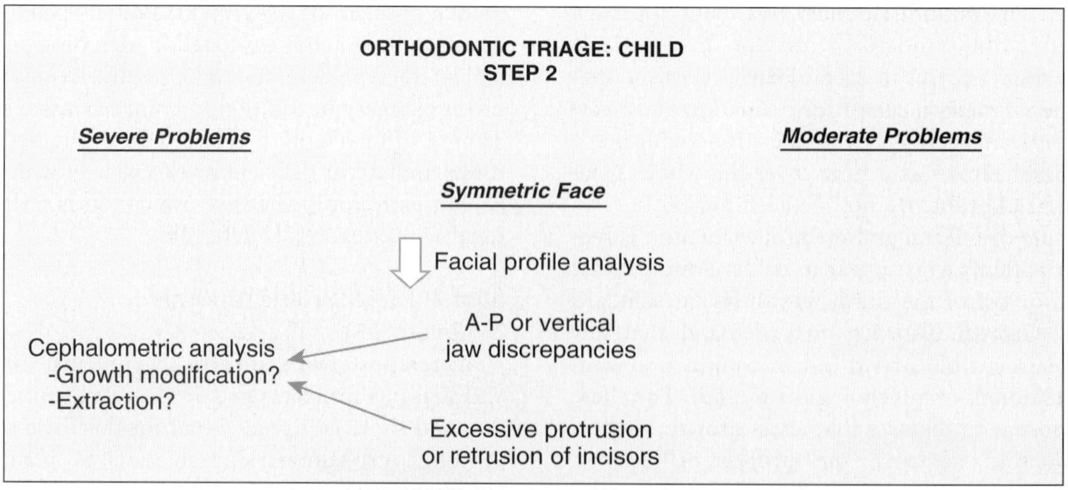

FIGURE 7-5 Orthodontic triage, Step 2.

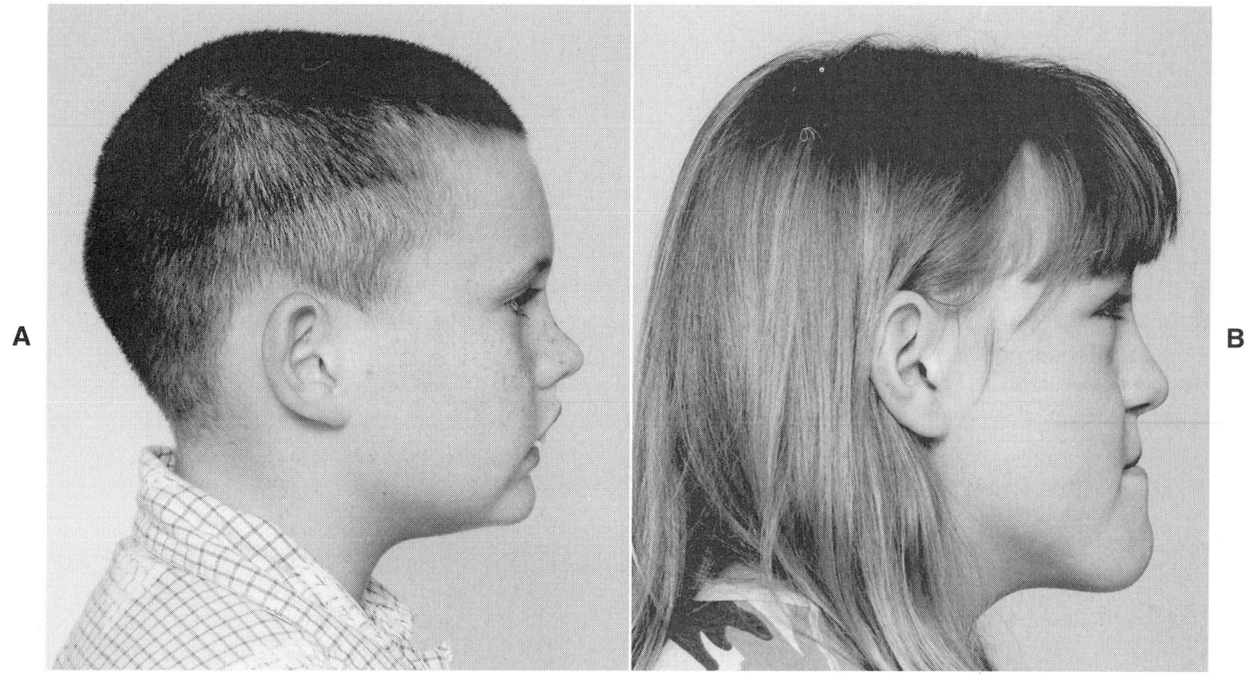

FIGURE 7-6 Patients with a skeletal problem of even moderate severity (**A,** Skeletal Class II due to mandibular deficiency; **B,** Skeletal Class III with a component of both maxillary deficiency and mandibular excess) can be picked up from examination of the profile. A cephalometric radiograph is not necessary.

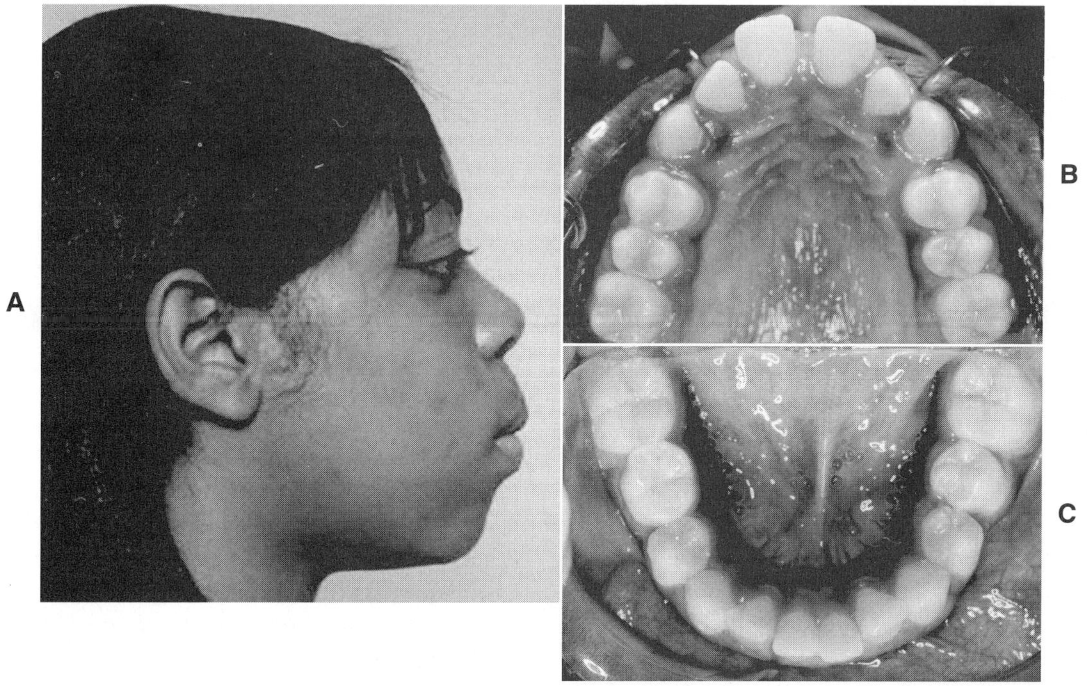

FIGURE 7-7 **A,** Bimaxillary dentoalveolar protrusion. Note the lip strain to bring the lips together over the teeth. The lips were separated at rest by the protruding incisors. **B, C,** Occlusal views. Note the spacing in the upper arch and very mild crowding in the lower arch. For this girl, potential crowding of the teeth is expressed almost completely as protrusion.

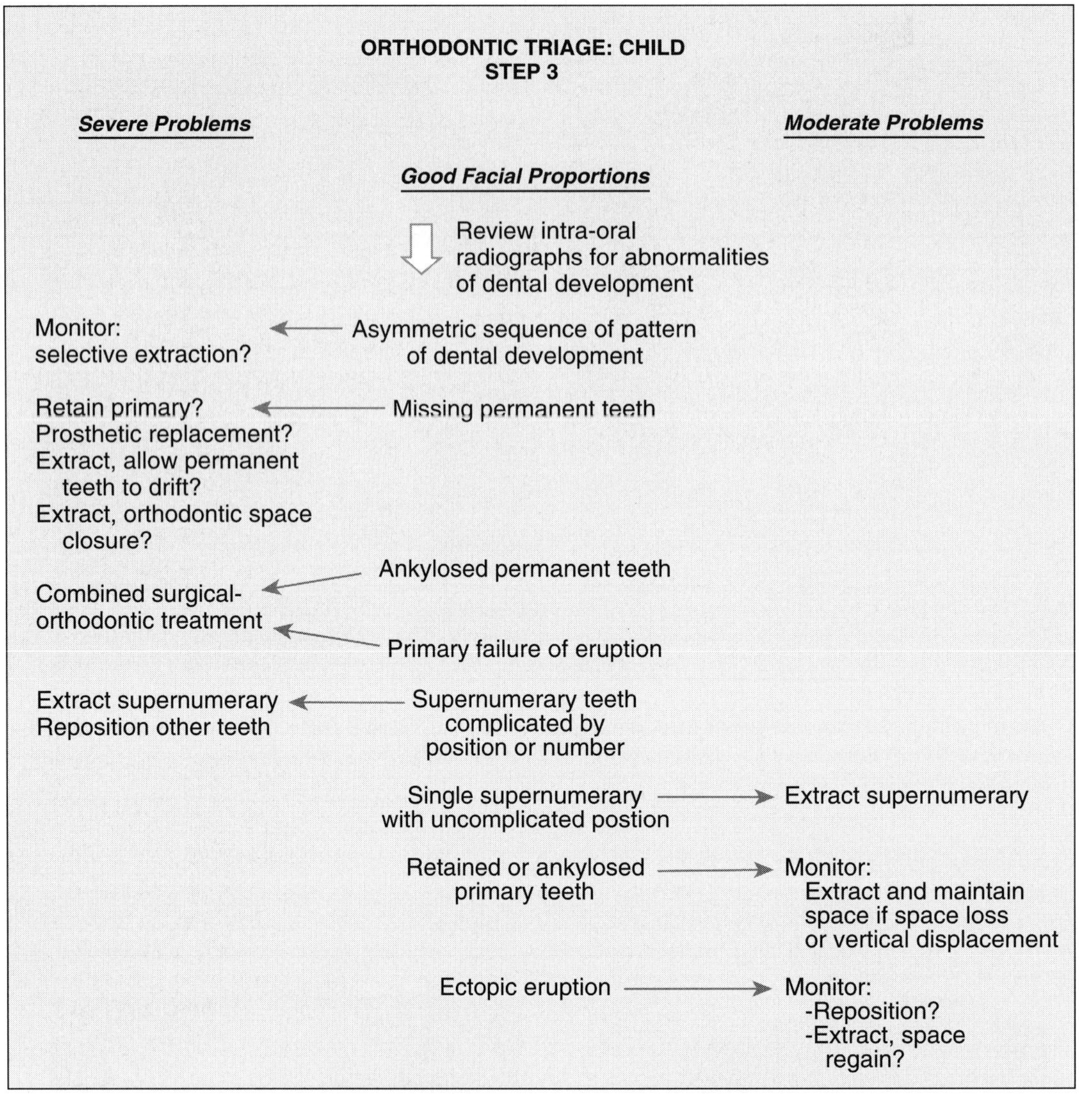

Figure 7-8 Orthodontic triage, Step 3.

selective extraction of primary or permanent teeth. Early intervention to promote more symmetric development of the dental arches, as for example the early extraction of the left mandibular primary canine after the right canine has been lost prematurely, can circumvent the need for treating a severe asymmetry problem at a later time (Figure 7-9), but such a step must be taken only after careful consideration of the total problem list for an individual patient.

A few patients with asymmetric dental development have a history of childhood radiation therapy to the head and neck. These patients often have extremes of delayed or asymmetric dental development. Surgical and orthodontic treatment for these patients must be planned and timed carefully with their medical treatment providers and definitely falls into the complex category.

Missing Permanent Teeth. A congenitally missing permanent tooth is an actual (if the primary predecessor is missing or lost) or potential (if the primary tooth is still present) problem of arch asymmetry. The permanent teeth most likely to be missing are the mandibular second premolars and the maxillary lateral incisors, but the treatment possibilities are the same whatever the missing tooth: (1) maintenance of the primary tooth or teeth; (2) replacement of the missing teeth prosthetically or perhaps by transplantation or implant; (3) extraction of the overlying primary teeth, and then allowing the permanent teeth to drift; or (4) extraction of the primary teeth followed by immediate orthodontic treatment. As with other growth problems, early evaluation and planning is essential, even if the decision is against aggressive treatment at that time, so early referral is indicated. Making the correct decision requires a careful assessment of facial profile, incisor position, space requirements, and the status of the primary teeth. Treatment of missing tooth problems in mixed dentition children is discussed in more detail in Chapter 12.

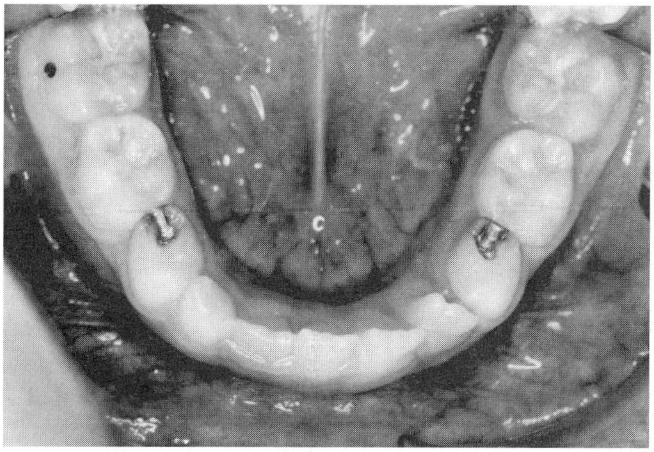

Figure 7-9 After early loss of the mandibular left primary canine (almost surely because of root resorption as the left permanent lateral incisor erupted), the permanent incisors have tipped toward the left side. As a general rule, when one mandibular primary canine is lost early for any reason, intervention by the dentist is needed to maintain symmetry within the arch. (The KISS rule can also be expressed for orthodontic purposes as Keep It Symmetric, Stupid.)

For all practical purposes, ankylosed permanent teeth at an early age or teeth that fail to erupt for other reasons (like primary failure of eruption) fall into the same category as missing teeth. These severe problems often require a combination of surgery and orthodontics, if indeed the condition can be treated satisfactorily at all. Usually there is little choice but to extract the affected teeth, and then the choices are orthodontic space closure (if enough alveolar bone exists to allow it) or prosthetic replacement (more likely).

Supernumerary Teeth. Ninety percent of all supernumerary teeth are found in the anterior part of the maxilla (see Figure 5-13). Multiple or inverted supernumeraries and those that are malformed often displace adjacent teeth or cause problems in eruption. The presence of multiple supernumerary teeth indicates a complex problem and perhaps a syndrome or congenital abnormality like cleidocranial dysplasia. Early removal is indicated, but this must be done carefully to minimize damage to adjacent teeth. If the permanent teeth have been displaced, surgical exposure, adjunctive periodontal surgery, and possibly mechanical traction are likely to be required to bring them into the arch after the supernumerary has been removed.

Single supernumeraries that are not malformed often erupt spontaneously, causing crowding problems. If these teeth can be removed before they cause distortions of arch form, or if the supernumerary tooth erupts outside the line of the arch, extraction may be all that is needed. Similarly, if an unusually large tooth (usually, a maxillary lateral incisor or mandibular second premolar) can be reduced in size before its presence causes displacement of other teeth, reduction of enamel may be all that is required.

Other Eruption Problems. Ectopic eruption often leads to early loss of a primary tooth, but in severe cases resorption of permanent teeth can result. Orthodontic repositioning of the ectopically erupting tooth may be indicated. A dramatic variation of ectopic eruption is transposition of teeth. Early intervention can reduce the extent to which teeth are malpositioned. These severe problems often require a combination of surgery and orthodontics and may be genetically linked to other anomalies.

Step 4: Space Problems?

Orthodontic problems in a child with good facial proportions must involve crowding, irregularity, or malposition of the teeth (Figure 7-10). At this stage, regardless of whether crowding is apparent, the results of space analysis are essential for planning treatment. The presence or absence of adequate space for the teeth must be taken into account when other treatment is planned.

In interpreting the results of space analysis for patients of any age, remember that if space to align the teeth is inadequate, either of two conditions may develop. One possibility is for the incisor teeth to remain upright and well positioned over the basal bone of the maxilla or mandible, and then rotate or tip labially or lingually. In this instance, the potential crowding is expressed as actual crowding and is difficult to miss (Figure 7-11). The other possibility, however, is for the crowded teeth to align themselves completely or partially at the expense of the lips, displacing the lips forward and separating them at rest (see Figure 7-7). Even if the space discrepancy and therefore the potential crowding are extreme, the teeth can always align themselves at the expense of the lip, interfering with lip closure. This must be detected on profile examination. If there is already a degree of protrusion in addition to the crowding, it is safe to presume that the natural limits of anterior displacement of incisors have been reached.

Space discrepancies of 5 mm or more, with or without incisor protrusion, or discrepancies smaller than 4 mm in the presence of incisor protrusion, constitute complex treatment problems. Depending on the circumstances, the appropriate response to space deficiencies of 4 mm or less can be treatment to regain lost space after early loss of a primary molar or ectopic eruption, management of transitional crowding and repositioning of the permanent incisors during the mixed dentition, or deferral of treatment until adolescence. Treatment planning for these moderate problems is outlined below in the preadolescent section of this chapter.

Step 5: Other Occlusal Discrepancies

Whether other problems of dental alignment and occlusion should be classified as moderate or severe is determined for most children by the facial form and space analysis results (Figure 7-12). A skeletal posterior crossbite, revealed by a narrow palatal vault, is a severe problem, but a dental posterior crossbite falls into the moderate category if no other complicating factors (like severe crowding) are present. In a

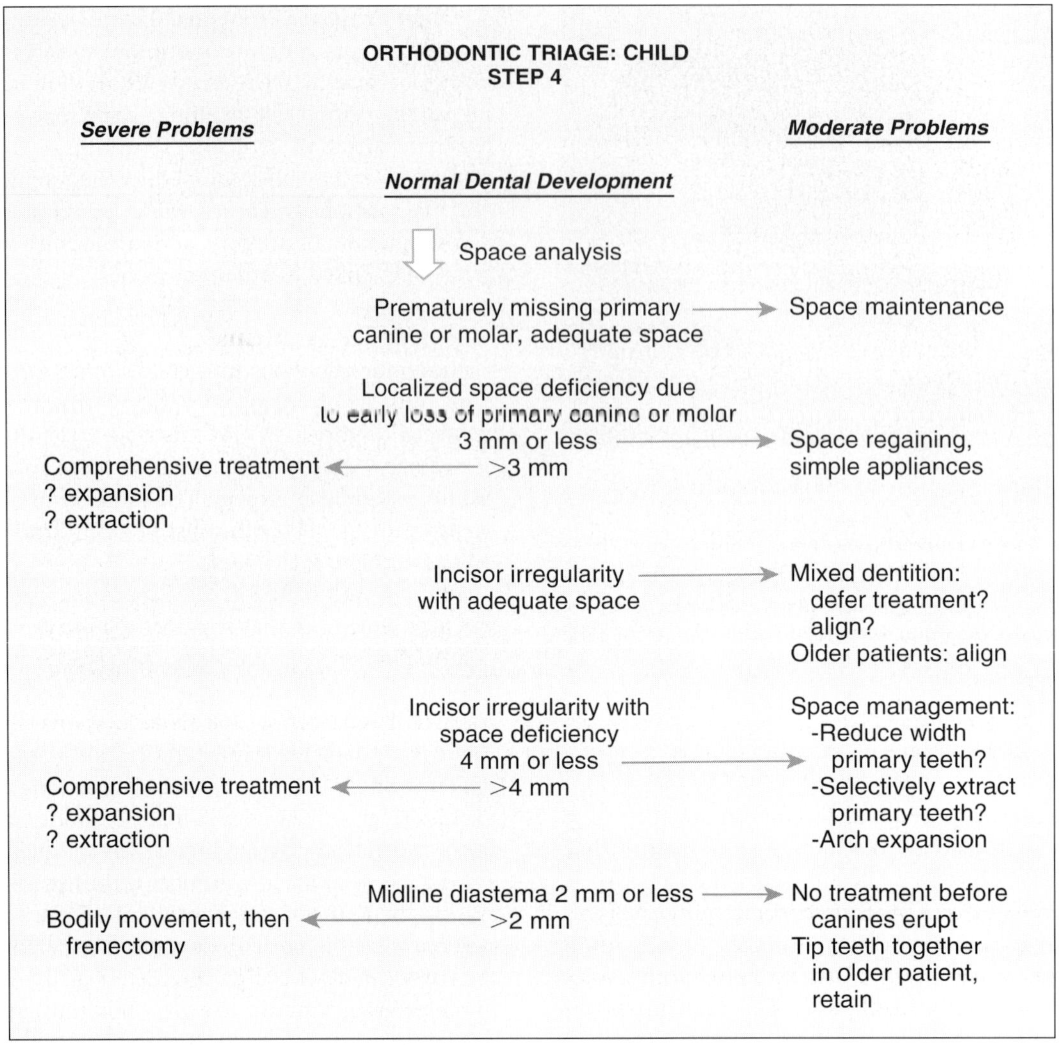

Figure 7-10 Orthodontic triage, Step 4.

skeletal posterior crossbite, it is possible to widen the maxilla itself by opening the midpalatal suture, provided the patient is young enough to allow suture opening. This topic is discussed further in Chapter 8. If the crossbite is caused by maxillary posterior teeth that are tipped lingually, it is possible to tip the teeth outward into proper position with a variety of simple appliances (see Chapter 12).

Anterior crossbite usually reflects a jaw discrepancy but can arise by lingual tipping of the incisors as they erupt. Treatment planning for the use of removable versus fixed appliances to correct these simple crossbites is discussed later under mixed dentition treatment. Excessive overjet, with the upper incisors flared and spaced, often reflects a skeletal problem but also can develop in patients with good jaw proportions. If adequate vertical clearance is present, the teeth can be tipped lingually and brought together with a simple removable appliance when the child is at almost any age. If a deep overbite is present, however, the protruding maxillary incisors can be retracted only if adequate vertical clearance is provided. Remember that deep overbite may reflect a skeletal vertical problem even if anteroposterior facial proportions are normal. Even if skeletal vertical also is normal, mixed dentition treatment usually involves placing a fixed orthodontic appliance on both maxillary and mandibular incisors and can rapidly become complex.

Anterior open bite in a young child with good facial proportions usually needs no treatment, because there is a good chance of spontaneous correction, especially if the open bite is related to an oral habit like finger sucking. A complex open bite (one with skeletal involvement or posterior manifestations), or any open bite in an older patient, is a severe problem, as is deep bite at all ages.

Traumatically displaced incisors pose a special problem because of the risk of ankylosis after healing occurs. Immediate treatment is needed, and the long-term prognosis must be guarded. Treatment planning after trauma is discussed later in the preadolescent section of this chapter.

This triage scheme is oriented toward helping the family practitioner decide which children with orthodontic problems to treat and which to refer. A triage scheme to help dis-

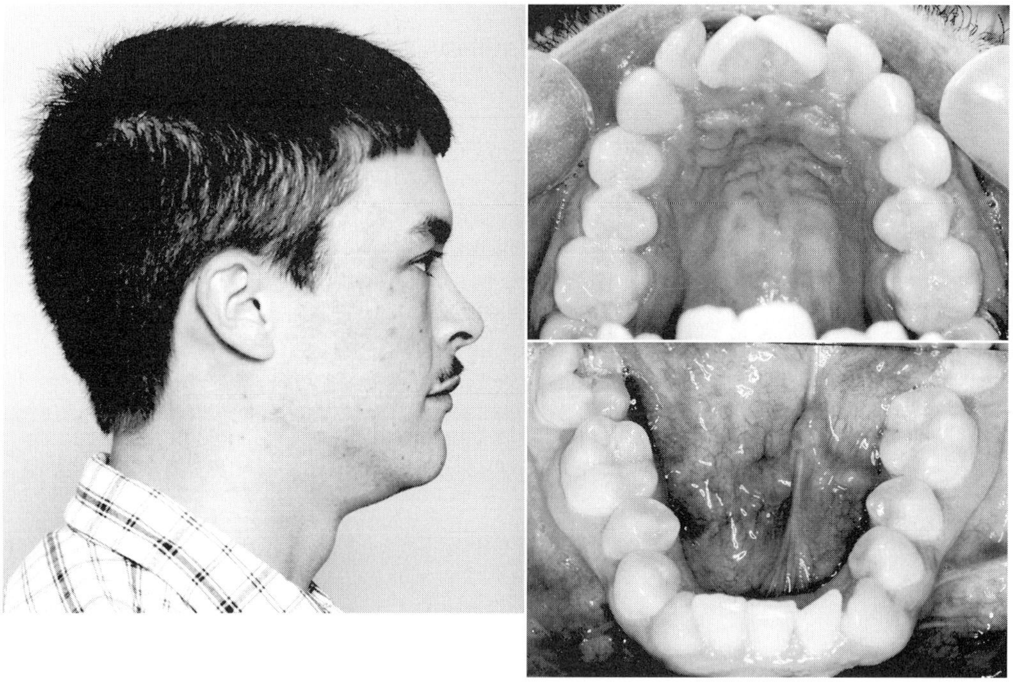

Figure 7-11 In some patients, as in this individual **(A)**, potential crowding is expressed completely as actual crowding **(B, C)** with no compensation in the form of dental and lip protrusion. In others (see Figure 7-7), potential crowding is expressed as protrusion. The teeth end up in a position of equilibrium between the tongue and lip forces against them (see Chapter 5).

tinguish moderate from severe orthodontic problems in adults is presented in Chapter 18.

Now let's review treatment planning for children with moderate problems, those selected for treatment in family practice using the triage scheme. Treatment planning for these non-skeletal problems is discussed in this section, and treatment procedures are described in Chapter 12.

Planning Treatment for Moderate Problems

Space Problems

Missing Primary Teeth With Adequate Space: Space Maintenance

If a primary first or second molar is missing, if there will be more than a 6-month delay before the permanent premolar erupts, and if there is adequate space (because there has been no space loss or because space regaining has been completed) (see later in this section); then space maintenance is needed. Otherwise the space is likely to close spontaneously before the premolar can come into position.

Although space maintenance can be done with either fixed or removable appliances, fixed appliances are preferred in most situations because they eliminate the factor of patient cooperation. If the space is unilateral, it can be managed by a unilateral fixed appliance (Figure 7-13). If molars on both sides have been lost and the lateral incisors have erupted, it is usually better to place a lingual arch rather than two unilateral appliances.

Early loss of a single primary canine in the mixed dentition requires space maintenance or extraction of the contralateral tooth to eliminate midline changes and the loss of arch symmetry (see Figure 7-9). In this circumstance, arch length shortens as the incisor teeth drift distally and lingually. If the contralateral canine is extracted, a lingual arch space maintainer may still be needed to prevent lingual movement of the incisors.

Localized Space Loss (3 mm or less): Space Regaining

Potential space problems can be created by drift of permanent incisors or molars after premature extraction of primary canines or molars. In children who meet the criteria for moderate problems (i.e., no skeletal or dentofacial involvement), lost space can be regained by repositioning the teeth that have drifted. Then, after the space discrepancy has been reduced to zero, a space maintainer is necessary to prevent further drift and space loss until the succedaneous teeth have erupted. A space maintainer alone is not adequate treatment for a space deficiency.

Space regaining is most likely to be needed when primary maxillary or mandibular second molars have been lost prematurely because of decay (Figure 7-14) or, less frequently, because of ectopic eruption of the permanent first molar.

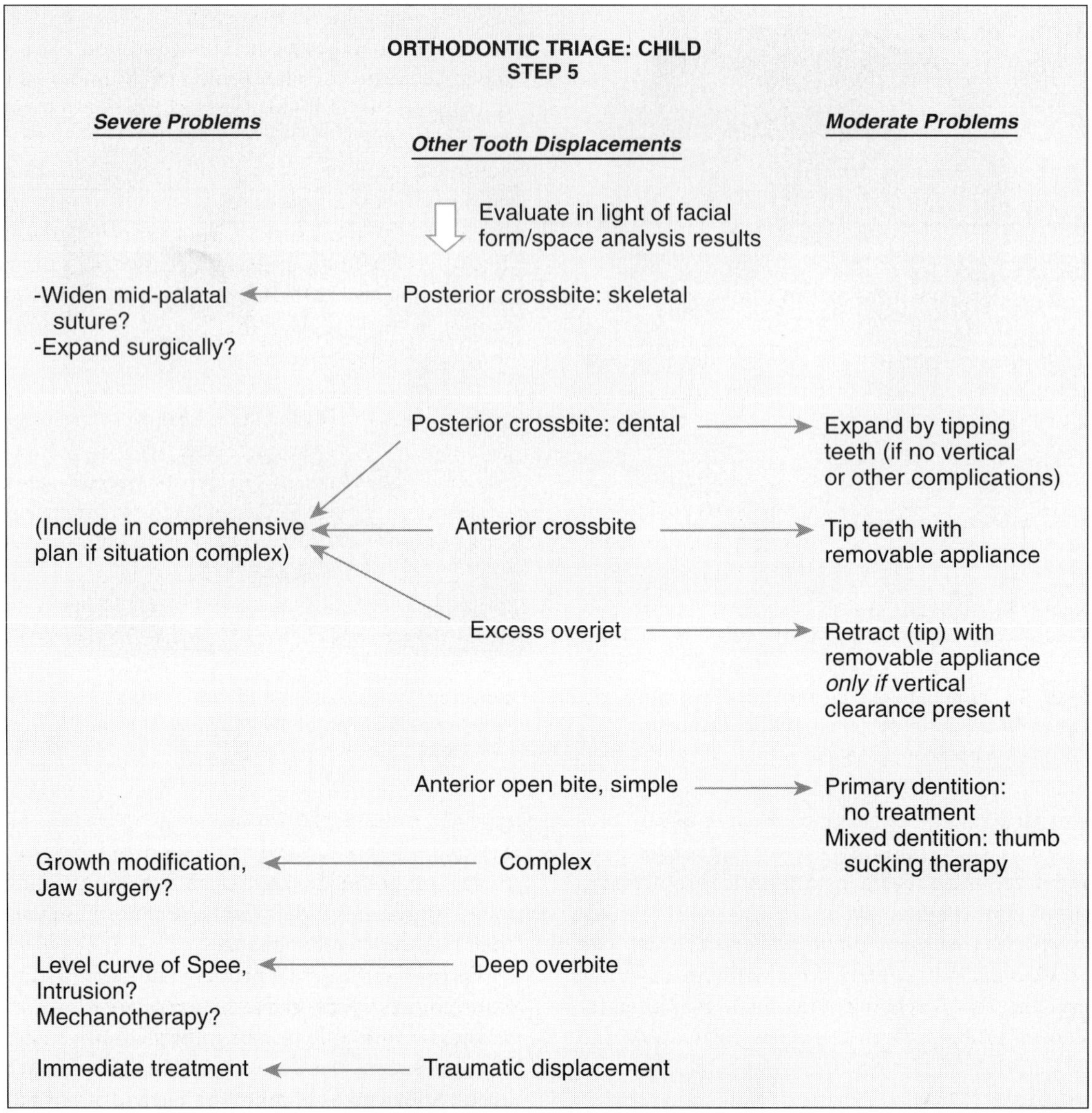

Figure 7-12 Orthodontic triage, Step 5.

A,B

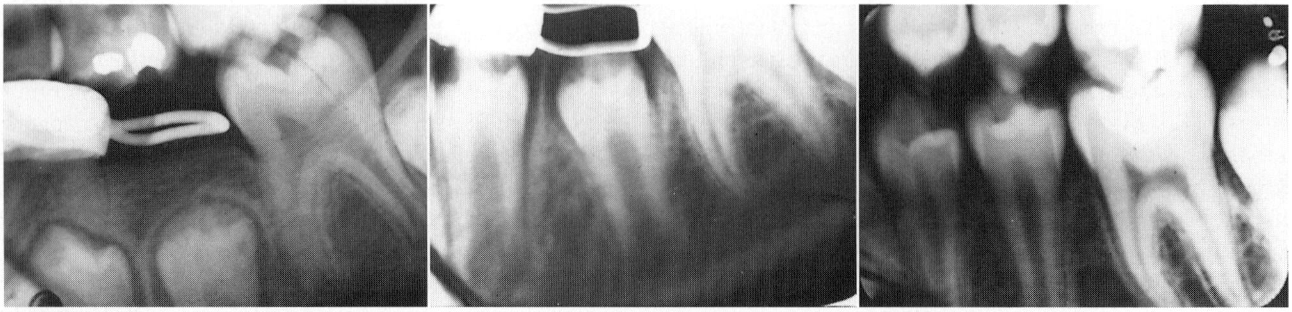

C

Figure 7-13 Space maintenance after early loss of a second primary molar. **A,** Band and loop space maintainer at age 8; **B,** Same patient, age 11; **C,** Same patient, age 12.

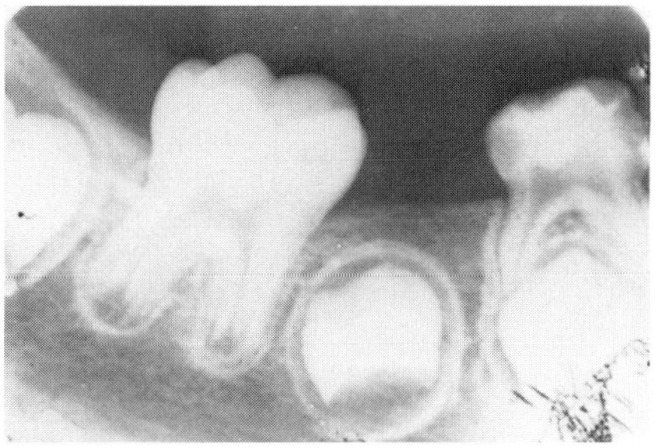

Figure 7-14 After early loss of a primary second molar, mesial drift of the permanent first molar nearly always occurs rapidly, as in this child.

The permanent first molar usually migrates mesially quite rapidly when the primary second molar has been lost, and in the extreme case may totally close the primary second molar extraction site. If the primary second molar has been lost prematurely in a single quadrant, up to 3 mm of space may be regained by tipping the molar back distally. If space loss is bilateral, the limit of space regaining is 5-6 mm for the total arch.

Space regaining also may be indicated after early loss of one mandibular primary canine, because space tends to close as the incisors drift lingually and toward the affected side (see Figure 7-9). Asymmetric activation of a lower lingual arch is one approach. Loss of a primary canine usually occurs because of root resorption caused by erupting lateral incisors without enough space, so it is important to be aware of the overall space deficiency, which should not exceed 4 mm.

Techniques for using space regaining appliances are presented in Chapter 12.

Generalized Moderate Crowding

A child with a generalized arch length discrepancy of 2-4 mm and no prematurely missing primary teeth can be expected to have moderately crowded incisors. Unless the incisors are severely protrusive, the long-term plan would be generalized expansion of the arch to align the teeth. The major advantage of doing this in the mixed dentition is esthetic, and the benefit is largely for the parents, not the child.

If the parents strongly desire early treatment for moderate crowding, in the mandibular arch an adjustable lingual arch is the appliance of choice for simple expansion. In the maxilla, either a removable or fixed appliance can be employed. Keep in mind that rotated incisors usually will not correct spontaneously even if space is provided, so early correction would require bonded attachments for these teeth.

Other Tooth Displacements

Spaced and Flared Maxillary Incisors

In children with spaced and flared maxillary incisors who have Class I molar relationships and good facial proportions, space analysis should show that the space available is excessive rather than deficient. This condition often is found in the mixed dentition after prolonged thumb-sucking and frequently occurs in connection with some narrowing of the maxillary arch. A thumb or finger habit should be eliminated before attempting to retract the incisors. Physiologic adaptation to the space between the anterior teeth requires that the tongue be placed in this area to seal off the gap for successful swallowing and speech. This "tongue thrust" is not the cause of the protrusion or open bite and should not be the focus of therapy. If the teeth are retracted, the tongue thrust will disappear.

If the upper incisors are flared forward and there is no contact with the lower incisors, the protruding upper incisors can be retracted quite satisfactorily with a removable appliance (see Chapter 13). On the other hand, if there is a deep overbite anteriorly, protruding upper incisor teeth cannot be retracted until it is corrected. The lower incisors biting against the lingual of the upper incisors prevents the upper teeth from being moved lingually. Even if anteroposterior jaw relationships are Class I, a skeletal vertical problem may be present, and complex treatment is likely to be required.

Maxillary Midline Diastema

A maxillary midline diastema (Figure 7-15) can pose a special management problem. Small spaces between the maxillary incisors are normal before eruption of the maxillary canines (see Chapter 4 and the discussion of the "ugly duckling" stage of development). In the absence of deep overbite, these spaces normally close spontaneously. If the space between the maxillary central incisors is greater than 2 mm, however, spontaneous closure is unlikely.[4] Persistent spacing between the incisors correlates with a cleft in the alveolar process between the central incisors into which fibers from the maxillary labial frenum insert. For larger diastemas, it may be necessary to surgically remove the frenal attachment to obtain a stable closure of the midline diastema.

The best approach, however, is to do nothing until the permanent canines erupt (unless crowding or the appearance of the teeth becomes a major issue). If the diastema does not close spontaneously at that time, an appliance can be used to move the teeth together, and a frenectomy should be considered then if there is excessive tissue bunched up in the midline. Early frenectomy should be avoided.

Posterior Crossbite

Posterior crossbites in mixed dentition children usually result from a narrowing of the maxillary arch and are often observed in children who have had prolonged sucking habits. If the child shifts on closure or the constriction is severe enough to significantly reduce space within the arch, early correction is indicated. If not, especially if other problems suggest that comprehensive orthodontics will be needed later, treatment can be deferred until adolescence.

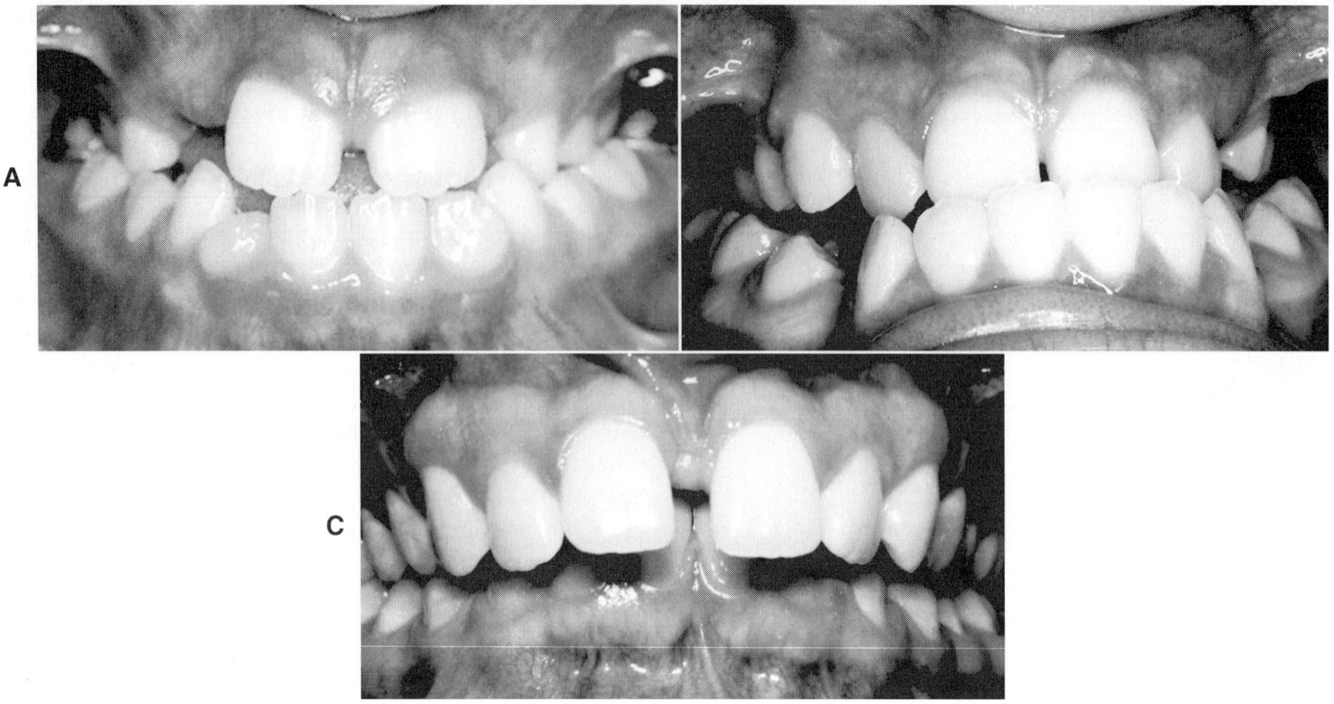

Figure 7-15 A diastema between the maxillary central incisors often is present when these teeth first erupt, and closes or reduces in size as the permanent canines erupt. **A,** Age 8 and **(B)** age 12 in a girl with a developing Class III problem who had no treatment during this period. Note the change in inclination of the central incisors and closure of the diastema. For a diastema of more than 2 mm, which is unlikely to completely close spontaneously, surgical removal of excessive tissue between the teeth may be needed. The preferred treatment approach is to move the teeth together at about the time the permanent canines are erupting and decide about frenum surgery at that point. **C,** A diastema of this severity in an older patient will require surgery to reposition the frenum. This surgery is most effective if done after the teeth have been brought together so they can be held together while healing occurs.

Both removable and fixed appliances can be effective in correcting posterior crossbites. Whether a fixed or removable appliance is used, the maxillary arch should be slightly overexpanded and then held passively in this overexpanded position for approximately 3 months before the appliance is removed. Techniques for both removable and fixed appliances to expand the maxillary arch are illustrated in Chapter 12.

Anterior Crossbite

Anterior crossbite, particularly crossbite of all the incisors, is rarely found in children who do not have a skeletal Class III jaw relationship. A crossbite relationship of one or two anterior teeth, however, may develop in a child who has good facial proportions. The maxillary lateral incisors tend to erupt to the lingual and may be trapped in that location, especially if there is not enough space (Figure 7-16). In this situation, extracting the adjacent primary canine prior to complete eruption of the lateral incisor usually leads to spontaneous correction of the crossbite. Lingually positioned incisors limit lateral jaw movements and they or their mandibular counterparts sometimes suffer significant incisal abrasion, so early correction of the crossbite is indicated.

It is important to evaluate the space situation before attempting to correct any anterior crossbite. The prognosis for successfully pushing a 7 mm maxillary lateral incisor into a 4 mm space is not good. Frequently, even if there is enough space overall within the arch, it is necessary to remove the maxillary primary canines prematurely to bring lateral incisors out of crossbite. If enough space is available, a maxillary removable appliance to tip the upper incisor(s) facially is usually the best mechanism to correct a simple anterior crossbite. Rotational changes and bodily movement are not effectively produced by removable appliances and require fixed appliance therapy.

Anterior Open Bite

A simple anterior open bite is one that is limited to the anterior region in a child with good facial proportions. The major cause of such an open bite is prolonged thumbsucking, and the most important step in obtaining correction is to stop sucking habits if they are present. For this purpose, behavior modification techniques are appropriate.

A

B

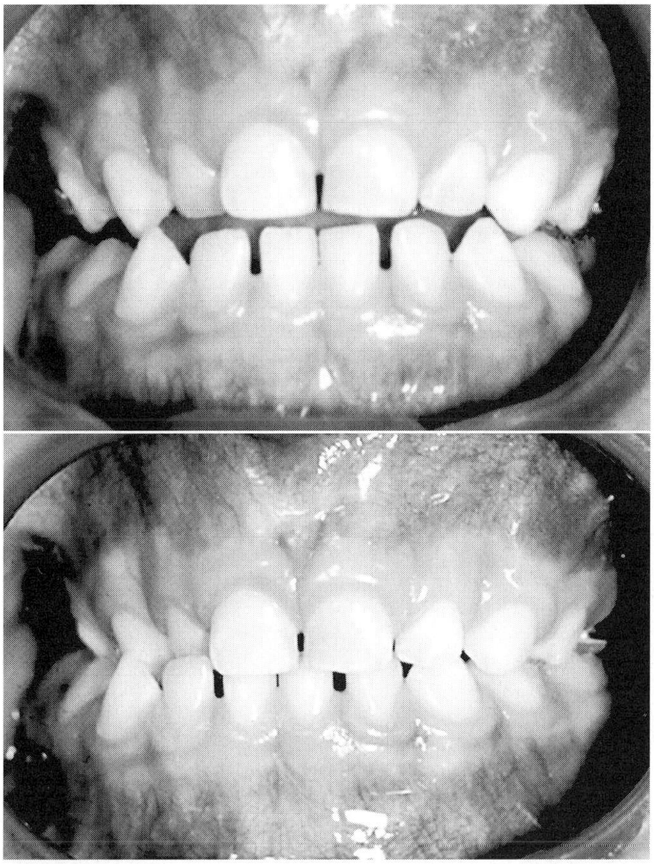

Figure 7-16 In a child with a narrow maxillary arch, interferences on initial contact of the incisors **(A)** often lead to a shift laterally and anteriorly **(B)** that leaves one incisor in crossbite. It is better to correct the shift before an erupting permanent incisor is trapped in a lingual position. Often relieving premature contacts on the primary canines is all that is required.

Several approaches are possible (see Chapter 12). When the sucking habit stops, the open bite usually gradually closes without the need for intra-oral appliances (Figure 7-17).

If an intra-oral appliance is needed, the preferred method is a maxillary lingual arch with an anterior crib device, making it extremely difficult for the child to place the thumb or other object in the mouth (Figure 7-17, *E*). It is important to present such a device to the child as an aid, not as a punishment, and to provide psychological support to help him or her adjust to it.

In about half of the children for whom such a crib is made, thumb-sucking stops immediately and the anterior open bite usually begins to close relatively rapidly thereafter. In the remaining children, thumb-sucking persists for a few weeks, but the crib device is eventually effective in extinguishing thumb-sucking in 85% to 90% of patients.[5] It is a good idea to leave the crib in place for 6 months after the habit has apparently been eliminated. Further details on fabrication and use of this appliance are provided in Chapter 12.

Over-Retained Primary Teeth and Ectopic Eruption

The eruption of a permanent tooth can be delayed if its primary predecessor is retained too long. When this happens, the obvious treatment is to remove the primary tooth. As a general guideline, a permanent tooth should erupt when approximately three-fourths of its root is completed. If root formation of the permanent successor has reached this point while a primary tooth still has considerable root remaining, the primary tooth should be extracted. This problem is most likely to arise when the permanent tooth bud is slightly displaced away from its primary predecessor (as in the canine ectopic eruption problems discussed next). In some children, the pace of resorption of the primary teeth is slow, for whatever reason, and occasionally almost all the primary teeth have to be removed to allow timely eruption of their permanent successors.

If a primary tooth is removed quite prematurely, a layer of relatively dense bone and soft tissue may form over the unerupted permanent tooth (see Figures 7-13 and 7-14). This usually delays but does not prevent the eruption of the permanent tooth, and intervention is rarely indicated. If eruption of a permanent tooth has been delayed until its root formation is complete, it may still erupt on its own and should be given a chance to do so. It may be necessary, however, to place an attachment on it and gently pull it into the arch (Figure 7-18).

The eruption of permanent molars and canines can be delayed by malposition of the permanent tooth (ectopic eruption). The most common site is the maxillary molar region, where the second primary molar blocks the first permanent molar and suffers root resorption in the process (Figure 7-19).[6] If the permanent molar does not self-correct (often it does), it should be repositioned as described in Chapter 12 or, if all else fails, the primary molar extracted. If the primary molar is extracted, rapid space loss will result in a need for space regaining or premolar extraction.

Ectopic eruption of maxillary canines, which occurs relatively frequently, can permanently damage the roots of lateral incisors (Figure 7-20). The abnormal eruption path may also leave the unerupted canine in a lingual position nearer the midline than normal. It is much easier to prevent these problems than to correct them later. Research has shown that extracting the maxillary primary canines when radiographs disclose that the permanent canines are overlapping the permanent lateral incisor roots is likely to have a positive influence on the permanent tooth's eruption path (although the more the overlap, the less the chance of eventual normal eruption).[7]

Adjunctive Treatment for Adults. A triage scheme for adults, and the treatment of moderate problems selected from its use, are discussed in Chapter 18. For these patients, orthodontic treatment almost always is an adjunct to treatment for other problems. Adjunctive orthodontic treatment is often within the scope of general dental practice and can be of considerable importance in the management of adults with periodontal disease and restorative needs.

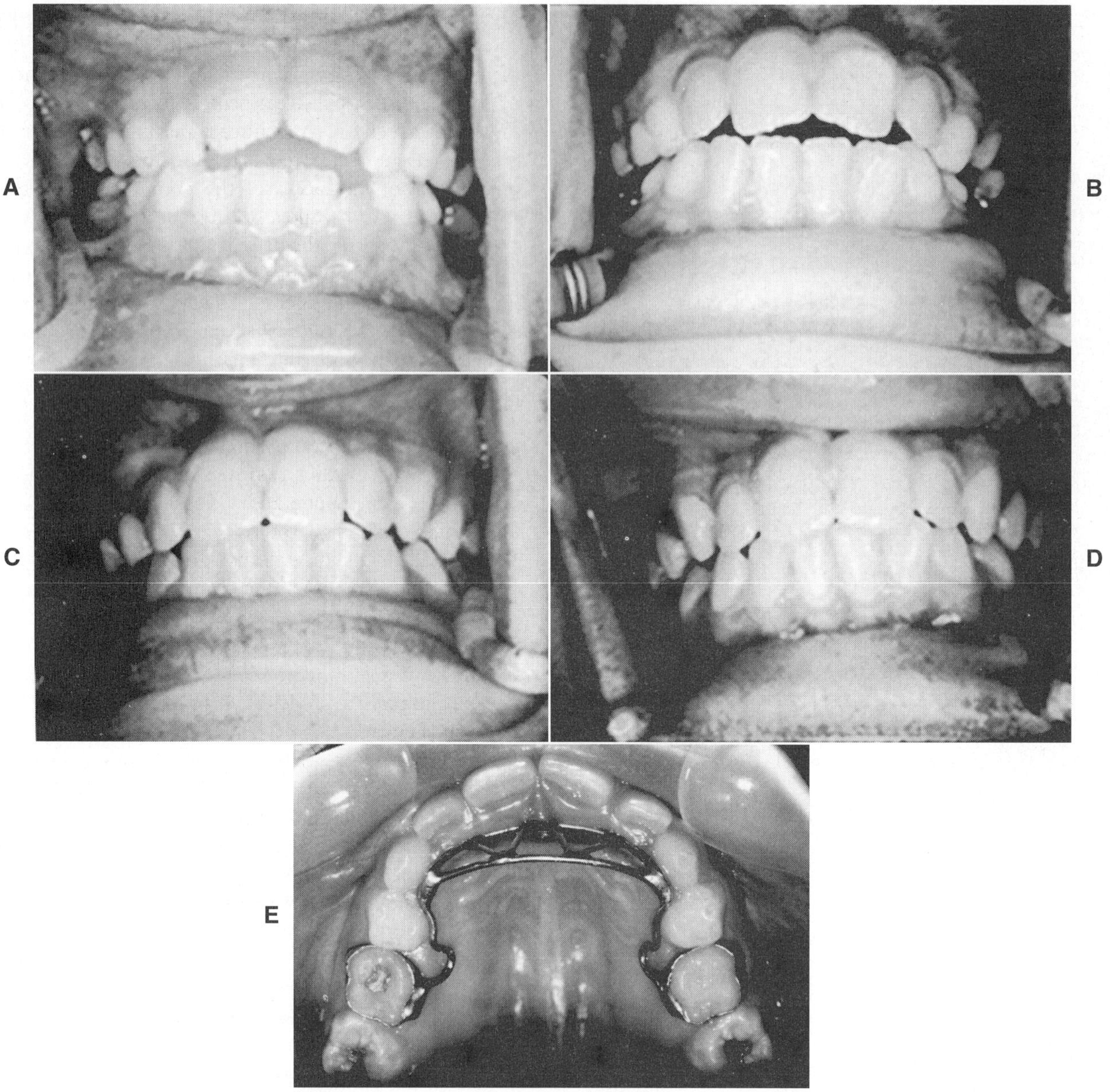

FIGURE 7-17 **A** to **D,** Photos at 1-year intervals of a child who stopped sucking his thumb at the time the first photo was taken. Gradual closure of the open bite, without a need for further intervention, usually occurs in patients with normal facial proportions after habits stop. **E,** If a sucking habit persists, a crib of this type can be used to help extinguish the habit. A crib is most effective in a child who wants to stop the thumb- or finger-sucking and accepts the crib as a reminder not to do so.

PLANNING COMPREHENSIVE ORTHODONTIC TREATMENT

Steps in Planning Complex Treatment

Diagnosis results in a comprehensive list of the patient's problems. Although any number of pathologic problems might be noted, if the five characteristics of malocclusion are used to structure the problem list, there can be a maximum of five major developmental problems. Most patients will not have that many. As the problem list is developed, the findings related to malocclusion can and should be grouped as the classification scheme suggests, to make the treatment planning process work efficiently. Having too many overlapping problems on the problem list only creates confusion.

The goal of treatment is to deal with the problems in a way that creates maximum benefit to the patient—not just to straighten the teeth. Using a logical sequence of steps on the way from the problem list to the final plan, keeping this goal in mind, is strongly recommended. The steps are (see Figure 7-1):

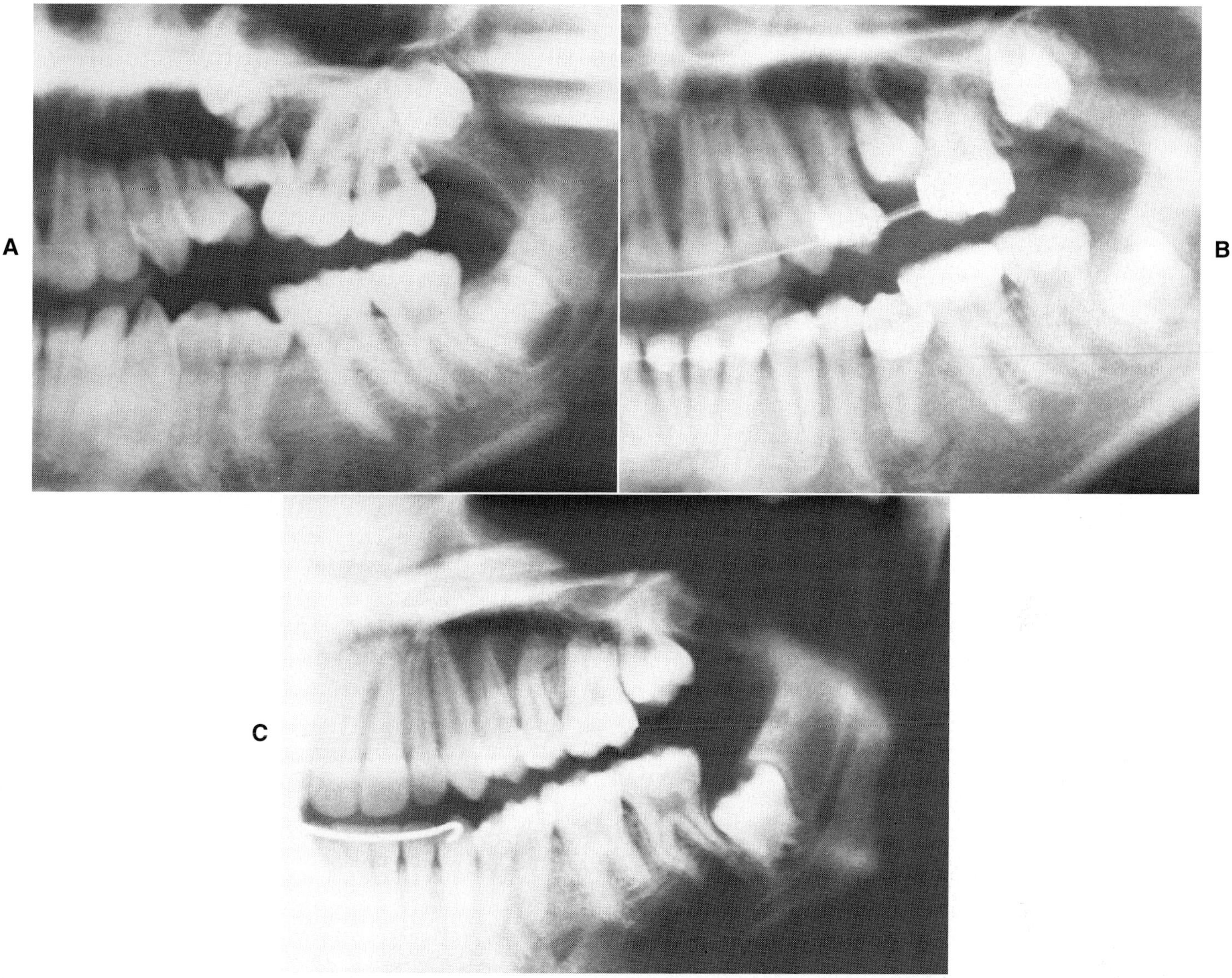

FIGURE 7-18 **A,** Extreme displacement of the maxillary left second premolar at age 13, after long-term ankylosis of the secondary primary molar. Note the space loss as the first molar has tipped mesially over the extraction of the ankylosed primary molar. **B,** The upper left second molar has been extracted to allow the first molar to be moved distally, opening space for the premolar now erupting; **C,** Second premolar in place at age 15, despite the root dilaceration.

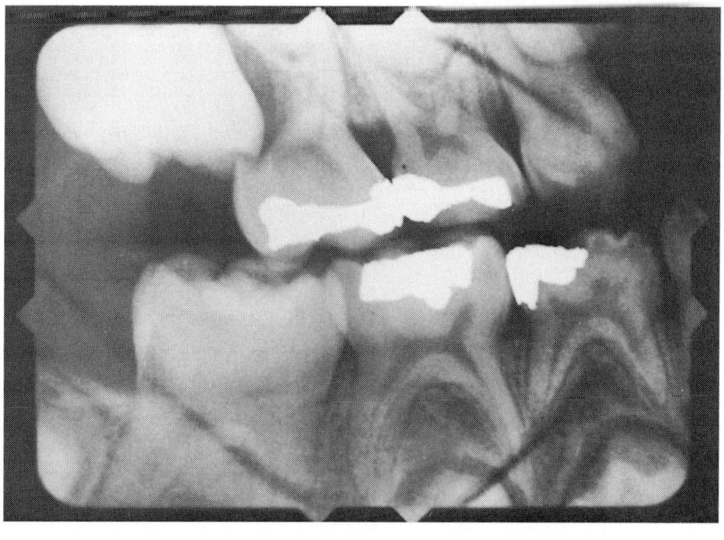

FIGURE 7-19 Ectopic eruption of the permanent first molar produces resorption of the distal root of the primary second molar. This occurs much more frequently in the upper arch but can happen in the lower arch.

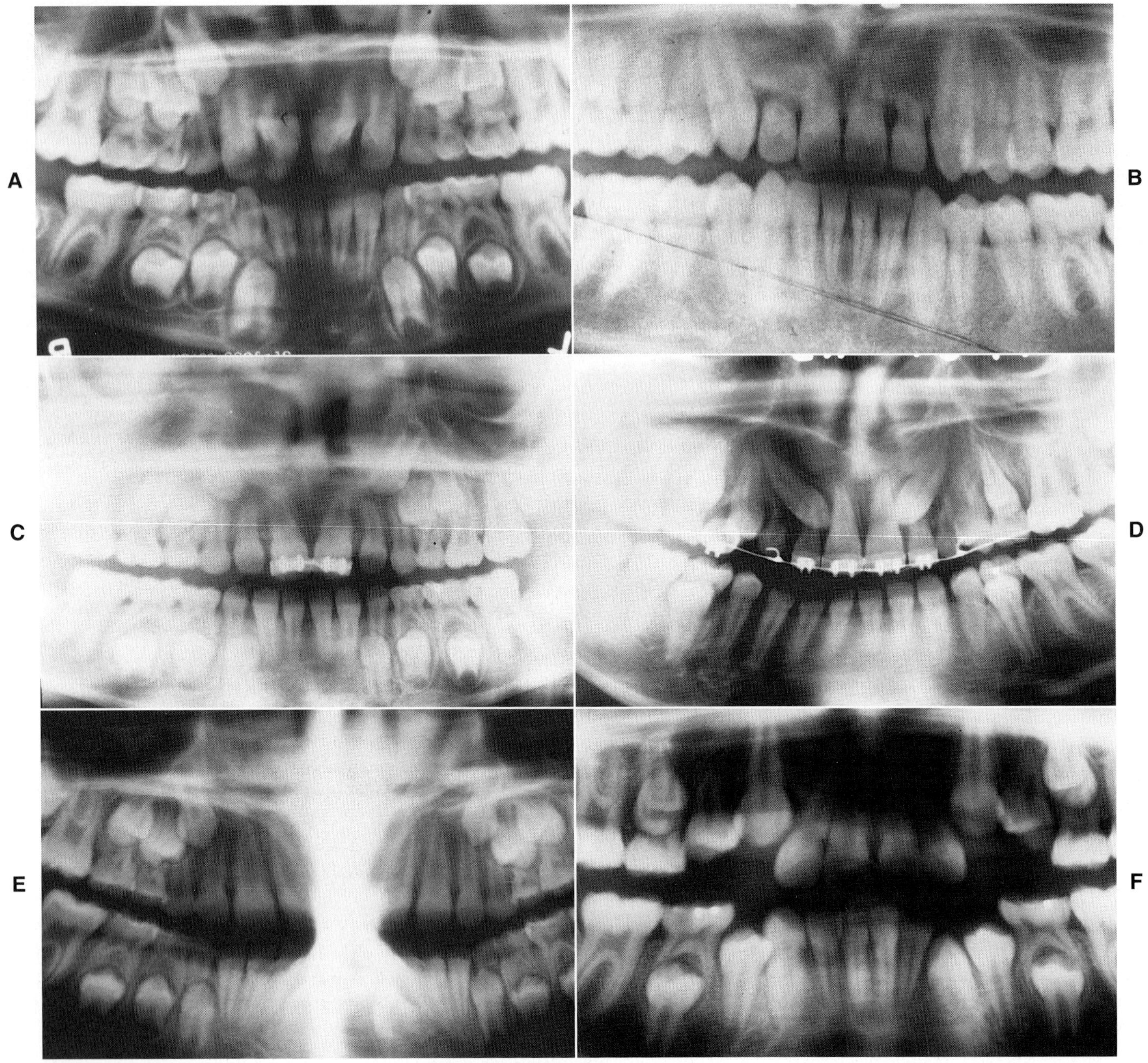

FIGURE 7-20 When maxillary canines erupt mesial to the roots of the primary canines, as often occurs, there is a risk of damage to the lateral incisors. Early extraction of the primary canines is recommended when the permanent canines are mesial to the midline of the primary canine crowns. **A,** Age 8 and **(B)** age 12 in a child who had no intervention until the erupting canines had severely damaged the lateral incisors. **C,** Age 8 and **(D)** age 10 in a child in whom mesial movement of the permanent canines continued and led to severe damage. **E,** Age 9, mesial position of canines that indicates early extraction of the primary canines. **F,** Age 11 in same patient, showing reasonably normal eruption of the canines without damage to the lateral incisors, after the early extraction of the primary canines. **(A-D,** Courtesy Dr. K. Lieberman.)

1. Separation of pathologic from developmental (orthodontic) problems
2. Prioritization of the items on the orthodontic problem list, so that the most important problem receives highest priority for treatment
3. Consideration of possible solutions to each problem, with each problem evaluated for the moment as if it were the only problem the patient had
4. Evaluation of the interactions among possible solutions to the individual problems

Box 7-1

PATIENT F.P.: PROBLEM LIST (DIAGNOSIS)

In the order they appeared in the evaluation sequence
- Mild gingivitis, mild gingival overgrowth
- Hypoplastic area maxillary left premolar
- Mandibular deficiency
- Maxillary incisors tipped lingually, short crowns
- Moderate maxillary incisor crowding
- Class II buccal segments, minimal overjet
- Deep bite, excessive eruption mandibular incisors

Box 7-2

PATIENT F.P.: PATHOLOGIC PROBLEMS/PLAN

- Mild gingivitis
  Hygiene instruction
- Hypoplastic area, upper left first premolar
  Restore at end of orthodontic treatment

Box 7-3

PATIENT F.P.: PRIORITIZED PROBLEM LIST

Tentative: awaiting parent/patient interaction
- Malaligned and unesthetic maxillary incisors
- Skeletal Class II, excess overjet—mandibular deficiency
- Anterior deep bite—excessive eruption of mandibular incisors

5. Development of alternative treatment approaches, with consideration of benefits to the patient vs. risks, costs, and complexity
6. Determination of a final treatment concept, with input from the patient and parent, and
7. Selection of the specific therapeutic approach (appliance design, mechanotherapy) to be used.

Interaction with the patient is required to develop the plan in this way and to obtain true consent for treatment. Let us now consider this sequence, and the logic behind it, in some detail.

Pathologic versus Developmental Problems

An important principle is that a patient does not have to be in perfect health to have orthodontic treatment, but any problems related to disease and pathology must be under control (i.e., the progression of any acute or chronic conditions must be stopped). For this reason, pathologic problems must be addressed before treatment of orthodontic (developmental) problems can begin. Thus in a treatment sequence, orthodontic treatment must appear after control of systemic disease, periodontal treatment (at least to the extent of bringing periodontal disease under control), and restoration of dental lesions. The sequencing of orthodontics with other types of treatment and the implications of certain types of systemic and oral pathology are discussed in Chapter 8. Multi-disciplinary treatment of adults with complex problems is illustrated in Chapters 18 and 19.

Let us continue with treatment planning for the patient whose initial records, diagnostic evaluation and development of a problem list are illustrated at the end of Chapter 6 (see Figures 6-71 to 6-74). Her problem list, which is the diagnosis, is repeated here in Box 7-1.

The first step in treatment planning is to separate pathologic from developmental (orthodontic) problems. Even when pathologic problems are as mild as those for this girl, they must not be overlooked in the treatment plan. For this patient (Box 7-2), the plan for the pathologic problems would be oral hygiene instruction, monitoring of the hyperplastic gingiva during orthodontic treatment and scheduling gingival surgery toward the end of treatment if it is needed, and restoration of the hypoplastic premolar after orthodontics is completed. For patients with more complex disease-related problems, the plan often is appropriate referral to another practitioner, which must be done in a timely manner.

Setting Priorities for the Orthodontic Problem List

Putting the patient's orthodontic (developmental) problems in priority order is the most important single step in the entire treatment planning process. In order to maximize benefit to the patient, the most important problems must be identified, and the treatment plan must focus on what is most important for that particular patient. The patient's perception of his or her condition is important in setting these priorities. For example, if a patient's major reason for seeking dental treatment is protruding and irregular incisors, this condition probably should receive higher priority than missing molar teeth needing prosthetic replacement. On the other hand, if the protruding and irregular incisors are no problem to the patient but difficulty in chewing is, replacing the missing teeth should receive higher priority.

It is always difficult for the clinician to avoid imposing his or her own feelings at this stage, and it is not totally inappropriate to do so; but ignoring the patient's chief complaint can lead to serious errors in planning treatment. For instance, consider the patient who complains of a protruding chin and who has a Class III malocclusion. If the clinician formulates the problem as Class III malocclusion and concentrates on bringing the teeth into correct occlusion while ignoring the chin, it is not likely that the patient will be happy with the treatment result. The plan did not deal with the patient's problem.

The prioritized problem list for the patient whose case we are following is shown in Box 7-3. Note that on the prioritized list, the most important problem is not exactly what

Box 7-4

PATIENT F.P.: POSSIBLE SOLUTIONS

Malaligned and unesthetic maxillary incisors
- *Align, lingual root torque, reduce overjet and overbite*
- *Remove excess gingiva?*

Skeletal Class II

Growth modification: Differential forward growth of mandible
- *Headgear?*
- *Herbst appliance?*
- *If unfavorable growth: Orthodontic camouflage? Orthognathic surgery??*

Anterior deep bite
- *Absolute intrusion: If needed, only for lower incisors*
- *Relative intrusion: Allow lower molar eruption as mandible grows vertically, prevent further lower incisor eruption*

the patient and her parents identified as their chief complaint. Her mandibular deficiency is a key element in making the upper incisors unattractive, and that must be recognized at the planning stage. The doctor does not have to agree with the patient's initial thoughts as to what is most important. Indeed, as in this case, often it is necessary to educate the patient about the nature of the problems. But the importance of various problems must be discussed, and informed consent to treatment has not been obtained unless the patient agrees that the focus of the plan is what he or she wants (see below).

Treatment Possibilities

The next step in the planning process is to list the possibilities for treatment of each of the problems, beginning with the highest priority problem. At this stage each problem is considered individually, and for the moment the possible solutions are examined as if this problem were the only one the patient had. Broad possibilities, not details of treatment procedures, are what is sought at this stage. The more complex the total situation, the more important it is to be sure no possibilities are overlooked.

Possible solutions to our example patient's problems are shown in Box 7-4. As we continue to develop her treatment plan, references to aspects of treatment that have not yet been presented in the text are inevitable. The first-time reader is urged to follow the logic rather than concentrate on details that will be discussed more fully in the following chapters.

Consider the possible solutions to this patient's most important problem, the appearance of the maxillary incisors and unattractive smile. Correcting this will require alignment of the teeth, but proper anterior tooth relationships cannot be achieved until overjet is reduced and the deep bite is corrected. The best solution to the first problem, therefore, can be determined only after the impact of possible solutions to overjet and overbite have been considered.

There are three ways that the Class II jaw relationship and overjet can be treated (Figure 7-21): (1) differential forward growth of the mandible, which is ideal if it can be achieved; (2) orthodontic camouflage, retracting the maxillary incisors and proclining the mandibular incisors to make the teeth fit even though the jaws do not; and (3) orthognathic surgery to correct the jaw position. Since our patient has not yet reached the adolescent growth spurt, growth modification would be the primary possibility, with camouflage and surgery as possibilities if growth modification did not succeed.

Class II growth modification can be done in several ways, which are discussed in detail in Chapter 8. For the patient whose work-up we have been following, differential forward growth of the mandible, while maintaining vertical control of the maxillary posterior teeth and bringing the maxillary incisors downward and facially, would increase the display of the maxillary incisors and the prominence of the chin (Figure 7-22). The two most effective ways to do that would be high pull headgear or a fixed functional appliance like the Herbst appliance. The functional appliance would be more likely to move the lower incisors forward, which is undesirable for this patient, so headgear would be preferred if she would agree to wear it.

There also are three ways to correct the anterior overbite (Figure 7-23): (1) absolute intrusion of the upper and lower incisors, moving their root apices closer to the nose and lower border of the mandible respectively; (2) relative intrusion of the incisors, keeping them where they are while the mandible grows and the posterior teeth erupt; and (3) extrusion of the posterior teeth, which would rotate the mandible downward and backward. Relative intrusion of incisors and extrusion of posterior teeth are identical in terms of the tooth movement. The difference is whether vertical growth of the ramus compensates for the increase in molar height (i.e., whether the mandibular plane angle is maintained [relative intrusion] or increases as the mandible rotates downward and backward [extrusion]).

In an immature 12-year-old like our patient, vertical growth can be expected, so relative intrusion would be the preferred approach. It is significant that in the absence of growth, leveling the arches by extrusion of posterior teeth would cause the mandible to rotate downward and backward, accentuating a Class II tendency (Figure 7-24), which would be highly undesirable for this patient. Controlling the vertical position of the maxillary posterior teeth, so that the vertical space between the jaws created by growth could be used largely for elongation of the lower molars, would facilitate leveling by relative intrusion. So the high pull headgear that appears to be the best approach to the skeletal Class II problem also would facilitate correction of the deep bite, if used along with a fixed appliance to level the lower arch.

Often, the same problem list prioritized differently results in a different treatment plan. For this patient, if the Class II malocclusion was considered the most important problem and the relationship of the upper incisors to the lip and

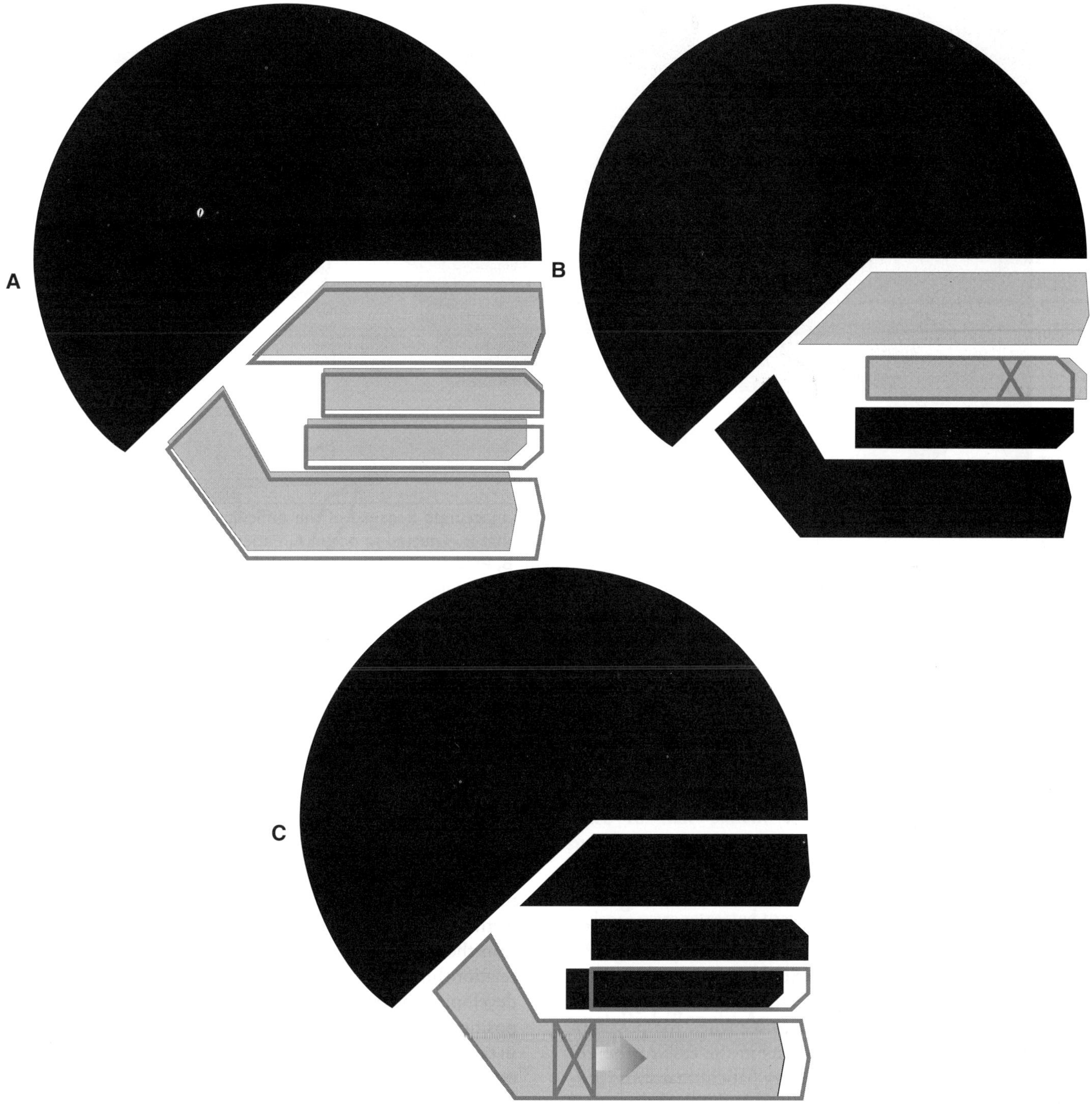

Figure 7-21 The possibilities for correction of a skeletal Class II problem include the following: **A,** Differential forward growth of the mandible, which is the ideal method if the patient has not yet gone through the adolescent growth spurt; **B,** Camouflage by retraction of the maxillary incisors, which can be quite successful *if* the other facial features allow it; and **C,** Orthognathic surgery to move the mandible forward to a normal relationship. In the absence of growth, camouflage and surgery are the only possibilities.

gingiva was not considered important, Class II camouflage might be chosen as the most efficient approach to treatment. Class II elastics, with or without premolar extraction, would correct the malocclusion but might harm rather than enhance the dental and facial appearance.

The objective at this stage of treatment planning is to be sure that no reasonable possibilities are overlooked. It is easy to develop the mindset that "For this problem, we always . . ." Sometimes an alternate approach would be better, but is overlooked unless a conscious effort is made to keep an open

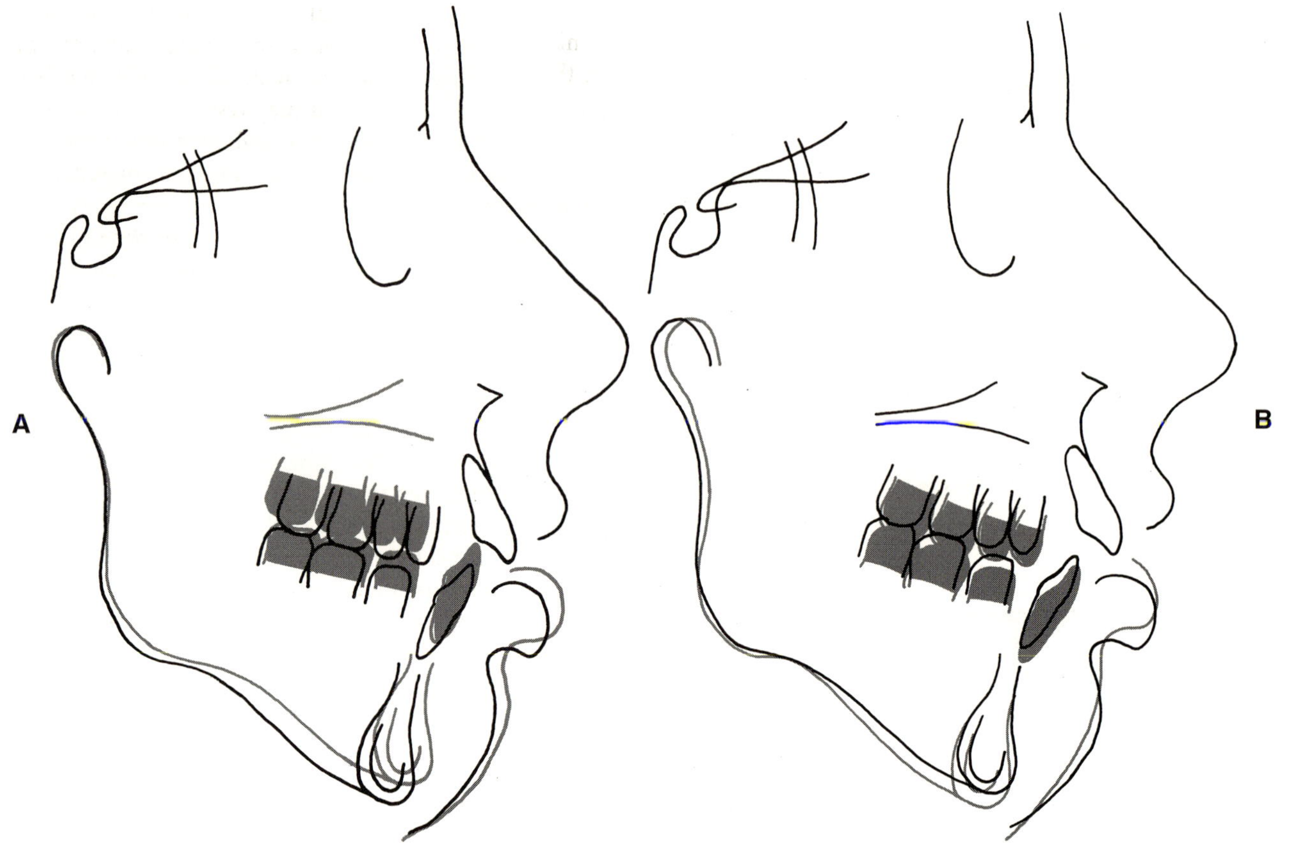

Figure 7-24 There is a strong interaction between the vertical position of the maxilla and both the anteroposterior and vertical positions of the mandible, because the mandible rotates backward as it moves downward **(A)** and forward as it moves upward **(B).** The superimposition in **A** is the actual growth of this particular patient in whom excessive vertical growth of the maxilla and downward-backward rotation of the mandible occurred. The superimposition in **B** shows what would happen if the maxilla were moved upward (this would require surgery). Note that this would improve the apparent mandibular deficiency.

surgery would provide considerable benefit, the cost-risk/benefit analysis might still favor the more difficult procedure. "Is it worth it?" is a question that must be answered not only from the point of view of what is involved, but in terms of the benefit to the patient.

Other Considerations

At this stage, it is important to take into account any pertinent special considerations about the individual patient. Should the treatment time be minimized because of possible exacerbation of periodontal disease? Should treatment options be left open as long as possible because of uncertainty of the pattern of growth? Should visible orthodontic appliances be avoided because of the patient's vanity, even if it makes treatment more difficult? Such questions must be addressed from the perspective of the individual patient. Rational answers can be obtained only when the treatment possibilities and other important factors influencing the treatment plan have been considered.

For our example patient, interactions, thoughts about necessary compromises, and other considerations (which in her case are quite minor) are shown in Box 7-5. The infor-

Box 7-5

PATIENT F.P.: INTERACTION OF TREATMENT POSSIBILITIES

- Repositioning the maxillary incisors for better appearance will increase overjet and require greater use of the mechanics for Class II correction.
- Extrusive mechanics to correct the deep bite may lead to a more vertical growth direction for the mandible, compromising the Class II correction.
- Correcting the deep bite with any intrusion of the maxillary incisors would compromise the smile arc, which is excellent now.

Other Considerations in Planning Treatment

- Patient is immature, growth modification will be more efficient if timed with growth spurt.
- Rotating the maxilla down anteriorly will improve incisor display and smile appearance.

Box 7-6

PATIENT F.P.: OUTLINE OF CASE PRESENTATION

Goal: To appropriately involve the patient and parents in the treatment decisions, which is necessary to obtain informed consent. The points to be discussed (in this sequence) are:

General and Oral Health

- There are three minor problems with oral health:
  - *Mild gingivitis: Better oral hygiene is required to prevent damage to the teeth during orthodontic treatment*
  - *Hypoplastic area in first premolar: May require restoration in the future, no treatment needed now*
  - *Overgrowth of maxillary gingiva: May require surgical removal at the end of orthodontic treatment if it does not resolve spontaneously*

Orthodontic Problems

- Appearance of upper incisors: Tipped back and not aligned properly, which partially conceals their relative protrusion
- Lower jaw has not grown forward properly, which is the reason the upper incisors appear to protrude
- Overbite: Lower front teeth have erupted too much, into the palate

Most Important Problem

- Upper incisor protrusion and crowding (do you agree?)
  - *This is largely due to lower jaw that has not grown as much as the upper jaw*

Plan to Correct the Most Important Problem

- Restrain downward and forward growth of the upper jaw during the adolescent growth spurt to maxilla so the mandible can catch up
  - *Requires favorable growth and cooperation*

Correction of Other Problems

- Alignment of teeth and correction of bite
  - *Requires braces on all the teeth*
- Overgrowth of gums
  - *May require surgery for correction later*

Benefits from Treatment

- Improved facial and dental appearance
  - *For an adult patient, this is the place to show computer image predictions*
- More normal jaw movements and incisor function

Risks of Treatment

- Discomfort after appliance adjustment
- Decalcification if hygiene is inadequate
- Root resorption, especially maxillary incisors
- Any other pertinent items
  - *A signed form acknowledging this discussion is strongly recommended*

Treatment Schedule, Costs, etc.

(Included with the presentation of the final treatment plan (Box 7-7)
(Schedule and costs will vary in individual practices)

mation now has been assembled and treatment possibilities are ready to be discussed with the patient and parents in order to finalize the treatment plan (Box 7-6).

Patient-Parent Consultation: Obtaining Informed Consent

Paternalism versus Patient Autonomy

Not so long ago, it was taken for granted that the doctor should analyze the patient's situation and should prescribe what he or she had determined to be the best treatment—with little or no regard for whether that treatment was what the patient desired. This is best described as a paternalistic approach to patient care: the doctor, as a father figure, knows best and makes the decisions.

At present, that approach is not defensible, ethically and legally or practically.[8,9] From an ethical perspective, patients have the right to determine what is done to them in treatment, and increasingly they demand that right. It is unethical not to inform patients of the alternatives, including the likely outcome of no treatment, that are possible in their case. The modern doctrine of informed consent has made the ethical imperative a legal one as well. Legally, the doctor now is liable for problems arising from failure to fully inform the patient about the treatment that is to be performed. Informed consent is not obtained just from a discussion of the risks of treatment. Patients must be told what their problems are, what the treatment alternatives are, and what the possible outcomes of treatment or no treatment are likely to be, in a way they can understand. Simply providing a brochure, video tape or written consent form that uses complex language often does not lead the patient to really comprehend the treatment and its consequences.

The problem-oriented method of diagnosis and treatment planning lends itself very well to the patient involvement that modern treatment planning requires.[10] A discussion with the patient and parents should begin with an outline of the patient's problems, and patient involvement begins with the prioritization of the problem list. Perhaps the doctor's single most important question in obtaining informed consent is, "Your most important problem, as I see it, is. . . . Do you agree?" When problems related to informed consent for orthodontic treatment arise, almost always they result from treatment that failed to address what was most important to the patient, or from treatment that focused on what was not an important problem to the patient.

The problem-oriented method requires examining the possible solutions to the patient's problems, starting with the most important one. This is exactly the way in which a discussion with the patient and parents is structured most effectively (see Box 7-6). Interactions, unavoidable compromises, and practical considerations must not only be considered by the doctor, they must be shared with the patient as the treatment plan is developed. Under most circumstances, there are advantages and disadvantages to the possible treatment approaches. The doctor's role is to clarify this to the best of his or her ability, involving the patient in the final decision as to the treatment approach that will be employed.

From a practical perspective, involving the patient and parents in decisions about treatment has important advantages. It places the responsibility where it belongs, on a patient who has been led to understand the uncertainties involved. The problems, after all, belong to the patient, not the doctor. A patient who "owns" the problems and recognizes that this is the case, is more likely to be cooperative and oriented toward helping with his or her treatment, than someone who takes the attitude that it's all up to the doctor.[11]

Several specific situations in orthodontics particularly require interaction between the doctor and the patient and parent in choosing the final treatment plan. Perhaps the most frequent revolves around the issue of arch expansion versus extraction in solving crowding problems.

To Expand or Extract?

From the beginning of the specialty, orthodontists have debated the limits of expansion of the dental arches, and whether the advantages of extraction of some teeth to provide space for the others outweigh the disadvantages. With extraction, a disadvantage is the loss of a tooth or teeth; an advantage is likely to be greater stability of the result; and there may be positive or negative effects on facial esthetics. But in fact for any individual patient the decision is a value judgment. It is not only appropriate but necessary to discuss the pros and cons with the patient and parent before making the expansion-extraction decision. Obviously, if camouflage requiring extractions was proposed (as it might be if she refused to cooperate with headgear or a fixed functional appliance), this would be an important item for discussion with our example patient and her parents. The issue of extraction in orthodontics is reviewed in detail in Chapter 8.

Type and Timing for Skeletal Problems

A second frequent problem requiring input from the patient is whether to begin treatment for a skeletal problem prior to adolescence or wait until the adolescent growth spurt. In this situation, two aspects must be discussed: the efficacy of beginning treatment early versus waiting for adolescence, and if early treatment is chosen, the mode of treatment.

The clearest indication for early treatment is a Class III problem due primarily to maxillary deficiency. Reverse pull headgear (face mask) is effective only at younger ages than comprehensive orthodontics usually is undertaken. The chance of significant change in the position of the maxilla is greatest with treatment prior to age 8, even though some treatment effects occur as late as age 11 (see Chapter 14). In contrast, excessive mandibular growth is almost impossible to control, and early treatment for a Class III child with this problem is unlikely to be of long term benefit.

Early treatment for severe deep bite, which is seen most frequently in a child with a short face and Class II tendency, is indicated if trauma to the soft tissues is occurring. In some of these children a spurt of mandibular growth occurs after the bite is opened, but this is unpredictable. The long face pattern of growth, usually accompanied by anterior open bite, is similar to mandibular prognathism in that it is very difficult to control, so that there is little to be gained by starting early.

There is no doubt that successful Class II treatment for most patients is possible either by beginning early or waiting. Current data, reviewed in detail in Chapter 8, suggest that the benefits of early treatment are not compelling in many cases, but a child experiencing psychosocial problems because of teasing about protruding teeth is a candidate for early treatment. A second phase of treatment during adolescence almost always is required, so a major disadvantage is a longer treatment time, with greater demands on cooperation and often greater cost.

The child's desire for treatment and potential cooperation also must be taken into account when treatment timing is considered. This affects both the decision as to treat now or wait and the selection of the appliance to be used if early treatment is chosen. There is little reason to proceed with headgear or functional appliance treatment for a child who has no intention of wearing the device. Treatment results with the two methods are not precisely the same but can be considered more similar than different, and if the child would wear one but not the other, it would be wise to select the one the child would prefer. For our example patient, it would be more efficient to wait for the adolescent growth spurt, and headgear is the preferred approach, but the patient and parent need to understand why these are the recommendations and what alternatives exist.

Considerations in the optimal timing of treatment timing are discussed in greater depth in Chapter 8.

Orthodontic Camouflage versus Orthognathic Surgery

A third frequent issue for discussion with the patient and parents when a severe skeletal problem exists, is whether orthodontic treatment alone would produce an acceptable result for a skeletal malocclusion, or whether orthognathic surgery should be selected. Sometimes this difficult decision revolves around whether jaw function would be satisfactory with displacement of the incisor teeth to compensate for a jaw malrelationship, versus function with the jaws in the correct position. In most instances, however, it is primarily an esthetic decision. The facial appearance is likely to be better if the jaw relationship is corrected. Is that improvement worth the additional risk, cost, and morbidity of surgery? In the final analysis, only the patient and parents can—or should—make that decision.

Recent advances in computer prediction of alternative outcomes, so that the likely effects on facial appearance from various treatment procedures can be simulated, have made it easier to communicate with patients. Especially in decisions like surgery versus orthodontic camouflage but also in deciding whether to expand the dental arches or extract, a picture is worth a thousand words (see Figure 7-22). Good evidence now shows that communication is improved when computer images of the likely outcome of alternative treatment procedures are shown to the patient.[12] Image predictions are much more accurate when growth is not involved, but this method can help parents understand the options for children and adolescents as well.

Patient Interaction in Treatment Planning Decisions

Sometimes involving patients in treatment planning discussions is interpreted as allowing the patient and parent to make all the decisions. Clearly this is not the case. It is the doctor's responsibility to explain the options to the patient and parents, and to negotiate with them the final treatment plan. It is not the doctor's responsibility to do anything the patient wants. Just as any patient has the right to refuse to accept treatment, the doctor has the right to refuse to carry out treatment that he or she considers not in the patient's best interest. At one time, the doctor decided what was to be done, and that was that. Now, establishing the concept of the final treatment plan is, and must be, an interactive process between the doctor and the patient.

In our example case, the patient and her parents understood the importance of correcting the Class II malocclusion and deep bite if a better facial appearance was to be achieved, accepted the suggestion that headgear would be the best approach but should be delayed until she was closer to adolescence, and acknowledged that a change in the treatment plan to include extraction or even orthognathic surgery might be needed if the patient did not respond well to the more conservative initial treatment plan. They also reviewed the anticipated risks of treatment in her case, the primary concerns being root resorption (especially of the maxillary incisors) and the possibility of damage to the teeth from inadequate hygiene. The result was both informed consent in the broad (and correct) sense and approval of the treatment plan concept (Box 7-7).

Box 7-7

PATIENT F.P.: FINAL TREATMENT PLAN

Treatment Concept

- During adolescent growth, headgear to correct skeletal Class II, reduce overjet
- Align maxillary incisors and correct their inclination without increasing overjet
- Correct anterior deep bite by controlling lower incisor eruption as vertical growth occurs
- Adjunctive gingival surgery if needed
- Observe asymmetry to be sure it is not getting worse

Treatment Details

- Delay start of treatment until level of maturation indicates onset of adolescent growth
- High-pull headgear
- Level mandibular arch with reverse curve arch wires
- Torque to maxillary incisors
- Class II elastics as needed
- Gingival surgery, if needed, before appliances are removed

The Detailed Plan: Specifying Orthodontic Mechanotherapy

What is established in the patient-parent consultation is the treatment plan in conceptual form—Class II treatment by growth modification with headgear and a complete fixed appliance to align the teeth and correct the deep bite, as in our example patient. The final step in planning treatment is specification of the details of the treatment method—in orthodontics, the mechanotherapy—that is to be used. This detailed plan would be what the doctor refers to during treatment, to guide the sequence of procedures and maintain a focus on correcting this specific patient's problems.

The detailed plan for our example patient is shown in Box 7-7. Note that for this patient, the conceptual plan leads directly to the mechanotherapy—which usually is the case. For any patient, the selected treatment procedures must meet two criteria: *effectiveness* in producing the desired result and *efficiency* in doing so without wasting either doctor or patient time. Progress and completion of this case are shown in Figures 7-25 to 7-28.

For a relatively simple treatment plan, the associated mechanotherapy is also reasonably simple or at least straightforward. Nevertheless, choices must be made and

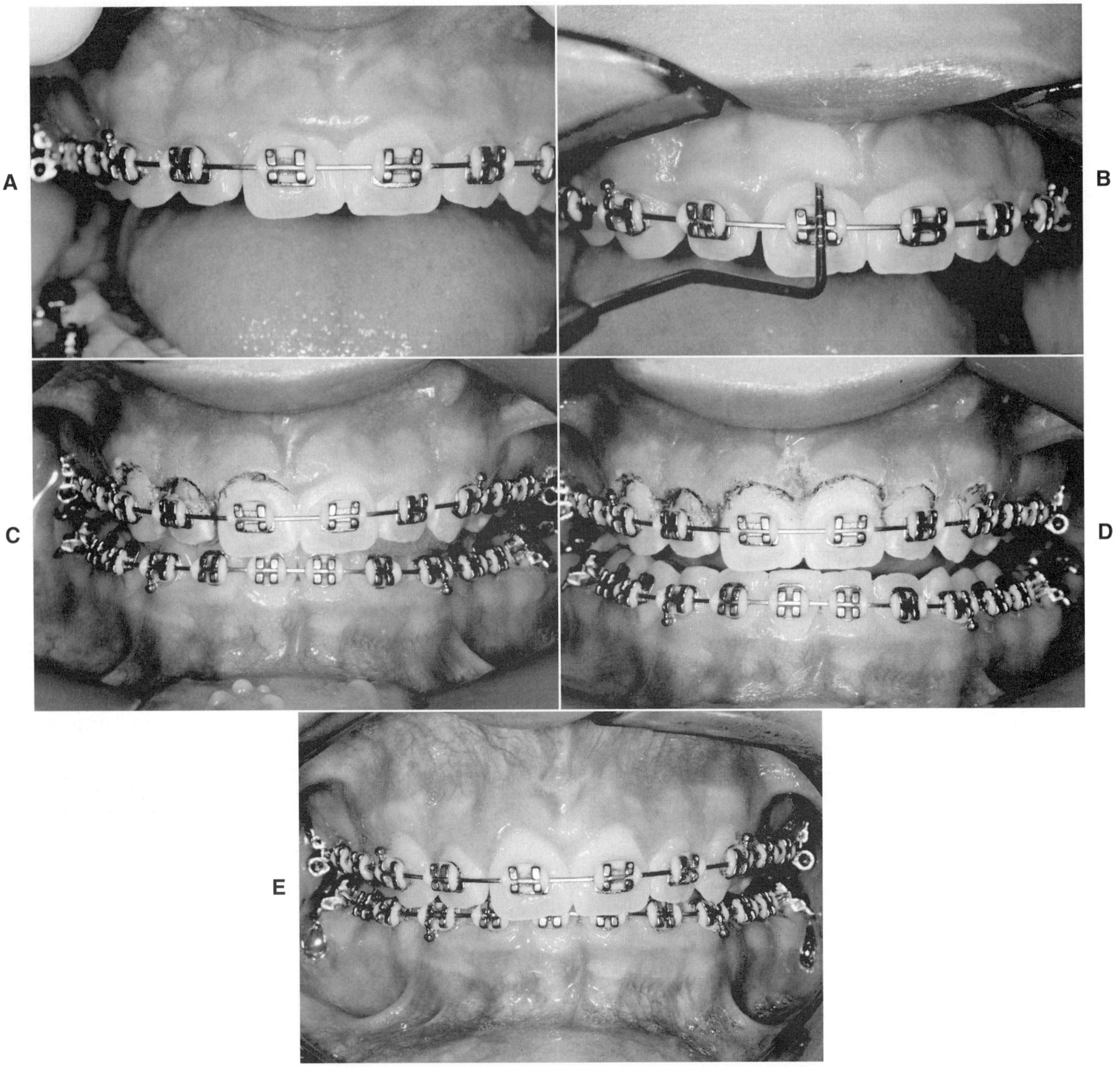

FIGURE 7-25 For patient F.P., whose diagnostic work-up is illustrated in Figures 6-71 to 6-74 (see Figure 7-22 for computer image predictions), treatment was deferred until she was entering her adolescent growth spurt. A fixed appliance was placed at age 12-5, and high-pull headgear was started at age 12-10. Dentally and skeletally, she responded well to treatment, but the gingival overgrowth of the maxillary incisors worsened rather than improved **(A)**. A diode laser now offers a painless and efficient way to manage problems of this type, and she was scheduled for gingival recontouring at age 13-11. A periodontal probe was used to establish the depth of the gingival sulcus **(B)**, and the laser was used to recontour the tissue (**C,** One side done; **D,** Gingival recontouring completed). Because the tissue is ablated (vaporized) and the heat of the laser seals the ablation site, no bleeding occurs and no periodontal dressing is needed. Healing occurs within a few days. **E,** The greatly improved tissue contours 4 weeks later.

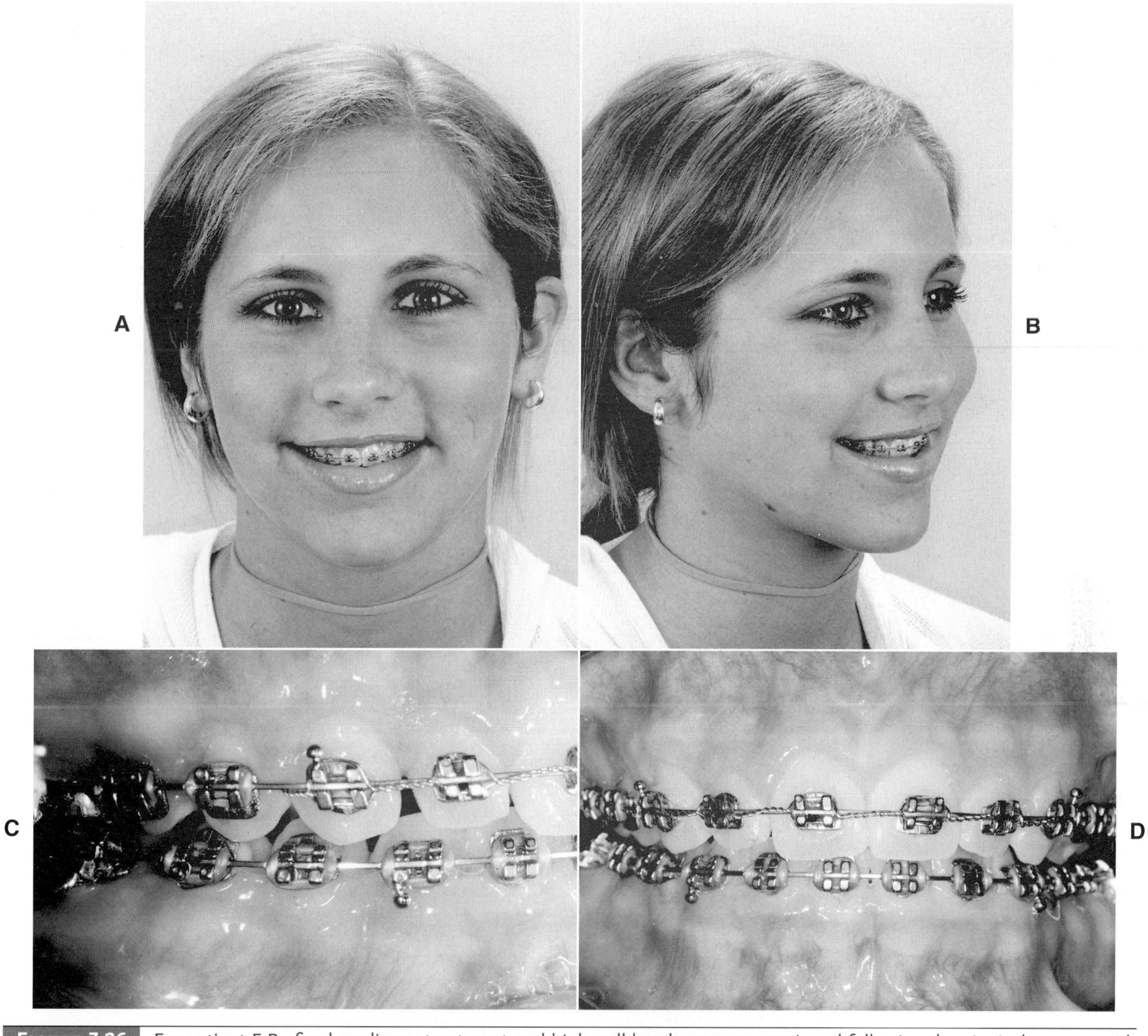

Figure 7-26 For patient F.P., fixed appliance treatment and high pull headgear were continued following the gingival surgery, with an effort to elongate the maxillary incisors for better display on smile while maintaining the overbite correction. **A, B,** Progress records at age 14-5 showed good incisor display and **(C, D)** a nearly corrected malocclusion.

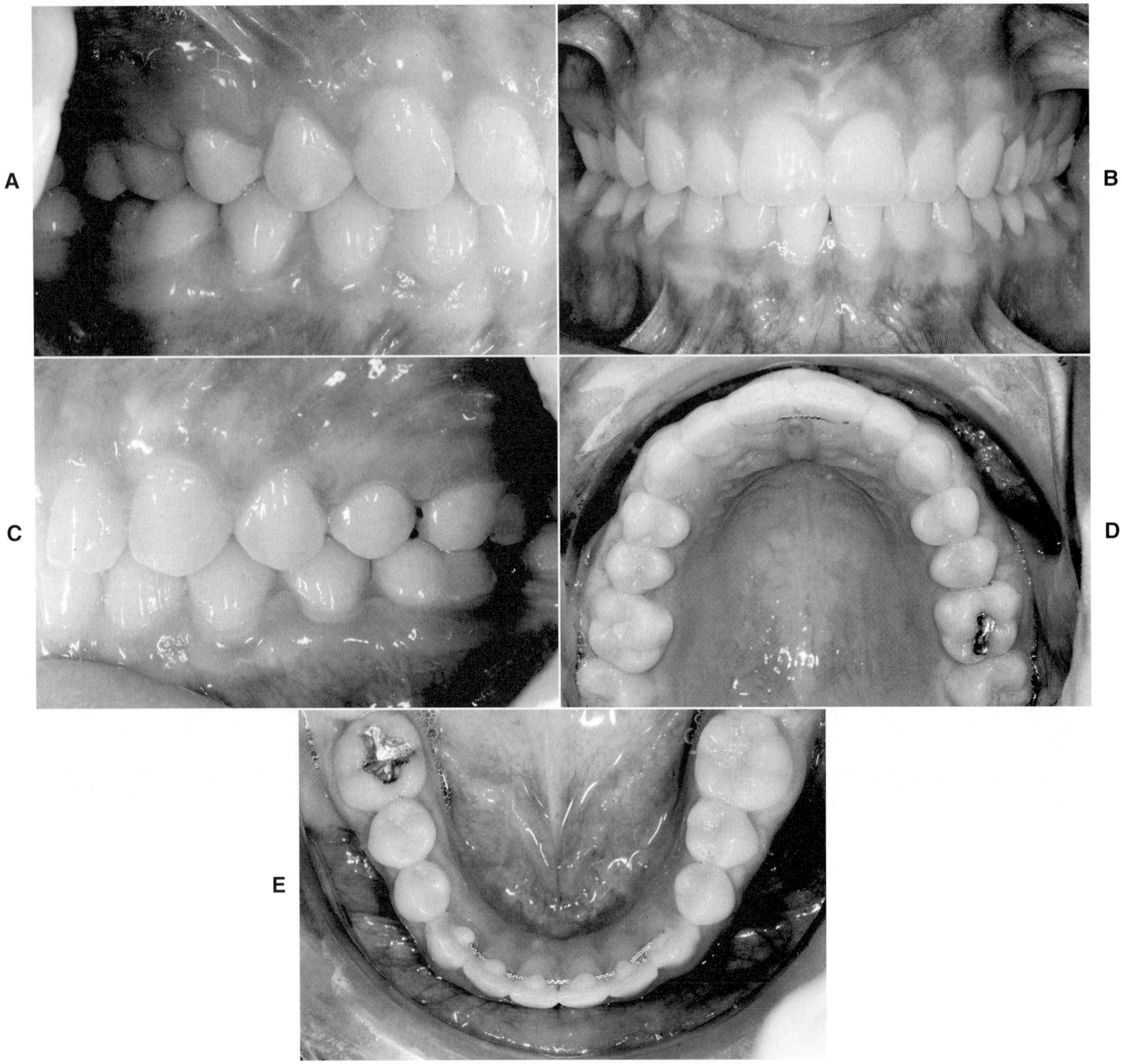

FIGURE 7-27 Patient F.P.: the orthodontic appliance was removed at age 14-9, 23 months after treatment began. The intra-oral views and panoramic radiograph **(A-F)** show excellent alignment and occlusion, with normal gingival contours. Note **(D)** the bonded maxillary retainer to maintain the rotation correction and space closure for the maxillary central incisors and **(E)** the bonded canine-to-canine retainer for the lower arch. In the close-up smile images **(G, H),** note the consonant smile arc and improved maxillary incisor display.

F

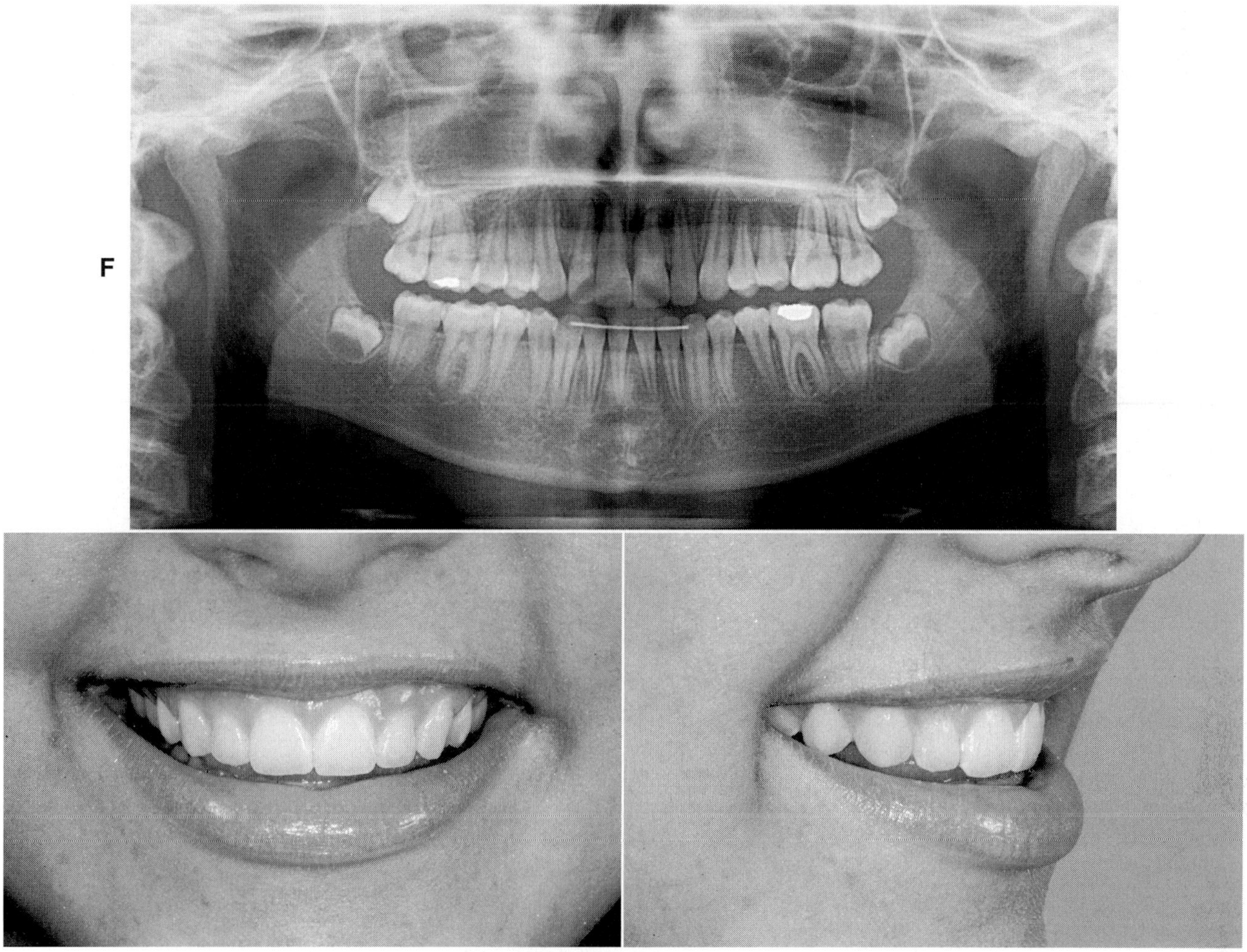

G H

Figure 7-27 cont'd

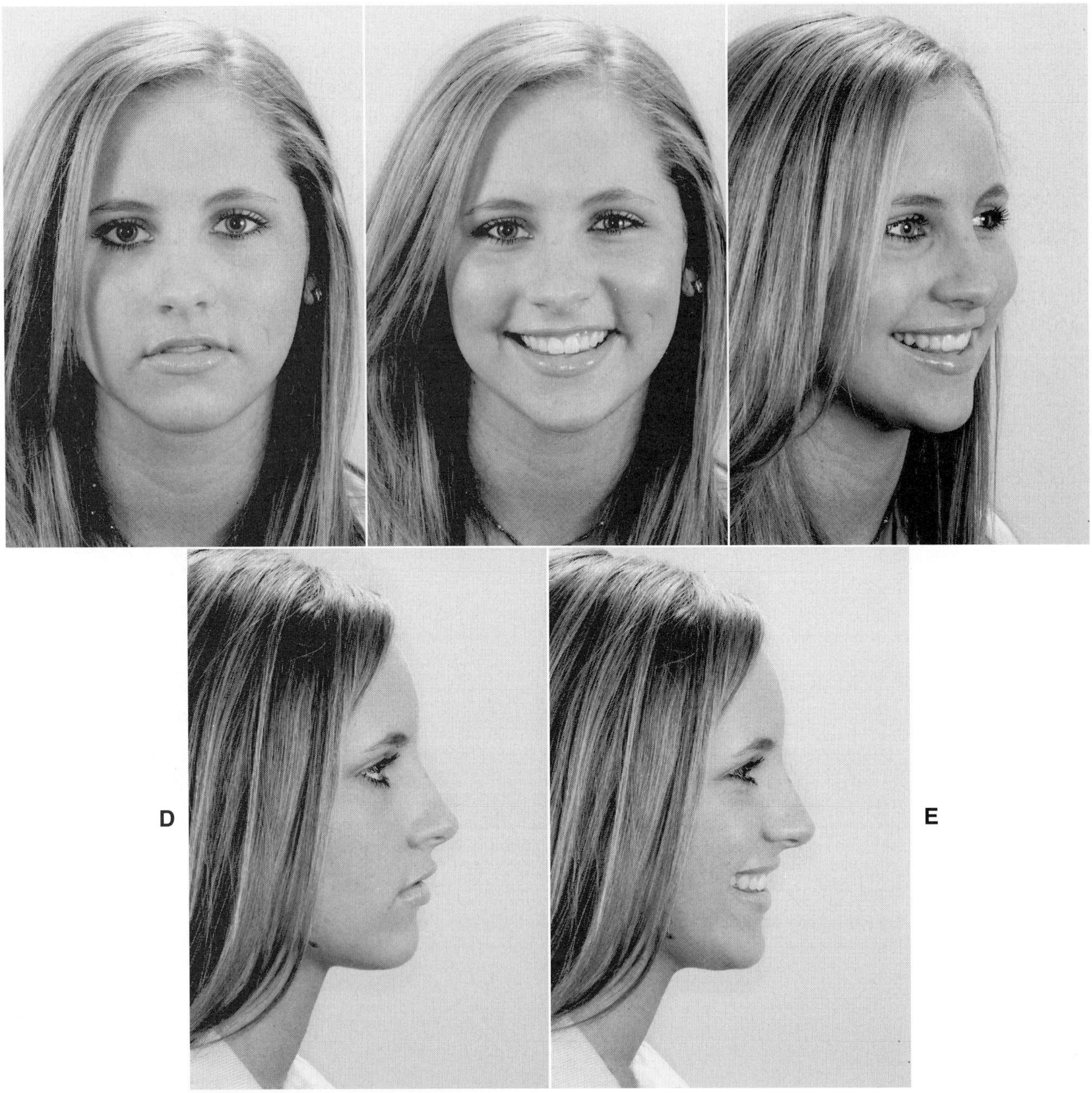

Figure 7-28 Patient F.P.: **A** to **E,** The post-treatment facial appearance. **F,** The post-treatment cephalometric radiograph, and **(G)** a cephalometric superimposition showing the changes during treatment. In the superimposition tracing, note the improvement in upper incisor angulation through palatal root torque, without intrusion or facial tipping of the incisors that would have elevated their incisal edges. One potential solution to a "gummy smile" is intrusion of the maxillary incisors, but in this case that would have flattened the smile arc and decreased incisor display, both of which were undesirable. Downward and forward growth of the mandible relative to the maxilla, while the vertical position of the maxillary molars was maintained, was the desired result from use of high pull headgear.

F

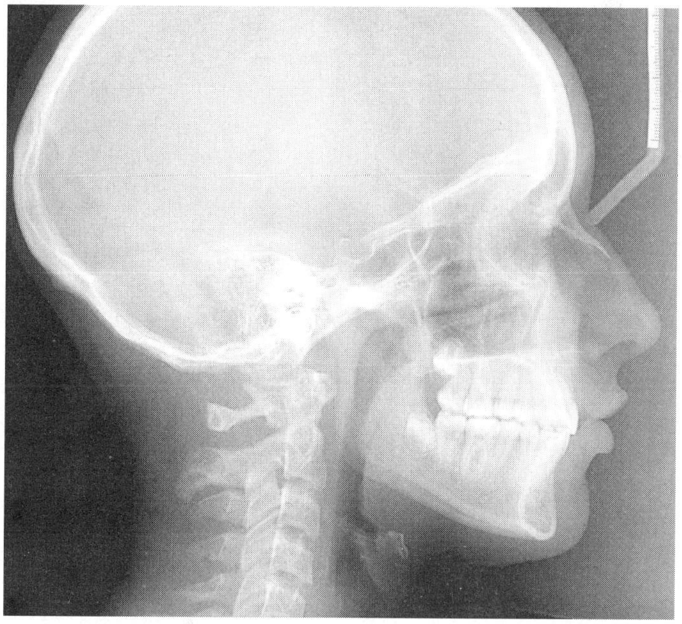

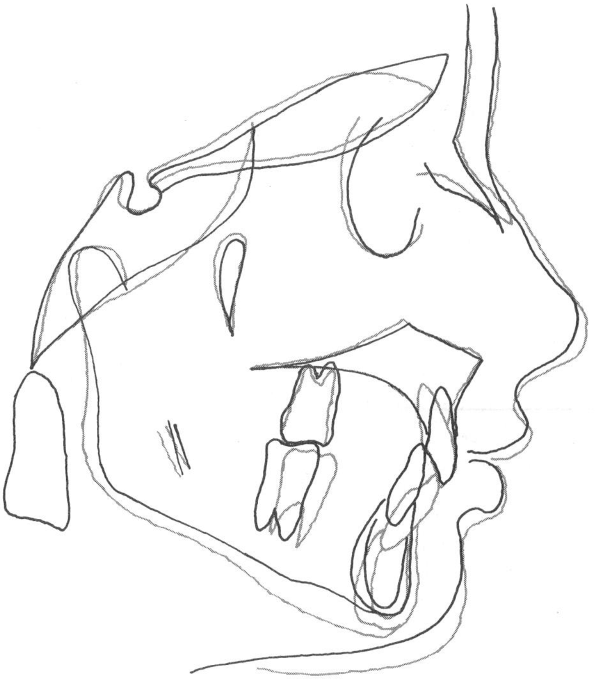

G

Figure 7-28 cont'd

clearly specified in the treatment plan. For example, if the plan is to expand a narrow maxillary arch, it would be possible to do this with an expansion lingual arch, an expansion labial arch, or a banded or bonded maxillary palatal expander. The treatment plan must specify which, and the effectiveness and efficiency of the various possibilities must be considered. There is a time and a place for everything, and this last step is the place for the practical considerations of which treatment method and what orthodontic therapy to use.

The most serious errors in orthodontic treatment planning are those that result from first thinking of which appliance to use, not what the appliance is supposed to accomplish. The treatment mechanics should not be allowed to determine the treatment result. It is an error to establish the treatment mechanics before establishing the broader goal of treatment. The treatment procedures should be manipulated to produce the desired result, not the other way around.

References

1. Gesch D, Bernhardt O, Kocher T, et al. Association of malocclusion and functional occlusion with signs of TMD in adults: Results of the population-based study of health in Pomerania. Angle Orthod 74:512-520, 2004.
2. Sackett DL. On identifying the best therapy. In: Trotman CA, McNamara JA, eds. Orthodontic Treatment: Outcome and Effectiveness. Ann Arbor, Mich: University of Michigan Center for Human Growth and Development; 1995.
3. American Cleft Palate Association: Membership-Team Directory (2006), ACPA/CPF National Office, 1504 E. Franklin St., Suite 102, Chapel Hill, NC,
4. Edwards JC. The diastema, the frenum, the frenectomy: A clinical study, Am J Orthod 71:489-508, 1977.
5. Villa NL, Cisneros GJ. Changes in the dentition secondary to palatal crib therapy in digit-suckers. Pediatric Dent 19:323-326, 1997.
6. Chintakanon K, Boonpinon P. Ectopic eruption of the first permanent molars: Prevalence and etiologic factors. Angle Orthod 68:153-160, 1998.
7. Ericson S, Kurol J. Resorption of maxillary lateral incisors caused by ectopic eruption of the canines. Am J Orthod Dentofacial Orthop 94:504-513, 1988.
8. Sfikas PM. A duty to disclose: Issues to consider in securing informed consent. J Am Dent Assoc 134:1329-1333, 2003.
9. Mortensen MG, Kiyak HA, Omnell L. Patient and parent understanding of informed consent in orthodontics. Am J Orthod Dentofac Orthop 124:541-550, 2003.
10. Ackerman JL, Proffit WR. Communication in orthodontic treatment planning: Bioethical and informed consent issues. Angle Orthod 65:253-262, 1995.
11. Bandura A, Barbaranelli C, et al. Self-efficacy beliefs as shapers of children's aspirations and career trajectories. Child Development 72:187-206, 2001.
12. Phillips C, Hill B, Cannac C. The influence of video imaging on patients' perceptions and expectations. Angle Orthod 65:263-270, 1995.

CHAPTER

8

Orthodontic Treatment Planning: Limitations, Controversies, and Special Problems

CHAPTER OUTLINE

THE EVIDENCE FOR CLINICAL DECISIONS

Orthodontics traditionally has been a specialty in which the opinions of leaders were important, to the point that professional groups coalesced around a strong leader. Angle, Begg, and Tweed societies still exist, and new ones whose primary purpose is to promulgate its leader's opinions were formed as late as the 1980s. As any professional group comes of age, however, there must be a focus on evidence-based rather than opinion-based decisions. The current trend in orthodontics in that direction is an encouraging indication of professional maturity.

Some important clinical decisions, however, must be made without solid data on which to base them. In that circumstance the clinician must use his or her best judgment, which requires some understanding of the quality of existing data. This important subject is reviewed in some detail immediately below.

Study Designs

Retrospective versus Prospective Data

Decisions about treatment are based on some combination of a theoretical understanding of the patient's circumstances (whether or not the theory is correct) and knowledge of the outcome of previous treatment in similar cases. Poorly conceived views of how the patient's condition developed lead to poor treatment decisions, which is why the discussion of etiology in Chapter 5 is an important background for rational treatment planning. The other part of the equation is equally important: We need to know as thoroughly as possible what really happens when various treatment procedures are used. Clinical experience provides important information, but progress occurs only if treatment regimens are applied systematically and the results are analyzed logically, carefully and thoughtfully.

As Box 8-1 illustrates, a hierarchy of quality exists in the evidence on which clinical decisions are based. Clinical data become available as reports of treatment outcomes. In the simplest form this is a case report, showing (usually in considerable detail) what happened in the treatment of a particular patient. A case series requires distilling the information, to separate the general trend among the patients from individual idiosyncrasies. The more patients for whom information is available, the more accurately the general trend can be discerned—but only if the sample of patients being reported is a reasonable representation of the larger population who might receive treatment of that type and if the data are analyzed appropriately. The hierarchy of quality in clinical data reflects, more than anything else, the probability that an accurate conclusion can be drawn from the group of patients who have been studied.

Box 8-1

EVIDENCE OF CLINICAL EFFECTIVENESS: A HIERARCHY OF QUALITY

Randomized clinical trial

↑

Prospective study, non-random assignment

↑

Retrospective study, inclusion based only on pretreatment characteristics

↑

Retrospective study, inclusion based on treatment response

↑

Case report(s)

↑

Unsupported opinion of expert

The unsupported opinion of an expert is the weakest form of clinical evidence. Often the expert opinion is supported by a series of cases that were selected retrospectively from practice records. The problem with that, of course, is that the cases are likely to have been selected because they show the expected outcome. A clinician who becomes an advocate of a treatment method is naturally tempted to select illustrative cases that show the desired outcome, and if even he or she tries to be objective, it is difficult to avoid introducing bias. When outcomes are variable, picking the cases that came out the way they were supposed to and discarding the ones that didn't is a great way to make your point. Information based on selected cases, therefore, must be viewed with considerable reserve.

It's much better, if retrospective cases are used in a clinical study, to select them on the basis of their characteristics when treatment began, not on the outcome. It's better yet to select the cases prospectively before treatment begins. Even then, it is quite possible to bias the sample so that the "right" patients are chosen. After experience with a treatment method, doctors tend to learn subtle indications that a particular patient is or is not likely to respond well, although they may have difficulty verbalizing exactly what criteria they used. But identifying the criteria associated with success is extremely important if the treatment method is to work well for others, and a biased sample makes that impossible. One important way to control bias in reporting the outcomes of treatment is to be sure that *all* of the treated cases are included in the report.

For this reason, the gold standard for evaluating clinical procedures is the randomized clinical trial, in which patients are randomly assigned in advance to alternative treatment procedures. The great advantage of this method is that random assignment, if the sample is large enough, should result in a similar distribution of all variables between (or among) the groups. Even variables that were not recognized in advance should be controlled by this type of patient assignment—and in clinical work, often important variables are identified only after the treatment has been started or even completed.

An important aspect of any prospective study is keeping track of *all* the patients once they have been assigned to a treatment regimen. The other major source of bias in prospective studies comes from drop-outs, who are likely to be the very patients who were not responding well to the treatment. Unless these patients are accounted for, the same bias produced by initially selecting only the "good" patients arises. Random assignment of patients, as in a randomized clinical trial, avoids the first source of selection bias but does nothing to control the second one. Data from randomized trials, therefore, must be reviewed on an "intent to treat" basis that includes all the subjects, using statistical techniques to estimate data for the ones who dropped out.

Data from randomized clinical trials now determine many clinical approaches in medicine and are beginning to do so in dentistry. The clinical trials in orthodontics that have been reported will be referred to in some detail later in this book. Many important clinical questions, however, do not lend themselves to clinical trial methodology, and inevitably many issues must be evaluated without randomized controls and/or from retrospective data. Let's now consider some important issues in evaluating such data.

Historical Control Groups

The best way to know—often the only way to know—whether a treatment method really works is to compare treated patients with an untreated control group. For such a comparison to be valid, the two groups must be equivalent before treatment starts. If the groups were different to start with, you cannot with any confidence say that differences afterward were due to the treatment.

There are a number of difficulties in setting up control groups for orthodontic treatment. The principal ones are that the controls must be followed over a long period of time, equivalent to the treatment time, and that sequential radiographs usually are required for the controls and the patients. Radiation exposure for untreated children is problematic. At present it is very difficult to get permission to expose children to x-rays that will be of no benefit to them personally. The growth studies carried out in the 1935-65 era in Burlington (Ontario) in association with the University of Toronto, Ann Arbor by the University of Michigan, and Cleveland by the Bolton Foundation provide reasonably large archives of sequential radiographs of untreated children (some of whom had malocclusion). Several smaller data bases from the same time period also exist.

This historical material is still being used as control data for evaluations of orthodontic treatment procedures, especially those involving growth modification. How valid is this? Are children seeking orthodontic treatment more than 50 years later, especially in other areas of the United States or even in other countries, really comparable with these historical samples? Probably not as much as one would like. The composition of current population groups often differs from the relatively homogenous growth study groups, especially when a current project focuses on children with a particular type of malocclusion but the comparison is with the mostly normal growth study groups. In addition, the secular trend in growth over 50 years almost surely has affected expected growth increments. When historical controls are the best that are available, it is better to have them than nothing, but the limitations must be kept in mind.

Sample Sizes and Composition

How many subjects does it take to demonstrate a treatment effect? That depends, of course, on the size of the effect to be detected. The bigger the difference between two groups, the fewer the subjects that are needed to show it (if variability remains the same). Statistical analysis calculates the probability that differences are due to chance alone when the null hypothesis is true. When that probability becomes small enough, we accept the hypothesis that the groups are different.

In orthodontics, the data for clinical decisions often are from cephalometric analysis. The differences created by orthodontic treatment usually are not very large and are about the same magnitude as the variability within the sample. For this reason, although small cephalometric samples can be analyzed, conclusions based on sample sizes under 20 must be regarded with considerable suspicion, regardless of the statistics. With sample sizes of 25-30 patients, often it is possible to discern differences that would be important clinically, and almost always such differences can be demonstrated in sample sizes of 50 or so.

Sample size becomes particularly important when the composition of the groups being studied is not homogenous. Heterogeneity of the group can relate to age, gender, maturity, racial/ethnic origin, and other demographic characteristics. It also can relate to characteristics of the malocclusion being treated. Heterogeneity tends to increase the observed variability, making it more difficult to detect differences of clinical interest within a small sample. Angle classification is inadequate not only for orthodontic diagnosis but also for sorting research subjects. For instance, if you're studying Class II malocclusion, it's not enough to just select Class II subjects. It will be important to note face height as an important variable, because subjects with short and long faces grow differently and are likely to respond differently to treatment aimed at the overjet and Class II occlusion they share (Figure 8-1). Other characteristics of the malocclusion also may need to be controlled if sample sizes are to be kept reasonably small.

ISSUES IN DATA ANALYSIS

Clinical versus Statistical Significance

Statistical analysis can never flatly confirm or reject the truth of an experimental hypothesis. It merely calculates the odds that the null hypothesis should be accepted or rejected. If the analysis shows less than a 5% chance that a difference between groups could have arisen due to random variation ($p < .05$), the research hypothesis often is accepted (or, in terms of the test procedure, the null form of that hypothesis is not accepted).

There are many possible sources of error in statistical analysis. For clinical studies, the most likely error arises from

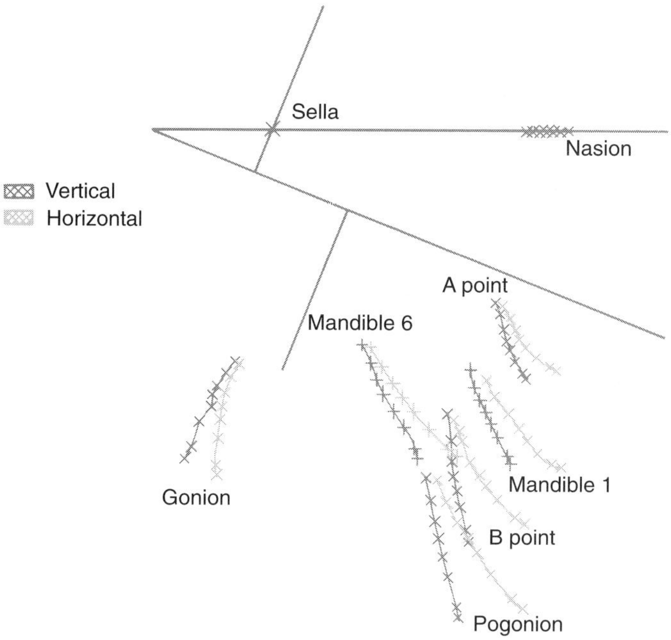

FIGURE 8-1 The varying growth direction of selected maxillary and mandibular landmarks is shown in this drawing derived from the templates of the Burlington (Ontario) growth study. The mean tracks for patients with a vertical vs. a horizontal growth pattern show clearly that both the direction and magnitude of growth at various locations are quite different, and the track for individuals with the usual horizontal-vertical pattern is intermediate between these two. For accuracy in growth prediction it would be important to place the patient in the correct group—which, unfortunately, can be quite difficult.

applying statistics based on the normal distribution to a data set that is not distributed like this bell-shaped curve. Wrongly applied statistics tend to generate incorrect probability values that can lead to incorrect interpretations—in other words, bad statistics lead to bad conclusions. Transforming the data before analyzing it (by performing the same mathematical operation on each datum, for instance, taking the logarithm of each number) often can make normal-distribution (parametric) statistics more applicable. Many clinical studies, however, require statistics not based on the normal distribution (often called nonparametric statistics because the data are noncontinuous).

Orthodontics is an excellent example of a clinical area in which both the theoretical framework for treatment and many treatment techniques have changed dramatically during the last 25 years. Similar progress has been made in statistics, especially in the analysis of clinical data. At this point, the use only of t-tests in a clinical study would be analogous to orthodontic treatment using gold bands and archwires—not wrong but not the best you could do. The modern clinician should be suspicious of conclusions based on superficial testing. Fortunately, clinical journals increasingly demand adequate statistical analysis, but that cannot be taken for granted, and the statistics that appear in some nonreviewed presentations (prominent on the Internet but often found in the report of presentations at a meeting and the "clinical" journals) must be examined carefully indeed.

It is important to remember that statistical significance and clinical significance are not the same. Tests of statistical significance ask questions like, "Is it probable that the difference between these groups is due only to chance?" Clinical significance asks, "Does that make any difference in treatment outcome?" Sometimes studies demonstrate statistically significant differences that are so small that they have no clinical significance. For example, studies of the size of the mandible with or without treatment aimed at stimulating its growth almost always show small differences in the ultimate size of the jaws. In some publications the differences are reported as statistically significant, in others as not significant. At that level, the argument is over whether average differences of 1-2 mm in the size of a 120 mm mandible are treatment-related. The more important consideration is whether it would make any real difference clinically if they were. The clinician's question is, "Can you stimulate mandibular growth?" The answer has to be based on the magnitude of the changes as well as the result of statistical analysis. It seems to be, "If you can, not much."

Can clinically significant differences escape detection by statistical analysis? Certainly that is possible, especially when samples are small and/or not well selected. The likelihood is in the other direction, however. If statistical analysis fails to confirm what the clinician is convinced is true, the clinician probably is wrong. It's a human characteristic to remember the unusual, not the usual. Reports of treatment outcomes tend to focus on very good or very poor results, making most doctors think both extremes are more frequent than they really are. Reports of statistically significant differences that may not be clinically significant are more frequently encountered in the literature than clinically significant differences missed statistically.

Variability in Outcomes and the Presentation of Data

How do you report what happened to a group of patients? Almost always, by reporting the central tendency of the data set (the average, or perhaps the median) and by presenting some measure of the dispersion of the group (standard deviation or percentile spread, range). The focus tends to be on the central tendency, so a typical report says, "On average, group A showed significantly [whatever] compared with group B."

The problem with that type of data reporting can be illustrated by comparing Table 8-1 and Figure 8-2, which show exactly the same data but produce (for most clinicians, at least) a different sense of what is happening with this treatment. The data are taken from a randomized clinical trial of early Class II treatment, from which children with

TABLE 8-1

Class II RCT: Skeletal Effects: ANB Angle (S.D.)

Visit	Control	Bionator	Headgear
Initial	6.29 (1.98)	6.26 (2.06)	6.04 (1.82)
End Ph 1	6.11 (1.90)	5.14 (1.99)	4.72 (1.82)
Ph 1 Change	−0.17	−1.12	−1.31
End Ph 2	4.28 (2.04)	3.93 (1.94)	4.10 (1.97)
Ph 2 Change	−1.83	−1.21	−0.62
Total Change	−2.00	−2.33	−1.93

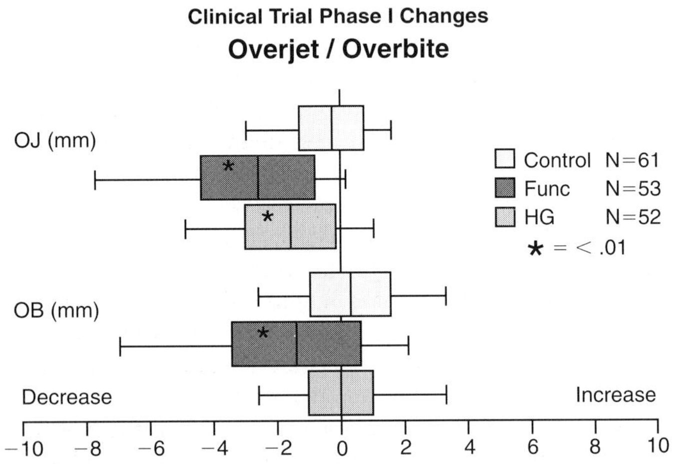

FIGURE 8-2 In this graphic display (called a 5-box plot) of data from the UNC Class II clinical trial, the median value for each group is shown as the line toward the center of each box; the box dimensions reflect the 25th and 75th percentiles for the group; and the line shows the range. The variability within the groups can be appreciated more readily from a display of this type than from a table (see Table 8-2). Note that although the median change in overjet without treatment was almost zero, some children in the untreated control group had a reduction in overjet while others had an increase. Although the decrease in overjet in both treated groups was statistically significant compared with the controls, not all treated children responded favorably.

abnormally long or short faces were excluded. (This important study is reviewed further below and in Chapter 13). Many doctors, looking at the table, would conclude that as they expected, nothing happened to the untreated children. The table shows that headgear produced some reduction in overjet but no change in overbite, while the functional appliance produced nearly twice as much change in overjet and also reduced overbite.

Figure 8-2 confirms that is true, on the average, but shows the variability within the groups as clearly as the central tendency. The variability was shown in the table too, but the standard deviation and range numbers just do not have the same impact, at least to the untrained eye. What you see in the figure is that many of the untreated children had a reduction in overjet, and about the same number had an increase, so that the average was zero although most children had changes. Some of the headgear patients had great improvement, while others had no response and a few got worse. There also was great variability among the functional appliance patients. It's important to comprehend the variations in response to treatment procedures, not just the average change, and particularly important not to be seduced into thinking that the average response is what you ought to expect to happen for every patient. The graphic form for presenting data (this type is called a 5-box plot) helps clinicians perceive the variability as well as the average changes.

Syndrome Recognition: Sensitivity versus Specificity in Diagnostic Records

By definition, a syndrome is a set of concurrent clinical findings that form an identifiable pattern. Many syndromes of developmental abnormalities have been recognized, and new ones are being noted all the time. Syndrome recognition is important in clinical studies, because patients who can be grouped by identifiable patterns are more predictable than those who have not been classified at that level. For example, you're much more likely to obtain a useful answer to the question, "How do patients with Crouzon syndrome respond to reverse-pull headgear?" than to the question, "How do patients with maxillary deficiency respond to reverse-pull headgear?", simply because there are several types of maxillary deficiency, Crouzon syndrome being one, that are likely to differ in their response.

Clinical progress requires the recognition of patterns of abnormalities, whether or not they are formally grouped as named syndromes. We already have commented on the importance of going beyond the Angle classification in orthodontic diagnosis. One way to view the Ackerman-

Proffit classification is that in grouping patients by their five major characteristics, it places them in more homogenous and therefore more predictable groups.

From that perspective, it is important to consider two additional scientific terms, *sensitivity* and *specificity,* as they apply to diagnostic criteria and criteria for evaluating treatment response. Sensitivity refers to the ability of a given criterion (ANB angle, for example) to differentiate degrees of severity or extent of change (for ANB: diagnostically, the severity of a Class II jaw relationship; as an indicator of treatment response, the amount of improvement or worsening of the Class II condition). Specificity refers to the extent to which the criterion reflects only what it is supposed to, vs. being influenced by other things—in the case of the ANB angle, how well it shows the anteroposterior jaw relationships without being influenced by the vertical position of the jaws, protrusion or retrusion of the incisor teeth, or other factors. An extremely sensitive measure is always positive in the presence of the condition. Specificity sometimes particularly refers to how well a criterion can separate normal (acceptable) from abnormal (unacceptable)—for ANB, its ability to separate skeletal Class II from normal jaw relationships. An extremely specific measure is always negative in the absence of the condition.

Why are these distinctions important? From what you know about ANB, you could deduce that it is sensitive to changes in the anteroposterior jaw relationship (i.e., only small changes in the anteroposterior position of either jaw will produce a measurable change in ANB). Its specificity is not so good, because the ANB angle changes as face height shortens or lengthens even though the anteroposterior position of the jaws stays the same. It also can change if the incisor teeth are moved forward or back because of bone remodeling in the area of points A and B. Could you uncritically accept changes in the ANB angle as showing skeletal change in Class II patients undergoing alternative types of treatment? Only if you could be sure that there were no major vertical changes and no changes in the position of the roots of the anterior teeth. Obviously, the same type of thinking applies to whatever the major indicators are, in any clinical study. The more sensitive and more specific the indicators, the easier it is to interpret the results—and vice versa. No single criterion is likely to be both sensitive and specific enough to indicate all you'd want to know about patient groupings or treatment response.

Computer Records and the Possibility of Meta-analysis

Clinical data exist in the form of careful records of treatment outcomes in many if not most private practices, not just in university or other clinical settings. Getting enough data about enough patients always is difficult in clinical studies. The widespread use of computers for storage of practice information, and the growing trend in orthodontics toward placing diagnostic as well as practice management information into electronic memory, offers an opportunity to widen the horizons of clinical research in a way that was hardly imaginable only a few years ago.

Most practitioners have had two problems in putting together data from their practices to obtain an honest answer to clinical questions: It is difficult and time-consuming to pull information from handwritten charts, manually analyze radiographs, and take measurements from dental casts or other records; and for most people, no clear protocol exists to show how to do this properly.

Computerization has the potential to solve both problems. If electronic entries replace chart notes and these are stored using a standard protocol (as most will be, because the format is established by the supplier of the practice software), and if x-rays, photographs and casts are obtained digitally or scanned for entry into the computer system (as they are, more and more, so they are accessible for communication with referring dentists as well as for analysis), then the information becomes readily available instead of having to be dug out of charts. One of the greatest problems with most existing data sets is the selective nature of the patients who are included. Often a major reason for selecting only some patients is that it is too much work to include everyone who was treated. But with routine electronic entry for all patients, there would be no reason to include only specially selected patients. In addition, it would be quite possible for a standard protocol for data collection to be established by a research group at a central facility, to which data could be transferred electronically from private practice. It would even be possible to add data to the research file via the Internet at the same time the clinical files were updated, and in fact this already is being done in some studies in medicine as "Internet trials." Only with this type of cooperative input of data from multiple practice locations will it be possible to pull together enough data to answer many important clinical questions. By the same token, the very availability of the data will make it almost unconscionable not to seek solid answers to questions that have drawn only opinion for so long. The greatest hurdle will be standardizing the data entry method so that all sites demonstrate the same reliability of the methods.

An additional way to gain better data for treatment responses is to group the data from several studies of the same phenomenon. This draws on the recently-developed method of meta-analysis, which allows statistical techniques to be applied across multiple studies.[1] Orthodontic research is an excellent example of an area in which numerous small studies have been carried out toward similar ends, often with protocols that were at least somewhat similar but different enough to make comparisons difficult. Meta-analysis is no substitute for new data collected with precise protocols, and including poorly-done studies in a meta-analysis carries with it a risk of confusing rather than clarifying the issue. Nevertheless, applying it to clinical questions has considerable potential to reduce uncertainty about the best treatment methods. Several recent reviews have taken advantage of this method to improve the quality of evidence about the outcomes of orthodontic treatment procedures.[2-7]

The era of orthodontics as an opinion-driven specialty clearly is at an end. In the future, it will be evidence-driven—which is all for the best. In the meantime, clinical decisions still must be made using the best information currently available. When the latest new method appears with someone's strong recommendation and a series of case reports in which it worked very well, it is wise to remember the aphorism "Enthusiastic reports tend to lack controls; well-controlled reports tend to lack enthusiasm."

REDUCING UNCERTAINTY IN PLANNING TREATMENT

Even when excellent data from clinical trials are available, it is difficult to predict how any one individual will respond to a particular plan of treatment. Variability must be expected. In orthodontics, two interrelated factors contribute most of the variability: the patient's growth pattern and the effect of treatment on the expression of growth. At present, in the absence of growth, treatment responses are reasonably predictable. Growth is not predictable.

Growth Prediction

Because predicting facial growth would be of great benefit in planning orthodontic treatment, repeated efforts have been made to develop methods to do this from cephalometric radiographs. Successful prediction requires specifying both the *amount* and the *direction* of growth, in the context of a baseline or reference point. The serial cephalometric radiographs obtained during the Burlington, Michigan, and Bolton growth studies have been treated statistically to allow their use in growth prediction, by grouping the data to provide a picture of average, normal growth changes. A convenient way to show average growth changes is with templates that show the expected direction and increment of growth at specified points or ages, or as a series of complete templates from which change at given points can be deduced (the same templates that also can be used diagnostically—see Chapter 6).

The more the individual whose growth one is attempting to predict is representative of the sample from which the average changes were derived, the more accurate one would expect the prediction to be, and vice versa. Ideally, separate growth standards would be established for the two sexes, the major racial groups, and important subgroups within each of the major categories (such as patients with skeletal Class II or Class III malocclusions). An Italian data set for untreated Class III children has been very helpful as a control for treated Class III patients (see below). No such data exist for untreated Class II individuals, and because it is no longer ethically acceptable to take repeated x-rays of children who will not be treated, it is unlikely that the necessary quantity of data ever will be available.

Data from the Bolton study[8] are not subdivided in any way. The Michigan data[9] are subdivided by sex, providing different male and female predictive values; the Burlington data[10] have been subdivided on the basis of facial pattern, with different growth predictions for individuals with short, normal, and long vertical facial dimensions (see Figure 8-1). All three data sets are derived from whites of northern European descent.

The major difficulty with growth prediction based on average changes is that a patient may have neither the average amount nor direction of growth, and thus there is the possibility of significant error. The growth samples were composed mostly of normal children. In clinical application, growth prediction is really needed for a child who has a skeletal malocclusion. His or her problem developed because of growth that deviated from the norm, and for such a child, deviant growth is likely to continue in the future—which means that average increments and directions are unlikely to be correct. Our ability to predict facial growth, therefore, is poorest for the very patients in whom it would be most useful.

The new clinical trial data offer hope of some improvement in this regard, in that the control groups do provide serial cephalometric radiographs of untreated children with specific types of malocclusion. It may be possible to detect characteristics that predict certain favorable or unfavorable patterns of growth. At present, however, accurate growth predictions simply are not possible for the children who need it most.

Predicting Treatment Outcomes

Visualized Treatment Objectives

A visualized treatment objective (VTO) is a cephalometric tracing representing the changes that are expected (desired) during treatment. In the 1980s, manually-prepared VTOs were advocated as a treatment planning tool. For a child, the VTO would have to incorporate the expected growth, any growth changes induced by treatment, and any repositioning of the teeth from orthodontic tooth movement. In a child with normal facial proportions, average growth increments are reasonably likely and growth modification is not likely to be part of treatment, so growth changes can be predicted fairly well. The effects of tooth movement of various types are much more predictable than growth, although assumptions about the orthodontic therapy are required. For a skeletally normal child, preparing a VTO using average growth increments can be quite helpful in understanding the amount of tooth movement needed to correct the malocclusion. For a child with a skeletal problem, given the uncertainty of both the growth pattern and the response to treatment, a VTO often is more a presentation of what is hoped for than what is likely to happen.

When the variables associated with growth are not present, as in treatment for adults and late adolescents with

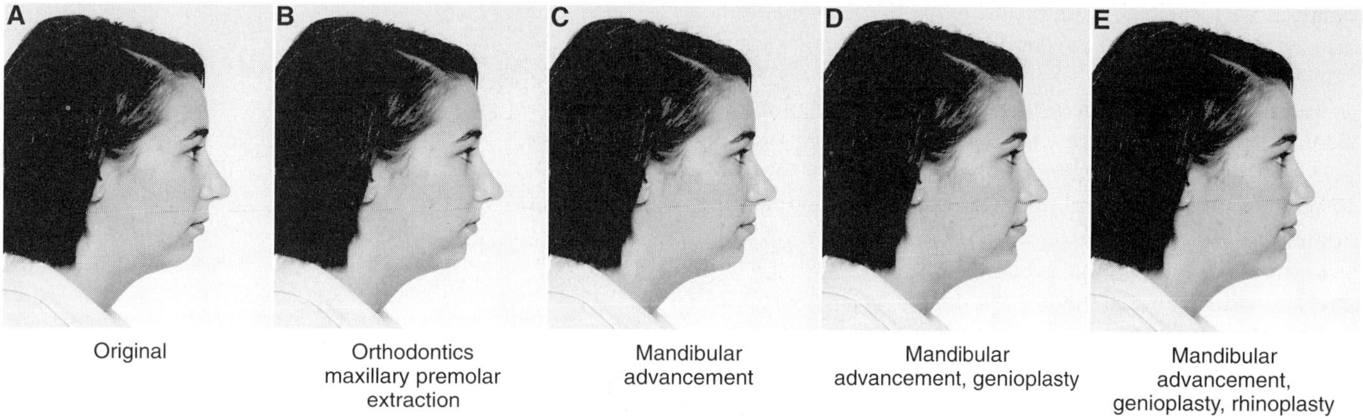

FIGURE 8-3 Presenting a computer-generated simulation of the post-treatment profile can greatly help patients understand the differences between alternative treatment approaches, in this case, the probable profile outcome of orthodontic camouflage of a skeletal Class II problem versus orthognathic surgery to correct the jaw relationship. Although showing patients these simulations heightens their esthetic awareness, it does not seem to create unrealistic expectations.[6]

little or no remaining growth, predicting treatment effects becomes easier and more reliable. Cephalometric prediction of possible outcomes of orthodontic camouflage and orthognathic surgery has been used routinely since the early 1980s. Although these are not usually called VTOs, there is no real difference except that growth is not considered.

With modern computer technology, it is possible to link cephalometric tracings and digital facial images, so that when the teeth or jaws are repositioned on the tracing, a corresponding change in the facial appearance is produced. At this point, manual cephalometric predictions or VTOs have been superseded by computer prediction programs.

Computer Image Predictions

Placing cephalometric information into computer memory is conveniently accomplished by digitizing points on the cephalometric tracing (see Chapter 6). Automatic recognition of cephalometric landmarks already can be accomplished by experimental computer programs and is likely to replace manual identification of landmarks in the future.

At present, all the commercially available cephalometric programs allow superimposition of the profile image (preferably, a direct digital image) onto the tracing, so that the doctor and patient can more readily visualize treatment effects (Figure 8-3). All the programs perform well for the less complex cases, but there are differences in the prediction quality with more difficult patients, which relate to the method by which the profile and x-ray are linked and to the prediction algorithms incorporated in the program.[11] Although presenting computer simulations to patients heightens their esthetic goals for treatment, it does not seem to create unrealistic expectations, and this helps patients make an informed decision between alternative treatment possibilities.[12] The computing algorithms for predictions of surgical or orthodontic changes in the absence of growth have improved remarkably in the last few years, and probably will continue to do so.

Does this mean that computerization will solve the problems of growth prediction? No, because the data on which the growth-prediction algorithms would have to be based simply do not exist. Computer images for growing children are just as inaccurate as VTO tracings, and potentially more misleading to parents. There is no reason to believe that the same kind of prediction that can be done with adults will be possible for children any time soon.

Treatment Response as an Aid in Treatment Planning

A practical problem in treatment planning for children, then, is how to reduce the uncertainty related to growth. What do you do, for instance, with a rather mature 12-year-old boy with a moderately severe skeletal Class II problem? Should you use the estimates underlying a VTO or computer prediction to make the decision, ignoring the possibility of serious error? Proceed with growth modification, regardless of a questionable prognosis? Go ahead with extractions for camouflage, on the theory that this would assure success whatever the patient's growth? Each of these approaches has been advocated by respected orthodontic clinicians, and would be the best approach to some patients—and a serious error for others.

One way to reduce the amount of uncertainty in planning treatment for children is to use the initial treatment response as an aid in treatment planning, deferring the adoption of a definitive treatment plan until some experience has been achieved with the patient. This approach, sometimes called "therapeutic diagnosis," allows a better evaluation of both growth response and cooperation with treatment than can be obtained by prediction alone. It is especially applicable to children with skeletal Class II and Class III problems, but also can be quite useful in Class I patients who are borderline extraction cases.

In practice, therapeutic diagnosis involves implementing a conservative (i.e., nonextraction or nonsurgical) treatment plan initially and reevaluating the patient after a few months to observe the response to this treatment. For example, an adolescent with a skeletal Class II malocclusion might be placed on a functional appliance or extraoral force to the maxilla, with minimal use of fixed appliances for tooth movement initially, to see if favorable growth reduces the jaw discrepancy. If a good response is observed after 6 to 9 months, this treatment approach is continued, with the odds of long-term success greatly improved. On the other hand, if a poor response is observed, whether because of poor cooperation or poor growth, the growth modification therapy might be dropped in favor of surgery to advance the mandible or extractions and a fixed appliance, camouflage-oriented approach. The disadvantage of the evaluation period in the latter instance is that treatment may take longer than it would have if the surgery or extraction decision had been made initially. The advantage is a decrease in the number of incorrect decisions. Whatever the treatment plan, it is important at all stages of all types of treatment to carefully monitor the patient's response and make appropriate adjustments in the original plan to deal with variations in response.

In the sections of this chapter immediately below, the goal is to review what is known about controversial areas, put it into perspective based on the quality of available data, and draw the best conclusions about treatment possibilities that are possible today. Better data in the not-too-distant future should allow a more confident emphasis on specific treatment approaches.

TO EXTRACT OR NOT TO EXTRACT: A LONG-RUNNING CONTROVERSY

"To extract or not to extract" may not have quite the significance of "To be or not to be," but for over 100 years it has been a key question in planning orthodontic treatment. In orthodontics, there are two major reasons to extract teeth: (1) to provide space to align the remaining teeth in the presence of severe crowding, and (2) to allow teeth to be moved (usually, incisors to be retracted) so protrusion can be reduced or so skeletal Class II or Class III problems can be camouflaged. The alternative to extraction in treating dental crowding is to expand the arches; the alternative for skeletal problems is to correct the jaw relationship, by modifying growth or surgery. All other things being equal, it is better not to extract—but in some cases extraction provides the best treatment. Opinions as to the indications for extraction have changed remarkably over the years, from one extreme to the other and back (Figure 8-4), and this particular pendulum appears to still be swinging.

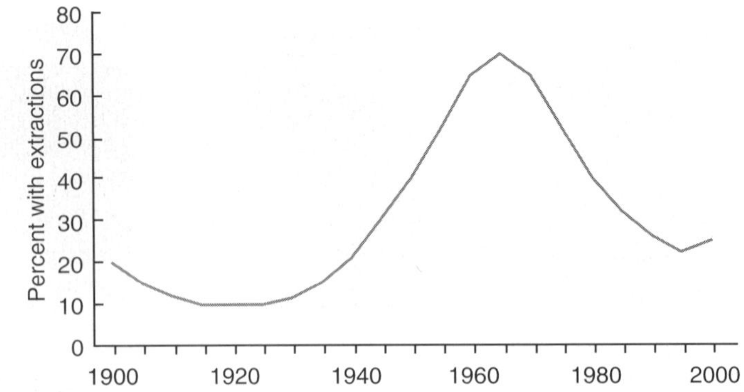

FIGURE 8-4 In general, extraction of teeth for orthodontic purposes was rare in the early 20th century, peaked in the 1960s with extraction occurring in a majority of orthodontic patients, declined to about the levels of the early 1950s by the 1990s, and has remained there for the first few years of the 21st century. Will it increase in the near future? Perhaps, but almost surely not to the previous maximum.

Changing Views of Indications for Extraction

Edward Angle and the Non-Extraction Philosophy

As the occlusal concepts that culminated in his definition of normal occlusion were developed, Edward Angle struggled with both facial esthetics and stability of result as potential complications in his efforts to achieve an idealized normal occlusion.[13] It is difficult to recreate the thought processes of a brilliant man many years ago, but it seems clear that Angle was influenced by both the philosophy of Rousseau and the biologic concepts of his time. Rousseau emphasized the perfectibility of man. His strong belief that many of the ills of modern man could be traced to the pernicious influences of civilization struck a responsive chord in Angle, who joined other progressive young dentists of the 1890s in their reaction to the casual attitude of that time toward extraction of teeth. In an era when teeth could be saved by dental treatment, extraction of teeth for orthodontic purposes seemed particularly inappropriate, especially if the patient was inherently capable of having a perfect dentition. Perfection, it appeared, required only diligent efforts to achieve it. It became an article of faith for Angle and the early orthodontists that every person had the potential for an ideal relationship of all 32 natural teeth, and therefore that extraction for orthodontic purposes was never needed.

Secondly, Angle was impressed by the discovery that the architecture of bone responds to the stresses placed on that part of the skeleton. In the early 1900s, the German physiologist Wolff demonstrated that bone trabeculae were arranged in response to the stress lines on the bone. The internal architecture of the head of the femur is the classic example, but the condylar process of the mandible shows the same effect of "Wolff's law of bone" (Figure 8-5). This led Angle to two key concepts. The first was that skeletal growth could be influenced readily by external pressures. If bone

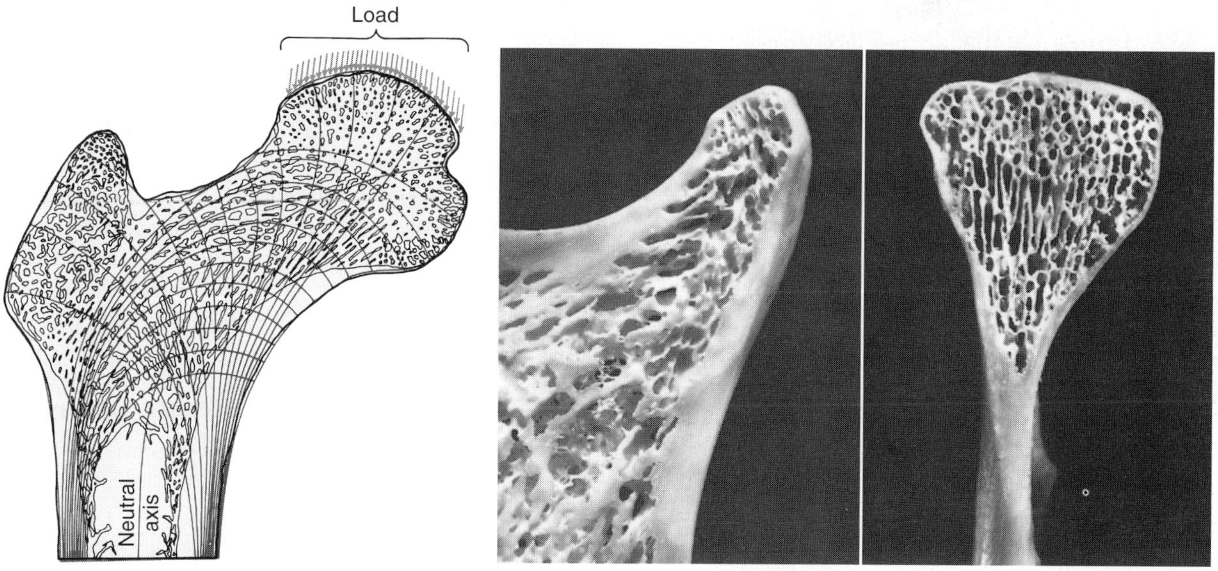

A B,C

Figure 8-5 **A,** Bone trabeculae in the head of the femur follow the calculated stress lines. This observation by the German physiologist Wolff at the end of the 19th century led to "Wolff's law of bone" that the internal architecture of bones represents the stress pattern on them. **B,** Frontal section through the head of the mandibular condyle. **C,** Sagittal section through the head of the condyle. Note the arrangement of bony trabeculae, indicating a similar arrangement for resistance to stress as seen in the head of the femur. (**B** and **C,** From DuBrul EL. Sicher's Oral Anatomy, ed 7. St Louis: Mosby; 1980.)

remodeled when stressed, the etiology of Class II or Class III problems must be abnormal stresses on the jaws, but different patterns of pressure associated with treatment could change growth so as to overcome the problem. Angle came to believe that skeletal structures were so adaptable that just rubber bands connecting the upper to the lower teeth could overcome improper jaw relationships, stimulating growth where it was needed.

The second concept was that proper function of the dentition would be the key to maintaining teeth in their correct position. Angle reasoned that if the teeth were placed in proper occlusion, forces transmitted to the teeth would cause bone to grow around them, thus stabilizing them in their new position even if a great deal of arch expansion had occurred. He soon saw that merely tipping the teeth to a new position might be inadequate and sought ways to move the teeth bodily. He described his edgewise appliance, the first appliance capable of fully controlling root position (see Chapter 11), as the "bone growing appliance."

To Angle and his followers, relapse after expansion of the arches or rubber bands to correct overjet and overbite meant only that an adequate occlusion had not been achieved. This too became an article of faith: If a correct occlusion had been produced, the result would be stable; therefore if the orthodontic result was not stable, the fault was that of the orthodontist, not the theory.

Finally, the problem of dentofacial esthetics was solved, at least for Angle, through his interaction with a famous artist of the day, Professor Wuerpel. Early in his career, Angle devoted much effort to a search for the ideal facial form, in parallel with his search for the ideal dental occlusion (Figure 8-6). When he consulted the art professor for advice about the perfect face, he was ridiculed—the artist's response was that the tremendous variety in human faces makes it impossible to specify any one facial form as the ideal. Reflecting on this, Angle had a moment of insight: The relationship of the dentition to the face, and with it the esthetics of the lower face, would vary, but for each individual, ideal facial esthetics would result when the teeth were placed in ideal occlusion. Whether the patient liked the outcome or not, by definition the best facial appearance for him or her would be achieved when the dental arches had been expanded so that all the teeth were in ideal occlusion.

Therefore, for Angle, proper orthodontic treatment for every patient involved expansion of the dental arches and rubber bands as needed to bring the teeth into occlusion, and extraction was not necessary for stability of result or esthetics. These concepts did not go unchallenged. Angle's great professional rival, Calvin Case, argued that although the arches could always be expanded so that the teeth could be placed in alignment, neither esthetics nor stability would be satisfactory in the long term for many patients. The controversy culminated in a widely publicized debate between Angle's student Dewey and Case, carried out in the dental literature of the 1920s.[14]

Reading these papers from a current perspective leaves the impression that Case had the better argument by far. Yet Angle's followers won the day, and extraction of teeth for

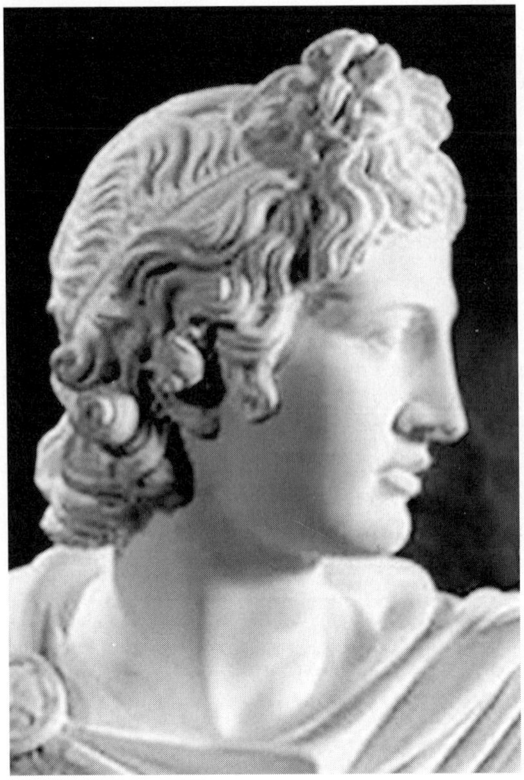

FIGURE 8-6 Angle sought an ideal profile, in parallel to his search for an ideal occlusion, and initially favored this classic Greek profile, which is often incompatible with non-extraction treatment.

orthodontic purposes essentially disappeared from the American orthodontic scene in the period between World Wars I and II. Even those who did not agree with Angle's appliance systems, particularly in the American South where removable (Crozat) or partially banded appliances (labiolingual, twin wire) were commonly used, accepted the non-extraction approach and its philosophic underpinnings.

The Re-introduction of Extraction in the Mid-20th Century

By the 1930s, relapse after non-extraction treatment was frequently observed. At this time soon after Angle's death, one of his last students, Charles Tweed, decided to re-treat with extraction a number of his patients who had experienced relapse. Four first premolar teeth were removed and the anterior teeth were aligned and retracted. After the re-treatment, Tweed observed that the occlusion was much more stable. Tweed's dramatic public presentation of consecutively treated cases with premolar extraction caused a revolution in American orthodontic thinking and led to the widespread reintroduction of extraction into orthodontic therapy by the late 1940s. Independently of Tweed but simultaneously, another of Angle's students, Raymond Begg in Australia, also concluded that non-extraction treatment was unstable. Like Tweed, he modified the Angle-designed appliance he was using (in his case, the ribbon arch) adapting it for extraction treatment and producing what is now called the Begg appliance (see Chapter 11).

The acceptance of extraction and the repudiation of Angle's ideas were made easier by an intellectual climate in which the limitations of human adaptation, both socially and physically, were emphasized. Breeding experiments with animals, of which Stockard's widely publicized results from crossbreeding dogs were most influential, seemed to show conclusively that malocclusion could be inherited (see Chapter 5). Rather than developing the (nonexistent) potential within each patient, it appeared that it was necessary for the orthodontist to recognize genetically determined disparities between tooth size and jaw size, or to acknowledge that the lack of proximal wear on teeth produced tooth size–jaw size discrepancies during development. In either case, extraction frequently was necessary.

By the early 1960s, more than half the American patients undergoing orthodontic treatment had extraction of some teeth, usually but not always first premolars. Since the accepted concept was that orthodontic treatment could not affect facial growth, extraction was considered necessary to accommodate the teeth to discrepancies in jaw position as well as to overcome crowding caused by tooth-jaw discrepancies, and was done for either or both purposes.

Recent Trends Toward Non-extraction

Extraction rates always have varied among doctors and regions, so no specific example of changes in extraction patterns can be taken totally as typical. Experience in the orthodontic clinic at the University of North Carolina (Figure 8-7), however, shows well the type of change over time that has occurred widely. At its inception in the 1950s, treatment in the clinic was strongly influenced by attitudes like Angle's. By the 1960s the Tweed/Begg view had been accepted, and extraction rates increased dramatically. From then until the early 1990s there was a continuing decline in extraction rates, which has stabilized or increased slightly recently.

The UNC patients can be grouped into three extraction categories: four first premolars, the usual extraction pattern for treatment of Class I crowding/protrusion (sometimes used also for Class II camouflage); upper first premolars only or upper first-lower second premolars, a pattern that indicates Class II camouflage; and all other extraction patterns (asymmetric extractions, impossibly impacted teeth, one lower incisor, etc.). As Figure 8-7 illustrates, the change over the years occurred mostly in the four first premolar group, with smaller changes in the camouflage extraction rate. For the "other" group, the rate has been remarkably constant over the period of 50 years. Decisions in this clinic always have been made by individual attending faculty. It is clear, therefore, that this group of orthodontists (a mix of full- and part-time faculty) showed remarkable changes in their decisions about extraction in the treatment of dental crowding, with much less change in extraction for other reasons. Why?

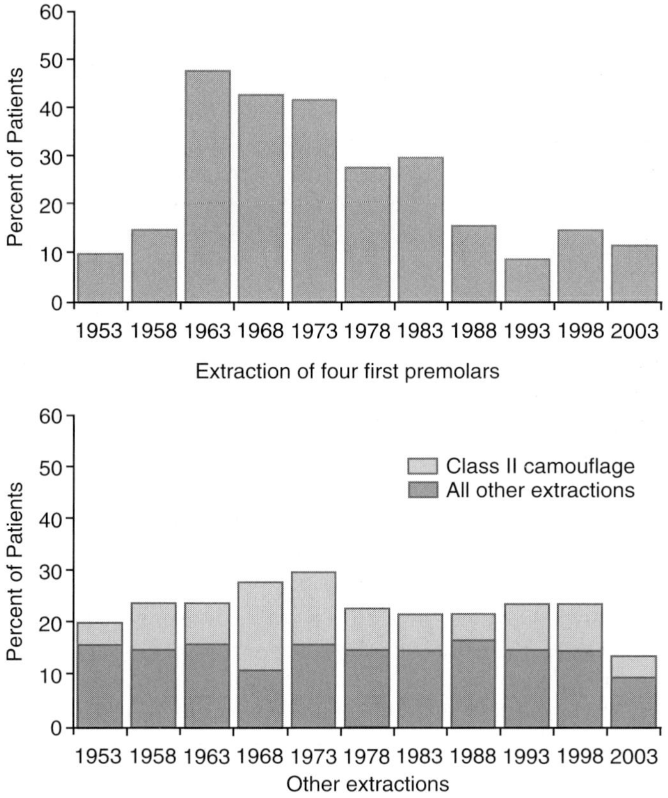

Figure 8-7 Extraction percentages in the Department of Orthodontics at the University of North Carolina over a 50-year period, 1953-2003. Extraction of first premolars usually is done for treatment of crowding/protrusion; extraction of upper first or upper first/lower second premolars indicates Class II camouflage; other extractions are done for a variety of purposes related to impaction, asymmetry, and tooth-size discrepancy. Note that the number of patients with extraction of four first premolars increased sharply in the 1960s, declined to the 1953 level in 1993, and has remained at approximately that level since then. The number of patients with extraction for Class II camouflage also increased in the 1960s and decreased thereafter, but did not change nearly as much. The number of patients with other all other extractions has been remarkably constant for 50 years.

The reasons for the increase in extraction have been discussed above, but it is important to put this in perspective: Premolar extraction was, more than anything else, a search for stability. In the earlier nonextraction era, collapse of expanded arches and relapse into crowding were frequently observed (but, it must be said, not well documented scientifically), and it became clear that perfection of the occlusion did not necessarily lead to stability. Extraction as a strategy was adopted, however, without evidence beyond selected cases that it produced stable results.

Why the decline in extraction rates more recently? There are several reasons. Experience has shown that premolar extraction does not necessarily guarantee stability of tooth alignment,[15,16] and one could argue that if the results are not very stable either way, there is no reason to sacrifice teeth. It also can be argued that even if extraction cases often are unstable, non-extraction would be worse. Nothing remotely like a randomized clinical trial of extraction vs nonextraction treatment of Class I crowding has ever been done, and there simply are no good data that really allow comparison of the outcomes of extraction and non-extraction treatment in similar groups of patients.

In addition, dentists have realized that standards for facial attractiveness are largely culturally determined, and change over time. At this point, the general public often prefer fuller and more prominent lips than the orthodontic standards of the 1950s and 1960s. The facial appearance in "borderline cases" generally is considered better without extraction by both dentists and others. The change from fully banded to largely bonded appliances made it easier to expand the arches by eliminating the need for band space. In the 1980s, claims were made that temporomandibular dysfunction (TMD) problems could be attributed to extraction of upper first premolars, and although this association has been refuted, for a time it also affected extraction rates, at least by some doctors.

The result, however, is two-fold: It is possible, perhaps even likely, that non-extraction treatment and expansion of the dental arches once again are being carried to an extreme. If so, stability problems once more are likely to become prominent. Controversy over the role of extraction continues because there are no good data to settle the issue. At present every shade of opinion and practice relative to extraction can be found. These range from an absolute rejection of the possibility of a need for extraction, supported by arguments that seem taken word-for-word from Angle's era, to a rejection of the possibilities of arch expansion and growth guidance along with a continued high percentage of extraction. The amount of change in treatment of dental crowding, the most frequent orthodontic problem—in the almost total absence of data—illustrates how far orthodontics still has to go in becoming an evidence-driven specialty. In this, as with so much else, it is necessary to understand the pertinent history to avoid repeating it.

A Contemporary Perspective: Expansion versus Extraction

In a rational contemporary view, the majority of patients, but by no means all, can be treated without removal of teeth. In addition to those who fall into the rather constant "other" category described above, some will require extraction to compensate for crowding, incisor protrusion that affects facial esthetics, or jaw discrepancy. Their number varies, depending on the population being treated. Extraction for camouflage is considered separately later in the chapter. The section immediately below is a discussion of the limits of expansion, and therefore the indications for extraction, for patients with normal jaw relationships.

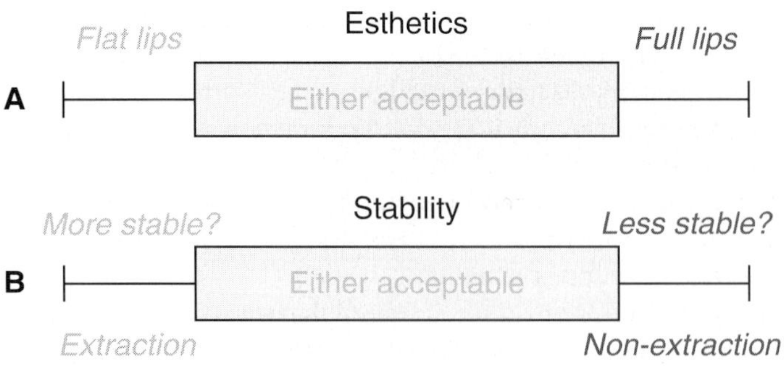

FIGURE 8-8 Expansion of the dental arches tends to make the teeth more prominent and extraction makes them less prominent. The choice between extraction and non-extraction (expansion) treatment is a critical esthetic decision for some patients who are toward the extremes of incisor protrusion or retrusion initially, but because there is an acceptable range of protrusion, many if not most can be treated with satisfactory esthetics either way. This is especially true if expansion is managed so as not to produce too much protrusion, or space closure after extraction is controlled so as not to produce too much incisor retraction. Similarly, expansion tends to make arches less stable and extraction favors stability, but the extraction–non-extraction decision probably is a critical factor in stability largely for patients who are toward the extremes of the protrusion-retrusion distribution. There are no data to show the number of patients who could be treated satisfactorily with either approach, versus the number for whom the extraction–non-extraction decision is critical in determining a satisfactory outcome.

Esthetic Considerations

If the major factors in extraction decisions are stability and esthetics, it is worthwhile to review existing data that relate these factors to expansion and extraction. Consider esthetics first. The conceptual relationship between expansion/extraction and esthetics is illustrated in Figure 8-8. All other things being equal, expansion of the arches moves the patient in the direction of more prominent teeth, while extraction tends to reduce the prominence of the teeth. Facial esthetics can become unacceptable on either the too-protrusive or too-retrusive side.

At what point have the incisors been moved too far forward, so that facial appearance is compromised? The answer is found in soft tissue, not hard tissue relationships: When the prominence of the incisors creates excessive lip separation at rest, so that the patient must strain to bring the lips together, the teeth are too protrusive, and retracting the incisors improves the facial appearance (Figure 8-9). Note that this has nothing to do with the prominence of the teeth relative to the supporting bone. An individual with thick, full lips looks good with incisor prominence that would not be acceptable in someone with thin, tight lips. Cephalometric measurements of incisor position that attempt to establish the esthetic limits of protrusion go all the way back to Tweed, but there is no way to determine the esthetic limit of expansion from tooth–bone relationships alone.

The size of the nose and chin has a profound effect on relative lip prominence. For a patient with a large nose and/or a large chin, if the choices are to treat without extraction and move the incisors forward, or extract and retract the incisors at least somewhat, moving the incisors forward is better, provided it does not diminish the labiomental sulcus too much. Lack of a well-defined labiomental sulcus, which usually is related to lip strain in gaining lip seal, can be due either to increased lower face height or protrusion of the teeth, and this also can be taken as evidence that the incisors are too prominent.

At what point are the incisors retracted to the point of adversely affecting facial esthetics? That too depends largely on the soft tissues. A concave profile with thinning of the lips, so that there is little vermilion border, is an unesthetic trait. In a patient with thin lips, proclining the incisors tends to create fuller lips with more vermilion display, and this is likely to be perceived as more attractive. Since the face tends to flatten with age and the lips become less full with aging, retracting teeth in a patient with thin lips can prematurely age the face. The upper incisors are too far lingually if the upper lip inclines backward—it should be slightly forward from its base at soft tissue point A (Figure 8-10, *A*). For best esthetics, the lower lip should be at least as prominent as the chin. Another cause of a poorly-defined labiomental sulcus is retroclined mandibular incisors (Figure 8-10, *B*). Variations in chin morphology may put the proper incisor–chin relationship beyond the control of orthodontics alone, in which case chin surgery perhaps should be considered (see the sections in this chapter on Class II camouflage and maximizing esthetic changes in treatment, and Chapter 19).

Stability Considerations

For stable results, how much can arches be expanded? The lower arch is more constrained than the upper, and so its limitations for stable expansion may be somewhat tighter than the upper arch. Current guidelines for the limits of expansion of the lower arch, admittedly based on limited data, are presented in Figure 8-11. The 2 mm limitation for forward movement of the incisors obviously is subject to considerable individual variation, but makes sense in light of the observation that lip pressure increases sharply 2 mm out into space usually occupied by the lip (see Chapter 5). If lip pressure is the limiting factor in forward movement, as it probably is, the initial position of the incisors relative to the lip would be a consideration in how much movement could be tolerated. This suggests, and clinical observation seems to confirm (again, limited data!) that incisors that are tipped lingually away from the lip can be moved farther forward than upright incisors. Incisors that are tipped labially and crowded probably represent the equivalent of a titrated end point in a chemical reaction, in that they have already

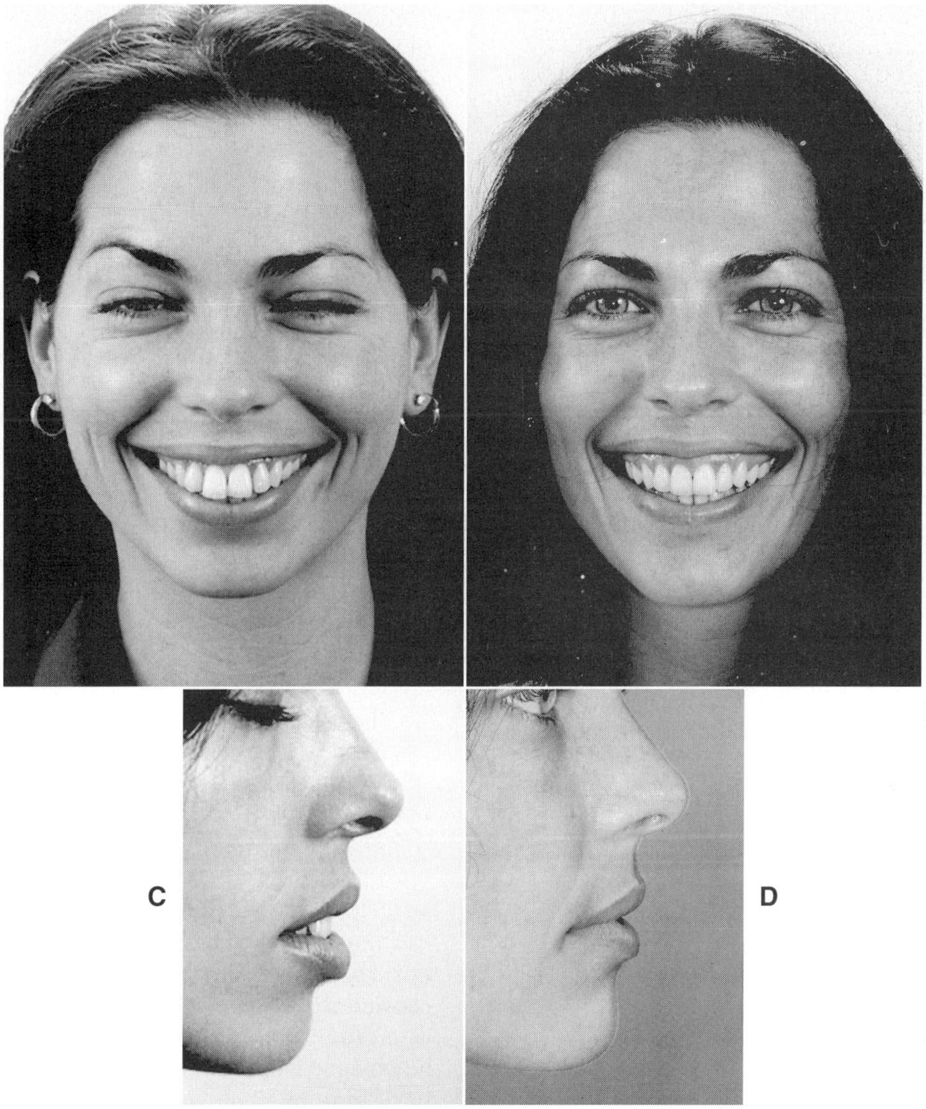

A B C D

Figure 8-9 In patients with excessive incisor protrusion, retracting the incisors improves facial esthetics. This young woman sought treatment because of dissatisfaction with the appearance of her teeth. After orthodontic treatment with premolar extraction and incisor retraction, dental and facial appearance were significantly improved. **A, B,** Appearance on smile before and after treatment; **C, D,** Profile before and after treatment.

become as protrusive as the musculature will allow. Moving them any further forward carries great risk of instability.

There also is a soft tissue limitation in how far the incisors, especially the lower incisors, can be moved facially: Fenestration of the alveolar bone and stripping of the gingiva become increasingly likely as the incisors are advanced. The amount of attached gingiva is a critical variable. It is important to carefully monitor patients who have a marginal amount of attached gingiva, so that they can be treated promptly if a problem arises (Figure 8-12). Pretreatment consultation with a periodontist often is advisable, and placing a gingival graft before orthodontic treatment begins is the best plan for some patients.

Figure 8-11 suggests that there is more opportunity to expand transversely than anteroposteriorly—but only posterior to the canines. Numerous reports show that transverse expansion across the canines is almost never maintained, especially in the lower arch. In fact, intercanine dimensions typically decrease as patients mature, whether or not they had orthodontic treatment, probably because of lip pressures at the corners of the mouth. Expansion across the premolars and molars is much more likely to be maintained, presumably because of the relatively low cheek pressures.

One approach to arch expansion is to expand the upper arch by opening the midpalatal suture. If the maxillary base is narrow, that is appropriate treatment (see the discussion

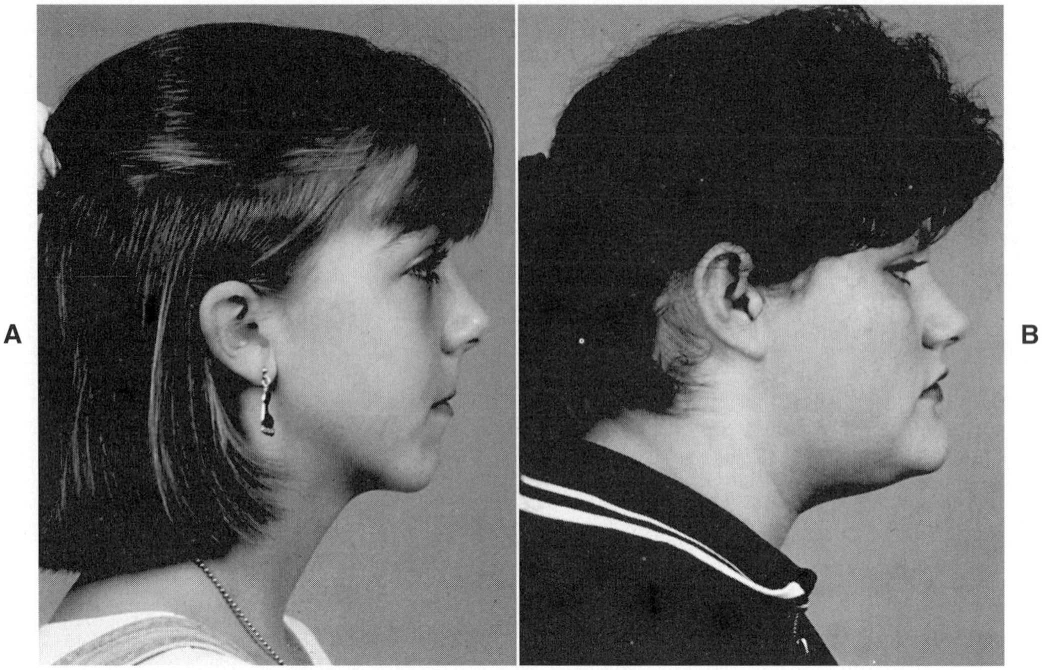

FIGURE 8-10 **A,** An upper lip that inclines backward relative to the true vertical line, which can result from retraction of upper incisors to correct excessive overjet, tends to compromise facial esthetics, as does a poorly-defined labiomental sulcus when lip strain is required to bring the lips together. **B,** Retroclined mandibular incisors, as in this patient with a prominent chin and dental compensation for a skeletal Class III jaw relationship, are another cause of a poorly-defined labiomental sulcus.

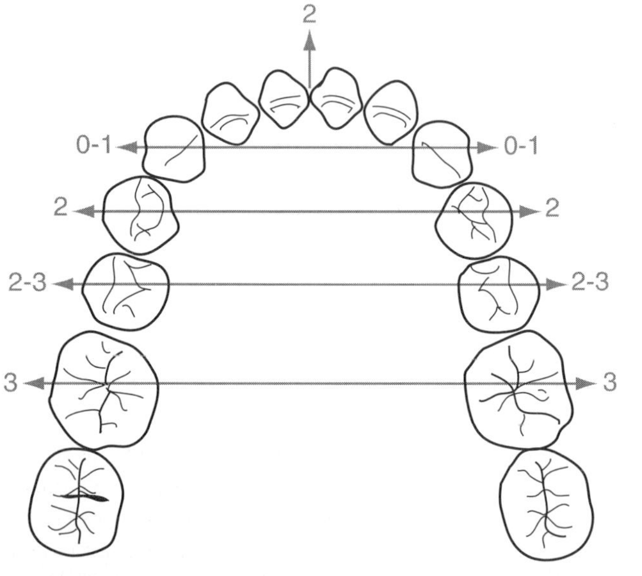

FIGURE 8-11 Because the lower arch is more constrained, the limits of expansion for stability seem to be tighter for it than the maxillary arch. The available data suggest that moving lower incisors forward more than 2 mm is problematic for stability, probably because lip pressure seems to increase sharply at about that point. A considerable body of data shows that expansion across the canines is not stable, even if the canines are retracted when they are expanded. Expansion across the premolars and molars, in contrast, can be stable.

of transverse maxillary deficiency, below). Some clinicians theorize (with no supporting evidence) that generously expanding the upper arch by opening the suture, temporarily creating a buccal crossbite, allows the lower arch then to be expanded more than otherwise would have been possible. If the limiting factor is cheek pressure, it seems unlikely that the method of expansion would make any difference. Excessive expansion carries the risk of fenestration of premolar and molar roots through the alveolar bone. There is an increasing risk of fenestration beyond 3 mm of transverse tooth movement.[17]

Summary of Contemporary Extraction Guidelines

Contemporary guidelines for orthodontic extraction in Class I crowding cases can be summarized as follows:

- Less than 4 mm arch length discrepancy: Extraction rarely indicated (only if there is severe incisor protrusion or in a few instances, a severe vertical discrepancy). In some cases this amount of crowding can be managed without arch expansion by slightly reducing the width of selected teeth, being careful to coordinate the amount of reduction in the upper and lower arch.
- Arch length discrepancy 5 to 9 mm: Non-extraction or extraction treatment possible. The extraction/non-extraction decision depends on both the hard- and soft-tissue characteristics of the patient and on how the

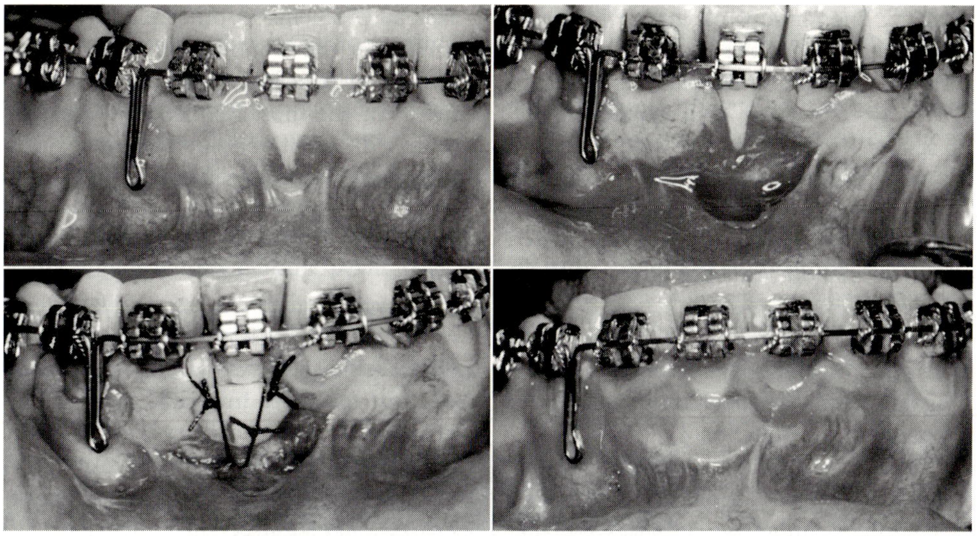

Figure 8-12 A, Gingival recession beginning to appear in a patient whose crowded lower incisors were aligned with some advancement despite premolar extraction to provide space; **B,** Preparation of a bed for a free gingival graft; **C,** The graft (tissue taken from the palate) sutured in position; **D,** 2 weeks later. (Courtesy Dr. John Moriarty, Department of Periodontics, University of North Carolina, Chapel Hill, NC.)

Table 8-2

Space From Various Extractions*

Extraction	Relief of Incisor Crowding	Incisor Retraction† Maximum	Incisor Retraction† Minimum	Posterior Forward† Maximum	Posterior Forward† Minimum
Central incisor	5	3	2	1	0
Lateral	5	3	2	1	0
Canine	6	5	3	2	0
First premolar	5	5	2	5	2
Second premolar	3	3	0	6	4
First molar	3	2	0	8	6
Second molar	2	1	0	—	—

Values in millimeters.
*With typical anchorage management (not skeletal anchorage).
†Anteroposterior plane of space in absence of crowding.

final position of the incisors will be controlled; any of several different teeth could be chosen for extraction. Non-extraction treatment usually requires transverse expansion across the molars and premolars.

- Arch length discrepancy 10 mm or more: extraction almost always required. The extraction choice is four first premolars or perhaps upper first premolars and mandibular lateral incisors; second premolar or molar extraction rarely is satisfactory because it does not provide enough space in severely crowded patients (Table 8-2).

The presence of protrusion in addition to crowding, of course, complicates the extraction decision. If the incisors need to be retracted to reduce lip prominence, space will be required for that. The effect is to increase the amount of arch length discrepancy. With that adjustment, the guidelines above can be applied. As a general rule, the lips will move two-thirds of the distance that the incisors are retracted, i.e., 3 mm of incisor retraction will reduce lip protrusion by 2 mm, but only until lip competence is reached. Beyond that point, further retraction of the incisors will not further reduce lip prominence.

It is interesting, but not surprising, that retrospective studies of changes in dental arch dimensions and facial appearance in extraction versus non-extraction cases show highly variable changes in both groups. The idea that extraction leads to incisor retraction and narrower arches, and that non-extraction leads to incisor protrusion and wider arches,

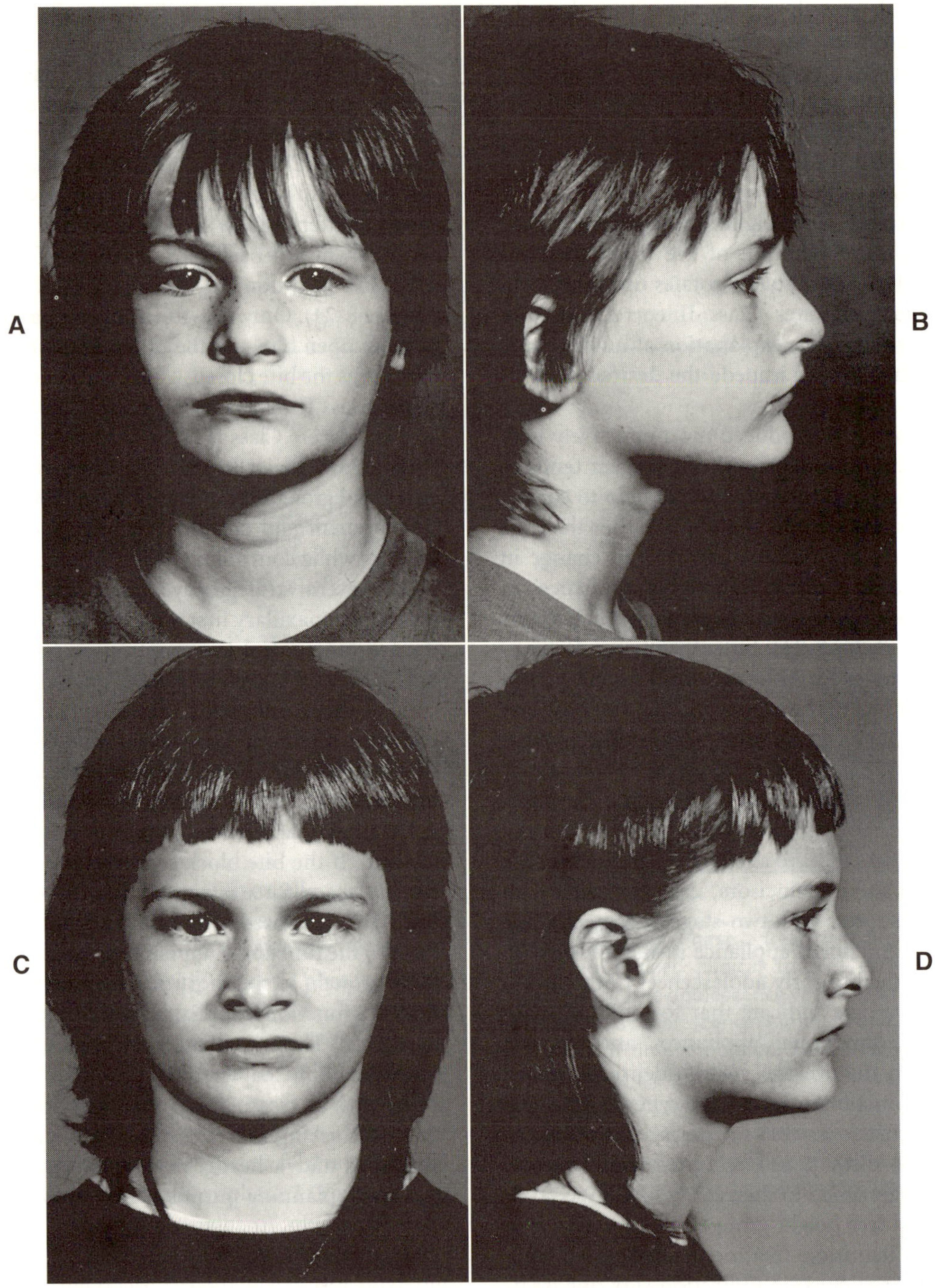

Figure 8-22 Facial changes produced by functional appliance treatment in a boy with a short face, skeletal deep bite malocclusion. **A, B,** Age 10 prior to treatment; **C, D,** Age 12 after 26 months of treatment. Note the increase in anterior face height and decrease in the labiomental fold.

prognosis is not as good as with less complex problems, even in a cooperative child.

In an older patient whose face height exceeds acceptable adult dimensions, it is not enough to prevent further eruption of posterior teeth; intrusion is needed. Neither bite blocks nor magnets have proven to be successful in accomplishing posterior intrusion, but using implants or bone screws as anchorage for an intrusive force now makes intrusion possible. The patients, many of whom had previous headgear treatment, report minimal pain from the implant placement and indicate that they much prefer implants to headgear.[35] Although the techniques for most effective use of bone anchors are still being worked out (see Chapter 12), already it is clear that skeletal open bites of mild to

A

B

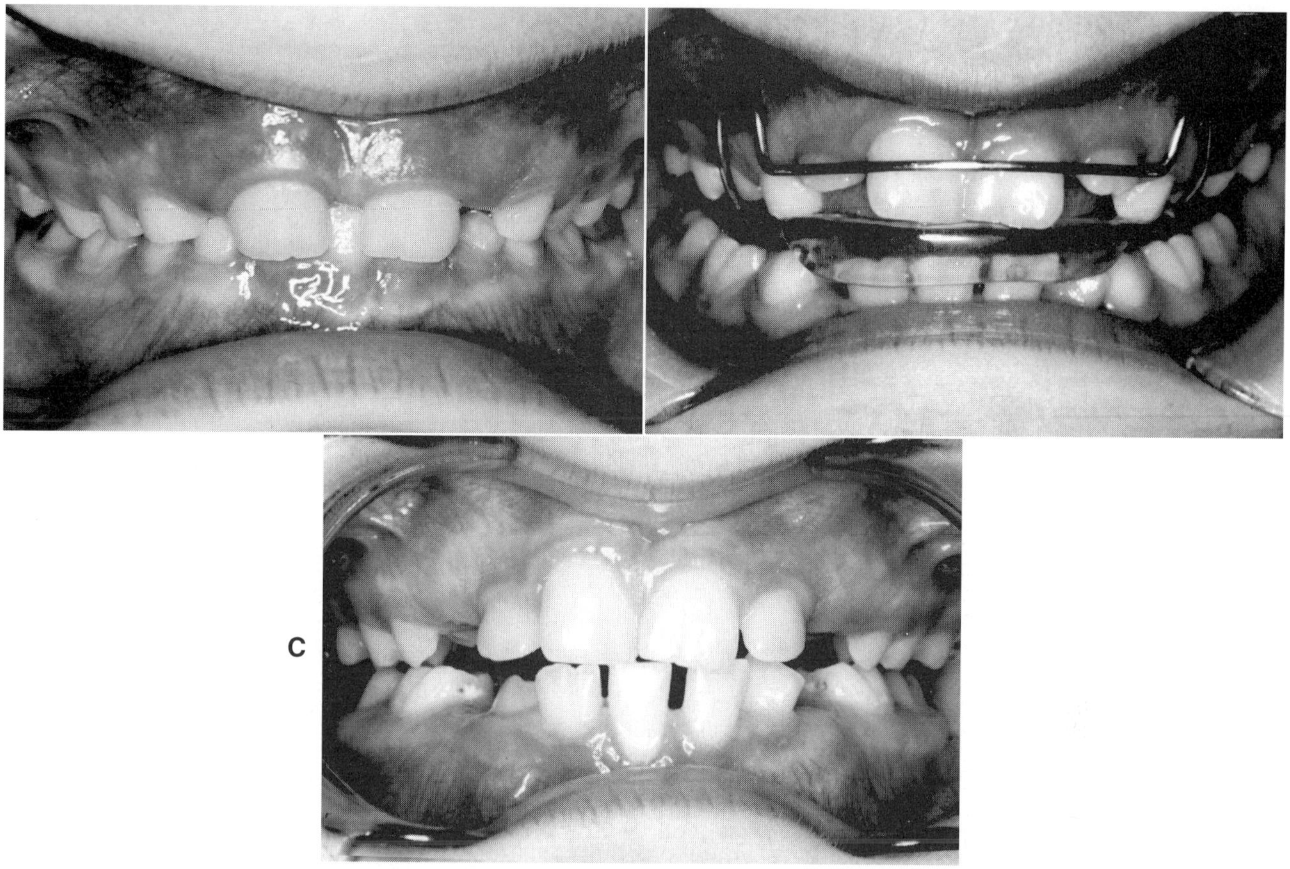

C

FIGURE 8-23 Dental changes with functional appliance treatment, same patient as figure 8-22. **A,** Prior to treatment. Note the gingival inflammation around the maxillary right central incisor resulting from palatal trauma from the deep bite. **B,** Deep bite bionator, constructed to allow eruption of lower posterior teeth and block eruption of incisors and upper posterior teeth. **C,** Dental relationships at the conclusion of phase 1 treatment, age 12. A second stage of treatment will be needed when the remaining succedaneous teeth erupt.

moderate severity can be corrected in this way. The more severely affected long face patients, however, will need orthognathic surgery.

The long face patient described as "Class III rotated to Class I" is a particularly difficult problem, and the one who is still Class III although the mandible is rotated down and back is even worse. Any treatment that decreases the excess face height tends to make the Class III condition worse by rotating the mandible upward and forward. Conversely, almost all therapy to control Class III growth tends to increase face height. It is not surprising that most of these patients eventually require orthognathic surgery.

Class II Treatment in Adolescents

The goal of treatment for Class II problems in adolescents (in addition to correcting any other problems that are present) is to establish the correct overjet and buccal segment occlusion. Exactly how this was expected to occur has been viewed differently at different times. Edward Angle was confident that if Class II elastics were used, differential growth of the mandible would produce most if not all the correction. When early cephalometric data showed that this rarely occurred and that most of the correction was produced by tooth movement, skeletal changes were discounted and it was expected that most of the correction would have to be produced by moving the teeth. More recently, the demonstration of growth modification by headgear and functional appliances led to renewed optimism about growth in adolescents contributing to the correction. The questions now are whether enough growth to make a difference can be expected in this age group and what mix of treatment responses can be expected.

There are no data from clinical trials of adolescent Class II treatment. The outcomes of treatment with different methods, however, have been evaluated by many investigators, so that a reasonable body of data exists for comparison of alternatives. Lysle Johnston has proposed a method of cephalometric analysis designed to specifically address the question of exactly what does happen in Class II treatment.[36] His "pitchfork analysis" (Figure 8-25) sums the skeletal and

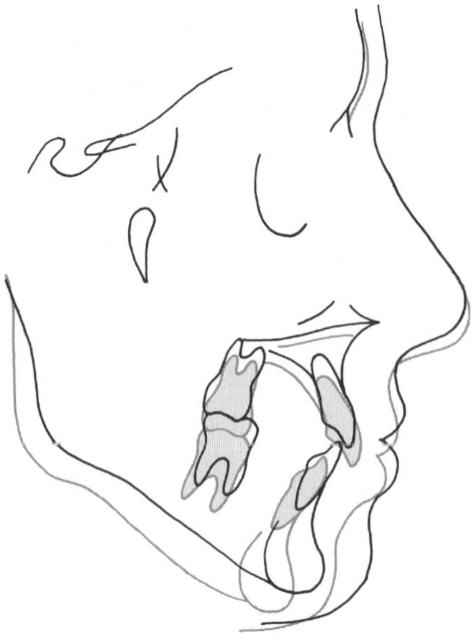

FIGURE 8-24 Cephalometric superimposition for a patient who experienced significant vertical maxillary growth after the completion of orthodontic treatment, without equivalent mandibular growth so that the mandible rotated downward and backward. *Black* = age 14; *red* = age 19. The effect was to produce Class II malocclusion by rotating the mandible down and back.

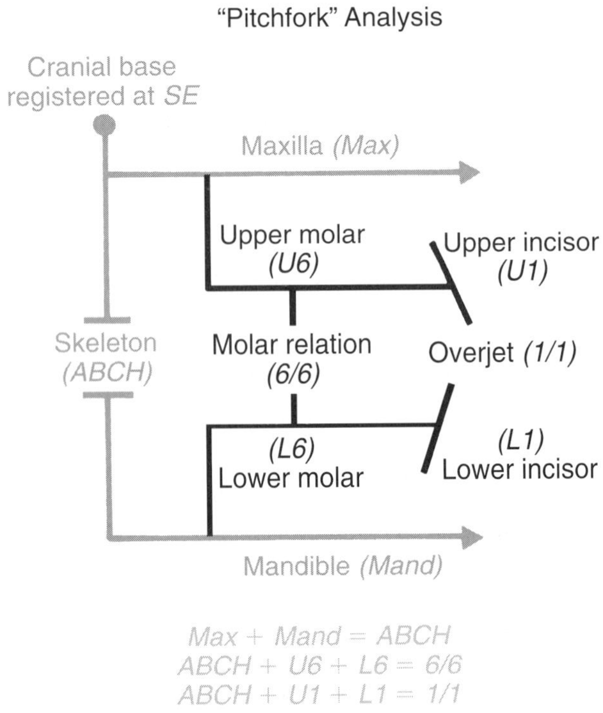

FIGURE 8-25 The "pitchfork analysis," which projects changes related to Class II correction to the occlusal plane, is a convenient way to show how dental and skeletal changes in both arches sum to produce the total change in occlusal relationships. As one might expect, a mix of dental and skeletal changes occur during treatment of almost any type, but apparently similar total changes can be produced in a variety of ways. (Redrawn from Johnston.[36])

dental components of Class II correction along the occlusal plane so that it is easy to see how the end result was obtained. To the extent possible, this thinking is used in the following discussion of the relative merits of various treatment plans for adolescent Class II problems.

There are four major approaches to Class II problems in adolescents:

- Growth modification with headgear or functional appliance
- Three variations of tooth movement:
  - Distal movement of maxillary molars, and eventually the entire upper dental arch
  - Retraction of maxillary incisors into a premolar extraction space
  - A combination of retraction of the upper teeth and forward movement of the lower teeth.

Growth Modification in Adolescents

The guiding principle is that growth can only be modified when it is occurring. Because dental and skeletal development are not tightly linked (see Chapter 2), treatment starting with the eruption of the permanent teeth could come almost anywhere from the beginning to the end of the adolescent growth spurt. Obviously, growth modification would be more successful during the adolescent growth spurt.

As a general guideline, even in the most favorable circumstances it is unlikely that more than half of the long-term changes needed to correct Class II malocclusion in an adolescent would be gained by differential jaw growth (i.e., a 3-4 mm contribution from growth to the total Class II correction would be as much as one could hope for). The more mature the patient, the less growth change should be expected. Both the phase 2 results from the UNC clinical trial and data from retrospective analyses show that favorable growth often occurs in adolescents and that early (preadolescent) treatment is not routinely superior in guiding growth. Because growth can be so unpredictable, often it is necessary to plan adolescent treatment so that the amount of tooth movement can be adjusted in compensation for whatever growth did occur.

An additional factor in the selection of a growth modification appliance comes into play with adolescents, its compatibility with a fixed appliance on the teeth. A complete fixed appliance cannot be used in the mixed dentition, so this does not affect the choice of headgear vs. a functional appliance for early treatment. In adolescents there is no reason to delay aligning the teeth, and a growth modification appliance that makes this difficult or impossible is a disadvantage. Headgear is compatible with fixed appliances but most removable functional appliances are not. If a functional appliance is desired for adolescent treatment, a fixed functional that allows brackets on the incisor teeth usually is the best choice.

To be successful, a functional appliance must displace the condyles (or stimulate the patient to displace them) a critical distance for a critical amount of time. The distance of condylar displacement rarely is considered, simply because almost any functional appliance repositions the condyles enough to be effective if it is worn enough. This becomes important, however, when we examine the growth modification effect of Class II elastics or flexible fixed units (like those described in Chapter 16). Both elastics and flexible fixed units have little growth effect and mostly move teeth, probably because they do not displace the condyles far enough, and should not be considered a substitute for headgear or a functional appliance.

Camouflage by Tooth Movement?

Nonextraction Treatment With Retraction of the Upper Teeth and Forward Movement of the Lower Teeth. If forward movement of the lower arch can be accepted, a Class II malocclusion can be corrected just with the use of Class II elastics (or their equivalent in the form of fixed connectors). The correction is achieved, however, much more by forward movement of the lower arch than by moving the upper teeth back. Rarely, excess overjet and Class II buccal segments are due to a distally positioned lower arch, and then moving it forward is exactly what is needed. Almost always, however, moving the lower incisors anteriorly more than 2 mm leads to instability and relapse. Lip pressure that moves the lower incisors lingually leads to incisor crowding, return of overjet, and return of overbite (because the incisors tend to erupt back into occlusal contact from their lingual position).

If non-extraction treatment of adolescent Class II problems is accomplished primarily with prolonged use of Class II elastics or the equivalent, the result is likely to be a convex profile with protrusive lower incisors and a prominent lower lip. This is best described as relapse waiting to occur. In addition, the elastics may produce an unesthetic elongation of the upper incisors. A lower border osteotomy to bring the chin forward can improve both the stability of the result and the facial appearance (see Chapter 19).

Retraction of the Upper Incisors Into a Premolar Extraction Space. A straightforward way to correct excessive overjet is to retract the protruding incisors into space created by extracting the maxillary first premolars. Without lower extractions, the patient would have a Class II molar relationship, but normal overjet, at the end of treatment. If mandibular first or second premolars also are extracted, Class II elastics can be used to bring the lower molars forward and retract the upper incisors, correcting both the molar relationship and the overjet.

Premolar extraction for Class II correction can produce excellent occlusion, but there are potential problems with this approach. If the patient's Class II malocclusion is primarily due to mandibular deficiency, retracting the maxillary incisors would create a maxillary deformity to go with the mandibular one—which is difficult to justify as correct treatment (see the discussion of Class II camouflage in adults in Chapter 18). Extractions in the lower arch allow the molars to come forward into a Class I relationship, but it would be important to close the lower space without retracting the lower incisors. If Class II elastics are used, the upper incisors are elongated as well as retracted, which can produce an undesirable "gummy smile."

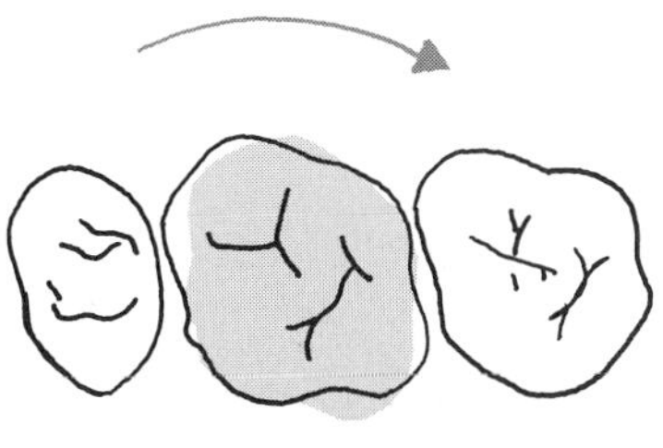

FIGURE 8-26 In a patient with Class II malocclusion, the upper first molar usually is rotated mesio-lingually. Correcting this rotation, which is necessary to obtain proper occlusion with the lower first molar, moves the buccal cusps distally. This improves the buccal occlusal relationship and creates at least a modest amount of space for retraction of other maxillary teeth.

Distal Movement of the Upper Teeth. If the upper molars could be moved posteriorly, this would correct a Class II molar relationship and provide space into which the other maxillary teeth could be retracted. If the maxillary first molars are rotated mesio-lingually, as they often are when a Class II molar relationship exists, correcting the rotation moves the buccal cusps posteriorly and provides at least a small space mesial to the molar (Figure 8-26). Tipping the crowns distally to gain space is more difficult, and bodily distal movement is more difficult still. There are two problems: (1) It is difficult to maintain the first molar in a distal position while the premolars and anterior teeth are moved back, so especially if it is tipped distally, it must be moved back a considerable distance; and (2) the further it must be moved, the more the second and third molars are in the way.

From this perspective it is easy to understand that the most successful way to move a maxillary first molar distally is to extract the second molar, which creates space for the tooth movement. Until quite recently, the anchorage created by a transpalatal lingual arch was accepted as the best way to undertake distalization of the maxillary dentition. Palatal anchorage for the molar movement can be created by splinting the maxillary premolars and including an acrylic pad in the splint so that it contacts the palatal mucosa. In theory, the palatal mucosa resists displacement; in clinical use, tissue irritation is likely. Even with the more elaborate appliances of this type (Figure 8-27), not more than half the total Class II correction can be expected from distal movement of the maxillary dentition. The molars can be tipped back farther than that initially, but they tend to come forward again when the other maxillary teeth are retracted. The ideal patient for treatment with this approach, therefore, is one with minimal growth potential, a reasonably good jaw relationship (not severely mandibular deficient) and a half-cusp Class II molar relationship.

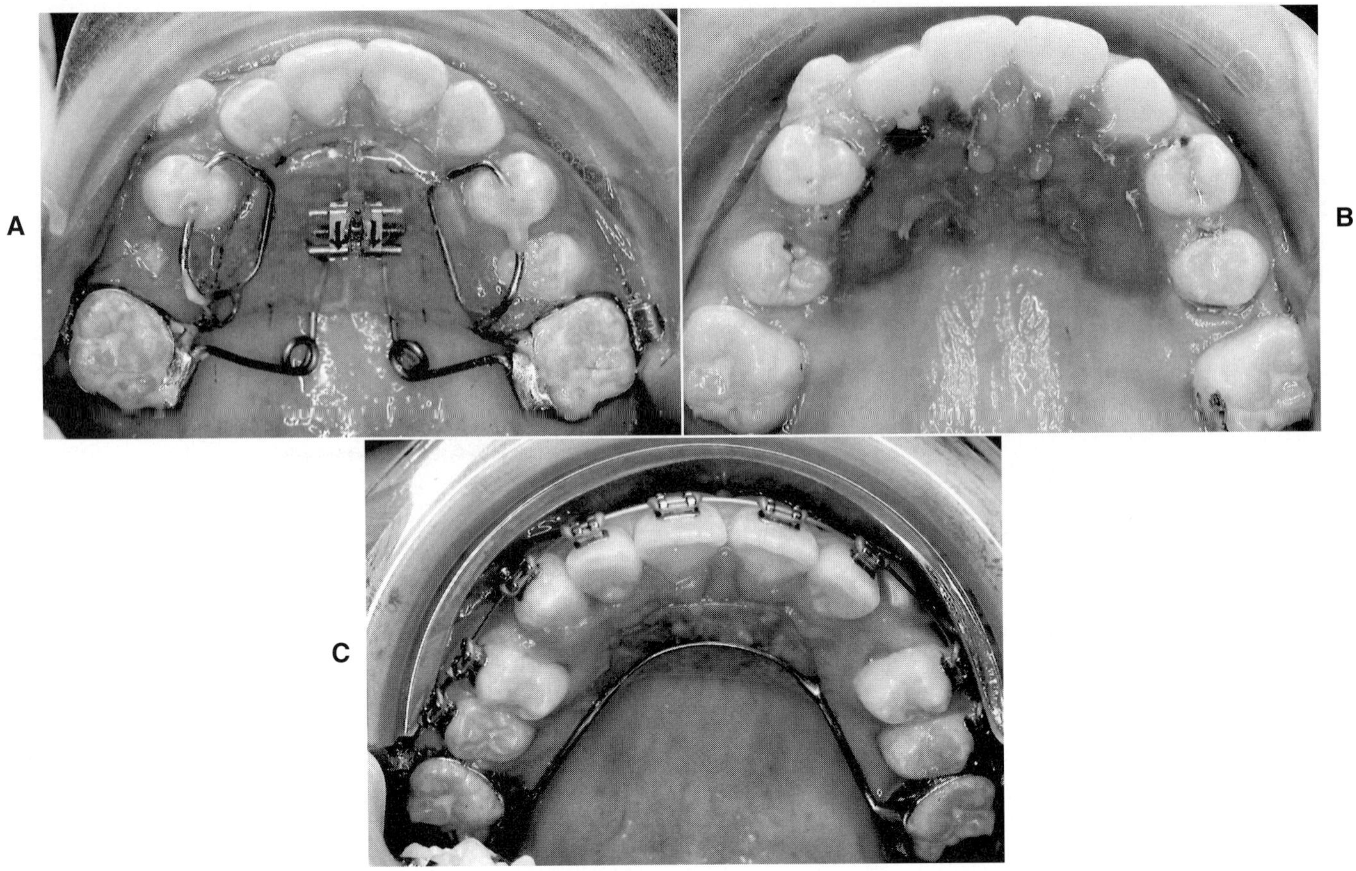

FIGURE 8-27 Molar distalization can be carried out with a variety of appliances that depend on the anterior teeth and the palate for anchorage. **A,** Combination distalization-expansion appliance (Pendex) at initial application; **B,** Appearance at appliance removal. Note the successful opening of space, but the tissue irritation caused by contact with the palatal mucosa; **C,** Nance holding arch with palatal button later in the same patient, to maintain the molar position while alignment of the other teeth is completed.

Using implants for anchorage greatly improves the amount of true distal movement of the maxillary dentition that can be achieved, and makes it possible to distalize both the second and first molars. It still is necessary to create some space in the tuberosity region, so removal of third molars will be required later if it is not done immediately. In typical treatment, a bone screw or better, a bone anchor is placed bilaterally in the vicinity of the base of the zygomatic arch (Edward Angle's "key ridge"). A nickel-titanium spring, either pulling from a screw or pushing from the anterior arm of a bone anchor (Figure 8-28), generates the force needed for distalization. Although good data for typical treatment outcomes still do not exist, in some patients it has been possible to produce up to 6 mm of distal movement.

The caveat, of course, is that moving the upper arch back that far may not be compatible with an acceptable facial appearance. If a Class II malocclusion is due to maxillary dental protrusion, moving the upper teeth back is a logical treatment approach. But if there is a significant component of mandibular deficiency, retraction of the maxillary incisors after distal movement of the molars and premolars has the same potential problem that can arise with first premolar extraction to allow retraction of the incisors: Correcting the malocclusion in that way may detract from rather than enhance facial appearance.

Summary. In the absence of favorable growth, the review above makes it apparent that treating a Class II relationship in adolescents is difficult. Compromises may have to be accepted in order to correct the occlusion. Fortunately, even though growth modification cannot be expected to totally correct an adolescent Class II problem, some forward movement of the mandible relative to the maxilla does contribute to successful treatment of the average patient. The rest of the correction must occur from some combination of retraction of the upper incisors and forward movement of the lower arch.

The easiest way to retract upper incisors is to extract the maxillary first premolars to create space for the tooth movement. Extraction of premolars in adolescent Class II treatment has been criticized in recent years on two grounds: that it leads to TM joint problems because the incisors are likely

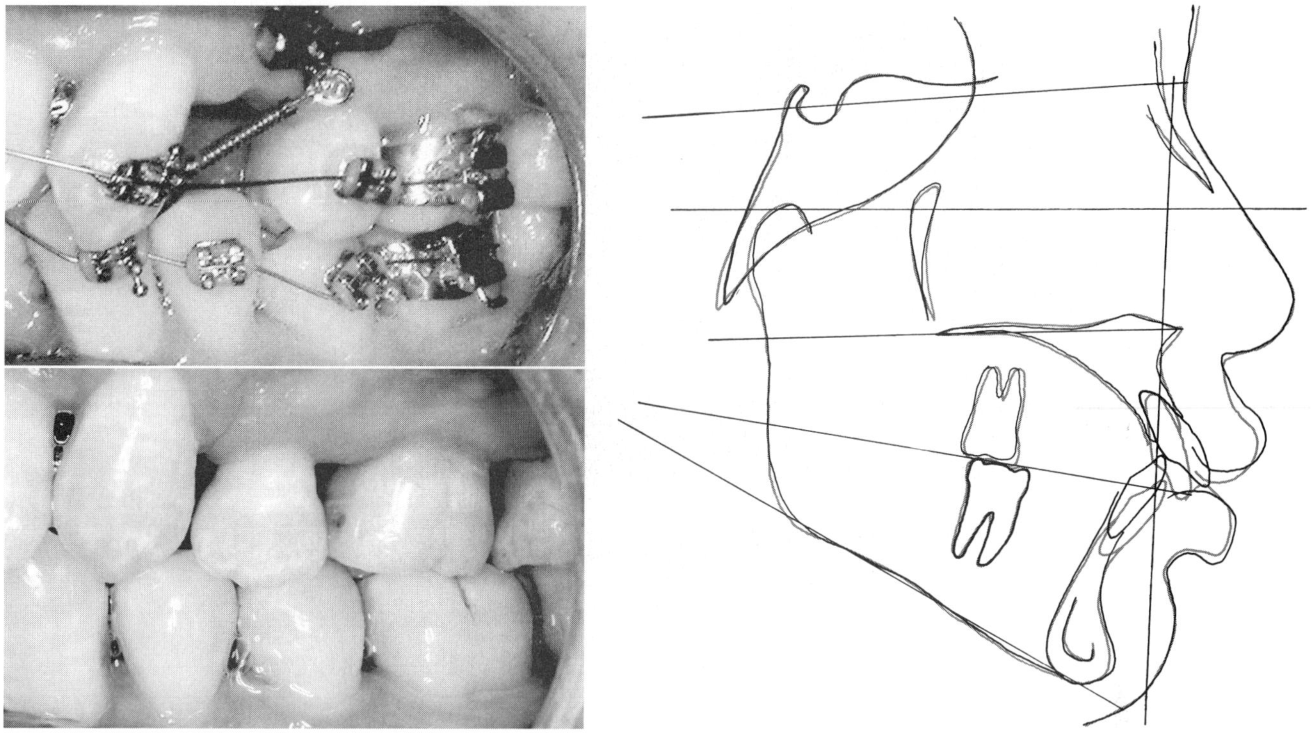

Figure 8-28 **A,** Bone anchor for retraction of severely protrusive maxillary incisors in a young adult with bone loss from periodontal disease (so that the maxillary posterior teeth had little anchorage value); **B,** Retraction completed. Note that the Class I molar relationship has been maintained, which would not have been possible without skeletal anchorage; **C,** Cephalometric superimpositions on cranial base and maxilla, showing the extent of maxillary incisor retraction without any forward movement of the posterior teeth. For this amount of tooth movement in an adult, a bone anchor placed in the zygomatic buttress and held with at least two screws (preferably three) is the best choice (see Chapter 11). There is a risk that a single screw in the alveolar process on each side would become loose before the tooth movement was completed.

to be retracted too much and that it compromises the facial appearance.

The relationship, if any, between TM dysfunction and premolar extraction is difficult to assess because data from well-controlled studies are not available. No relationships between symptoms of TMD and the type of orthodontic treatment were noted in any of a considerable series of reports in the early 1990s. The best data come from a study in which a careful compilation of retrospective data was used to create two groups of patients whose "borderline" Class II malocclusions could have been treated equally plausibly with or without premolar extraction. One group had extractions, the other did not. Both groups had low scores for signs or symptoms of dysfunction, and there was no difference between them in any aspect of TM joint function.[37] There is simply no evidence to support the allegation that premolar extraction causes TMD.

The effect of premolar extraction on facial esthetics is even more difficult to assess, because extraction is only one determinant of where the incisors end up. The extraction decision in Class II adolescents often is influenced by the degree of crowding or protrusion, not just by considerations of anteroposterior movement of teeth. For example, a Class II patient with incisor crowding that might not be an indication for extraction in a Class I patient might need extraction to tolerate even a modest amount of Class II elastics. When discriminant analysis based on consideration of crowding and protrusion was used to create clear-cut extraction and non-extraction groups within a large retrospective sample of adolescent Class II patients, extraction did reduce lip prominence more than non-extraction, but the non-extraction patients had less prominent lips on long-term recall.[38] One cannot automatically assume, therefore, that premolar extraction flattens the profile too much in adolescent Class II patients—but clearly it has the potential to do so, if the incisors are retracted too much.

Long-term results with distalization of the entire maxillary arch, using implant anchorage, are not yet available. It seems likely, however, that the outcomes would be similar to first premolar extraction: no increase in the chance of TMD, and a risk of bringing the maxillary incisors too far back in patients with mandibular deficiency. Because the primary indication for retracting the upper incisors in adolescent Class II patients is a lack of mandibular growth, this leads directly to further consideration of treatment in late adolescence and adult life, when little or no growth can be expected

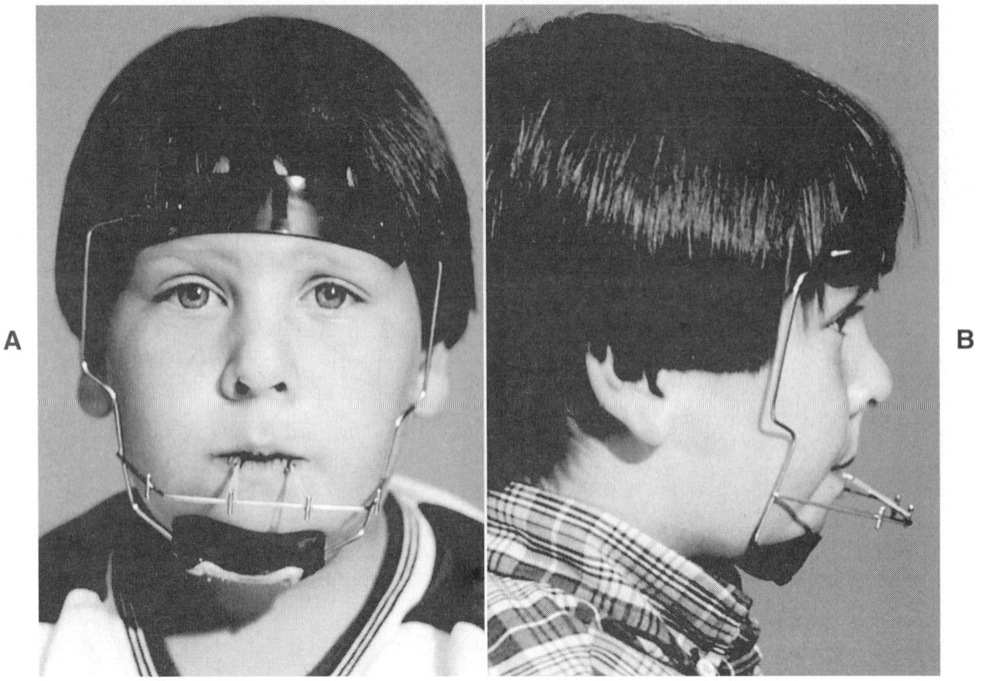

FIGURE 8-29 Delaire-type facemask (sometimes called reverse headgear) used to place forward traction against the maxilla. Because the maxilla often is deficient vertically as well as antero-posteriorly, a downward and forward direction of force usually is needed.

and orthognathic surgery may be necessary to achieve a satisfactory result.

Class III Problems

Growth modification for Class III problems is just the reverse of Class II: What is needed is differential growth of the maxilla relative to the mandible. Edward Angle's concept was that Class III malocclusion was due exclusively to excessive mandibular growth. In fact, almost any combination of deficient maxillary growth and excessive mandibular growth can be found in Class III patients, and maxillary deficiency and mandibular excess are about equally likely. The realization that maxillary deficiency is so frequently a component of skeletal Class III, and new possibilities for correcting it, have led recently to a great increase in treatment aimed at promoting maxillary growth. Unfortunately, data from randomized clinical trials are not available, and treatment recommendations must be based on reports from small and often poorly controlled studies.

Horizontal-Vertical Maxillary Deficiency

If headgear force compressing the maxillary sutures can inhibit forward growth of the maxilla, reverse (forward-pull) headgear separating the sutures should stimulate growth. Until Delaire and coworkers in France showed that forward positioning of the maxilla could be achieved with reverse headgear, *if* treatment was begun at an early age,[39] reverse pull headgear (Figure 8-29) was remarkably unsuccessful in producing anything but movement of the upper teeth. The French results suggested that successful forward repositioning of the maxilla can be accomplished before age 8, but after that orthodontic tooth movement usually overwhelms skeletal change, and more recent studies comparing untreated Class III children to those treated with maxillary protrusion have confirmed this outcome.[40] For this reason, a child with maxillary deficiency should be referred for complete evaluation as early as possible. Meta-analysis, pooling the results of multiple studies of face mask effects, suggests that for a reasonable chance of success, treatment must begin by age 10 at the latest.[41] The chance of successful forward movement is essentially zero by the time sexual maturity is achieved.

Even in young patients, two side effects of treatment are almost inevitable when reverse headgear that attaches to the teeth is used (Figure 8-30): forward movement of maxillary teeth relative to the maxilla and downward and backward rotation of the mandible. For this reason, in addition to being quite young, the ideal patients for treatment with this method would have both:

- Normally positioned or retrusive, but not protrusive, maxillary teeth
- Normal or short, but not long, anterior facial vertical dimensions

An obvious way to decrease the amount of tooth movement in face mask treatment would be to place the traction force to skeletal anchors in the maxilla (see Figure 8-16). As with all applications of skeletal anchorage, only preliminary reports with this technique are available as yet, but already it is clear that skeletal anchorage can be used to help bring the maxilla forward. Treatment using reverse-pull headgear is discussed in detail in Chapter 13.

Mandibular Excess

Although extraoral force applied via a chin cup is an old idea (Figure 8-31), this is not analogous to the use of extraoral force against the maxilla because there are no mandibular sutures to influence. If the cartilage of the mandibular condyle were a growth center with the capacity to grow independently, one would not expect chin cup therapy to be particularly successful. From the opposite and more contemporary view that condylar growth is largely a response to translation as surrounding tissues grow, a more optimistic view of the possibilities for growth restraint would be warranted. Research in recent years (see Chapter 2) indicates that the second view of mandibular growth is more correct. Nevertheless, results from chin cup therapy are usually discouraging.

There are two major ways to direct force against the mandible (Figure 8-32). The first is to apply it on a line directly through the mandibular condyle, with the intent of impeding mandibular growth in exactly the same way that extraoral force against the maxilla impedes its growth. This works in experimental animals,[42] but in humans the changes are considerably less impressive. It appears that human children will not tolerate the amount of force and/or number of hours per day that are required to impede growth of the mandible.

A second approach to chin cup therapy is to orient the line of force application below the mandibular condyle, so that the chin is deliberately rotated downward and backward. Less force is applied than when direct growth restriction is the objective. In essence, an increase in facial height is traded for a decrease in the prominence of the chin. This can be quite effective within the limits established by excessive face height. Obviously, it would work best in

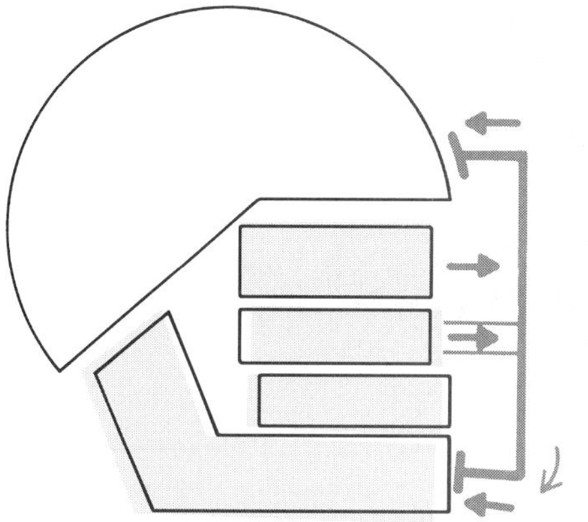

FIGURE 8-30 Forward traction against the maxilla typically has three effects: (1) some forward movement of the maxilla, the amount depending to a large extent on the patient's age; (2) forward movement of the maxillary teeth relative to the maxilla; and (3) downward and backward rotation of the mandible because of the reciprocal force placed against the chin.

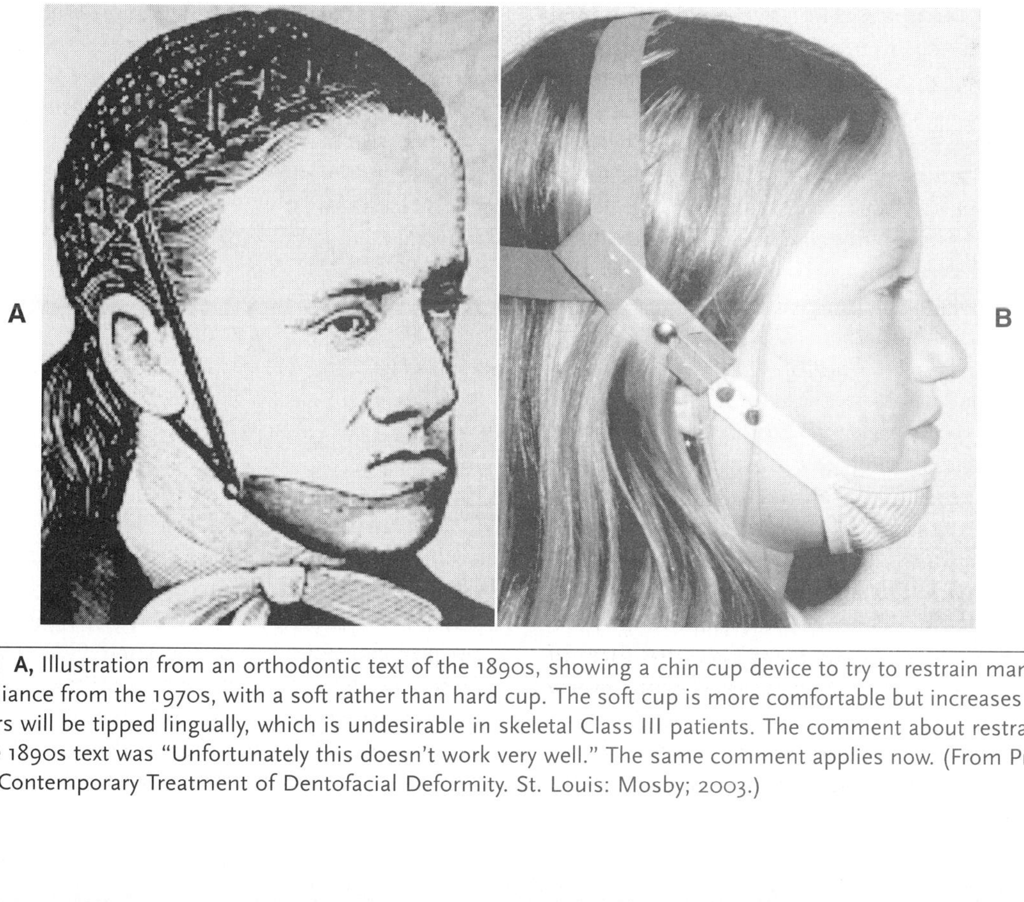

FIGURE 8-31 **A,** Illustration from an orthodontic text of the 1890s, showing a chin cup device to try to restrain mandibular growth; **B,** Chin cup appliance from the 1970s, with a soft rather than hard cup. The soft cup is more comfortable but increases the chance that the lower incisors will be tipped lingually, which is undesirable in skeletal Class III patients. The comment about restraining mandibular growth in the 1890s text was "Unfortunately this doesn't work very well." The same comment applies now. (From Proffit WR, White RP, Sarver DM. Contemporary Treatment of Dentofacial Deformity. St. Louis: Mosby; 2003.)

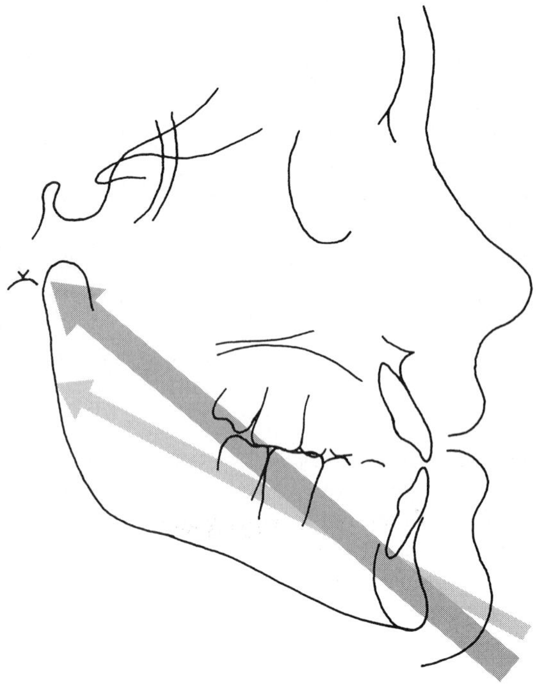

FIGURE 8-32 There are two main approaches to chin cup therapy, as shown diagrammatically here: heavy force aimed directly at the condylar area, or lighter force aimed below the condyle to produce downward rotation of the mandible.

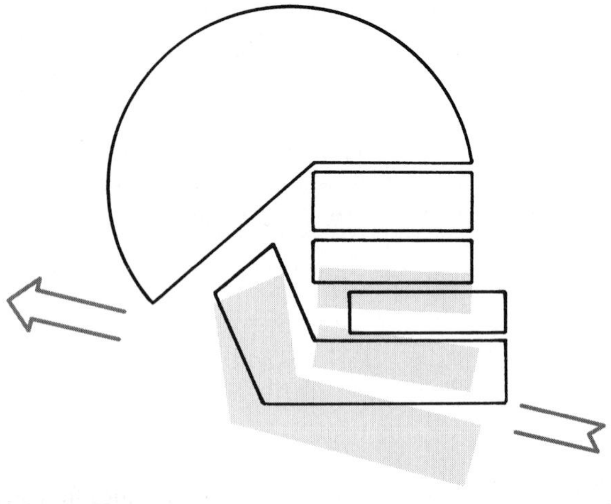

FIGURE 8-33 Diagrammatic representation of a typical response to chin cup therapy, showing the downward and backward rotation of the mandible accompanied by an increase in facial height.

individuals who had short facial vertical dimensions initially (Figure 8-33).

When extraoral force is applied against the chin, it is difficult to avoid tipping the lower incisors lingually. An elastic type of chin cup (the sort worn by football players, adapted for orthodontic use) transfers a significant amount of force to the base of the alveolar process and causes uprighting of the lower incisors. Even when a more rigid chin cup is used, a component of dental displacement in addition to the desired skeletal change is usually observed. If the mandibular dentition was protrusive initially, of course, uprighting of the incisors is desirable. In most cases, however, the incisor uprighting is an undesirable side effect and can cause crowding.

Functional appliances for mandibular prognathism work in exactly the same way as the second approach to chin cup therapy: They rotate the mandible downward and backward. The construction bite for Class III functional appliances is based on opening the mandible on a hinge, creating additional vertical space into which eruption of the teeth is guided. Just the reverse of the eruption pattern in Class II treatment is desired: The upper molars should erupt more than the lower. Although there are several types of Class III functional appliances, none of these create any direct force to restrain the mandible.

The ideal patient for chin cup or functional appliance treatment of excessive mandibular growth has:

- A mild skeletal problem, with the ability to bring the incisors end-to-end or nearly so
- Short vertical face height
- Normally positioned or protrusive, but not retrusive, lower incisors

It is possible to combine maxillary protraction and chin cup force against the mandible, which accentuates downward-backward rotation of the mandible, but patients with severe Class III problems, especially those with mandibular prognathism, will eventually require surgical correction (see Chapter 19). Modification of excessive mandibular growth can be successful only within narrow limits and usually is transitory, whatever the appliance system. Maxillary deficiency is somewhat more treatable, but bringing the maxilla forward more than a few millimeters is unlikely. As a guideline, more than 4 mm reverse overjet in a preadolescent child indicates that surgery eventually will be needed.

SKELETAL PROBLEMS IN OLDER PATIENTS: CAMOUFLAGE VERSUS SURGERY

Considerations in Camouflage Treatment

Beyond the adolescent growth spurt, even though some facial growth continues, too little remains to correct skeletal problems. The possibilities for treatment, therefore, are either displacement of the teeth relative to their supporting bone, to compensate for the underlying jaw discrepancy, or surgical repositioning of the jaws (Figure 8-34). Displacement of the teeth, as in retraction of protruding incisors, often is termed *camouflage*. The name is well chosen, because the objective of the treatment is to correct the malocclusion while making the underlying skeletal problem less apparent.

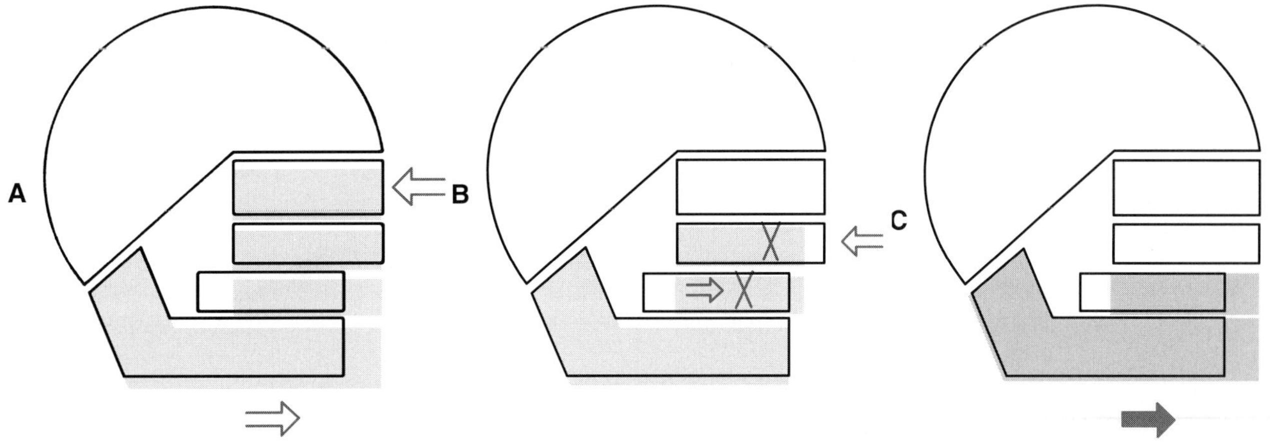

FIGURE 8-34 There are three major possibilities for correction of skeletal mandibular deficiency. **A,** Differential growth of the lower jaw, bringing the dentition forward with it; **B,** Camouflage, achieved in most cases by extracting premolars and then closing the space by retracting the maxillary anterior teeth while bringing the mandibular posterior teeth forward (at least a small amount of vertical growth is needed because most aspects of the orthodontic mechanotherapy tend to extrude the teeth); **C,** Surgical advancement of the mandible. Growth modification is most successful in preadolescent patients; camouflage is most useful for adolescents with moderately severe problems; jaw surgery is most useful for patients with no remaining growth potential and severe problems.

Because skeletal Class II problems often can be camouflaged rather well, most camouflage treatment is for Class II patients. Class III and long face problems, in contrast, do not camouflage well, in the sense that correcting the occlusion does not conceal the skeletal problem and may make it worse.

With extraction of teeth to provide space for the necessary tooth movement, often it is possible to obtain correct molar and incisor relationships despite an underlying skeletal Class II or Class III jaw relationship. For Class II correction, the extraction of upper first premolars alone or upper first and lower second premolars often is the choice; for Class III, lower first premolars alone or lower first and upper second premolars might be chosen. The method was developed as extraction treatment was reintroduced into orthodontics in the mid-20th century. In that era, it was the major approach to treating skeletal problems. At the time that extraction for camouflage became popular, growth modification as a treatment approach had been largely rejected as ineffective, and surgical techniques to correct skeletal problems had barely begun to be developed. It seemed appropriate, therefore, for the orthodontist to accept the limitations in skeletal relationships and concentrate on the dental occlusion.

Camouflage implies that repositioning the teeth will have a favorable, or at least not a detrimental, effect on facial esthetics. For patients with mild to moderate skeletal Class II problems, displacement of the teeth relative to their bony bases to achieve good occlusion is compatible with reasonable facial esthetics, and the camouflage can be quite successful (Figure 8-35). In more severe Class II problems, it may be possible to obtain good occlusion only at considerable expense to facial esthetics. If the upper incisors must be displaced far distally and the lower incisors proclined to compensate for mandibular deficiency, the esthetic result is increased prominence of the nose and an overall appearance of mid- and lower face deficiency. Even if the occlusion is corrected, such a result is unacceptable for two reasons—it did not address the patient's major problem of facial appearance and social acceptability, and the lower incisors are likely to relapse lingually and become crowded (Figure 8-36).

Camouflage also can be used in patients with mild skeletal Class III problems, in whom adjustment of incisor position can achieve acceptable occlusion and reasonable facial esthetics (Figure 8-37). Unfortunately, in even moderately severe skeletal Class III problems, camouflage is much less successful. Extraction of lower premolars combined with Class III elastics and extraoral force can improve the dental occlusion for many Class III patients, but the treatment rarely produces successful camouflage and frequently makes the facial appearance worse. Even minimal retraction of the lower incisors often magnifies the chin prominence that was a major reason for seeking treatment initially (Figure 8-38).

Because extractions provide space to displace the remaining teeth only in the anteroposterior plane of space, camouflage rarely succeeds with skeletal vertical problems. The force systems used to reposition dental segments tend to extrude posterior teeth and are likely to make both the occlusion and the facial appearance worse. In long face patients with excessive vertical development, implant anchorage can make it possible to intrude rather than extrude posterior teeth, and therefore has the potential to allow successful camouflage that would not otherwise be possible.

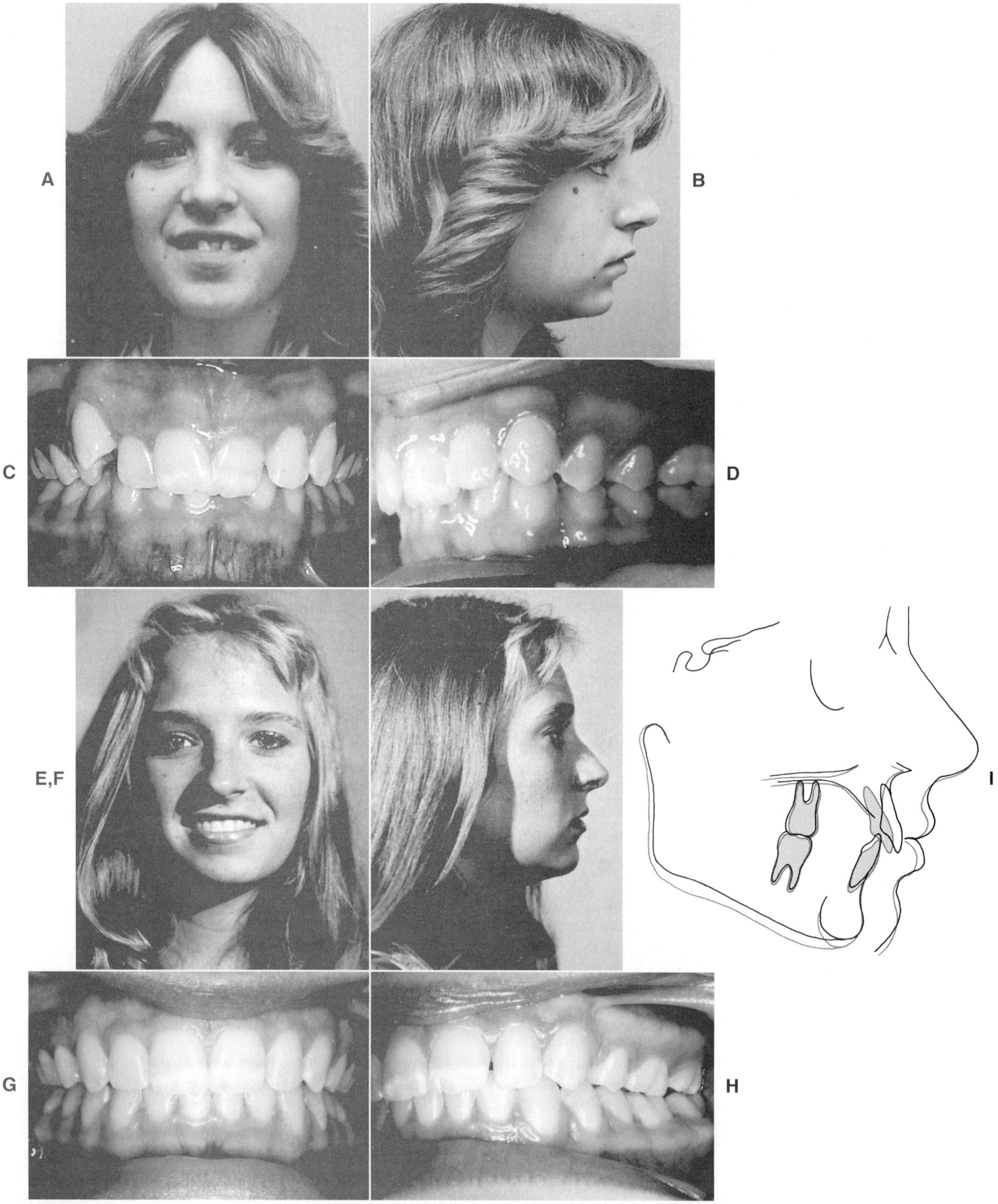

FIGURE 8-35 In skeletal Class II malocclusion of moderate severity, camouflage of the problem by displacement of the incisor teeth can be quite successful, as in this girl who was age 16 at the beginning of treatment. **A** and **B,** Facial appearance before treatment; occlusal relationships before (**C** and **D**) and after (**E** and **F**) treatment with extraction of maxillary first premolars; **G** and **H,** Facial appearance at age 18, after treatment; **I,** Cephalometric superimposition showing the retraction of the upper incisors.

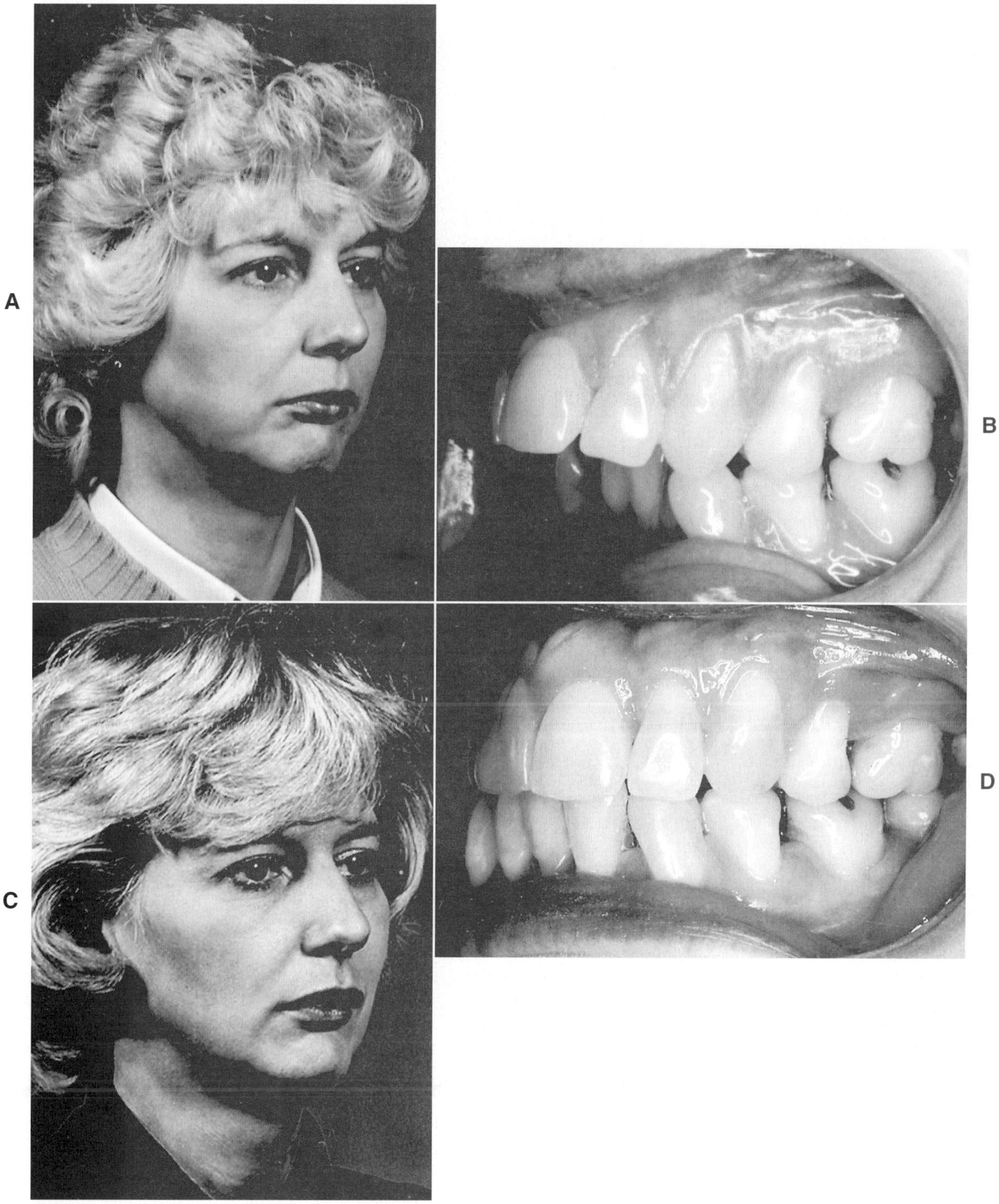

FIGURE 8-36 If mandibular deficiency is severe, orthodontic treatment for Class II malocclusion may result in reasonably satisfactory occlusal relationships but poor facial esthetics (i.e., a failure of camouflage). **A,** Facial appearance and **(B)** dental occlusion 15 years after premolar extractions and 4 years of orthodontic treatment; **C,** Facial appearance and **(D)** dental occlusion after re-treatment with surgical advancement of the mandible. The term *camouflage* is chosen to emphasize that successful treatment must produce acceptable facial esthetics as well as acceptable dental occlusion.

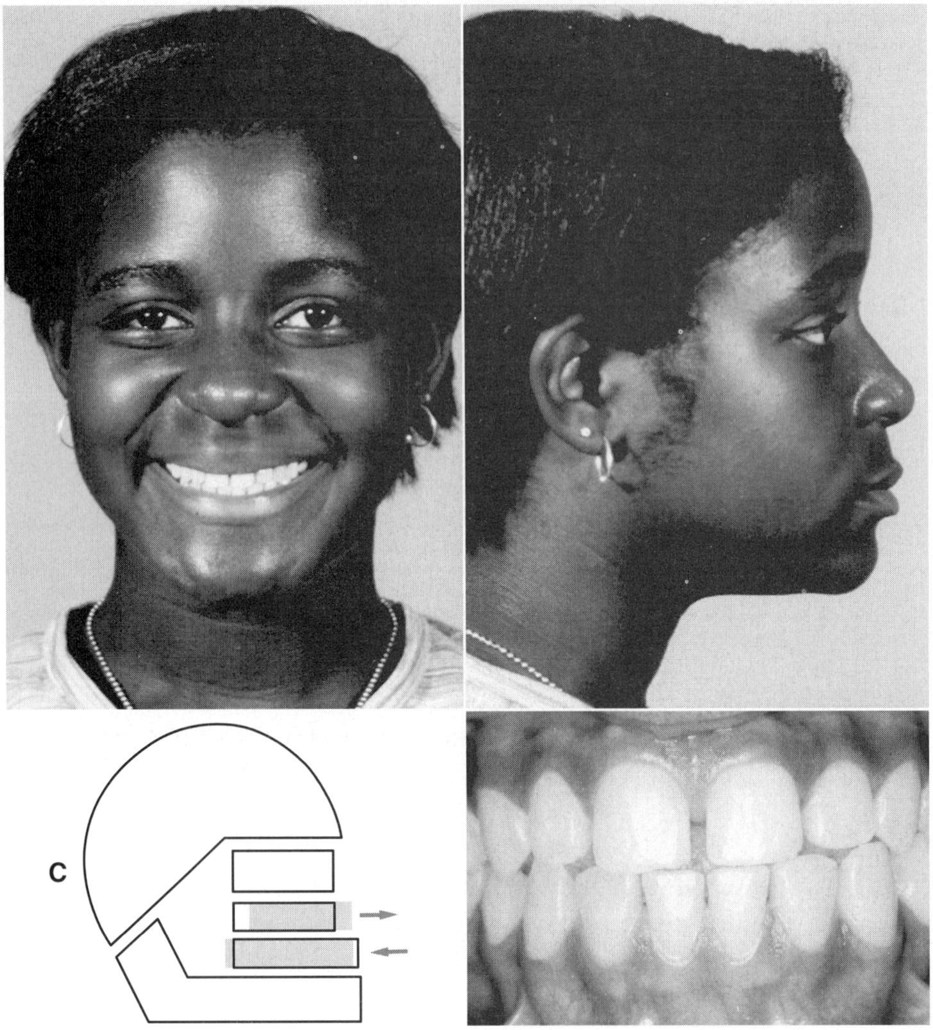

FIGURE 8-37 **A,** Camouflage treatment for patients with mild skeletal Class III malocclusion involves some combination of proclining the upper incisors and retracting the lower incisors. This must be approached carefully, because excessive retraction of lower incisors can produce the reverse of camouflage by making the chin more, not less prominent. **B, C,** At age 11-8, this girl had an acceptable facial and dental appearance, with **(D)** lower incisors in an edge-to-edge relationship. She was quite mature for her age and was considered not at great risk of developing true mandibular prognathism. The treatment plan was comprehensive orthodontics with extraction of one lower incisor, which **(E)** would provide space for modest retraction of the other incisors. **F, G,** Age 15-2, 18 months after the completion of treatment, showing the maintenance of acceptable facial esthetics. **H,** Cephalometric superimposition. (**B-H,** From Proffit WR, White RP, Sarver DM. Contemporary Treatment of Dentofacial Deformity. St. Louis: Mosby; 2003.)

Because of the extrusive nature of most orthodontic mechanics, it helps to have some vertical growth during treatment to avoid downward and backward rotation of the mandible. For that reason, camouflage works best in late adolescents who are past the pubertal growth spurt but still have some growth remaining. Although this type of treatment is possible for nongrowing adults, it is more difficult because the potentially extrusive components of any mechanical system must be much more carefully controlled. That means that implant anchorage for camouflage treatment is more likely to be required in patients beyond their late teens (see Chapter 18).

The characteristics of a patient who would be a good candidate for camouflage treatment are:

- Too old for successful growth modification
- Mild to moderate skeletal Class II or mild skeletal Class III
- Reasonably good alignment of teeth (so that the extraction spaces would be available for controlled anteroposterior displacement and not used to relieve crowding)
- Good vertical facial proportions, neither extreme short face (skeletal deep bite) nor long face (skeletal open bite)

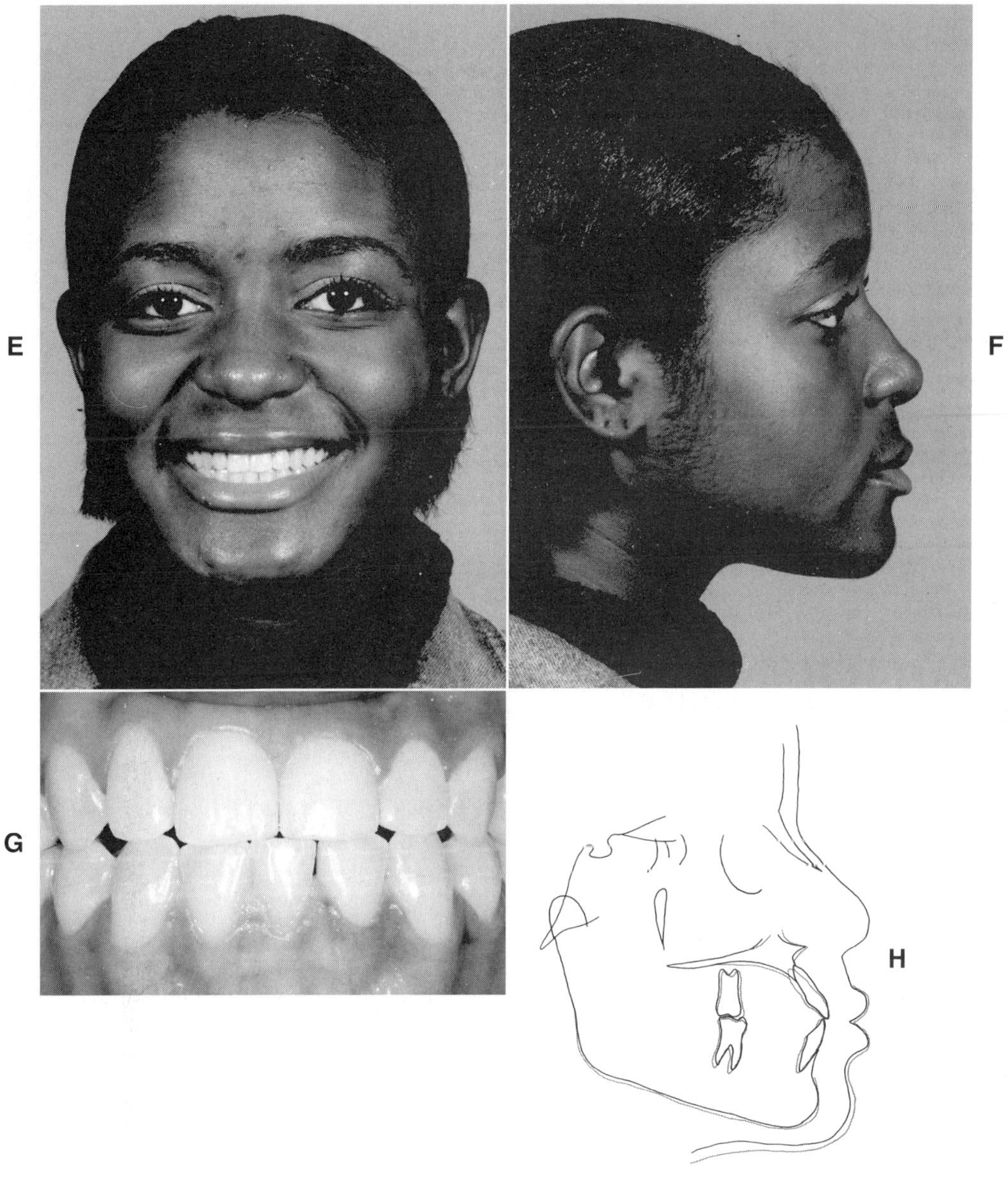

Figure 8-37 **cont'd** See previous page for legend.

Conversely, camouflage treatment designed to correct the occlusion despite jaw relationship problems should be avoided in:

- Severe Class II, moderate or severe Class III, and vertical skeletal discrepancies
- Patients with severe crowding or protrusion of incisors, in whom space created by extractions will be required to achieve proper alignment of the incisors
- Adolescents with good growth potential (in whom growth modification should tried first) or non-growing adults with more than mild discrepancies (in whom orthognathic surgery usually offers better long-term results)

Surgical Correction

Although surgical procedures to correct mandibular prognathism date back to the beginning of the 20th century, contemporary orthognathic surgery was developed quite recently. Surgical techniques now exist to correct severe problems of any type. Excellent results require careful coordination of the orthodontic and surgical phases of treatment. The principles of combined surgical and orthodontic treatment are discussed in some detail in Chapter 19, and further references to the literature on this subject are found there.

The characteristics of a patient who would be treated best by surgically repositioning the jaws are:

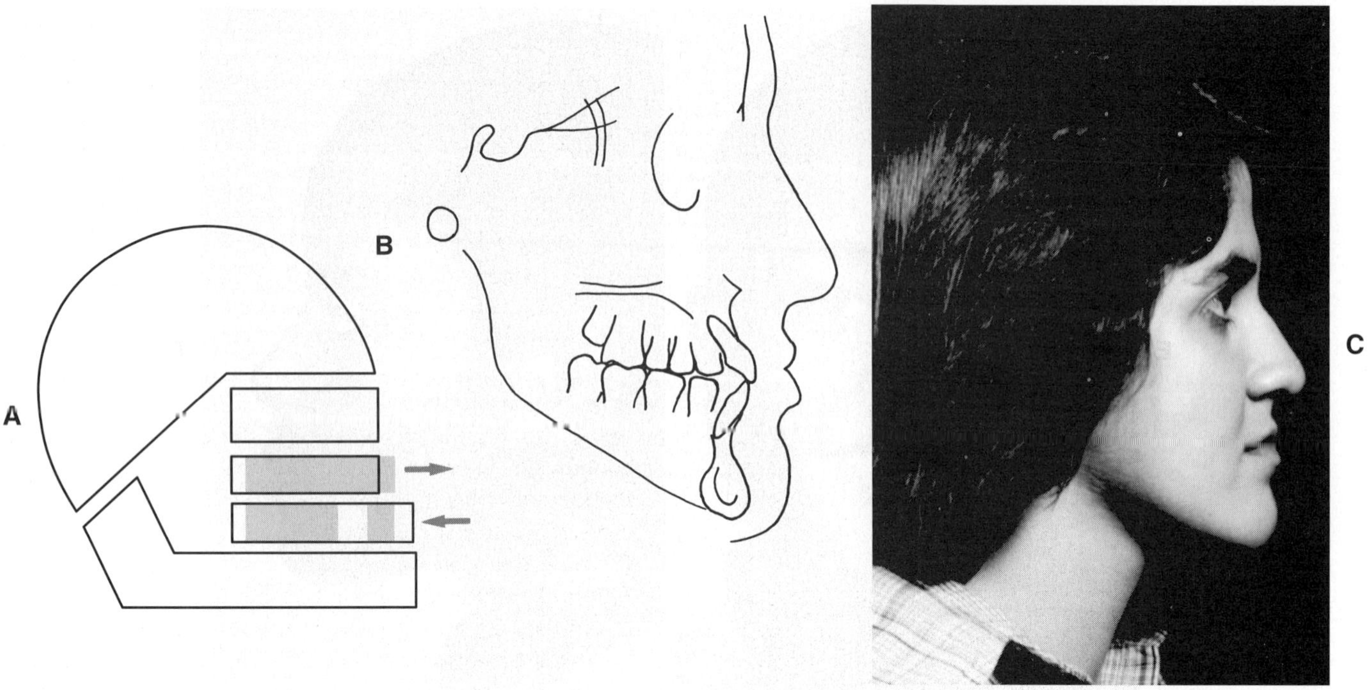

FIGURE 8-38 **A,** Diagrammatic representation of attempted camouflage for a more severe skeletal Class III problem, showing the obvious chin prominence created by retracting mandibular incisor teeth; **B,** Cephalometric tracing and **(C)** profile relationships for a patient after treatment in which lower but not upper premolars were retracted, lower incisors were retracted and upper incisors were tipped forward. She was unhappy with the prominence of her chin and sought further surgical treatment to correct it.

- Severe skeletal discrepancy or extremely severe dentoalveolar problem
- Adult patient (little if any remaining growth), or younger patient with extremely severe or progressive deformity
- Good general health status (mild, controlled systemic disease acceptable)

An important principle of treatment planning is that orthodontic camouflage and orthodontic preparation for surgery often require exactly opposite tooth movements. The reason is found in the concept of "dental compensation for skeletal discrepancy." This can occur naturally as well as being created by orthodontic camouflage treatment. In mandibular prognathism, for instance, as the individual grows the upper incisors tend to protrude while the lower incisors incline lingually. By the time growth is completed, the dental discrepancy usually is smaller than the jaw discrepancy. Tooth position has compensated at least partially for the jaw discrepancy. Some degree of dental compensation accompanies most skeletal jaw discrepancies, even without treatment.

If the jaws are to be repositioned surgically, this dental compensation must be removed. Otherwise, when the teeth are placed in normal occlusion, the jaw discrepancy will not be totally corrected, and dental interferences make it almost impossible to put the jaws in their proper relationship to each other (see Chapter 19). Orthodontic preparation for surgery usually involves removing, not creating, dental compensation and therefore the tooth movement is just the opposite of orthodontic camouflage. The result is that vigorous orthodontic treatment to correct the malocclusion in a patient with a difficult skeletal problem may eventually make surgical correction all but impossible without another session of orthodontic treatment to undo the original orthodontics. The patient, of course, is not likely to be pleased by this news. For that reason, an attempt at camouflage in a patient who may well need surgery should be avoided unless a successful outcome can be clearly predicted. Therapeutic diagnosis is a good way to evaluate the response to conservative orthodontic treatment but is not applicable to treatment based on extreme tooth movements for attempted camouflage.

The boundary between orthodontic and surgical treatment is particularly troublesome for teenagers with Class II problems. Given the risk of camouflage failure vs. the greater cost and morbidity of orthognathic surgery, what do you do with the rather mature 14 year old with a full cusp Class II malocclusion, 10 mm overjet, and an obvious mandibular deficiency? The choices are retraction of the upper incisors (with maxillary premolar extraction or implant anchorage) or surgical mandibular advancement. Although no clinical trial has occurred (and probably never will, given the problems in randomly assigning patients to surgery), some data now are available to more clearly indicate the limits of

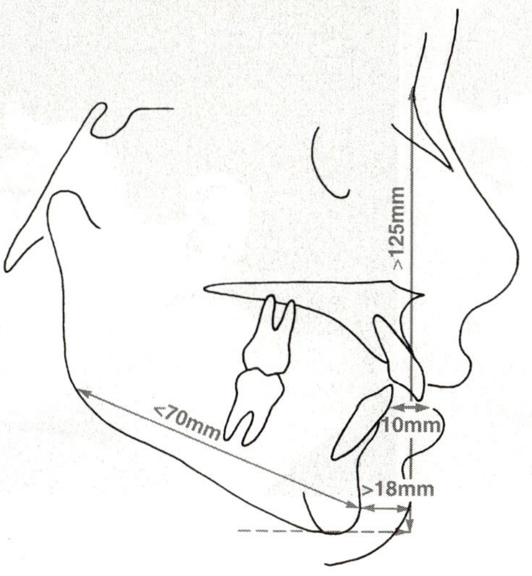

Figure 8-39 For adolescent Class II patients, the best indicator of the limits of satisfactory orthodontic correction is the simplest thing one can measure—overjet. More than 10 mm overjet in a patient who is past the peak of the adolescent growth spurt suggests that surgical correction probably would be needed, especially if the lower incisors are protrusive relative to a deficient mandible (Pg-Nperp >18 mm), the mandible is short (mandibular body length <70 mm), and/or face height is long (>125 mm). Mandibular body length (GoPg) is a more reliable indicator than total length (CoPg), probably because of the difficulty in accurately locating condylion and variations in chin morphology. (From Proffit et al[43].)

camouflage and therefore the indications for surgery for postadolescent Class II patients.[43,44]

In an individual who is past the adolescent growth spurt, the best single indicator of a problem too severe for likely success with camouflage is >10 mm overjet. That is particularly true if the mandible is short, the lower teeth already protrude relative to the mandible so that the chin is well behind the teeth, and/or the face is long (Figure 8-39).

Two other factors to consider in the decision for orthodontics vs. surgery are the possible role of augmentation genioplasty as an adjunct to Class II camouflage and the risk of root resorption with camouflage treatment. A limiting factor in orthodontic Class II treatment is the extent to which the lower teeth can be moved forward relative to the mandible. Moving the lower incisors forward more than 2 mm is highly unstable unless they were severely tipped lingually, but this is likely to occur during camouflage treatment when Class II elastics are used unless lower premolars were extracted. Often it is undesirable esthetically to retract the upper incisors to the extent that would be necessary if the lower incisors were not advanced significantly. If orthodontic treatment would otherwise move the lower incisors too far forward for reasonable esthetics or stability, a lower border osteotomy to reposition the chin can both improve facial balance and decrease lip pressure against the lower incisors, improving their stability (Figure 8-40). The lower border osteotomy is no more extensive a surgical procedure than premolar extraction would be, it can be done as an outpatient or day-op procedure at much less cost than mandibular advancement, and if it is done prior to age 19, remodeling of the lingual cortex is better than at older ages.[45]

The relationship between root resorption and camouflage treatment also should be kept in mind. A major risk factor for severe resorption of maxillary incisor roots during orthodontic treatment is contact of the roots with the lingual cortical plate (Figure 8-41). The best data (see Chapter 9) suggest that the risk of resorption increases twenty-fold when lingual plate contact occurs. What causes the roots to contact the lingual cortical plate? Two circumstances, primarily: torquing the upper incisors back during Class II camouflage and tipping them facially in Class III camouflage (because the roots go lingually as the crowns go facially). Camouflage failure, in both Class II and Class III patients, often is accompanied by incisor root resorption that can complicate surgical retreatment—but fortunately, further orthodontic tooth movement without additional resorption is possible if lingual contact is avoided during retreatment (see Chapter 19).

Planning Treatment for Maximal Esthetic Improvement

Careful clinical examination of the patient, so that important data related to facial and dental esthetics are incorporated into the database, is the key to planning treatment to obtain maximal improvement in appearance. In Chapter 6, a systematic approach to evaluation of facial proportions (macro-esthetics), the smile framework (mini-esthetics), and tooth-gingival characteristics (micro-esthetics) was described. The discussion here is of ways to deal with these esthetic issues.

Macro-esthetic Considerations: Correcting Facial Disproportions

Computer Imaging in the Decision for Camouflage versus Orthognathic Surgery

The ultimate judgment as to whether orthodontic treatment alone, to camouflage a skeletal problem, would be an acceptable result, or whether orthognathic surgery to correct the jaw discrepancy would be required, must be made by the patient and parents. The orthodontist's role is to supply the information they need to make that decision—and in that context, computer image predictions of the outcome without and with surgery are an important tool to help the patient and parents understand.

For the doctor, there are two possible attitudes toward the use of computer predictions: (1) this is dangerous because the predicted outcome may not be obtained, or (2) this is

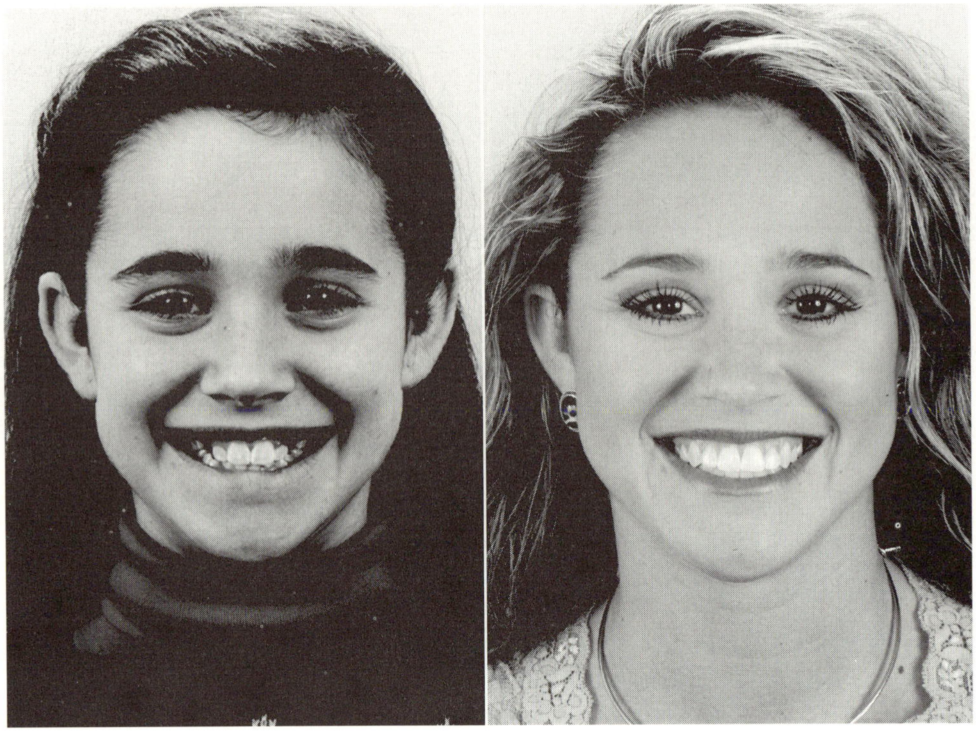

A B

FIGURE 8-45 For patients with wide buccal corridors, transverse expansion of the maxilla can improve smile esthetics. **A,** Age 12, prior to treatment; **B,** Age 15, after orthodontic treatment with widening of the maxillary arch.

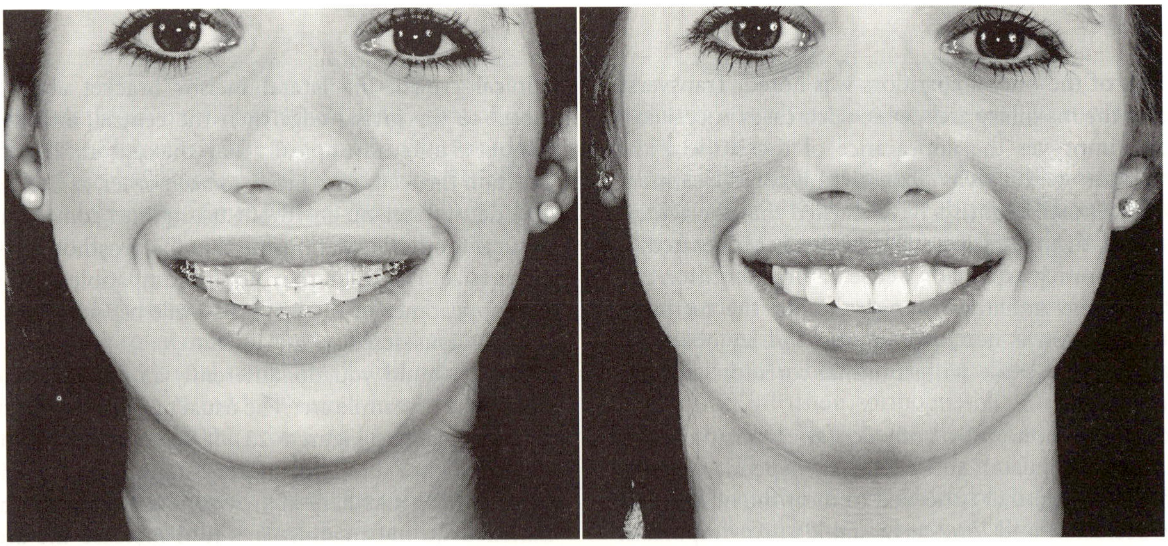

A B

FIGURE 8-46 For best appearance, the position of the maxillary incisors relative to the lower lip on smile (the smile arc) must be evaluated during treatment. **A,** Flattening of the smile arc was noted toward the end of orthodontic treatment. **B,** Before treatment was completed, the maxillary incisors were elongated to produce an appropriate smile arc. Placing the maxillary incisors properly relative to the lip sometimes requires intruding the lower incisors.

of the teeth or different crown heights on one side, and if so repositioning the teeth or changing the gingival contours should be included in the treatment plan. Often, however, greater elevation of the lip on one side on smile, which is an innate characteristic that cannot be changed, gives the appearance of a cant to the maxillary dentition when it really is symmetric. For a patient who complains about smile asymmetry, this becomes an important informed consent issue—the patient must understand that the asymmetric lip movements will not be changed by treatment.

Micro-esthetic Considerations: Enhancing the Appearance of the Teeth

Treatment plans for problems relating directly to the appearance of the teeth fall into three major categories: (1) reshaping teeth to change tooth proportions and/or correct "black triangles" between the teeth; (2) orthodontic preparation for restorations to replace lost tooth structure and correct problems of tooth shade and color; and (3) reshaping of the gingiva.[47]

Reshaping Teeth

Often it is desirable to do minor reshaping of the incisal edges of anterior teeth, to remove mamelons or smooth out irregular edges from minor trauma. When minor reshaping is planned, it must be taken into account when brackets are placed, and it may be easier to do this before beginning fixed appliance treatment.

Changing Tooth Proportions. Extensive changes in tooth proportions are needed primarily when one tooth is to substitute for another, and the most frequent substitution is substituting maxillary canines for congenitally missing maxillary lateral incisors. When a lateral incisor is missing, the treatment alternatives always are closing the space and substituting the canine, or prosthetic replacement of the missing tooth with a single-tooth implant or fixed bridge. Closing the space and reshaping the canine to look like a lateral incisor can provide an excellent esthetic result, perhaps superior to an implant in the long run.[48]

The technique for reshaping a canine is illustrated in Figure 8-47. It requires significant removal of facial, occlusal, interproximal and lingual enamel. In some patients, composite build-ups of ceramic laminates are needed to obtain good tooth color.

Canine substitution works best, however, when the dental arch was crowded anyway, and may not be compatible with excellent occlusion and smile esthetics if closing the lateral incisor space would result in significant retraction of the central incisors. In that circumstance, encouraging the permanent canine to erupt into the lateral incisor position so that alveolar bone is formed in the area of the missing tooth, and then moving the canine distally to open space, is the best way to prepare for an eventual implant.[49]

Correcting Black Triangles. Decreasing or eliminating spaces between teeth above the contact points, which are unsightly if they are not filled with an interdental papilla, can be accomplished most readily by removing enamel at the contact point so the teeth can be moved closer together (see Figure 6-30). Moving the contact area apically eliminates much if not all the space. When this is done, however, care is required not to distort the proportional relationships of the teeth to each other, and if possible the progression of connector heights (see below) should be maintained. Clinically, that means that if the central incisors are narrowed, it may be necessary also to slightly narrow the lateral incisors and move their contact area more apically to maintain a good dental appearance.

Interaction Between Orthodontist and Restorative Dentist

When the teeth are small or if tooth color or appearance is to be improved by restorative dentistry, during orthodontic treatment it is necessary to position them so that the restorations will bring them to normal size and position. In modern practice, the restorations are either composite build-ups or ceramic laminates, laminates being used particularly when it is desirable to change tooth color and shade in addition to the size of the crown (see Figures 1-4 to 1-7).

There are two ways to manage the orthodontic-restorative interaction. The first is to carefully plan where the teeth are to be placed, place a vacuum-formed retainer immediately after the orthodontic appliance is removed that the patient wears full-time, and send the patient to the restorative dentist for completion of the treatment. A new retainer is needed as soon as the restorations have been completed. This has the advantages that the restorative work can be scheduled at everyone's convenience after the orthodontic treatment is completed and any gingival swelling related to the orthodontic treatment has time to resolve, and the major disadvantage that excellent patient cooperation is required to maintain the precise spacing needed for the best restorations.

An alternative, which is most applicable when composite build-ups rather than laminates are planned, is for the orthodontist to deliberately provide slightly more space than the restorative dentist requires to bring the teeth to just the right size, remove the brackets from the teeth to be restored, send the patient immediately to the restorative dentist, replace the brackets the same day after the restorations are completed, and close any residual space before removing the orthodontic appliance (Figure 8-48). This has the advantage of eliminating compromises in the restorative work, but the disadvantage that careful coordination of the appointments is required.

Reshaping Gingival Contours: Applications of a Soft Tissue Laser

Appropriate display of the teeth requires removal of excessive gingiva covering the clinical crown, and is enhanced by

A,B C D,E F G,H I

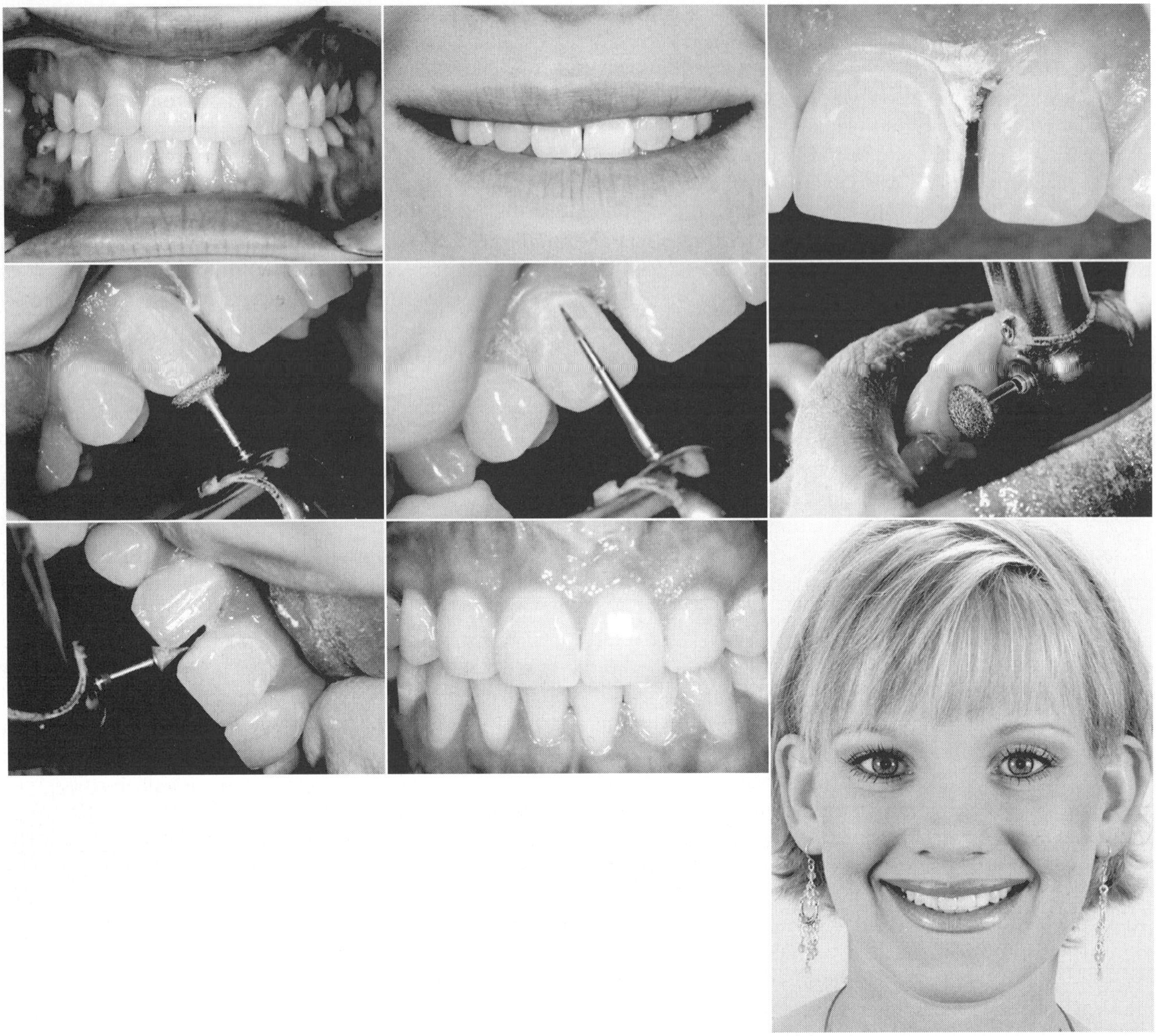

FIGURE 8-47 Reshaping a maxillary canine that is to substitute for a missing maxillary lateral incisor is necessary for a normal appearance of the dentition. As a general rule, the canine needs reduction in cingulum thickness, narrowing, and flattening of the tip and across the facial surface. If the gingival margin of the canine is visible, it can be brought down by elongating the tooth and increasing the amount of gingival reduction. Recontouring of the gingiva over the first premolar that becomes a substitution for the canine also enhances appearance. **A,** Dental appearance in a young woman who was dissatisfied with the appearance of her teeth after previous orthodontic treatment to substitute maxillary canines for congenitally missing lateral incisors; **B,** The initial frontal smile; **C,** Interproximal reduction to narrow the canines; **D,** Reduction of the incisal tip, which both improves appearance of the tooth and allows it to be extruded to bring the gingival margin down; **E,** Reduction in facial convexity; **F,** Reduction of the cingulum; **G,** Reshaping the corners. At this point, a lateral bracket can be placed on the canine during orthodontic treatment. **H,** Close-up after completion of treatment. Note that the gingival margin of the first premolar has been reshaped (with a diode laser) to make it look more like a canine. **I,** Smile at completion of treatment.

correcting the gingival contours. Treatment of this type now can be carried out effectively with the use of a diode laser (see Figure 7-25). A laser of this type, in comparison to the CO_2 or erbium-YAG lasers also used now in dentistry, has two primary advantages: (1) it does not cut hard tissue, so that there is no risk of damage to the teeth or alveolar bone if it is used for gingival contouring, and (2) it creates a "biologic dressing" because it coagulates, sterilizes and seals the soft tissue as it is used. There is no bleeding, no other dressing is required, and there is no waiting for a healing period.

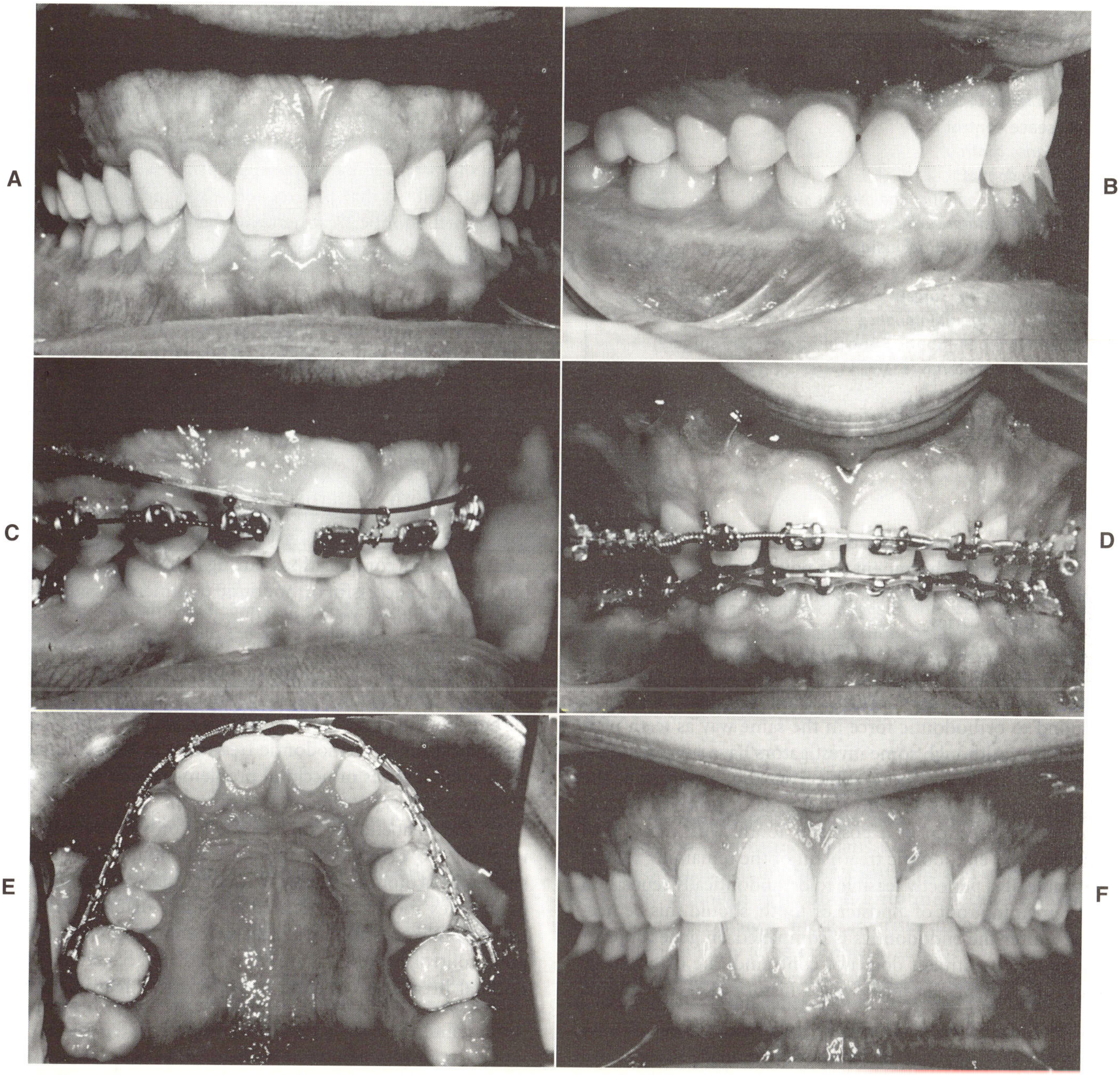

FIGURE 8-48 **A, B,** This patient's complaint was the appearance of his upper incisors. The central incisors were elongated and quite upright; the lateral incisors were small, and the excess space was seen as a maxillary midline diastema. **C,** Intrusion archwire to central incisors; **D, E,** After intrusion and spacing of the incisors to allow build-ups of the lateral incisors; **F,** Completion of orthodontic and restorative treatment.

TREATMENT PLANNING IN SPECIAL CIRCUMSTANCES

Sequence of Treatment for Patients With Multiple Dental Problems

For patients with multiple dental problems including malocclusion, the appropriate sequencing of treatment is important (Box 8-3). Although these patients usually are adults, the principles are the same for adults or children:

- Dental disease should be brought under control initially
- Orthodontic treatment, including skeletal as well as dental changes, should be carried out next
- Definitive restorative and periodontal treatment should be completed after the orthodontic phase of treatment

Control of dental disease includes a number of treatment procedures: tooth extractions if necessary, endodontic

A B C D E F G H

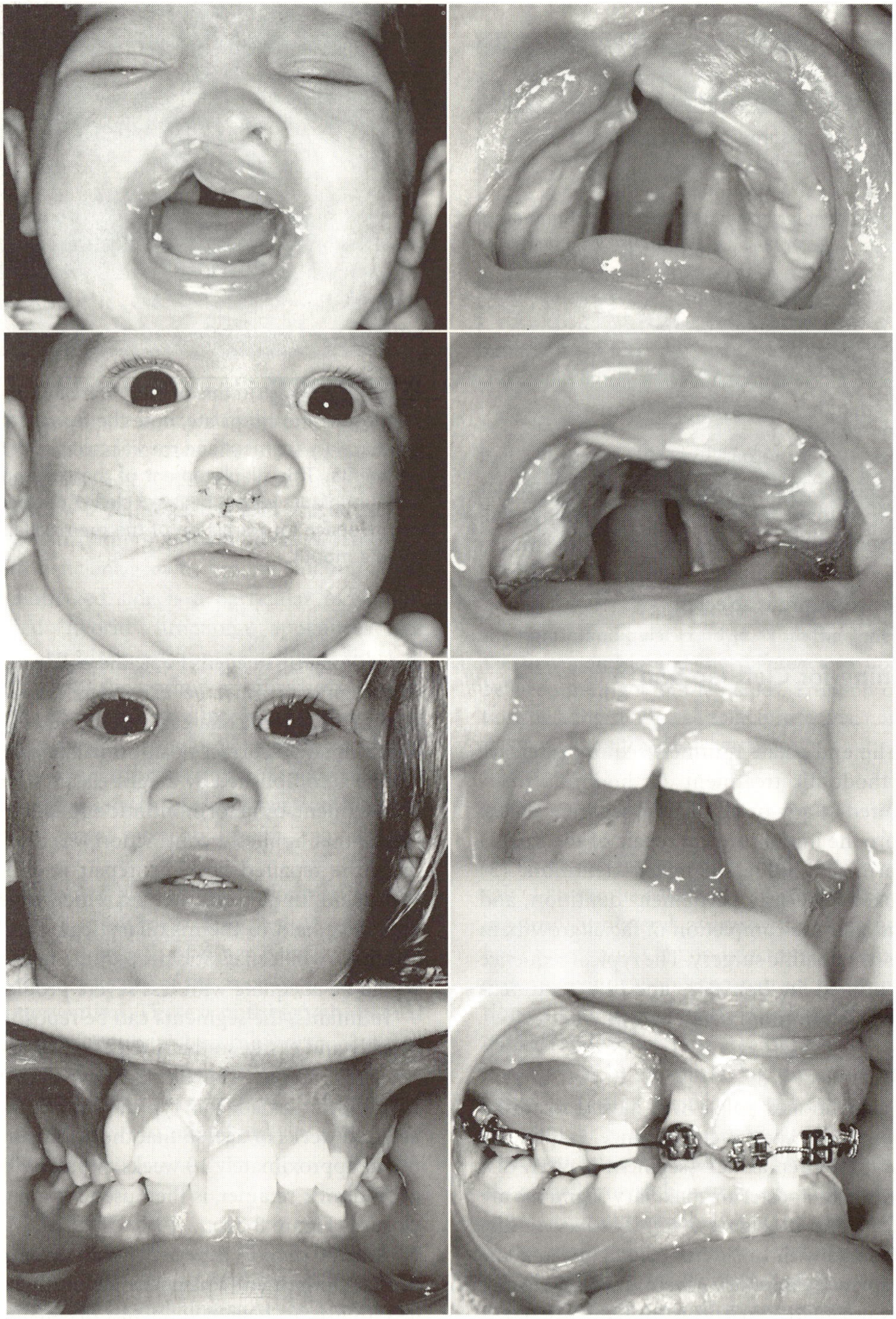

FIGURE 8-53 Long-term observation of treatment of a girl with unilateral cleft lip and palate (through Figure 8-57). **A, B,** Age 8 weeks prior to lip repair. Note the displacement of the alveolar segments at the cleft site. **C, D,** Age 9 weeks after lip closure. A palatal plate has been pinned into position to control the alveolar segments while lip pressure molds them into position. This type of infant orthopedics, popular in the 1970s, is used less now than previously because its long-term efficacy is questionable. **E, F,** Age 2, prior to palate closure. **G,** Age 8, after eruption of maxillary incisors; **H,** Age 9, incisor alignment in preparation for alveolar bone graft.

I

J

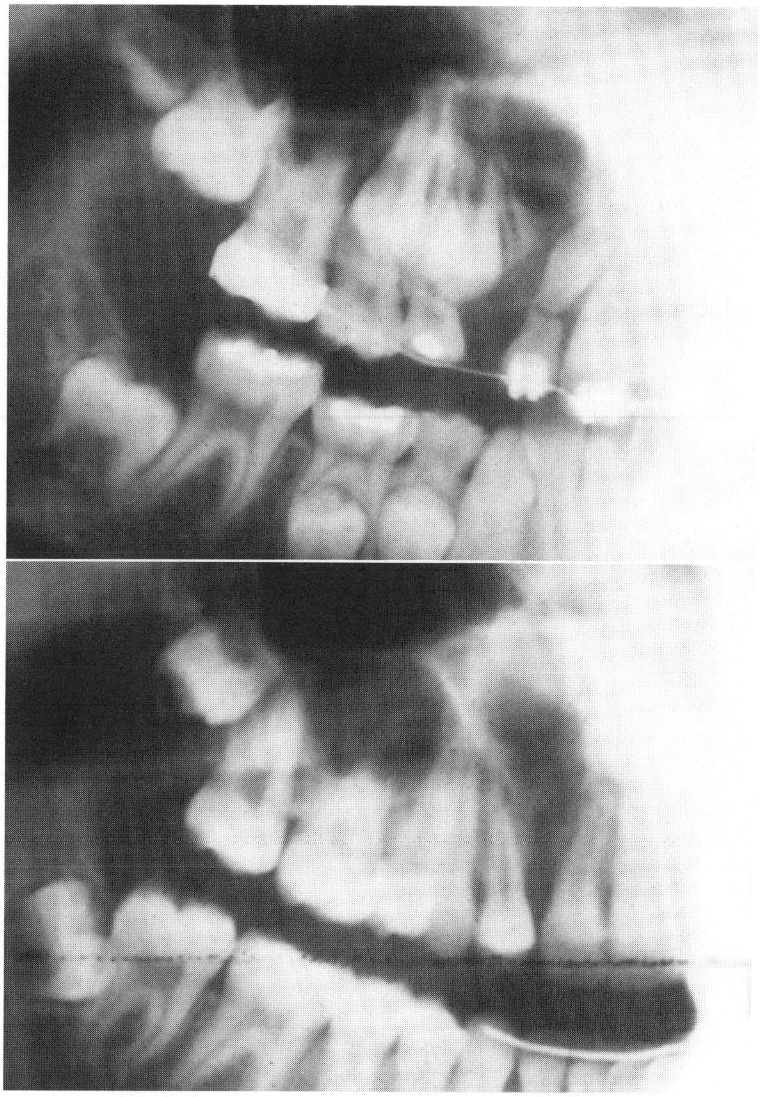

Figure 8-53 cont'd **I,** Panoramic radiograph, age 9, just prior to bone graft; **J,** Panoramic radiograph age 12, at completion of orthodontic treatment, showing bone fill-in at the cleft site.

majority of patients with cleft lip or palate, however, the orthodontist is no longer called to reposition segments in infants. Instead, if the segments protrude, the lip repair may be carried out in two stages, first with a lip adhesion to provide an elastic force from the lip itself, followed at a somewhat later stage by definitive lip repair. Rather than presurgical orthopedics being recommended for nearly all infants with cleft lip or palate, at present a minority are treated with presurgical orthopedics.

At some centers, bone grafts were placed across the cleft alveolus soon after the infant orthopedics to stabilize the position of the segments. Although a few clinicians still advocate this procedure, the consensus is that early grafting of the alveolar process is contraindicated because it tends to interfere with later growth.[53] Alveolar bone grafts are better deferred until the early mixed dentition.

Late Primary and Early Mixed Dentition Treatment

Many of the orthodontic problems of cleft palate children in the late and early mixed dentition result not from the cleft itself, but from the effects of surgical repair. Although the techniques for repair of cleft lip and palate have improved tremendously in recent years, closure of the lip inevitably creates some constriction across the anterior part of the maxillary arch, and closure of a cleft palate causes at least some degree of lateral constriction. As a result, surgically treated cleft palate patients have a tendency toward both anterior and lateral crossbite, which is not seen in patients with untreated clefts. This result is not an argument against surgical repair of the lip and palate, which is necessary for esthetic and functional (speech) reasons. It simply means that orthodontic treatment must be considered a necessary part of the habilitation of such patients.

Orthodontic intervention is often unnecessary until the permanent incisor teeth begin to erupt but is usually imperative at that point (Figure 8-54). As the permanent teeth come in, there is a strong tendency for the maxillary incisors to erupt rotated and often in crossbite. The major goal of orthodontic treatment at this time is to correct incisor

CHAPTER

9

The Biologic Basis of Orthodontic Therapy

CHAPTER OUTLINE

Orthodontic treatment is based on the principle that if prolonged pressure is applied to a tooth, tooth movement will occur as the bone around the tooth remodels. Bone is selectively removed in some areas and added in others. In essence, the tooth moves through the bone carrying its attachment apparatus with it, as the socket of the tooth migrates. Because the bony response is mediated by the periodontal ligament, tooth movement is primarily a periodontal ligament phenomenon.

Forces applied to the teeth can also affect the pattern of bone apposition and resorption at sites distant from the teeth, particularly the sutures of the maxilla and bony surfaces on both sides of the temporomandibular joint. Thus the biologic response to orthodontic therapy includes not only the response of the periodontal ligament but also the response of growing areas distant from the dentition. In this chapter, the response of periodontal structures to orthodontic force is discussed first, and then the response of skeletal areas distant from the dentition is considered briefly, drawing on the background of normal growth provided in Chapters 2 through 4.

PERIODONTAL AND BONE RESPONSE TO NORMAL FUNCTION

Periodontal Ligament Structure and Function

Each tooth is attached to and separated from the adjacent alveolar bone by a heavy collagenous supporting structure, the periodontal ligament (PDL). Under normal circumstances, the PDL occupies a space approximately 0.5 mm in width around all parts of the root. By far the major component of the ligament is a network of parallel collagenous

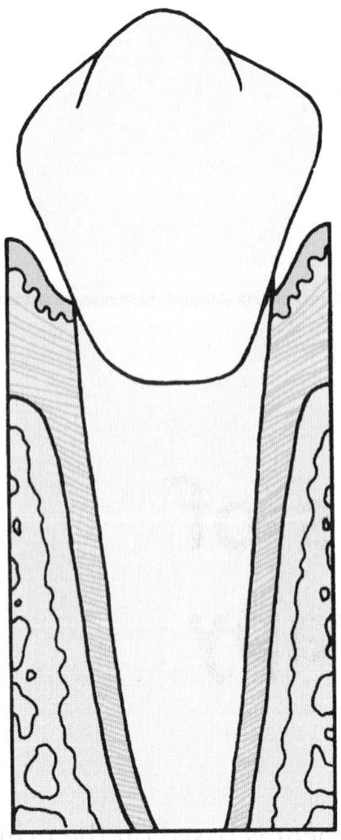

FIGURE 9-1 Diagrammatic representation of periodontal structures (bone in *pale red*). Note the angulation of the PDL fibers.

fibers, inserting into cementum of the root surface on one side and into a relatively dense bony plate, the lamina dura, on the other side. These supporting fibers run at an angle, attaching farther apically on the tooth than on the adjacent alveolar bone. This arrangement, of course, resists the displacement of the tooth expected during normal function (Figure 9-1).

Although most of the PDL space is taken up with the collagenous fiber bundles that constitute the ligamentous attachment, two other major components of the ligament must be considered. These are (1) the cellular elements, including mesenchymal cells of various types along with vascular and neural elements; and (2) the tissue fluids. Both play an important role in normal function and in making orthodontic tooth movement possible.

The principal cellular elements in the PDL are undifferentiated mesenchymal cells and their progeny in the form of fibroblasts and osteoblasts. The collagen of the ligament is constantly being remodeled and renewed during normal function.[1] The same cells can serve as both fibroblasts, producing new collagenous matrix materials, and fibroclasts, destroying previously produced collagen. Remodeling and recontouring of the bony socket and the cementum of the root is also constantly being carried out, though on a smaller scale, as a response to normal function.

Fibroblasts in the PDL have properties similar to osteoblasts, and new bone probably is formed by osteoblasts that differentiated from the local cellular population.[2] Bone and cementum are removed by specialized osteoclasts and cementoclasts, respectively. These multinucleated giant cells are quite different from the osteoblasts and cementoblasts that produce bone and cementum. Despite years of investigation, their origin remains controversial. Most are of hematogenous origin; some may be derived from stem cells found in the local area.[3]

Although the PDL is not highly vascular, it does contain blood vessels and cells from the vascular system. Nerve endings are also found within the ligament, both the unmyelinated free endings associated with perception of pain and the more complex receptors associated with pressure and positional information (proprioception).

Finally, it is important to recognize that the PDL space is filled with fluid; this fluid is the same as that found in all other tissues, ultimately derived from the vascular system. A fluid-filled chamber with retentive but porous walls could be a description of a shock absorber, and in normal function, the fluid allows the PDL space to play just this role.

Response to Normal Function

During masticatory function, the teeth and periodontal structures are subjected to intermittent heavy forces. Tooth contacts last for 1 second or less; forces are quite heavy, ranging from 1 or 2 kg while soft substances are chewed up to as much as 50 kg against a more resistant object. When a tooth is subjected to heavy loads of this type, quick displacement of the tooth within the PDL space is prevented by the incompressible tissue fluid. Instead, the force is transmitted to the alveolar bone, which bends in response.

The extent of bone bending during normal function of the jaws (and other skeletal elements of the body) is often not appreciated. The body of the mandible bends as the mouth is opened and closed, even without heavy masticatory loads. Upon wide opening, the distance between the mandibular molars decreases by 2 to 3 mm. In heavy function, individual teeth are slightly displaced as the bone of the alveolar process bends to allow this to occur, and bending stresses are transmitted over considerable distances. Bone bending in response to normal function generates piezoelectric currents (Figure 9-2; see further discussion below) that appear to be an important stimulus to skeletal regeneration and repair. This is the mechanism by which bony architecture is adapted to functional demands.

Very little of the fluid within the PDL space is squeezed out during the first second of pressure application. If pressure against a tooth is maintained, however, the fluid is rapidly expressed, and the tooth displaces within the PDL space, compressing the ligament itself against adjacent bone. Not surprisingly, this hurts. Pain is normally felt after 3 to 5 seconds of heavy force application, indicating that the fluids are expressed and crushing pressure is applied against the PDL in this amount of time (Table 9-1). The resistance provided by tissue fluids allows normal mastication, with its force applications of 1 second or less, to occur without pain.

Although the PDL is beautifully adapted to resist forces of short duration, it rapidly loses its adaptive capability as

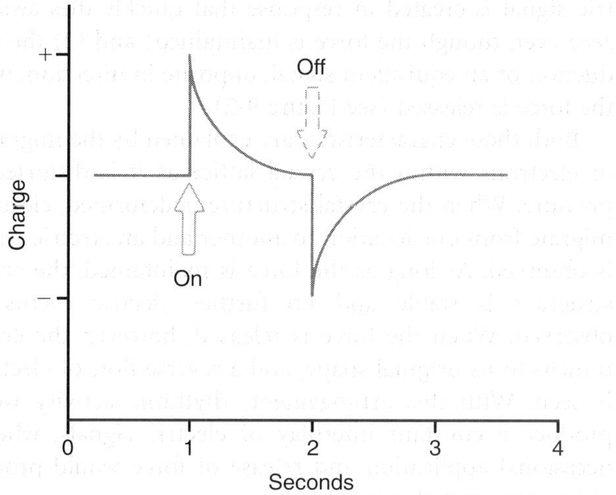

Figure 9-2 Resting pressures from the lips or cheeks and tongue are usually not balanced. In some areas, as in the mandibular anterior, tongue pressure is greater than lip pressure. In other areas, as in the maxillary incisor region, lip pressure is greater. Active stabilization produced by metabolic effects in the PDL probably explains why teeth are stable in the presence of imbalanced pressures that would otherwise cause tooth movement.

Table 9-1

Physiologic Response to Heavy Pressure Against a Tooth

Time (seconds)	Event
<1	PDL* fluid incompressible, alveolar bone bends, piezoelectric signal generated
1-2	PDL fluid expressed, tooth moves within PDL space
3-5	PDL fluid squeezed out, tissues compressed; immediate pain if pressure is heavy

*PDL, periodontal ligament.

the tissue fluids are squeezed out of its confined area. Prolonged force, even of low magnitude, produces a different physiologic response—remodeling of the adjacent bone. Orthodontic tooth movement is made possible by the application of prolonged forces. In addition, light prolonged forces in the natural environment—forces from the lips, cheeks, or tongue resting against the teeth—have the same potential as orthodontic forces to cause the teeth to move to a different location (see the discussion of equilibrium factors in Chapter 5).

Role of the Periodontal Ligament in Eruption and Stabilization of the Teeth

The phenomenon of tooth eruption makes it plain that forces generated within the PDL itself can produce tooth

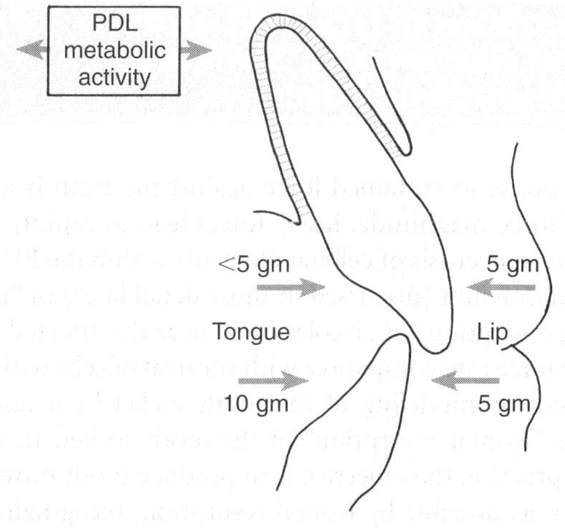

Figure 9-3 When a force is applied to a crystalline structure (like bone or collagen), a flow of current is produced that quickly dies away. When the force is released, an opposite current flow is observed. The piezoelectric effect results from migration of electrons within the crystal lattice.

movement. The eruption mechanism appears to depend on metabolic events within the PDL, including but perhaps not limited to formation, cross-linkage and maturational shortening of collagen fibers (see Marks[4] for a comprehensive review). This process continues, although at a reduced rate, into adult life. A tooth whose antagonist has been extracted will often begin to erupt again after many years of apparent quiescence.

The continuing presence of this mechanism indicates that it may produce not only eruption of the teeth under appropriate circumstances but also active stabilization of the teeth against prolonged forces of light magnitude. It is commonly observed that light prolonged pressures against the teeth are not in perfect balance, as would seem to be required if tooth movement were not to occur (Figure 9-3). The ability of the PDL to generate a force and thereby contribute to the set of forces that determine the equilibrium situation, probably explains this (see the discussion of equilibrium in Chapter 5).

Active stabilization also implies a threshold for orthodontic force, since forces below the stabilization level would be expected to be ineffective. The threshold for outside force, of course, would vary depending on the extent to which existing soft tissue pressures were already being resisted by the stabilization mechanism. In some experiments, the threshold for orthodontic force, if one existed at all, appeared extremely low. In other circumstances, a somewhat higher threshold, but still one of only a few grams, seems to exist. The current concept is that active stabilization can overcome prolonged forces of a few grams at most, perhaps up to the 5 to 10 gm/cm^2 often observed as the magnitude of unbalanced soft tissue resting pressures.

Periodontal Ligament and Bone Response to Sustained Orthodontic Force

The response to sustained force against the teeth is a function of force magnitude: heavy forces lead to rapidly developing pain, necrosis of cellular elements within the PDL, and the phenomenon (discussed in more detail later) of "undermining resorption" of alveolar bone near the affected tooth. Lighter forces are compatible with survival of cells within the PDL and a remodeling of the tooth socket by a relatively painless "frontal resorption" of the tooth socket. In orthodontic practice, the objective is to produce tooth movement as much as possible by frontal resorption, recognizing that some areas of PDL necrosis and undermining resorption will probably occur despite efforts to prevent this.

Biologic Control of Tooth Movement

Before discussing in detail the response to orthodontic force, it is necessary to consider the biologic control mechanisms that lead from the stimulus of sustained force application to the response of orthodontic tooth movement. Two possible control elements, biologic electricity and pressure-tension in the PDL that affects blood flow, are contrasted in the two major theories of orthodontic tooth movement. The bioelectric theory relates tooth movement at least in part to changes in bone metabolism controlled by the electric signals that are produced when alveolar bone flexes and bends. The pressure-tension theory relates tooth movement to cellular changes produced by chemical messengers, traditionally thought to be generated by alterations in blood flow through the PDL. Pressure and tension within the PDL, by reducing (pressure) or increasing (tension) the diameter of blood vessels in the ligament space, could certainly alter blood flow. The two theories are neither incompatible nor mutually exclusive. From a contemporary perspective, it appears that both mechanisms may play a part in the biologic control of tooth movement.[5]

Electric signals that might initiate tooth movement initially were thought to be piezoelectric. Piezoelectricity is a phenomenon observed in many crystalline materials in which a deformation of the crystal structure produces a flow of electric current as electrons are displaced from one part of the crystal lattice to another. The piezoelectricity of many inorganic crystals has been recognized for many years and has been used in everyday technology (e.g., the crystal pickup found in inexpensive phonographic systems). Organic crystals can also have piezoelectric properties. Not only is bone mineral a crystal structure with piezoelectric properties, collagen itself is piezoelectric, and stress-generated potentials in dried bone specimens can be attributed to piezoelectricity.

Piezoelectric signals have two unusual characteristics: (1) a quick decay rate (i.e., when a force is applied, a piezoelectric signal is created in response that quickly dies away to zero even though the force is maintained) and (2) the production of an equivalent signal, opposite in direction, when the force is released (see Figure 9-2).

Both these characteristics are explained by the migration of electrons within the crystal lattice as it is distorted by pressure. When the crystal structure is deformed, electrons migrate from one location to another and an electric charge is observed. As long as the force is maintained, the crystal structure is stable and no further electric events are observed. When the force is released, however, the crystal returns to its original shape, and a reverse flow of electrons is seen. With this arrangement, rhythmic activity would produce a constant interplay of electric signals, whereas occasional application and release of force would produce only occasional electric signals.

Ions in the fluids that bathe living bone interact with the complex electric field generated when the bone bends, causing temperature changes as well as electric signals. As a result, both convection and conduction currents can be detected in the extracellular fluids, and the currents are affected by the nature of the fluids. The small voltages that are observed are called the "streaming potential." These voltages, though different from piezoelectric signals in dry material, have in common their rapid onset and alteration, as changing stresses are placed on the bone. There is also a reverse piezoelectric effect. Not only will the application of force cause distortion of crystalline structure and with it an electric signal, application of an electric field can cause a crystal to deform and produce force in doing so. Reverse piezoelectricity has no place in natural control systems, at least as far as is presently known, but there are intriguing possibilities for using external electric fields to promote bone healing and regeneration after injury.[6]

There is no longer any doubt that stress-generated signals are important in the general maintenance of the skeleton. Without such signals, bone mineral is lost and general skeletal atrophy ensues—a situation that has proved troublesome for astronauts whose bones no longer flex in a weightless environment as they would under normal gravity. Signals generated by the bending of alveolar bone during normal chewing almost surely are important for maintenance of the bone around the teeth. On the other hand, sustained force of the type used to induce orthodontic tooth movement does not produce prominent stress-generated signals. When the force is applied, a brief signal is created; when it is removed, the reverse signal appears. As long as the force is sustained, however, nothing happens. If stress-generated signals were important in producing the bone remodeling associated with orthodontic tooth movement, a vibrating application of pressure would be advantageous. Experiments indicate little or no advantage in vibrating over sustained force for the movement of teeth[7]; in fact, there may be disadvantages. It appears that stress-generated signals, important as they may be for normal skeletal function, probably have little if anything to do with the response to orthodontic tooth movement.

One should not conclude from this that all types of electric signals are unimportant in the control of tooth movement. A second type of endogenous electric signal, which is called the "bioelectric potential," can be observed in bone that is not being stressed. Metabolically active bone or connective tissue cells (in areas of active growth or remodeling) produce electronegative charges that are generally proportional to how active they are; inactive cells and areas are nearly electrically neutral. Although the purpose of this bioelectric potential is not known, cellular activity can be modified by adding exogenous electric signals. The effects, presumably, are felt at cell membranes. Membrane depolarization triggers nerve impulses and muscle contraction, but changes in membrane potentials accompany other cellular responses as well. The external electric signals probably affect cell membrane receptors, membrane permeability, or both.[8] Both animal and human experiments indicate that when low voltage direct current is applied to the alveolar bone, modifying the bioelectric potential, a tooth moves faster than its control in response to an identical spring.[9]

Electromagnetic fields also can affect cell membrane potentials and permeability, and thereby trigger changes in cellular activity. In animal experiments, a pulsed electromagnetic field increased the role of tooth movement, apparently by shortening the initial "lag phase" before tooth movement begins.[10] Electromagnetic fields can be induced within tissues by adjacent magnets, without the contact required by electrodes, and bone healing has been shown to be enhanced by certain types of fields. It is possible that this effect can be utilized in the future to enhance orthodontic tooth movement and/or alter jaw growth. Perhaps a fair conclusion is that even though stress-generated electrical signals do not explain tooth movement, electric and electromagnetic influences can modify the bony remodeling on which tooth movement depends and may yet prove useful therapeutically. It seems highly unlikely, however, that the fields generated by small magnets attached to the teeth to generate tooth-moving forces (see Chapter 10) could change the basic biology of the response to force. Claims that magnetic force generation reduces pain and mobility are not supported by evidence.

Pressure-Tension Theory

The pressure-tension theory, the classic theory of tooth movement, relies on chemical rather than electric signals as the stimulus for cellular differentiation and ultimately tooth movement. There is no doubt that chemical messengers are important in the cascade of events that lead to remodeling of alveolar bone and tooth movement. Because this theory does explain the course of events reasonably well, it remains the basis of the following discussion.

In this theory, an alteration in blood flow within the PDL is produced by the sustained pressure that causes the tooth to shift position within the PDL space, compressing the ligament in some areas while stretching it in others. Blood flow is decreased where the PDL is compressed (Figure 9-4), while it usually is maintained or increased where the PDL is under tension (Figure 9-5). If regions of the PDL are overstretched, blood flow may be decreased transiently. Alterations in blood flow quickly create changes in the chemical environment. For instance, oxygen levels certainly would fall in the compressed area, but might increase on the tension side, and the relative proportions of other metabolites would also change in a matter of minutes. These chemical changes, acting either directly or by stimulating the release of other biologically active agents, then would stimulate cellular differentiation and activity. In essence, this view of tooth movement shows three stages: (1) alterations in blood flow associated with pressure within the PDL, (2) the formation and/or release of chemical messengers, and (3) activation of cells (Table 9-2).

Effects of Force Magnitude

The heavier the sustained pressure, the greater should be the reduction in blood flow through compressed areas of the PDL, up to the point that the vessels are totally collapsed and no further blood flows (Figure 9-6). That this theoretic sequence actually occurs has been demonstrated in animal experiments, in which increasing the force against a tooth causes decreasing perfusion of the PDL on the compression side (see Figures 9-4 and 9-5).[11] Let us consider the time course of events after application of orthodontic force, contrasting what happens with heavy vs. light force (see Table 9-2).

When light but prolonged force is applied to a tooth, blood flow through the partially compressed PDL decreases as soon as fluids are expressed from the PDL space and the tooth moves in its socket (i.e., in a few seconds). Within a few hours at most, the resulting change in the chemical environment produces a different pattern of cellular activity. Animal experiments have shown that increased levels of cyclic adenosine monophosphate (AMP), the "second messenger" for many important cellular functions including differentiation, appear after about 4 hours of sustained pressure.[12] This amount of time to produce a response correlates rather well with the human response to removable appliances. If a removable appliance is worn less than 4 to 6 hours per day, it will produce no orthodontic effects. Above this duration threshold, tooth movement does occur.

What happens in the first hours after sustained force was placed against a tooth, between the onset of pressure and tension in the PDL and the appearance of second messengers a few hours later? Experiments have shown that prostaglandin and interleukin-1 beta levels increase within the PDL within a short time after the application of pressure, and it is clear now that prostaglandin E is an important mediator of the cellular response.[13] Changes in cell shape probably play a role. There is some evidence that prostaglandins are released when cells are mechanically deformed (i.e., prostaglandin release may be a primary rather than a secondary response to pressure).[14] It is likely that mobilization of membrane phospholipids, which leads

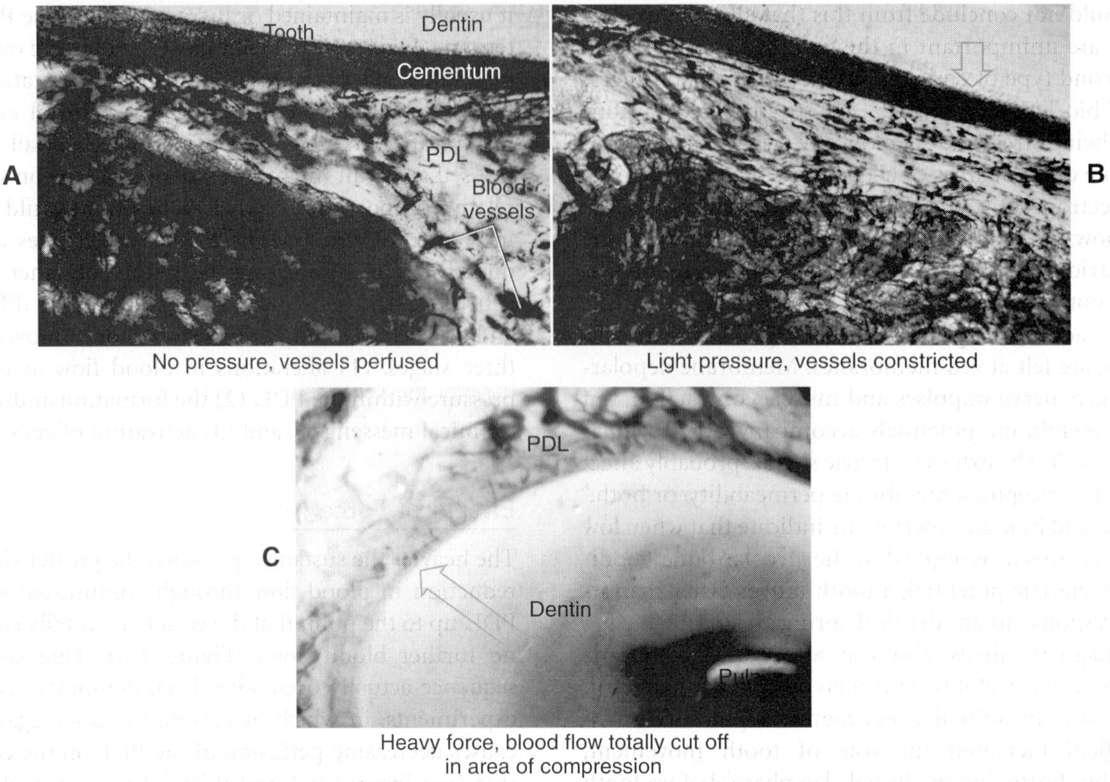

FIGURE 9-4 In experimental animals, changes in blood flow in the PDL can be observed by perfusing India ink into the vascular system while the animal is being sacrificed. The vessels are filled with India ink, so that their size can be seen easily. **A,** Normal perfusion of the PDL—note the dark areas indicating blood flow. **B,** 50 gm force compressing the PDL. Note the decreased amount of perfusion but there still is blow flow through the compressed area. **C,** Heavy force with almost complete obliteration of blood flow in the compressed area. This specimen is seen in horizontal section, with the tooth root on the left and the pulp chamber just visible in the upper left. The PDL is below and to the right. Cells disappear in the compressed areas, and the area is sometimes said to be hyalinized because of its resemblance to hyaline cartilage. (Courtesy Dr. F. E. Khouw.)

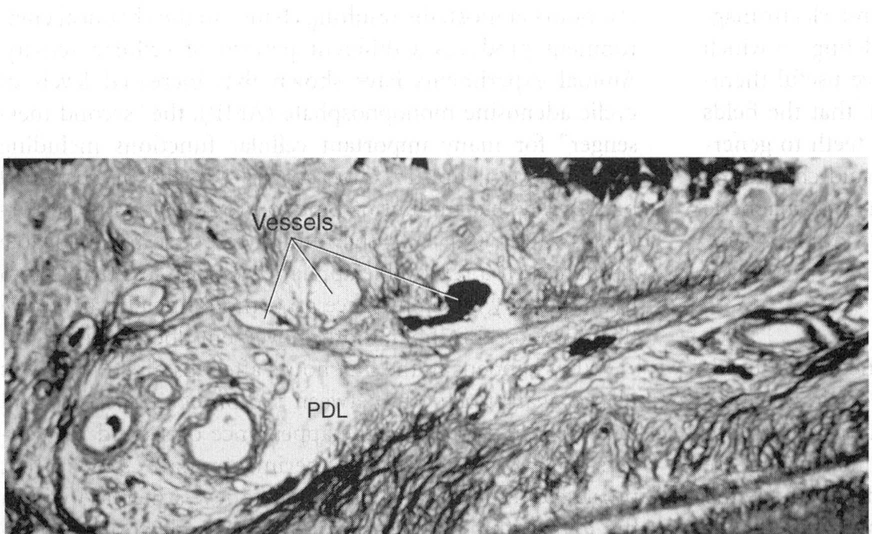

FIGURE 9-5 On the side away from the direction of tooth movement, the PDL space is enlarged and blood vessels dilate. Expanded vessels that are only partially filled can be seen on the tension side of the PDL. (Courtesy Dr. F. E. Khouw.)

TABLE 9-2

Physiologic Response to Sustained Pressure Against a Tooth

TIME		
Light pressure	**Heavy pressure**	**Event**
<1 sec		PDL* fluid incompressible, alveolar bone bends, piezoelectric signal generated
1-2 sec		PDL fluid expressed, tooth moves within PDL space
3-5 sec		Blood vessels within PDL partially compressed on pressure side, dilated on tension side; PDL fibers and cells mechanically distorted
Minutes		Blood flow altered, oxygen tension begins to change; prostaglandins and cytokines released
Hours		Metabolic changes occurring: Chemical messengers affect cellular activity, enzyme levels change
~4 hours		Increased cAMP levels detectable, cellular differentiation begins within PDL
~2 days		Tooth movement beginning as osteoclasts/osteoblasts remodel bony socket
	3-5 sec	Blood vessels within PDL occluded on pressure side
	Minutes	Blood flow cut off to compressed PDL area
	Hours	Cell death in compressed area
	3-5 days	Cell differentiation in adjacent narrow spaces, undermining resorption begins
	7-14 days	Undermining resorption removes lamina dura adjacent to compressed PDL, tooth movement occurs

*PDL, periodontal ligament.

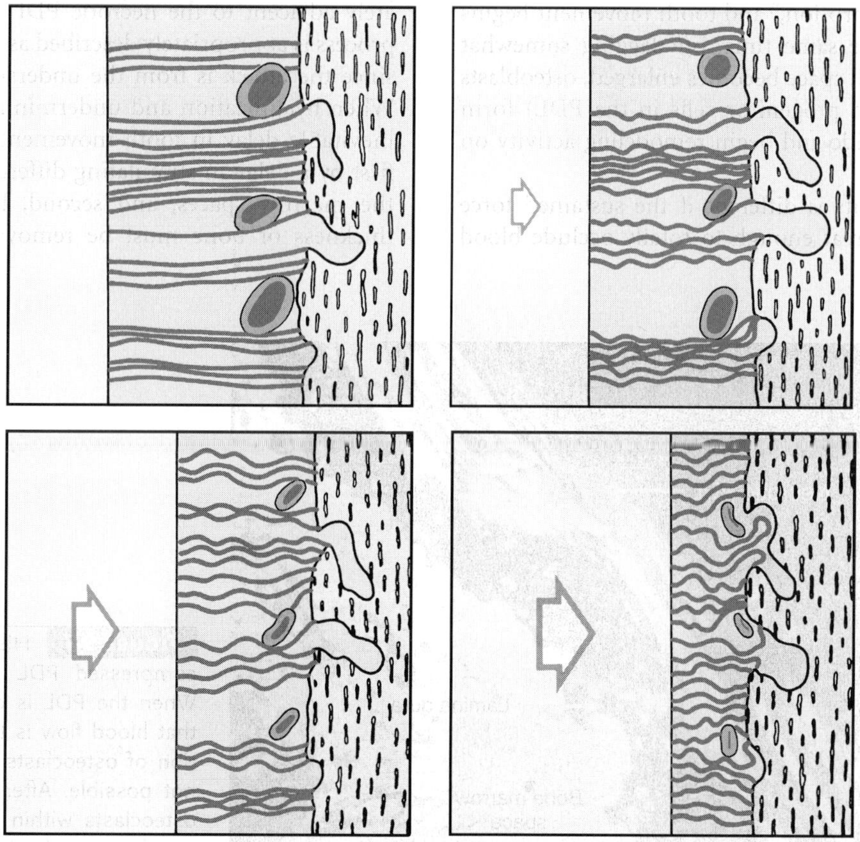

FIGURE 9-6 Diagrammatic representation of the increasing compression of blood vessels as pressure increases in the PDL. At a certain magnitude of continuous pressure, blood vessels are totally occluded and a sterile necrosis of PDL tissue ensues.

to the formation of inositol phosphates, is another pathway toward the eventual cellular response. Other chemical messengers, particularly members of the cytokine family but also nitric oxide (NO) and other regulators of cellular activity, also are involved.[15] Since drugs of various types can affect both prostaglandin levels and other potential chemical messengers, it is clear that pharmacologic modification of the response to orthodontic force is more than just a theoretic possibility (see the discussion on p. 343 of drug interactions with orthodontic treatment).

For a tooth to move, osteoclasts must be formed so that they can remove bone from the area adjacent to the compressed part of the PDL. Osteoblasts also are needed to form new bone on the tension side and remodel resorbed areas on the pressure side. Prostaglandin E has the interesting property of stimulating both osteoclastic and osteoblastic activity, making it particularly suitable as a mediator of tooth movement. If parathyroid hormone is injected, osteoclasts can be induced in only a few hours, but the response is much slower when mechanical deformation of the PDL is the stimulus, and it can be up to 48 hours before the first osteoclasts appear within and adjacent to the compressed PDL. Studies of cellular kinetics indicate that they arrive in two waves, implying that some (the first wave) may be derived from a local cell population, while others (the larger second wave) are brought in from distant areas via blood flow.[16] These cells attack the adjacent lamina dura, removing bone in the process of "frontal resorption," and tooth movement begins soon thereafter. At the same time, but lagging somewhat behind so that the PDL space becomes enlarged, osteoblasts (recruited locally from progenitor cells in the PDL) form bone on the tension side and begin remodeling activity on the pressure side.

The course of events is different if the sustained force against the tooth is great enough to totally occlude blood vessels and cut off the blood supply to an area within the PDL. When this happens, rather than cells within the compressed area of the PDL being stimulated to develop into osteoclasts, a sterile necrosis ensues within the compressed area. In clinical orthodontics it is difficult to avoid pressure that produces at least some avascular areas in the PDL, and it has been suggested that releasing pressure against a tooth at intervals, while maintaining the pressure for enough hours to produce the biologic response, could help in maintaining tissue vitality. At present, however, there is no practical way to implement this approach. It is possible in the future that interrupted force of this type will become clinically useful, if methods for activating and de-activating springs can be worked out.

Because of its histologic appearance as the cells disappear, an avascular area in the PDL traditionally has been referred to as *hyalinized* (see Figure 9-4). Despite the name, the process has nothing to do with the formation of hyaline connective tissue but represents the inevitable loss of all cells when the blood supply is totally cut off. When this happens, remodeling of bone bordering the necrotic area of the PDL must be accomplished by cells derived from adjacent undamaged areas.

After a delay of several days, cellular elements begin to invade the necrotic (hyalinized) area. More importantly, osteoclasts appear within the adjacent bone marrow spaces and begin an attack on the underside of the bone immediately adjacent to the necrotic PDL area (Figure 9-7). This process is appropriately described as *undermining resorption*, since the attack is from the underside of the lamina dura. When hyalinization and undermining resorption occur, an inevitable delay in tooth movement results. This is caused first by a delay in stimulating differentiation of cells within the marrow spaces, and second, because a considerable thickness of bone must be removed from the underside

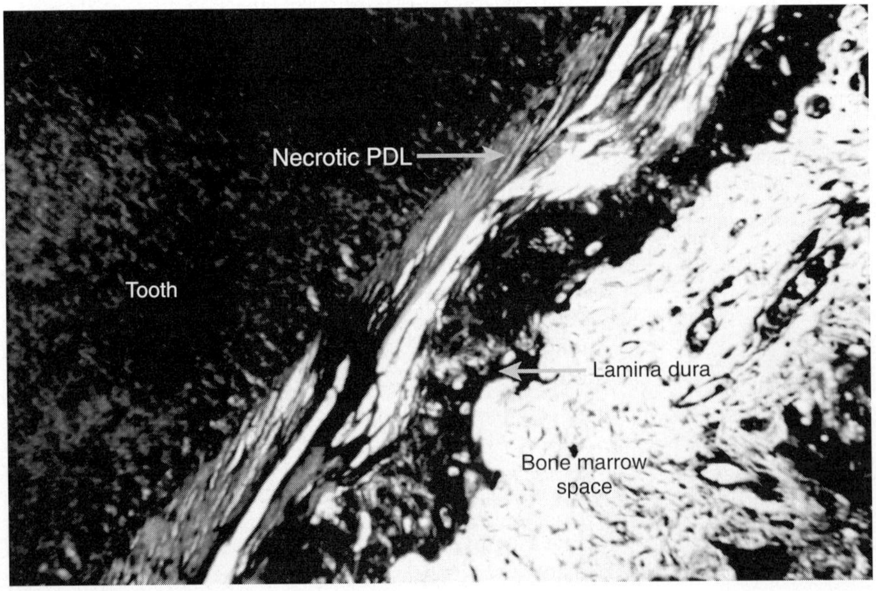

Figure 9-7 Histologic specimen of compressed PDL area after several days. When the PDL is compressed to the point that blood flow is totally cut off, differentiation of osteoclasts within the PDL space is not possible. After a delay of several days, osteoclasts within adjacent marrow spaces attack the underside of the lamina dura in the process called *undermining resorption*. (Courtesy Dr. F. E. Khouw.)

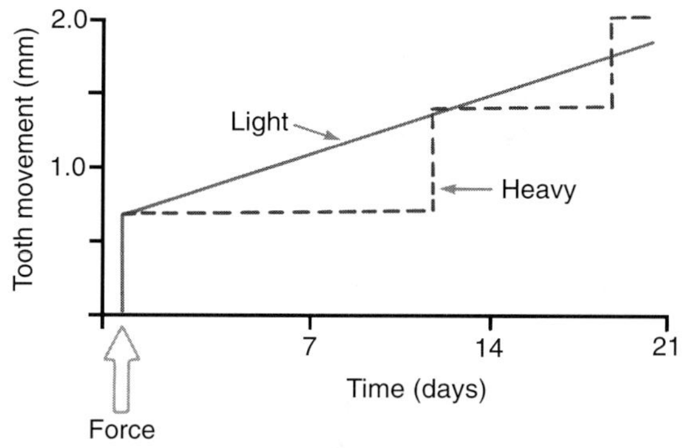

FIGURE 9-8 Diagrammatic representation of the time course of tooth movement with frontal resorption vs. undermining resorption. With frontal resorption, a steady attack on the outer surface of the lamina dura results in smooth continuous tooth movement. With undermining resorption, there is a delay until the bone adjacent to the tooth can be removed. At that point, the tooth "jumps" to a new position, and if heavy force is maintained, there will again be a delay until a second round of undermining resorption can occur.

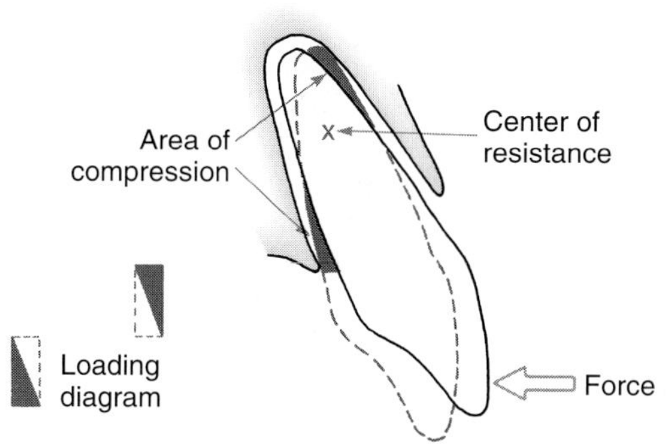

FIGURE 9-9 Application of a single force to the crown of a tooth creates rotation around a point approximately halfway down the root. Heavy pressure is felt at the root apex and at the crest of the alveolar bone, but pressure decreases to zero at the center of resistance. The loading diagram, therefore, consists of two triangles as shown.

before any tooth movement can take place. The different time course of tooth movement when frontal resorption is compared with undermining resorption is shown graphically in Figure 9-8.

Not only is tooth movement more efficient when areas of PDL necrosis are avoided but pain is also lessened. However, even with light forces, small avascular areas are likely to develop in the PDL and tooth movement will be delayed until these can be removed by undermining resorption. The smooth progression of tooth movement with light force shown in Figure 9-8 may be an unattainable ideal when continuous force is used. In clinical practice, tooth movement usually proceeds in a more stepwise fashion because of the inevitable areas of undermining resorption. Nevertheless, too much force is not helpful.

Effects of Force Distribution and Types of Tooth Movement

From the previous discussion, it is apparent that the optimum force levels for orthodontic tooth movement should be just high enough to stimulate cellular activity without completely occluding blood vessels in the PDL. Both the amount of force delivered to a tooth and also the area of the PDL over which that force is distributed are important in determining the biologic effect. The PDL response is determined not by force alone, but by force per unit area, or pressure. Since the distribution of force within the PDL, and therefore the pressure, differs with different types of tooth movement, it is necessary to specify the type of tooth movement as well as the amount of force in discussing optimum force levels for orthodontic purposes.

The simplest form of orthodontic movement is tipping. Tipping movements are produced when a single force (e.g., a spring extending from a removable appliance) is applied against the crown of a tooth. When this is done, the tooth rotates around its "center of resistance," a point located about halfway down the root. (A further discussion of the center of resistance and its control follows in Chapter 10.) When the tooth rotates in this fashion, the PDL is compressed near the root apex on the same side as the spring and at the crest of the alveolar bone on the opposite side from the spring (Figure 9-9). Maximum pressure in the PDL is created at the alveolar crest and at the root apex. Progressively less pressure is created as the center of resistance is approached, and there is minimum pressure at that point.

In tipping, only one-half the PDL area that could be loaded actually is. As shown in Figure 9-9, the "loading diagram" consists of two triangles, covering half the total PDL area. On the other hand, pressure in the two areas where it is concentrated is high in relation to the force applied to the crown. For this reason, forces used to tip teeth must be kept quite low. Both experiments with animals and clinical experience with humans suggest that tipping forces should not exceed approximately 50 gm.

If two forces are applied simultaneously to the crown of a tooth, the tooth can be moved bodily (translated) (i.e., the root apex and crown move in the same direction the same amount). In this case, the total PDL area is loaded uniformly (Figure 9-10). It is apparent that to produce the same pressure in the PDL and therefore the same biologic response, twice as much force would be required for bodily movement as for tipping. To move a tooth so that it is partially tipped and partially translated would require forces intermediate between those needed for pure tipping and bodily movement (Table 9-3).

In theory, forces to produce rotation of a tooth around its long axis could be much larger than those to produce other

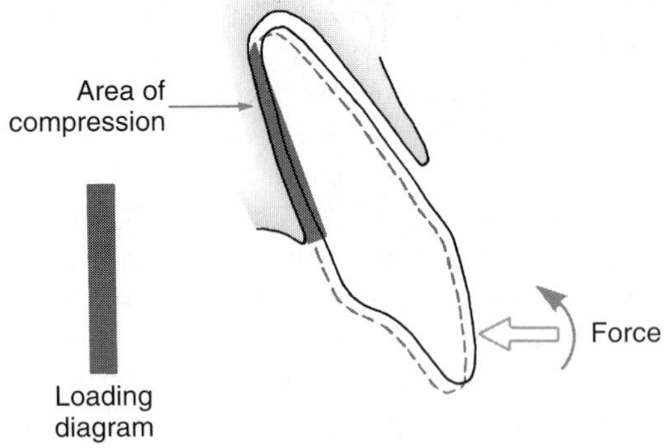

FIGURE 9-10 Translation or bodily movement of a tooth requires that the PDL space be loaded uniformly from alveolar crest to apex, creating a rectangular loading diagram. Twice as much force applied to the crown of the tooth would be required to produce the same pressure within the PDL for bodily movement as compared with tipping.

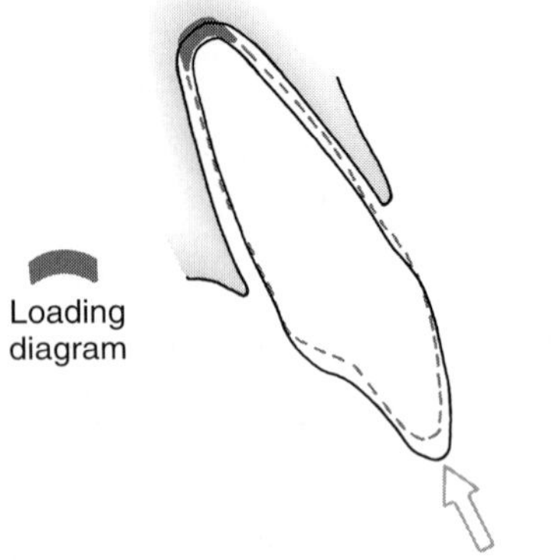

FIGURE 9-11 When a tooth is intruded, the force is concentrated over a small area at the apex. For this reason, extremely light forces are needed to produce appropriate pressure within the PDL during intrusion.

TABLE 9-3

Optimum Forces for Orthodontic Tooth Movement

Type of movement	Force* (gm)
Tipping	35-60
Bodily movement (translation)	70-120
Root uprighting	50-100
Rotation	35-60
Extrusion	35-60
Intrusion	10-20

*Values depend in part on the size of the tooth; smaller values appropriate for incisors, higher values for multirooted posterior teeth.

tooth movements, since the force could be distributed over the entire PDL rather than over a narrow vertical strip. In fact, however, it is essentially impossible to apply a rotational force so that the tooth does not also tip in its socket, and when this happens, an area of compression is created just as in any other tipping movement. For this reason, appropriate forces for rotation are similar to those for tipping.

Extrusion and intrusion are also special cases. Extrusive movements ideally would produce no areas of compression within the PDL, only tension. Like rotation, this is probably more a theoretic than a practical possibility, since if the tooth tipped at all while being extruded, areas of compression would be created. Even if compressed areas could be avoided, heavy forces in pure tension would be undesirable unless the goal was to extract the tooth rather than to bring alveolar bone along with the tooth. Extrusive forces, like rotation, should be of about the same magnitude as those for tipping.

For many years it was considered essentially impossible to produce orthodontic intrusion of teeth. It has become clear that clinically successful intrusion can be accomplished, but only if very light forces are applied to the teeth. Light force is required for intrusion because the force will be concentrated in a small area at the tooth apex (Figure 9-11). As with extrusion, the tooth probably will tip somewhat as it is intruded, but the loading diagram nevertheless will show high force concentration at the apex. Only if the force is kept very light can intrusion be expected.

Effects of Force Duration and Force Decay

The key to producing orthodontic tooth movement is the application of sustained force, which does not mean that the force must be absolutely continuous. It does mean that the force must be present for a considerable percentage of the time, certainly hours rather than minutes per day. As we have noted previously, animal experiments suggest that only after force is maintained for approximately 4 hours do cyclic nucleotide levels in the PDL increase, indicating that this duration of pressure is required to produce the "second messengers" needed to stimulate cellular differentiation.

Clinical experience suggests that there is a threshold for force duration in humans in the 4-8 hour range, and that increasingly effective tooth movement is produced if force is maintained for longer durations. Although no firm experimental data are available, a plot of efficiency of tooth movement as a function of force duration would probably look like Figure 9-12. Continuous forces, produced by fixed appliances that are not affected by what the patient does, produce more tooth movement than removable appliances unless the removable appliance is present almost all the time. Removable appliances worn for decreasing fractions of time produce decreasing amounts of tooth movement. If the idea of providing brief intervals of no pressure and resumed blood flow (to improve the vitality of PDL tissues) is ever to be used clinically, it will be necessary to modify fixed appliances to do this. With removable appliances, not only are

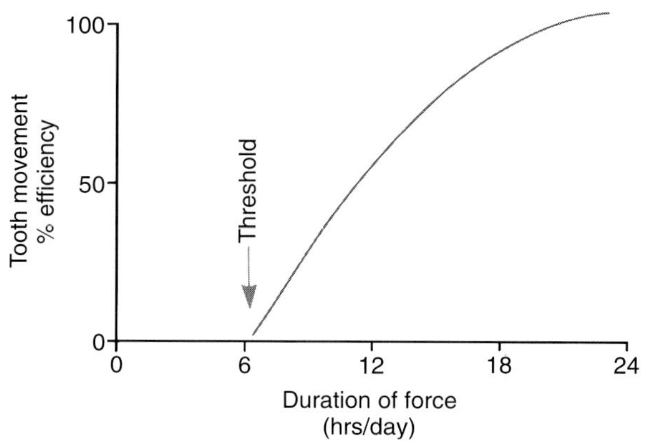

FIGURE 9-12 Theoretic plot of tooth movement efficiency versus duration of force in hours per day. Continuous force, 24 hours per day, produces the most efficient tooth movement, but successful tooth movement can be produced by shorter durations, with a threshold at about 6 hours.

patients too unreliably compliant, the two-point contacts on teeth that are needed to control tooth movement (see Chapter 10) are too difficult to produce.

Duration of force has another aspect, related to how force magnitude changes as the tooth responds by moving. Only in theory is it possible to make a perfect spring, one that would deliver the same force day after day, no matter how much or how little the tooth moved in response to that force. In reality, some decline in force magnitude (i.e., force decay) is noted with even the springiest device after the tooth has moved a short distance (though with the superelastic nickel-titanium materials discussed in Chapter 10, the decrease is amazingly small). With many orthodontic devices, the force may drop all the way to zero. From this perspective, orthodontic force duration is classified (Figure 9-13) by the rate of decay as:

- Continuous—force maintained at some appreciable fraction of the original from one patient visit to the next
- Interrupted—force levels decline to zero between activations

Both continuous and interrupted forces can be produced by fixed appliances that are constantly present.

- Intermittent—force levels decline abruptly to zero intermittently, when the orthodontic appliance is removed by the patient or perhaps when a fixed appliance is temporarily deactivated, and then return to the original level some time later. When tooth movement occurs, force levels will decrease as they would with a fixed appliance (i.e., the intermittent force can also become interrupted between adjustments of the appliance).

Intermittent forces are produced by all patient-activated appliances, such as removable plates, headgear, and elastics. Forces generated during normal function (chewing, swallowing, speaking, etc.) can be viewed as a special case of intermittently applied forces, most of which are not maintained for enough hours per day to have significant effects on the position of the teeth.

There is an important interaction between force magnitude and how rapidly the force declines as the tooth responds. Consider first the effect of a nearly continuous force. If this force is quite light, a relatively smooth progression of tooth movement will result from frontal resorption. If the continuous force is heavy, however, tooth movement will be delayed until undermining resorption can remove the bone necessary to allow the tooth movement. At that time, the tooth will change its position rapidly, and the constant force will again compress the tissues, preventing repair of the PDL and creating the need for further undermining resorption, and so on. Such a heavy continuous force can be quite destructive to both the periodontal structures and the tooth itself (as we discuss in more detail below).

Consider now the effect of forces that decay fairly rapidly, so that the force declines to zero after the tooth moves only a short distance. If the initial force level is relatively light, the tooth will move a small amount by frontal resorption and then will remain in that position until the appliance is activated again. If the force level is heavy enough to produce undermining resorption, the tooth will move when the undermining resorption is complete. Then, since the force has dropped to zero at that point, it will remain in that position until the next activation. Although the original force is heavy, after the tooth moves there is a period for regeneration and repair of the PDL before force is applied again.

Theoretically, there is no doubt that light continuous forces produce the most efficient tooth movement. Despite the clinician's best efforts to keep forces light enough to produce only frontal resorption, some areas of undermining resorption are probably produced in every clinical patient. The heavier forces that produce this response are physiologically acceptable, only if force levels decline so that there is a period of repair and regeneration before the next activation, or if the force decreases at least to the point that no second and third rounds of undermining resorption occur.

Heavy continuous forces are to be avoided; heavy intermittent forces, though less efficient, can be clinically acceptable. To say it another way: the more perfect the spring in the sense of its ability to provide continuous force, the more careful the clinician must be that only light force is applied. Some of the cruder springs used in orthodontic treatment have the paradoxic virtue of producing forces that rapidly decline to zero and are thus incapable of inflicting the biologic damage that can occur from heavy continuous forces. Several clinical studies have indicated that heavy force applications may produce more tooth movement than lighter ones, an apparently paradox that can be understood from consideration of force decay characteristics.

Experience has shown that orthodontic appliances should not be reactivated more frequently than at 3-week intervals. A 4- to 6-week appointment cycle is more typical in clinical practice. Undermining resorption requires 7 to 14 days

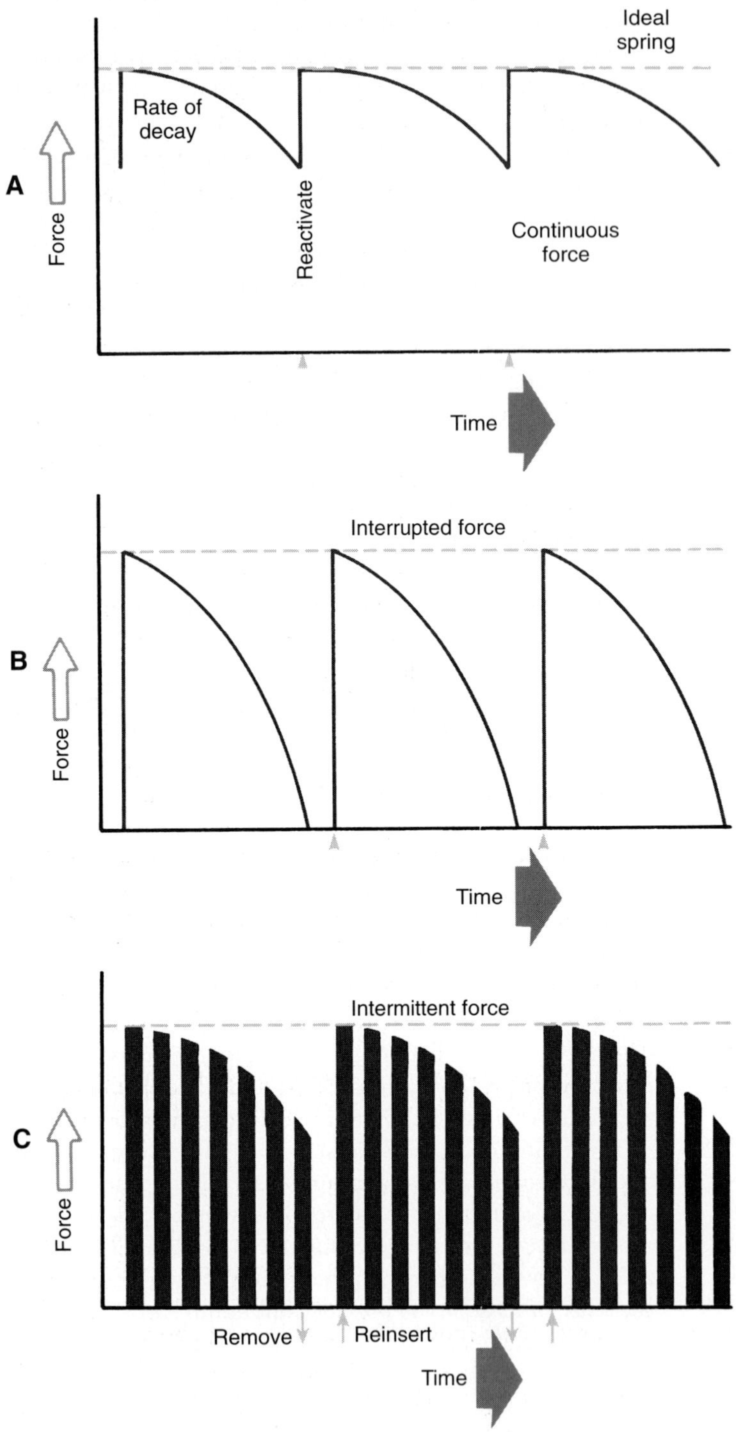

FIGURE 9-13 Diagrammatic representation of force decay. **A,** An ideal spring would maintain the same amount of force regardless of distance a tooth had moved, but with real springs the force decays at least somewhat as tooth movement occurs. Forces that are maintained between activations of an orthodontic appliance, even though the force declines, are defined as continuous. In contrast, **B,** Interrupted forces drop to zero between activations. **C,** Intermittent forces fall to zero when a removable appliance is taken out, only to resume when the appliance is reinserted into the mouth. These forces also decay as tooth movement occurs.

(longer on the initial application of force, shorter thereafter). When this is the mode of tooth movement and when force levels decline rapidly, tooth movement is essentially complete in this length of time. The wisdom of the interval between adjustments now becomes clear. If the appliance is springy and light forces produce continuous frontal resorption, there is no need for further activation. If the appliance is stiffer and undermining resorption occurs, but then the force drops to zero, the tooth movement occurs in the first 10 days or so, and there is an equal or longer period for PDL regeneration and repair before force is applied again. This repair phase is highly desirable and needed with many appliances. Activating an appliance too frequently, short circuiting the repair process, can produce damage to the teeth or bone that a longer appointment cycle would have prevented or at least minimized.

Drug Effects on the Response to Orthodontic Force

It is quite possible that pharmacologic agents to manipulate tooth movement in both directions will come into common use. At present, agents that stimulate tooth movement are unlikely to be encountered, although under some circumstances vitamin D administration can enhance the response to orthodontic force. Direct injection of prostaglandin into the periodontal ligament has been shown to increase the rate of tooth movement, but this is quite painful (a bee sting is essentially an injection of prostaglandin) and not very practical. Drugs that inhibit tooth movement, however, already are encountered frequently, though not yet prescribed for their tooth-stabilizing effect.

Two types of drugs are known to depress the response to orthodontic force and may influence current treatment: the bisphosphonates used in treatment of osteoporosis (e.g., alendronate [Fosamax] or risedronate [Actonel]), and prostaglandin inhibitors (especially the more potent members of this group that are used in treatment of arthritis, like indomethacin).

Osteoporosis is a problem particularly in postmenopausal females but is associated with aging in both sexes. Medication for this purpose, therefore, is encountered almost entirely in older adult orthodontic patients. Estrogen therapy (usually Evista), which is used frequently to prevent loss of bone in older women, has little or no impact on orthodontic treatment, but pharmacologic agents that inhibit bone resorption are a potential problem. At present bisphosphonates, synthetic analogues of pyrophosphate that bind to hydroxyapatite in bone, are the major class of drugs of this type. They act as specific inhibitors of osteoclast-mediated bone resorption, so it is not surprising that the bone remodeling necessary for tooth movement is slower in patients on this medication. If orthodontic treatment were necessary in an older woman taking one of these agents, it would be worthwhile to explore with her physician the possibility of switching to Evista, at least temporarily.

If prostaglandin E plays an important role in the cascade of signals that leads to tooth movement, one would expect inhibitors of its activity to affect tooth movement. Drugs that affect prostaglandin activity fall into two categories: (1) corticosteroids and nonsteroidal antiinflammatory drugs (NSAIDs) that interfere with prostaglandin synthesis, and (2) other agents that have mixed agonistic and antagonistic effects on various prostaglandins. In the body, prostaglandins are formed from arachidonic acid, which in turn is derived from phospholipids. Corticosteroids reduce prostaglandin synthesis by inhibiting the formation of arachidonic acid; NSAIDs inhibit the conversion of arachidonic acid to prostaglandins.

Both children and adults on chronic steroid therapy may be encountered, and the possibility of difficult tooth movement in these patients must be kept in mind. The fact that analgesics often are prostaglandin inhibitors raises the interesting possibility that the medication used by many patients to control pain after orthodontic appointments could interfere with tooth movement. Fortunately, although potent prostaglandin inhibitors like indomethacin can inhibit tooth movement,[17] the common analgesics (ibuprofen, aspirin) seem to have little or no inhibiting effect on tooth movement at the dose levels used with orthodontic patients.

Several other classes of drugs can affect prostaglandin levels, and therefore could affect the response to orthodontic force. Tricyclic antidepressants (doxepin, amitriptyline, imipramine), antiarrhythmic agents (procaine), antimalarial drugs (quinine, quinidine, chloroquine), and methyl xanthines fall into this category. In addition, the anticonvulsant drug phenytoin has been reported to decrease tooth movement in rats, and some tetracyclines (e.g., doxycycline) inhibit osteoclast recruitment, an effect similar to bisphosphonates. It is possible that unusual responses to orthodontic force could be encountered in patients taking any of these medications.

Recently, the possibility that locally applied prostaglandin inhibitors could be used to decrease the response of specific teeth has been explored.[18] It now is possible in periodontal therapy to place miniature spheres that release a specific antibiotic into the gingival sulcus and in periodontal pockets. If a prostaglandin inhibitor were placed in similar mini-spheres and could be maintained in the sulcus around teeth that were to serve as anchors, the improved anchorage would allow more effective movement of the teeth whose movement was desired. This, of course, leads us directly to a discussion of anchorage.

ANCHORAGE AND ITS CONTROL

Anchorage: Resistance to Unwanted Tooth Movement

The term *anchorage,* in its orthodontic application, is defined in an unusual way: the definition as "resistance to unwanted tooth movement" includes a statement of what the dentist desires. The usage, though unusual, is clearest when presented this way. The dentist or orthodontist always constructs an appliance to produce certain desired tooth movements. For every (desired) action there is an equal and opposite reaction. Inevitably, reaction forces can move other teeth as well if the appliance contacts them. Anchorage, then, is the resistance to reaction forces that is provided (usually) by other teeth, (sometimes) by the palate, head or neck (via extraoral force) and (less frequently) by anchors screwed to the jaws.

At this point, let us focus first on controlling unwanted tooth movement when some teeth are to serve as anchors. In

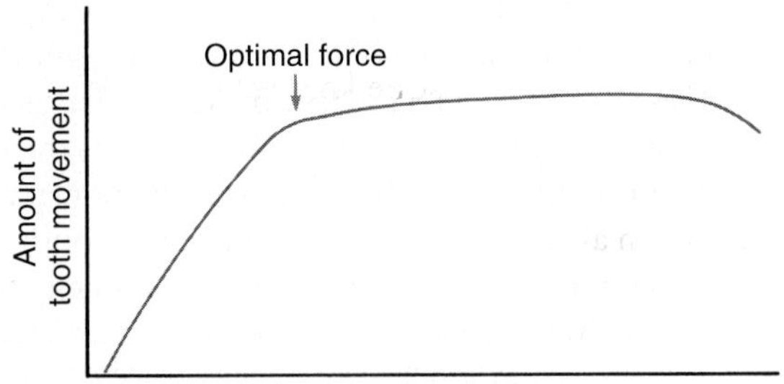

FIGURE 9-14 Theoretic representation of the relationship of pressure within the periodontal ligament to the amount of tooth movement. Pressure in the PDL is determined by the force applied to a tooth divided by the area of the PDL over which that force is distributed. The threshold for tooth movement is very small. Tooth movement increases as pressure increases up to a point, remains at about the same level over a broad range, and then may actually decline with extremely heavy pressure. The best definition of the optimum force for orthodontic purposes is the lightest force that produces a maximum or near-maximum response (i.e., that brings pressure in the PDL to the edge of the nearly-constant portion of the response curve). The magnitude of the optimum force will vary depending on the way it is distributed in the PDL (i.e., is different for different types of tooth movement [tipping, bodily movement, intrusion, etc.]).

planning orthodontic therapy, it is simply not possible to consider only the teeth whose movement is desired. Reciprocal effects throughout the dental arches must be carefully analyzed, evaluated, and controlled. An important aspect of treatment is maximizing the tooth movement that is desired, while minimizing undesirable side effects.

Relationship of Tooth Movement to Force

An obvious strategy for anchorage control would be to concentrate the force needed to produce tooth movement where it was desired, and then to dissipate the reaction force over as many other teeth as possible, keeping the pressure in the PDL of anchor teeth as low as possible. A threshold, below which pressure would produce no reaction, could provide perfect anchorage control, since it would only be necessary to be certain that the threshold for tooth movement was not reached for teeth in the anchorage unit. A differential response to pressure, so that heavier pressure produced more tooth movement than lighter pressure, would make it possible to move some teeth more than others even though some undesired tooth movement occurred.

In fact, the threshold for tooth movement appears to be quite low, but there is a differential response to pressure, and so this strategy of "divide and conquer" is reasonably effective. As Figure 9-14 indicates, teeth behave as if orthodontic movement is proportional to the magnitude of the pressure, up to a point. When that point is reached, the amount of tooth movement becomes more or less independent of the magnitude of the pressure, so that a broad plateau of orthodontically effective pressure is created.[19] The optimum force level for orthodontic movement is the lightest force and resulting pressure that produces a near-maximum response (i.e., at the edge of the plateau). Forces greater than that, though equally effective in producing tooth movement, would be unnecessarily traumatic and, as we will see, unnecessarily stressful to anchorage.

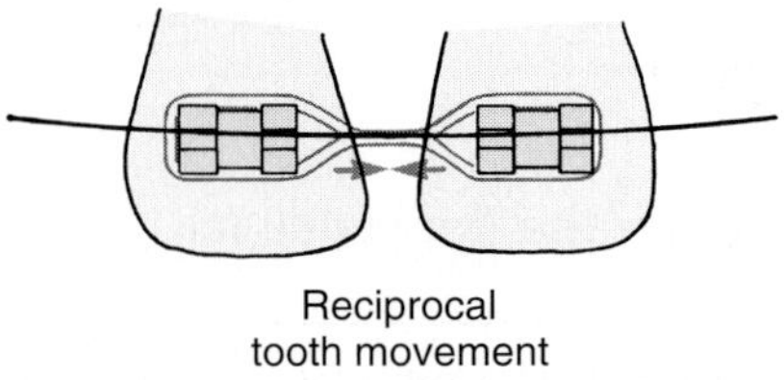

FIGURE 9-15 Reciprocal tooth movement is produced when two teeth or resistance units of equal size pull against each other, as in this example of the reciprocal closure of a maxillary midline diastema.

Anchorage Situations

From this background, we can now define several anchorage situations.

Reciprocal Tooth Movement

In a reciprocal situation, the forces applied to teeth and to arch segments are equal, and so is the force distribution in the PDL. A simple example is what would occur if two maxillary central incisors separated by a diastema were connected by an active spring (Figure 9-15). The essentially identical teeth would feel the same force distributed in the same way through the PDL and would move toward each other by the same amount.

A somewhat similar situation would arise if a spring were placed across a first premolar extraction site, pitting the central incisor, lateral incisor and canine in the anterior arch segment against the second premolar and first molar posteriorly. Whether this technique would really produce reciprocal tooth movement requires some thought. Certainly the same force would be felt by the three anterior teeth and the two posterior teeth, since the action of the spring on one segment has an equal and opposite reaction on the other. Reciprocal movement would require the same total PDL area over which the force was distributed.

Conceptually, the "anchorage value" of a tooth, that is, its resistance to movement, can be thought of as a function of its root surface area, which is the same as its PDL area. The larger the root, the greater the area over which a force can be distributed, and vice versa. As Figure 9-16 shows, the PDL area for the two posterior teeth in this example is slightly larger than the total anterior PDL area. Therefore with a simple spring connecting the segments, the anterior teeth would move slightly more than the posterior teeth. The

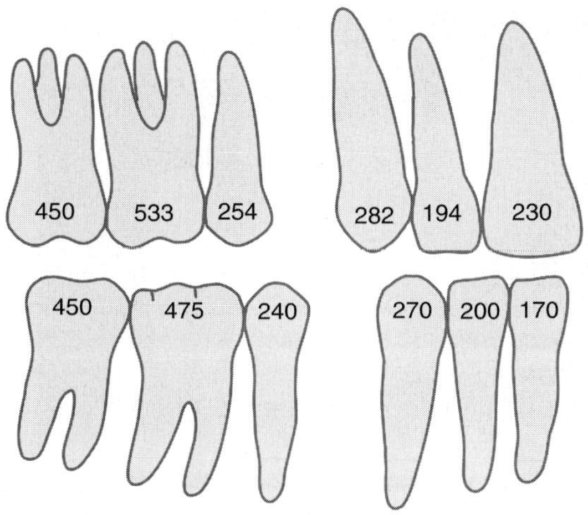

FIGURE 9-16 The "anchorage value" of any tooth is roughly equivalent to its root surface area. As this diagram shows, the first molar and second premolar in each arch are approximately equal in surface area to the canine and two incisors. (Modified from Freeman DC. Root Surface Area Related to Anchorage in the Begg Technique. Memphis: University of Tennessee Department of Orthodontics, M.S. Thesis, 1965.)

movement would not be truly reciprocal but would be close to it.

Reinforced Anchorage

Continuing with the extraction site example: if it was desired to differentially retract the anterior teeth, the anchorage of the posterior teeth could be reinforced by adding the second molar to the posterior unit (see Figure 9-16). This would change the ratio of the root surface areas so that there would be relatively more pressure in the PDL of the anterior teeth, and therefore relatively more retraction of the anterior segment than forward movement of the posterior segment.

Note that reinforcing anchorage by adding more resistance units is effective because with more teeth (or extraoral structures) in the anchorage, the reaction force is distributed over a larger PDL area. This reduces the pressure on the anchor units, moving them down the slope of the pressure-response curve. Now the shape of the pressure-response curve becomes important. Keeping the force light has two virtues. Not only does it minimize trauma and pain but also it makes it possible to create anchorage by taking advantage of different PDL areas in the anchor segments. As Figure 9-17 illustrates, too much force destroys the effectiveness of reinforced anchorage by pulling the anchor teeth up onto the flatter portion of the pressure-response curve. Then the clinician is said to have slipped, burned or blown the anchorage by moving the anchor teeth too much.

Stationary Anchorage

The term *stationary anchorage,* traditionally used though inherently less descriptive than the term *reinforced anchorage,* refers to the advantage that can be obtained by pitting

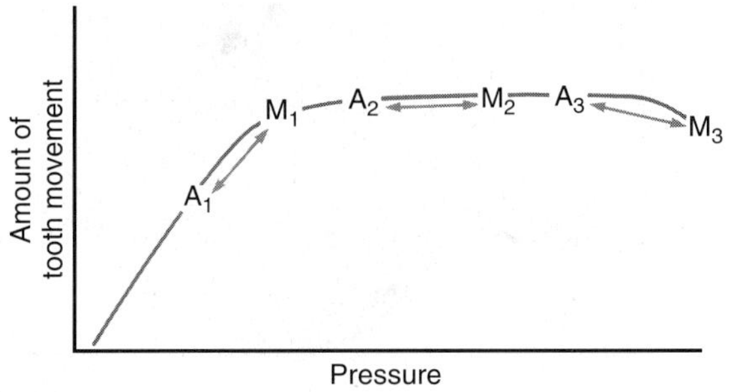

FIGURE 9-17 Consider the response of anchor teeth (**A** on the chart) and teeth to be moved *(M)* in three circumstances. In each case, the pressure in the PDL of the anchor teeth is less than the pressure in the PDL of the teeth to be moved because there are more teeth in the anchor unit. In the first case *(A1-M1),* the pressure for the teeth to be moved is optimal, whereas the pressure in the anchor unit is suboptimal, and the anchor teeth move less (anchorage is preserved). In the second case *(A2-M2),* although the pressure for the anchor teeth is less than for the teeth to be moved, both are on the plateau of the pressure-response curve, and the anchor teeth can be expected to move as much as the teeth that are desired to move (anchorage is lost). With extremely high force *(A3-M3),* the anchor teeth might move more than the teeth it was desired to move. Although the third possibility is theoretic and may not be encountered clinically, both the first and second situations are seen in clinical orthodontics. This principle explains the efficacy of light forces in controlling anchorage, and why heavy force destroys anchorage.

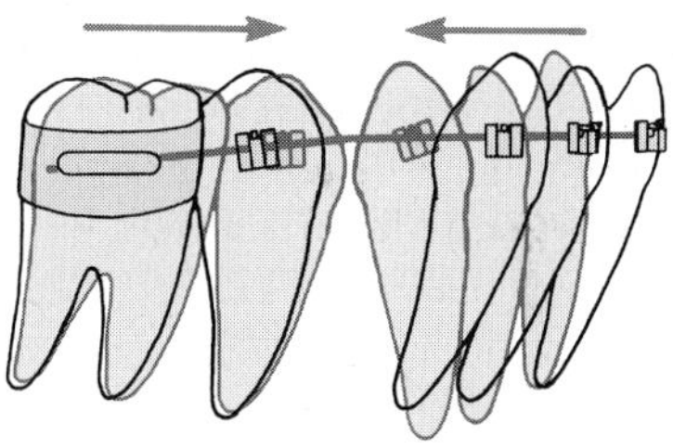

FIGURE 9-18 Displacement of anchor teeth can be minimized by arranging the force system so that the anchor teeth must move bodily if they move at all, while movement teeth are allowed to tip, as in this example of retracting incisors by tipping them posteriorly. The approach is called "stationary anchorage." In this example, treatment is not complete because the roots of the lingually tipped incisors will have to be uprighted at a later stage, but two-stage treatment with tipping followed by uprighting can be used as a means of controlling anchorage. Distributing the force over a larger PDL area of the anchor teeth reduces pressure there.

bodily movement of one group of teeth against tipping of another (Figure 9-18). Using our same example of a premolar extraction site, if the appliance were arranged so that the anterior teeth could tip lingually while the posterior teeth could only move bodily, the optimum pressure for the anterior segment would be produced by about half as much force as if the anterior teeth were to be retracted bodily. This

A
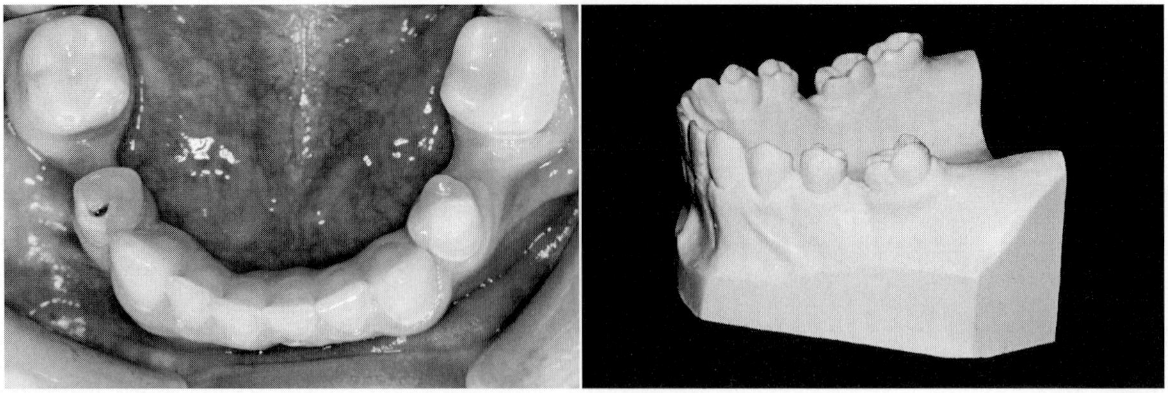
B

Figure 9-19 Loss of alveolar bone at an old extraction site can create an area of cortical bone between adjacent teeth, as the alveolar process resorbs and narrows. **A,** This child lost second primary molars early and was congenitally missing the second premolars. The greater ridge resorption on the right than the left side indicates that the right 2nd primary molar was lost first. This is one situation in which "cortical anchorage" definitely can be a factor. Closing such an extraction site is extremely difficult because of the resistance of cortical bone to remodeling. **B,** In adults who "lost" permanent first molar in adolescence, the second molar tips mesially, but resorption of alveolar bone at the extraction site narrows the ridge. Closing these spaces orthodontically also is difficult and slow, because remodeling of cortical bone is required.

would mean that the reaction force distributed over the posterior teeth would be reduced by half, and as a consequence, these teeth would move half as much.

If PDL areas were equal, tipping the anterior segment while holding the posterior segment for bodily movement would have the effect of doubling the amount of anterior retraction compared with posterior forward movement. It is important to note again, however, that successful implementation of this strategy requires light force. If the force were large enough to bring the posterior teeth into their optimum movement range, it would no longer matter whether the anterior segment tipped or was moved bodily. Using too much force would disastrously undermine this method of anchorage control.

Differential Effect of Very Large Forces

If tooth movement were actually impeded by very high levels of pressure, it might be possible to structure an anchorage situation so that there was more movement of the arch segment with the larger PDL area. This result could happen, of course, if such high force were used that the smaller segment was placed beyond the greatest tooth movement range, while the larger segment was still in it (see Figure 9-17). Because the effect would be highly traumatic, it would be an undesirable way to deliberately manage anchorage.

In fact, it is not certain that the amount of tooth movement in response to applied force really decreases with very high force levels in any circumstance, and so this type of differential movement may not really exist. By using too much force, however, it is certainly possible to produce more movement of the anchor segment than was expected, even if the mechanism is merely a differential movement of the anchor segment up the slope of the pressure-response curve rather than a decline in the response of the movement segment. Differential force is understood best in terms of the plateau portion of the curve in Figures 9-14 and 9-17, not the questionable decline at the far right.

Cortical Anchorage

Another consideration in anchorage control is the different response of cortical compared with medullary bone. Cortical bone is more resistant to resorption, and tooth movement is slowed when a root contacts it. Some authors have advocated torquing the roots of posterior teeth outward against the cortical plate as a way to inhibit their mesial movement when extraction spaces are to be closed.[20] Since the mesial movement would be along rather than against the cortical plate, it is doubtful that this technique greatly augments anchorage (although it has the potential to create root resorption). However, a layer of dense cortical bone that has formed within the alveolar process can certainly affect tooth movement. This situation may be encountered at an old extraction site, for example, in an adult in whom a molar or premolar was lost many years previously (Figure 9-19). It can be very difficult to close such an extraction site, because tooth movement is slowed to a minimum as the roots encounter cortical bone along the resorbed alveolar ridge.

As a general rule, torquing movements are limited by the facial and lingual cortical plates. If a root is persistently forced against either of these cortical plates, tooth movement is greatly slowed and root resorption is likely, but penetration of the cortical bone may occur. Although it is possible to torque the root of a tooth labially or lingually out of the bone (Figure 9-20), fortunately, it is difficult to do so.

Skeletal (Absolute) Anchorage

It has long been realized that if structures other than the teeth could be made to serve as anchorage, it would be pos-

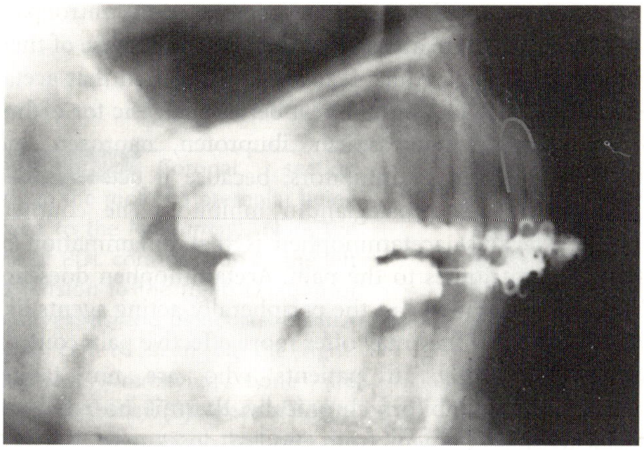

Figure 9-20 Extreme tipping of maxillary incisor teeth from excessive and poorly controlled orthodontic forces. In this patient, the apices of all four maxillary incisors were carried through the labial cortical plate, and pulp vitality was lost.

sible to produce tooth movement or growth modification without unwanted side effects. Until recently, extra-oral force (headgear) was the only way to obtain anchorage that was not from the teeth. Although headgear can be used to augment anchorage, there are two problems: (1) it is impossible for a patient to wear headgear all the time, and most wear it half the time at best; and (2) when headgear is worn, the force against the teeth is larger than optimal. The result is a force system that is far from ideal. Heavy intermittent force from headgear is simply not a good way to counterbalance the effect of light continuous force from the orthodontic appliance. It is not surprising that headgear to the anchor segment of a dental arch usually does not control its movement very well.

With the development of successful bone implant techniques, the potential existed for what could be described as *absolute anchorage*, with no tooth movement except what was desired. Experiments in recent years showed that implants could be used as anchorage for orthodontic tooth movement, and that they made it possible to do things that were previously impossible, for example, intrusion of maxillary posterior teeth in the treatment of anterior open bite. Recently, it has become apparent that the osseointegration needed for long-term implant success is not necessary, and perhaps not desirable, for temporary attachments to bone to provide orthodontic anchorage. A number of options for absolute anchorage exist at present, the principal ones being titanium screws that penetrate through the gingiva into alveolar bone (Figure 9-21, *A;* see also Figure 8-16) and bone anchors placed beneath the soft tissue, usually in the zygomatic buttress area of the maxilla (Figure 9-21, *B*).

At this point, temporary skeletal anchorage is an exciting new aspect of clinical orthodontics. The application of absolute anchorage to various clinical problems is discussed in Chapter 8, the devices are reviewed in the fixed appliance section of Chapter 11, and clinical applications of temporary skeletal anchorage are described in Chapter 18.

A

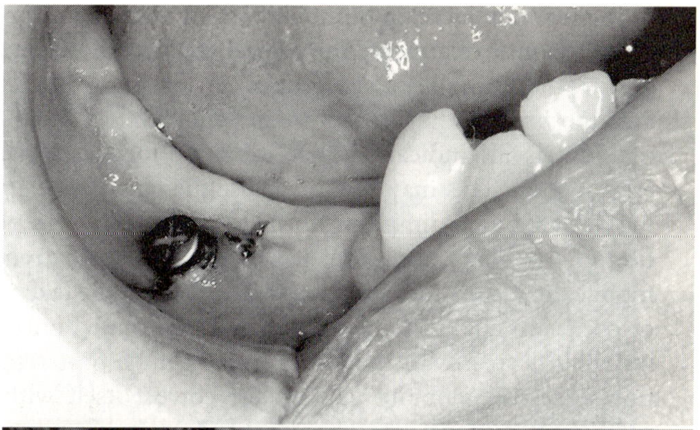

B

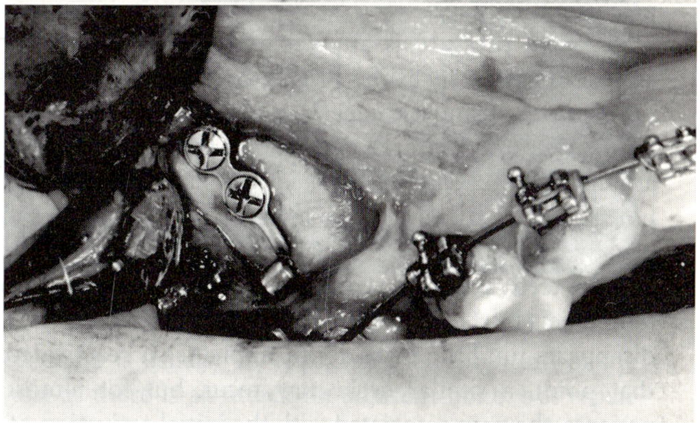

Figure 9-21 Skeletal (absolute) anchorage can be provided in two major ways. **A,** Screws placed through the gingiva into the alveolar bone, as in this patient in whom the screw will be used for anchorage so that the lower incisors can be aligned before prosthodontic replacement of the missing teeth; or **B,** Bone anchors placed beneath the soft tissue, usually at the base of the zygomatic arch, so that the posterior teeth can be intruded or the anterior teeth retracted. After soft tissues are sutured back over the plate and screws, only the tube for attachment of springs will extend into the oral cavity.

Deleterious Effects of Orthodontic Force

Mobility and Pain Related to Orthodontic Treatment

Orthodontic tooth movement requires not only a remodeling of bone adjacent to the teeth, but also a reorganization of the PDL itself. Fibers become detached from the bone and cementum, then reattach at a later time. Radiographically, it can be observed that the PDL space widens during orthodontic tooth movement. The combination of a wider ligament space and a somewhat disorganized ligament means that some increase in mobility will be observed in every patient.

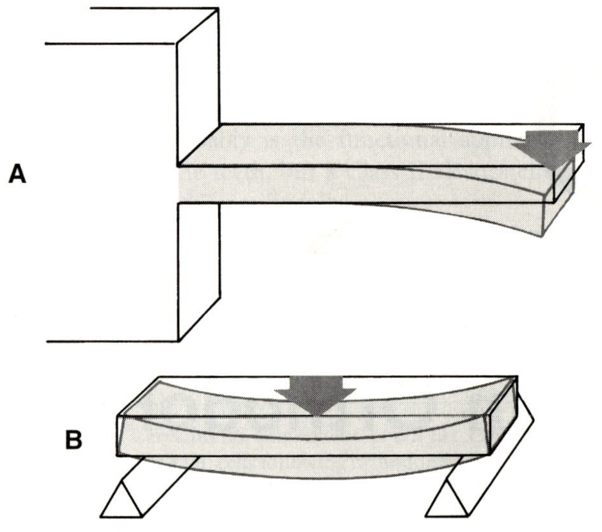

Figure 10-1 Cantilever **(A)** and supported beams **(B)**.

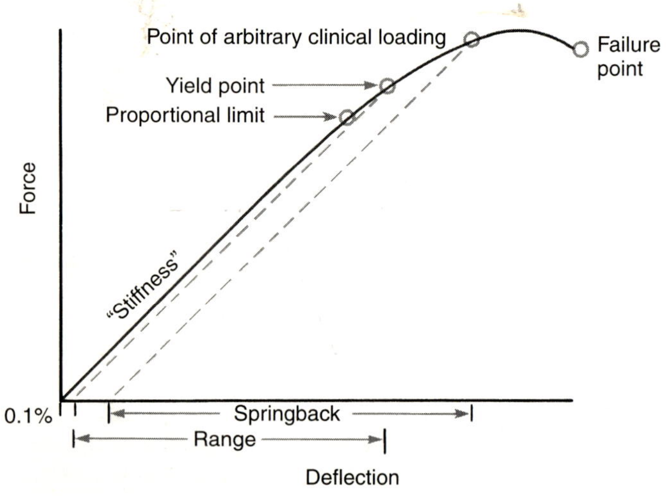

Figure 10-2 A typical force-deflection curve for an elastic material like an orthodontic arch wire. The stiffness of the material is given by the slope of the linear portion of the curve. The range is the distance along the X-axis to the point at which permanent deformation occurs (usually taken as the yield point, at which 0.1% permanent deformation has occurred). Clinically useful springback occurs if the wire is deflected beyond the yield point (as to the point indicated here as "arbitrary clinical loading"), but it no longer returns to its original shape. At the failure point, the wire breaks.

from force and deflection by considering the area and length of the beam.

For orthodontic purposes, three major properties of beam materials are critical in defining their clinical usefulness: strength, stiffness (or its inverse, springiness), and range. Each can be defined by appropriate reference to a force-deflection or stress-strain diagram (Figures 10-2 and 10-3).

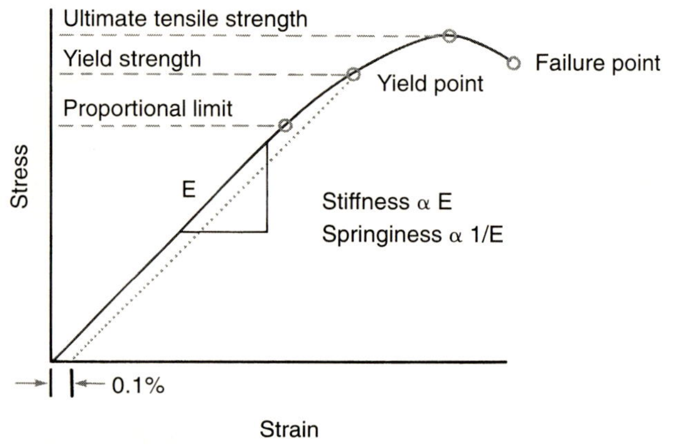

Figure 10-3 Stress and strain are internal characteristics that can be calculated from measurements of force and deflection, so the general shapes of force-deflection and stress-strain curves are similar. Three different points on a stress-strain diagram can be taken as representing the strength. The slope of the stress-strain curve *(E)* is the modulus of elasticity, to which stiffness and springiness are proportional.

Three different points on a stress-strain diagram can be taken as representative of the strength of a material (see Figure 10-3). Each represents, in a somewhat different way, the maximum load that the material can resist. The most conservative measure is the proportional limit, the point at which any permanent deformation is first observed. (Although there is a slight difference in the engineering definition of the term *elastic limit,* it is essentially the same point, and elastic and proportional limit may be used interchangeably.) A more practical indicator is the point at which a deformation of 0.1% is measured; this is defined as the yield strength. The maximum load the wire can sustain—the ultimate tensile strength—is reached after some permanent deformation and is greater than the yield strength. Since this ultimate strength determines the maximum force the wire can deliver if used as a spring, it is important clinically, especially since yield strength and ultimate strength differ much more for the newer titanium alloys than for steel wires. Strength is measured in stress units (gm/cm^2).

Stiffness and springiness are reciprocal properties:

Springiness = 1/Stiffness

Each is proportional to the slope of the elastic portion of the force-deflection curve (see Figure 10-2). The more horizontal the slope, the springier the wire; the more vertical the slope, the stiffer the wire.

Range is defined as the distance that the wire will bend elastically before permanent deformation occurs. This distance is measured in millimeters (or other length units) (see Figure 10-2). If the wire is deflected beyond its yield strength, it will not return to its original shape, but clinically useful springback will occur unless the failure point is reached. This springback is measured along the horizontal axis as shown in Figure 10-2. In many clinical situations, orthodontic wires

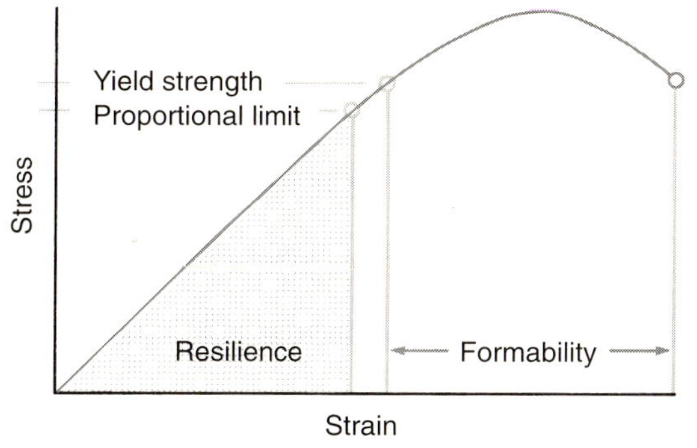

FIGURE 10-4 Resilience and formability are defined as an area under the stress-strain curve and a distance along the X-axis respectively, as shown here. Because the plastic deformation that makes a material formable also may be thought of as cold work, formability alternatively can be interpreted as the area under that part of the stress-strain curve.

are deformed beyond their elastic limit. Their springback properties in the portion of the load-deflection curve between the elastic limit and the ultimate strength, therefore, are important in determining clinical performance.

These three major properties have an important relationship:

Strength = Stiffness × Range

Two other characteristics of some clinical importance also can be illustrated with a stress-strain diagram: resilience and formability (Figure 10-4). Resilience is the area under the stress-strain curve out to the proportional limit. It represents the energy storage capacity of the wire, which is a combination of strength and springiness. Formability is the amount of permanent deformation that a wire can withstand before failing. It represents the amount of permanent bending the wire will tolerate (while being formed into a clinically useful spring, for instance) before it breaks.

The properties of an ideal wire material for orthodontic purposes can be described largely in terms of these criteria: it should possess (1) high strength, (2) low stiffness (in most applications), (3) high range, and (4) high formability. In addition, the material should be weldable or solderable, so that hooks or stops can be attached to the wire. It should also be reasonable in cost. In contemporary practice, no one arch wire material meets all these requirements, and the best results are obtained by using specific arch wire materials for specific purposes.

In the United States, orthodontic appliance dimensions, including wire sizes, are specified in thousandths of an inch. For simplicity in this text, they are given in mils (i.e., .016 inch = 16 mils). In Europe and many other areas of the world, appliance dimensions are specified in millimeters. For the range of orthodontic sizes, a close approximation of sizes in millimeters can be obtained by dividing the dimensions in mils by 4 and placing a decimal point in front (i.e., 16 mils = 0.4 mm).

Orthodontic Arch Wire Materials

Precious Metal Alloys

In the first half of the 20th century, precious metal alloys were used routinely for orthodontic purposes, primarily because nothing else would tolerate intraoral conditions. Gold itself is too soft for nearly all dental purposes, but alloys (which often included platinum and palladium along with gold and copper) could be useful orthodontically. The introduction of stainless steel made precious metal alloys obsolete for orthodontic purposes even before precious metals became prohibitively expensive. Only the Crozat appliance is still occasionally made from gold, following the original design of the early 1900s (see Chapter 11).

Stainless Steel and Cobalt-Chromium Alloys

Stainless steel, or on a cobalt-chromium alloy (Elgiloy; Rocky Mountain Co.) with similar properties, replaced precious metal in orthodontics because of considerably better strength and springiness with equivalent corrosion resistance. Stainless steel's rust resistance results from a relatively high chromium content. A typical formulation for orthodontic use has 18% chromium and 8% nickel (thus the material is often referred to as an 18-8 stainless steel).

The properties of these steel wires can be controlled over a reasonably wide range by varying the amount of cold working and annealing during manufacture. Steel is softened by annealing and hardened by cold working. Fully annealed stainless steel wires are soft and highly formable. The steel ligatures used to tie orthodontic arch wires into brackets on the teeth are made from such "dead soft" wire. Steel arch wire materials are offered in a range of partially annealed states, in which yield strength is progressively enhanced at the cost of formability. The steel wires with the most impressive yield strength ("super" grades) are almost brittle and will break if bent sharply. The "regular" grade of orthodontic steel wire can be bent to almost any desired shape without breaking. If sharp bends are not needed, the super wires can be useful, but it is difficult to show improved clinical performance that justifies either their higher cost or limited formability.

Elgiloy, the cobalt-chromium alloy, has the advantage that it can be supplied in a softer and therefore more formable state, and then can be hardened by heat treatment after being shaped. The heat treatment increases strength significantly. After heat treatment, the softest Elgiloy becomes equivalent to regular stainless steel, while harder initial grades are equivalent to the "super" steels.

Nickel-Titanium (NiTi) Alloys

The first of the titanium alloys introduced into orthodontics in recent years, a nickel-titanium alloy marketed as Nitinol (Unitek Corp.), was developed for the space program (Ni, nickel; Ti, titanium; NOL, Naval Ordnance Laboratory) but has proved very useful in clinical orthodontics because of its exceptional springiness. In this book, the term *NiTi* is used subsequently to refer to the family of nickel-titanium wire

TABLE 10-4

Wires of Equivalent Stiffness—Bending

WIRE TYPE			
M-NiTi	Beta-Ti	Stainless steel	Relative springiness
16		17.5 (3 × 8)	6.6
19	16	12	3.3
	18	14	1.9
17 × 25		16	1.0
21 × 25		18	0.70
	19 × 25		0.37
		19 × 26	0.12

TABLE 10-5

A Sequence of Increasingly Stiff Wires in Torsion

Wire	Stiffness index
18 × 18 M-NiTi	1.0
17 × 25 M-NiTi	1.7
21 × 25 M-NiTi	2.8
17 × 25 beta-Ti	3.5
19 × 25 beta-Ti	4.6
21 × 25 beta-Ti	5.7
16 × 22 steel	8.0
17 × 25 steel	12
19 × 25 steel	16
21 × 25 steel	21

2. Stiffness of the small round M-NiTi and beta-Ti wires also is similar, less than one-third that of steel.
3. TMA has nearly twice the range of steel, and M-NiTi has twice the range of TMA and nearly four times the range of steel. The A-NiTi alloys quickly move into the nonlinear portion of the force-deflection curve and so in the strict definition of the term do not have much range, but as Figure 10-5 shows, they have tremendous springback and behave clinically as if they have very large range.

Table 10-3 shows that properties of rectangular wire in bending and torsion are quite different. Note that at this common wire size, both beta-Ti and M-NiTi have greater springiness and range than steel. M-NiTi in torsion must bend more than twice as far as TMA to deliver the same load (because of its great springiness), and thus is at a disadvantage when small precise adjustments are needed. A-NiTi would be at an even greater disadvantage in this application. Beta-Ti or steel (depending on wire size) would be a better choice for making final adjustments in tooth inclination (torque).

Table 10-4 shows wires of equivalent stiffness, with 16 mil stainless steel as the index value, i.e., 16 steel = 1. Table 10-5 illustrates a sequence of rectangular wires that are increasingly stiff in torsion. The application of this information to the selection of arch wires at various stages of fixed appliance treatment is covered in detail in Chapters 14 to 16.

A more graphic and efficient method for comparing different wire materials and sizes (within the limitations described above) is the use of nomograms—fixed charts that display mathematical relationships via appropriately adjusted scales. In the preparation of a nomogram, a reference wire is given a value of 1, and many other wires can then be located appropriately in reference to it. Nomograms developed by Kusy to provide generalized comparisons of stainless steel, M-NiTi, and beta-Ti in bending and torsion are shown in Figures 10-10 and 10-11. Note that because the nomograms of each set are all drawn to the same base, wires of different materials as well as different sizes can be compared.

The nomograms are particularly helpful in allowing one to assess at a glance a whole set of relationships that would require pages of tables. For example, using Figure 10-11 to compare 21 × 25 M-NiTi to 21 × 25 beta-Ti in torsion (the appropriate comparison if the wires would be used to produce a torquing movement of the root of a tooth): 21 × 25 beta-Ti has a stiffness value of 6, while 21 × 25 M-NiTi has a value of 3, so the beta-Ti would deliver twice the force at a given deflection; the strength value for 21 × 25 beta-Ti wire is 4, while the value for this size M-NiTi wire is 6, so the NiTi wire is less likely to become permanently distorted if twisted into a bracket; the range value for 21 × 25 beta-Ti is 0.7, while the same size M-NiTi has a range value of 1.9, so the NiTi could be twisted nearly three times as far. The nomograms contain the information to allow a similar comparison of any one of the wire sizes listed to any other wire shown on the chart, in bending (see Figure 10-10) or torsion (see Figure 10-11).

Effects of Size and Shape on Elastic Properties

Each of the major elastic properties—strength, stiffness, and range—is substantially affected by a change in the geometry of a beam. Both the cross-section (whether the beam is circular, rectangular, or square) and the length of a beam are of great significance in determining its properties. Changes related to size and shape are independent of the material. In other words, decreasing the diameter of a steel beam by 50% would reduce its strength to a specific percentage of what it had been previously (the exact reduction would depend on how the beam was supported, as we discuss below). Decreasing the diameter of a TMA beam by 50% would reduce its strength by exactly the same percentage. But keep in mind that the performance of a beam, whether beneath a highway bridge or between two teeth in an orthodontic appliance, is determined by the combination of material properties and geometric factors.

A,B

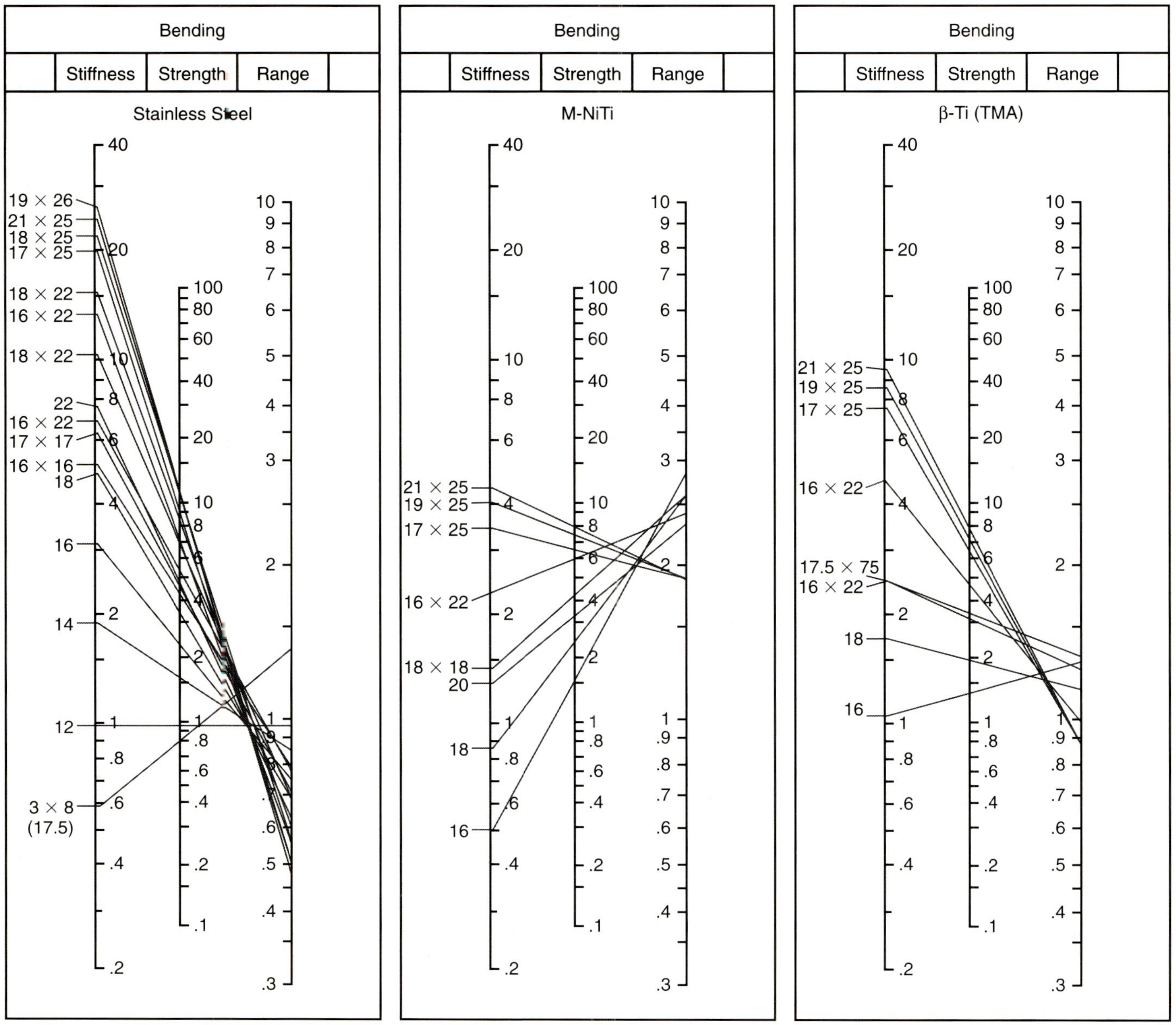

C

FIGURE 10-10 Bending nomograms for stainless steel **(A)**, M-NiTi (Nitinol) **(B)**, and beta-titanium (TMA) wires **(C)**. The index for all three nomograms, with an assigned value of 1, is 12 mil steel, so all values on the three nomograms are comparable. (Redrawn from Kusy RP.[6])

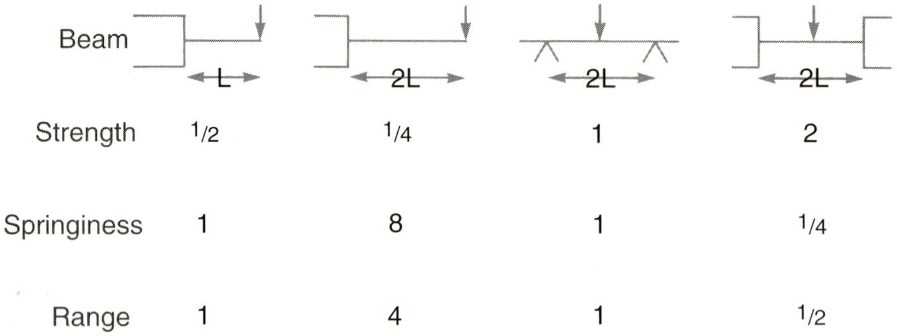

FIGURE 10-13 Changing either the length of a beam or the way in which it is attached dramatically affects its properties. Doubling the length of a cantilever beam cuts its strength in half, but makes it 8 times as springy and gives it 4 times the range. More generally, strength varies inversely with length, whereas springiness varies as a cubic function of the length ratios, and range as a second power function. Supporting a beam on both ends makes it much stronger but also much less springy than supporting it on only one end. Note that if a beam is rigidly attached on both ends, it is twice as strong but only one fourth as springy as a beam of the same material and length that can slide over the abutments. For this reason, the elastic properties of an orthodontic arch wire are affected by whether it is tied tightly or held loosely in a bracket.

but not as strong. Their useful sizes therefore are larger than steel and quite close to the sizes for gold.

Effects of Length and Attachment

Changing the length of a beam, whatever its size or the material from which it is made, also dramatically affects its properties (Figure 10-13). If the length of a cantilever beam is doubled, its bending strength is cut in half, but its springiness increases eight times and its range four times. More generally, when the length of a cantilever beam increases, its strength decreases proportionately, while its springiness increases as the cubic function of the ratio of the length and its range increases as the square of the ratio of the length. Length changes affect torsion quite differently from bending: springiness and range in torsion increase proportionally with length, while torsional strength is not affected by length.

Changing from a cantilever to a supported beam, though it complicates the mathematics, does not affect the big picture: as beam length increases, there are proportional decreases in strength but exponential increases in springiness and range.

The way in which a beam is attached also affects its properties. An arch wire can be tied tightly or loosely, and the point of loading can be any point along the span. As Figure 10-12 shows, a supported beam like an arch wire is four times as springy if it can slide over the abutments (in clinical use, through a bracket into which it is loosely tied) rather than if the beam is firmly attached (tied tightly). With multiple attachments, as with an arch wire tied to several teeth, the gain in springiness from loose ties of an initial arch wire is less dramatic but still significant.[7]

Controlling Orthodontic Force by Varying Materials and Size-Shape

Obtaining enough orthodontic force is never a problem. The difficulty is in obtaining light but sustained force. A spring or arch wire strong enough to resist permanent deformation may be too stiff, which creates two problems: the force is likely to be too heavy initially and then decay rapidly when the tooth begins to move. A wire with excellent springiness and range may nevertheless fail to provide a sustained force if it distorts from inadequate strength the first time the patient has lunch. The best balance of strength, springiness, and range must be sought among the almost innumerable possible combinations of beam materials, diameters, and lengths.

The first consideration in spring design is adequate strength: the wire that is selected must not deform permanently in use. As a general rule, finger springs for removable appliances are best constructed using steel wire. Great advantage can be taken of the fact that finger springs behave like cantilever beams: springiness increases as a cubic function of the increase in length of the beam, while strength decreases only in direct proportion. Thus a relatively large wire, selected for its strength, can be given the desired spring qualities by increasing its length.

In practice, this lengthening often means doubling the wire back on itself or winding a helix into it to gain length while keeping the spring within a confined intraoral area (Figure 10-14). The same technique can be used with arch wires, of course; the effective length of a beam is measured along the wire from one support to the other, and this does not have to be in a straight line (Figure 10-15). Bending loops in arch wires can be a time-consuming chairside procedure, which is the major disadvantage.

Another way to obtain a better combination of springiness and strength is to combine two or more strands of a small, and therefore springy, wire. Two 10 mil steel wires in tandem, for instance, could withstand twice the load as a single strand before permanently deforming, but if each strand could bend without being restrained by the other, springiness would not be affected. The genesis of the "twin

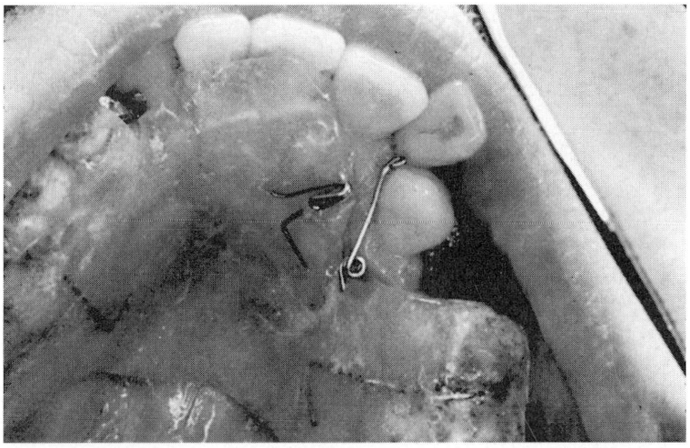

FIGURE 10-14 A removable appliance incorporating a cantilever springs for initial tipping of a maxillary canine toward a premolar extraction site. Note that a helix has been bent into the base of the cantilever spring, effectively increasing its length to obtain more desirable mechanical properties.

wire" appliance system (see Chapter 12) was just this observation, that a pair of 10 mil steel wires offered excellent springiness and range for aligning teeth, and that two wires gave adequate strength although one did not. Later, three or more strands of smaller steel wires, twisted into a cable, came into common use (see Figure 10-15). The properties of the multistrand wire depend both on the characteristics of the individual wire strands and on how tightly they have been woven together. Multistrand wires offer an impressive combination of strength and spring qualities, but now have been displaced for most applications by NiTi wires.

The exceptional springiness of A-NiTi makes it a particularly attractive alternative to steel wires in the initial phases of treatment when the teeth are severely malaligned. A continuous NiTi arch wire of either type will have better properties than multistrand steel wires and properties similar to a steel arch wire with loops. TMA, as an intermediate between NiTi and steel, is less useful than either in the first stage of full-appliance treatment. Its excellent overall properties, however, make it quite useful in the later stages of

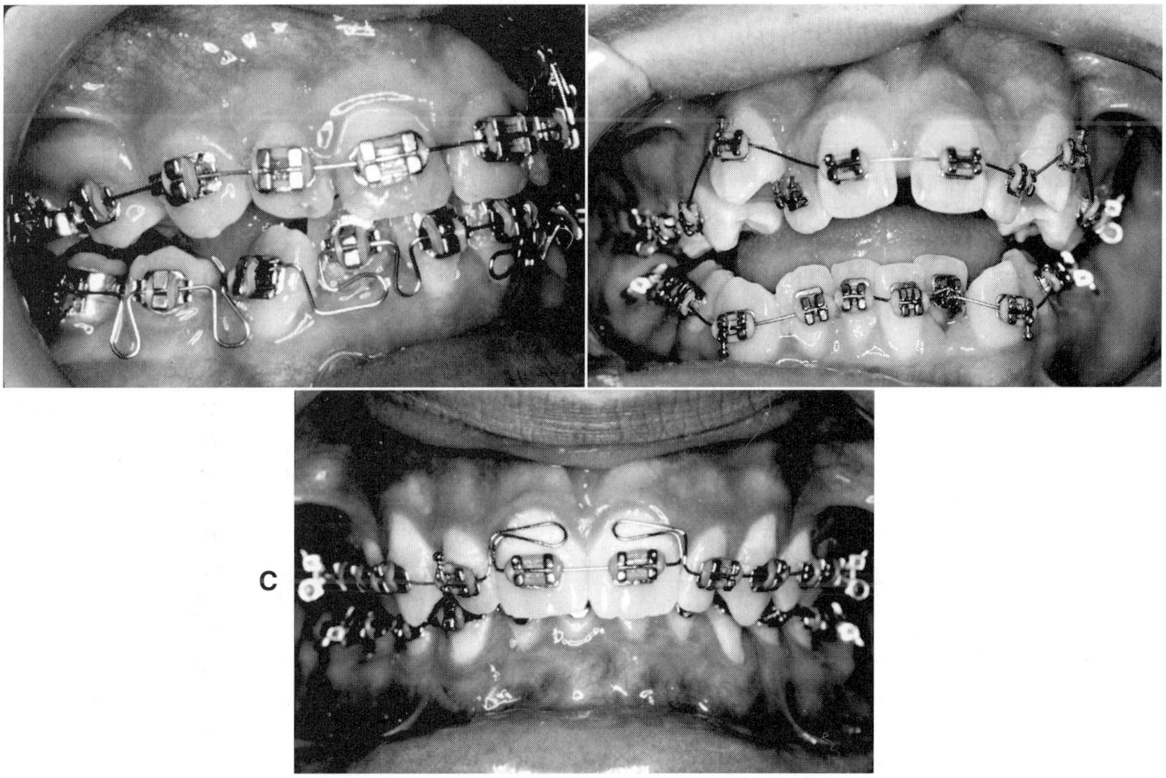

FIGURE 10-15 **A,** Improved springiness and range with steel arch wires can be obtained by either of two strategies: Bending loops into the arch wire, as shown in the lower arch here, to increase the length of the beam segments between adjacent teeth; or using multistranded or small diameter steel wires, as shown in the upper arch. **B,** The exceptional range and flat force-deflection curve of modern superelastic A-NiTi wire make it possible to use a single strand of 14 or 16 mil wire for initial alignment. Using these wires is more efficient than using multi-strand steel wires because of the greater range of A-NiTi, and takes less clinical time than bending loops, so A-NiTi has almost totally replaced both the steel alternatives. **C,** A round steel wire can be used advantageously to change the axial inclination of incisors if this is needed at the initial stage of treatment (as it may be in Class II division 2 patients), by bending loops that contact the gingival area of the teeth when the wire is tied in place. If the end of the wire is free to slide forward, the result is facial tipping of the incisors; if it is bent over so that the teeth cannot tip facially, the result is torque.

treatment. It is possible, and frequently desirable, to carry out orthodontic treatment with a series of wires of approximately the same size, using a sequence from NiTi to TMA to steel. Arch wire selection in varying circumstances is discussed in more detail later in this chapter and in Chapters 14 through 16.

Rubber and Plastic Sources of Elastic Force

From the beginning, rubber bands were used in orthodontics to transmit force from the upper arch to the lower. Rubber has the particularly valuable quality of a great elastic range, so that the extreme stretching produced when a patient opens the mouth while wearing rubber bands can be tolerated without destroying the appliance. Rubber bands are also easier for a patient to remove and replace than, for instance, a heavy coil spring would be. More recently, rubber and plastic elastomers also have been used to close spaces within the arches.

From a materials point of view, the greatest problem with all types of rubber is that they absorb water and deteriorate under intraoral conditions. Gum rubber, which is used to make the rubber bands commonly used in households and offices, begins to deteriorate in the mouth within a couple of hours, and much of its elasticity is lost in 12 to 24 hours. Although orthodontic elastics once were made from this material, they have been superseded by latex elastics, which have a useful performance life 4 to 6 times as long. In contemporary orthodontics, only latex rubber elastics should be used.

Elastomeric plastics for orthodontic purposes are marketed under a variety of trade names. Small elastomeric modules replace wire ligature ties to hold archwires in the brackets in many applications (Figure 10-16), and also can be used to apply a force to close spaces within the arches. Like rubber, however, these elastomers tend to deteriorate in elastic performance after a relatively short period in the mouth. This feature does not prevent them from performing quite well in holding arch wires in place, nor does it contraindicate their use to close small spaces. It simply must be kept in mind that when elastomers are used, the forces decay rapidly, and so can be characterized better as interrupted rather than continuous. Although larger spaces within the dental arch can be closed by sliding teeth with rubber bands or elastomeric chains, the same tooth movement can be done much more efficiently with A-NiTi springs that provide a nearly constant force over quite a large range.

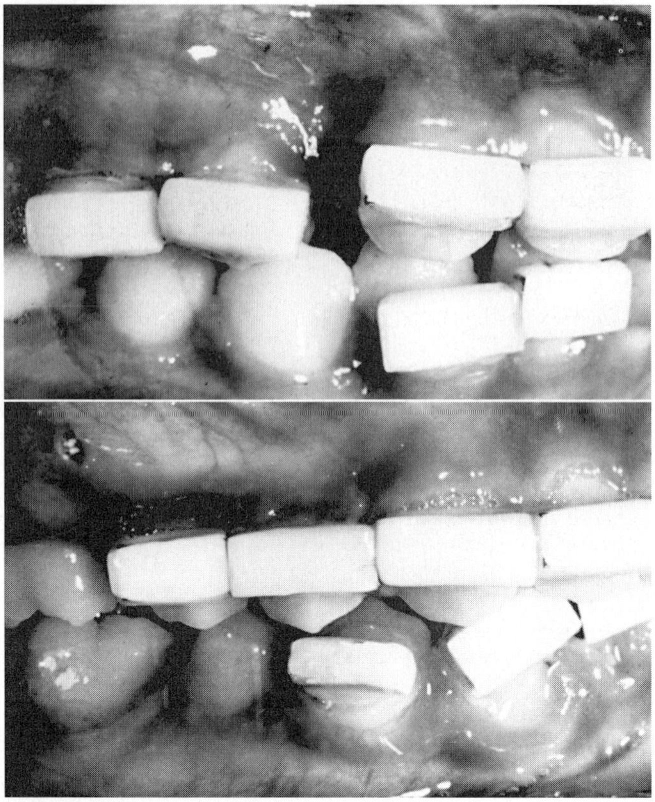
A
B

Figure 10-16 **A, B,** Magnets bonded to individual teeth can be used to close spaces and bring teeth into better alignment. (Courtesy Dr. M. A. Darendeliler.)

Magnets as a Source of Orthodontic Force

Magnets in attraction or repulsion could generate forces of the magnitude needed to move teeth and would have the advantage of providing predictable force levels without direct contact or friction. Until rare earth magnets were developed in the 1980s, magnetic devices with enough force at reasonable separation distances were simply too bulky for orthodontic purposes. In the 1990s, with smaller and more powerful magnets available, there was considerable interest in the possibility of using magnetic force in orthodontics.

The two key questions with magnets as a source of force are their biological implications and their clinical effectiveness.[9] Although the rare earth materials are potentially toxic, direct cytotoxic effects have not been observed when magnets in sealed cases are placed intraorally. If a magnetic field increased the rate of bone remodeling and tooth movement, this would be a compelling reason to use magnets, but careful research has shown little if any biologic effect from the small magnets used to generate orthodontic force. Biologically, it appears that safety is not a problem, but the magnets are just another device to produce orthodontic force.[10]

There is no doubt that magnets can be clinically effective. A particularly attractive potential application is bringing impacted teeth into the arch, because if a magnet were attached to an impacted tooth when it was exposed, it would not be necessary to maintain a physical connection (see Figure 10-16). There are two major problems with magnets for general orthodontic use. First, even the smallest magnets still are quite bulky compared with, for instance, a NiTi spring. Second, the force follows the inverse square law (i.e., the force changes as the square of the distance between the magnets). Force decay (or increase) as teeth move can be a problem if the magnets were close together initially. For both reasons, it is unlikely that magnetic force will become an important part of orthodontic treatment.

DESIGN FACTORS IN ORTHODONTIC APPLIANCES

Two Point Contact and Control of Root Position

Definition of Terms

Before beginning to discuss control of root position, it is necessary to understand some basic physical terms that must be used in the discussion:

- *Force*—a load applied to an object that will tend to move it to a different position in space. Force, though rigidly defined in units of Newtons (mass times the acceleration of gravity), is usually measured in weight units of grams or ounces.
- *Center of resistance*—a point at which resistance to movement can be concentrated for mathematical analysis. For an object in free space, the center of resistance is the same as the center of mass. If the object is partially restrained, as is the case for a fence post extending into the earth or a tooth root embedded in bone, the center of resistance will be determined by the nature of the external constraints. The center of resistance for a tooth is at the approximate midpoint of the embedded portion of the root (i.e., about halfway between the root apex and the crest of the alveolar bone) (Figure 10-17).
- *Moment*—a force acting at a distance. A moment is defined as the product of the force times the perpendicular distance from the point of force application to the center of resistance, and thus is measured in units of gm-mm (or equivalent). If the line of action of an applied force does not pass through the center of resistance, a moment is necessarily created. Not only will the force tend to translate the object, moving it to a different position, it also will tend to rotate the object around the center of resistance. This, of course, is precisely the situation when a force is applied to the crown of a tooth (see Figure 10-17). Not only is the tooth displaced in the direction of the force, it also rotates around the center of resistance—thus the tooth tips as it moves.
- *Couple*—two forces equal in magnitude and opposite in direction. The result of applying two forces in this way is a pure moment, since the translatory effect of the forces cancels out. A couple will produce pure rotation, spinning the object around its center of resistance, while the combination of a force and a couple can change the way an object rotates while it is being moved (Figure 10-18).
- *Center of rotation*—the point around which rotation actually occurs when an object is being moved. If a force

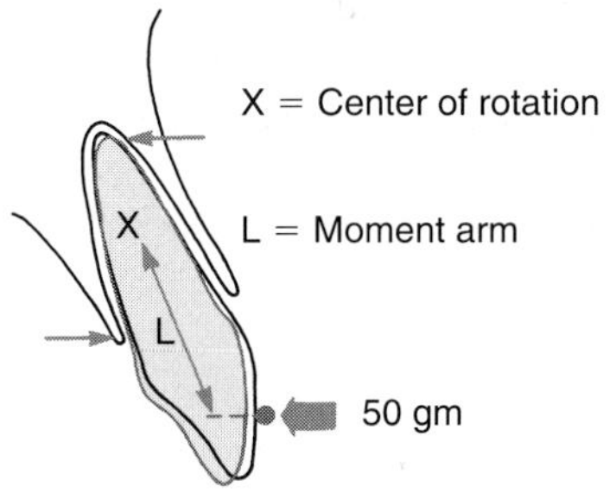

FIGURE 10-17 The center of resistance (C_R) for any tooth is at the approximate midpoint of the embedded portion of the root. If a single force is applied to the crown of a tooth, the tooth will not only translate but also rotate around C_R (i.e., the center of rotation and center of resistance are identical), because a moment is created by applying a force at a distance from C_R. The perpendicular distance from the point of force application to the center of resistance is the moment arm. Pressure in the periodontal ligament will be greatest at the alveolar crest and opposite the root apex (see Figure 9-9).

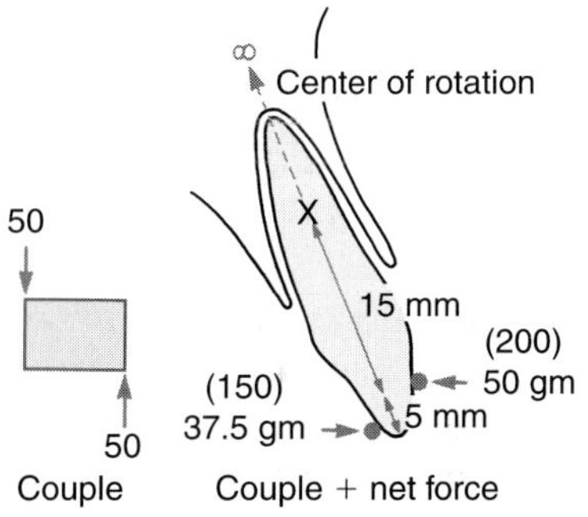

FIGURE 10-18 A couple, as shown on the left, is defined as two forces equal in magnitude and opposite in direction. The application of a couple produces pure rotation. In clinical application, two unequal forces applied to the crown of a tooth to control root position can be resolved into a couple and a net force to move the tooth. If a 50 gm force were applied to a point on the labial surface of an incisor tooth 15 mm from the center of resistance, a 750 gm-mm moment (the moment of the force, or M_F) would be produced, tipping the tooth. To obtain bodily movement, it is necessary to apply a couple, to create a moment (the moment of the couple, or M_C) equal in magnitude and opposite in direction to the original movement. One way to do this would be to apply a force of 37.5 gm pushing the incisal edge labially at a point 22 mm from the center of resistance. This creates a 750 gm-mm moment in the opposite direction, so the force system is equivalent to a couple with a 12.5 gm net force to move the tooth lingually. With this force system, the tooth would not tip, but with so light a net force, there would be only a small amount of movement. To achieve a net 50 gm for effective movement, it would be necessary to use 200 gm against the labial surface and 150 gm in the opposite direction against the incisal edge. Controlling forces of this magnitude without a fixed appliance is difficult.

and a couple are applied to an object, the center of rotation can be controlled and made to have any desired location. The application of a force and a couple to the crown of a tooth, in fact, is the mechanism by which bodily movement of a tooth, or even greater movement of the root than the crown, can be produced.

Forces, Moments, and Couples in Tooth Movement

Consider the clinical problem posed by a protruding maxillary central incisor. If a single force of 50 gm is applied against the crown of this tooth, as might happen with a spring on a maxillary removable appliance, a force system will be created that includes a 750 gm-mm moment (see Figure 10-18). The result will be that the crown will be retracted more than the root apex, which might actually move slightly in the opposite direction. (Remember that a force will tend to displace the entire object, despite the fact that its orientation will change via simultaneous rotation around the center of resistance.) If it is desired to maintain the inclination of the tooth while retracting it, it will be necessary to overcome the moment inadvertently created when the force was applied to the crown.

One way to decrease the magnitude of the moment is to apply the force closer to the center of resistance. In orthodontics, it is impractical to apply the force directly to the root, but a similar effect could be achieved by constructing a rigid attachment that projected upward from the crown. Then the force could be applied to the attachment such that its line of action passed near or through the center of resistance. If the attachment were perfectly rigid, the effect would be to reduce or eliminate the moment arm and thereby the tipping (Figure 10-19). Since it is difficult to make the arms long enough to totally eliminate tipping, this procedure is only a partial solution at best, and it creates problems with oral hygiene.

Another way to control or eliminate tipping is to create a second moment opposite in direction to the first one. If a second counterbalancing moment could be created equal in magnitude to the moment produced by the first force application, the tooth would remain upright and move bodily. A moment can be created only by application of a force at a distance, however, so this would require that a second force be applied to the crown of the tooth.

In our example of the protruding central incisor, the tendency for the incisor to tip when it was being retracted could be controlled by applying a second force to the lingual surface of this tooth, perhaps with a spring in a removable appliance pushing outward from the lingual edge near the incisal edge (see Figure 10-18). As a practical matter, it can be difficult to maintain removable appliances in place against the displacing effects of a pair of springs with heavy activation. The usual orthodontic solution is a fixed attachment on the tooth, constructed so that forces can be applied at two points. With round wires, an auxiliary spring is needed (Figure 10-20). A rectangular arch wire fitting into a rectangular bracket slot on the tooth is most widely used

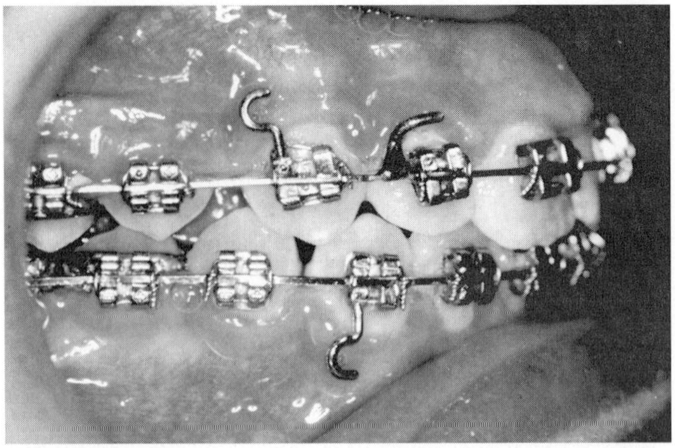

Figure 10-19 Attachments extending toward the center of resistance, seen here as hooks integrated into the canine brackets, can be used to shorten the moment arm and thereby decrease the amount of tipping when elastics or springs are used to slide teeth mesiodistally along an arch wire. This idea from the 1920s was reintroduced as part of the early straight-wire appliance. Unfortunately, the longer the hook the more effective it is mechanically but the greater the chance of oral hygiene problems leading to gingival irritation and/or decalcification. Other methods for controlling tipping are more practical.

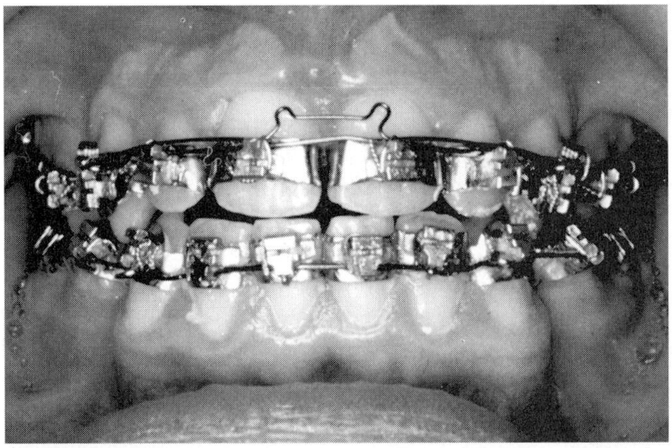

Figure 10-20 Auxiliary root positioning springs and auxiliary torquing springs were used routinely with the Begg appliance, and both can be seen in the maxillary arch of this patient being treated with a Begg-edgewise combination appliance. The torquing spring contacts the facial surface of the central incisors; uprighting springs are present bilaterally on the canines. Note that the base wires are pinned in the Begg slot, while the edgewise slot is not used at this point in treatment. (Courtesy Dr. W. J. Thompson.)

because the entire force system can be produced with a single wire (Figure 10-21).

It should be noted that with this approach, the two points of contact are the opposite edges of the rectangular wire. The moment arms of the couple therefore are quite small, which means that the forces at the bracket necessary to create a countervailing moment are quite large. If a rectangular arch

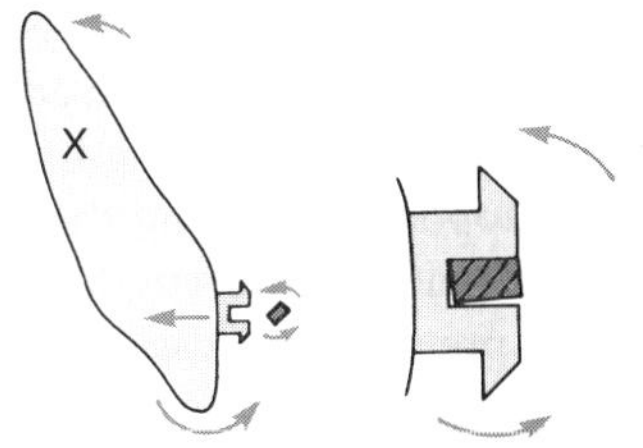

Figure 10-21 A rectangular arch wire fitting into a rectangular slot can generate the moment of a couple necessary to control root position. The wire is twisted (placed into torsion) as it is put into the bracket slot. The two points of contact are at the edge of the wire, where it contacts the bracket. The moment arm therefore is quite small, and forces must be large to generate the necessary M_C. Using the same tooth dimensions indicated in Figure 10-18, a 50 gm net lingual force would generate a 750 gm-mm moment. To balance it by creating an opposite 750 gm-mm moment within a 0.5 mm bracket, a torsional force of 1500 gm is required.

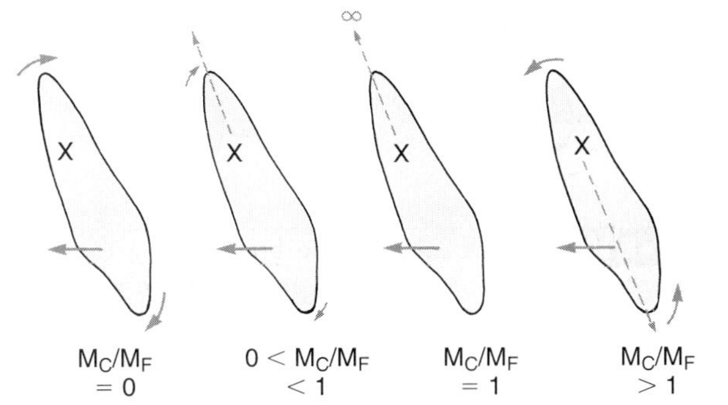

Figure 10-22 The ratio between the moment produced by the force applied to move a tooth (M_F) and the counterbalancing moment produced by the couple used to control root position (M_C) determines the type of tooth movement. With no M_C, ($M_C/M_F = 0$), the tooth rotates around the center of resistance (pure tipping). As the moment-to-force ratio increases ($0 < M_C/M_F < 1$), the center of rotation is displaced further and further away from the center of resistance, producing what is called controlled tipping. When $M_C/M_F = 1$, the center of rotation is displaced to infinity and bodily movement (translation) occurs. If $M_C/M_F > 1$, the center of rotation is displaced incisally and the root apex will move more than the crown, producing root torque.

wire is to be used to retract a central incisor bodily, the net retraction force should be small, but the twisting forces on the bracket must be large in order to generate the moment.

Moment-to-Force Ratios and Control of Root Position

The previous analysis demonstrates that control of root position during movement requires both a force to move the tooth in the desired direction, and a couple to produce the necessary counterbalancing moment for control of root position. The heavier the force, the larger the counterbalancing movement must be to prevent tipping, and vice-versa.

Perhaps the simplest way to determine how a tooth will move is to consider the ratio between the moment created when a force is applied to the crown of a tooth (the moment of the force, or M_F), and the counterbalancing moment generated by a couple within the bracket (the moment of the couple, or M_C). Then it can be seen (Figure 10-22) that the following possibilities exist:

$M_C/M_F = 0$	Pure tipping (tooth rotates around center of resistance)
$0 < M_C/M_F < 1$	Controlled tipping (inclination of tooth changes but the center of rotation is displaced away from the center of resistance, and the root and crown move in the same direction)
$M_C/M_F = 1$	Bodily movement (equal movement of crown and root)
$M_C/M_F > 1$	Torque (root apex moves further than crown)

The moment of the force is determined by the magnitude of the force and the distance from the point of force application to the center of resistance. For most teeth, this is 8 to 10 mm, so M_F will be 8 to 10 times the force. In other words, if a 100 gm net force were used to move a tooth, a balancing moment of 800 to 1000 gm-mm (depending on root length and alveolar bone support) would be needed to obtain bodily movement. In the orthodontic literature, the relationship between the force and the counterbalancing couple often has been expressed in this way, as the "moment-to-force" ratio. In those terms, moment-to-force ratios of 1 to 7 would produce controlled tipping, ratios of 8 to 10 (depending on the length of the root) would produce bodily movement, and ratios greater than 10 would produce torque. Because the distance from the point of force application to the center of resistance can and does vary, moment-to-force ratios must be adjusted if root length, amount of alveolar bone support or point of force application differs from the usual condition. M_C/M_F ratios more precisely describe how a tooth will respond.

Remember that when a force is applied to a bracket to slide it along an arch wire, as often is the case in clinical orthodontics, the force felt by the tooth will be less than the force applied to the bracket because of frictional resistance (see further discussion, below). The *net* force, after frictional resistance is subtracted, and the moment associated with the net force, are what is important. In contrast, when a couple is created within a bracket, friction rarely is a factor.

It is easy to underestimate the magnitude of the forces needed to create the balancing couple. In the example presented previously, if a 50 gm net force was used to retract a central incisor, a 500 gm-mm moment would be needed to keep it from tipping as the crown moved lingually. To produce a moment of this magnitude within the confines of an 18 mil (0.45 mm) bracket would require opposite forces

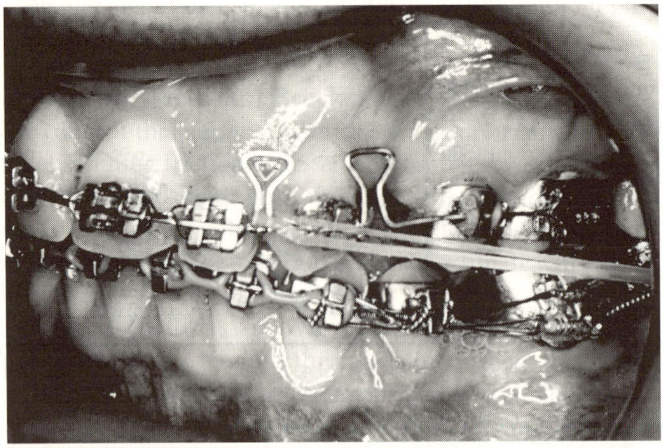

Figure 10-28 A closing loop is being used to retract the maxillary incisors, while a spring to slide the arch wire through the molar tube is used for space closure in the lower arch. In contemporary use, closing loops are bent into (preformed) steel archwires, and teeth slide along steel wires, but the coil spring is A-NiTi. The Class II elastic from lower posterior to upper anterior also provides force to close both upper and lower spaces.

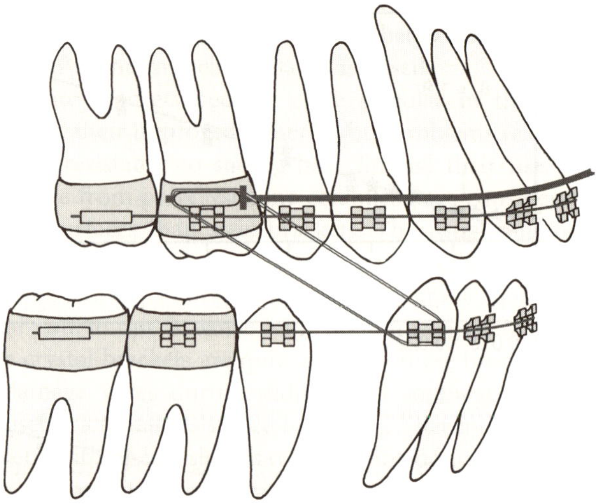

Figure 10-29 Reinforcement of anchorage can be produced by adding additional teeth within the same arch to the anchor unit, or by using elastics from the opposite arch to help produce desired tooth movement, as with the interarch elastic shown here. Additional reinforcement can be obtained with extraoral force, as with addition of a facebow to the upper molar to resist the forward pull of the elastic.

response. It is difficult to avoid the temptation to estimate friction generously and add enough force to be certain that tooth movement will occur. The effect of any force beyond what was really needed to overcome friction is to bring the anchor teeth up onto the plateau of the tooth movement curve (see Figure 9-17). Then either unnecessary movement of the anchor teeth occurs, or additional steps to maintain anchorage are necessary (such as headgear or bone screws).

Friction in the appliance system can be avoided if a spring loop is bent into the arch wire, so that arch wire segments move, taking the teeth with them instead of the teeth moving relative to the wire. Springs of this type are called *retraction springs* if they attach to only one tooth, or *closing loops* if they connect two arch wire segments (Figure 10-28). Incorporating springs into the arch wire makes the appliance more complex to fabricate and to use clinically but eliminates the difficulty in anchorage control caused by frictional resistance.

Methods to Control Anchorage

From the previous discussion, of both the biologic aspects of anchorage in Chapter 9 and the review above of frictional effects, it is apparent that several potential strategies can be used to control anchorage. Nearly all the possible approaches are actually used in clinical orthodontics, and all are affected by whether friction will be encountered and if so, how much. Considering them in more detail:

Reinforcement

The extent to which anchorage should be reinforced (by adding teeth to the anchorage unit) depends on the tooth movement that is desired. In practice, this means that anchorage requirements must be established individually in each clinical situation. Once it has been determined that reinforcement is desirable, however, this typically involves including as many teeth as possible in the anchorage. For significant differential tooth movement, the ratio of PDL area in the anchorage unit to PDL area in the tooth movement unit should be at least 2 to 1 without friction, 4 to 1 with it. Anything less produces something close to reciprocal movement. Obviously, larger ratios are desirable if they can be obtained.

Satisfactory reinforcement of anchorage may require the addition of teeth from the opposite dental arch to the anchor unit. Reinforcement may also include forces derived from structures outside the mouth. For example, to close a mandibular premolar extraction site, it would be possible to stabilize all the teeth in the maxillary arch so that they could only move bodily as a group, and then to run an elastic from the upper posterior to the lower anterior, thus pitting forward movement of the entire upper arch against distal movement of the lower anterior segment (Figure 10-29). This addition of the entire upper arch would greatly alter the balance between retraction of the lower anteriors and forward slippage of the lower posteriors.

This anchorage could be reinforced even further by having the patient wear an extraoral appliance (headgear) placing backward force against the upper arch. The reaction force from the headgear is dissipated against the bones of the cranial vault, thus adding the resistance of these structures to the anchorage unit. The only problem with reinforcement outside the dental arch is that springs within an arch provide constant forces, whereas elastics from one arch to the other

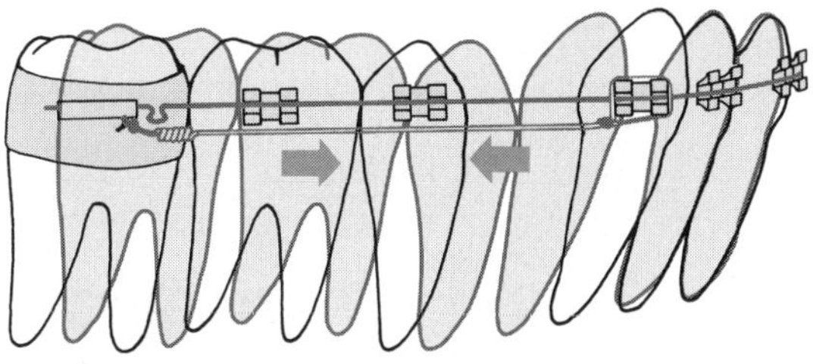

Figure 10-30 Retraction of the canine by itself, as the first step in a two-stage space closure, often is used to conserve anchorage, particularly when sliding teeth along an arch wire.

tend to be intermittent, and extra-oral force is likely to be even more intermittent. Although this time factor can significantly decrease the value of cross-arch and extraoral reinforcement, both can be quite useful clinically.

Subdivision of Desired Movement

A common way to improve anchorage control is to pit the resistance of a group of teeth against the movement of a single tooth, rather than dividing the arch into more or less equal segments. In our same extraction site example, it would be perfectly possible to reduce the strain on posterior anchorage by retracting the canine individually, pitting its distal movement against mesial movement of all other teeth within the arch (Figure 10-30). After the canine tooth had been retracted, one could then add it to the posterior anchorage unit and retract the incisors. This approach would have the advantage that the reaction force would always be dissipated over a large PDL area in the anchor unit. Its disadvantage is that closing the space in two steps rather than one would take nearly twice as long.

Subdivision of tooth movement improves the anchorage situation regardless of whether friction is involved and where a space in the arch is located. If it is desired to slip all the posterior teeth forward (in which case the anterior teeth are the anchor unit), bringing them forward one at a time is the most conservative way to proceed. Moving them one at a time without friction, of course, will put less strain on anchorage than sliding them one at a time.

Tipping/Uprighting

Another possible strategy for anchorage control is to tip the teeth and then upright them, rather than moving them bodily. In our familiar extraction site example, this would again require two steps in treatment. First, the anterior teeth would be tipped distally by being pitted against mesial bodily movement of the posterior segment (see Figure 9-18). As a second step, the tipped teeth would be uprighted, moving the canine roots distally and torquing the incisor roots lingually, again with stationary anchorage in the posterior segments. It would be extremely important to keep forces as light as possible during both steps, so that the teeth in the posterior segment were always below the optimum force range while the anterior teeth received optimum force.

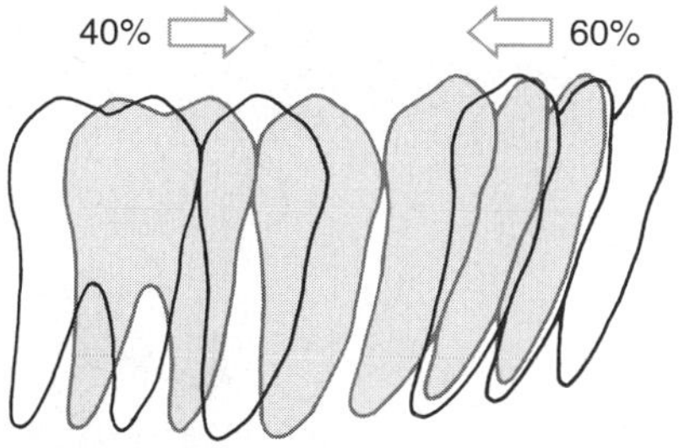

Figure 10-31 Closure of a premolar extraction site often is desired in a ratio of 60% retraction of incisors, 40% forward movement of molar and second premolar. This result can be obtained straightforwardly in three ways: (1) One-step space closure with a frictionless (closing loop) mechanism; (2) two-step space closure with sliding mechanics, retracting the canine individually, and then retracting the four incisors in a second step (the classic Tweed approach); or (3) two-step sliding space closure with distal tipping of the canine and incisors initially, followed by uprighting of these teeth (the classic Begg approach). Good clinical results can be obtained with all three methods. The cost of friction in space closure, with well-managed orthodontic appliances, is paid more in increased treatment time than in decreased quality of result.

Friction and Anchorage Control Strategies

Anchorage control is particularly important when protruding incisors are to be retracted. The goal is to end up with the teeth in the correct position, not necessarily to retract them as much as possible. The desired amount of incisor retraction for any patient should be carefully planned, and the mechanotherapy should be selected to produce the desired outcome. This subject is discussed in considerably more detail in Chapter 15.

At this point, however, it is interesting to consider a relatively typical extraction situation, in which it is desired to close the extraction space 60% by retraction of the anterior teeth and 40% by forward movement of the posterior segments (Figure 10-31). This outcome would be expected from any of three possible approaches: (1) one-step space closure with a frictionless appliance; (2) a two-step closure sliding the canine along the arch wire, then retracting the incisors (as in the original Tweed technique); or (3) two-step space closure, tipping the anterior segment with some friction, then uprighting the tipped teeth (as in the Begg technique). (See Chapters 11 and 14 through 17 for a detailed discussion of these techniques.) The example makes the cost of friction in a clinical setting more apparent: the greater strain on anchorage when brackets slide along an arch wire must be compensated by a more conservative approach to anchorage control. The price is usually paid therefore in increased treatment time. The frictionless appliance, though more difficult to fabricate and manipulate, will result in the same space closure significantly faster.

Note that strategies for anchorage control are associated with particular orthodontic appliances, indeed are literally built into the appliance in many instances. The

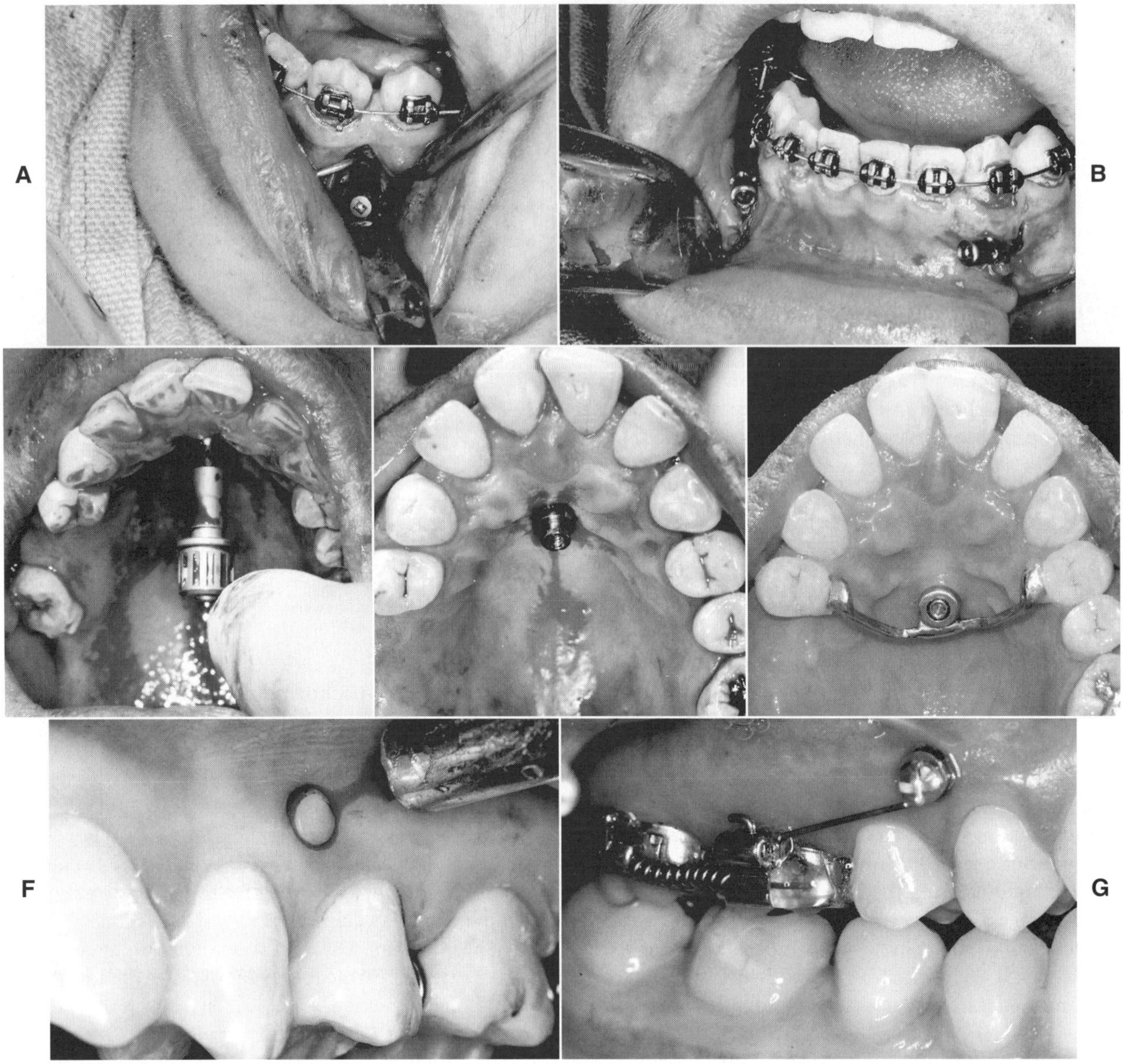

FIGURE 10-32 Bone anchors retained by screws or screws with a head that extends into the mouth can be placed in both the mandibular and maxillary arches to provide skeletal anchorage for tooth movement. This method makes it possible to produce tooth movement that otherwise would be impossible. **A,** Placement of screws to hold a bone anchor in the mandible; **B,** anchors in place bilaterally; **C,** surgical placement of a palatal anchor; **D,** anchor (Straumann OrthoSystem) in position; **E,** stabilizing lingual arch attached to the anchor, in preparation for retraction of the protruding maxillary incisors; **F,** removal of a small area of mucosa over the site where a bone screw is to be placed in the maxillary alveolar process; **G,** TOMAS screw (Dentarum) with a stabilizing wire attached to a channel in the screw head, being used to stabilize the maxillary first molar as the second molar is moved distally. (**C-E,** Courtesy Drs. S. Cunnigham and P. Thomas; **F, G,** Courtesy Prof. A. Bumann.)

mechanical design principles discussed in this chapter have shaped the development of contemporary fixed appliances, but appliance designers have also had to consider anchorage as a design factor of considerable importance. The approach to anchorage control that is implicit in the appliance design is sometimes called the *appliance philosophy,* not quite so strange a term when viewed in this way.

Skeletal Anchorage

Temporary skeletal anchorage is derived from implants, miniplates attached with screws to basal bone of the maxilla or mandible, or just a screw with a channel for attaching a spring that is placed into the alveolar process (Figure 10-32). Collectively these devices are referred as temporary anchorage devices (TADs). This approach makes it possible to accomplish tooth movement, especially in adults, that was very difficult or impossible previously (see Chapter 18). With skeletal anchorage there is no concern about moving teeth that were not intended to be moved, but the amount of force to teeth that are to be moved still must be determined with the amount of friction in mind.

Determinate versus Indeterminate Force Systems

The laws of equilibrium require not only that for every force there is an equal and opposite reactive force but also that the sum of the moments in any plane are equal to zero. In other words, the moments as well as the forces generated by an orthodontic appliance system must be balanced, in all three planes of space. It can be very difficult to visualize the total force system in orthodontics. Unexpected and unwanted tooth movement easily can result when an important component of the system is overlooked.

Force systems can be defined as statically *determinate*, meaning that the moments and forces can readily be discerned, measured and evaluated, or as *indeterminate*. Statically indeterminate systems are too complex for precisely measuring all forces and moments involved in the equilibrium. Typically, only the direction of net moments and approximate net force levels can be determined. This is more of a problem in orthodontics than in many engineering situations, because the eventual action of the system is determined by the biologic response. For instance, the amount of tooth movement will be determined to a large extent by the magnitude of the forces felt by anchor teeth and teeth whose movement is intended, not just by the differential between those forces. If the force applied to the anchor teeth is high enough to pull them up onto the plateau of the pressure-response curve, reciprocal tooth movement will occur despite a difference in PDL pressures (see Figure 9-17). Similarly, whether intrusion of incisor teeth or extrusion of posterior teeth occurs is almost totally a function of the magnitude of intrusive vs. extrusive forces, not their direction or the difference between them. Determinate force systems, therefore, are advantageous in orthodontics because they provide much better control of the magnitude of forces and couples.

For all practical purposes, determinate systems in orthodontics are those in which a couple is created at one end of an attachment, with only a force (no couple) at the other. This means that a wire that will serve as a spring can be inserted into a tube or bracket at one end, but must be tied so that there is only one point of contact on the other (Figure 10-33). When the wire is tied into a bracket on both ends, a statically indeterminate two-couple system has been created.

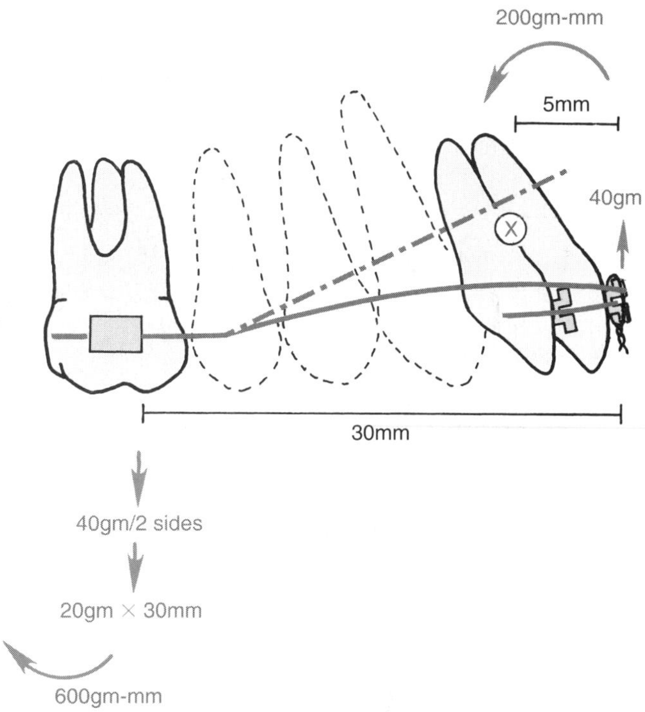

Figure 10-33 An intrusion arch made from rectangular wire, which fits into a rectangular tube on the molars and is tied to one point of contact on the incisor segment, is an example of a determinate one-couple system. If the arch wire is activated by pulling it down and tying it to the incisor segment so that it delivers 40 gm intrusion force (10 gm per tooth, 20 gm per side), and if the distance from the molar tube to the point of attachment is 30 mm, each molar will feel a 20 gm extrusive force in reaction and a 600 gm-mm moment to tip the crown distally. At the incisor segment, the force will create a 200 gm-mm moment to rotate the incisor crowns facially. At each molar, the extrusive force also would create a moment to roll the crown lingually. If the buccal tube were 4 mm buccal to the center of resistance, its magnitude would be 80 gm-mm.

One-Couple Systems

In orthodontic applications, one-couple systems are found when two conditions are met: (1) A cantilever spring or auxiliary arch wire is placed into a bracket or tube(s). It typically attaches to a tooth or teeth that is part of a stabilized segment (i.e., reinforced anchorage is being used); and (2) the other end of the cantilever spring or auxiliary arch wire is tied to a tooth or group of teeth that are to be moved, with a single point of force application.[17]

For analysis, the teeth in the anchor unit are considered as if stabilization had created a single large multirooted tooth, with a single center of resistance. It is important to tie teeth in an anchor unit tightly together with as rigid a stabilizing wire segment as possible. Often the posterior teeth on both sides are tied together with a rigid lingual arch, so that a single posterior stabilizing segment is created. If the goal is

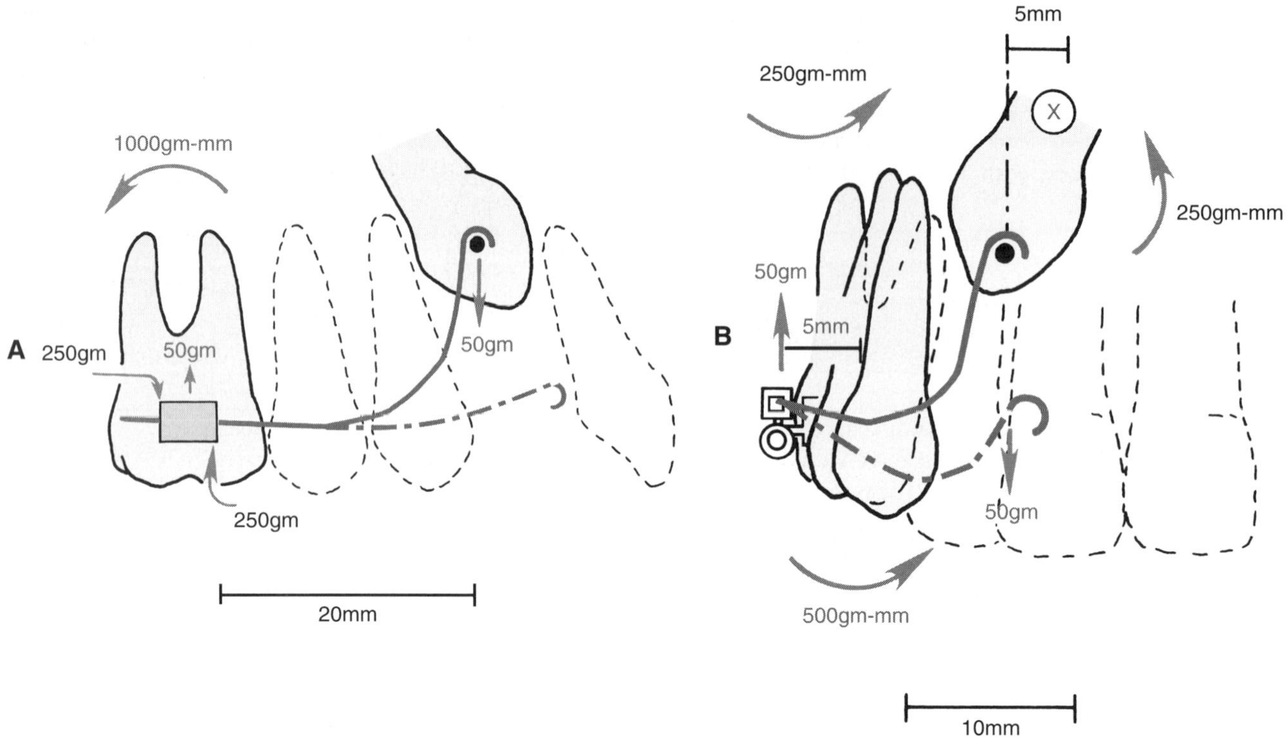

FIGURE 10-34 A cantilever spring, made from a rectangular wire that fits into a rectangular tube (or bracket) on one end and is tied to one point of contact on the other, produces a determinate one-couple system in which the forces and moments can be known precisely. **A,** Lateral view of the force system created by a cantilever spring to extrude an impacted maxillary canine. If the distance between the molar tube and a button on the canine to which the spring is tied is 20 mm, placing a 50 gm extrusive force on the canine creates a 50 gm intrusive force on the molar and also a 1000 gm-mm moment to rotate the molar crown forward around its center of resistance. If the molar tube is 4 mm in length, the moment would be created by a couple with 250 gm force upward on the mesial end of the tube and 250 gm downward on the distal end. **B,** Frontal view of the same force system. Consider the bucco-lingual (torque) moments created by the force on the molar and canine. If the center of resistance of the canine is 5 mm lingual to the button on its crown, a 50 gm extrusive force creates a 250 gm-mm moment to rotate the crown lingually (which usually is not desired). At the molar, if the center of resistance is 4 mm lingual to the tube on the buccal surface, the 50 gm intrusive force creates a 200 gm-mm moment to rotate the crown facially. But if the impacted canine is 10 mm lingual to the buccal surface of the molar, activating the spring also twists it, creating a 500 gm-mm torquing moment to rotate the molar crown lingually. The result at the molar is a net 300 gm-mm moment to torque the molar crown lingually and roots buccally. If the rectangular spring were tied into a bracket on the canine, a moment to torque its root facially could be generated, but the resulting two-couple system would be indeterminate—it would no longer be possible to know the forces and moments with certainty.

to move more than one tooth, the tooth movement segment similarly must be tied so the teeth become a single unit.

Cantilever Spring Applications

Cantilever springs are used most frequently to bring severely displaced (impacted) teeth into the arch (Figure 10-34). These springs have the advantage of a long range of action, with minimal decrease in force as tooth movement proceeds and excellent control of force magnitude. There are two disadvantages: (1) As with most devices with a long range of action, cantilever springs do not fail safely. If they are distorted by the patient, significant tooth movement in the wrong direction is quite possible; (2) the moment of the force on an unerupted tooth rotates the crown lingually as the tooth is brought toward the occlusal plane, which is likely to be undesirable. Although an additional force can be added to overcome this, the system rapidly can become complex. If the cantilever spring is tied into a bracket on the unerupted tooth so that a couple can be created for better control, the force system becomes statically indeterminate and force magnitudes are no longer known with certainty.

Auxiliary Intrusion/Extrusion Arches

The major use of one couple systems is for intrusion, typically of incisors that have erupted too much. For this purpose, light force against the teeth to be intruded is critical. An intrusion arch typically employs posterior (molar) anchorage against two or four incisors (Figure 10-35). Because the intrusive force must be light, the reaction force against the anchor teeth also is light, well below the force

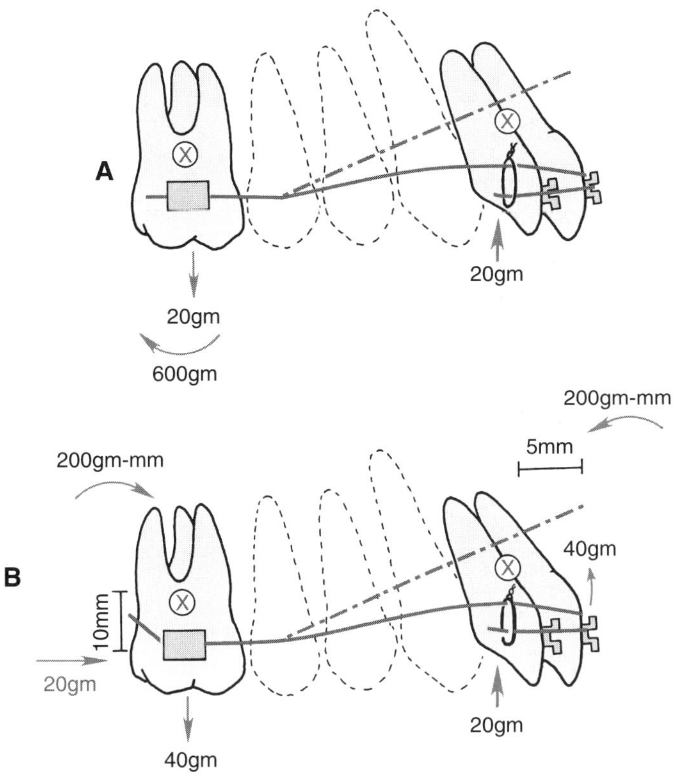

FIGURE 10-35 Two factors in the action of an intrusion arch are the relationship of the point of force application relative to the center of resistance of the incisor segment, and whether the incisor teeth are free to tip facially as they intrude or whether the arch is cinched back to produce lingual root torque. **A,** An intrusion arch can be tied at any point along the incisor segment. If it is tied behind the lateral incisor bracket, the force is applied in line with the center of resistance, and there is no moment to rotate the incisors facio-lingually. The effect on the anchor molar would be the same as if the intrusion arch were tied in the midline (see Figure 10-33). **B,** If the intrusion arch were tied in the midline and cinched back so it could not slide forward in the molar tube, the effect would be lingual root torque on the incisors as they intruded. Equilibrium requires that both moments and forces be balanced, so the moment on the incisors would be balanced by a similar moment on the anchor molars. Each would receive a 100 gm-mm moment to bring the crown mesially, which would require a 10 gm force at the distal of the molar tube if the distance from the tube to the molar's center of resistance is 10 mm.

levels needed for extrusion and tipping that would be the reactive movements of the anchor teeth. Tying the molar teeth together with a rigid lingual arch prevents buccal tipping of the molars. In adults, usually the premolar teeth also are added to the anchor unit.

It would be easy enough to activate an auxiliary arch wire to produce extrusion of incisors rather than intrusion. This is rarely done clinically, however. The force needed for extrusion is 4 to 5 times higher than intrusion, however, so the reactive force against the anchor teeth also would be higher and the anchor teeth would not be as stable. Perhaps more importantly, the precise control of force magnitude that is the major advantage of a one-couple system, is less critical when extrusion is desired. The additional complexity of stabilizing segments and an auxiliary arch wire may not be cost-effective if extrusion is the goal.

Two-Couple Systems

An easy way to see the effect of changing from a determinate one-couple to an indeterminate two-couple system is to observe the effect of tying an intrusion arch into brackets on incisor teeth, rather than tying it with one-point contact.[18] The utility arch, popularized by Ricketts and used most frequently for incisor intrusion, makes just this change. Like a one-couple intrusion arch, it is formed from rectangular wire so that it will not roll in the molar tubes. Also like a one-couple intrusion arch, it bypasses the canine and premolar teeth, i.e., it is a 2 × 4 arch wire (attached to 2 molars and 4 incisors). The resulting long span provides excellent load deflection properties so that the light force necessary for intrusion can be created. The difference comes when the utility arch is tied into the incisor brackets, creating a two-couple system.

When the utility arch is activated for intrusion, the moment of the intrusive force tips the crowns facially (Figure 10-36). One way to prevent the facial tipping is to apply a force to retract the incisors, which would create a moment in the opposite direction. This could be done by cinching or tying back the intrusion utility arch. Although the retraction force could be light, any force to bring the anchor teeth mesially is likely to be undesirable.

Another strategy to control the facial tipping is immediately apparent: Place a twist in the anterior segment of the utility arch, to torque the incisors lingually. Let us examine the effect of doing this (see Figure 10-36, *B*). An effect of the couple within the bracket is to increase the intrusive force on the incisors, and also the reactive extrusive force on the molars. Although one can be sure that the magnitude of the intrusive force would increase, it is impossible to know how much—but any increase would shift the balance of tooth movement away from the desired intrusion of the incisor, for which highly controlled light force is critical, toward extrusion of the anchor teeth.

Note that the "torque bend" in the utility arch wire produces two problems. The first is the reactive force generated by the couple within the bracket. An increase in the magnitude of the intrusive force often is not anticipated from such an apparently unrelated change in the arch wire. The second problem is that the magnitude of the reactive forces is not known with certainty, which makes it impossible to accurately adjust the arch wire even if you do anticipate the increase. Both effects help explain why utility arches often produce disappointing amounts of incisor intrusion relative to molar extrusion.

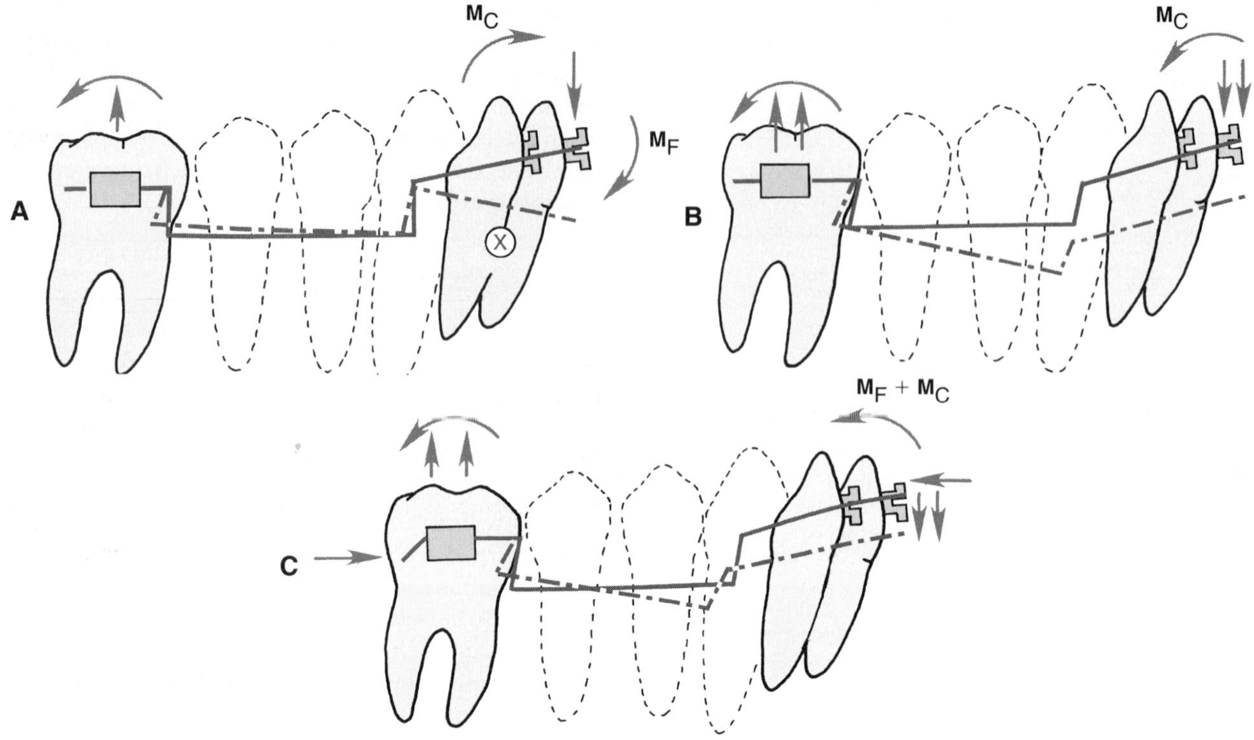

Figure 10-36 A utility arch often is an intrusion arch in a two-couple configuration, created by tying the rectangular intrusion arch into the brackets on the incisors. When this is done, the precise magnitude of forces and couples cannot be known, but the initial activation of the arch should be to provide about 40 grams to the incisor segment for intrusion. **A,** Activating the utility arch by placing it in the brackets creates the intrusion force, with a reactive force of the same magnitude on the anchor molar and a couple to tip its crown distally. At the incisors, a moment to tip the crowns facially (M_F) is created by distance of the brackets forward from the center of resistance, and an additional moment in the same direction is created by the couple within the bracket (M_C) as the inclination of the wire is changed when it is brought to the brackets. The moment of this couple cannot be known, but it is clinically important because it affects the magnitude of the intrusion force. **B,** Placing a torque bend in the utility arch creates a moment to bring the crown lingually, controlling the tendency for the teeth to tip facially as they intrude, but it also increases the magnitude of the intrusive force on the incisor segment and the extrusive force and couple on the molar. **C,** Cinching back the utility arch creates a force to bring the incisors lingually, and a moment of this force opposes the moment of the intrusion force. At the molar, a force to bring the molar mesially is created, along with a moment to tip the molar mesially. Especially if a torque bend still is present, it is difficult to be certain which of the moments will prevail, or whether the intrusion force is appropriate. With this two-couple system, the vertical forces easily can be heavier than desired, changing the balance between intrusion of the incisors and extrusion of the molars. (Redrawn from Davidovitch M, Rebellato J. Utility arches: A two-couple intrusion system. Semin Orthod 1: 25-30, 1995.)

Applications of Complex (Two-Couple) Force Systems

Symmetric and Asymmetric Bends

When a wire is placed into two brackets, the forces of the equilibrium always act at both brackets. There are three possibilities for placing a bend in the wire to activate it:

- Symmetric V-bend, which creates equal and opposite couples at the brackets (Figure 10-37). The associated equilibrium forces at each bracket also are equal and opposite, and therefore cancel each other out. A symmetrical V-bend is not necessarily halfway between two teeth or two groups of teeth. If two teeth are involved but one is bigger than the other (e.g., a canine and lateral incisor), equal and opposite moments would require placing the bend closer to the large tooth, to compensate for the longer distance from the bracket to its center of resistance. The same would be true if two groups of teeth had been created by tying them into the equivalent of a single large multi-rooted tooth, as when posterior teeth are grouped into a stabilizing segment and used for anchorage to move a group of four incisors. A symmetrical V-bend would have to be offset, to compensate for the greater resistance of one segment.
- Asymmetric V-bend, which creates unequal and opposite couples, and net equilibrium forces that would intrude one unit and extrude the other (Figure 10-38).

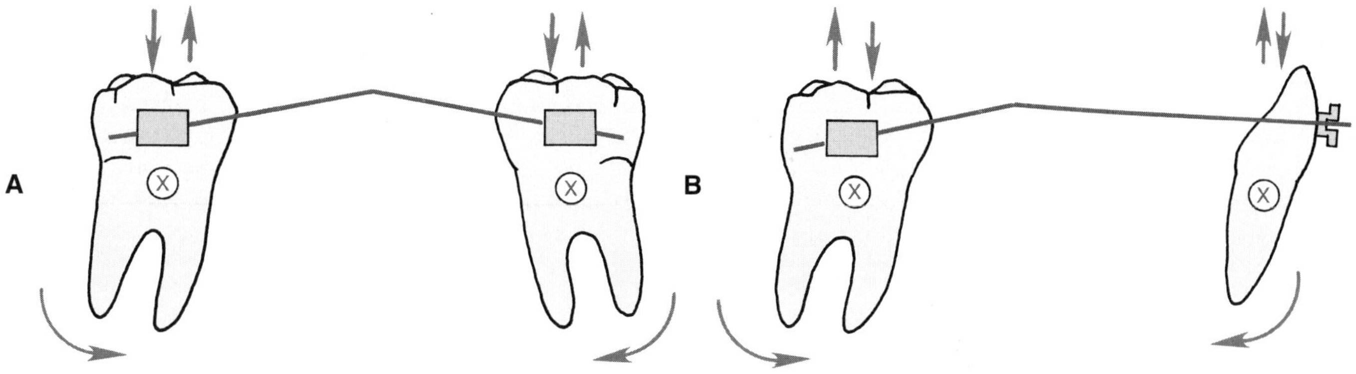

FIGURE 10-37 **A,** A symmetric V-bend is placed halfway between two units with equal resistance to movement. It creates equal and opposite moments, and the intrusive/extrusive forces cancel each other. **B,** To create equal and opposite couples, a V-bend must be displaced toward the unit with greater resistance to movement, so a symmetric V-bend between an incisor and molar would be offset toward the molar. One must know the approximate anchorage value of teeth or units of the dental arch to calculate the appropriate location of symmetric or asymmetric V-bends.

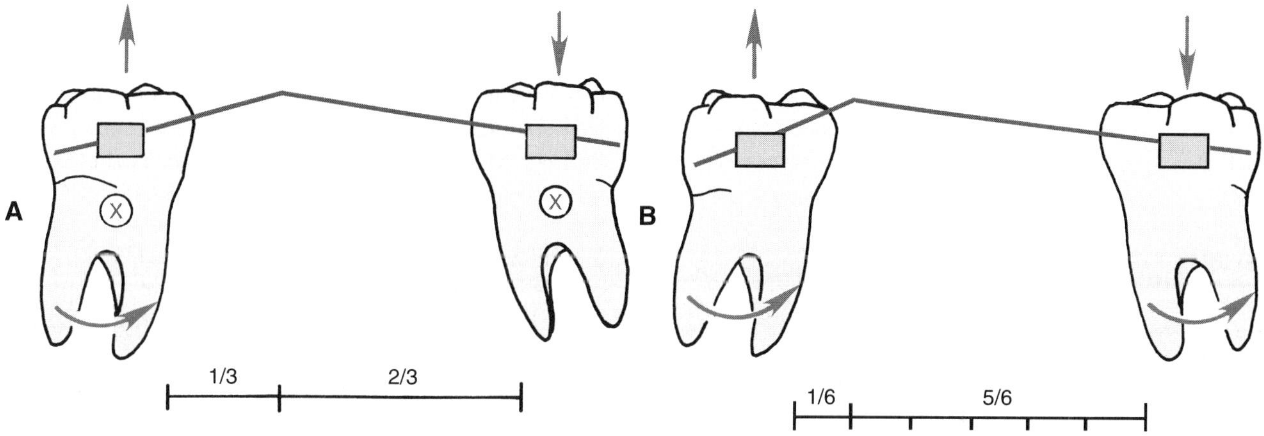

FIGURE 10-38 **A,** An asymmetric V-bend creates a greater moment on one tooth or unit than the other. As the bend moves toward one tooth, the moment on it increases and the moment on the distant tooth decreases. When the bend is one-third of the way along the interbracket span, the distant tooth receives only a force, with no moment. **B,** If the V-bend moves closer than the one-third point to one of the teeth, a moment in the same direction is created on both teeth, instead of opposite moments. A V-bend placed to parallel the roots of the adjacent teeth would not do so if the bend were too close to one of the teeth.

Although the absolute magnitude of the forces involved cannot be known with certainty (this is, after all, an indeterminate system), the relative magnitude of the moments and the direction of the associated equilibrium forces can be determined. The bracket with the larger moment will have a greater tendency to rotate than the bracket with the smaller moment, and this will indicate the direction of the equilibrium forces. As the bend moves closer to one of two equal units, the moment increases on the closer unit and decreases on the distant one, while equilibrium forces increase. When the bend is located one-third of the distance along the wire between two equal units, no moment is felt at the distant bracket, only a single force. When the bend moves closer than that to one bracket, moments at both brackets are in the same direction, and equilibrium forces increase further.

- Step bend, which creates two couples in the same direction regardless of its location between the brackets (Figure 10-39). The location of a V-bend is a critical variable in determining its effect, but the location of a step bend has little or no effect on either the magnitude of the moments or the equilibrium forces.

The general relationship between bend location and the forces and moments that are produced is shown in Table 10-7. Note that for V-bends, the force increases steadily as the beam moves off-center. For step bends, since both couples are in the same direction, the force is increased over what a symmetrical V-bend would produce.

Under laboratory conditions, the forces and couples created in a two-couple system can be evaluated experimentally.[19] With a 16 mil steel wire and an interbracket distance of 7 mm (about what would be found between central incisors with twin brackets or between narrow canine and premolar brackets), a step bend of only 0.35 mm would produce intrusive/extrusive forces of 347 grams and 1210 gm-mm couples in the same direction (see Table 10-7). Permanent distortion of the wire would occur with a step bend of 0.8 mm. Since this force magnitude is far too great for intrusion, it is clear that extrusion would prevail. The heavy vertical forces produced by what orthodontists would consider modest bends in a light arch wire explain why extrusion is the response to step bends in continuous arch wires. An asymmetric V-bend that places the apex of the bend 0.35 mm above the plane of the brackets, produces 803 gm-mm couples with no net intrusive/extrusive forces at the one-third position. At the one-sixth position, intrusive/extrusive forces over 900 grams occur, with very large moments (see Table 10-7), so the result here also would be extrusion in addition to root movement.

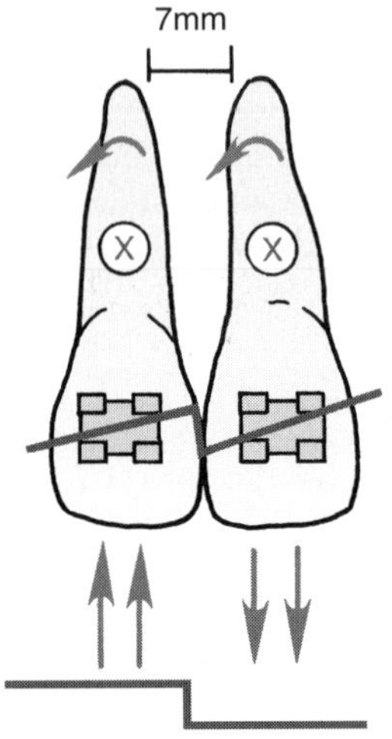

FIGURE 10-39 A step bend between two teeth produces intrusive force on one tooth, extrusive force on the other, and creates couples in the same direction. In contrast to V-bends, there is little effect on either the force or the couples when the step bend is moved off-center.

The moments and forces are greatly reduced as interbracket distances increase. For instance, the same 0.35 mm step bend that produced 347 grams with a 7 mm interbracket span, produces only 43 grams with a 14 mm span (which is still too high for intrusion). Even with flexible arch wires, an interbracket span equivalent to the distance from the first molar to the lateral incisor is needed to obtain the light force necessary for intrusion. Longer spans also make the location of V-bends less critical. With a 7 mm interbracket span, moving a V-bend only 1.2 mm from a centered position would put it at the one-third position that totally eliminates the moment on the distant bracket. With a 21 mm span, the same error would be almost negligible. It is much easier, therefore, to control two-couple systems when the distances between attachments are relatively large, as they are when wires connect only to molars and incisors in a 2 × 4 arrangement, or to anterior and posterior segments.

Still another level of complexity exists for a 2 × 4 two-couple wire, because three-dimensional effects are produced when the wire goes around the arch from the molars to the incisors. This makes the analysis of torque bends particularly difficult. Using finite analysis modeling, Isaacson et al have

TABLE 10-7

Force Systems From Step and V-Bends

	Percent of total span to closest bracket	Moment far tooth/ moment near tooth	Force general condition	Data from experiment 16 steel, 7 mm span, 0.35 mm bend: Force (gm)	Moment (gm-mm)
Step Bend					
	All	1.0	XX	347	1210/1210
V-Bend					
	0.5	−1.0	None	0	803/803
	0.4	−0.3	X		
	0.33	0	XX		
	0.29			353	2210/262
	0.2	0.3	XXX		
	0.14			937	4840/1720
	0.1	0.4	XXXX		

(From Burstone CJ, Koening HA: Am J Orthod Dentofac Orthop 93: 59-67, 1988.)

shown that the general principles of 2-D analysis remain valid when 3-D analysis is done.[20] In a long-span wire like a utility arch, however, a V-bend at the molar produces significantly less moment and associated equilibrium forces than the same V-bend located at the same distance from the incisor segment. In addition, the reversal of moments so that the moment is in the same direction on the molar and the incisor, does not occur in the 3-D analysis when the V-bend moves closer than one-third of the distance to the molar or incisors. The effect is to make the effect of utility arches with complex bends even less predictable.

Utility and 2 × 4 Arches to Change Incisor Positions

The use of a two-couple utility arch to change the vertical position of incisors, and the problems that arise in controlling intrusion with this method, have been briefly outlined above. Two-couple systems work better for other types of tooth movement in which force magnitudes do not have to be controlled so precisely.

A two-couple system to change the inclination of incisors can be arranged to produce either tipping or torque. If a wire spanning from the molars to the incisors is activated to rotate incisors around their center of resistance, the crowns will move facially when the wire is free to slide through the molar tube (Figure 10-40).[21] Occasionally, this provides a convenient way to tip maxillary incisors facially to correct anterior crossbite in the mixed dentition (see Chapter 14).

If the wire is cinched back, the effect will be to torque the incisor roots lingually, and a reaction force to bring the molar mesially is created. The incisors also will extrude, while the molars will intrude and roll lingually. For incisor root torque, the long range of action provided by a 2 × 4 two-couple system is not necessarily an advantage, particularly when there is nothing to control the vertical side effects on the incisors. In patients with severely upright maxillary central incisors (as in Class II division 2 malocclusion), a one-couple torquing arch can be used to advantage (Figure 10-41).

Transverse Movement of Posterior Teeth

Dental posterior crossbite, requiring expansion or constriction of molars, can be approached with two-couple arch wires.[22] Then the anterior segment becomes the anchorage and movement of one or both first molars is desired (Figure 10-42). Incorporating the canines into the anchor segment is a necessity (i.e., this requires a 2 × 6 rather than a 2 × 4 appliance). A long span bypassing the premolars still is needed for appropriate force levels and control of moments. Asymmetric expansion or constriction to correct unilateral crossbite is quite feasible and often is the indication for using this method. As with other applications of two-couple systems, the large range of the appliance means that teeth can be moved a considerable distance with a single activation of the appliance. The corresponding disadvantage, of course, is that the system has poor fail-safe properties.

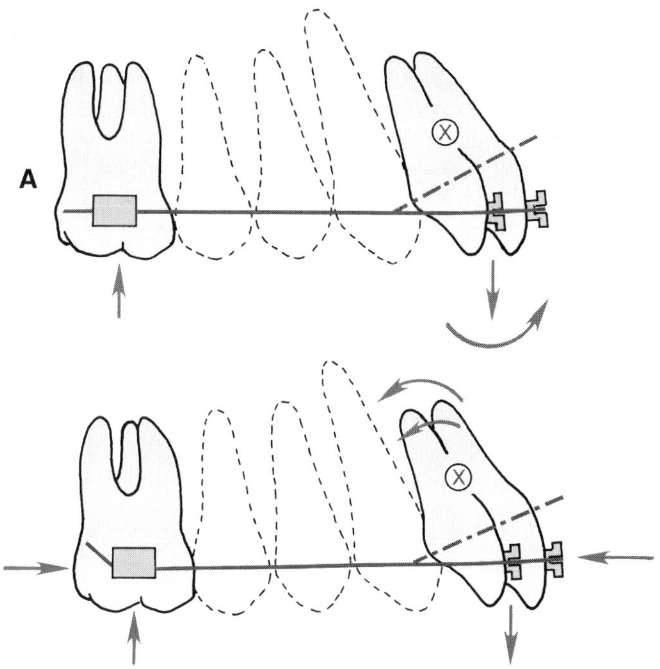

FIGURE 10-40 An asymmetric V-bend in a rectangular wire spanning from the first molars to the incisor segment produces a moment to rotate the incisors facio-lingually, with an intrusive force but no moment on the molars and an extrusive force on the incisors. **A,** If the arch wire is free to slide forward through the molar tube, the result is anterior tipping and extrusion of the incisors. Occasionally, this is desirable in the correction of anterior crossbite in the mixed dentition. **B,** If the arch wire is cinched behind the molar so that it cannot slide, the effect is lingual root torque and extrusion for the incisors and a mesial force on the molars.

Lingual Arches as Two-Couple Systems

Still another example of a two-couple appliance system is a transpalatal lingual arch (or a mandibular lingual arch that does not contact the anterior teeth).[23] Lingual arches often are employed to prevent tooth movement rather than create it. The need for a lingual arch to stabilize posterior segments in many situations has been noted above. When a lingual arch is used to move teeth, spring properties are required—which means that either a different wire size or different material is needed for an active rather than a stabilizing lingual arch. Often when a flexible lingual arch is used to reposition molars, a rigid one then is needed to stabilize them while other tooth movement occurs. Steel lingual arches usually are 30 mil when tooth movement is desired, 36 mil when stabilization is needed. Replacing one with the other would require changing the tube on the molar band. To prevent this, one possible approach is to use a 32 × 32

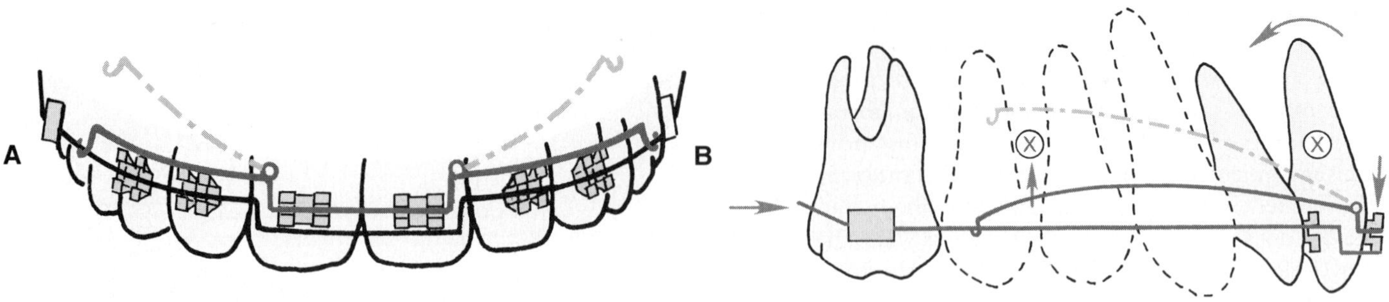

FIGURE 10-41 For torque of very upright maxillary central incisors (as in Class II division 2 malocclusion), a one-couple torquing arch designed by Burstone can be very effective. **A,** A heavy stabilizing arch is placed in all the teeth but the central incisors, contoured so that it steps below the brackets on the central incisors and contacts the facial surface of these teeth, is tied back against the molars. A wire tied into the central incisor brackets and activated by bending it down and hooking it between the first molar and second premolar, then produces the desired moment. **B,** Because the stabilizing arch wire prevents facial tipping and extrusion of the central incisors, the result is lingual root torque with optimum force over a long range. The reaction force to intrude the remaining teeth and bring them anteriorly is distributed over all the other teeth, minimizing the reaction.

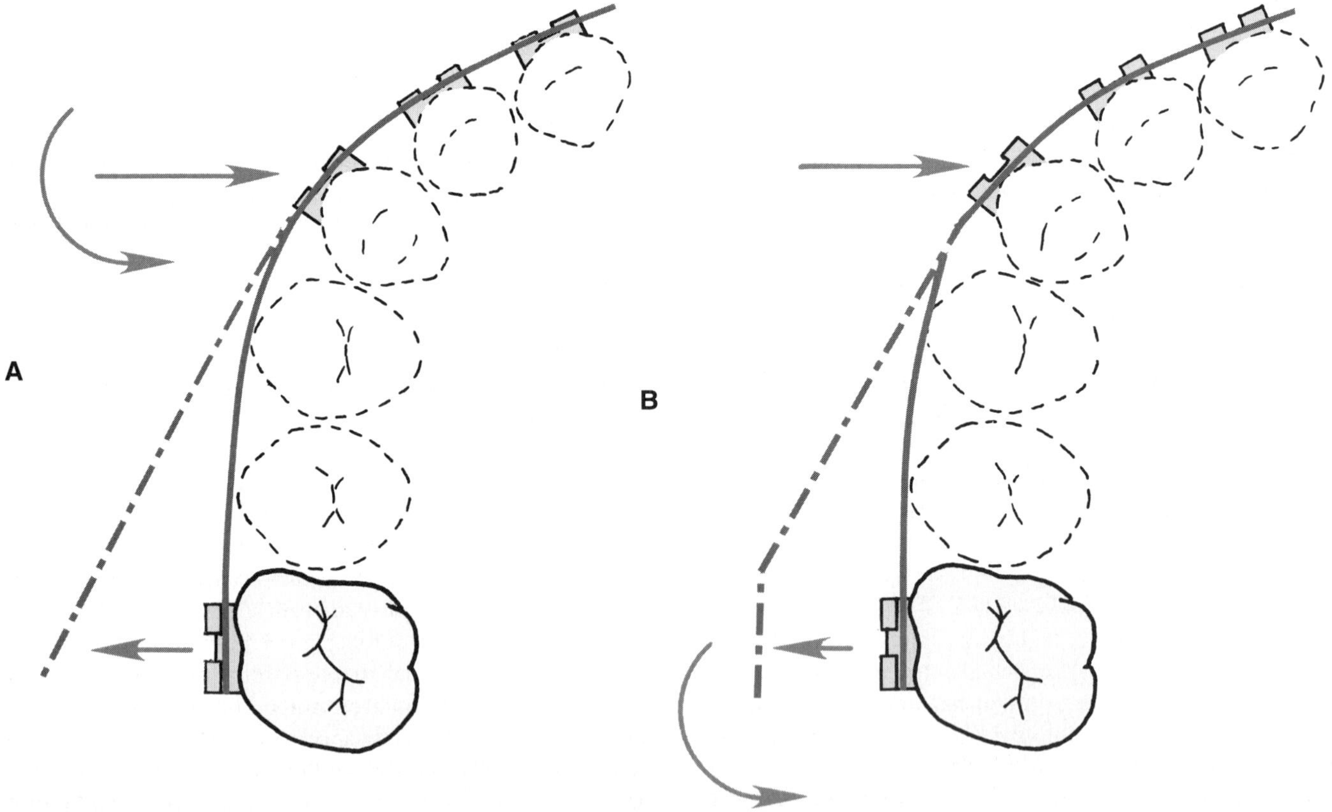

FIGURE 10-42 A 2 × 6 appliance can be used to produce transverse movement of first permanent molars. In this circumstance, the anterior segment becomes the anchorage, and it is important to add the canines to the anchor unit, but the premolars cannot be tied to the arch wire without destroying its effectiveness. The long span between the canine and molar is needed to produce the desired forces and moments in this two-couple system. **A,** An outward bend a few mm behind the canine bracket results primarily in expansion of the molar, with little or no rotation (with the unequal segments, this approximates the one-third position between the units of the two-couple system). **B,** An outward bend behind the canine combined with a toe-in bend at the molar results in expansion and mesial-out rotation of the molar. (Redrawn from Isaacson RJ, Rebellato J.[21])

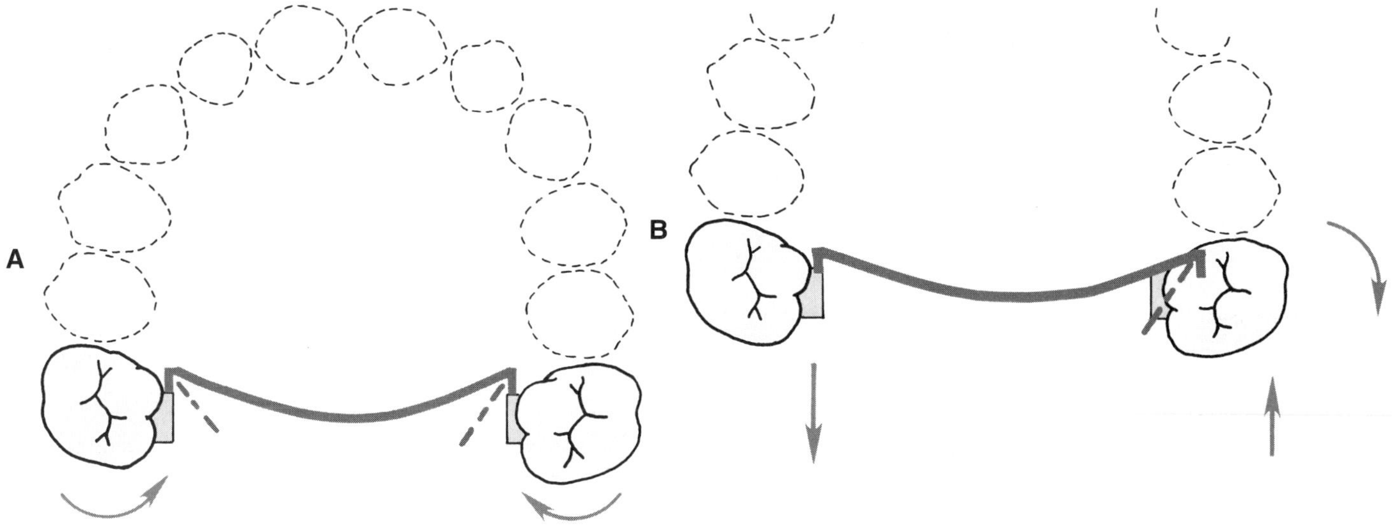

Figure 10-43 **A,** Bilateral toe-in bends at the first molars create equal and opposite couples, so the mesio-distal forces cancel and the teeth are rotated to bring the mesio-buccal cusp facially. When space has been lost in the maxillary arch or when a Class II molar relationship exists, this type of rotation often is desired, but a flexible rather than a rigid lingual arch is needed to obtain it. **B,** A unilateral toe-in bend rotates the molar on the side of the bend, and creates a force to move the other molar distally. Although mesial movement of the molar on the side of the bend is limited by contact with the other teeth, mesial movement may occur. Although net distalization of both molars has been claimed by bends of this type on first one side, then the other, significant distal movement of both teeth is unlikely.

TMA wire for active movement and 32 × 32 steel for stabilization, both of which will fit into the same rectangular lingual tube.[24] Lingual arches in general, and this approach in particular, are discussed in some detail in Chapter 11.

Whatever a lingual arch is made of, and however it is attached, its two-couple design predicts the effect of symmetric V, asymmetric V and step bends. Often it is desirable to rotate maxillary first molars so that the mesio-buccal cusp moves facially. This can be accomplished bilaterally with symmetric bends, or unilaterally with an asymmetric bend (Figure 10-43). An asymmetric activation tends to rotate the molar on the side closest to the bend and move it mesially, while the molar on the other side is displaced distally. It is tempting to think that net distal movement of upper molars can be accomplished routinely with this type of activation of lingual arches, and it has been suggested that a clinician can distalize one molar while rotating the other, then reverse the process, moving both of them back. However, the evidence indicates that significant distal movement beyond rotation of the buccal cusps is unlikely—mesial movement of the anchor molar is entirely possible.[25]

A lingual arch also can be activated to torque roots facially or lingually (Figure 10-44). Symmetric torque when molars are expanded provides bodily movement rather than tipping. An interesting approach to unilateral crossbite is the use of a lingual arch with buccal root torque (lingual crown torque) on one side pitted against buccal tipping on the other side. As Ingervall and co-workers have shown quite convincingly, significant expansion on the tipping side can be produced, perhaps more effectively if the appliance is converted to a one-couple device by placing a round rather than rectangular wire in the bracket on the tipping side.[26]

A somewhat unusual application of a lingual arch would be to tip one molar distally, uprighting it. The reciprocal, of course, would be mesial tipping of the opposite molar. This activation would require a twist in the lingual wire. The location of this twist bend is not critical. The relative moments on the molar teeth will be equal and opposite, wherever the twist bend is placed.

Segmented Arch Mechanics

What is often called segmented arch mechanics is best considered an organized approach to using one-couple and two-couple systems for most tooth movements, so as to obtain both more favorable force levels and better control.[11] The essence of the segmented arch system is the establishment of well-defined units of teeth, so that anchorage and movement segments are clearly defined. The desired tooth movement is accomplished with cantilever springs where possible, so that the precision of the one-couple approach is available, or with the use of two-couple systems through which at least net moments and the direction of equilibrium forces can be known.

In segmented arch treatment, lingual arches are used for stabilization in a majority of the patients, and stabilizing wire segments in the brackets of teeth in anchor units also are used routinely. The requirements for stabilization, of

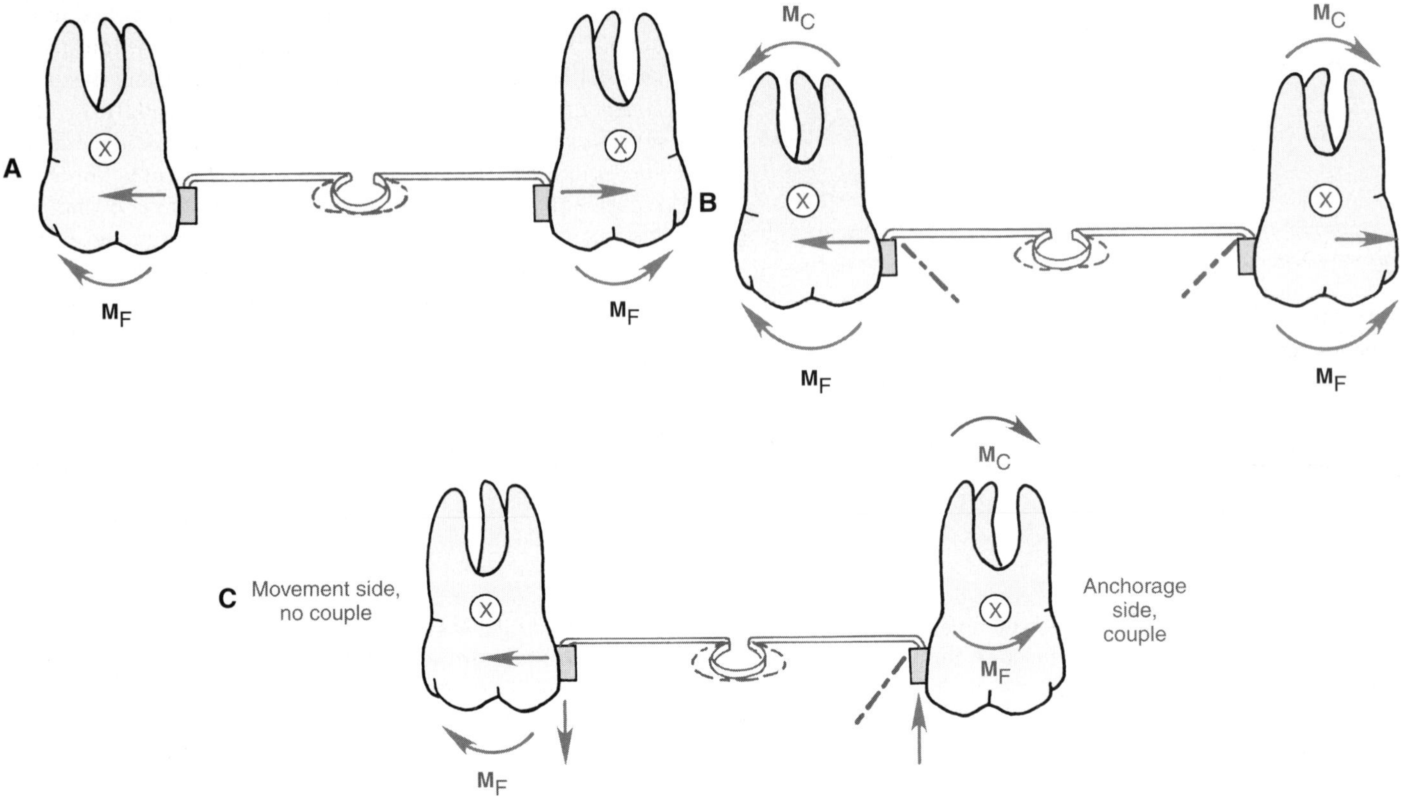

FIGURE 10-44 **A,** Bilateral expansion of molars can be created by expansion of a transpalatal arch, which typically is achieved by opening a loop in the mid-palate area. The moment of the expansion force tips the crowns facially. **B,** Placing a twist in the wire creates a moment to torque the roots facially. The moment of the couple must be greater than the moment of the force for this to occur. Unless a flexible wire is used for the lingual arch, it can be difficult to insert the activated lingual arch with enough twist to produce the desired torque. **C,** A twist in the wire on one side can be used to create stationary anchorage to tip the opposite molar facially. This is particularly effective if the wire is rounded on the movement side, so that a one-couple rather than two-couple system exists in the facio-lingual plane of space. (**A, B** redrawn from Rebellato[22]; **C,** Modified from Ingervall B et al.[26])

course, are just the opposite of those for tooth movement: the heaviest and most rigid available wires are desired. For this reason, the 22 slot edgewise appliance is favored for segmented arch treatment. The wires used for stabilizing segments usually are 21 × 25 steel, which is far too stiff for tooth movement. Until 32 × 32 steel wires became available, the stabilizing lingual arches usually were 36 steel, with doubled-over ends that fit into rectangular sheaths.

Typical segmented arch treatment would call for initial alignment within anterior and posterior segments, the creation of appropriate anchorage and tooth movement segments, vertical leveling using intrusion or extrusion as needed, space closure with differential movement of anterior and posterior segments, and perhaps the use of auxiliary torquing arches. Friction as wires slide through brackets is almost always avoided, because it hampers efforts to control anchorage and introduces almost intolerable uncertainties into the calculation of appropriate force levels. Continuous archwires, particularly rectangular wires, would be reserved for the final stages of treatment when quite small but precise movements are required.

The advantages of the segmented arch approach are the control that is available, and the possibility of tooth movements that would be impossible with continuous archwires. The disadvantage is the greater complexity of the orthodontic appliance, and the greater amount of the doctor's time needed to install, adjust and maintain it. It is an interesting paradox that simplifying the engineering analysis of the appliance, by dealing insofar as possible with identifiable one- and two-couple systems, complicates the appliance rather than making it simpler.

An excellent example of the segmented arch approach is the design of an appliance to simultaneously retract and intrude protruding maxillary central incisors. This is difficult to accomplish because lingual tipping of the incisors tends to move the crown downward as the tooth rotates around its center of resistance. Intrusion of the root apex is necessary to keep the crown at the same vertical level rela-

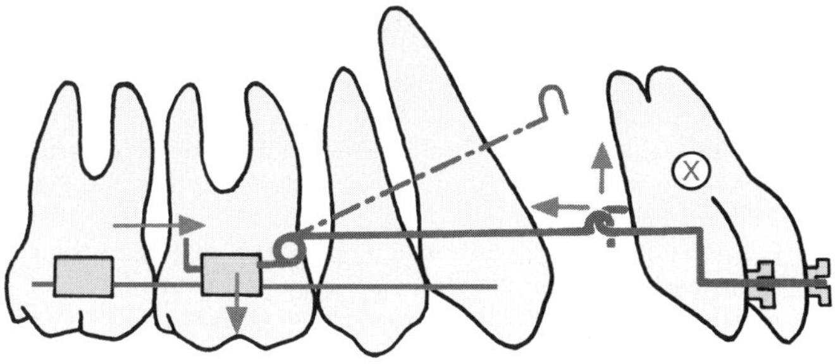

FIGURE 10-45 A segmented arch approach allows simultaneous retraction and intrusion of an anterior segment. A rigid bar in the anterior segment can be extended posteriorly so that the point of application of an intrusive force is at or distal to the center of resistance of the incisor segment. If a cantilever spring is used to apply an intrusive force at that point, the tendency of a retraction force to elongate the anterior segment can be overcome. (Redrawn from Shroff B et al.[28])

tive to the lip and other teeth. This problem can be solved by creating anterior and posterior segments, using a rigid bar to move the point of force application distal to the center of resistance of the incisor segment, and applying separate intrusion and retraction forces (Figure 10-45).[27] This could be done much more easily now, however, by using miniplates as illustrated in Chapter 15. Skeletal anchorage has the potential to replace many of the more complex applications of segmented arch treatment.

Complex segmented arch treatment carries with it two other potential disadvantages that must be kept in mind. First, even with the most careful engineering analysis, it can turn out that something was overlooked in the determination of the likely outcome. Obviously, that is more likely when two-couple rather than one-couple devices are employed, but occasionally the simplifications that are part of normal engineering practice (e.g., neglecting the torque that may be created within a lingual arch bracket as tooth movement starts) can lead to surprising outcomes. It remains true that the more often something has been attempted, the more predictable the outcome is likely to be. The application of engineering theory to orthodontics is imperfect enough that a unique force system for an individual patient may not produce the expected outcome.

Second, most segmented arch mechanisms contain little or nothing to control the distance that teeth can be displaced if something goes wrong. If precisely calibrated springs with a long range of action encounter something that distorts them (e.g., a sticky candy bar), major problems can occur. The mechanical efficiency of a segmented appliance can be both an advantage and a disadvantage.

Continuous Arch Mechanics

Analysis of the effects of a continuous arch wire, one that is tied into the brackets on all the teeth, is essentially impossible. All that can be said is that an extremely complex multicouple force system is established when the wire is tied into place. The initial result is a small movement of one tooth. As soon as that occurs, the force system is changed, and the new system causes a small movement of another tooth (or a different movement of the first tooth). Either way, the result is still another complex force system, which causes another movement, leading to another change in the system, and so forth. Sometimes orthodontic tooth movement is conceived as a slow, smooth transition of the teeth from one arrangement to another. Some thought about the force systems involved, particularly those with continuous arch mechanics, make it plain that this is far from the case. If it were possible to take time-lapse photographs of teeth being moved into position, we undoubtedly would see "the dance of the teeth," as the complex force systems formed and changed, producing varied effects in sequence. It is a saving grace that a continuous arch wire usually does not allow the teeth to move very far from the desired end point.

The advantages and disadvantages of the continuous arch approach are just the reverse of those with the segmented arch approach. Continuous arch treatment is not as well defined in terms of the forces and moments that will be generated at any one time, and certainly is less elegant from an engineering perspective. But continuous arch wires often take less chair time because they are simpler to make and install, and because they have excellent fail-safe properties in most applications. In modern orthodontics, often the clinician must evaluate the trade-off between segmented and continuous arch approaches to specific problems. For those who use primarily the segmented approach, some use of continuous arch wires simplifies life. For those who use primarily continuous arch wires, some use of the segmented approach is necessary to meet specific objectives. Quite literally, you consider the benefits vs. the cost (time) and risks, and take your choice.

The development of contemporary fixed appliances and their characteristics are discussed in Chapter 11. Clinical applications of the mechanical principles reviewed in this chapter, and further information about the use of specific treatment methods, are provided in some detail in Chapters 14 to 18.

REFERENCES

1. Burstone CJ, Qin B, Morton JY. Chinese NiTi wire: A new orthodontic alloy. Am J Orthod 87:445-452, 1985.
2. Miura F, Mogi M, Yoshiaki O, et al. The super-elastic property of the Japanese NiTi alloy wire for use in orthodontics. Am J Orthod 90:1-10, 1986.
3. Gurgel J, Kerr S, Powers JM, LeCrone V. Force-deflection properties of superelastic nickel-titanium archwires. Am J Orthod Dentofac Orthop 120:378-382, 2001.
4. Miura F, Mogi M, Okamoto Y. New application of superelastic NiTi rectangular wire. J Clin Orthod 24:544-548, 1990.
5. Freudenthaler JW, Tischler GK, Burstone CJ. Bond strength of fiber-reinforced composite bars for orthodontic attachment. Am J Orthod Dentofac Orthop 120:648-653, 2001.

6. Kusy RP. On the use of nomograms to determine the elastic property ratios of orthodontic archwires. Am J Orthod 83:374-381, 1983.
7. Adams DM, Powers JM, Asgar K. Effects of brackets and ties on stiffness of an arch wire. Am J Orthod Dentofac Orthop 91:131-136, 1987.
8. Josell SD, Leiss JB, Rekow ED. Force degradation in elastomeric chains. Semin Orthod 3:189-197, 1997.
9. Darendeliler MA, Darendeliler A, Mandurino M. Clinical application of magnets in orthodontics and biological implications: A review. Eur J Orthod 19:431-442, 1997.
10. Linder-Aronson A, Lindskog S, Rygh P. Orthodontic magnets: Effects on gingival epithelium and alveolar bone in monkeys. Eur J Orthod 14:255-263, 1992.
11. Jastrzebski ZD. The Nature and Properties of Engineering Materials, ed 3. New York: Wiley; 1987.
12. Kusy RP, Whitley JQ. Effects of surface roughness on the coefficients of friction in model orthodontic systems. J Biomech 23:913-925, 1990.
13. Kusy RP, Whitley JQ, Gurgel J. Comparisons of surface roughnesses and sliding resistances of 6 titanium-based or TMA-type archwires. Am J Orthod Dentofac Orthop 126:589-603, 2004.
14. Saunders CR, Kusy RP. Surface topography and frictional characteristics of ceramic brackets. Am J Orthod Dentofac Orthop 106:76-87, 1994.
15. Kusy RP, Whitley JQ. Assessment of second-order clearances between orthodontic archwires and bracket slots via the critical contact angle for binding. Angle Orthod 69:71-80, 1999.
16. Thorstenson GA, Kusy RP. Comparison of resistance to sliding between different self-ligating brackets with second-order angulations in the dry and saliva states. Am J Orthod Dentofac Orthop 121:472-482, 2001.
17. Lindauer SJ, Isaacson RJ. One-couple systems. Semin Orthod 1:12-24, 1995.
18. Davidovitch M, Rebellato J. Utility arches: A two-couple intrusion system. Semin Orthod 1:25-30, 1995.
19. Burstone CJ, Koenig HA. Creative wire bending—the force system from step and V bends. Am J Orthod Dentofac Orthop 93:59-67, 1988.
20. Isaacson RJ, Lindauer SJ, Conley P. Responses of 3-dimensional archwires to vertical V-bends: Comparisons with existing 2-dimensional data in the lateral view. Semin Orthod 1:57-63, 1995.
21. Isaacson RJ, Rebellato J. Two-couple orthodontic appliance systems: Torquing arches. Semin Orthod 1:31-36, 1995.
22. Rebellato J. Two-couple orthodontic appliance systems: Activations in the transverse dimension. Semin Orthod 1:37-43, 1995.
23. Rebellato J. Two-couple orthodontic appliance systems: Transpalatal arches. Semin Orthod 1:44-54, 1995.
24. Burstone CJ. Precision lingual arches: Active applications. J Clin Orthod 23:101-109, 1989.
25. Dahlquist A, Gebauer U, Ingervall B. The effect of a transpalatal arch for correction of first molar rotation. Eur J Orthod 18:257-267, 1996.
26. Ingervall B, Gollner P, Gebauer U, Frolich K. A clinical investigation of the correction of unilateral molar crossbite with a transpalatal arch. Am J Orthod Dentofac Orthop 107:418-425, 1995.
27. Marcotte MR. Biomechanics in Orthodontics. Philadelphia: Decker; 1990.
28. Shroff B, Yoon WM, Lindauer SJ, Burstone CJ. Simultaneous intrusion and retraction using a three-piece base arch. Angle Orthod 67:455-462, 1997.

CHAPTER

11

Contemporary Orthodontic Appliances

CHAPTER OUTLINE

REMOVABLE APPLIANCES

Removable orthodontic appliances have two immediately apparent advantages: (1) they are fabricated in the laboratory rather than directly in the patient's mouth, reducing the dentist's chair time, and (2) they can be removed on socially sensitive occasions if wires on the facial part of the teeth would be visible, or can be made almost invisible if fabricated from clear plastic materials. This makes them (at least initially) more acceptable to adult patients. In addition, removables allow some types of growth guidance treatment to be carried out more readily than is possible with fixed appliances. These advantages for both the patient and the dentist have ensured a continuing interest in removable appliances for both children and adults.

There are also two significant disadvantages: (1) the response to treatment is heavily dependent on patient compliance, since the appliance can be effective only when the patient chooses to wear it, and (2) it is difficult to obtain the two-point contacts on teeth necessary to produce complex tooth movements, which means that the appliance itself may limit the possibilities for treatment. Because of these limitations, removable appliances in children are most useful for the first of two phases of treatment, with fixed appliances used in the second phase; and if removable clear aligners are used in treatment of adults, some fixed attachments (which can be relatively small tooth-colored composites rather than brackets) often must be bonded in order to achieve effective tooth movement. For these reasons, contemporary comprehensive treatment for adolescents almost always requires fixed, non-removable appliances, and clear aligner therapy for adults is evolving toward the use of a combination of aligners and fixed appliances for the more complex cases.

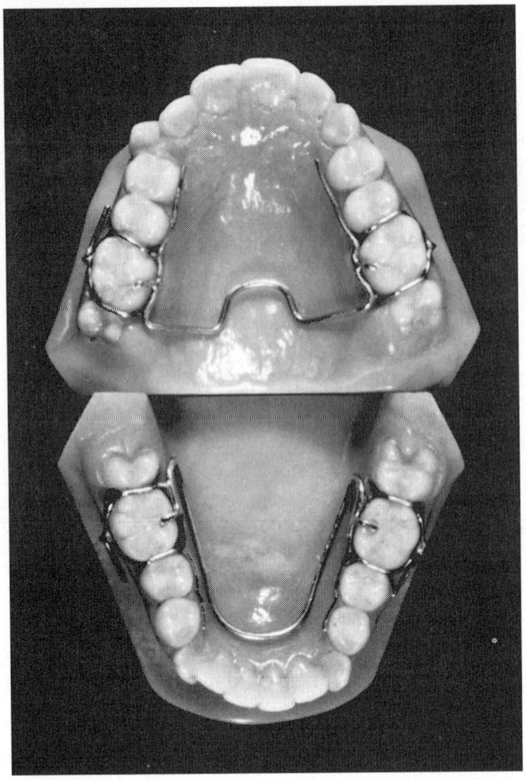

FIGURE 11-1 Crozat appliances for the upper and lower arch, showing the transverse connectors that allow lateral expansion. The Crozat clasps on the molars utilize fingers extending into the mesio-buccal and disto-buccal undercuts.

The Development of Removable Appliances

In the United States, the original removable appliances were rather clumsy combinations of vulcanite bases and precious metal or nickel-silver wires. In the early 1900s, George Crozat developed a removable appliance fabricated entirely of precious metal that is still used occasionally. The appliance consisted of an effective clasp for first molar teeth, heavy gold wires as a framework, and lighter gold finger springs to produce the desired tooth movement (Figure 11-1). The Crozat appliance attracted a small but devoted following, and still is used by some practitioners for comprehensive treatment. Its limitation is that, like almost all removables, it produces mostly tipping of teeth. It had little impact on the mainstream of American orthodontic thought and practice, however, which from the beginning was focused on fixed appliances.

For a variety of reasons, development of removable appliances continued in Europe despite their neglect in the United States. There were three major reasons for this trend: (1) Angle's dogmatic approach to occlusion, with its emphasis on precise positioning of each tooth, had less impact in Europe than in the United States; (2) social welfare systems developed much more rapidly in Europe, which tended to place the emphasis on limited orthodontic treatment for large numbers of people, often delivered by general practitioners rather than orthodontic specialists; and (3) precious metal for fixed appliances was less available in Europe, both as a consequence of the social systems and because the use of precious metal in dentistry was banned in Nazi Germany. This forced German orthodontists to focus on removable appliances that could be made with available materials. (Precision steel attachments were not available until long after World War II; fixed appliances required precious metal.)

The interesting result was that in the 1925 to 1965 era, American orthodontics was based almost exclusively on the use of fixed appliances (partial or complete banding), while fixed appliances were essentially unknown in Europe and all treatment was done with removables, not only for growth guidance but also for tooth movement of all types.

A major part of European removable appliance orthodontics of this period was functional appliances for guidance of growth. A functional appliance by definition is one that changes the posture of the mandible, holding it open or open and forward. Pressures created by stretch of the muscles and soft tissues are transmitted to the dental and skeletal structures, moving teeth and modifying growth. The monobloc developed by Robin in the early 1900s is generally considered the forerunner of all functional appliances, but the activator developed in Norway by Andresen in the 1920s (Figure 11-2) was the first functional appliance to be widely accepted.

Andresen's activator became the basis of the "Norwegian system" of treatment. Both the appliance system and its theoretic underpinnings were improved and extended elsewhere in Europe, particularly by the German school led by Haupl, who believed that the only stable tooth movement was produced by natural forces and that alterations in function produced by these appliances would give stable corrections of malocclusion. This philosophic approach was diametrically opposite to that espoused by Angle and his followers in the United States, who emphasized fixed appliances to precisely position the teeth. These opposing beliefs contributed to the great differences between European and American orthodontics at mid-20th century.

In the European approach at that time, removable appliances often were differentiated into "activators," or functional appliances aimed at modifying growth, and "active plates" aimed at moving teeth. In addition to the functional appliance pioneers, two European orthodontists deserve special mention for their contributions to removable appliance techniques for moving teeth. Martin Schwartz in Vienna developed and publicized a variety of "split plate" appliances, which could produce most types of tooth movements. Philip Adams in Belfast modified the arrowhead clasp favored by Schwartz into the Adams crib, which became the basis for English removable appliances and is still the most effective clasp for orthodontic purposes. (Both split plates and Adams clasps are pictured below.)

Functional appliances were introduced into American orthodontics in the 1960s, through the influence of

A

B

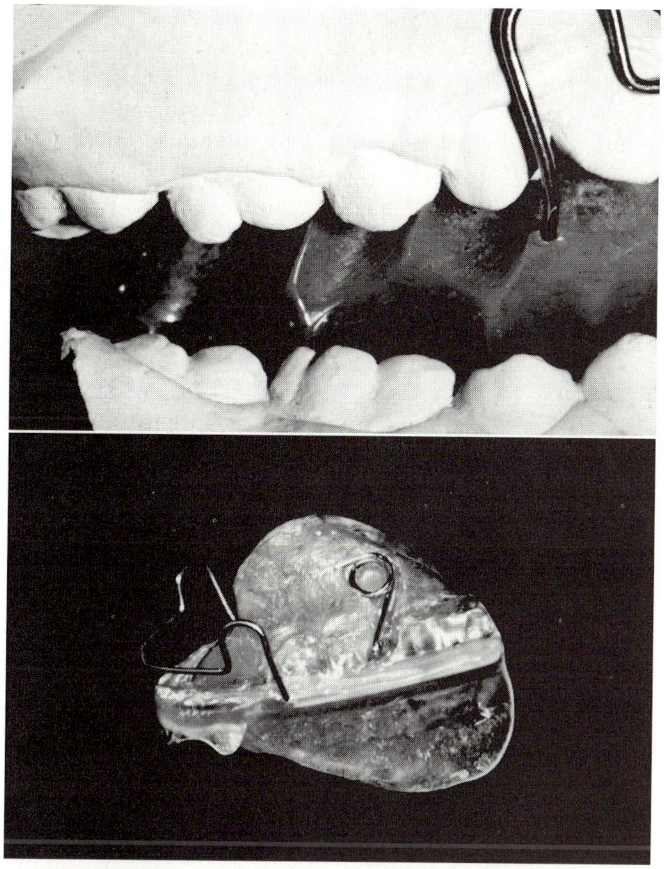

FIGURE 11-2 The Activator, a tooth-borne passive appliance, was the first widely used functional appliance. The appliance opens the bite, and the mandible is advanced for Class II correction. **A,** In the original Andresen activator, angled flutes in the acrylic were used to guide the path of eruption of the posterior teeth, usually so that the molars moved distally in the upper arch and mesially in the lower arch as the teeth erupted, and also to expand the dental arches if desired. **B,** The lingual flanges of an activator are the mechanism to advance the mandible. In this design, the maxillary posterior teeth are prevented from erupting by the acrylic shelf, while the mandibular posterior teeth are free to erupt; thus the appliance will induce a rotation of the occlusal plane, which usually is desirable in functional appliance treatment because it makes it easier to change a Class II to a Class I molar relationship. This appliance also has displacement springs on the upper first molars, which requires the patient to actively maintain the appliance in the proper position. It was once thought that a loosely-fitting appliance contributed to activation of the mandibular musculature, but research has not supported this concept, so modern activators are more likely to incorporate clasps than displacing springs.

orthodontic faculty members with a background in Europe (of whom Egil Harvold was prominent), and later from personal contact by a number of American orthodontists with their European counterparts. (Fixed appliances spread to Europe at the same time through similar personal contacts.) A major boost to functional appliance treatment in the United States came from the publication of animal experiment results in the 1970s showing that skeletal changes really could be produced by posturing the mandible to a new position and holding out the possibility that true stimulation of mandibular growth could be achieved (see Chapter 9). Although some of the enthusiasm for functional appliance treatment caused by the favorable animal experiments has faded in the light of less impressive results from clinical trials and retrospective clinical studies (see Chapter 8), functional appliances have achieved a major place in contemporary growth modification treatment.

At this point, the dichotomy between European and American orthodontics has largely disappeared. European-style removable appliances, particularly for growth modification during first-stage mixed dentition treatment, have become widely used in the United States, while fixed appliances have largely replaced removables for comprehensive treatment in Europe and elsewhere throughout the world.

Modern removable appliance therapy consists largely of the use of (1) various types of functional appliances for growth guidance in adolescents and, less frequently, in children; (2) active plates for tooth movement in preadolescents; and (3) clear plastic aligners for tooth movement in adults. The focus of this part of the chapter, accordingly, is on the characteristics of the appliances used for these purposes. The clinical use of removable appliances in mixed dentition treatment is covered in Chapter 13, and the application of clear aligner therapy to specific problems in adults is discussed in Chapter 18.

Functional Appliances for Growth Modification

The design and fabrication of many types of functional appliances are covered in detail in a text devoted to the subject.[1] The goal here is to put these devices in a contemporary perspective. They are understood best when viewed as falling into one of three broad categories, and as made up from a set of possible components that can be combined as needed in the design of an appliance for any individual patient.

Categories of Functional Appliances

Passive Tooth-Borne Appliances. These appliances have no intrinsic force-generating capacity from springs or screws and depend only on soft tissue stretch and muscular activity to produce treatment effects.

The original functional appliance design (see Figure 11-2) was a block of plastic covering the teeth of both arches and the palate. It was made to fit loosely, advance the mandible several millimeters for Class II correction, and open the bite 3-4 mm. In current activator designs, flutes to guide erupting teeth are replaced by a plastic shelf to impede eruption of upper posterior teeth while allowing eruption of lower posterior teeth, and lower incisors are capped to control forward displacement of the lower arch.

The bionator, originated by Balters and sometimes still bearing his name, is best described as a cut-down activator

A

B

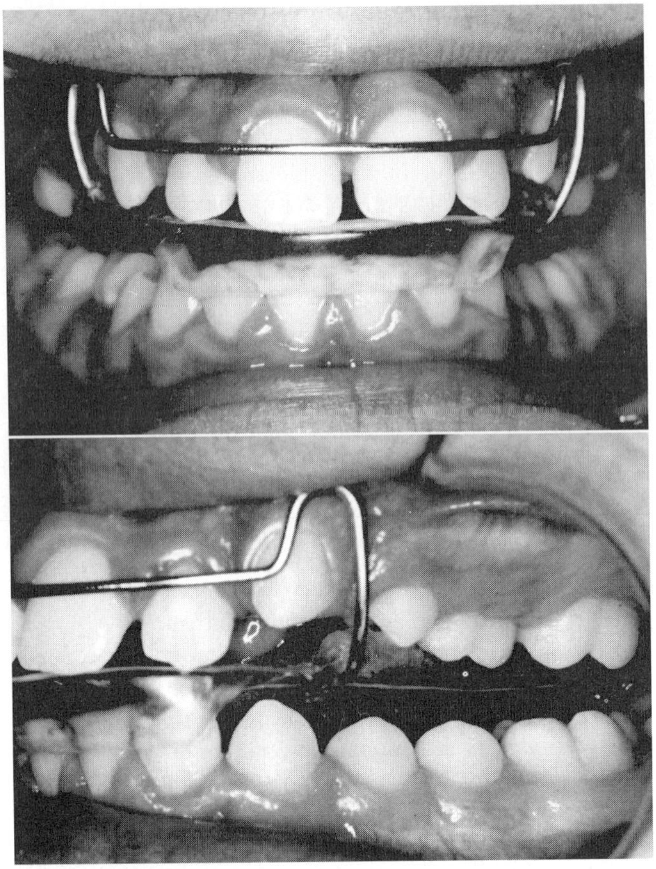

Figure 11-3 The bionator design, which removes much of the bulk of the activator, can include posterior facets or acrylic occlusal stops to control the amount and direction of eruption. Note that for this patient who is biting into the bionator so that his mandible is advanced, the lower incisors are capped with acrylic to prevent them from erupting and control their tendency to tip facially. Usually, the lower molars are free to erupt, while the upper molars are prevented from erupting by the acrylic shelf between the teeth. For this patient the upper molars are being allowed to erupt more than the lower molars.

with an inter-occlusal shelf and incisor capping if desired (Figure 11-3). Palatal coverage is eliminated. As with the activator, lingual flanges stimulate forward posturing of the mandible and shelves or blocks between the teeth provide vertical control.

The Herbst appliance (Figure 11-4) was developed in the early 1900s and reintroduced in the 1970s by Pancherz. The maxillary and mandibular arches are splinted with frameworks that usually are cemented or bonded but can be removable, and are connected with a pin-and-tube device that holds the mandible forward. Sometimes a modification of this appliance is superimposed on traditional fixed appliances (see Chapter 15).

The twin block appliance (Figure 11-5), like the Herbst, can be used as either a removable or fixed (cemented) device, but usually is removable. Its maxillary and mandibular portions are configured so the interaction of the two parts controls how much the mandible is postured forward and how much the jaws are separated vertically. This is similar to the Herbst appliance in that pressure against the teeth rather than the mucosa is employed to bring the jaw forward. The appliance has the advantage of allowing nearly a full range of mandibular movement, easy acclimation and reasonable

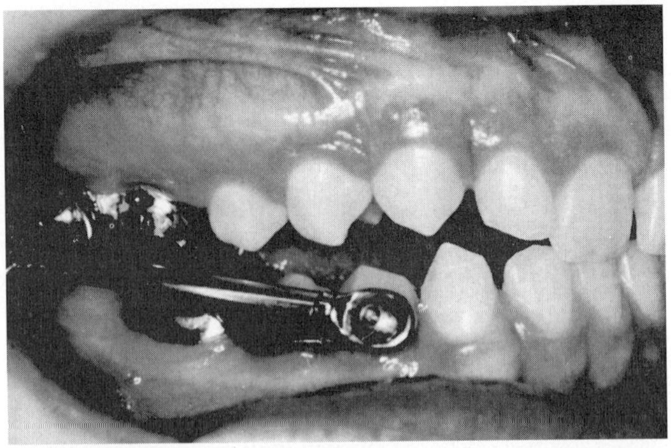

Figure 11-4 The Herbst appliance is the only fixed functional appliance. The maxillary and mandibular splints usually are cemented or bonded to the teeth (but can be removable and clasp-retained). The upper and lower splints are joined by the pin and tube apparatus that dictates the mandibular position.

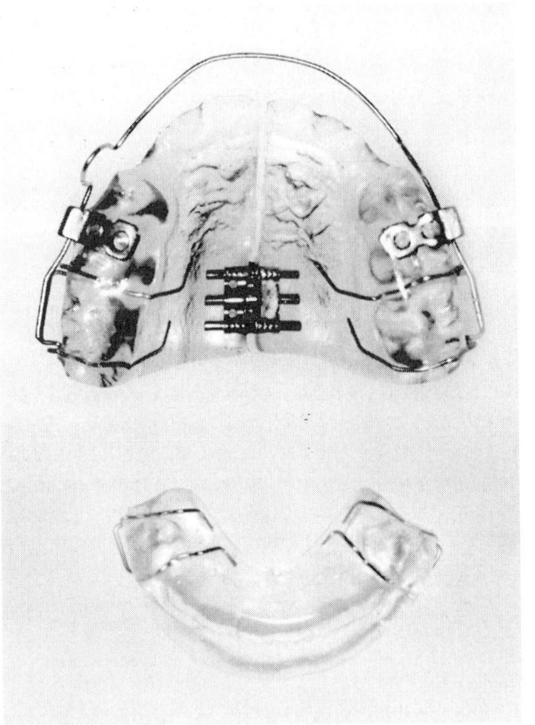

Figure 11-5 The twin-block appliance (also see Figure 13-26) consists of individual maxillary and mandibular plates with ramps that guide the mandible forward when the patient closes down. The maxillary plate incorporates tubes for attachment of a headgear, and often includes an expansion screw.

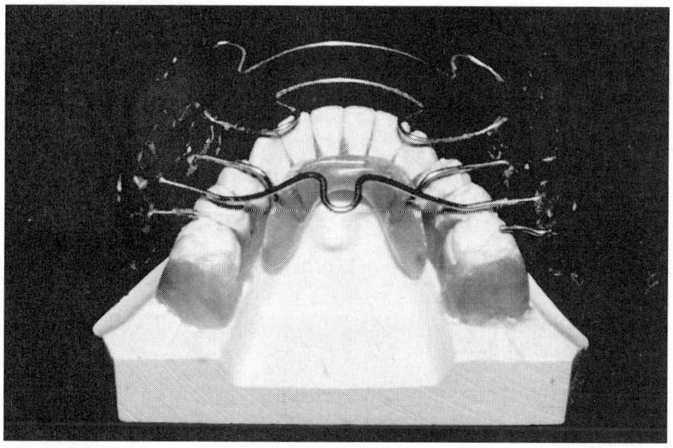

Figure 11-6 The Frankel appliance, shown here sitting on the lower cast, is the only functional appliance that is primarily tissue-borne rather than tooth-borne. The large buccal shields and lip pads reduce cheek and lip pressure on the dentition, and provide the expansion of the maxillary arch that usually is needed as part of Class II correction; the lingual pad dictates the mandibular position. The appliance looks bulky, but for the most part it is restricted to the buccal vestibule, and therefore it interferes less with speech and is more compatible with 24-hour wear than most other functional designs.

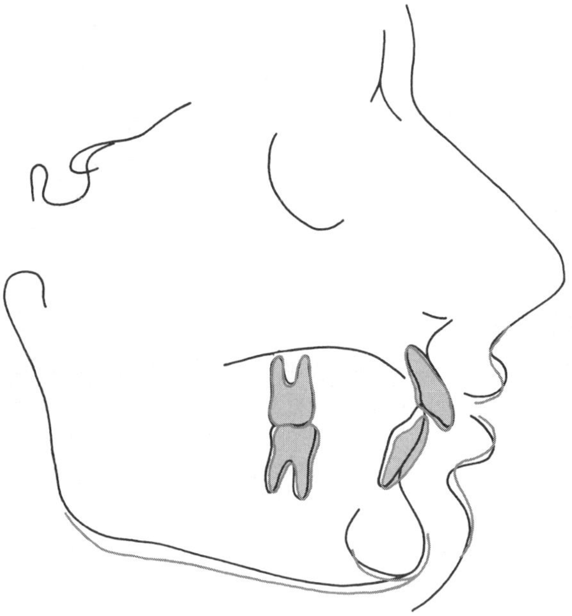

Figure 11-7 Cephalometric superimposition showing an unsatisfactory response to a removable functional appliance for a skeletal Class II malocclusion. Note the lack of skeletal response, but dental changes including forward movement of the lower incisors, slight retraction and elongation of the upper incisors, and downward and backward rotation of the mandible. Adding springs to a functional appliance, if it accentuates this pattern of tooth movement, makes the treatment response worse rather than better.

speech, so that it can be worn most of the time. The greatest disadvantage is that displacement of incisors can occur freely despite the absence of active springs or screws.

Tissue-Borne Appliances. The Frankel appliance (which Frankel called the function regulator) is the only tissue-borne functional appliance (Figure 11-6). A small pad against the lingual mucosa beneath the lower incisors stimulates mandibular repositioning. Much of the appliance is located in the vestibule, however, and it alters both mandibular posture and the contour of facial soft tissue. It serves as an arch expansion appliance in addition to its effects on jaw growth because the arches tend to expand when lip and cheek pressure is removed.

Active Tooth-Borne Appliances. These are largely modifications of activator and bionator designs that include expansion screws or springs to move teeth. This group includes the expansion activator, orthopedic corrector, sagittal appliance, any number of activators carrying the developer's name, and many other variations on the same theme. The springs and screws added to a functional appliance produce tooth movement that often detracts from correction of the underlying jaw discrepancy. During functional appliance treatment, every millimeter of incisor tipping (camouflage) is a millimeter of potential skeletal correction that has been lost. With any functional appliance, there is a tendency for the lower incisors to be moved facially (Figure 11-7), and springs and screws to move teeth magnify this undesirable side effect. For this reason, active tooth-borne appliances have little or no place in modern orthodontics, and now are used much less than previously.

Components Approach to Functional Appliances. Each functional appliance, no matter what name it carries, is simply a melding of wire and plastic components. If one understands the different component parts of these appliances and how the components translate into treatment effects, it is possible to plan functional appliance treatment by combining the appropriate components to deal with specific aspects of the patient's problems. This approach leads to custom-designed appliances for individual patients, so that the therapy is focused on that patient's specific problems. Appliance designs for asymmetry problems are particularly likely to end up quite different from any conventional design (Figure 11-8), but subtle variations in the appliance for common Class II problems can enhance treatment.

Functional and tooth-controlling components are listed and briefly annotated in Table 11-1. Although the functional components are the heart of the device, often they are only a small portion of the total appliance, the bulk of which is devoted to controlling the position of the teeth to minimize undesirable tooth movement.

The components approach suggests that there is no ideal appliance that can be used in all situations, nor is there necessarily a single optimum appliance design for a specific malocclusion. How the possible components should be put together is determined by two things: (1) exactly what is

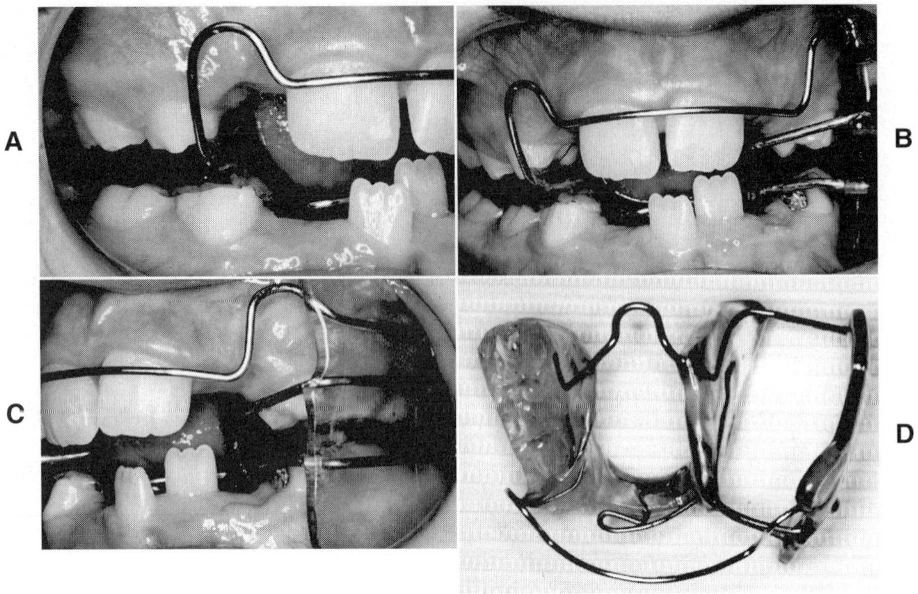

FIGURE 11-8 A hybrid functional appliance consists of the components of one type of functional on one side, and components of another type on the other. For a child with a facial asymmetry, an appliance of the type shown here can be effective in improving both the vertical and a-p aspects of the problem. Note that the teeth are free to erupt on the left side, while a bite block impedes eruption on the other. The bite is taken to bring the jaw to the midline, advancing the deficient side (here, the left) more than the other. (From Proffit WR, White RP, Sarver DM. Contemporary Treatment of Dentofacial Deformity. St. Louis: Mosby; 2003.)

desired in the treatment, and (2) practical considerations of cost, complexity, and acceptability of the appliance to the patient. As a general rule, it is better to use contact of lingual flanges with the soft tissue to produce forward posturing of the mandible, rather than pressure against the teeth. The reason is simple: pressure against the teeth leads to camouflage-type tooth movement, which is usually undesirable. For the same reason, active elements within a functional appliance must be considered as having the potential to diminish, not augment, the growth modification desired from treatment.

Clinical Acceptability of Functional Appliances. As a general rule, simple and sturdy functional appliance designs are more effective than complex and fragile ones. Children and adolescents are not known for their gentle treatment of removable appliances; if something can be broken easily, it will be. The original activators, and the twin block appliance, have a significant advantage from this perspective. The bionator is less sturdy, and its relative fragility is the greatest weakness of the Frankel appliance.

Vertical control always is a key element, and one of the advantages of functional appliances in general is the control of eruption they provide. Blocking the eruption of some teeth and allowing the eruption of others is the key to correcting deep bite or open bite problems. The activator and bionator designs are particularly easy to adjust so that some teeth can erupt while others are blocked.

Finally, acceptability to the patient is critical. One important factor in acceptability is the extent of interference with speech, which can make full-time wear impossible. The original activators do interfere with speech and for all practical purposes cannot be worn to school. Removing the palatal plastic and making the appliance into a less bulky bionator helps significantly (while also making the appliance more fragile, of course). Twin block appliances produce even less interference with speech and can be compatible with full-time wear, and the Frankel appliance (after a period of adaptation) does not interfere with normal speech, so that children can wear it to school routinely.

Removable Appliances for Tooth Movement in Children

Tooth movement with removable appliances in children almost always falls into one of two major categories: (1) arch expansion, in which groups of teeth are moved to expand the arch perimeter; and (2) repositioning of individual teeth within the arch.

Active Plates for Arch Expansion

The framework of an active plate is a baseplate that serves as a base in which screws or springs are embedded and to which clasps are attached. The active element almost always is a jackscrew placed so that it holds the parts of the plate together (Figure 11-9). Opening the screw with a key then separates the sections of the plate. The screw offers the advantage that the amount of movement can be controlled, and the baseplate remains rigid despite being cut into two

Table 11-1

Functional Appliance Components

Component	Comment
Functional Components	
Lingual flanges	Contact with mucosa; most effective
Lingual pad	Contact with mucosa; less effective
Sliding pin and tube	Contact with teeth; variable tooth displacement
Tooth-supported ramps	Contact with teeth; tooth displacement likely
Lip pads	Secondary effect only on mandibular position
Tooth-Controlling Components	
Arch Expansion	
Buccal shields	Passive, effective
Buccinator bow, other wire shield	Passive, less effective
Expansion screws and/or springs	Must activate slowly; questionable stability
Vertical Control	
Occlusal or incisal stops	Prevent eruption in discrete area
Bite blocks	Prevent eruption of all posterior teeth
Lingual shield	Facilitate eruption
Stabilizing Components	
Clasps	No effect on growth modification
Labial bow	Keep away from incisors, lingual tipping undesirable
Anterior torquing springs	Needed to control lingual tipping, especially with headgear-activator combination

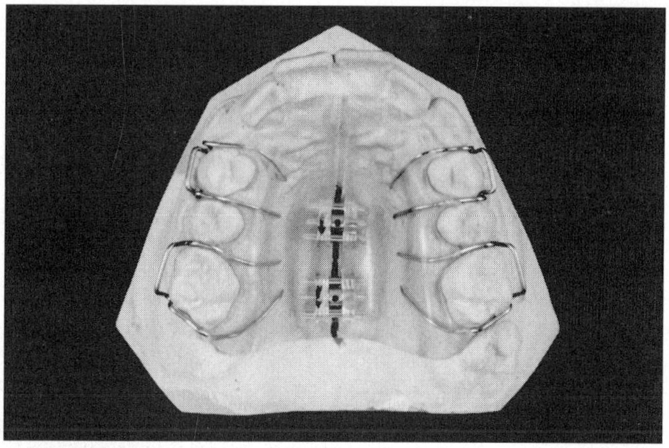

Figure 11-9 A split-plate expansion appliance of the type popularized by Martin Schwartz in Vienna, now usually called a Schwartz plate.

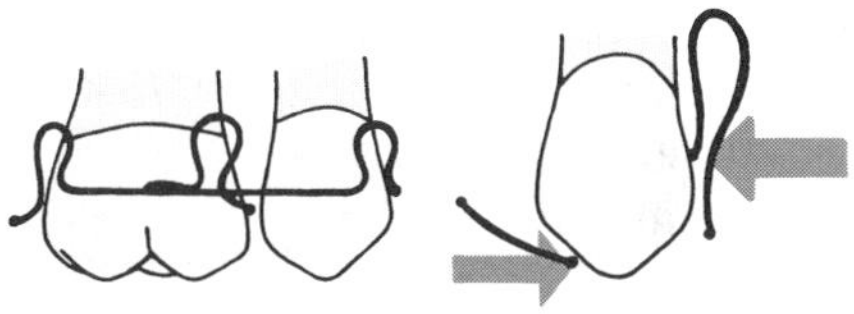

Figure 11-10 Diagrammatic representation of the spring assembly necessary for bodily retraction of a canine with a removable appliance. The spring on the mesial of the canine exerts a heavier force than the distal spring, leaving a net force to move the canine distally, while the couple necessary for control of root position is created by the opposing action of the two springs. Although bodily movement with a removable appliance is theoretically possible with spring arrangements of this type, the spring adjustments and clasp arrangements become too complex for practical clinical use. A fixed appliance is necessary for efficient bodily tooth movement.

parts. The disadvantage is that the force system is very different from the ideal one for moving teeth. Rather than providing a light but continuous force, activation of the screw produces a heavy force that decays rapidly, and rapid reactivation of the appliance has the potential of damaging the teeth.

If the force levels become too high, the appliance is likely to be displaced. This is the most common problem with expansion plates: activating the screw too rapidly results in the appliance being progressively displaced away from the teeth rather than the arch being expanded as desired.

Removable Appliances With Springs for Tooth Movement

In contrast to the heavy, rapidly decaying forces produced by a screw, nearly optimum light continuous forces can be produced by springs in a removable appliance. Like the edges of an active plate, however, these springs contact the tooth surface at only one point, and it is difficult to use them for anything but tipping tooth movements (Figure 11-10). The guideline for tooth movement with a spring from a removable appliance therefore is that this is acceptable for a few millimeters of tipping movement. Root control is needed for more than 3 to 4 mm of crown movement.

In designing springs for tooth movement, two important principles must be kept in mind: (1) the design must ensure adequate springiness and range while retaining acceptable strength. This usually means using recurved or looped wires for additional length (see Figure 10-14); and (2) the spring must be guided so that its action is exerted only in the appropriate direction.

Because smaller wires are not strong enough, it is unwise to fabricate springs for removable appliances from steel wire smaller than 20 mil (0.5 mm); larger diameter wires usually are preferred. In general, it is better to use a larger wire for its (considerably) greater strength, and then gain springiness

A

B

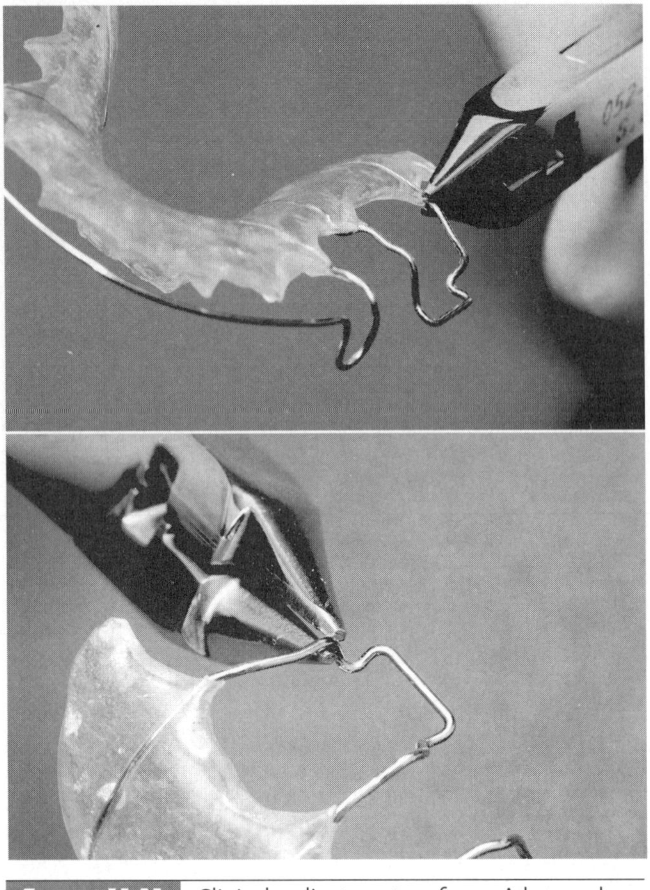

Figure 11-11 Clinical adjustments of an Adams clasp. **A,** Tightening the clasp by bending it gingivally at the point where the wire emerges from the baseplate. This is the usual adjustment for a clasp that has become loose after repeated insertions and removals of an appliance. **B,** Adjustment of the clasp by bending the retentive points inward. This alternative method of tightening a clasp is particularly useful during the initial fitting of an appliance.

and range by increasing the length of the spring, than to use a smaller wire initially.

Clasps

Retention of an active appliance is critical to its success. The best springs are ineffective if the appliance becomes displaced. It is probably fair to say that clasps are even more important than springs in determining how well a removable appliance performs clinically.

Adams Clasp. By far the most useful and versatile clasp for contemporary removable appliances is the Adams crib (Figure 11-11).[2] This clasp is made of 28 mil (0.7 mm) wire, except that 24 mil (0.6 mm) wire is preferred for clasps on canines. The retentive points of the clasp must fit well into the undercuts for good retention. When this clasp is used for children, it may be necessary for the points to slip slightly into the gingival crevice. This step is accomplished by trimming away stone interproximally on the laboratory cast, so that the clasp can fit far enough to engage undercuts below the height of contour.

When a new removable appliance is received from the laboratory, or when a patient returns for adjustments, it is often necessary for the dentist to tighten the clasps. Most of the time, this adjustment is done as illustrated in Figure 11-11, *A*, by simply bending the clasp slightly gingivally from its point of attachment. It is also possible to bend the retentive points inward to obtain better contact in the undercut areas (Figure 11-11, *B*), which really should be necessary only if the laboratory fabrication of the clasps was imperfect. As a general principle, the more active a removable appliance is to be and the greater the force applied during its use, the more clasping is required to hold it in place.

As treatment proceeds, three adjustments are necessary when an active removable appliance is being used appropriately: tightening of clasps when they become loose, activation of the spring or springs, and removal of material from the baseplate. Activation of the springs must be done carefully, and not more than approximately 1 mm at a time. The more the spring is activated, the more difficult it becomes to keep it in the proper position. Too much activation usually displaces either the spring or the whole appliance. Baseplate material must be removed from the path of a tooth that is to be moved. Failure to relieve the baseplate near a spring is a common error.

Clear Aligner Therapy (CAT)

The Development of Clear Aligners

The use of clear aligners in orthodontic treatment for adults became possible as vacuum-formed clear thermoplastic sheets to fit tightly over the teeth were introduced into orthodontics in the 1980s. These "suckdown" materials were used initially as retainers, and still are important for this purpose (see Chapter 17). It became apparent rather quickly, however, that if teeth were reset slightly and the vacuum-formed sheet was made to fit the reset teeth, a tooth moving device rather than a retainer would be the result. The device now could be, and quickly was called an "aligner" because the typical use was to bring mildly displaced teeth back into alignment, as for instance when mild irregularity of maxillary or mandibular incisors occurred in an orthodontic patient after retainers were discontinued.

Only small amounts of tooth movement are possible with a single aligner, however, because of the stiffness of the plastic material. To obtain more than minor changes, it was necessary either to reshape the aligner or make a new one, on a new cast with the teeth reset to a greater degree. Because the material is softened and becomes moldable when heated, it would be possible to alter the shape of an aligner with a heated instrument,[3] and in an attempt to extend the use of aligners, a special heated plier for this type of reshaping was offered as a way to avoid the cost and complexity of having to make multiple new aligners (Figure 11-12). This still allowed only minor tooth movement, and great skill was

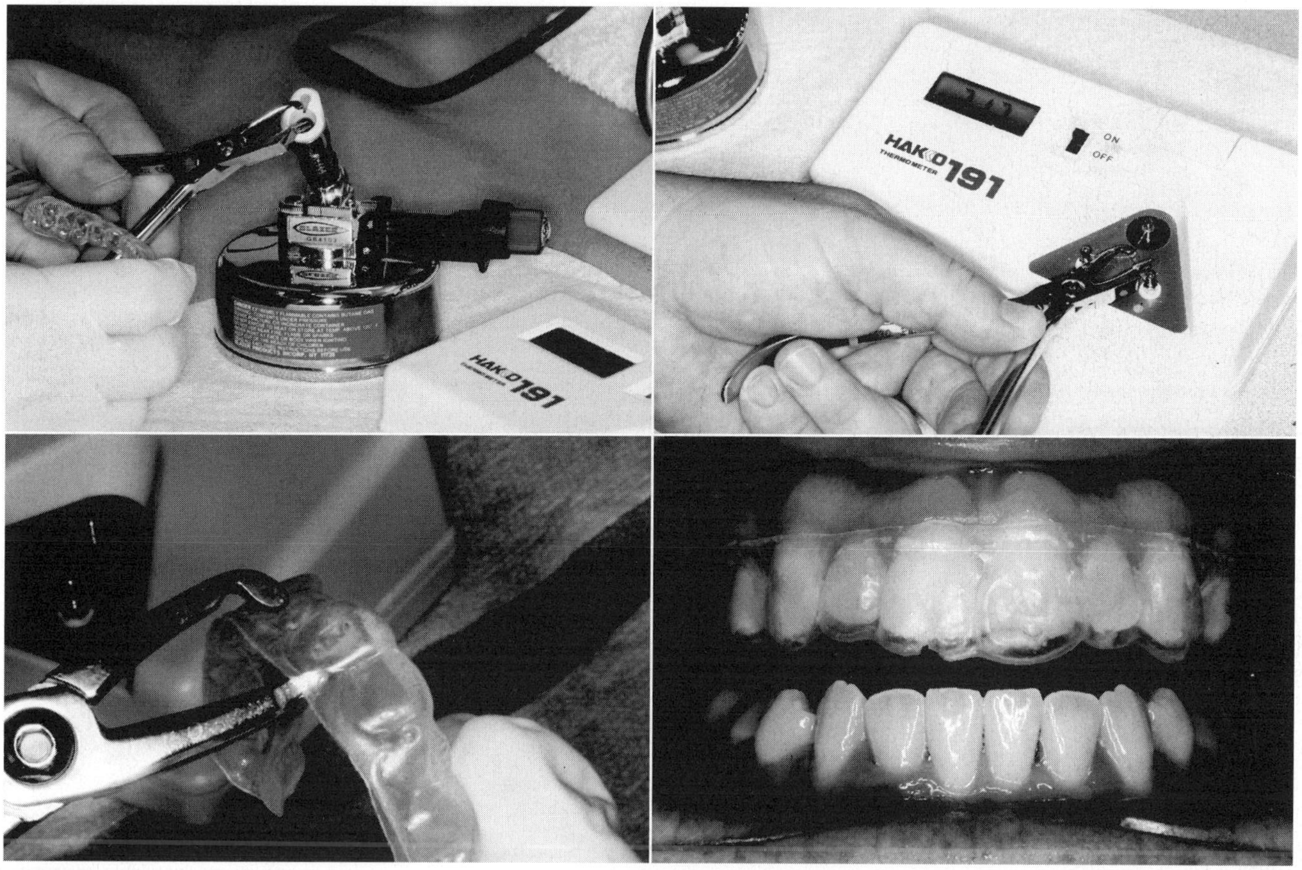

FIGURE 11-12 A plier heated to the correct temperature (which must be checked) can be used to create a divot in an aligner, to increase the amount of movement of a selected tooth without having to make a totally new aligner. **A,** Heating the special plier; **B,** checking the temperature; **C,** creating a divot in the aligner, in this case to increase movement of one maxillary central incisor; **D,** the modified aligner in place, with increased pressure against the central incisor.

required to obtain just the right amount of change in the aligner. A major limitation is that the plastic can only be stretched a maximum of about 3 mm (in 1 mm increments) before it becomes too thin to exert force. More recently, hard plastic bumps that snap into a hole in the aligner have been used to modify it for further tooth movement, which has the advantage that the plastic of the aligner is not stretched and thinned,[3] and a hot air jet now is suggested as the best way to soften the plastic of the aligner so that it can be thermoformed with another instrument.

Despite these improvements, reshaped aligners are not a practical way to manage orthodontic problems of any complexity. It became clear that a sequence of several aligners, made on a series of casts with reset teeth, each incorporating another small amount of tooth movement, would be needed to correct more severe alignment problems. Although a sequence of modified dental casts could be produced by hand in a standard dental laboratory, this was prohibitively time consuming and difficult if more than a few casts were required.

In the late 1990s, a new company with no ties to previous suppliers of dental and orthodontic materials, Align Technology, obtained venture capital to computerize the process of producing a sequence of casts with incremental changes, on which aligners could be fabricated. The approach (illustrated in more detail below) was to scan dental casts to create a digital model, make small changes in the position of the teeth on the digital model, produce a stereolithographic cast from the digital model on which an aligner could be made, then make a series of additional incremental changes on the digital model and produce a matching series of modified casts for aligner fabrication. With careful planning, this would result in a sequence of aligners that could correct more complex problems. From the beginning, it was recognized that since growth changes could not be predicted, the method would be useful only for treatment of adults or adolescents in whom growth modification was not needed, but these are the patients most interested in making an orthodontic appliance invisible or minimally visible.

This new approach was introduced with a blaze of television publicity for "Invisalign" that was designed to create consumer interest, before careful research evaluation had identified and solved problems in this type of treatment. Not surprisingly, problems appeared because staging of

A B C D

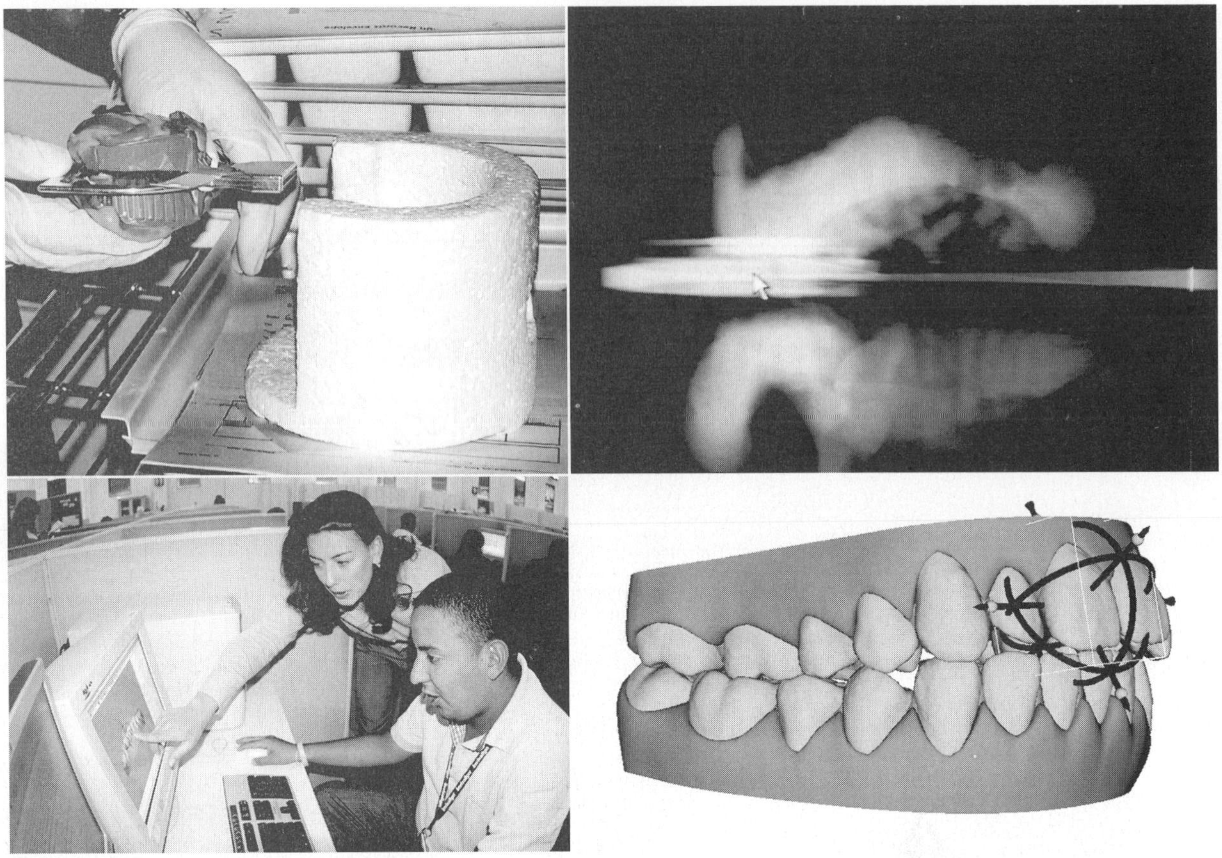

Figure 11-13 **A,** The first step in the production of a series of aligners using Invisalign's computer technology is a CT scan of the impressions submitted by the doctor. The impressions are placed in a container before going into the CT scanner. **B,** This produces a three-dimensionally-accurate digital image that is transmitted to a technology facility consisting entirely of computer work stations. **C,** In this view, the seated technician is conferring with one of the orthodontic advisors as the digital dental arches are displayed on the computer screen. **D,** Using the company's proprietary software, virtual tooth movement in three dimensions can be created and staged as desired.

treatment, optimal rates of tooth movement and indications for use of attachments on the teeth had not been worked out, and initial professional acceptance of the method was spotty. The technique has matured, however, as clinical evaluation by well-trained orthodontists has clarified the best sequence of steps in treatment and the amount of tooth movement in steps that should be attempted, and as the use of tooth-colored shapes bonded to the teeth has improved the appliance's grip on the teeth and ability to move them. Although remarkably little has been published about the outcomes of Invisalign treatment, there is no doubt now that for many adults, complex malocclusions can be successfully treated in this way (see Chapter 18). As patents expire or are challenged (which already is occurring), competitive companies will offer sequenced aligners based on modifications of the current techniques.

Invisalign Production Process

Steps in Preparing the Aligners. Diagnostic records for CAT therapy are not different from those for any other type of orthodontic treatment, but for Invisalign sequenced aligners, impressions and a bite registration (maximum intercuspation) are obtained with a highly stable material, typically PVS (poly-vinyl siloxane). The impressions, intraoral photographs and initial doctor's instructions are submitted to the company. The production process begins when the impressions are subjected to a CT scan to create an accurate three-dimensional digital model of each dental arch (Figure 11-13). Analog photos of the patient are scanned if digital photos were not submitted, and these records are transferred electronically to a computer work area (which can be anywhere).

At the computer facility, the teeth are digitally sectioned, cleaned up (obvious artifacts removed), the dental arches are related to each other, gingiva is added, movement is staged following the doctor's instructions, and this preliminary plan is placed online for the doctor's review on "ClinCheck" (see Chapter 18). After the doctor is satisfied with the planned sequence of aligners, the set of digital models for a patient are transferred to a cast production facility, where a stereolithographic model for each step is fabricated (Figure 11-14). Finally, the stereolithographic models are sent to a

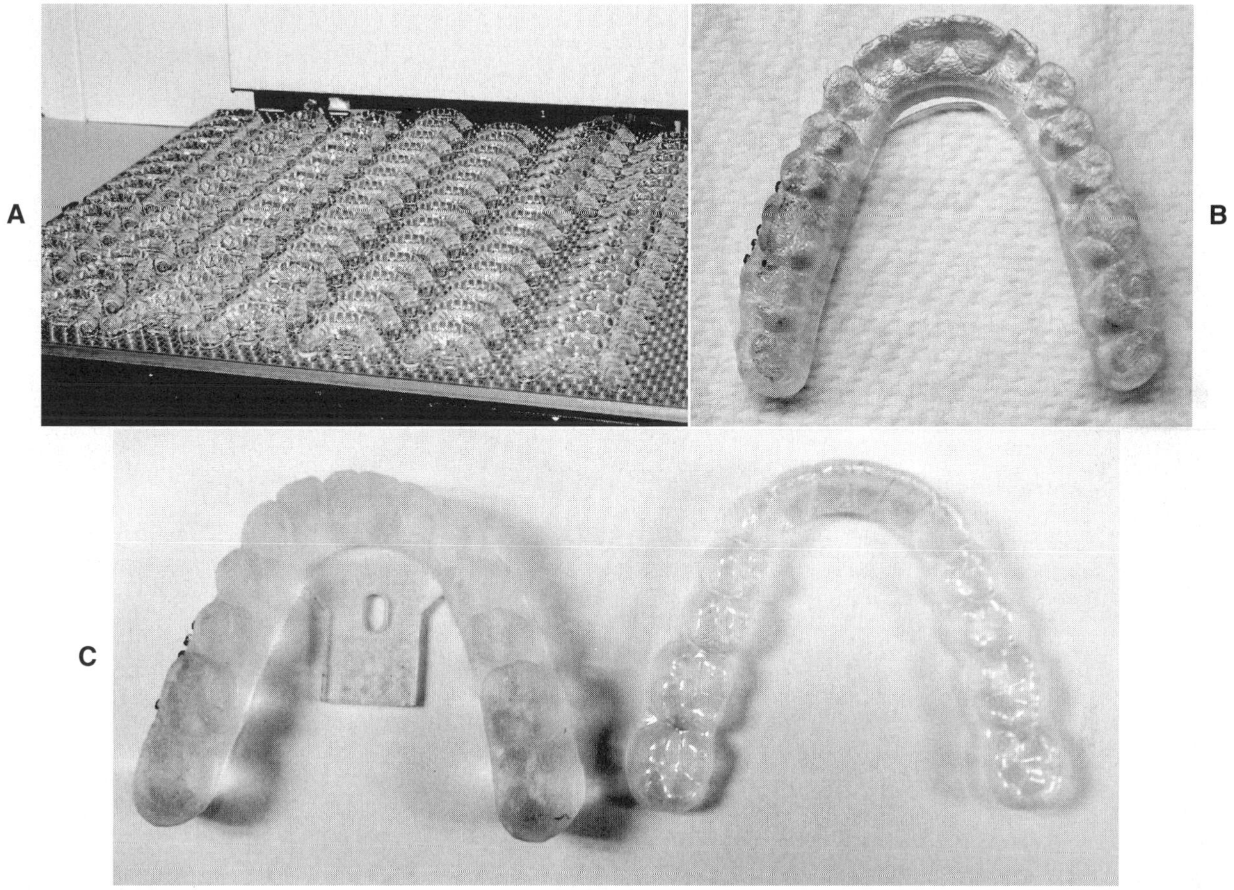

Figure 11-14 After the sequence of treatment steps has been adjusted if desired and approved by the doctor, who can access the digital models electronically after the preliminary treatment sequence has been put together, the models are used to fabricate a sequence of stereolithographic (SL) casts and a sequence of aligners are formed over the casts. **A,** SL casts emerging from the production machine; **B,** close-up of a single SL cast; **C,** SL cast and the aligner formed from it.

separate production facility, where the clear plastic aligners are formed over the models, and the set of aligners is sent directly to the doctor.

Clinician's Role in ClinCheck. With experience, doctors tend to be more specific in their initial prescription of what they want, but the sequence of steps and the amount of movement between steps is specified by the technician if this is not spelled out in detail in the prescription. In essence, when the ClinCheck is posted for the doctor to examine, the computer technician has sent a draft treatment plan for review (Figure 11-15). The software used by the computer technicians has default scenarios for different types of malocclusions and default rates of tooth movement (0.25 mm/aligner for anterior teeth, 0.33 mm/aligner for posterior teeth). These defaults are satisfactory for simpler cases but not for the more complex ones.

For complex treatment, the doctor must customize the plan in terms of the amount of interproximal reduction of teeth (if any) is to be done, the sequence of tooth movement steps, the rate of tooth movement with each subsequent aligner (often reducing the amount of movement at critical points), the extent to which bonded shapes are to be used to increase the aligner's grip on the teeth.

Considerations in Clinical Use of Clear Aligners. At this point, although a number of case reports have appeared, almost no data for the outcomes of Invisalign treatment have been published in refereed professional journals. How do success rates (in terms of PAR scores or other objective measures of alignment and occlusion) compare to fixed appliance treatment? No published data exist to allow the comparison.[5] To some extent this reflects the strong commercial orientation of the technique, and perhaps also its development, until recently, largely outside the mainstream of orthodontic thought. Based on information from the company itself and from experienced users, however, it seems clear that Invisalign, and clear aligners more generally, do some things well and others not so well (Box 11-1). The limitations should be kept in mind when CAT therapy is considered.

Several other considerations in the use of sequential aligners include the following:

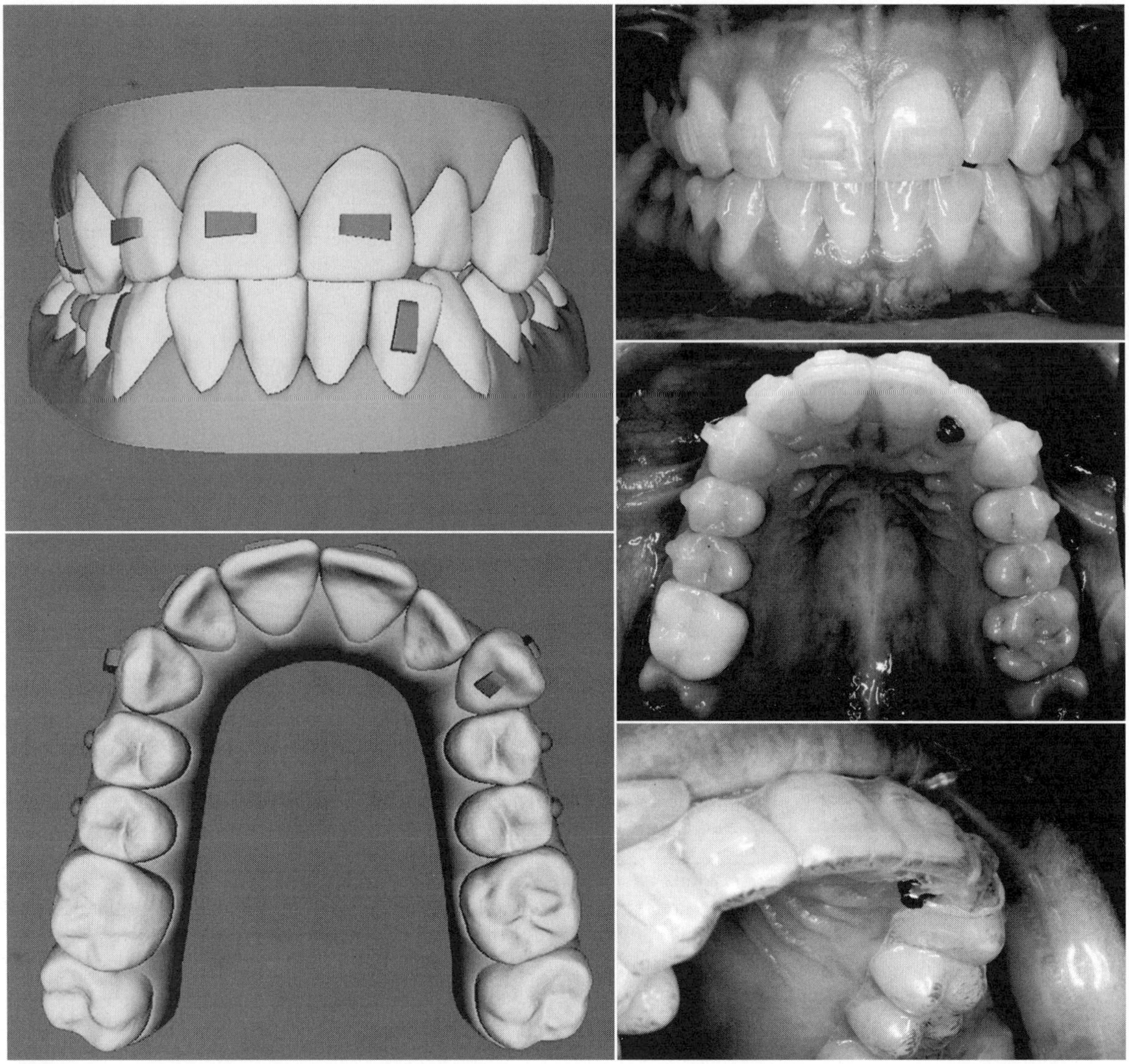

Figure 11-15 **A,** The Invisalign Clincheck form, as modified by the doctor, shows where bonded attachments are to be placed, the steps in the treatment sequence, and the amount of tooth movement at each step. For this patient, bonded attachments are to be placed as shown in the frontal and maxillary occlusal views. **B,** Bonded attachments on the facial surface of the teeth (same patient as the Clincheck form) are made of clear plastic in a variety of shapes. These are necessary to produce rotation or extrusion, and facilitate other types of tooth movement. **C, D,** It is possible to bond a button on the lingual side of a tooth that is proving difficult to rotate, and use a rubber band to rotate it along with the aligner.

- The use of attachments that are bonded to selected teeth greatly extends the possible tooth movement with aligners. In general, significant root movement (as in the closure of extraction sites) is almost impossible without the use of attachments, as is closure of open bites by elongation of incisor teeth; with attachments, both are possible (see Figure 18-22). Even with attachments, rotation of rounded teeth (canines and premolars) is so difficult that often it is wise to de-rotate these teeth prior to PVS impressions, using fixed auxiliaries such as buttons and elastomeric chains. It is possible to bond a button to a rotated tooth so that a rubber band can be used to rotate it while an aligner is being worn (see Figure 11-15). There is an increasing trend toward a combination approach to complex treatment, using a short phase of partial fixed appliances or auxiliaries in addition to the sequence of aligners.
- Interproximal enamel reduction (IPR) to obtain space of aligning crowded teeth often is part of the treatment plan. If IPR is planned, removal of interproximal enamel in the canine-premolar region to provide space can be used in addition to reduction in the width of incisors. The amount of interproximal reduction is part of the doctor's prescription (Figure 11-16).

Box 11-1

CLEAR ALIGNER THERAPY APPLICABILITY

CAT performs well:
- Mild-moderate crowding with IPR or expansion
- Posterior dental expansion
- Close mild-moderate spacing
- Absolute intrusion (1 or 2 teeth only)
- Lower incisor extraction for severe crowding
- Tip molar distally

CAT does not perform well:
- Dental expansion for blocked-out teeth
- Extrusion of incisors*
- High canines
- Severe rotations (particularly of round teeth)
- Leveling by relative intrusion
- Molar uprighting (any teeth with large undercuts)
- Translation of molars*
- Closure of premolar extraction spaces*

*Possible using attachments.

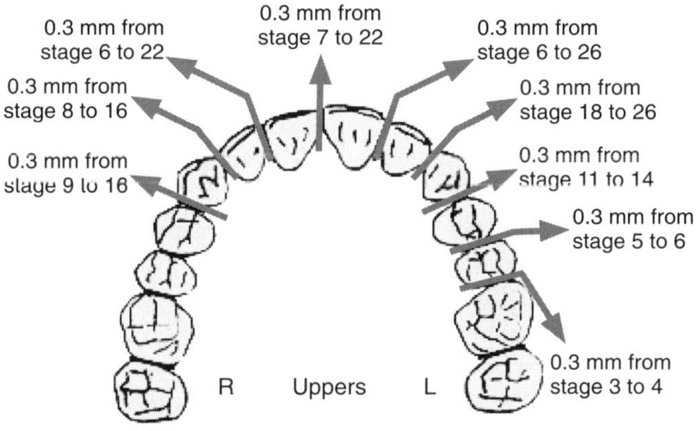

FIGURE 11-16 The Invisalign reproximation form (same patient as Figure 11-15), specifying how much enamel is to be removed from teeth and when in the sequence of aligners the reproximation will be done. For this patient, the upper incisors are to be reduced slightly in width to facilitate their alignment.

- Patients must be monitored carefully to verify that tooth movement is tracking with the series of aligners, i.e., that all teeth are seated completely in the aligner after it has been worn for the specified period of time. If the teeth are not tracking, there are several possibilities: not enough wear of the aligners by the patient, insufficient interproximal reduction, insufficient crown height or shape to allow a grip on the tooth or teeth to be moved, wrong type or position of bonded attachments, or movement created in ClinCheck that is too fast to be possible biologically. A refinement or mid-course correction, with a new set of PVS impressions and revision of the treatment plan, often is necessary in treatment of complex problems.
- Aligners cover the teeth like a bleaching tray, and they can be used to bleach during treatment (unless the patient has attachments on the anterior teeth). If this is done, it is important to remember that tooth movement causes transient pulpitis, and so does bleaching. The combination of the two procedures can lead to significant tooth sensitivity. This can be controlled by increasing the intervals between bleaching sessions.

The clinical use of CAT in adjunctive and comprehensive treatment is discussed in greater detail in Chapter 18.

FIXED APPLIANCES

Contemporary fixed appliances are predominantly variations of the edgewise appliance system. The only current fixed appliance system that does not use rectangular archwires in a rectangular slot is the Begg appliance, and practitioners using it have shown renewed interest in rectangular archwires at the finishing stage as the original Begg appliance has morphed into the Tip-Edge appliance. The focus in this and the succeeding chapters, therefore, is almost entirely on the contemporary edgewise appliance, with occasional reference to the modified Begg technique.

The Development of Contemporary Fixed Appliances

Angle's Progression to the Edgewise Appliance

Edward Angle's position as the "father of modern orthodontics" is based not only on his contributions to classification and diagnosis but also on his creativity in developing new orthodontic appliances. With few exceptions, the fixed appliances used in contemporary orthodontics are based on Angle's designs from the early 20th century. Angle developed four major appliance systems:

E-Arch. In the late 1800s, a typical orthodontic appliance depended on some sort of rigid framework to which the teeth were tied so that they could be expanded to the arch form dictated by the appliance. Angle's first appliance, the E-arch, was an improvement on this basic design (Figure 11-17). Bands were placed only on molar teeth, and a heavy labial archwire extended around the arch. The end of the wire was threaded, and a small nut placed on the threaded portion of the arch allowed the archwire to be advanced so that the arch perimeter increased. Individual teeth were simply ligated to this expansion arch. This appliance still could be found in the catalogs of some mail-order orthodontic laboratories as late as the 1980s, perhaps because of its simplicity, and despite the fact that it can deliver only heavy interrupted force.

Pin and Tube. The E-arch was capable only of tipping teeth to a new position. It was not able to precisely position any individual tooth. To overcome this difficulty, Angle began placing bands on other teeth and used a vertical tube

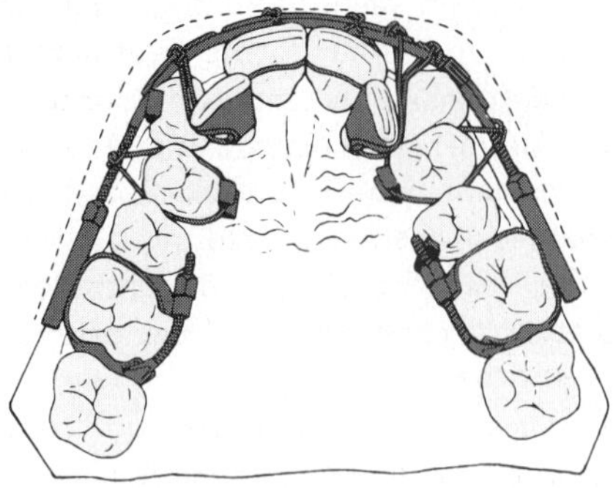

FIGURE 11-17 Edward Angle's E-arch, from the early 1900s. Ligatures from a heavy labial arch were used to bring malposed teeth to the line of occlusion.

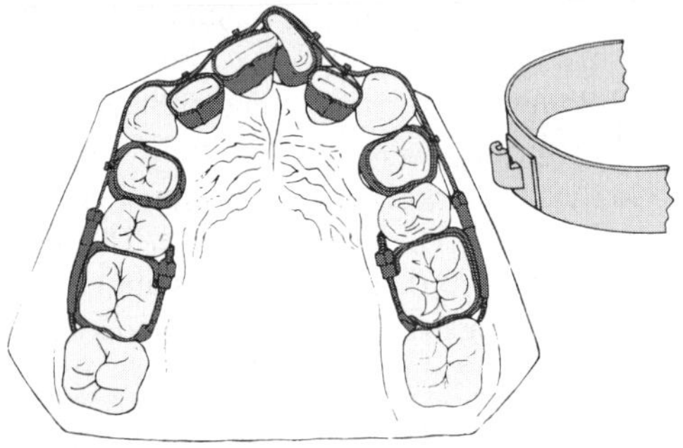

FIGURE 11-18 Angle's ribbon arch appliance, introduced about 1910, was well-adapted to bring teeth into alignment but was too flexible to allow precise positioning of roots.

on each tooth into which a soldered pin from a smaller archwire was placed. With this appliance, tooth movement was accomplished by repositioning the individual pins at each appointment.

An incredible degree of craftsmanship was involved in constructing and adjusting this pin and tube appliance, and although it was theoretically capable of great precision in tooth movement, it proved impractical in clinical use. It is said that only Angle himself and one of his students ever mastered the appliance. The relatively heavy base arch meant that spring qualities were poor, and the problem therefore was compounded because many small adjustments were needed.

Ribbon Arch. Angle's next appliance modified the tube on each tooth to provide a vertically positioned rectangular slot behind the tube. A ribbon arch of 10 × 20 gold wire was placed into the slot and held with pins (Figure 11-18). The ribbon arch was an immediate success, primarily because the archwire, unlike any of its predecessors, was small enough to have good spring qualities and was quite efficient in aligning malposed teeth. Although the ribbon arch could be twisted as it was inserted into its slot, the major weakness of the appliance was that it provided relatively poor control of root position. The resiliency of the ribbon archwire simply did not allow generation of the moments necessary to torque roots to a new position.

Edgewise. To overcome the deficiencies of the ribbon arch, Angle reoriented the slot from vertical to horizontal and inserted a rectangular wire rotated 90 degrees to the orientation it had with the ribbon arch—thus the name "edgewise" (Figure 11-19). The dimensions of the slot were altered to 22 × 28 mils, and a 22 × 28 precious metal wire was used. These dimensions, arrived at after extensive experimentation, did allow excellent control of crown and root position in all three planes of space.

After its introduction in 1928,[6] this appliance became the mainstay of multibanded fixed appliance therapy, although the ribbon arch continued in common use for another decade.

Other Early Fixed Appliance Systems

Labiolingual, Twin Wire. Before Angle, placing attachments on individual teeth simply had not been done, and Angle's concern about precisely positioning each tooth was not widely shared during his lifetime. In addition to a variety of removable appliances utilizing finger springs for repositioning teeth, the major competing appliance systems of the first half of the 20th century were the labiolingual appliance, which used bands on first molars and a combination of heavy lingual and labial archwires to which fingersprings were soldered to move individual teeth, and the twin-wire appliance. This appliance used bands on incisors as well as molars and featured twin 10 mil steel archwires for alignment of the incisor teeth. These delicate wires were protected by long tubes that extended forward from the molars to the vicinity of the canines. None of these appliances, however, were capable of more than tipping movements except with special and unusual modifications. They have disappeared from contemporary use.

Begg Appliance. Given Angle's insistence on expansion of the arches rather than extraction to deal with crowding problems, it is ironic that the edgewise appliance finally provided the control of root position necessary for successful extraction treatment. The appliance was being used for this purpose within a few years of its introduction. Charles Tweed, one of Angle's last students, was the leader in the United States in adapting the edgewise appliance for extraction treatment. In fact, little adaptation of the appliance was needed. Tweed moved the teeth bodily and used the subdivision approach for anchorage control, first sliding the canines distally along the archwire, then retracting the incisors (see Figure 10-31).

Raymond Begg had been taught use of the ribbon arch appliance at the Angle school before his return to Australia in the 1920s. Working independently in Adelaide, Begg also concluded that extraction of teeth was often necessary, and set out to adapt the ribbon arch appliance so that it could be used for better control of root position.

Begg's adaptation took three forms: (1) he replaced the precious metal ribbon arch with high-strength 16 mil stain-

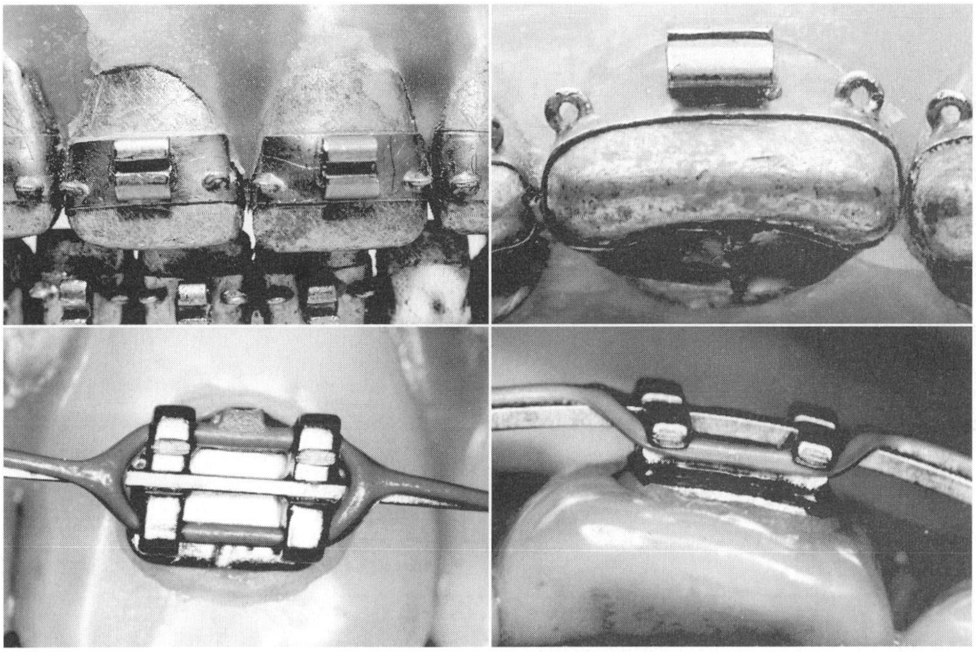

Figure 11-19 **A, B,** Angle's edgewise appliance received its name because the archwire was inserted at a 90-degree angle to the plane of insertion of the ribbon arch, which made it wider than it was tall. The rectangular wire could be twisted to create torque (see Figure 10-22). It was tied into a rectangular slot with wire ligatures, making excellent control of root position possible. The original appliance is seen here on a typodont. Note the narrow brackets (double width on the maxillary centrals, which are wider teeth), which were soldered to gold bands. Also note the eyelets soldered on the corners of the bands. These were used for ligature ties to the archwire as needed for rotational control. **C, D,** Close-up views of a modern edgewise twin bracket with a rectangular archwire in place. The wire is held in the bracket by an elastomeric ligature, here part of a chain of ligatures that also keep spaces closed between the teeth.

less steel wire as this became available in the late 1930s; (2) he retained the original ribbon arch bracket, but turned it upside down so that the bracket slot pointed gingivally rather than occlusally; and (3) he added auxiliary springs to the appliance for control of root position. In the resulting Begg appliance (Figure 11-20),[7] friction was minimized because the area of contact between the narrow ribbon arch bracket and the archwire was very small and the force of the wire against the bracket was also small. Begg's strategy for anchorage control was tipping/uprighting (see Figure 9-18).

Although the progress records with his approach looked vastly different, it is not surprising that Begg's overall result in anchorage control was similar to Tweed's, since both used two steps to overcome some frictional problems. The Begg appliance is still seen in contemporary use though it has declined in popularity and often appears now in a hybrid form, with brackets that allow the use of rectangular wires in finishing (Figure 11-21).[8] It is a complete appliance in the sense that it allows good control of crown and root position in all three planes of space.

Contemporary Edgewise

The Begg appliance became widely popular in the 1960s because it was more efficient than the edgewise appliance of that era, in the sense that equivalent results could be

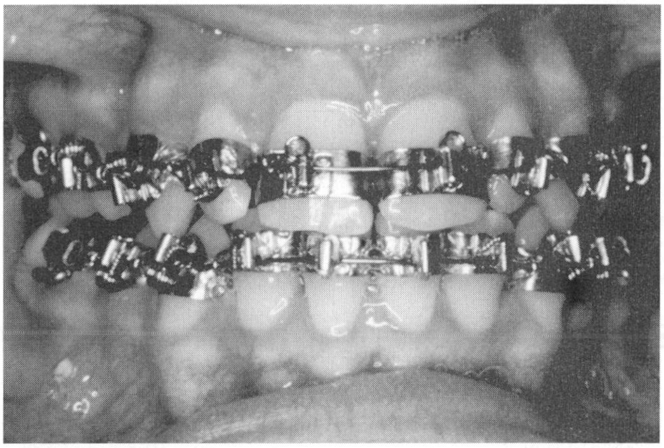

Figure 11-20 The Begg appliance uses a modification of the ribbon arch attachment, into which round archwires are pinned. A variety of auxiliary archwires are used in this system to obtain control of root position. For this patient late in treatment, the mandibular archwire is held in place in the central incisors with brass pins, and auxiliary springs (placed in the vertical slot and also serving as pins to retain the archwire) are being used to position the roots of several teeth (they are seen clearly in the maxillary central incisors, activated to move the roots distally).

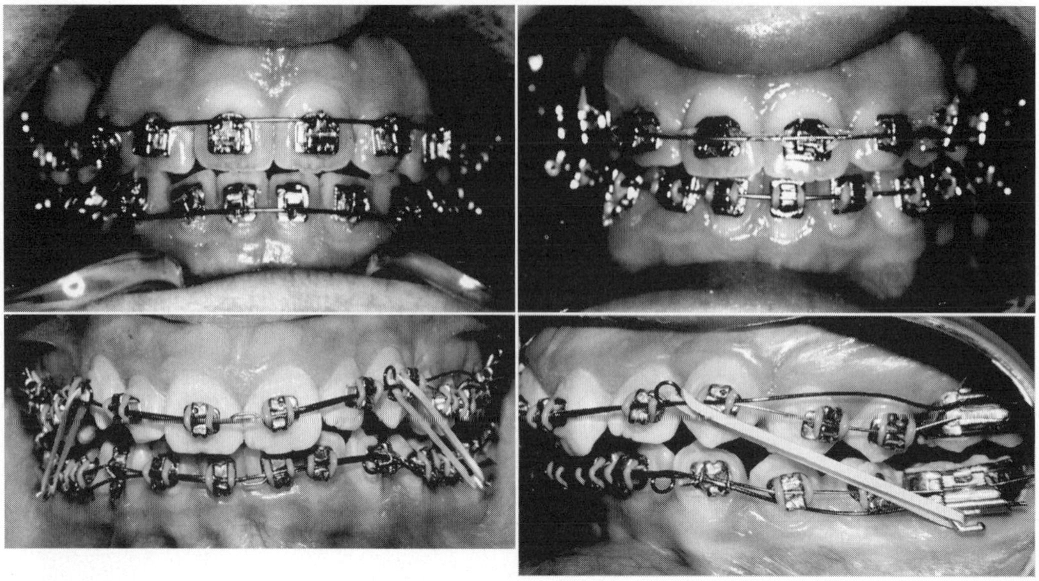

FIGURE 11-21 Modified brackets, such as this stage-4 bracket with both an edgewise slot (either 18 × 25 or 21 × 25) and a 22 × 32 gingival slot in which a wire can be pin-retained, allow a combination of Begg and edgewise mechanics. **A,** For this patient in the first stage of treatment, NiTi wires are pinned in place (which allows free movement in the slot as compared to holding them in the edgewise slot with a ligature). **B,** Later in treatment, heavier wires are tied into the edgewise slot. **C,** Tip-Edge bracket, which has a rectangular slot cut away on one side to allow crown tipping in that direction with no incisal deflection of the archwire. This allows the teeth to be tipped in the initial stage of treatment, but a rectangular wire can be used for torque in finishing. **D,** Tip-Edge brackets in the initial stage of treatment, with small diameter steel archwires. (**A, B,** Courtesy Dr. W. J. Thompson; **C, D,** Courtesy Dr. D. Grauer.)

produced with less investment of the clinician's time. Developments since then have reversed the balance: the contemporary edgewise appliance has evolved far beyond the original design while retaining the basic principle of a rectangular wire in a rectangular slot, and now is more efficient than the Begg appliance—which is the reason for its almost universal use now. Major steps in the evolution of the edgewise appliance include:

Automatic Rotational Control. In the original appliance, Angle soldered eyelets to the corners of the bands, so a separate ligature tie could be used as needed to correct rotations or control the tendency for a tooth to rotate as it was moved (see Figure 11-19). Now rotation control is achieved without the necessity for an additional ligature by using either twin brackets or single brackets with extension wings that contact the underside of the archwire (Lewis or Lang brackets) (Figure 11-22) to obtain the necessary moment in the rotational plane of space.

Alteration in Bracket Slot Dimensions. The significance of reducing Angle's original slot size from 22 to 18 mils and the implications of using the larger slot with undersize steel wires have been discussed in Chapter 10. In essence, there are now two modern edgewise appliances, because the 18 and 22 slot appliances are used rather differently. Chapters 14-16 focus on these differences.

Straight-Wire Prescriptions. Angle used the same bracket on all teeth, as did the other appliance systems. In the 1980s Andrews developed bracket modifications for specific teeth, to eliminate the many repetitive bends in archwires that were necessary to compensate for differences in tooth anatomy. The result was the "straight wire" appliance.[9] This was the key step in improving the efficiency of the edgewise appliance.

In the original edgewise appliance, faciolingual bends in the archwires (*first-order,* or *in-out, bends*) were necessary to compensate for variations in the contour of labial surfaces of individual teeth. In the contemporary appliance, this compensation is built into the base of the bracket itself.[9] This reduces the need for compensating bends but does not eliminate them, because of individual variations in tooth thickness.

Angulation of brackets relative to the long axis of the tooth is necessary to achieve proper positioning of the roots of most teeth. Originally, this mesio-distal root positioning required angled bends in the archwire, called *second-order,* or *tip,* bends. Angulating the bracket or bracket slot decreases or removes the necessity for these bends in archwires.

Because the facial surface of individual teeth varies markedly in inclination to the true vertical, in the original edgewise appliance it was necessary to place a varying twist (referred to as *third-order,* or *torque,* bends) in segments of each rectangular archwire, in order to make the wire fit passively. Torque bends were required for every patient in every rectangular archwire, not just when roots needed to be moved facially or lingually, in order to avoid inadvertent movements of properly positioned teeth. The bracket slots

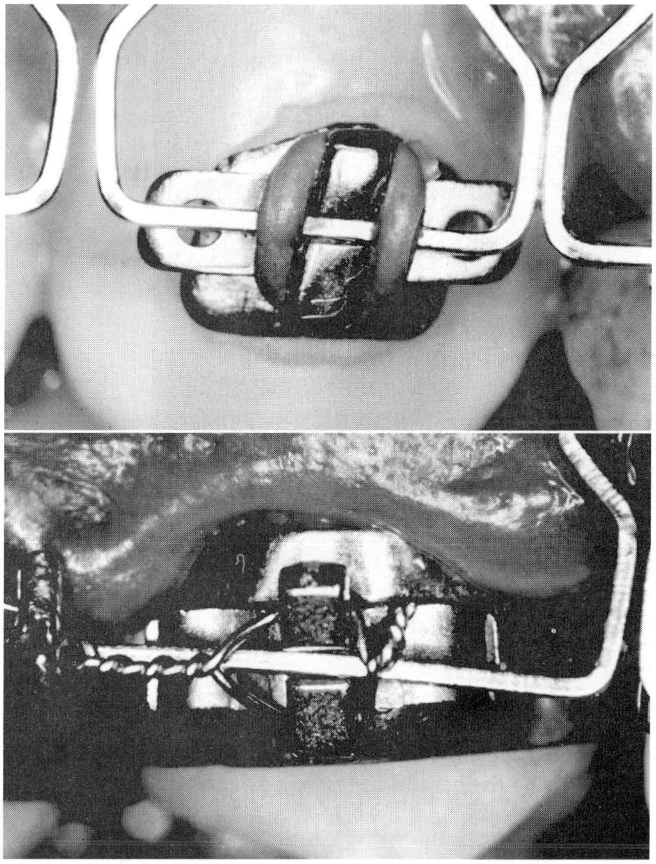

FIGURE 11-22 In contemporary edgewise appliances, the alternative methods for rotation control are twin brackets (as seen above) or single brackets with anti-rotation wings. **A,** Bonded single-wing (Lang) bracket with anti-rotation arms; **B,** Single-wing (Lewis) bracket welded to a premolar band. In both **A** and **B,** note that the end of an anti-rotation arm would contact the back of the archwire if the tooth began to rotate, creating the needed anti-rotation couple. Note also that the slightly undersized rectangular wire crosses the bracket at an angle, creating a moment to control the position of the roots.

in the contemporary edgewise appliance are inclined to compensate for the inclination of the facial surface, so that third-order bends are less necessary.

The angulation and torque values built into the bracket are often referred to as the *appliance prescription.* A generalized prescription to minimize second- and third-order bends is illustrated in Table 11-2. Obviously, this would precisely position the average tooth, but would not be exactly correct for any deviations from the average—and many teeth do deviate from the average.

The edgewise appliance continues to evolve. Current commercially-available edgewise appliances are reviewed in some detail at the end of this chapter. Before doing that, let us examine banding vs. bonding as the means of fixing the appliance in place.

Bands for Attachments

Indications for Banding

Until the 1980s, the only practical way to place a fixed attachment was to put it on a band that could be cemented to a tooth. The pioneer orthodontists of the early 1900s used clamp bands, which were tightened around molar teeth by screw attachments. Only with the advent of custom-fitted gold bands that were fabricated with special pliers, was it practical to place fixed attachments on more than a few teeth. Preformed steel bands came into widespread use during the 1960s, but are used now primarily for molar teeth.

There are many advantages to bonding brackets, so it is no longer appropriate to routinely place bands on all teeth. However, a number of indications still exist for use of a band rather than a bonded attachment, including:

1. Teeth that will receive heavy intermittent forces against the attachments. This is the primary indication for banding now. An excellent example is an upper first molar against which extraoral force will be placed via a headgear. The twisting and shearing forces often encountered

TABLE 11-2

A Generalized Angulation and/or Torque Prescription for "Straight-Wire" Edgewise Appliances

	MAXILLARY		MANDIBULAR	
	Angulation	Torque	Angulation	Torque
Central	+5°	+14°	0°	−1°
Lateral	+8°	+7°	0°	−1°
Canine	+10°	−3°	+6°	−7°
First premolar	0°	−7°	0°	−14°
Second premolar	0°	−7°	0°	−17°
First molar	+10°	−10°	0°	−25°
Second molar	+10°	−10°	0°	−30°

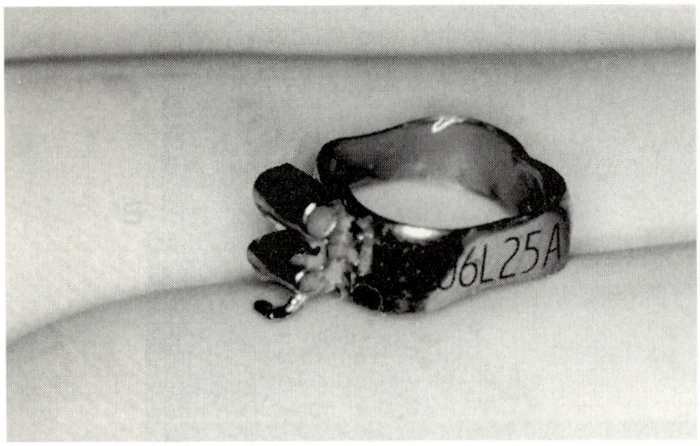

FIGURE 11-25 Molar band ready to cement. The cement must cover all the anterior surface of the band. We recommend placing a gloved finger over the top of the band when it is carried to place, to help in keeping cement on the gingival aspect of the band.

tend to be a composite of glass ionomer and resin materials, and usually are light-cured.[10] Their use has greatly reduced problems with leakage beneath bands that previously was a risk for decalcification of banded teeth.

All interior surfaces of an orthodontic band must be coated with cement before it is placed, so that there is no bare metal. As the band is carried to place, the occlusal surface should be covered so that cement is expressed from the gingival as well as the occlusal margins of the band (Figure 11-25).

Bonding Attachments

The Basis of Bonding

Bonding of attachments, eliminating the need for bands, was a dream for many years before rather abruptly becoming a routine clinical procedure in the 1980s. Bonding is based on the mechanical locking of an adhesive to irregularities in the enamel surface of the tooth and to mechanical locks formed in the base of the orthodontic attachment. Successful bonding in orthodontics, therefore, requires careful attention to three components of the system: the tooth surface and its preparation, the design of the attachment base, and the bonding material itself.

Preparation of the Tooth Surface. Before bonding an orthodontic attachment, it is necessary to remove the enamel pellicle and to create irregularities in the enamel surface. This is accomplished by gently cleaning and drying the enamel surface (avoiding heavy pumicing), then treating it with an etching agent, usually 35% to 50% unbuffered phosphoric acid for 20-30 seconds. The effect is to remove a small amount of the softer interprismatic enamel and open up pores between the enamel prisms, so the adhesive can penetrate into the enamel surface (Figure 11-26). At present, etching and sealing the tooth surface often are done in a single step. The tooth surface must not be contaminated with saliva, which promotes immediate remineralization, but the new tooth preparation materials now minimize the need to have a perfectly dry tooth surface.

Surface of Attachments. The base of a metal bonded bracket or tube must be manufactured so that a mechanical interlock between the bonding material and the attachment surface can be achieved. Either chemical bonding or mechanical interlocking can be used with ceramic brackets. The strength of chemical bonds can become high enough to create problems in debonding, so mechanical retention now is preferred for ceramic as well as metal brackets.

Bonding Materials. A successful bonding material must meet a set of formidable criteria: it must be dimensionally stable; it must be quite fluid, so that it penetrates the enamel surface; it must have excellent inherent strength; and it must be easy to use clinically.

At present, filled acrylic (bis-GMA) resins are the preferred bonding materials. These are available in a variety of formulations that differ mainly in the composition and extent of the fillers, in a variety of colors to make clean-up easier, and in the arrangement—chemical- or light-activation—to initiate polymerization of the resin. Although a number of fluoride-releasing bonding materials have been offered commercially, it has not yet been possible to develop one that has any lasting protective effects.[11]

Direct Bonding. Direct bonding of attachments can be used quite successfully as a routine clinical procedure, and even when most attachments are bonded indirectly, it is indicated whenever a single bracket must be changed or replaced. After preparation of the tooth surface, either a chemically-activated composite resin with a very rapid setting time or a light-activated material can be used.

The major difficulty with direct bonding is that the dentist must be able to judge the proper position for the attachment and must carry it to place rapidly and accurately. There is less opportunity for precise measurements of bracket position or detailed adjustments than there would be at the laboratory bench. It is generally conceded that for this reason, direct bonding does not provide as accurate a placement of brackets as indirect bonding. On the other hand, direct bonding is easier, faster (especially if only a few teeth are to be bonded), and less expensive (because the laboratory fabrication steps are eliminated).

Steps in the direct bonding technique, using an individual mix of chemically-activated resin for each bracket, are illustrated in Figure 11-27. Direct bonding with a light-cured resin, of course, also is possible, and is used more frequently now because the newer light-cured materials usually have higher bond strengths.

Indirect Bonding Technique. Indirect bonding is done by placing the brackets on a model in the laboratory, then using a template or tray to transfer the laboratory positioning to the teeth. The advantage is more precise location of brackets that is possible in the laboratory. An alginate impression, poured relatively rapidly, gives an accurate enough working cast for indirect bonding. Custom

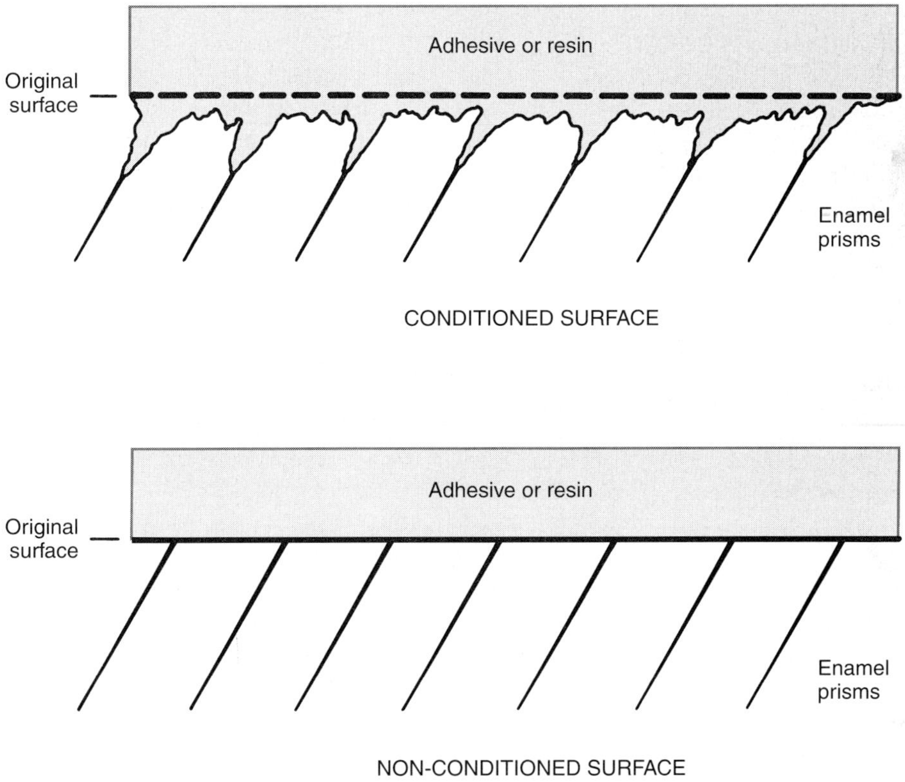

FIGURE 11-26 Diagrammatic representation of the effect of preparation of the enamel surface before bonding. Pretreatment with phosphoric acid creates minute irregularities in the enamel surface, allowing the bonding material to form penetrating "tags" that mechanically interlock with the enamel surface.

impression trays and silicone or rubber impressions are not necessary. Laboratory and clinical steps in indirect bonding are illustrated in Figure 11-28.

For indirect bonding, "no-mix" chemically-activated materials usually are employed. The composite resin is placed on the tooth surface in unpolymerized form, while the polymerization catalyst is placed on the back of the brackets. When the tray carrying the brackets is placed against the tooth surface, the resin immediately beneath the bracket is activated and polymerizes, but excess resin around the margins of the brackets does not polymerize and can easily be scaled away when the bracket tray is removed. This overcomes one of the greatest problems with indirect bonding, the difficulty of clean-up of excess bonding material when it has hardened. An alternative is to use a flowable light-cured material and a transparent tray, expecting only a thin layer of excess material and minimal clean-up.

At present, indirect bonding is used routinely by some practitioners, but is reserved for special circumstances by most. Custom brackets that were manufactured for an individual patient require the precision of indirect bonding. More generally, the poorer the visibility, the more difficult direct bonding becomes, and the greater the indication for an indirect approach. For this reason, indirect bonding is almost a necessity for lingual attachments. Bonding an isolated lingual hook or button is not difficult, but precisely positioning the attachments for a lingual appliance is, and even the placement of a fixed lingual retainer is done more easily with indirect technique and a transfer tray.

Debanding/Debonding. It is as important to remove a fixed appliance safely as to place it properly. Bands are largely retained by the elasticity of the band material as it fits around the tooth. This is augmented by the cement that seals between the band and the tooth, but a band retained only by cement was not fitted tightly enough. No orthodontic cement bonds strongly to enamel (which is why band cements cannot be used to bond brackets). When the band is distorted by force to remove it, the cement breaks away from the band or the tooth, and there is almost no chance of damaging the enamel surface.

The greater strength of bonding adhesives becomes a potential problem in debonding. When a bonded bracket is removed, failure at one of three interfaces must occur: between the bonding material and the bracket, within the bonding material itself, or between the bonding material and the enamel surface. If a strong bond to the enamel has been achieved, which is the case with the modern materials, failure at the enamel surface on debonding is undesirable, because the bonding material may tear the enamel surface as it pulls away from it. The interface between the bonding material

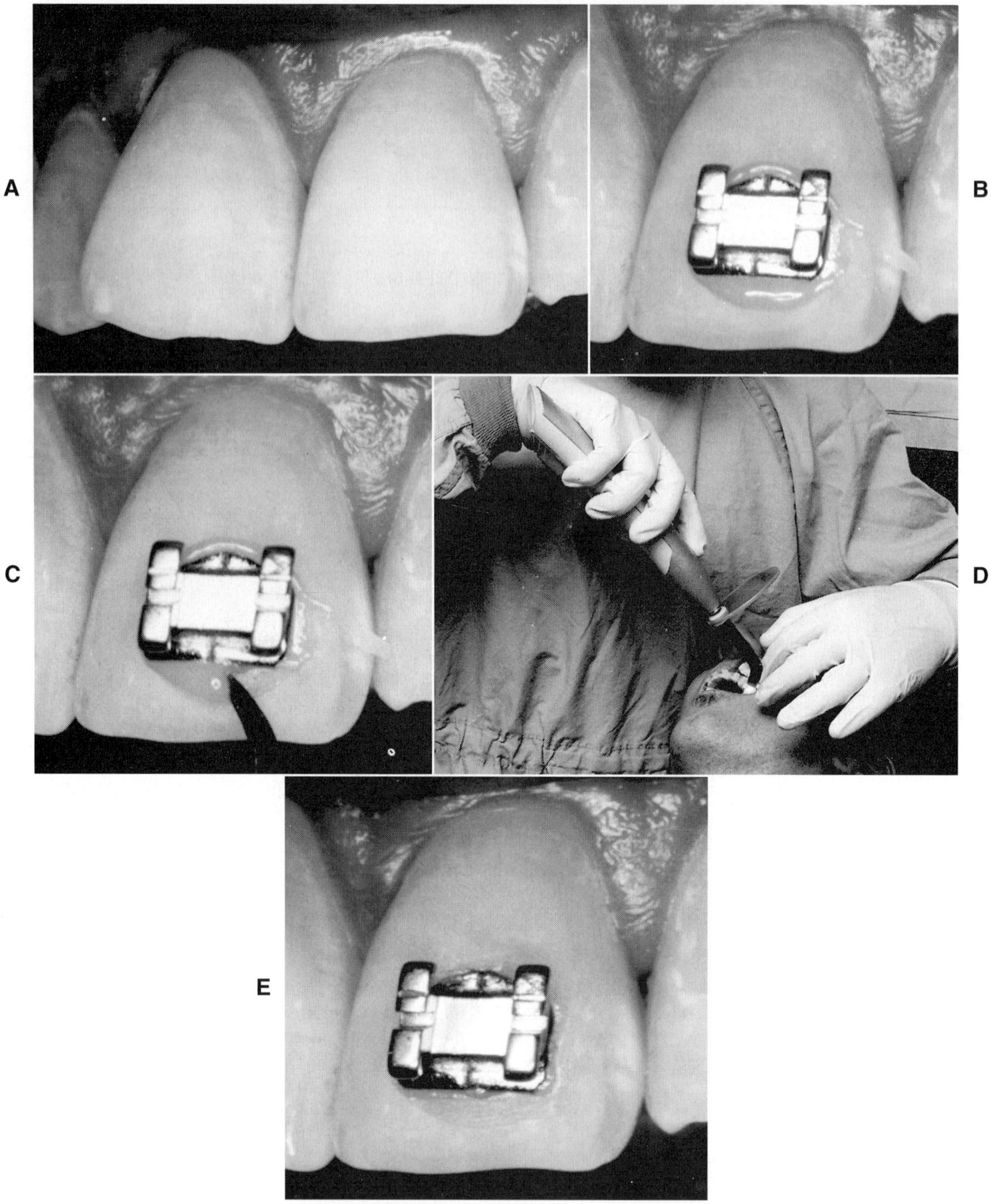

Figure 11-27 Steps in direct bonding. **A,** After etching, the tooth surface has a somewhat chalky or frosted appearance if dried (drying is no longer necessary with modern tooth preparation materials, but the tooth surface must be etched); **B,** a small amount of the bonding agent is squeezed into the mesh on the back of the bracket, and it is pressed to place on the tooth surface; **C,** excess bonding material is removed from around the bracket; **D,** for light-cured materials, a cordless light now is the most convenient way to activate the adhesive bonding process; **E,** the bracket bonded in place.

and the bracket is the usual, and preferred, site of failure when brackets are removed. The safest way to remove metal brackets is to distort the bracket base, which induces failure between it and the bonding adhesive. This damages the bracket so that it cannot be reused. The major reason for not recycling and reusing brackets is the possibility of enamel damage when they are removed without distorting the base. If brackets can be removed without damage they can be cleaned, sterilized, and reused without risk to the patient, in exactly the same way as other medical devices.

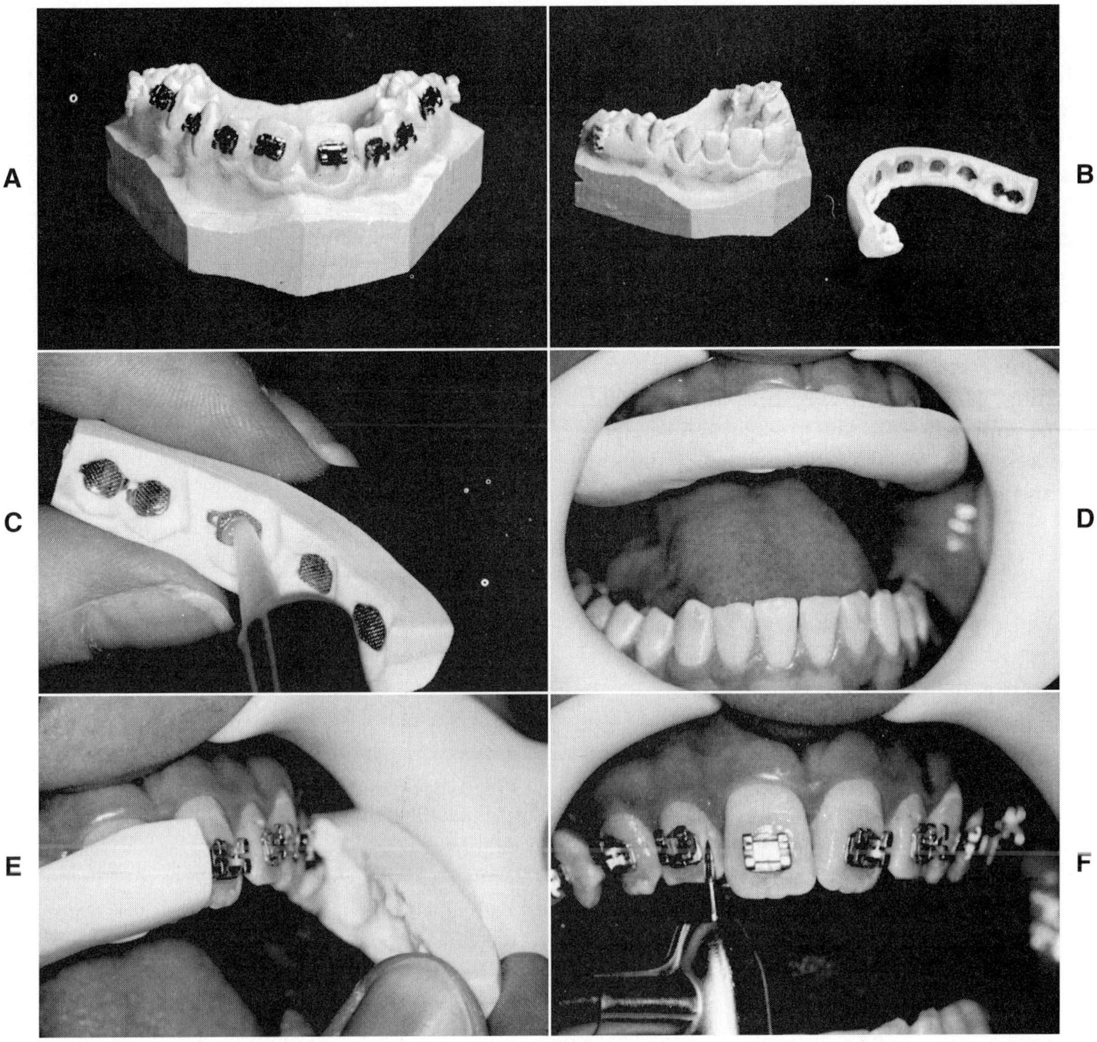

FIGURE 11-28 Steps in indirect bonding. **A,** Brackets are placed precisely as desired on a cast of the teeth and held in place with a temporary (water-soluble) adhesive; **B,** a transfer tray is formed by adapting a carrier material, usually silicone rubber, over the working cast and the adapted brackets. The tray is trimmed to remove excess material from the labial vestibule, but tray material is left extending onto the occlusal and incisal surfaces of the teeth. The completed tray is removed from the working cast by soaking in warm water, and the remaining temporary adhesive is washed away from the inner surface of the brackets with hot water; **C,** the adhesive material is applied to the back of each bracket in the transfer tray. The catalyst portion of a two-paste chemically-cured resin is placed on the tooth surface, so that mixing occurs when the two components contact each other when the tray is carried to the mouth; **D,** the tray or tray section is carried to place, and pressed firmly against the teeth. If a light-activated material is the bonding agent, a translucent transfer tray is needed. **E,** After the adhesive has set, the tray material is gently peeled away from the teeth. **F,** Excess bonding material is removed, with a carbide finishing bur if hardened adhesive is encountered, or with a scaler if unset material is present.

Ceramic brackets are a particular problem for debonding, because their base cannot be distorted. They break before they bend. There are two ways to create adhesion between a ceramic bracket and the bonding adhesive: mechanical retention through undercuts on the bracket base, as is done with metal brackets; or chemical bonding between the adhesive and a treated bracket base. It is quite possible to create such a strong bond between the adhesive and a chemically treated bracket base that failure will not occur there—but then when the bracket is removed, there is a real chance of enamel surface damage. Reports of enamel damage on debonding began to appear soon after ceramic brackets were introduced, and have been a problem ever since.

Modifications to ceramic brackets to enhance the chance of debonding at the right interface, and electro-thermal and laser techniques to weaken the adhesive during debonding, are discussed in the section below on modern bracket materials.

Characteristics of Contemporary Fixed Appliances

Appliance Materials

Stamped versus Cast Stainless Steel Brackets. The brackets and tubes for an edgewise appliance must be precisely manufactured so that the internal slot dimensions are accurate to at least 1 mil. Until the recent introduction of ceramic and titanium brackets, fixed appliances had been fabricated entirely from stainless steel for many years, and steel remains the standard material for appliance components.

There are two ways to produce steel edgewise brackets and tubes: from thin metal strip material that is stamped to shape, or by casting. Although stamped brackets and tubes were used almost routinely until the prescription straight-wire appliances were introduced, cast attachments are both more accurate and more durable, and clearly are superior. Most of the brackets and tubes for contemporary appliances now are castings, but some inexpensive appliances still use stamped brackets and tubes. Effective use of the straight-wire approach all but demands the precision of castings.

Titanium as an Alternative to Stainless Steel. Nickel is a potentially allergenic material. Given the significant nickel content of stainless steel, it is fortunate for orthodontists that mucosal allergic reactions to nickel are much less prevalent than cutaneous reactions. Cutaneous sensitization to nickel often develops from skin contact with cheap jewelry, and 10% or more of the population now have some degree of sensitivity to nickel.[12] Most patients who show skin reactions tolerate stainless steel orthodontic appliances quite satisfactorily, but a few do not, and there is concern that this number is increasing. Some European countries are now considering a ban on steel orthodontic appliances because of the risk of allergic responses.

The metal alternatives to steel are gold, long since abandoned because of performance and cost considerations, and titanium, which contains no nickel and is exceptionally biocompatible. Titanium archwires have been used since the 1980s, and the use of bonded titanium brackets and tubes has increased rapidly since the turn of the century. In addition to its hypoallergenic properties, titanium brackets and tubes seem to reduce the failure rate in bonding, perhaps because the material is more "wettable" and the bonding materials adhere better to the retention pad, perhaps because titanium is more resilient than steel and absorbs impacts better. For patients with nickel allergy, the choice would be between these brackets and non-metallic ones.

Non-Metallic Appliance Materials. Recurring efforts have been made to make fixed appliances more esthetic by eliminating their metallic appearance. A major impetus to the development of bonding for orthodontic attachments was elimination of the unsightly metal band. Tooth-colored or clear brackets for anterior teeth (Figure 11-29) became practical when successful systems for direct bonding were developed. Although plastic brackets were introduced with considerable enthusiasm in the 1980s and have remained on the market ever since, they suffer from three largely unresolved problems: (1) staining and discoloration, particularly in patients who smoke or drink coffee; (2) poor dimensional stability, so that it is not possible to provide precise bracket slots or build in all the straight-wire features; and (3) friction between the plastic bracket and metal archwires that makes it very difficult to slide teeth to a new position. Using a metal slot in the plastic bracket helps the second and third problems, but even with this modification, plastic brackets are useful only when complex tooth movements are not required.

Table 11-3

Ceramic Brackets

Material	Manufacturer, name
Polycrystalline alumina (PCA)	American, 20/20 Dentarum, Fascination GAC, Allure Rocky Mtn, Signature Unitek, Transcend and many others
PCA with metal slot	Unitek, Clarity
Monocystalline alumina	A Co., Starfire
Polycrystalline zirconia	Yamaura, Toray

Ceramic brackets, which were first made available commercially in the late 1980s, largely overcome the esthetic limitations of plastic brackets in that they are quite durable and resist staining. In addition, they can be custom-molded for individual teeth and are dimensionally stable, so that the precise bracket angulations and slots of the straight-wire appliance can be incorporated. Several different types of ceramic brackets currently are available (Table 11-3).

Ceramic brackets were received enthusiastically and immediately achieved widespread use, but problems with fractures of brackets, friction within bracket slots, wear on teeth contacting a bracket, and enamel damage from bracket removal soon became apparent. Fractures of ceramic brackets occur in two ways: loss of part of the brackets (e.g., tie wings) during archwire changes or eating,[13] and cracking of the bracket when torque forces are applied. Ceramics are a form of glass, and like glass, ceramic brackets tend to be brittle. Because the fracture toughness of steel is much greater, ceramic brackets must be bulkier than stainless steel brackets, and the ceramic design is much closer to a wide single bracket than is usual in steel.

Most currently-available ceramic brackets are produced from alumina, either as single-crystal or polycrystalline units. In theory, single-crystal brackets should offer greater strength, which is true until the bracket surface is scratched. At that point, the small surface crack tends to spread, and fracture resistance is reduced to or below the level of the polycrystalline materials. Scratches, of course, are likely to occur during the course of treatment.

A
B
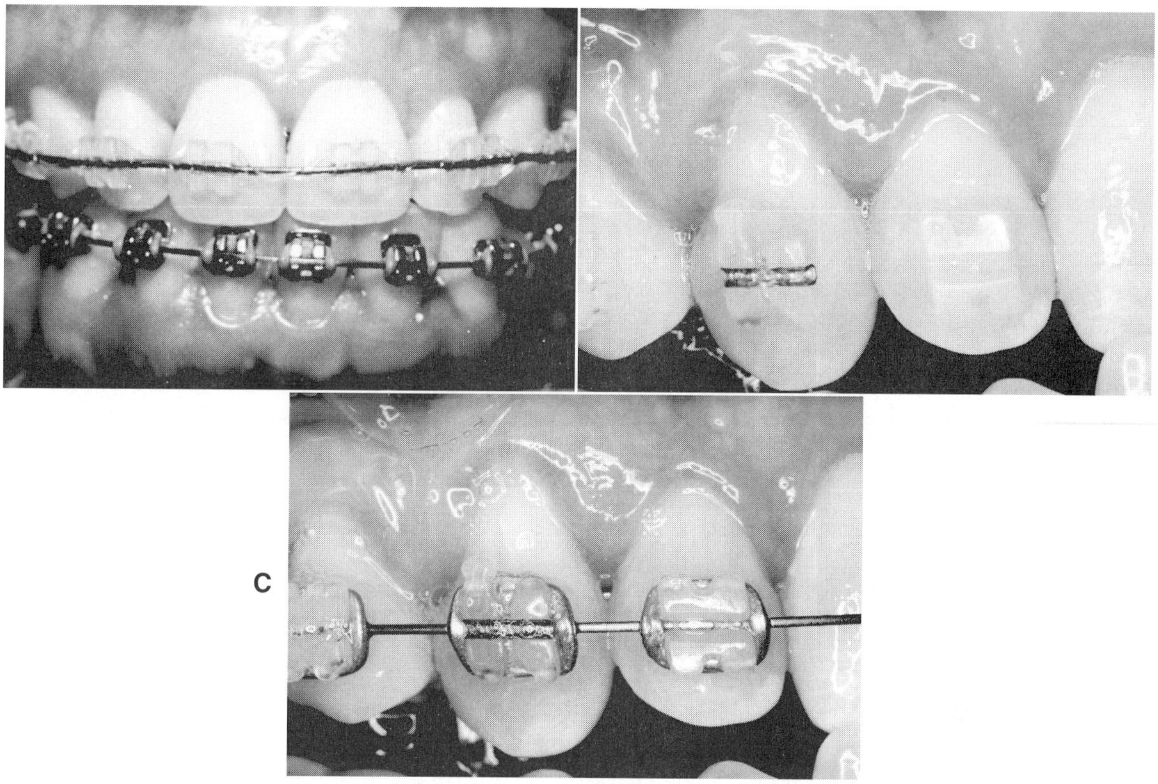
C

FIGURE 11-29 **A,** Ceramic twin brackets on the maxillary anterior teeth, with steel brackets on all teeth that are not highly visible. Using ceramic brackets in this way eliminates the possibility of enamel abrasion when teeth contact ceramic brackets in function while maintaining the esthetic benefit of using brackets of this type. **B,** Ceramic brackets with and without a metal slot, wire out; **C,** Same brackets with wire in place. Note the similarity of appearance when an archwire is present.

Although ceramic brackets are better in this regard than plastics, frictional resistance to sliding has proved to be greater with ceramic than with steel brackets. Because of the multiple crystals, polycrystalline alumina brackets have relatively rough surfaces (Figure 11-30). Even though monocrystalline alumina is as smooth as steel, these brackets also show greater friction than steel, perhaps reflecting a chemical interaction between the wire and bracket material. With ceramic as with steel brackets, friction is worst with beta-Ti wires (Figure 11-31).[14] The bracket surface can abrade the surface of the relatively soft beta-Ti wire, so that small pieces of the wire are pulled out and adhere to the bracket. Even with steel wires, nicks and cuts in the surface of the wire often are observed after movement of the wire against a ceramic bracket. Using a metal slot in a ceramic bracket has the potential to help this problem.

Many patients bite against a bracket or tube at some point in treatment. Contact against a steel or titanium bracket causes little or no wear of enamel, but ceramic brackets can abrade enamel quite rapidly. This risk is largely avoided if ceramic brackets are placed only on the upper anterior teeth, which is the location where improved esthetics is most important. Most patients who want the esthetic effect will accept ceramic brackets only where they are most visible and steel or titanium brackets elsewhere.

As noted above in the section on debonding, ceramic brackets also can be a problem when it comes time for bracket removal. Some recently introduced brackets have an additional interface at the bracket base that is designed to be the point of failure. Ceramic brackets with a metal slot are made to fracture at the slot, and this also facilitates removal.

In addition, the debonding technique is important. The current recommendation is to use a debonding instrument that concentrates force at the bracket-adhesive interface (sharp cutter), or an instrument that induces an asymmetric shearing rather than a torquing stress. An alternative is to use a thermal or laser instrument to weaken the adhesive by heating it, to induce failure within the bonding agent itself. Thermal debonding of this type is quite effective in reducing the chance of enamel damage. Unfortunately, it introduces the chance of damaging the tooth pulp unless the heat application is controlled quite precisely, and for that reason rarely is used now.

Just as composite plastic fibers are likely to replace metal archwires in clinical orthodontics (see Chapter 10), it seems highly probable that composite plastic brackets will become the standard in another few years. Composite plastics with better physical properties than any metal already exist. It is just a matter of overcoming the engineering problems to produce brackets with better mechanical properties, and

TABLE 11-4

Bracket/Tube Prescriptions: Incisors Through Premolars, Bracket Prescription

MAXILLARY	CENTRAL		LATERAL		CANINE		1ST PREMOLAR		2ND PREMOLAR	
	Torque	Tip	Torque	Tip	Torque	Tip	Torque	Tip	Torque	Tip
Roth	12	5	8	9	−2	9	−7	0	−7	0
Hilgers	22	5	14	8	7	10	−7	0	−7	0
Ricketts	22	0	14	8	7	5	0	0	0	0
Standard Edgewise	0	0	0	0	0	0	0	0	0	0
Alexander	14	5	7	8	−3	10	−7	0	−7	0
MBT	17	4	10	8	−7	8	−7	0	−7	0
Sprint	12	5	8	9	−2	11	−7	0	−7	0
Orthos	15	5	9	9	−3	10	−6	0	−8	4
Damon (Med Torque)	12	5	8	9	7	6	−7	2	−7	2
Andrews	7	5	3	9	−7	11	−7	2	−7	2

MANDIBULAR	CENTRAL		LATERAL		CANINE		1ST PREMOLAR		2ND PREMOLAR	
	Torque	Tip	Torque	Tip	Torque	Tip	Torque	Tip	Torque	Tip
Roth	0	0	0	0	−11	7	−17	0	−22	0
Hilgers	−1	0	−1	0	7	15	−11	0	−17	0
Ricketts	0	0	0	0	7	15	0	0	0	0
Standard Edgewise	0	0	0	0	0	0	0	0	0	0
Alexander	0	0	−5	0	−7	6	−11	0	−11	0
MBT	−6	0	−6	0	−6	3	−12	2	−17	2
Sprint	0	0	0	0	−10	7	−17	0	−22	0
Orthos	−5	2	−5	4	−6	6	−7	3	−9	3
Damon (Med Torque)	−1	2	−6	2	0	5	−12	2	−17	2
Andrews	−1	2	−1	2	−11	5	−17	2	−22	2

A,B

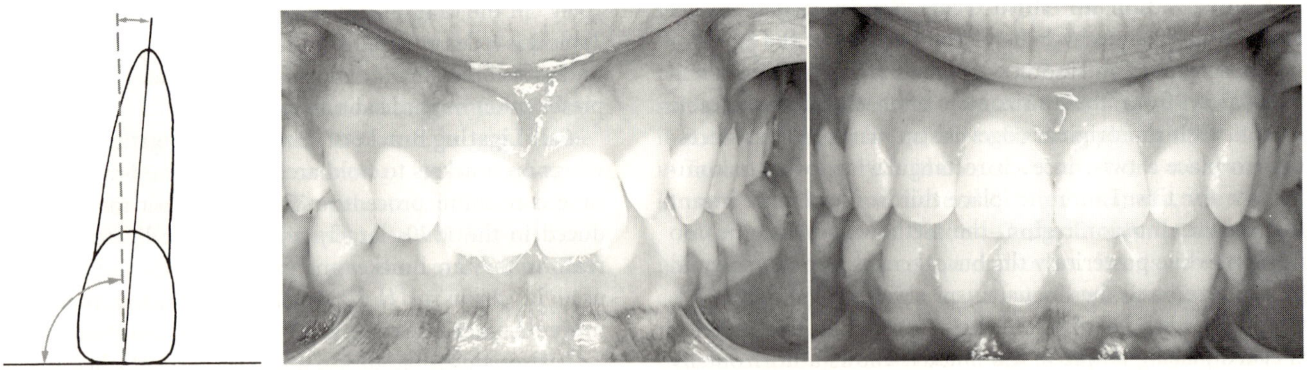

C

FIGURE 11-33 **A,** A second-order bend, or an inclination of the bracket slot to produce the same effect, is necessary for the maxillary incisors because the long axes of these teeth are inclined relative to the incisal edge. The smaller angle (shown above) is the bracket angulation or the tip. (Redrawn from Andrews LF. J Clin Orthod 12:179, 1976.) **B, C,** Malaligned maxillary incisors before and after treatment using straight-wire brackets to facilitate both mesio-distal (tip) and facio-lingual (torque) root positioning.

Table 11-5

Molar Tube/Bracket Prescriptions

MAXILLARY	1ST MOLAR			2ND MOLAR		
	Torque	Tip	Rotation	Torque	Tip	Rotation
Roth	−14	0	14	−14	0	14
Hilgers	−10	0	15	−10	0	12
Ricketts	0	0	0	0	0	0
Standard Edgewise	0	0	0	0	0	0
Alexander	−10	0	15	−10	0	6
MBT	−14	0	10	−14	0	10
Sprint	−10	0	8	−10	0	6
Orthos	10	0	15	−10	0	15
Damon (Med Torque)	−9	0	10	−10	0	5
Andrews	−9	5	10	−9	0	10

MANDIBULAR	1ST MOLAR			2ND MOLAR		
	Torque	Tip	Rotation	Torque	Tip	Rotation
Roth	−30	1	4	−30	0	4
Hilgers	−27	5	12	−27	0	12
Ricketts	0	0	0	0	0	0
Standard Edgewise	0	0	0	0	0	0
Alexander	−22	6	5	−27	0	6
MBT	−20	0	0	−10	0	0
Sprint	−25	0	6	−30	1	4
Orthos	−10	0	0	−10	0	5
Damon (Med Torque)	−30	2	0	−10	2	0
Andrews	−25	2	0	−30	0	0

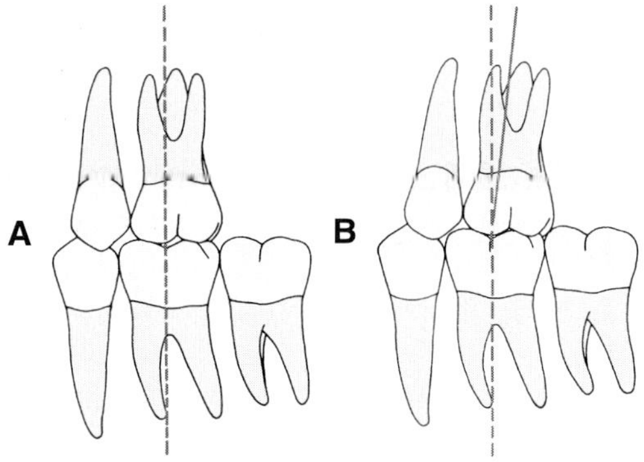

Figure 11-34 A distal inclination or tip of the maxillary first molar is important for proper posterior occlusal interdigitation. If the mesio-buccal cusp occludes in the mesial groove of the mandibular first molar, creating an apparently ideal Class I relationship, proper interdigitation of the premolars still cannot be obtained if the molar is positioned too upright **(A).** Tipping the molar distally **(B)** allows the premolars to interdigitate properly. (Redrawn from Andrews LF. Am J Orthod 62:296, 1972.)

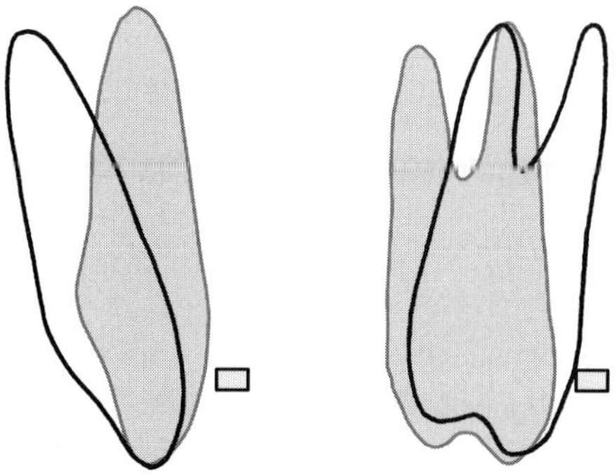

Figure 11-35 The plane of a flat rectangular archwire relative to a maxillary incisor and molar is shown in red. To produce the proper facio-lingual position of both anterior and posterior teeth, either a rectangular archwire must be twisted (torqued), or the bracket slot must be cut at an angle to produce the same torque effect. Otherwise, the improper inclination shown in red will be produced. Proper torque is necessary, not to move teeth, but to prevent undesired movement.

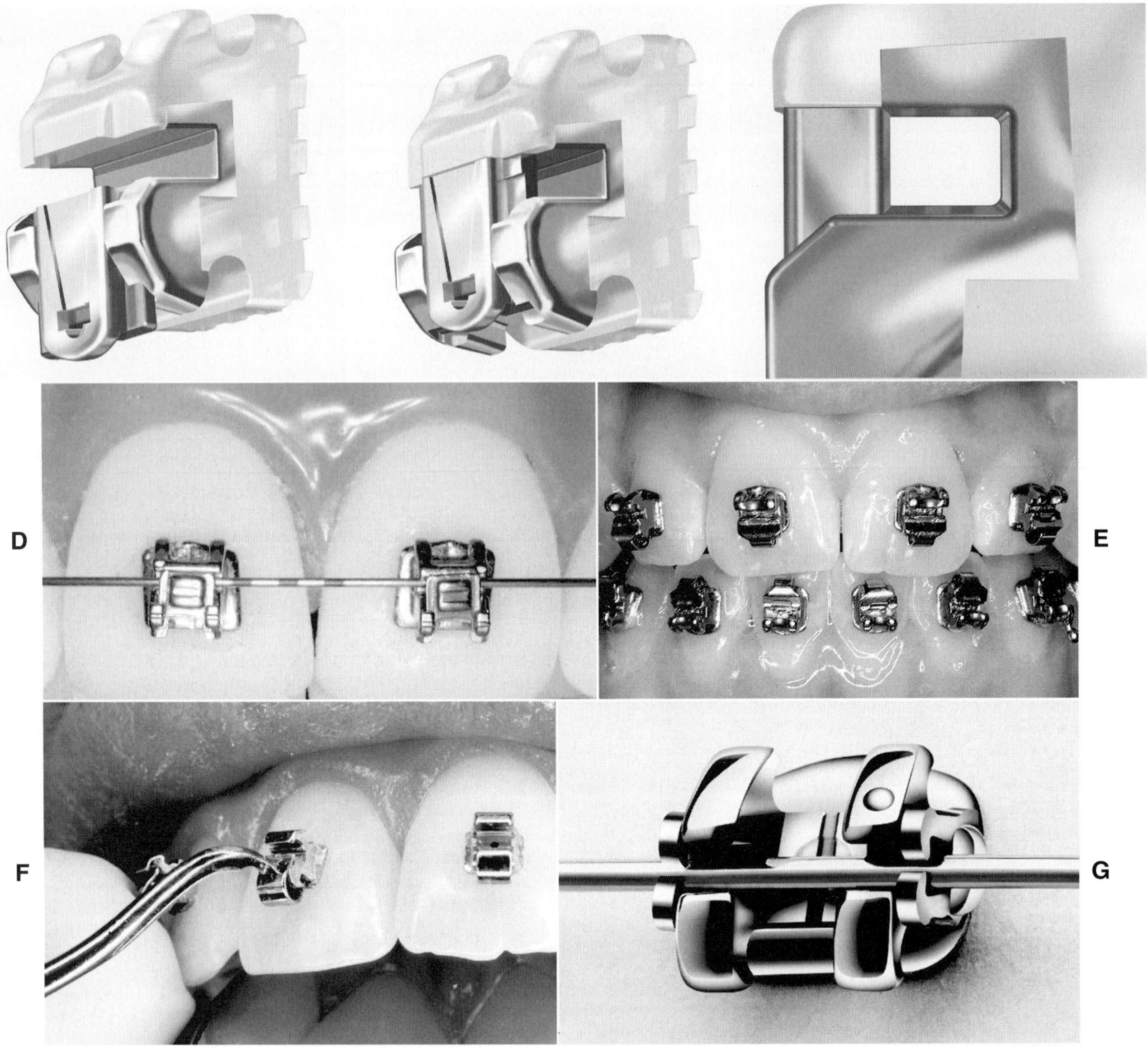

FIGURE 11-36 Self-ligating brackets have either a rigid (Damon, Innovation) or spring clip (Speed), or retaining springs (Smart-Clip) to hold an archwire in the bracket slot. The great advantage, especially with a rigid clip, is a reduction in friction as the bracket moves relative to the archwire, because there is no force pressing the wire against the bottom of the bracket slot. **A,** The Damon bracket (rigid clip) open; **B,** closed; **C,** side view; **D,** brackets closed, archwire in place; **E,** innovation bracket (rigid clip), with slots open; **F,** speed bracket (spring clip), with the spring clip open; **G,** SmartClip bracket (retaining springs), with a wire in place. The wire is simply pulled out of the bracket past the springs, or forced past the springs into the bracket. (**A-D,** Courtesy Ormco/Sybron; **E,** Courtesy GAC; **F,** Courtesy Speed Inc; **G,** Courtesy 3-M Unitek.)

and rigid latching caps (Figure 11-36). The principal advantage is a reduction of friction between the wire and bracket because the archwire is not pressed against the base of the bracket, as it is by a wire ligature or elastomeric module (see Chapter 10). This makes it easier to slide teeth along the archwire as spaces are opened or closed. Easier placement and removal of archwires may or may not be a secondary benefit, depending on how user-friendly the design is. However, what is an advantage for sliding is a disadvantage for frictionless space closure. The springy clips of both types may not hold a wire in place well enough to deliver adequate moments to prevent tipping when closing loops are used, and with rigid clips, it can be quite difficult to completely engage full-dimension wires in the finishing stage of treatment.

Individually Customized Brackets. Because of the marked individual variations in the contour of the teeth, no appliance prescription can be optimal for all patients, and compensatory bends in finishing archwires often are necessary. Custom brackets for the facial surface of teeth offer the

A

B

C

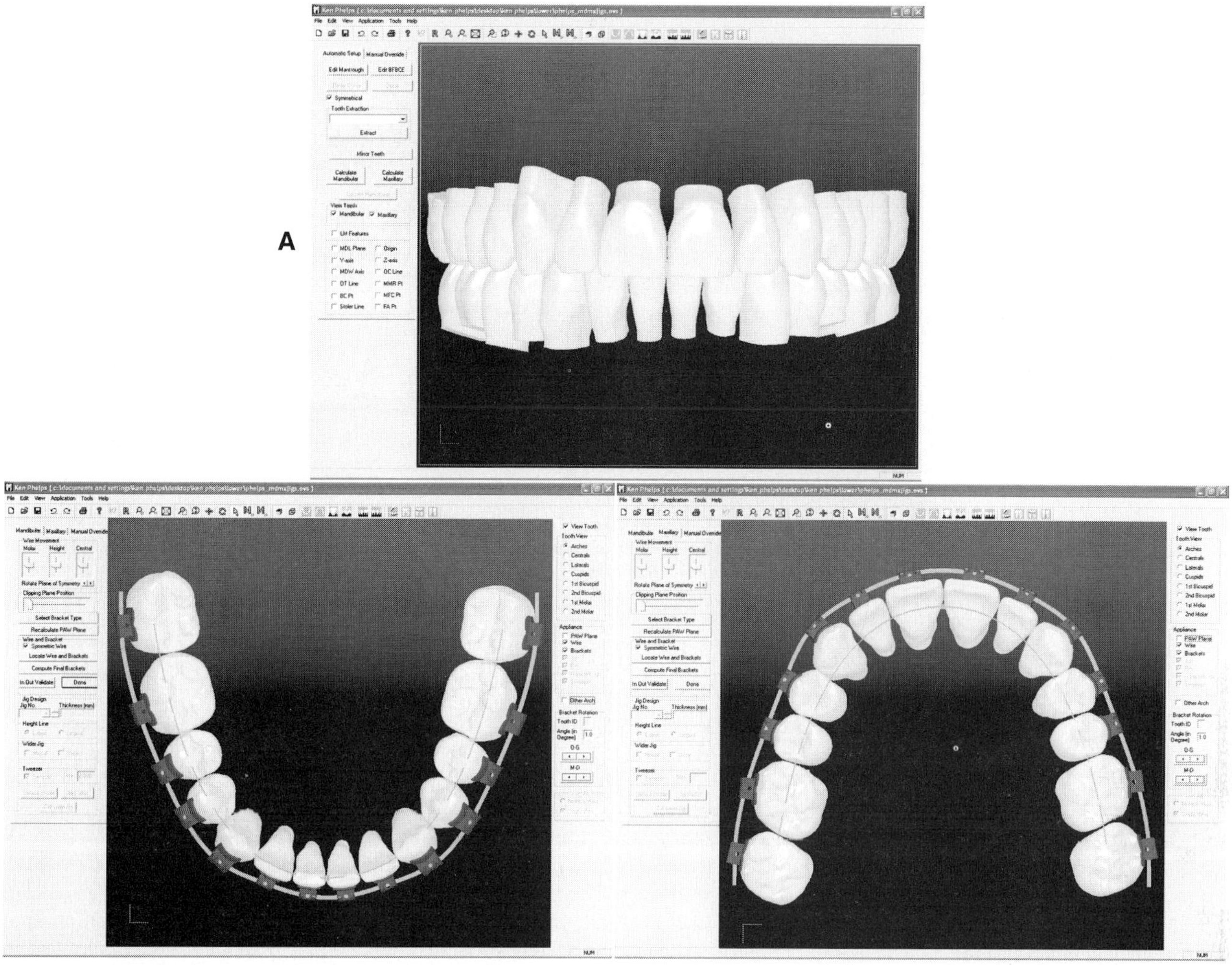

FIGURE 11-37 **A,** The preparation of Insignia custom facial brackets (Ormco) begins with a laser scan of the patient's dental casts, so that the contours of the individual teeth are captured in computer memory and the teeth are reset to ideal position. **B, C,** The base for each individual bracket is milled to fit a specific tooth, and the bracket slot is cut to match the ideal position of that tooth with a rectangular archwire in place. The goal is to have a final rectangular archwire that requires no chairside fabrication to produce ideal tooth positions. (Courtesy Ormco/Sybron.)

prospect of eliminating almost all archwire bending, i.e., they could provide the perfect straight wire appliance.

Whether custom brackets are to be made for the facial or lingual surfaces (see below), the technology is much the same. The first step is a 3-dimensional digital scan of casts of the patient's teeth on a laboratory bench, using a laser beam with a resolution at least as good as 50 microns. Direct intraoral scans have the potential to offer a more time-efficient way to obtain the dimensions, but at present this technology is not fully developed.

The current approach to custom labial brackets is to precisely cut each bracket using CAD-CAM technology, so that the base of each bracket is contoured for a particular place on the surface of a particular tooth, and the slot for each bracket has the appropriate thickness, inclination and torque needed for ideal positioning of that tooth (Figure 11-37). Using such brackets, it would be possible to place a sequence of a minimal number of archwires, each selected for optimal performance, so that treatment time would be minimized for the doctor and treatment duration minimized for the patient. The technology now exists to produce such brackets from laboratory or intraoral laser scans, with a 2-3 week turnaround time.

Individualized custom brackets must be attached to the teeth with precision equal to that used in making them—so an indirect bonding system with an accurate placement template is required. What happens when one of the custom brackets is lost and requires replacement and rebonding, or is loose and requires rebonding? Because the specifications for each bracket can be maintained in computer memory, it is possible to obtain a replacement bracket within 2-3 weeks (but of course not instantaneously), and a secondary

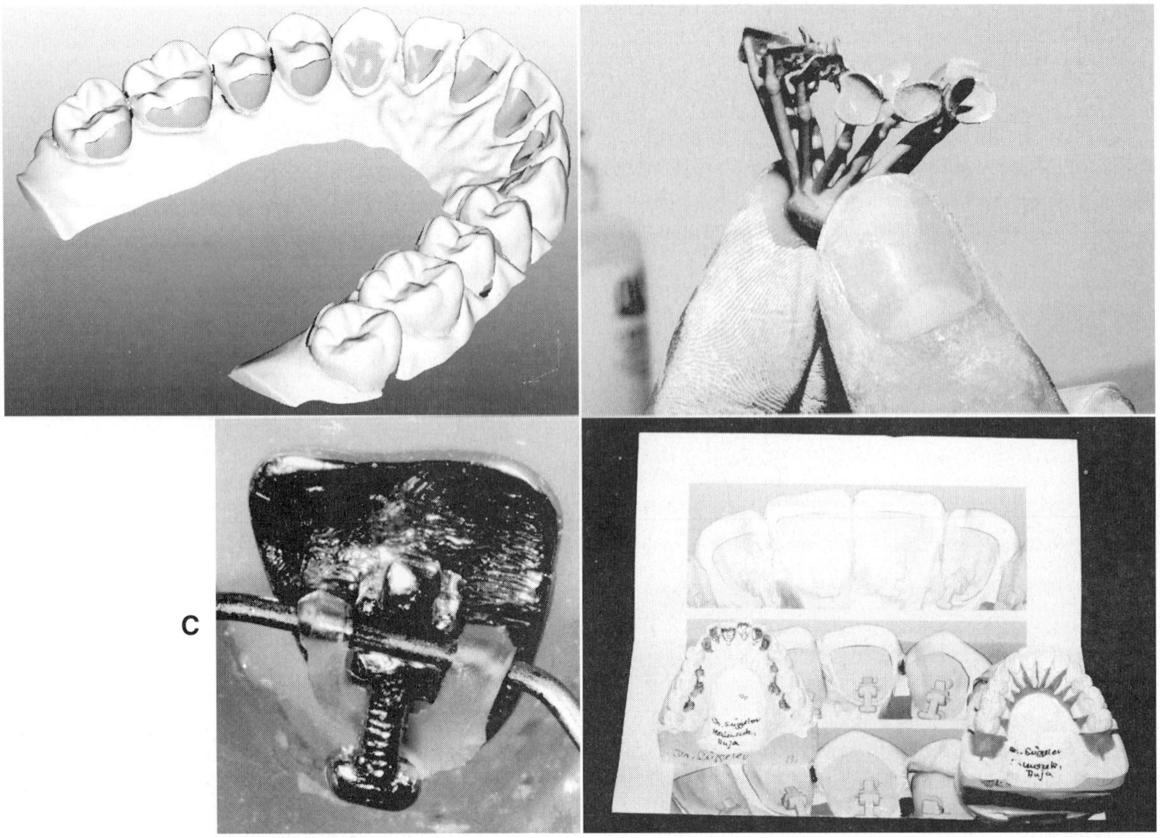

FIGURE 11-38 **A,** The approach for one successful custom lingual appliance (Incognito, TopService GMBH) is based on laser scans of casts after the teeth are separated and set in ideal position. The location of the custom bracket pad for each tooth is established, and wax patterns are made for **(B)** gold castings of custom bracket pads for each tooth. The use of these custom pads greatly improves retention of the bonded lingual brackets. A standard bracket (not individualized for each tooth) that allows vertical insertion of archwires and the use of elastomeric or wire ligatures **(C)** is attached to the custom pads, and the completed appliance **(D)** is supplied ready for indirect bonding. Note that extraction of maxillary first premolars is planned for this patient. (Courtesy Dr. D. Weichmann.)

template can be provided with it. Rebonding a loose bracket is done most efficiently by using the original bonding template, which should be kept with the patient's records for this possible re-use.

At present, however, that is not the biggest problem. Even a set of modern CAD-CAM brackets formed on individual dental casts is still focused only on dental relationships and so, for example, the Class II patient who requires slightly more upright maxillary incisors and more proclined lower incisors would still receive brackets with "ideal" incisor inclinations. It remains important to introduce coordination with the patient's individual skeletal and soft tissue pattern into this type of design. Attempts are being made now to integrate images of tooth-lip relationships into the data base for fabrication of the custom brackets.

Lingual Appliances. A major objection to fixed orthodontic appliances always has been their visible placement on the facial surface of the teeth. This is one reason for using removable appliances, and is the major reason for the current popularity of clear aligners in treatment of adults. The introduction of bonding in the 1970s made it possible to place fixed attachments on the lingual surface of teeth to provide an invisible fixed appliance. Brackets designed for the lingual surface were first offered soon after bonding was introduced. Although it is possible to obtain the same three-dimensional control of crown and root position from the lingual surface as the labial, the difficulty, duration and cost of treatment are all significantly increased. In the United States, most orthodontists who experimented with the lingual appliances available in the 1980s abandoned this approach as more trouble than it was worth, and lingual appliance treatment all but disappeared until quite recently.

Recent progress in Europe has made lingual orthodontics much more widely used there. One successful European approach is to fabricate a custom precious metal pad that covers as much as possible of the lingual surface of each tooth, and then attach low-profile brackets to the custom pads (Figure 11-38). These brackets, designed so the archwire can be inserted from the top, are the same for each tooth, so eliminating wire bending is not a major goal with this approach. Computer-controlled wire bending devices are particularly applicable to the fabrication of the lingual archwires and are a part of the more advanced applications of lingual techniques (see below).

Arch Form and Archwire Fabrication

Selection of Arch Form for Individual Patients. As another contributor to increased efficiency, preformed archwires are an important part of the modern appliance. When NiTi and beta-Ti wires are needed, there is no choice but to use preformed archwires, because these wires are almost impossible to shape to arch form without special tools. What arch form should be employed?

The concept that dental arch form varies among individuals is driven home to most dentists in full denture prosthodontics, where it is taught that the dimensions and shape of the dental arches are correlated with the dimensions and shape of the face. The same variations in arch form and dimensions of course exist in the natural dentition, and it is not the goal of orthodontic treatment to produce dental arches of a single ideal size and shape for everyone.

The basic principle of arch form in orthodontic treatment is that within reason, the patient's original arch form should be preserved. Most thoughtful orthodontists have assumed that this would place the teeth in a position of maximum stability, and long-term retention studies support the view that post-treatment changes are greater when arch form is altered than when it is maintained (see Chapter 17).

As a more general guideline, if the maxillary and mandibular arch forms are incompatible at the beginning of treatment, the mandibular arch form should be used as a basic guide. In many patients with Class II malocclusion, the maxillary arch is narrow across the canines and premolars, and should be expanded to match the lower arch as overjet is reduced. Obviously, this guideline would not apply when mandibular arch form is distorted. This can happen in a number of ways, the most common being lingual displacement of the mandibular incisors by habits or heavy lip pressures, and unilateral drift of teeth in response to early loss of primary canines or molars. Although some judgment is required, the arch form desired at the end of orthodontic treatment should be determined at the beginning, and the patient's occlusal relationships should be established with this in mind.

An excellent mathematical description of the natural dental arch form is provided by a catenary curve, which is the shape that a loop of chain would take if it were suspended from two hooks. The length of the chain and the width between the supports determine the precise shape of the curve. When the width across the first molars is used to establish the posterior attachments, a catenary curve fits the dental arch form of the premolar-canine-incisor segment of the arch very nicely for most individuals. For all patients, the fit is not as good if the catenary curve is extended posteriorly, because the dental arch normally curves slightly lingually in the second and third molar region (Figure 11-39,

A

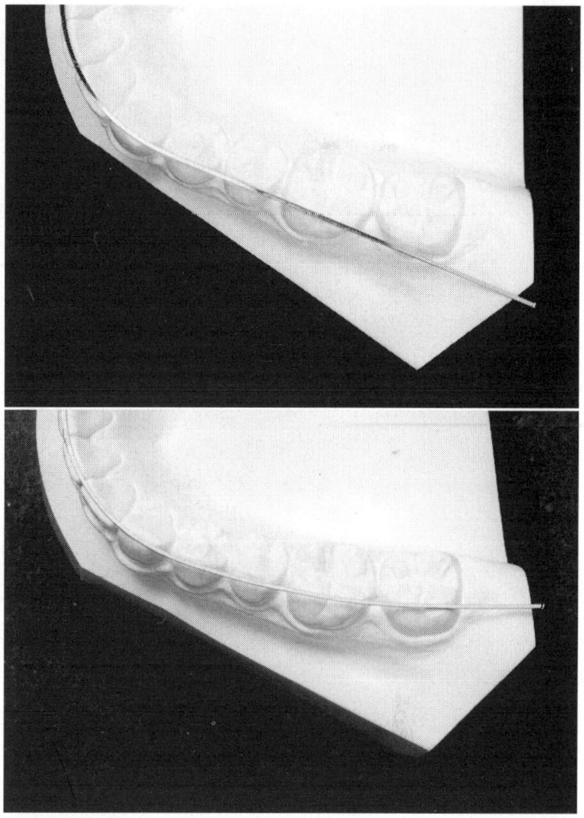

B

FIGURE 11-39 **A,** Preformed archwire with catenary arch form on a lower dental cast from an untreated patient. Note the good correspondence between the arch form and the line of occlusion, except for the second molars. **B,** The Brader arch form for preformed archwires is based on a trifocal ellipse, which slightly rounds the arch in the premolar region compared with a catenary curve and constricts it posteriorly. Note that an archwire formed to the Brader curve fits much better in the second molar region for this untreated patient than a catenary curve.

A). Most of the preformed archwires offered by contemporary manufacturers are based on a catenary curve, with average intermolar dimensions. Modifications to accommodate for a generally more tapering or more square morphology are appropriate, and the second molars must be "tucked in" slightly.

Another mathematical model of dental arch form, originally advocated by Brader and often called the *Brader arch form,* is based on a trifocal ellipse. The anterior segment of the trifocal ellipse closely approximates the anterior segment of a catenary curve, but the trifocal ellipse gradually constricts posteriorly in a way that the catenary curve does not (Figure 11-39, *B*). The Brader arch form, therefore, will more closely approximate the normal position of the second and third molars. It also differs from a catenary curve in producing somewhat greater width across the premolars.

Recently, several manufacturers have offered preformed archwires that appear to be variations of the Brader arch,

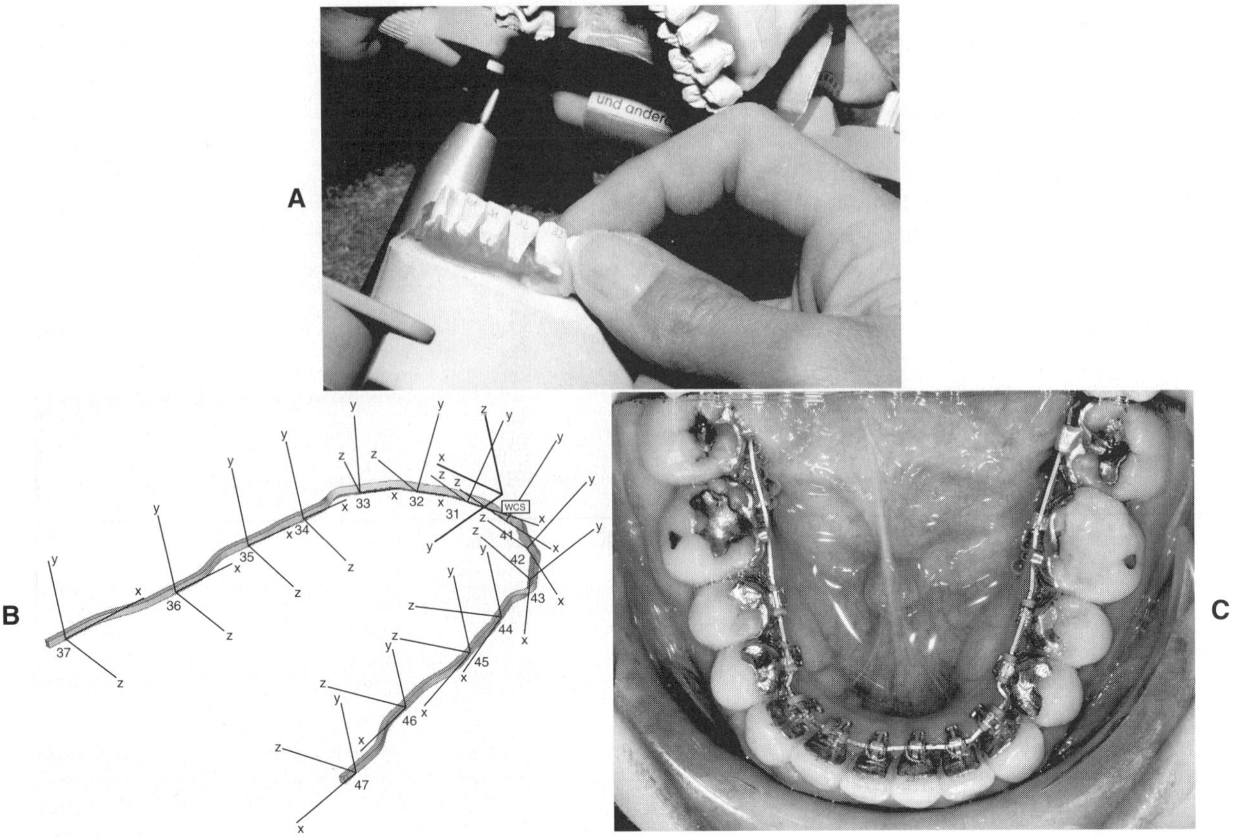

FIGURE 11-40 Archwires for the incognito lingual appliance are formed with a wire-bending robot, using an ideal setup of the teeth that were scanned in preparation of the bracket pads. **A,** Ideal setup in preparation on an articulator; **B,** archwire coordinates for bending an archwire; **C,** archwire in place after robotic fabrication. See Figure 11-41, *B* for a view of a robot in action. (Courtesy Dr. D. Weichmann.)

with advertisements that suggest these wires are more compatible with expansion therapy than conventional arch forms. Expansion across the premolars often is thought to have esthetic advantages; whether the modified arch form to produce this has any effect on stability is unknown. More refined mathematical descriptions of typical human arch forms now are available,[15-17] and it is likely that better mathematical models will improve the preformed archwires available in the near future.

It is important to keep in mind that the adjustments placed in brackets for all of the straight-wire edgewise systems have nothing to do with arch form, which is still established by the shape of the archwires connecting the brackets. Arch form is particularly important during the finishing stage of treatment, when heavy rectangular archwires are employed. Preformed archwires are often listed in the catalogs as "arch blanks" and the name is appropriate, since this properly implies that a degree of individualization of the shape of the preformed archwires will be required to accommodate the needs of patients.

Wire Bending Robots. Another approach to the goal of reducing the amount of clinical time spent bending archwires is to use a computer-controlled machine to shape the archwire as desired. If the effort to fabricate a complex archwire were eliminated, "plain vanilla" brackets without all the straight wire compensations could be used instead of going to the trouble of producing custom brackets with elaborate prescriptions.

In lingual orthodontics, the laser-scanned casts needed for fabrication of custom bracket pads also can provide the data needed to generate computer-fabricated archwires (Figure 11-40). For labial archwires, the data can be accomplished via an intraoral scan that is done using a charged-couple device (CCD) video camera connected to a projector (Figure 11-41). The projector illuminates the teeth with a strobe light that is synchronized with the video signal, and a digital encrypted pattern is projected sequentially onto the dentition. The reflected pattern is captured (the exposure time for an image is 0.0001 second, which virtually eliminates image blurring) and a three-dimensional image of the dentition is the result. The patient's teeth are scanned whenever an archwire is to be fabricated, and straight lengths of wire are placed in the beaks of the robot, which then completes the steps of shaping the wire to the desired arch form and adjusting it at each bracket to provide correct in-out, angulation and torque bends. The difficulty is that the robot

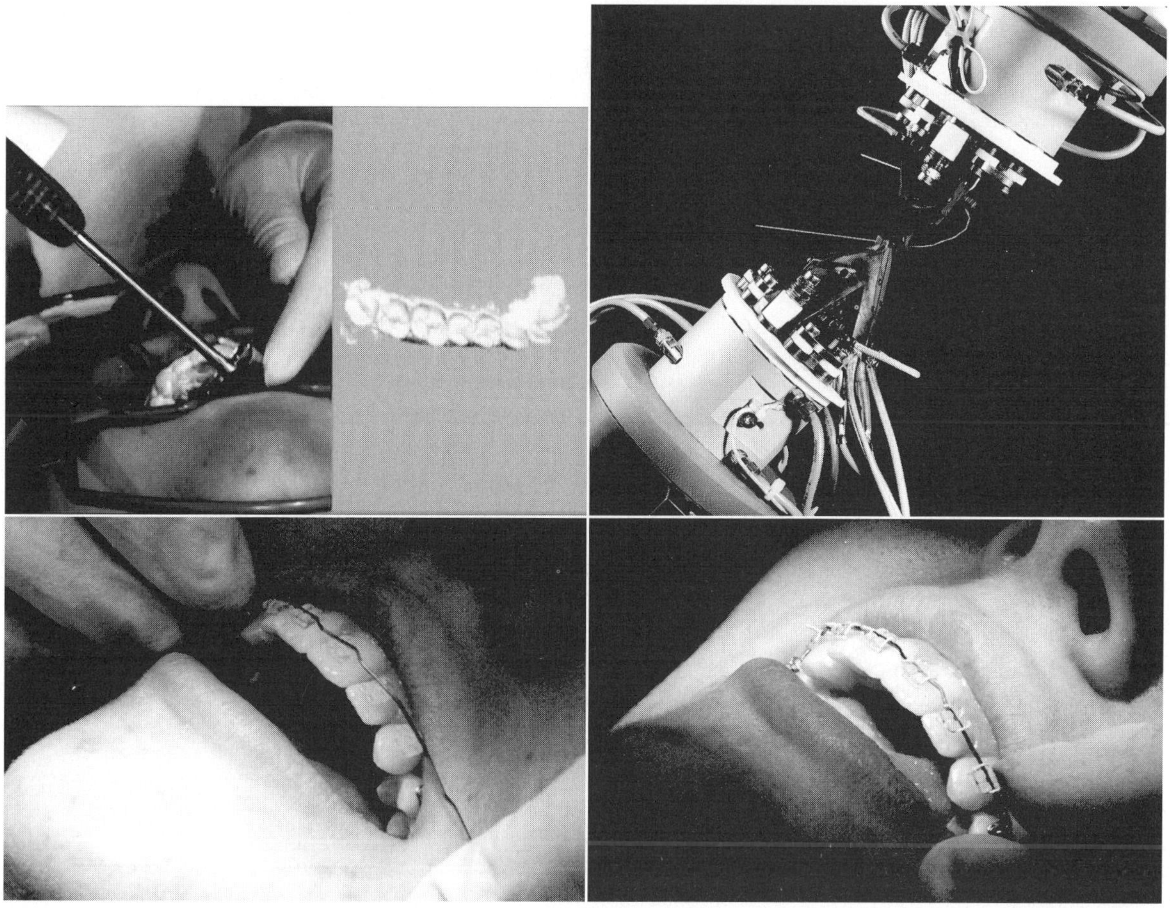

FIGURE 11-41 In the SureSmile system, a CCD scan of the patient's teeth is used (instead of a scan of dental casts) to provide information for archwire preparation. **A,** The intraoral scanning device and its output on a computer screen; **B,** a wire-bending robot making the precise bends in a custom archwire. In this system, precise positioning of brackets and special bracket prescriptions are not necessary because the robot can bend the wire as desired. For this patient **(C, D),** bends compensating for discrepancies in bracket height and root positioning bends for the maxillary central incisors can be seen before and after the archwire is tied in. (Courtesy Dr. R. Sachdeva.)

is expensive, so except in very large practices, the archwires have to be fabricated in a distant laboratory and cannot be supplied immediately. Nevertheless, distant computer-controlled fabrication of custom wires already is offered commercially.

At this point, it seems likely that computer technology will be applied so that most orthodontic appliances of the not-too-distant future will be individualized using laser scans of the tooth surfaces. It is too soon to tell, however, whether the usual approach will be custom brackets that allow the use of preformed archwires with little or no manual wire bending, or minimally compensated (and less expensive) brackets that are used in connection with a wire bending robot.

REFERENCES

1. Graber TM, Rakosi T, Petrovic AG, eds. Dentofacial Orthopedics with Functional Appliances. St. Louis: Mosby; 1997.
2. Adams CP. The Design and Construction of Removable Appliances, ed 4. Bristol, England: John Wright & Sons; 1970.
3. Sheridan JJ, Ledoux W, McMinn R. Essix appliances: Minor tooth movement with divots and windows. J Clin Orthod 28:659-665, 1994.
4. Sheridan JJ, Armbruster P, Nguyen P, Pulitzer S. Tooth movement with Essix mounding. J Clin Orthod 38:435-441, 2004.
5. Turpin DL. Clinical trials needed to answer questions about Invisalign. Am J Orthod Dentofacial Orthop 127:157-158, 2005.
6. Angle EH. The latest and best in orthodontic mechanisms. Dent Cosmos 70:1143-1158, 1928.
7. Begg PR, Kesling PC. Begg Orthodontic Theory and Technique, ed 3. Philadelphia: WB Saunders; 1977.
8. Parkhouse RC. Tip-Edge Orthodontics. Edinburg/New York: Mosby; 2003.
9. Andrews LF. Straight Wire: The Concept and Appliance. San Diego: LA Wells; 1989.
10. Ewoldsen N, Demke RS. A review of orthodontic cements and adhesives. Am J Orthod Dentofacial Orthop 120:45-48, 2001.
11. Derks A, Katsaros C, Frencken JE, van't Hof MA, Kuijpers-Jagtman AM. Caries-inhibiting effect of preventive measures during orthodontic treatment with fixed appliances. A systematic review. Caries Res 38:413-420, 2004.

12. Menezes LM, Campos LC, Quintao CC, Bolognese AM. Hypersensitivity to metals in orthodontics. Am J Orthod Dentofacial Orthop 126:58-64, 2004.
13. Johnson G, Walker MP, Kula K. Fracture strength of ceramic bracket tie wings subjected to tension. Angle Orthod 75:95-100, 2005.
14. Thorstenson GA, Kusy RP. Effect of archwire size and material on the resistance to sliding of self-ligating brackets with second-order angulation in the dry state. Am J Orthod Dentofacial Orthop 122:295-305, 2002.
15. Braun S, Hnat WH, Fender WE, Legan HL. The form of the human dental arch. Angle Orthod 68:29-36, 1998.
16. Begole EA, Lyew RC. A new method for analyzing change in dental arch form. Am J Orthod Dentofacial Orthop 113:394-401, 1998.
17. Taner TU, Ciger S, Germec D, et al. Evaluation of dental arch width and form changes after orthodontic treatment and retention with a new computerized method. Am J Orthod Dentofacial Orthop 2004 126:464-475; discussion 475-476, 2004.

SECTION

V

Treatment in Preadolescent Children

Although most orthodontic problems can be resolved during the transition from the mixed to permanent dentitions when most children are still growing and reasonably cooperative, orthodontic treatment during the preadolescent years sometimes provides a real benefit to the patient. Some of this earlier-than-usual treatment has been described as "preventive" or "interceptive" and during recent years it has become increasingly popular. In reality few early interventions really prevent a malocclusion from developing, and most treatment will require follow-up care during the adolescent years with a second phase of treatment. Essentially, appropriate early treatment lessens the severity of the problems rather than eliminating the need for later treatment.

Orthodontic problems in children can be divided conveniently into nonskeletal (dental) and skeletal problems, which are treated by tooth movement and by growth modification, respectively. Treatment of nonskeletal problems is described in Chapter 12 and skeletal problems are discussed in Chapter 13. The complexity of the treatment procedures varies. Some are definitely within the scope of the general practitioner, whereas others rarely should be attempted outside specialty practice.

Even the simplest treatment in children requires continuous reevaluation to be sure that the expected response is occurring. The transition of the dentition, coupled with rapid growth, means that rapid changes can and do occur. In children, appliance therapy tends to be simpler than in adults, where all changes that occur must be caused by tooth movement, but treatment planning and monitoring are more complex. Whether treatment in children involves skeletal or nonskeletal problems, the totality of changes must be considered. Although diagnosis and treatment planning are not discussed in this section, which focuses on treatment, careful analysis and planning are imperative before any treatment begins. These issues, as they apply to preschool children, have been addressed in Chapters 7 and 8. ■

CHAPTER 12

Treatment of Nonskeletal Problems in Preadolescent Children

Our approach to treatment of dental problems in preadolescent children is built around the triage scheme presented in some detail in Chapter 6 and the treatment planning considerations outlined in Chapters 7 and 8. The triage makes two critical distinctions: first between nonskeletal and skeletal orthodontic problems, then by severity among the nonskeletal problems. For the family dentist, the decision to treat or refer depends on one's education and experience, but generally, we would expect that as the triage scheme indicates, the more straightforward problems would be addressed by generalists and the more difficult problems by specialists. In each of the three sections of the chapter on treatment procedures, clinical problems and appropriate treatment are presented in a sequence of increasing treatment complexity.

SPECIAL CONSIDERATIONS IN EARLY TREATMENT

Some issues only present themselves or take on special importance during early treatment. Among the important points to consider when early treatment is considered are these:

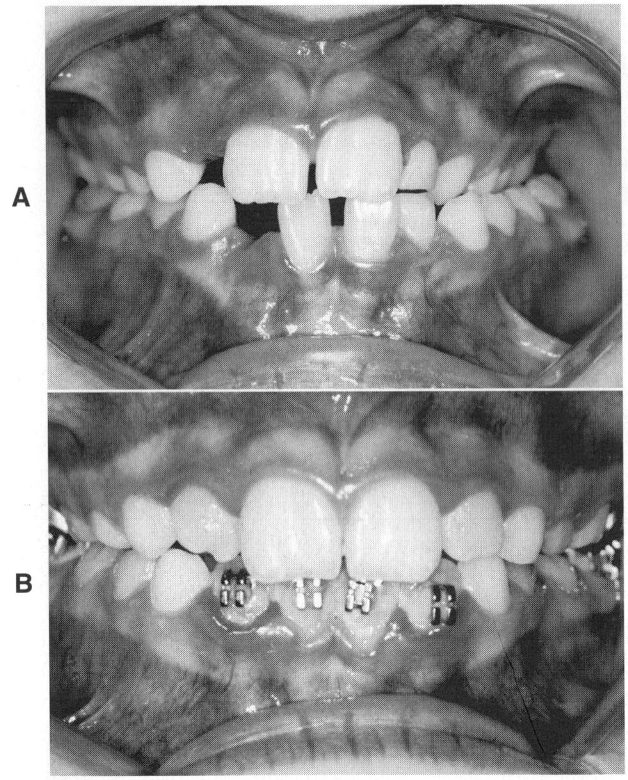

FIGURE 12-1 Limited treatment in the mixed dentition requires objectives, but does not require comprehensive objectives. **A,** This patient has lower incisor spacing and a posterior crossbite. Both were addressed in the first phase of treatment, but **(B)** detailed tooth positioning was not attempted and probably is not generally required because additional teeth will erupt and cause potential problems.

The Goals of the Treatment Must Be Clearly Outlined and Understood

For a child with a complex problem, it is highly likely that a second stage of treatment in the early permanent dentition will be required, even if early treatment is carried out effectively and properly (Figure 12-1). There is a limit to the time and cooperation that patients and parents are willing to devote to treatment. Unless appropriate end points are set in advance, it is easy for mixed dentition treatment to extend over several years and result in one extremely long period of treatment instead of defined segments of treatment that are more advantageous. If mixed dentition treatment takes too long, there are two problems: (1) patients can be "burned out" by the time they are ready for comprehensive treatment in the early permanent dentition, and (2) the chance of damage to the teeth increases as treatment time goes up.

This means that the diagnosis and treatment planning for early treatment are just as demanding and important as in comprehensive treatment. If the treatment goals are not clear, setting appropriate endpoints will be impossible. In early treatment, all aspects of the occlusion usually are not modified to ideal or near ideal. Final tooth and root positions are not required in most cases unless this is all the treatment the child will ever encounter—a prediction that is hard to make.

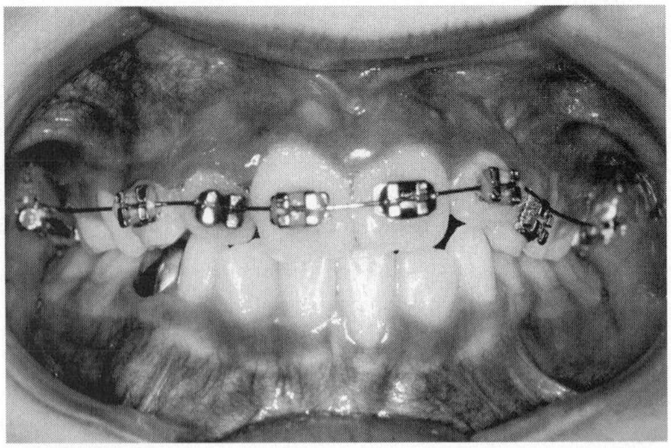

FIGURE 12-2 This patient has a "2 by 6" appliance in place that includes 2 molars and 6 anterior teeth. The "2 by 4" appliance includes 2 molars and 4 anterior teeth. This is a typical appliance for the mixed dentition and can include both primary and permanent teeth.

Fewer Options Are Available, and Patient Cooperation Is More Critical

In mixed dentition treatment with a partial appliance, there simply are fewer options available. For instance, if a child does not wear a headgear as prescribed in limited treatment, you are out of luck—starting over with a different approach, usually with full appliances, is about the only option. In comprehensive treatment, there are the options of Class II elastics, interarch springs, fixed interarch connectors, Herbst attachments or guide planes. Although some of these options also require cooperation, one of the alternatives may catch the imagination of a recalcitrant patient and allow treatment to be completed in an acceptable manner. In limited treatment, the options are not there.

There Are Important Biomechanical Differences Between Complete and Partial Appliances

The typical fixed appliance for mixed dentition treatment is a "2 × 4" or "2 × 6" arrangement (2 molar bands, 4 or 6 bonded anterior teeth) (Figure 12-2). When a fixed appliance includes only some of the teeth, archwire spans are longer, large moments are easy to create, and the wires themselves are more springy and less strong (see Chapter 10).

This can provide some biomechanical advantages. For example, intrusion of teeth is easier with long spans of wire that keep forces light and allow the appropriate moments to be generated. On the other hand, the wires are more prone to breakage, distortion and displacement from the molar tubes. There is little indication for use of the newer superelastic wires when long unsupported spans exist. Wires with intermediate flexibility and looped stainless steel configurations are more effective. Because the available permanent teeth are grouped in anterior (incisor) and posterior (molar) segments, a segmented arch approach to mechanics often is required. The apparently simple fixed appliances used in the mixed dentition can be quite complex to use appropriately (see Chapter 10). They are better described as deceptively simple.

Anchorage Control Is Both More Difficult and More Critical

With only the first molars available as anchorage in the posterior segment of the arch, there are limits to the amount of tooth movement that should be attempted in the mixed dentition. Extraoral support from headgear and facemasks can be used, but implant-supported anchorage usually is not practical due to the presence of unerupted teeth and the reduced density of the bone. In addition, stabilizing maxillary and mandibular lingual arches are more likely to be necessary as an adjunct to anchorage.

Beware of Unerupted Teeth

Although radiographic images of the developing dentition are obtained routinely when early treatment is considered, the effect of tooth movement on unerupted teeth often escapes continued consideration. This is a particular risk when moving lateral incisors that are adjacent to unerupted canines. Care must be taken so the roots of the lateral incisors are not inadvertently tipped into the path of the erupting canines. Failure to pay attention to this can lead to resorption of considerable portions of the lateral incisor root (Figure 12-3).

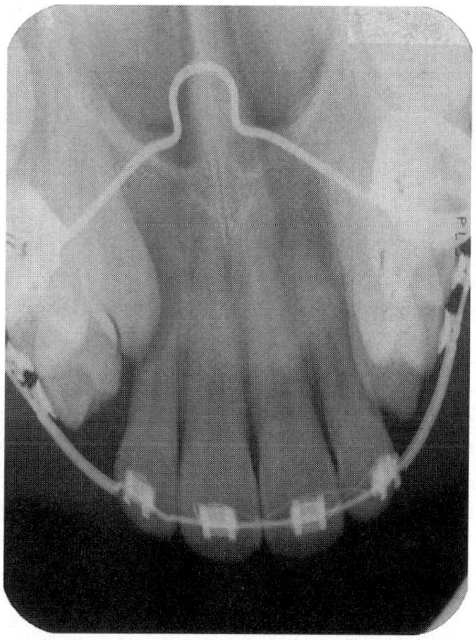

Figure 12-3 This patient has resorption of the maxillary right lateral incisor prior to eruption of the maxillary right canine with appliances in place. This can occur if the canine position is more mesial than normal or the lateral incisor has excessive or even normal distal root tip.

Space Closure Must Be Managed with Particular Care

Otherwise, when all teeth are not banded or bonded, the teeth without attachments will tend to be displaced and squeezed out of the arch. Teeth without attachments may move facially or lingually, or in some instances occlusally. Unanticipated side effects of space closure that would not be encountered with a complete fixed appliance often are a problem in mixed dentition treatment.

Interarch Mechanics Must Be Used Sparingly If At All

The side effects of Class II, Class III, or vertical elastics, such as widening or constriction of the dental arches and alteration of the occlusal plane, make them risky with partial fixed appliances like the typical mixed dentition 2 × 4 arrangement. Interarch forces are not recommended under most circumstances unless a complete fixed appliance is present with one exception: cross elastics can be employed in the mixed dentition in the treatment of unilateral crossbite. This also subjects the treatment result to the limitations of not using interarch mechanics (Figure 12-4).

Final Results Are Dictated Largely by the Untreated Arch

If early treatment is carried out in only one dental arch, the final result is dictated by the untreated teeth and arch. For instance, if the lower arch is not ideally aligned, it will be difficult to ideally align the upper arch and have proper coordination of the teeth without interferences. Likewise, if there is a substantial curve of Spee in the lower arch and only the upper arch is leveled, the overbite and overjet will be excessive. Despite this, early treatment in only one arch, and the associated delay in obtaining ideal tooth positions, can be quite acceptable if the remainder of the total correction is to be accomplished later (Figure 12-5).

Retention Often Is Needed Between Mixed Dentition Treatment and Eruption of the Permanent Teeth

After any significant tooth movement, it is important to maintain the teeth in their new position until a condition of stability is reached. That is as true in the mixed dentition as

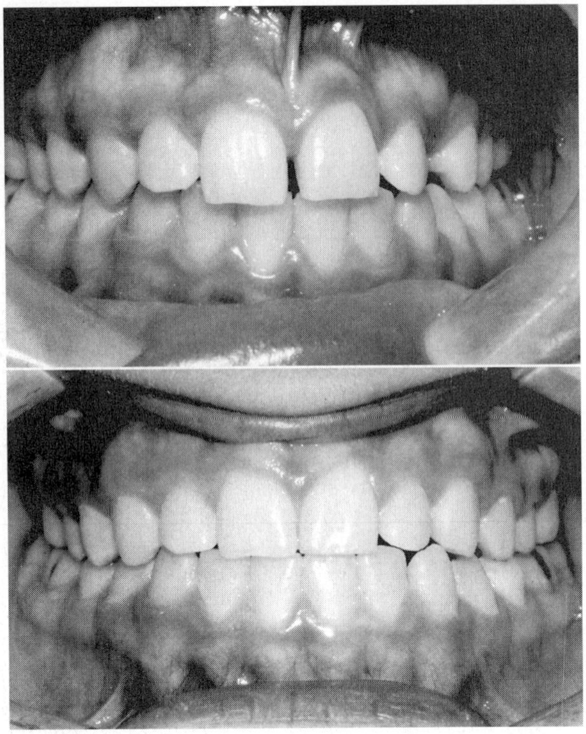

FIGURE 12-4 This shows the limitations of not using inter-arch mechanics for limited treatment. **A,** This patient had limited overbite on the left side where an impacted canine was located. **B,** The patient still has limited overbite after extrusion of the canine because appliances were only used on the maxillary, so no inter-arch vertical elastics could be used.

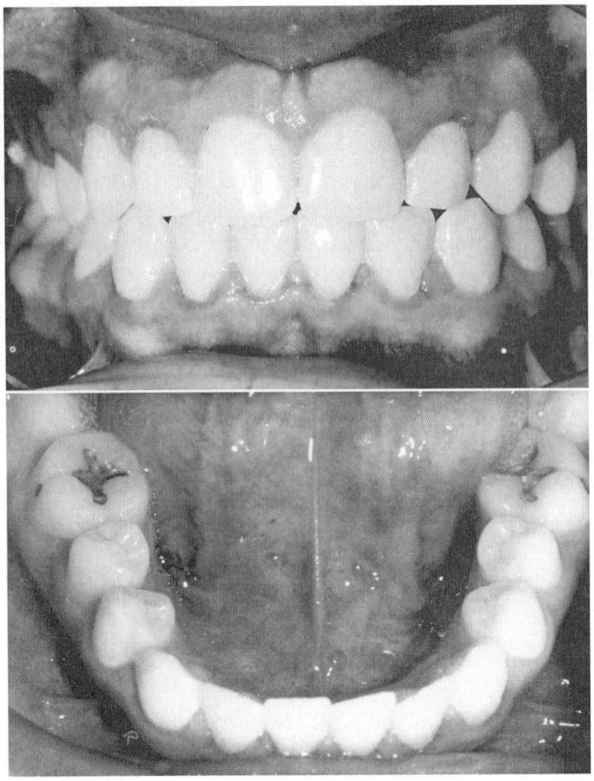

FIGURE 12-5 When limited treatment is attempted in the mixed dentition, it is highly likely that a second stage of treatment will be required later, or a less-than-ideal result will have to be accepted. **A,** This completed patient shows limited overbite and overjet in the maxillary left incisor region. **B,** Because only the maxillary arch had a fixed appliance, the pretreatment irregular alignment in the lower arch was accepted. It is difficult to have ideal alignment and occlusion when only one arch is treated.

later. In fact, careful retention may be even more necessary after early treatment. The final stage of transition from the mixed to the permanent dentition is a particularly unstable time. For instance, mesial drift of molars that shortens arch length normally occurs then, but this must be prevented if arch expansion was the goal of early treatment.

In mixed dentition patients, retention must be planned with two things in mind: the patient's current vs. initial condition and subsequent changes in the dentition and occlusion that will occur as the child matures (Figure 12-6). With removable retainers, the location and design of clasps, wires and labial bows should make them either modifiable or removable. Wires through edentulous areas can interfere with eruption of the permanent teeth in that area, and clasps on primary teeth will be of limited use because these teeth will be lost. Preadolescent children, even those who were quite cooperative with active treatment, may not be reliable patients for removable retainers—but the greater control provided by fixed retainers must be balanced against their greater hygiene risk and lower modifiability as teeth erupt. A prolonged period of retention before comprehensive treatment begins also increases the chance of patient burn-out.

OCCLUSAL RELATIONSHIP PROBLEMS

Crossbites of Dental Origin

By definition, crossbites of dental origin are due solely to displacement of teeth. They usually affect only some of the teeth in an area of the arch, and as a rule are less severe than crossbites due to jaw discrepancies—but this means that occlusal interferences often are present, increasing the chance of a shift on closure. For both posterior and anterior crossbites, the distinction between skeletal and dental etiology is important. Full-cusp bilateral posterior crossbite is quite likely to have a skeletal component. A unilateral posterior crossbite usually is due to displaced teeth, but it may result from maxillary or mandibular skeletal asymmetry. If multiple teeth are in anterior crossbite, it is quite likely that the problem is a jaw discrepancy, not just displacement of teeth.

Correction of dental crossbites in the mixed dentition is recommended because it eliminates functional shifts and

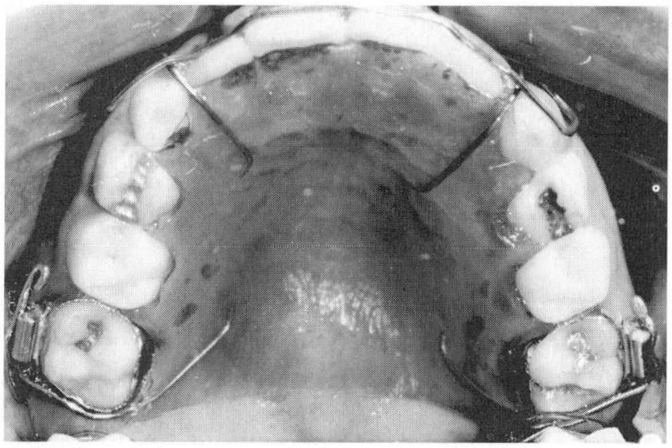

Figure 12-6 When retention is used between early (phase 1) and later (phase 2) treatment, creative planning of bow and clasp positions is required to avoid interference with erupting teeth and maintain the effectiveness of clasps. Note that the labial bow crosses the occlusion distal to the lateral incisors rather than in the area where the canines will erupt, and the molar clasps adapt to the bands and headgear tubes.

wear on the erupted permanent teeth, and possibly dentoalveolar asymmetry.[1] This usually also increases arch circumference[2] and provides more room for the permanent teeth. Relapse into crossbite is unlikely in the absence of a skeletal problem, so early correction also simplifies future treatment by eliminating at least that problem from the list.

Posterior Crossbite

Theoretically, treatment of posterior crossbite differs depending on its underlying cause. Skeletal crossbites, usually resulting from a narrow maxilla but occasionally from an excessively wide mandible, generally are treated by heavy forces to open the midpalatal suture and make the maxilla wider (as discussed in Chapter 13). Dental crossbites are treated by moving the teeth with lighter forces. Heavy force and rapid expansion are not indicated in the primary or early mixed dentition. There is a significant risk of distortion of the nose if this is done in younger children (see Figure 8-14).

There are three basic approaches to the treatment of moderate posterior crossbites in children: equilibration to eliminate mandibular shift, expansion of a constricted maxillary arch, and repositioning of individual teeth to deal with intra-arch asymmetries.

In a few cases, mostly observed in the primary or early mixed dentition, a shift into posterior crossbite will be due solely to interference caused by the primary canines (Figure 12-7). These patients can be diagnosed by careful positioning of the mandible. They require only limited equilibration of the primary canines to eliminate the interference and the resulting lateral shift into crossbite.

A greater maxillary constriction will allow the maxillary teeth to fit inside the mandibular teeth and will not be accompanied by a shift on closure (Figure 12-8). These patients often have reduced arch circumference so that crossbite correction will provide more space and improve the chances that the permanent teeth will not erupt in crossbite.[3] More commonly, a bilateral maxillary constriction does cause a mandibular shift. Even a small constriction creates dental interferences that force the mandible to shift to a new position for maximum intercuspation (Figure 12-9). Whether or not a mandibular shift is present, a crossbite due to a narrow maxilla should be corrected when it is noted, in the primary or mixed dentition, unless the permanent first molars are expected to erupt in less than 6 months. In that situation, it is better to allow the permanent molars to erupt so that correction can include these teeth if necessary. Although it is possible to treat posterior crossbite with a split-plate type of removable appliance (see Figure 11-9), there are two problems: this relies on patient compliance for success, and the appliance can be displaced easily. This approach is less successful and less cost-effective than an expansion lingual arch.[4]

The preferred appliance for modest expansion of the maxillary arch to correct a posterior crossbite in a preadolescent child is an adjustable lingual arch that requires little

A

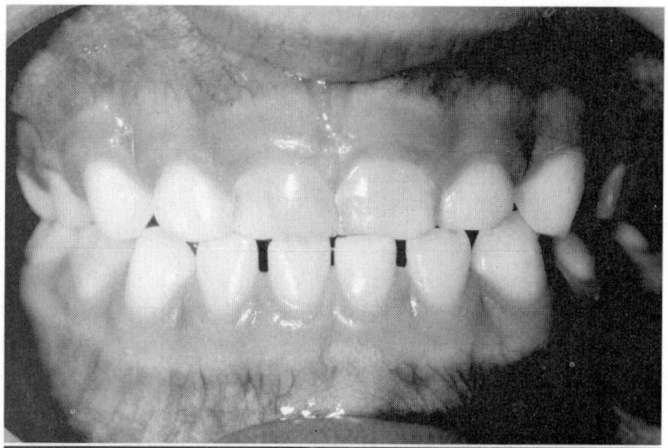

B

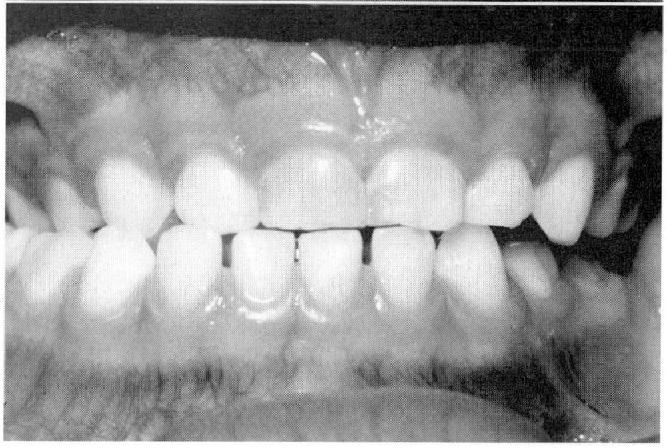

Figure 12-7 Minor canine interferences leading to a mandibular shift. **A,** Initial contact; **B,** shift into centric occlusion. The slight lingual position of the primary canines can lead to occlusal interferences and an apparent posterior crossbite. This cause of posterior crossbite is infrequent and is best treated by occlusal adjustment of the primary canines.

A
B
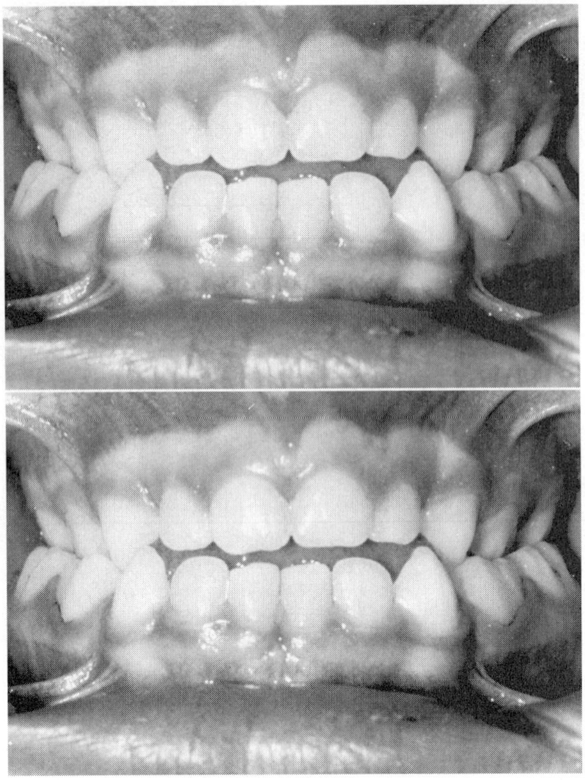

FIGURE 12-8 Marked bilateral maxillary constriction. **A,** Initial contact; **B,** centric occlusion (no shift). Severe constriction often produces no interferences upon closure, and the patient has a bilateral posterior crossbite in centric relation. This problem is best treated by bilateral maxillary expansion.

A
B
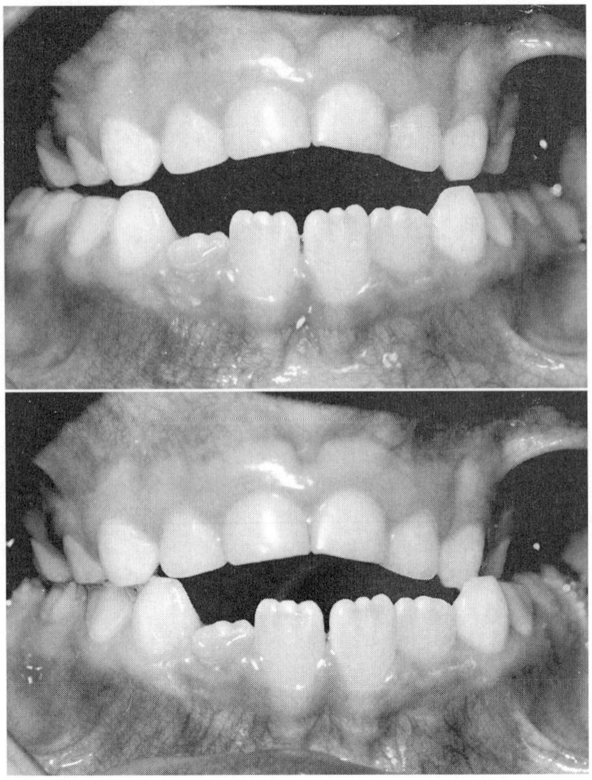

FIGURE 12-9 Moderate bilateral maxillary constriction. **A,** Initial contact; **B,** shift into centric occlusion. Moderate bilateral maxillary constriction often leads to posterior interferences upon closure and a lateral shift of the mandible into an apparent unilateral posterior crossbite. This problem also is best treated by bilateral maxillary expansion.

patient cooperation. Both the W-arch and the quad helix are reliable and easy to use. The W-arch is a fixed appliance constructed of 36 mil steel wire soldered to molar bands (Figure 12-10). It is activated simply by opening the apices of the W and is easily adjusted to provide more anterior than posterior expansion, or vice versa, if this is desired. The appliance delivers proper force levels when opened 4-5 mm wider than the passive width and should be adjusted to this dimension before being inserted. It is not uncommon for the teeth and maxilla to move more on one side than the other, so precise bilateral expansion is the exception rather than the rule, but acceptable correction and tooth position are almost always achieved.

The quad helix (Figure 12-11) is a more flexible version of the W-arch. The helices in the anterior palate are bulky, which can effectively serve as a reminder to aid in stopping a finger habit. The combination of a posterior crossbite and a finger-sucking habit is the best indication for this appliance. The extra wire incorporated in this appliance gives it slightly greater range of action than the W-arch, but the forces are equivalent. Attention to soft tissue irritation is also recommended with this appliance. Both the W-arch and the quad helix leave an imprint on the tongue, about which the parents and child should be warned. This will disappear when the appliance is removed.

With both types of expansion lingual arches, some opening of the midpalatal suture can be expected in a young child, so the expansion is not solely dental.[5] This is of no consequence and will require no difference in either treatment or retention. Expansion should continue at the rate of 2 mm per month (1 mm tooth movement on each side) until the crossbite is slightly overcorrected. In other words, the lingual cusps of the maxillary teeth should occlude on the lingual inclines of the buccal cusps of the mandibular molars at the end of active treatment (Figure 12-12). Intraoral appliance adjustment is possible but may lead to unexpected changes. For this reason, removal and recementation are recommended at each active treatment visit. Most posterior crossbites require 2 to 3 months of active treatment and 3 months of retention (during which the lingual arch is left passively in place).

Some children do have true unilateral crossbites due to unilateral maxillary constriction of the upper arch (Figure 12-13). In these cases the ideal treatment is to move selected teeth on the constricted side. To a limited extent, this goal can be achieved by using different length arms on a W-arch

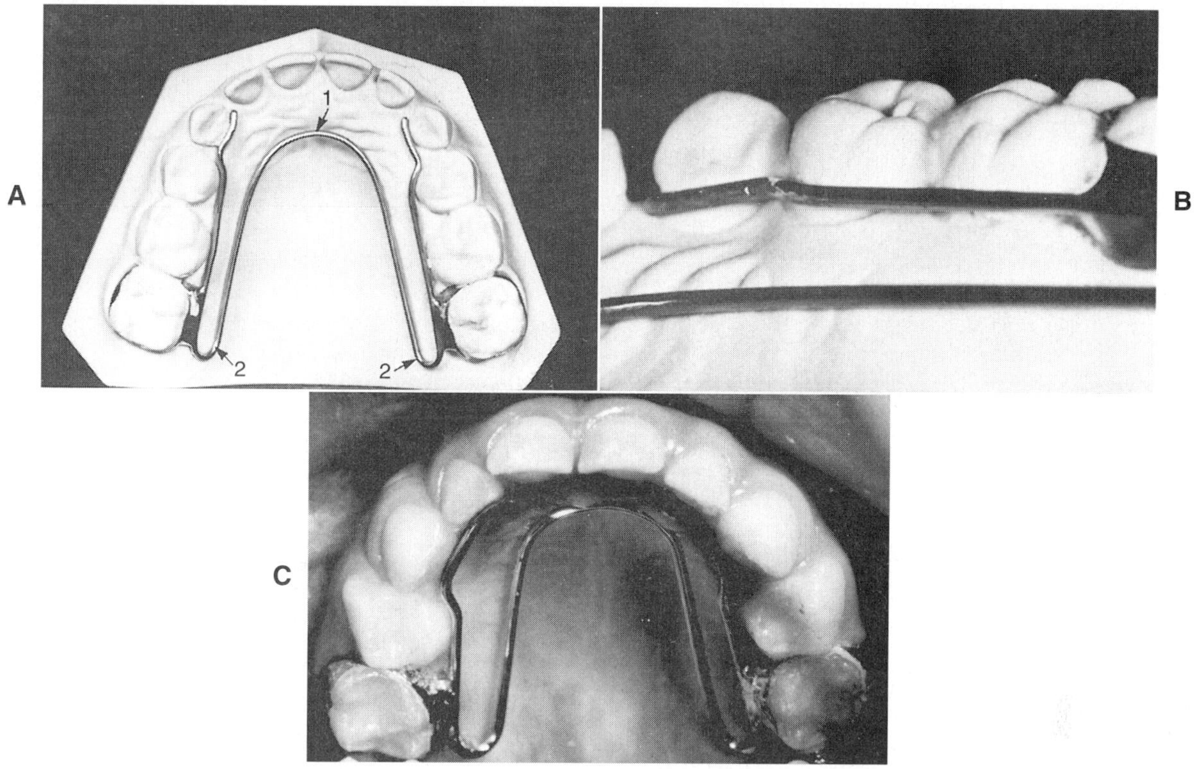

Figure 12-10 The W-arch appliance is ideal for bilateral maxillary expansion. **A,** The appliance is fabricated from 36 mil wire and soldered to the bands. The lingual wire should contact the teeth involved in the crossbite and extend not more than 1 to 2 mm distal to the banded molars to eliminate soft tissue irritation. Activation at point 1 produces posterior expansion and activation at point 2 produces anterior expansion. **B,** The lingual wire should remain 1 to 1.5 mm away from the marginal gingiva and the palatal tissue. **C,** This W-arch is being used to correct a bilateral constriction in the primary dentition.

or quad helix (Figure 12-14), but some bilateral expansion must be expected. An alternative is to use a mandibular lingual arch to stabilize the lower teeth and attach cross-elastics to the maxillary teeth that are at fault. This is more complicated and requires cooperation to be successful, but is more unilateral in its effect. A third alternative is to use a removable appliance similar to the one in Figure 11-9, but sectioned asymmetrically. This has the effect of pitting more teeth against fewer teeth and results in asymmetric movement. Of course, this appliance has the same restrictions as all removable appliances: its success depends on both the quality of its retentive clasps and the patient's cooperation.

All of the appliances described here are aimed at correction of teeth in the maxillary arch, which is usually where the problem is located. If teeth in both arches contribute to the problem, cross-elastics between banded or bonded attachments in both arches (Figure 12-15) can reposition both upper and lower teeth. The force from the elastics is directed vertically as well as faciolingually, which will extrude the posterior teeth and reduce the overbite. Therefore cross-elastics should be used with caution in children with increased lower face height or limited overbite. Crossbites treated with elastics should be overcorrected, and the bands or bonds left in place immediately after active treatment. If there is relapse, the elastics can be reinstated without rebanding or rebonding. When the occlusion is stable after several weeks without elastic force, the attachments can be removed. The most common problem with this form of crossbite correction is lack of cooperation from the child.

A flowchart is provided to help guide decision making for posterior crossbites (Figure 12-16).

Anterior Crossbites

In planning treatment for anterior crossbites, it is critically important to differentiate skeletal problems of deficient maxillary or excessive mandibular growth from crossbites due only to displacement of teeth.[6] Most children with anterior crossbite, especially if more than one or two teeth are in crossbite, have a skeletal problem (see Chapter 13).

The most common etiologic factor for nonskeletal anterior crossbites is lack of space for the permanent incisors, and it is important to focus the treatment plan on management of the total space situation, not just the crossbite. If the developing crossbite is discovered before eruption is complete and overbite has not been established, the adjacent primary teeth can be extracted to provide the necessary space (Figure 12-17).

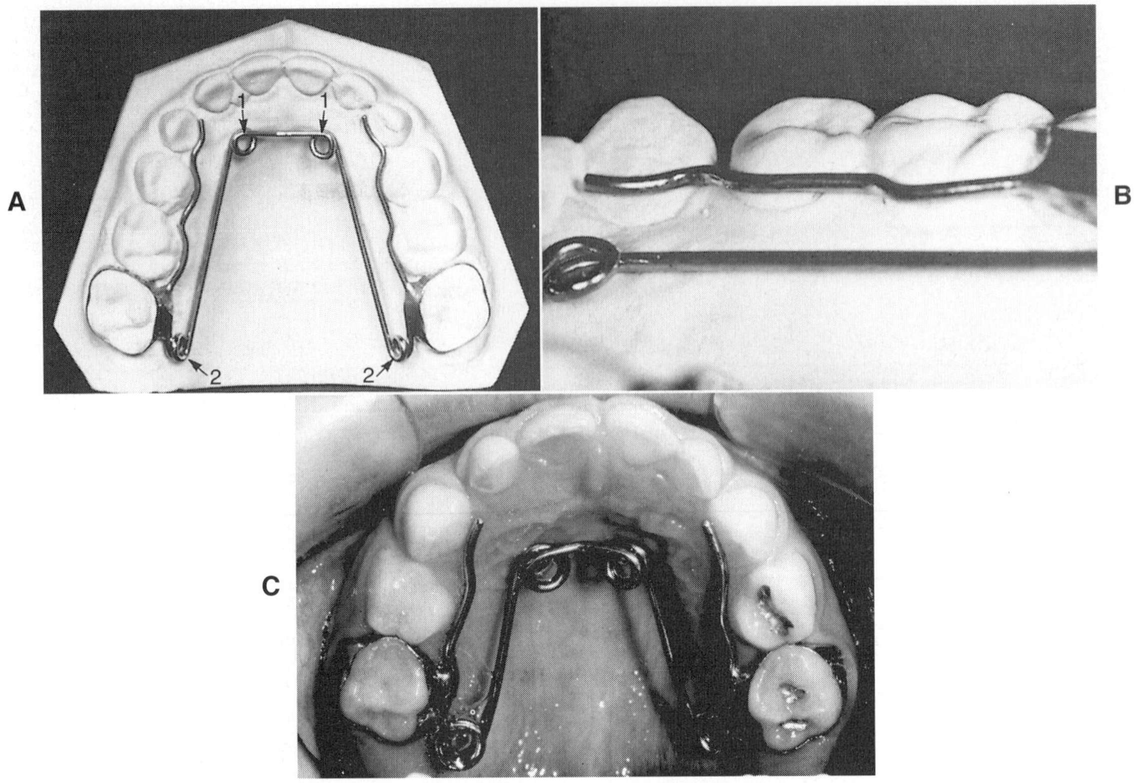

FIGURE 12-11 The quad helix used to correct bilateral maxillary constriction. **A,** The appliance is fabricated from 38 mil wire and soldered to the bands. The lingual wire should contact the teeth involved in the crossbite and extend no more than 1 to 2 mm distal to the banded molars to eliminate soft tissue irritation. Activation at point 1 produces posterior expansion, while activation at point 2 produces anterior expansion. **B,** The lingual wire should remain 1 to 1.5 mm away from the marginal gingiva and palatal tissue. **C,** This quad helix is being used to correct a bilateral maxillary constriction in the primary dentition.

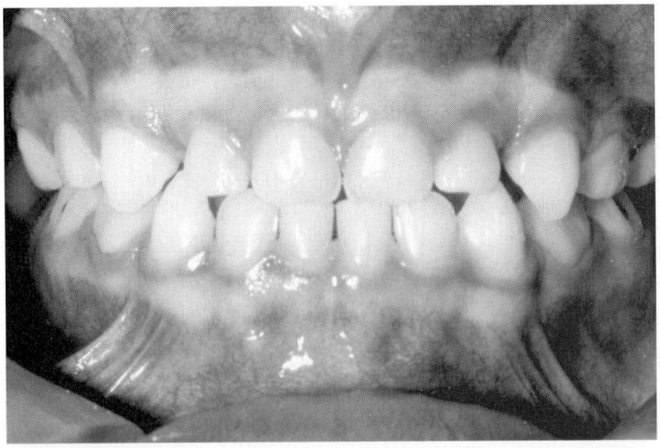

FIGURE 12-12 A posterior crossbite should be overcorrected until the maxillary posterior lingual cusps occlude with the lingual inclines of the mandibular buccal cusps, as shown here, and then retained for approximately 3 months. After retention, slight lingual movement of the maxillary teeth results in a stable result.

Only occasionally is it indicated to correct anterior crossbite in the primary dentition by moving the primary teeth, because crowding severe enough to cause it is rare. Skeletal problems require a different treatment approach (see Chapter 13). Dental anterior crossbites typically develop as the permanent incisors erupt. Those diagnosed after overbite is established require appliance therapy for correction. The first concern is adequate space for tooth movement, which usually requires bilateral disking, extraction of the adjacent primary teeth, or opening space for tooth movement. The diagnostic evaluation should determine whether tipping will provide appropriate correction. Often it will, because the problem arose as eruption paths were deflected. If teeth are tipped when bodily movement is required, stability of the result is questionable. In a young child, the best method for tipping maxillary and mandibular anterior teeth out of crossbite is a removable appliance using fingersprings for facial movement of maxillary incisors (Figure 12-18) or (less frequently) an active labial bow for lingual movement of mandibular incisors. Two maxillary anterior teeth can be moved facially with one 22 mil double helical cantilever

A

B

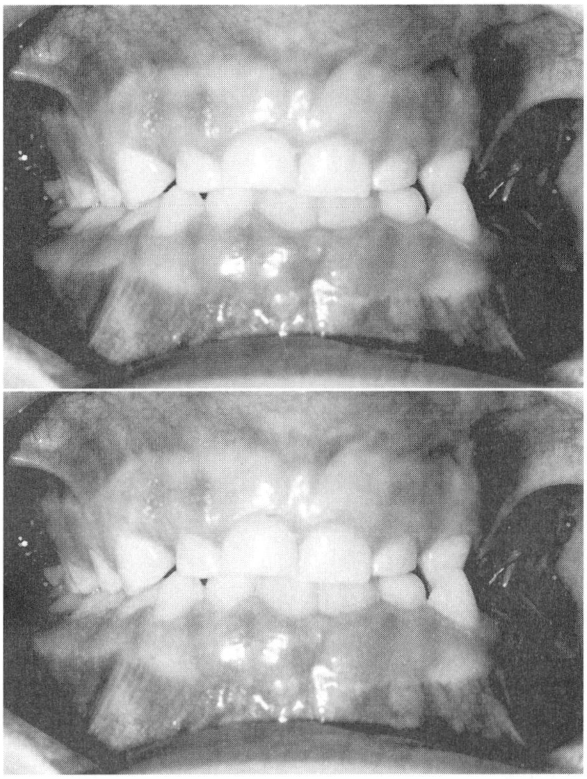

FIGURE 12-13 True unilateral maxillary posterior constriction. **A,** Initial contact. **B,** Full occlusion (no shift). True unilateral constriction has a unilateral posterior crossbite in centric relation and in centric occlusion, without a lateral shift. This problem is best treated with unilateral posterior expansion.

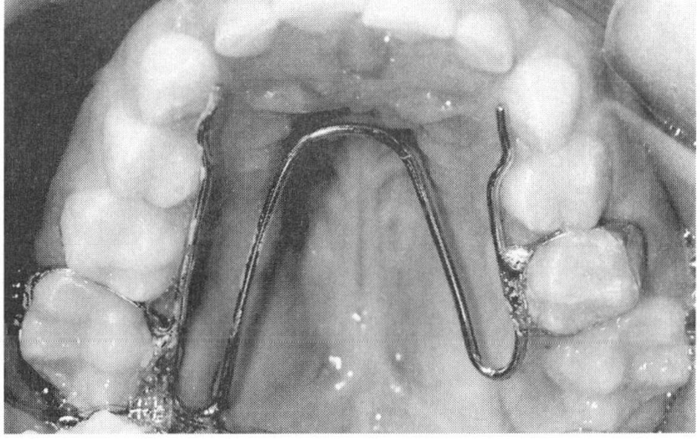

FIGURE 12-14 An unequal W-arch used to correct a true unilateral maxillary constriction. The side of the arch to be expanded has fewer teeth against the lingual wire than the anchorage unit. Even with this arrangement, both sides can be expected to show some expansion movement.

spring. The appliance should have multiple clasps for retention, but a labial bow is usually contraindicated because it can interfere with facial movement of the incisors and would add little or no retention.

An anterior or posterior biteplate to reduce the overbite while the crossbite is being corrected usually is unnecessary

A

B

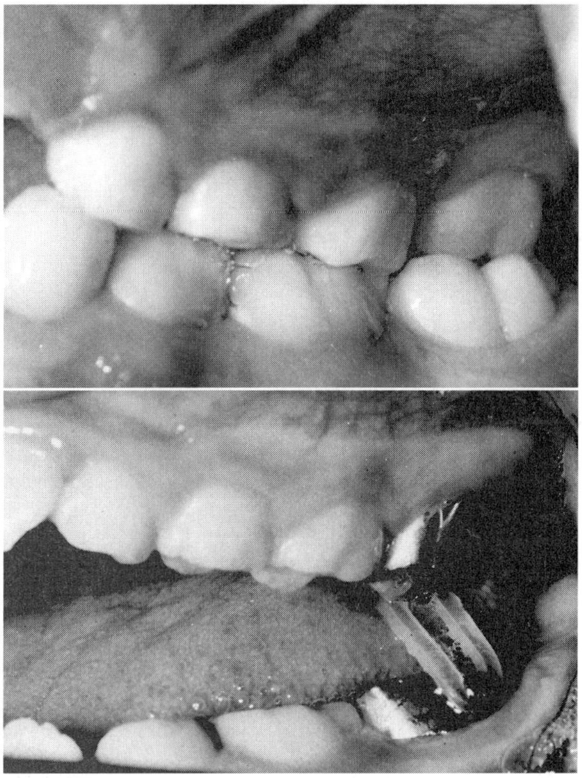

FIGURE 12-15 **A,** This patient has the permanent maxillary left first molar displaced lingually and the permanent mandibular left first molar displaced facially, which resulted in a posterior crossbite between these teeth. **B,** A short and relatively heavy cross-elastic is placed between the buttons welded on the bands. The elastic can be challenging for some children to place, but should be worn full-time and changed frequently.

in children. Unless the overbite is exceptionally deep, a biteplate would be needed only in a child with a clenching or grinding habit. A reasonable approach is to place the removable appliance without a biteplate and attempt tooth movement. If, after 2 months, the teeth in the opposing arch are moving in the same direction as the teeth to which the force is being applied, a biteplate is indicated and can be added to the appliance. Using a biteplate risks the chance that teeth not in contact with the appliance or the opposing arch will erupt excessively.

A removable appliance of this type requires nearly full-time wear to be effective and efficient. If the lingual finger-springs are activated 1.5 to 2 mm, they will produce approximately 1 mm of tooth movement in a month. The offending teeth should be slightly overcorrected and retained until overbite is adequate to retain the corrected tooth positions. One or two months of retention with a passive appliance is usually sufficient. The most common problems associated with these simple removable appliances are lack of patient cooperation, poor design leading to lack of retention, and improper activation.

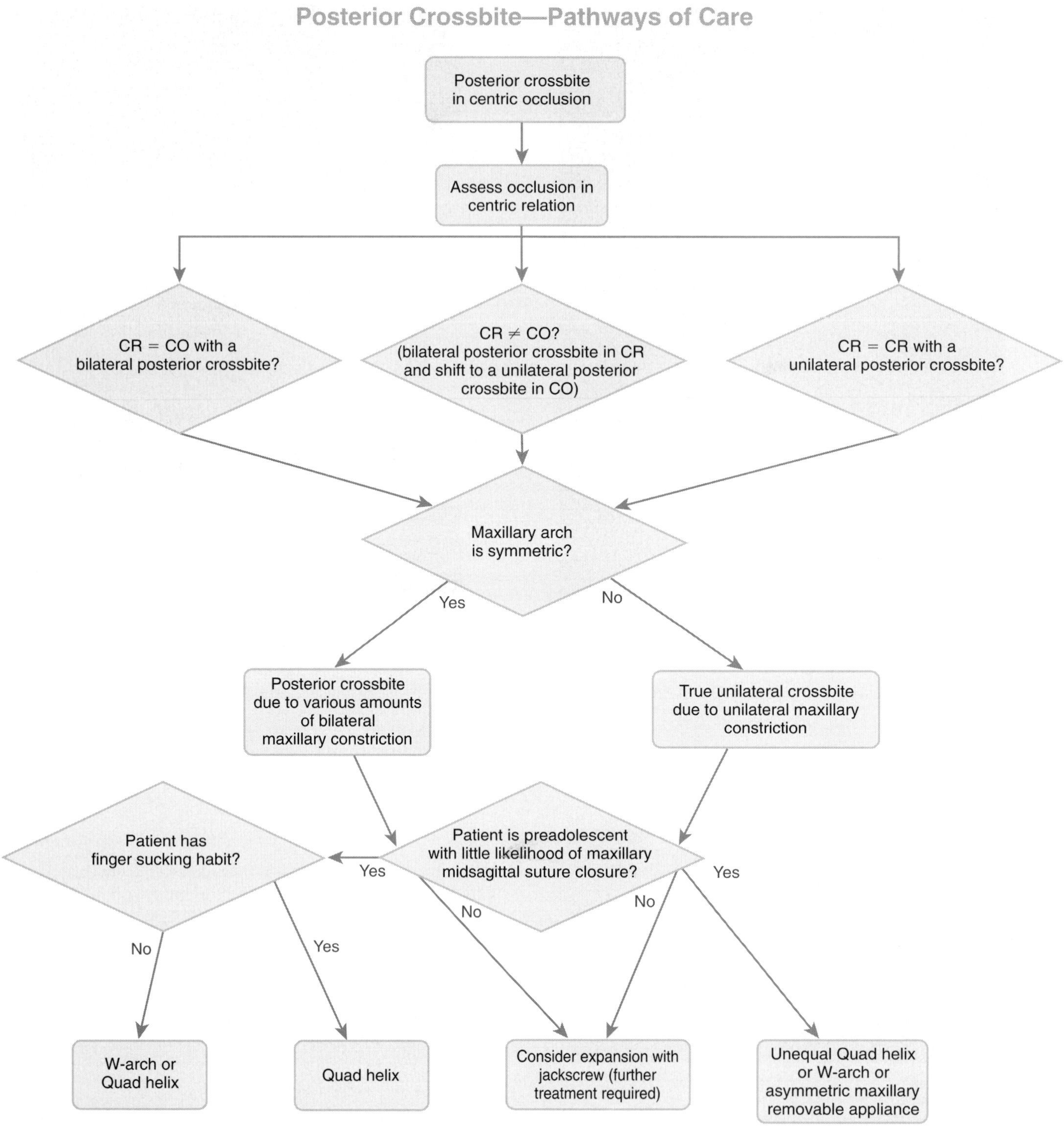

Figure 12-16 This flowchart can be used to aid decision making regarding possible options for posterior crossbite correction in the primary and mixed dentitions. Answers to the questions posed in the chart should lead to successful treatment pathways. The approaches to skeletal correction of posterior crossbites are described in Chapter 13.

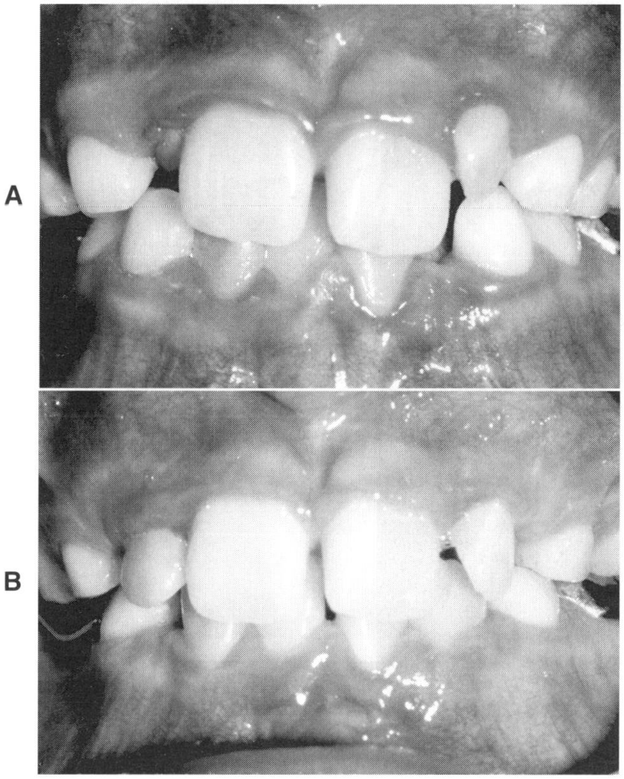

Figure 12-17 Anterior crossbite that is developing as erupting permanent incisors are deflected lingually can be treated by extracting adjacent primary teeth if space is not available for the erupting permanent teeth. **A,** The permanent maxillary right lateral incisor is beginning to erupt lingual to the other anterior teeth. **B,** Extraction of both primary maxillary canines has allowed spontaneous correction of the crossbite although all the irregularity has not been resolved.

One of the simplest fixed appliances for correction of crowded maxillary incisors with a moderate anterior crossbite is a maxillary lingual arch with fingersprings (sometimes referred to as whip springs). This appliance (Figure 12-19) is indicated for a child with whom compliance problems are anticipated. The springs usually are soldered on the opposite side of the arch from the tooth to be corrected, in order to increase their length. They are most effective if they are approximately 15 mm long. When these springs are activated properly at each monthly visit (advancing the spring about 3 mm), they produce tooth movement at the optimum rate of 1 mm per month. The greatest problems are distortion and breakage from poor patient cooperation and poor oral hygiene, which can lead to decalcification and decay.

It also is possible to tip the maxillary incisors forward with a 2 × 4 appliance (2 molar bands, 4 bonded incisor brackets). This may be the best choice for a somewhat older mixed dentition patient with crowding, rotations, and more permanent teeth in crossbite (Figure 12-20). An especially efficient method, which takes advantage of the forces and moments produced on the anterior teeth by a rectangular archwire, is to use a 17 × 25 beta-titanium maxillary archwire with increased lingual root torque bent into the wire, and active coil springs from the molars to the lateral incisors. The archwire is not tied back. Both the torque and the coil springs tip the incisors facially. Multiple incisors can be readily corrected with this method in a short time (Figure 12-21), but of course the correction is not likely to be maintained if the crossbite is skeletal rather than dental. When the anterior teeth are bonded and moved prior to permanent canine eruption, it is best to place the lateral incisor brackets with some increased mesial root tip so that the roots of the lateral incisors are not repositioned into the canine path of eruption, with resultant resorption of the lateral incisor roots. If the torque or bodily repositioning is needed for these teeth, finishing with a rectangular wire is required even in early mixed dentition treatment. Otherwise, the teeth will tip back into crossbite again.

A flowchart is provided to help guide decision making for anterior crossbites (Figure 12-22).

Oral Habits and Open Bites

Open bite in a preadolescent child has several possible causes: the normal transition as primary teeth are replaced by the permanent teeth; a habit like finger sucking; tooth displacement by resting soft tissue; or a skeletal problem (excessive vertical growth and rotation of the jaws). Most of the transitional and habit problems resolve with either time or cessation of the sucking habit. Open bites that persist until adolescence or those that involve more than just the incisors almost always have a significant skeletal component, and careful diagnosis of the contributing factors is required.[7] The treatment of more complex and persistent open bites is discussed in Chapter 13.

Effects of Sucking Habits

During the primary dentition and early mixed dentition years, many children engage in digit and pacifier sucking.[8] Although it is possible to deform the alveolus and dentition during the primary dentition years with a prolonged and intense habit, much of the effect is on eruption of the permanent anterior teeth. Girls are more likely than boys to continue sucking habits after beginning school. The effect of such a habit on the hard and soft tissues depends on its frequency (hours per day) and duration (months/years) (see Chapter 5). With frequent and prolonged sucking, maxillary incisors are tipped facially, mandibular incisors are tipped lingually, and eruption of some incisors is impeded. As one would expect, overjet increases and overbite decreases. In some instances, maxillary intercanine and intermolar width may be narrowed, resulting in a posterior crossbite.

When the effect of digit sucking is compared to pacifier use, there is some evidence for increased prevalence of posterior crossbites with pacifiers.[9] Pacifier shapes that are designed to produce a more physiologic sucking pattern have not been proven to be beneficial when compared with other pacifiers or to finger sucking.[10]

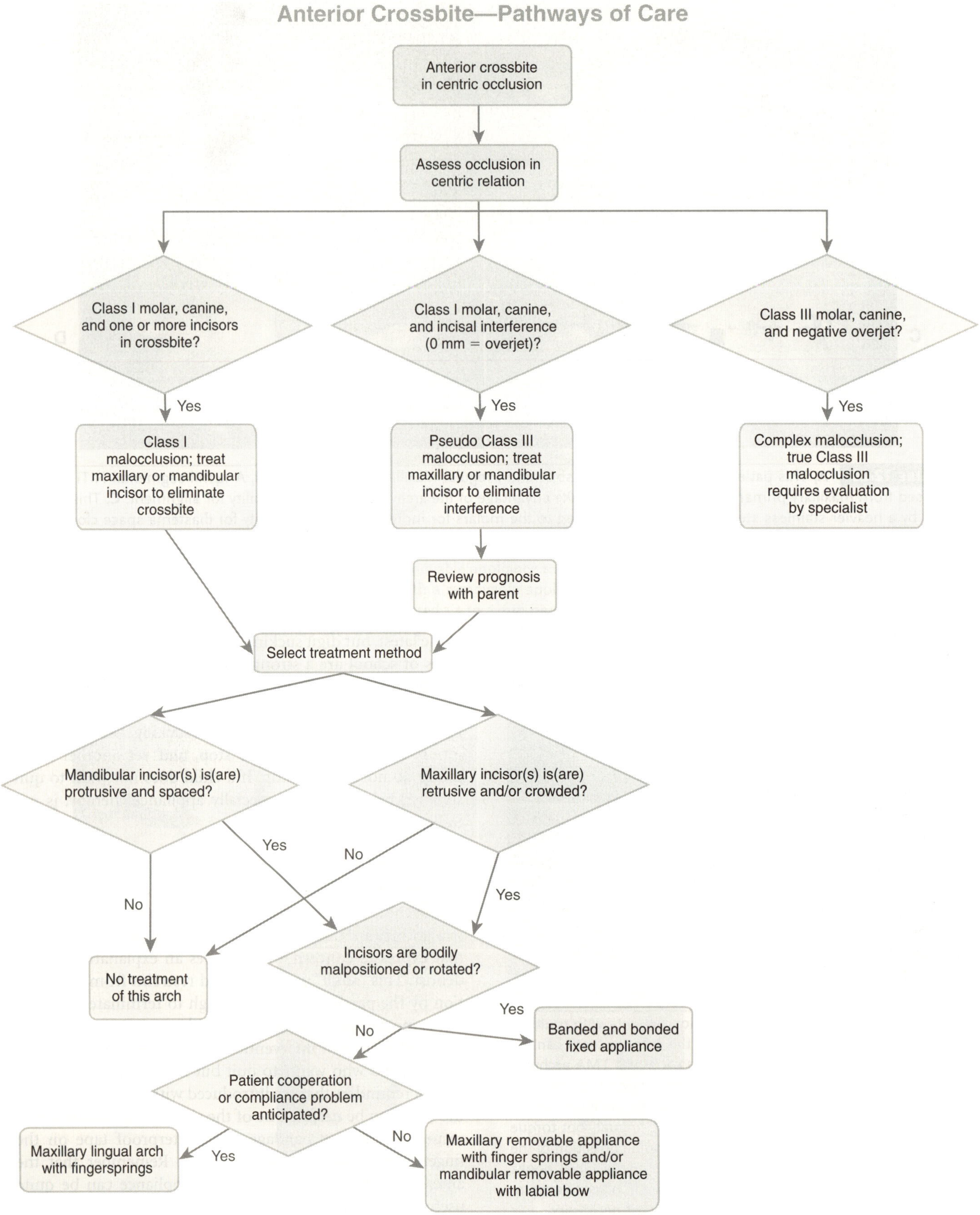

Figure 12-22 This flowchart can be used to aid decision making regarding possible options for anterior crossbites in the primary and mixed dentitions. Answers to the questions posed in the chart should lead to successful treatment pathways.

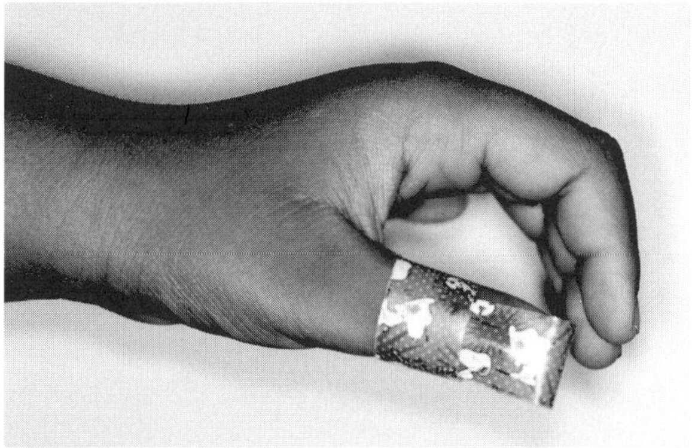

Figure 12-23 An adhesive bandage can be applied over the end of the finger to remind the child not to suck and to reduce the enjoyment. The bandage should be anchored at its base for retention with waterproof tape, so that it will stay in place if sucking is still attempted. (Courtesy Dr. B. Joo.)

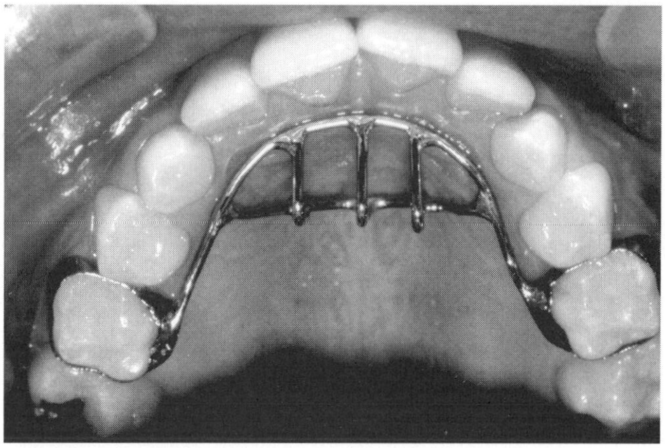

Figure 12-24 A cemented habit crib made of 38 to 40 mil wire can be used as a reminder to interrupt a finger-sucking habit. The appliance can be cemented to either primary or permanent molars and should be extended anteriorly to interfere with the finger position during sucking. The amount of overbite will also help determine the appliance position.

not engaging in the habit. In some cases, a large reward must be negotiated for complete cessation of the habit.

If all the above fail and the child really wants to quit, an elastic bandage loosely wrapped around the elbow prevents the arm from flexing and the fingers from being sucked. If this is necessary, it is usually only at nights and 6 to 8 weeks of intervention should be sufficient. The child should understand that this is not punishment.

Appliance Therapy

If the previous methods have not succeeded in eliminating the habit, a removable appliance is contraindicated because lack of compliance is part of the problem. The child who wants to stop can be fitted with a cemented reminder appliance that also actively impedes sucking (Figure 12-24). These appliances can be deformed and removed by children who are not compliant and do not truly wish to stop the habit, so cooperation still is important. If this is understood by the child as a "helping hand" rather than punishment, the treatment will be successful and psychological problems will not result.[11] When sucking apparently ceases, the appliance should be retained in place for approximately 6 months to ensure the habit has truly stopped. Commonly these cemented reminders leave an imprint on the tongue that will resolve when the appliance is removed. The appliances also trap food and can lead to mouth odor, so excellent oral hygiene is beneficial.

The open bites associated with sucking in children with normal jaw relationships often resolve after sucking stops and the remaining permanent teeth erupt (Figure 12-25). An appliance to laterally expand a constricted maxillary arch or retract flared and spaced incisors may be needed, but the open bite should require no further treatment in children with good skeletal proportions.

A flowchart is provided to help guide decision making for open bite problems (Figure 12-26).

A

B

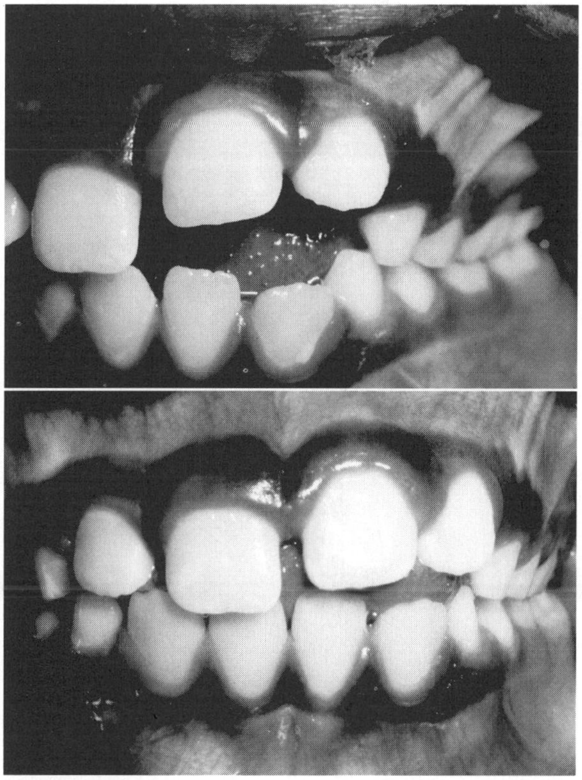

Figure 12-25 Open bites observed during the transitional dentition years or due to previous habits often close spontaneously. **A,** This patient had good skeletal relationships and an open bite during the early mixed dentition years. **B,** Several months later, without appliance therapy, the open bite has spontaneously closed.

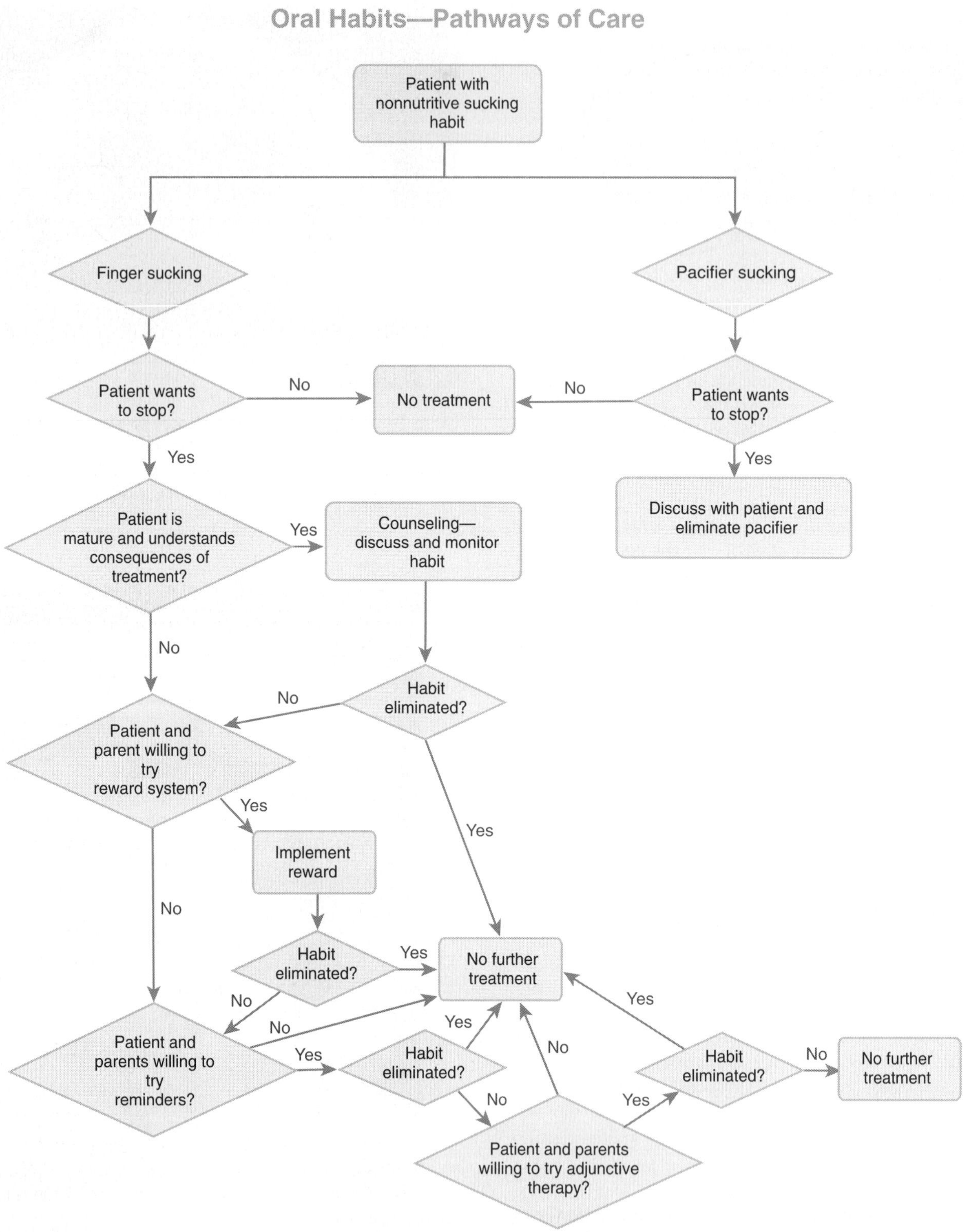

Figure 12-26 This flowchart can be used to aid decision making regarding possible options for nonnutritive sucking habits during the primary and mixed dentitions. Answers to the questions posed in the chart should lead to successful treatment pathways.

Deep Bite

Before treating a deep bite, it is necessary to establish its cause. The problem may result from reduced lower face height and lack of eruption of posterior teeth, or from over-eruption of the anterior teeth. The possible treatments that attack these two causes are quite different and mutually exclusive.

Removable biteplate appliances to reduce the overbite can be used for children who have less than normal eruption of the posterior teeth (which is usually associated with reduced face height). An anterior biteplate is incorporated into a removable appliance so that the mandibular incisors occlude with the plastic plane lingual to the maxillary incisors. This prevents the posterior teeth from occluding and encourages their eruption, which may take several months. The appliance must be worn full-time during this phase of treatment. Posterior eruption is hard to regulate, and once the proper vertical dimension has been established, the biteplate must continue to be worn at night as a retainer, or the anterior teeth will erupt and the deep bite will return.

A more challenging approach to deep bite is necessary when the maxillary or mandibular anterior teeth have erupted excessively. For these patients the task is to stop the eruption (relatively intrude) or actually intrude the incisors. This type of tooth movement requires light continuous forces and careful management of the posterior teeth that provide anchorage. Realistically, although bite depth changes can be made in the mixed dentition by intrusion of anterior teeth, intrusion is difficult to retain—even in later phases of full appliance therapy. For this reason, intrusion as a part of early treatment is seldom indicated. It is often better to defer this treatment until the early permanent dentition, using an intrusion arch during the first stage of comprehensive fixed appliance therapy (see Chapter 14).

A

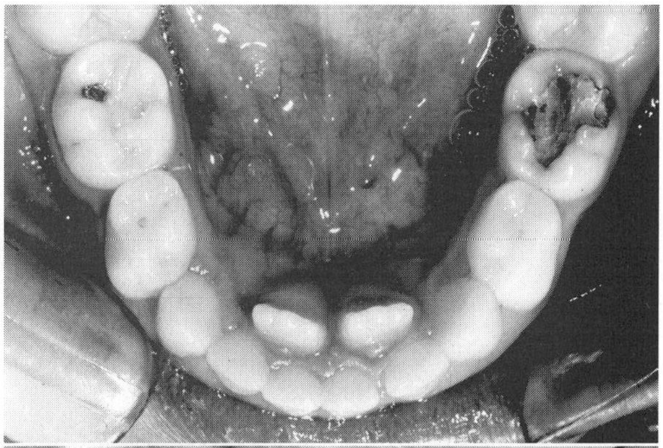

B

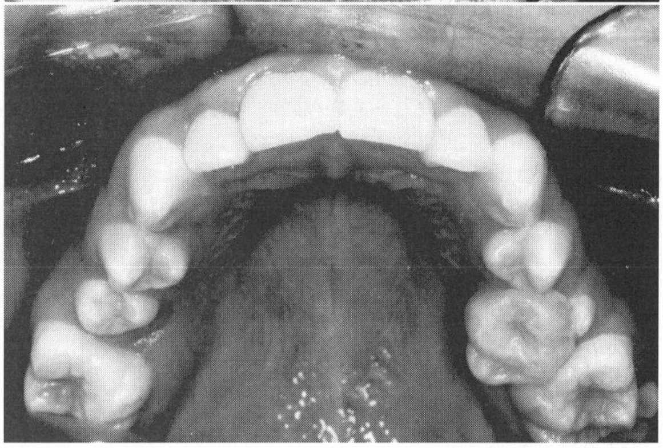

Figure 12-27 Permanent teeth often erupt in abnormal positions as a result of retained primary teeth. **A,** These lower central incisors erupted lingually because the permanent incisors have not been lost and their tooth buds are positioned lingual to the primary incisors. This is a common occurrence in this area and is the main reason lingual arches should not be placed until after lower incisors erupt. **B,** This maxillary premolar has been deflected facially because of the retained primary molar. In both the circumstances shown here, removal of the retained primary tooth or teeth will allow some spontaneous alignment.

Eruption Problems

Over-Retained Primary Teeth

A permanent tooth should replace its primary predecessor when approximately three fourths of the root of the permanent tooth has formed, whether or not resorption of the primary roots is to the point of spontaneous exfoliation. A primary tooth that is retained beyond this point should be removed. An over-retained primary tooth leads to gingival inflammation and hyperplasia that cause pain and bleeding, and sets the stage for deflected eruption paths that can result in irregularity, crowding, and crossbite. If a portion of the permanent tooth crown is visible and the primary tooth is mobile to the extent that the crown will move 1 mm in the facial and lingual direction, it is probably advisable to encourage the child to "wiggle" the tooth out. If that cannot be accomplished, extraction is indicated. Most over-retained primary maxillary molars have either the buccal roots or the large lingual root intact; most over-retained primary mandibular molars have either the mesial or distal root still intact and hindering exfoliation.

Once the primary tooth is out, if space is adequate, moderately abnormal facial or lingual positioning will usually be corrected by the equilibrium forces of the lip, cheeks and tongue. Generally, incisors will erupt lingually and then move facially when the primary tooth exfoliates (Figure 12-27). If spontaneous correction has not occurred when overbite is achieved, however, further alignment is unlikely in either the anterior or posterior quadrants, and active tooth movement will be required.

Supernumerary Teeth

Supernumerary teeth can disrupt both the normal eruption of other teeth and their alignment and spacing.[12] Treatment is aimed at extraction of the supernumeraries before problems arise, or at minimizing the effect if other teeth have already been displaced.

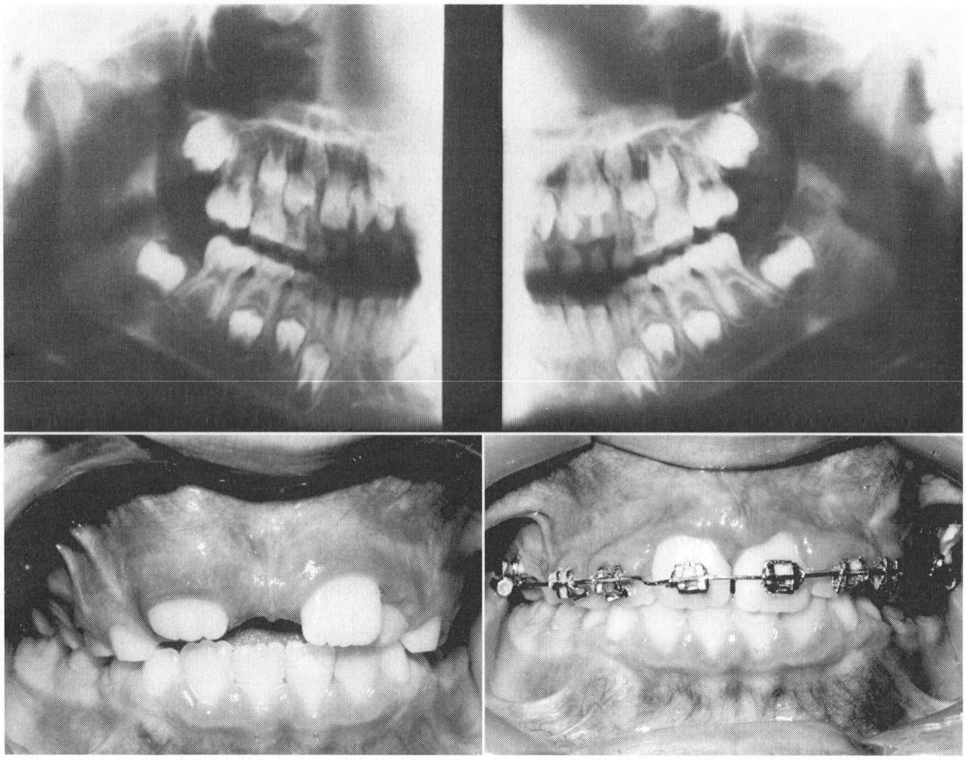

FIGURE 12-28 Multiple supernumerary teeth in the maxilla are often the cause of spacing and delayed eruption of anterior teeth. **A,** This patient has an exceptionally wide diastema and delayed eruption of the maxillary lateral incisors. **B,** The panoramic radiograph reveals three supernumeraries of various shapes and orientations. Conical and noninverted supernumeraries usually erupt, whereas tubercle-shaped and inverted ones do not. **C,** The supernumeraries were removed, the diastema closed, and the incisors were aligned with fixed appliances after they erupted.

The most common location for supernumerary teeth is the anterior maxilla. These teeth are often discovered on a panoramic or occlusal radiograph when a child is about 6 to 7 years of age, either during a routine examination or when permanent incisors fail to erupt. The simple cases are those in which a single supernumerary tooth is present and superficially located. If the tooth is not inverted, it will often erupt before the normal tooth and can be extracted before it interferes with the adjacent teeth.[13] In a few instances, multiple supernumerary teeth will be located superficially, and uncomplicated extractions can be performed without interfering appreciably with the normal teeth.

As a general rule, the more supernumeraries, the more abnormal their shape and the higher their position, the harder it will be to manage the situation. Several abnormal supernumeraries are likely to have disturbed the position and eruption timing of the normal teeth before their discovery, and tubercle teeth are unlikely to erupt (Figure 12-28). Extractions should be completed as soon as the supernumerary teeth can be removed without harming the developing normal teeth. The surgeon may wish to delay extraction until continued growth has improved both access and the child's ability to tolerate surgery, and until further root development has improved the prognosis for the teeth that will remain. This is reasonable, but the earlier the supernumeraries can be removed, the more likely that the normal teeth will erupt without further intervention. Conversely, the later the extractions, the more likely that the remaining normal teeth will need surgical exposure, orthodontic traction or both to bring them into the arch.

Delayed Incisor Eruption

Sometimes incisors fail to erupt even when there is no retained or overlying primary tooth or supernumerary teeth present. Changes in the overlying keratinized tissue occur in long-standing edentulous regions,[14] and this contributes to slow eruption of a permanent incisor when its predecessor was lost prematurely. If the delayed incisor is located superficially, it can be exposed with a simple soft tissue excision and usually will erupt rapidly (Figure 12-29). When the tooth is more deeply positioned, the overlying and adjacent tissue can be repositioned apically and the crown exposed, which usually leads to normal eruption or the tooth can have an attachment placed and repositioned orthodontically (Figure 12-30). If the tooth is even more deeply positioned, an attachment can be bonded and traction immediately applied using a fixed appliance (Figure 12-31).

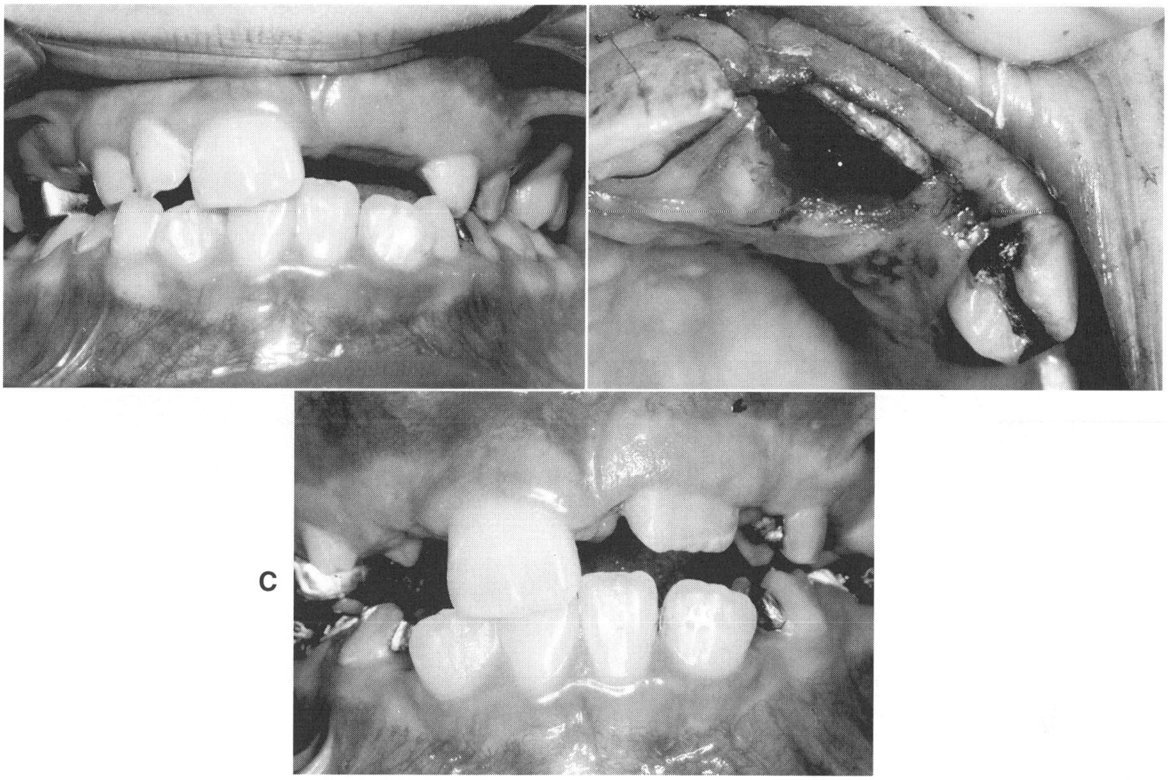

Figure 12-29 Overlying soft tissue may be the cause of delayed eruption after surgical intervention to remove primary or supernumerary teeth. **A,** This unerupted permanent maxillary left central incisor is covered by only soft tissue. **B,** Removal of a limited amount of the tissue while maintaining a band of keratinized tissue on the facial area **(C)** usually results in rapid eruption.

If it is likely that unerupted teeth will have to be moved orthodontically, because of the distance they have been displaced by a supernumerary or for other reasons, an attachment should be bonded to each unerupted tooth as it is exposed. Then a wire ligature or (better) a precious metal chain is attached to the bracket or button and extended out of the tissue so traction can be applied using a fixed appliance. Attachments sometimes are difficult to bond because of contamination of the tooth surface by saliva and hemorrhage, but the alternative approach of looping a wire around the cervical part of the crown is no longer recommended. That requires more extensive bone removal and increases the risk of ankylosis. A small undercut preparation to provide mechanical retention to aid in bonding is better than pin placement in a tooth with a large pulp chamber.

To obtain the necessary anchorage, a fixed appliance to bring an unerupted incisor into the arch should extend from molar to molar, attaching to as many other teeth as feasible, which during the mixed dentition years may mean some primary molars and canines. Before the unerupted tooth is clinically visible, the extruding force can be delivered by an elastomeric module, helical cantilever spring, or NiTi auxiliary (piggyback) wire. Any of these devices can be extended from a relatively stiff archwire to the attachment on the unerupted tooth. Elastomeric materials produce a force that is relatively high initially but decays rapidly, so theoretically they are less desirable than springs that produce light continuous force. Despite this, because the unerupted tooth often is high in the vestibule, the inefficient but non-bulky elastomeric modules are often less irritating than springs and can be an excellent starting point (Figure 12-32).

The best option at present is to use the flexibility of a superelastic auxiliary archwire (A-NiTi) while stabilizing across the edentulous area with another stiffer wire to control the reciprocal forces (see Figure 12-31). This is accomplished by tying the superelastic wire over the base archwire except in the area of the unerupted tooth, and deflecting it gingivally there to provide the traction. This combination of wires offers a simple and efficient method for moving unerupted teeth. Final root positioning can be left until a second stage of treatment during the permanent dentition if one is anticipated.

Ankylosed Primary Teeth

Ankylosed primary teeth with permanent successors, especially ankylosed primary molars, constitute a potential alignment problem for the permanent teeth. Although these teeth usually resorb without creating long-term problems,[15,16] occasionally they fail to resorb or are retained by an attachment in the cervical region. This delays the erupting permanent tooth and can deflect it from the normal eruption path.

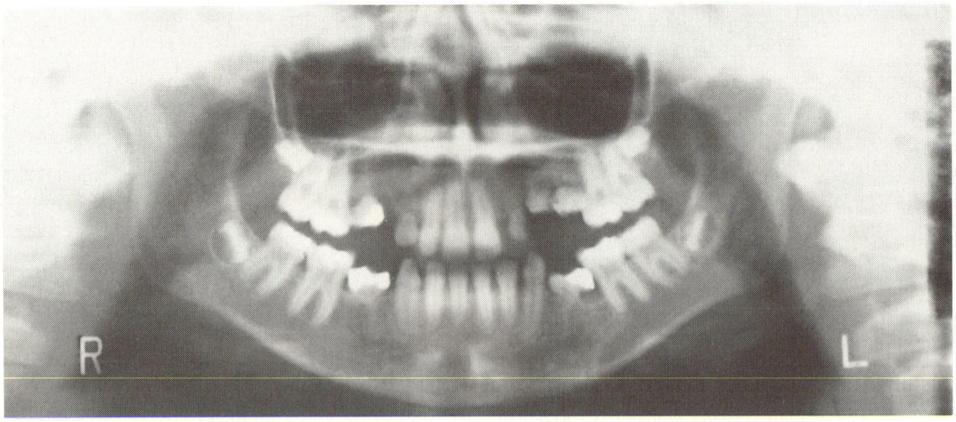

FIGURE 12-34 If they have no successors, ankylosed primary teeth should be carefully removed when vertical discrepancies begin to develop. It is better to allow permanent teeth to drift into the edentulous space and bring bone with them, and then reposition the teeth prior to implant or prosthetic replacement, so that large periodontal defects such as those adjacent to the primary molars in this patient do not develop.

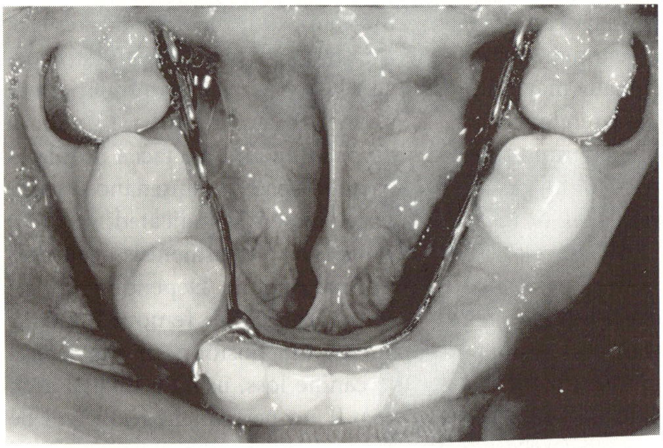

FIGURE 12-35 A spur on a lingual arch can be used in the mixed dentition either to maintain a correct midline when a primary canine is lost, or to retain a corrected midline.

skeletal relationships.[19] When only small amounts of resorption are observed (Figure 12-36), a period of watchful waiting is indicated because self-correction is possible. If the blockage of eruption persists for 6 months or if resorption continues to increase, treatment is indicated. Lack of timely intervention may cause loss of the primary molar and space loss as the permanent molar erupts mesially.

Several methods can be helpful when intervention is necessary.[20] The basic approach is to move the ectopically erupting tooth away from the primary molar it is resorbing. If a limited amount of movement is needed but little or none of the permanent first molar is visible clinically, a 20 mil brass wire looped and tightened around the contact between the primary second molar and the permanent molar is suggested (Figure 12-37). It may be necessary to anesthetize the soft tissue to place the brass wire, and depending on the tooth position and depth of the contact between the permanent and primary molars, it can be difficult to successfully direct the brass wire subgingivally. The brass wire should be tightened approximately every 2 weeks. Treatment is slow but reliable.

A steel spring clip separator, available commercially, may work if only a small amount of resorption of the primary molar roots exists. These clips are difficult to place if the point of contact between the permanent and primary molars is much below the cementoenamel junction of the primary molar, although some are available that have greater vertical distances for just these situations (Figure 12-38). They can be activated on a biweekly basis. Elastomeric separators wedged mesial to the first molar also can be used to push it distally so it can erupt, but are not recommended. They have the potential to become dislodged in an apical direction and cause periodontal irritation. If this occurs, the separators are hard to locate and retrieve, especially if the material is not radiopaque.

If resorption is more severe and more distal movement is required than can be provided by these simple appliances, the situation becomes more complex. If access can be gained to the occlusal surface of the molar, a simple fixed appliance can be fabricated to move the molar distally. The appliance consists of a band on the primary molar (which can be further stabilized with a lingual arch) with a soldered spring that is bonded to the permanent molar (Figure 12-39). In lieu of using a soldered appliance that must be fabricated in the laboratory, a similar but alternative appliance can be fabricated intraorally (Figure 12-40). Using either appliance, if the movement is not sufficient in two weeks, the loop can be reactivated.

Occasionally it is difficult to bond to the partially erupted tooth because the occlusal surface is contaminated by saliva. This may make it necessary to cut a preparation in its occlusal surface so the end of the spring can lodge in the preparation and grip the tooth. The tooth is restored

A

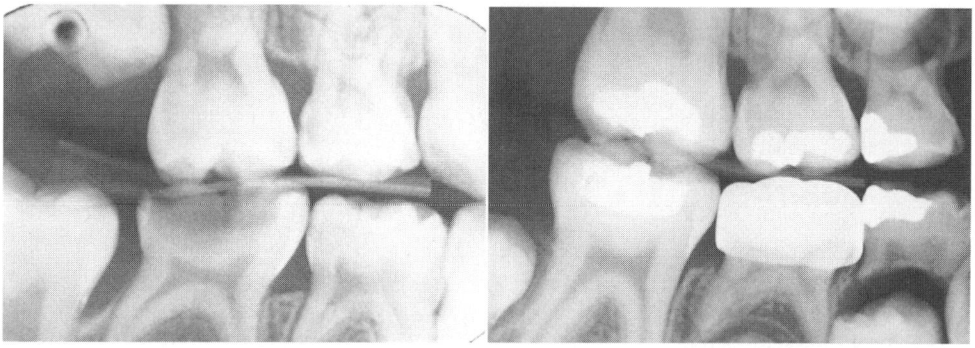

B

Figure 12-36 Ectopic eruption of the permanent first molar is usually diagnosed from routine bitewing radiographs. If the resorption is limited, immediate treatment is not required. **A,** The distal root of the primary maxillary second molar shows minor resorption from ectopic eruption. **B,** This radiograph taken approximately 18 months later illustrates that the permanent molar was able to erupt without treatment.

A

B

C

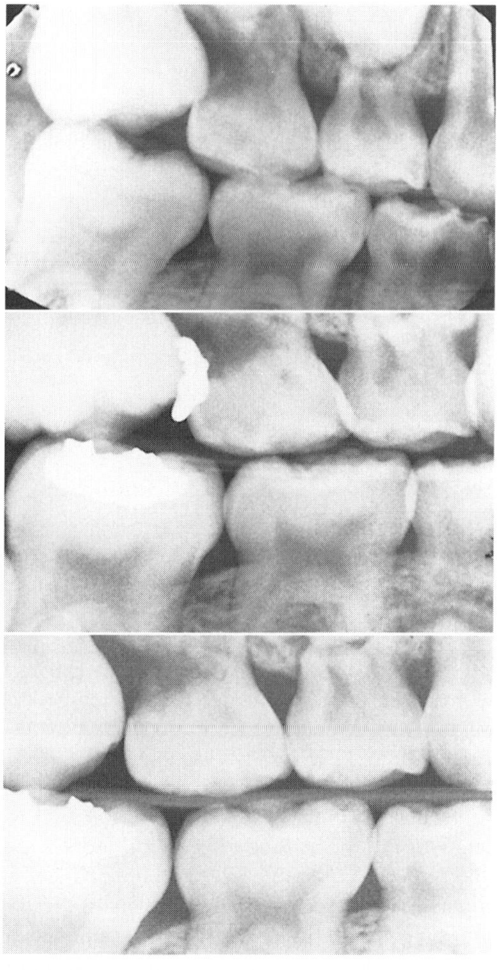

Figure 12-37 Moderately advanced resorption from ectopic eruption of the permanent maxillary first molar requires active intervention. **A,** This distal root of the primary maxillary second molar shows enough resorption that self-correction is highly unlikely. **B,** A 20 mil dead soft brass wire is looped around the contact between the teeth and tightened at approximately 2-week intervals; **C,** the permanent tooth is dislodged distally and erupts past the primary tooth that is retained.

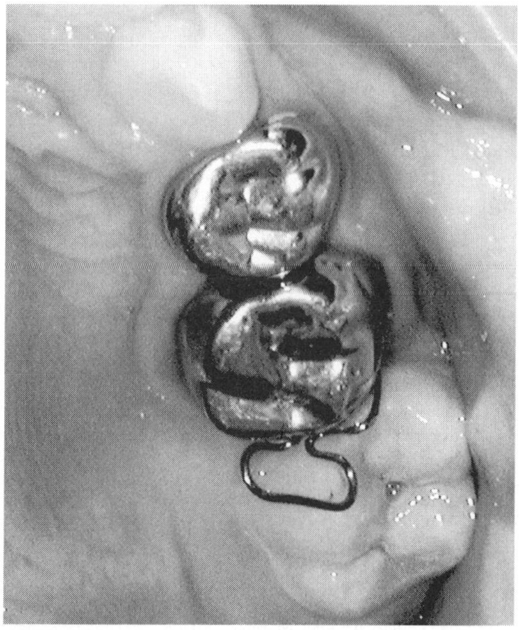

Figure 12-38 An Arkansas spring, a scissors-like spring that extends below the contact point, can be effective in tipping a permanent first molar distally so that it can erupt.

following tooth movement. If the permanent molar has caused extensive resorption of the primary molar, there may be no choice but to extract the primary tooth, which allows the permanent molar to continue to move mesially and shorten the arch length. Unless the second premolar is missing and the arch length is purposefully to be reduced, or unless considerable mesial molar movement is tolerable and later premolar extraction is planned, a distal shoe that guides the erupting molar (see Space Maintainers, pp. 472-476) should be placed after the extraction. Even if this technique is used, some space has already been lost and the permanent molar will have to be repositioned distally, using headgear or

A B C D

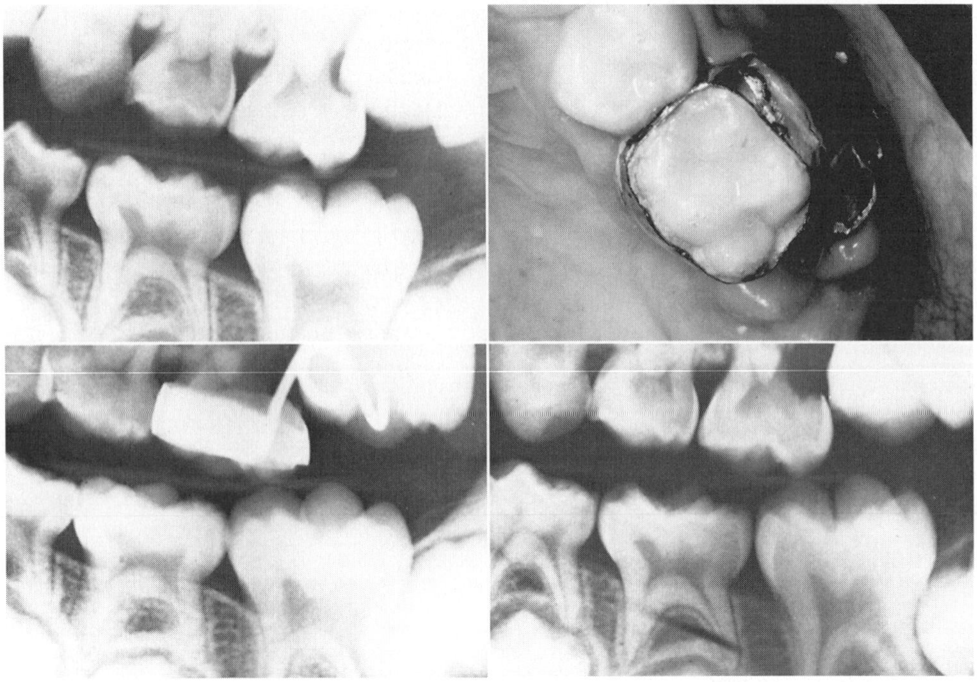

FIGURE 12-39 Ectopic eruption with severe resorption may require appliance therapy. **A,** This primary maxillary second molar shows severe resorption. **B,** If the occlusal surface of the permanent molar is accessible, the primary molar can be banded and a 20 mil spring soldered to the band. **C,** The permanent molar is tipped distally out of the resorption defect and **(D)** once disengaged, is free to erupt.

A B

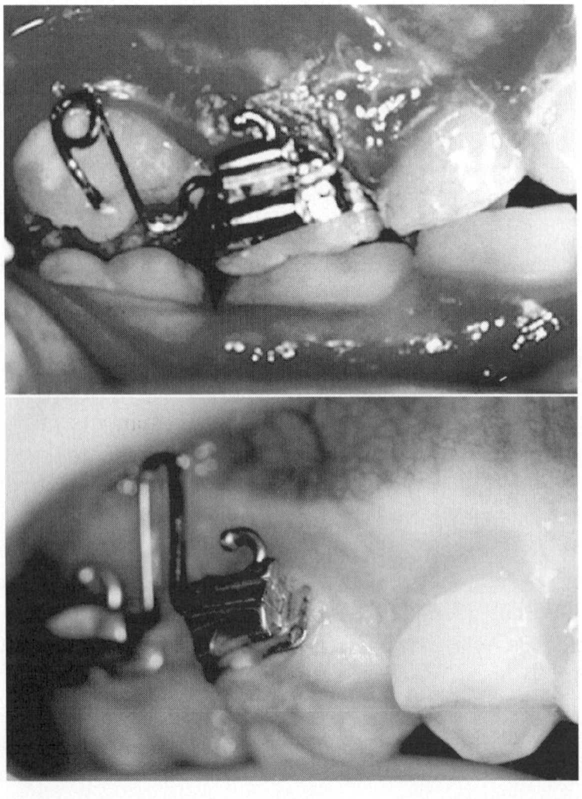

FIGURE 12-40 **A,** A band and spring appliance can be fabricated intraorally with a savings of time and laboratory expense. A band with an attachment having a buccal tube is cemented on the primary second molar. Next a large omega-shaped loop and a helical loop are bent distal to the primary molar. The spring is activated, the wire inserted into the primary molar tube from the distal and secured with a bend anterior to the molar tube. The helical loop is compressed during bonding to the occlusal surface of the permanent first molar. The appliance is reactivated intraorally by opening the omega loop with a loop-forming plier with the round beak positioned superior to the wire. **B,** Another option for repositioning an ectopically-erupting first molar is to bond archwire tubes on both the primary second molar and the permanent first molar. Then, bend an opening loop from either rectangular beta-titanium or stainless steel wire, and compress it to seat from the distal into the primary molar tube and from the mesial into the permanent molar tube. The force from the activated loop will retain the rectangular wire, which can be carefully positioned adjacent to the soft tissue. This avoids banding and laboratory procedures.

another type of space regaining appliance as described later in this chapter.

A flowchart (modified from Kennedy and Turley[20]) summarizes the decision making for ectopic eruption of permanent first molars (Figure 12-41).

Maxillary Canines

Ectopic eruption of maxillary canines occurs relatively frequently and can lead to either or both of two problems: (1) impaction of the canine[21] and/or (2) resorption of permanent lateral incisor roots.[22] There appears to be a genetic basis for this eruption phenomenon, and in some cases it is related to small or missing maxillary lateral incisors and missing second premolars (Figure 12-42).[23]

At age 10, if the primary canine is not mobile and there is no observable or palpable facial canine bulge, a panoramic, occlusal, or periapical radiograph is indicated.[24] When a mesial position of the erupting permanent canine is detected and incisor root resorption is threatened but has not yet occurred, the treatment of choice is to extract the overlying primary canine (Figure 12-43). Ericson and Kurol found that if the permanent canine crown was overlapping less than half of the root of the lateral incisor, there was an excellent chance (91%) of normalization of the path of eruption. When more than half of the lateral incisor root was overlapped, early extraction of the primary tooth resulted in a 64% chance of normal eruption and likely improvement in the position of the canine even if it was not totally corrected (Figure 12-44).[25] If the canine is not redirected by this procedure, it most likely will remain unerupted in a palatal position or erupt lingual to the maxillary incisors, but another consequence can be the beginning of resorption of the permanent incisor roots. If that occurs, usually it is necessary to surgically expose the permanent canine and use orthodontic force to bring it to its correct position (Figure 12-45). This comprehensive treatment will extend into the early permanent dentition period (see Chapter 14).

Transposition

Transposition is a positional interchange of two adjacent teeth. There appears to be a genetic component to this problem as well.[26] In the early mixed dentition years, transposition can develop when distally-directed eruption of the permanent mandibular lateral incisor leads to loss of the primary mandibular canine and primary first molar (Figure 12-46). If left untreated, this will result in a true transposition of the permanent lateral incisor and canine.[27] Treatment requires repositioning the lateral incisor mesially (Figure 12-46, *C*), which eliminates the possibility of the complete transposition with the canine. One possible adverse consequence of this early repositioning is resorption of the lateral incisor root, because it may be brought into contact with the unerupted canine. This is unlikely but should be discussed with the patient and parents prior to treatment. Beginning treatment before the canine is actively erupting is important.

Later in the transitional years, the more prevalent transpositions of the maxillary canine and first premolar and maxillary canine and lateral incisor can occur.[28] Treatment of transpositions involving the maxillary canine is quite challenging. Moving the teeth to their natural positions can be difficult because this requires bodily repositioning, translating the canine facially or lingually past the other tooth. Careful consideration of alveolar width and the integrity of the attached supporting tissue is required. Often the best approach is to move a partially transposed tooth to a total transposed position, or to leave fully transposed teeth in that position.[29] This requires careful finishing, reshaping the transposed teeth to improve both their appearance and fit within the dental arch. Although this can be difficult, the time and difficulty in correcting the transposition is even more challenging.

Primary Failure of Eruption

Diagnosis of primary failure of eruption often occurs in the late mixed dentition period when some or all the permanent first molars still have not erupted (see Chapter 6). Incomplete eruption of other teeth in the same quadrant, even though their eruption path has been cleared, confirms the diagnosis (Figure 12-47).[30] A family history of teeth that did not erupt is further indication that the problem is primary failure of eruption, because there is a genetic component to this problem.[31]

The affected teeth are not ankylosed, but do not erupt and do not respond normally to orthodontic force. If tooth movement is attempted, usually the teeth will ankylose after 1-1.5 mm of movement in any direction, so the correct diagnosis is important in preventing what would be futile orthodontic treatment. In the long term, prosthetic replacement of the teeth that failed to erupt is almost the only treatment possibility.

Roots Shortened by Radiation Therapy

Due to the increased prevalence of successful radiation therapy to treat malignancies of the head and neck in children, some patients with shortened roots due to radiation inevitably will be encountered. Because these patients have high survival rates, they seek orthodontic treatment. Some of the irradiated teeth fail to develop, others fail to erupt, and some may erupt even though they have extremely limited root development. Although the roots are short, light forces can be used to reposition these teeth and achieve better occlusion without fear of tooth loss (Figure 12-48).

TRAUMATIC DISPLACEMENT OF TEETH

Immediately following a traumatic injury, teeth that have not been irreparably damaged usually are repositioned with finger pressure and stabilized (with a light wire or nylon

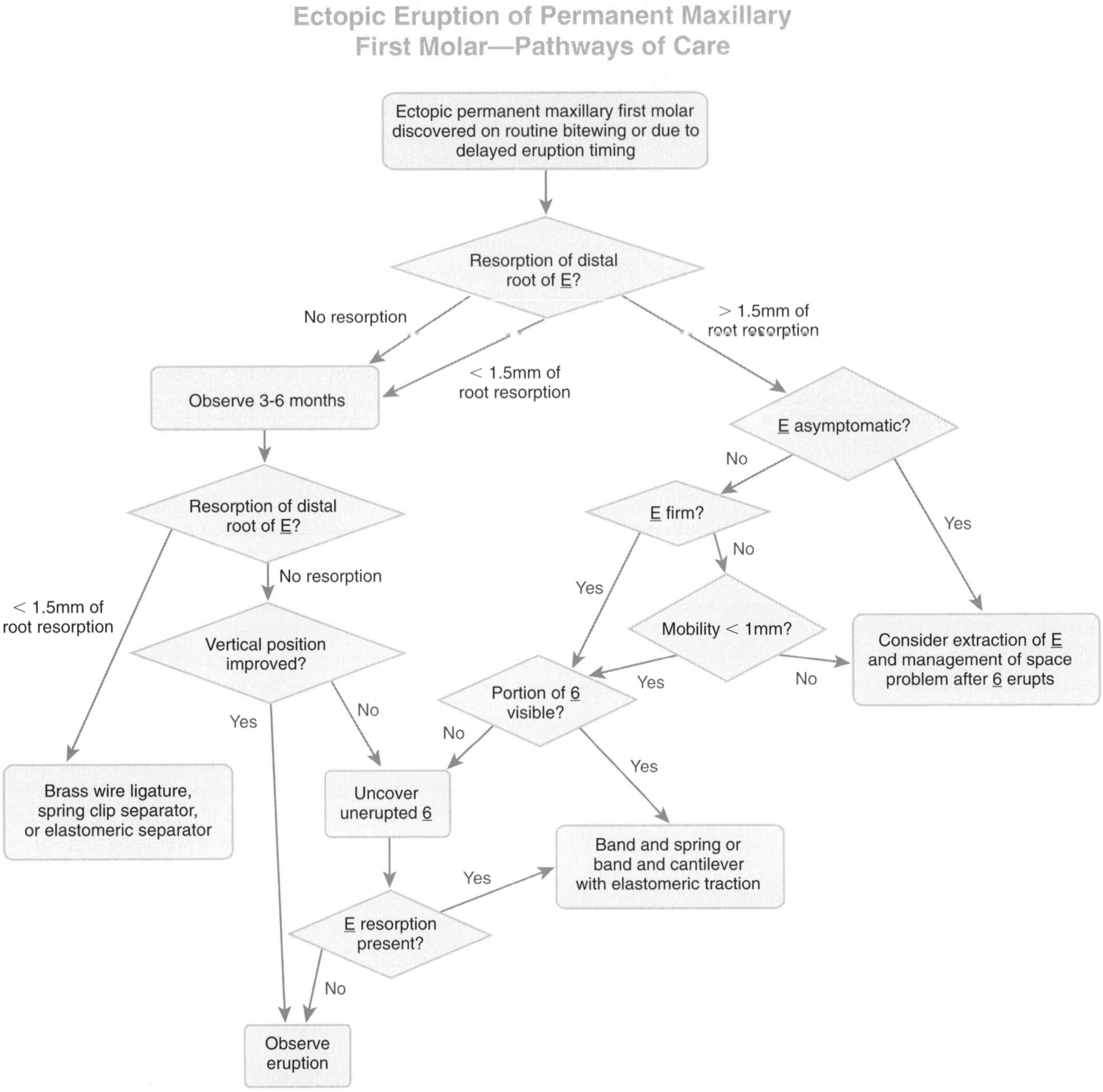

FIGURE 12-41 This flowchart can be used to aid decision making regarding possible options when a permanent molar is ectopically erupting during the mixed dentition. Answers to the questions posed in the chart should lead to successful treatment pathways.

filament) for 7 to 10 days. At this point, the teeth usually exhibit physiologic mobility, and the prognosis is better if they are not splinted any longer. If the teeth are not in ideal positions and orthodontic treatment to reposition them is indicated, it should begin at that time, using light force. Prior to treatment, multiple radiographs at numerous vertical and horizontal angulations should be obtained to rule out vertical, and horizontal root fractures that may make it impossible to save the tooth or teeth.

Vertical displacement of teeth is a major indication for post-trauma orthodontics (Figure 12-49). All severely intruded teeth with mature apices become nonvital and fail to erupt.[32] Early repositioning (using the methods described above in the section on supernumerary teeth) is critical to reduce the chance of ankylosis, improve access for

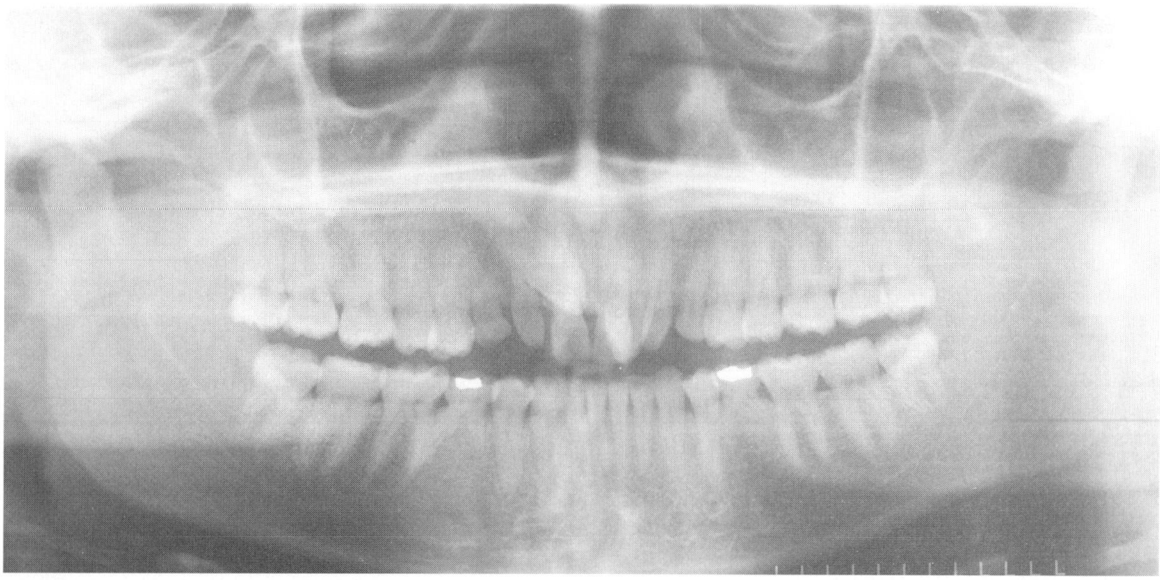

Figure 12-42 This panoramic radiograph shows ectopic eruption of maxillary canines, small maxillary lateral incisors and missing mandibular second premolars. This constellation of findings appears to have a genetic basis.

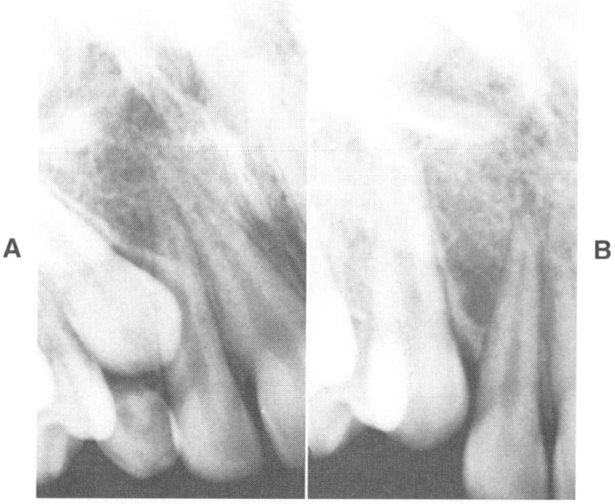

Figure 12-43 This patient demonstrates an ectopic position of the unerupted maxillary right canine relative to the adjacent lateral incisor that is associated with an increased risk of resorption of the incisor. **A,** Note the overlap of the canine and the incisor root. **B,** Following extraction of the primary canine the permanent canine's eruption path changed, and the tooth erupted in a normal position.

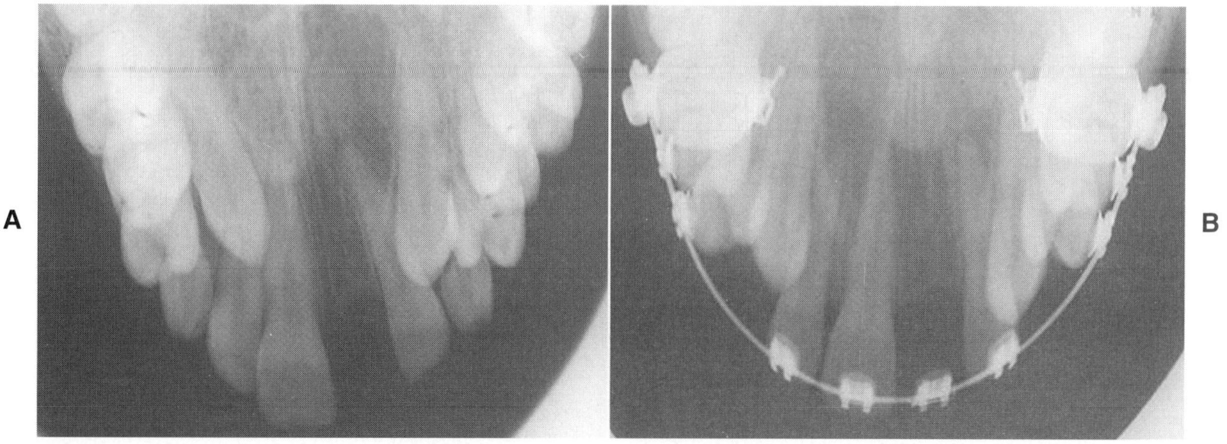

Figure 12-44 **A,** This patient has a maxillary right canine positioned over the root of the maxillary right lateral incisor with more than 50% overlap. Some improvement can be expected with early extraction of the primary canine and **(B)** in this patient the canine migrated into the correct position, which probably would not have occurred without the intervention.

A,B

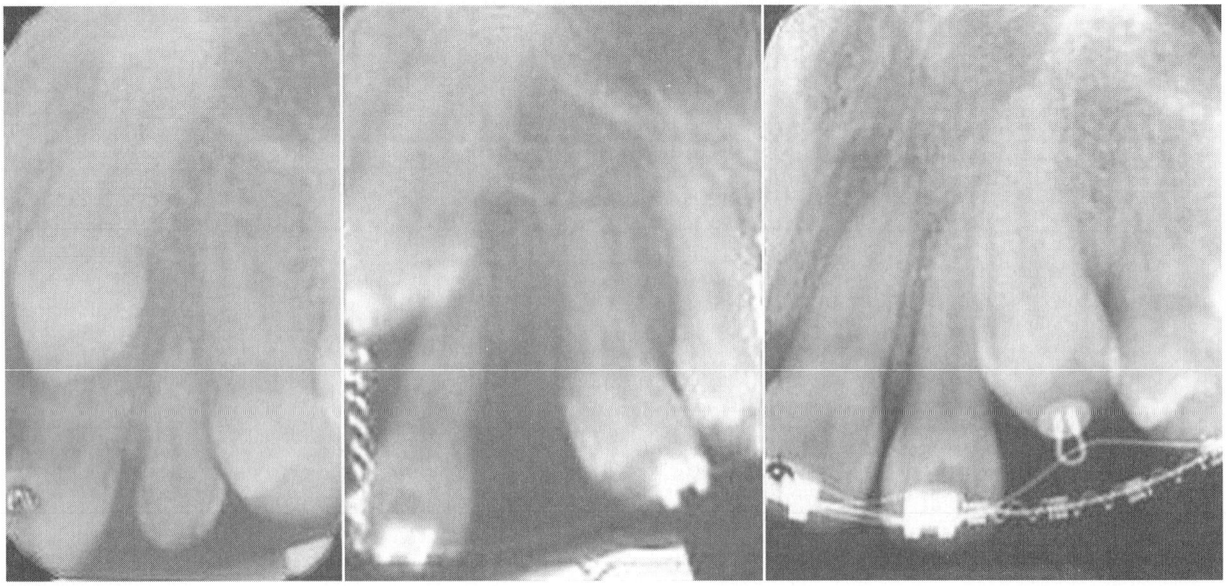

C

FIGURE 12-45 A, The maxillary left canine is positioned over the root of the adjacent lateral incisor and causing some initial root resorption. B, The canine was exposed surgically, and an attachment and precious metal chain were bonded to its crown and ligated to the archwire. C, Subsequently, the canine was repositioned distally away from the lateral incisor and into its correct position. This limited the continued resorption of the lateral incisor.

A

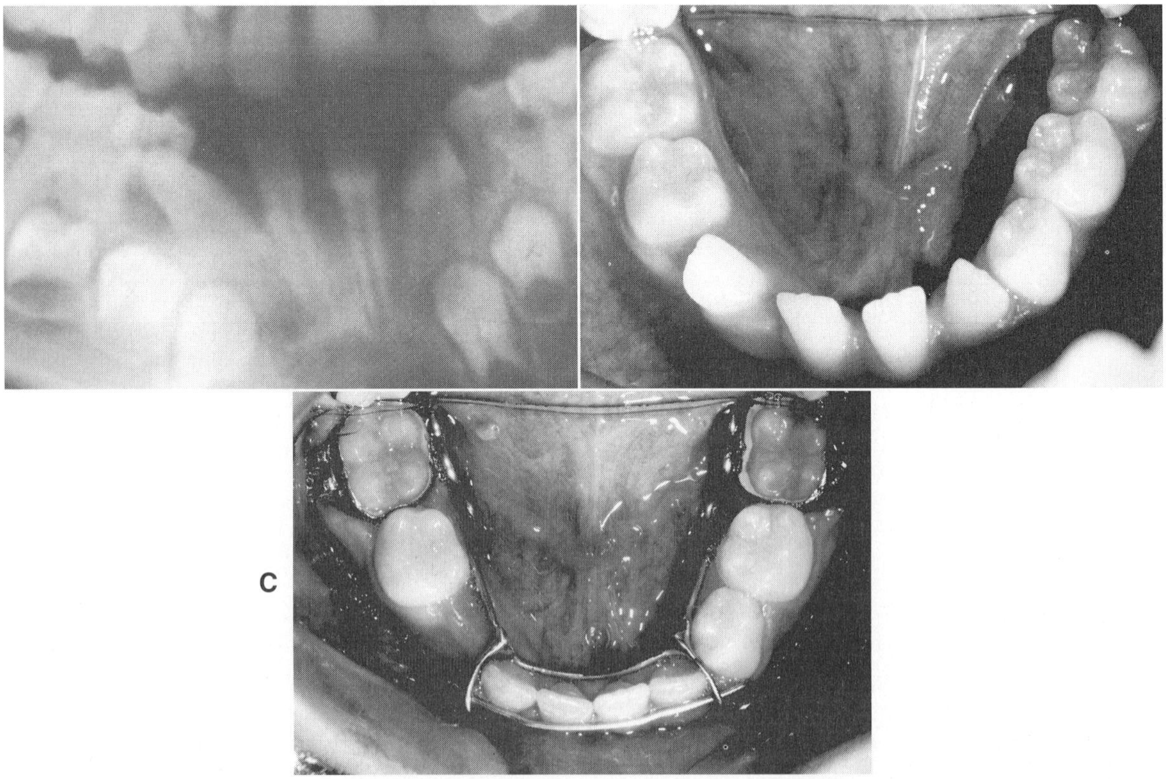

B

C

FIGURE 12-46 A, This radiograph shows that the mandibular lateral incisor is erupting ectopically and has resorbed the roots of the primary canine and first molar. B, Failure to reposition the lateral incisor will lead to true transposition of the permanent lateral and canine. C, The lateral incisors have been repositioned with fixed appliances and are now retained.

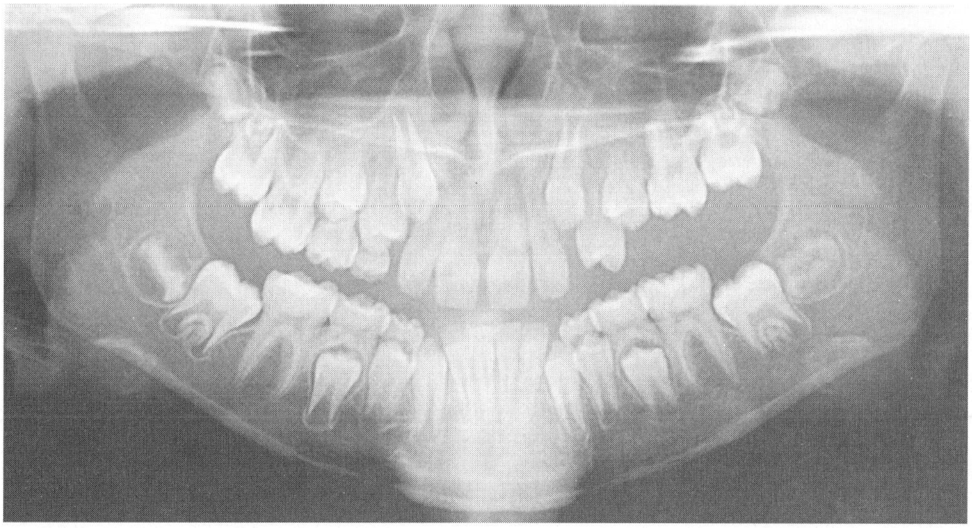

FIGURE 12-47 Primary failure of eruption is characterized by posterior open bite due to failure of some or all posterior permanent teeth to erupt even though their eruption path has been cleared. It can involve any or all posterior quadrants. In this patient, the maxillary left quadrant from second premolar posteriorly is affected. The cause is a failure of the eruption mechanism, apparently due to an abnormal periodontal ligament. Because of the PDL abnormality, the unerupted permanent teeth do not respond to orthodontic force and cannot be moved into the dental arch even though they are not ankylosed.

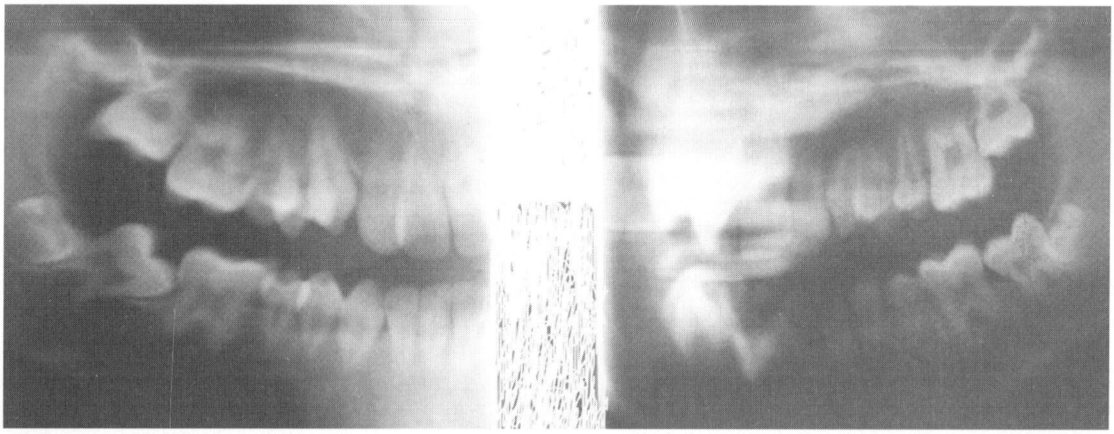

FIGURE 12-48 This patient's panoramic radiograph shows shortening of the roots of multiple permanent teeth following radiation therapy. Using light forces and limiting the extent of movement, the treatment was successful and the compromised teeth were retained. (Courtesy Dr. D. Grosshandler.)

endodontics, and complete the diagnosis; crown and root fractures can remain undiagnosed even following extensive radiographs. Within 2 weeks of the injury, the intruded tooth should have been moved enough to allow endodontic access—ideally, it would be at or near the pre-trauma position. Pulp therapy is best instituted within 2 weeks to reduce the possibility of resorption.[33] If further tooth movement of an endodontically-treated tooth will be needed during a second stage of comprehensive treatment, calcium hydroxide can be retained in the pulp chamber until active tooth movement is completed, as a hedge against root resorption (see Figure 18-39).

The other major problem following trauma is faciolingual displacement of teeth that produces crossbite and occlusal interferences, and orthodontic repositioning should be done immediately after the period of initial healing. The prognosis for pulp vitality is better in teeth that were not intruded when they were displaced, and in teeth with open apices. Nevertheless, any tooth can become nonvital following a traumatic injury. For this reason, follow-up periapical

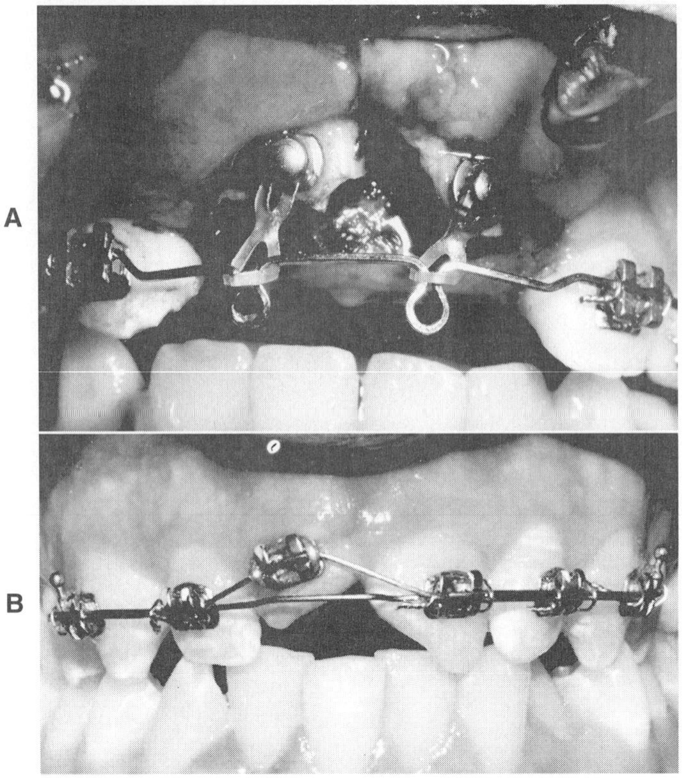

FIGURE 12-49 **A,** Early traction following intrusion of mature permanent teeth is critical to prevent ankylosis, and ensure adequate endodontic access if necessary. To begin, elastomeric chain can be used. **B,** A more efficient method is to use a heavy base archwire complemented by a NiTi overlay wire for rapid tooth movement. Note that the base archwire has been stepped facially to allow the bracketed tooth to pass on its lingual side.

radiographs should be taken at 2 to 3 weeks, 6 to 8 weeks, and 1 year post-injury to check for pathologic changes (Figure 12-50).

Teeth that were extruded at the time of injury and not immediately reduced pose a difficult problem. These teeth have reduced bony support and a poor crown root ratio. Attempts to intrude them result in bony defects between the teeth, so orthodontic intrusion is not a good plan. When the discrepancy is minor to moderate, reshaping the elongated tooth by crown reduction may be the best plan (Figure 12-51).

Another consideration for patients with traumatically injured anterior teeth that offer no restorative option is to retain the root of the compromised tooth until a later time when an implant can be placed into the area.[34] This adjunctive procedure reduces the chance of ridge resorption and the later need for bone grafting. If the tooth is compromised and can still be moved orthodontically, it can be repositioned and the root buried. Root burial entails decorination (removal of the clinical crown and root structure to below the soft tissue level) and closure of the soft tissue. The root can subsequently be removed or the implant placed through it (Figure 12-52).

SPACE-RELATED PROBLEMS

Irregular and malaligned teeth in the early mixed dentition arise from two major causes: (1) lack of adequate space for alignment, which causes an erupting tooth to be deflected from its normal position in the arch; and (2) interferences with eruption, which prevent a permanent tooth from erupting on a normal schedule and secondarily can lead to space problems because other teeth drift to improper positions. A

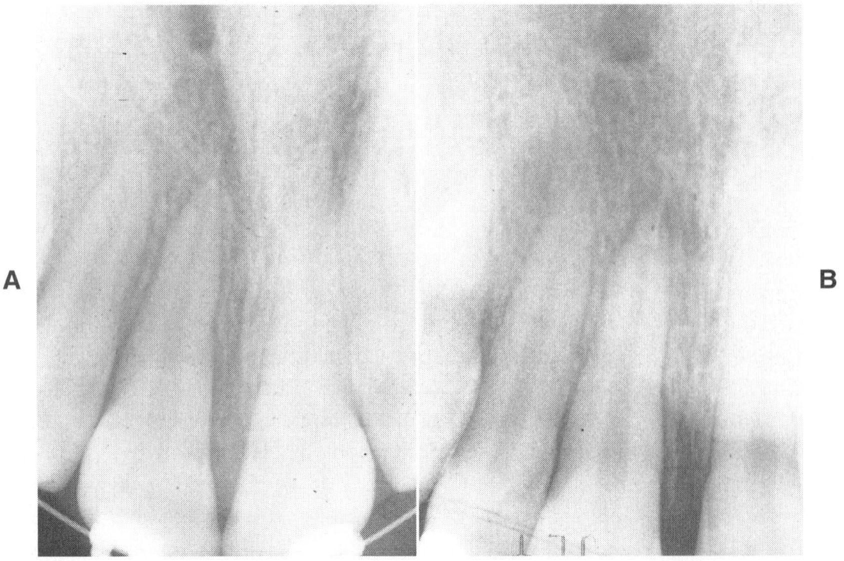

FIGURE 12-50 Multiple vertically-positioned radiographs are required for an adequate diagnosis of previously traumatized teeth. **A,** This radiograph displays no periapical pathology 2 weeks after the trauma to the central incisors, but **(B)** this radiograph exposed at the same time from a different vertical position shows a periapical radiolucency at the apex of the maxillary right central incisor.

A
B
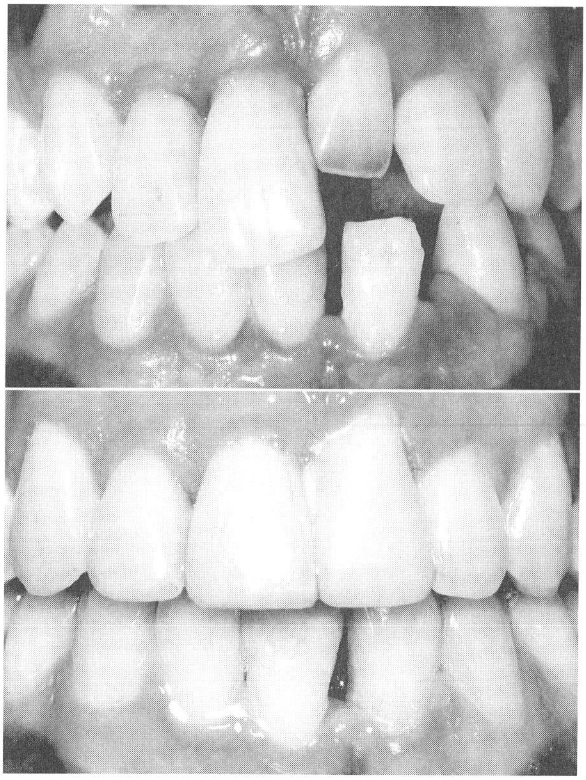

Figure 12-51 **A,** This patient had extrusive displacement injuries to the permanent incisors. **B,** Because it is difficult to intrude these teeth and there is a risk of a subsequent bony defect, the crowns of these teeth were reduced to provide a better crown-root ratio and improve the appearance.

A
B
C
D
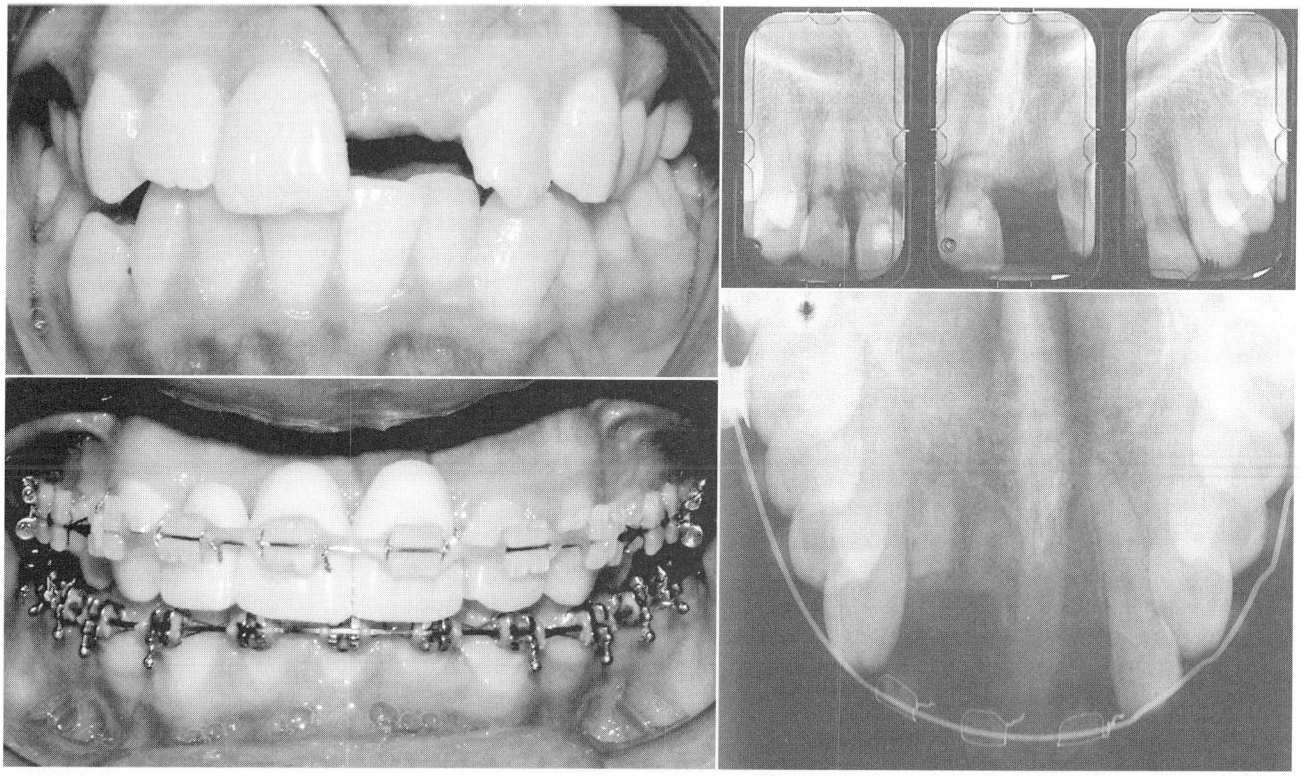

Figure 12-52 This patient had root burial to retain the maxillary anterior alveolar bone. **A,** The maxillary left central incisor was avulsed. **B,** The maxillary radiograph shows severe resorption of the roots of the maxillary right central and lateral incisors. Instead of extracting these two teeth, they were de-corinated (crowns removed and roots covered with soft tissue) to maintain the ridge. **C,** The pontics are in place during orthodontic treatment for space control and esthetics, while **(D)** the roots maintain the ridge as seen on the radiograph.

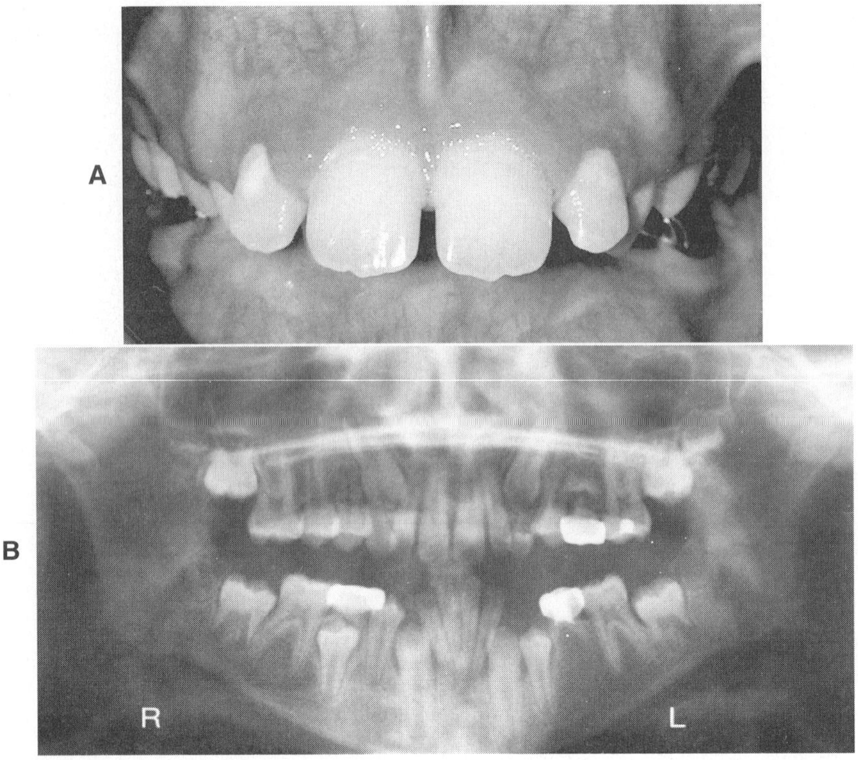

Figure 12-53 The "Ugly Duckling" phase of dental development. **A,** Spacing and mesial root position of the maxillary incisors results from the position of the unerupted permanent canines. **B,** This panoramic radiograph shows that the canines are erupting and in close proximity to the roots of the lateral incisors. The spaces between the incisors, including the midline diastema, decrease and often completely disappear when the canines erupt.

major goal of early treatment is to prevent molars or incisors from drifting after premature loss of primary teeth, reducing the space available for unerupted teeth. Early treatment to align crowded incisors when space ultimately would be adequate, or to create some additional space when a space deficiency exists, may or may not be indicated. The decision as to whether this should be done in the mixed dentition and how it will be accomplished depends more than anything else on the parents' view of the severity of the problem.

Excess Space

Generalized Spacing of Permanent Teeth

Excess space is not a frequent finding in the mixed dentition in the absence of incisor protrusion. It can result from either small teeth in normal-sized arches or normal-sized teeth in large arches. Unless the space presents an esthetic problem, it is reasonable to allow eruption of the remaining permanent teeth before closing the space with fixed appliances (see Chapter 14). There is little or no advantage to early treatment.[35]

Maxillary Midline Diastema

A small maxillary midline diastema, which is present in many children, is not necessarily an indication for orthodontic treatment. The unerupted permanent canines often lie superior and distal to the lateral incisor roots, which forces the lateral and central incisor roots toward the midline while their crowns diverge distally (Figure 12-53). In its extreme form, this condition of flared and spaced incisors is called the "ugly duckling" stage of development (see Chapter 4). These spaces tend to close spontaneously when the canines erupt and the incisor root and crown positions change. Until the canines erupt, it is difficult to be certain whether the diastema will close completely or only partially.

A small but unesthetic diastema (2 mm or less) can be closed in the early mixed dentition by tipping the central incisors together. A maxillary removable appliance with clasps, fingersprings, and possibly an anterior bow will successfully complete this type of treatment (Figure 12-54). Under no circumstances should an unsupported elastic be looped around the central incisors—there is a high probability that the elastic will slip apically and destroy the periodontal attachment. The elastic can become an effective way to extract the teeth.

When a larger diastema (>2 mm) is present, a midline supernumerary tooth or intrabony lesion must always be suspected. A maxillary occlusal or periapical radiograph will reveal whether a pathologic condition exists in the area. Missing permanent lateral incisors also can lead to a large space between the central incisors because the permanent central incisors frequently move distally into the available space. Some digit-sucking habits can lead to diastemas and spacing.

Whatever its cause, a diastema greater than 2 mm is unlikely to close spontaneously. In most instances, closing a large unesthetic diastema requires bodily repositioning of

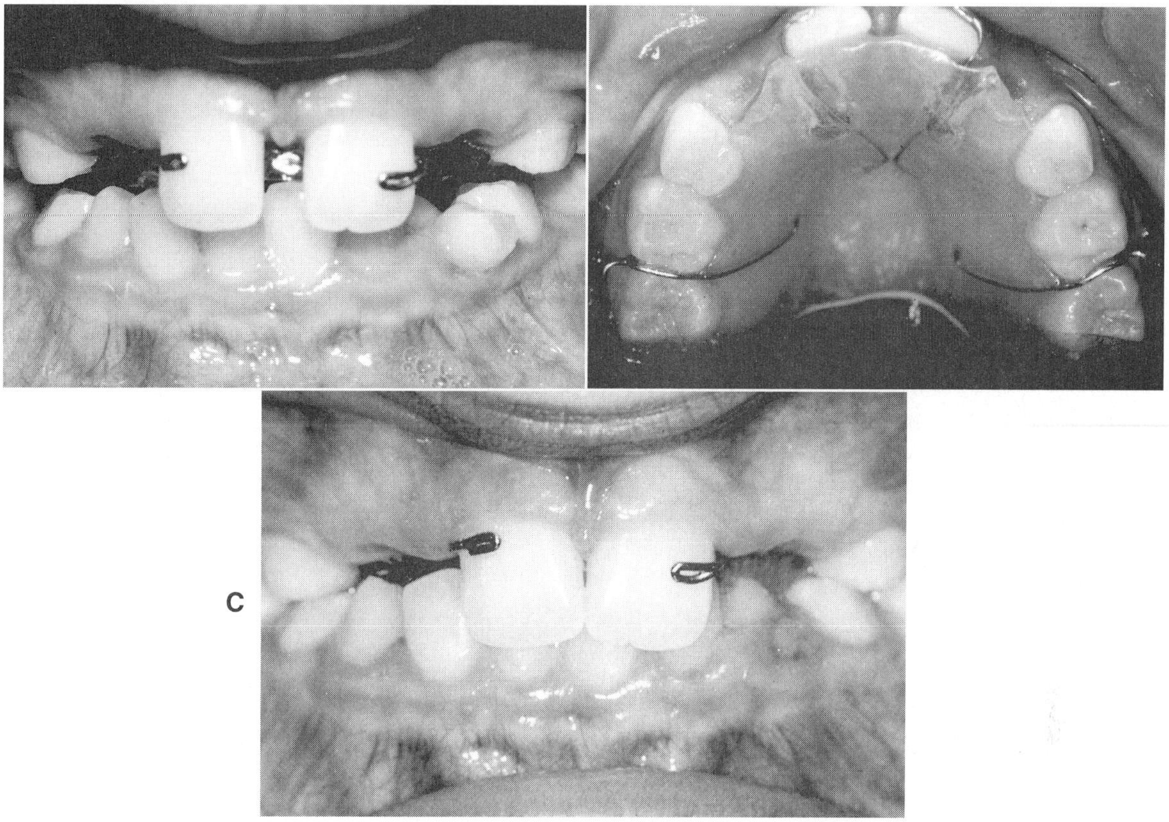

Figure 12-54 **A,** Closure of a midline diastema can be accomplished with a removable appliance and fingersprings to tip the teeth mesially. **B,** The 28 mil helical fingersprings are activated to move the incisors together. **C,** The final position can be maintained with the same appliance.

the central incisors to maintain proper inclinations of the teeth. Mesial root movement also provides more space for the eruption of the lateral incisors and canines. When the situation demands bodily mesiodistal movement, an anterior segmental archwire from central to central incisor or the classic 2 × 4 appliance can be quite satisfactory. Initial alignment of the incisors with a flexible wire is required. Then a stiffer archwire can be employed as the teeth slide together (18 mil round or 16 × 22 mil steel are good choices during the space closure) (Figure 12-55). The force to move the incisors together can be provided by an elastomeric chain tying these teeth together, or by a coil spring compressed over the archwire between the first molar and lateral incisors. The diastema closure is more predictable if only mesiodistal movement is required. If protruding incisors are to be retracted as the space closes, careful attention to the posterior anchorage is required.

The experienced clinician's desire to close diastemas at an early age is tempered by knowledge of how difficult it can be to keep the space closed as the other permanent teeth erupt. If the lateral incisors and canines have not erupted when the diastema is closed, a removable retainer will require constant modification. If the overbite is not prohibitively deep, an alternative approach for retention is to bond a 17.5 mil multistranded archwire to the linguocervical portion of the incisors (Figure 12-56). This provides excellent retention with less maintenance.

The retention problem is due primarily to failure of the gingival elastic fibers to cross the midline when a large diastema is present, but may be aggravated by the presence of a large or inferiorly attached labial frenum. A frenectomy after space closure and retention may be necessary in some cases, but it is difficult to determine the potential contribution of the frenum to retention problems from its pretreatment morphology. Therefore a frenectomy before treatment is contraindicated, and a post-treatment frenectomy should be done only if unresolved bunching of tissue between the teeth shows that it is necessary.[36]

Maxillary Dental Protrusion and Spacing

Treatment for maxillary dental protrusion during the early mixed dentition is indicated only when the maxillary incisors protrude with spaces between them and are esthetically objectionable or in danger of traumatic injury. When this condition occurs in a child who has no skeletal discrepancies, it is often a sequel to prolonged thumbsucking. Eliminating the thumb habit prior to tooth movement is advisable (see the earlier section in this chapter). The more common

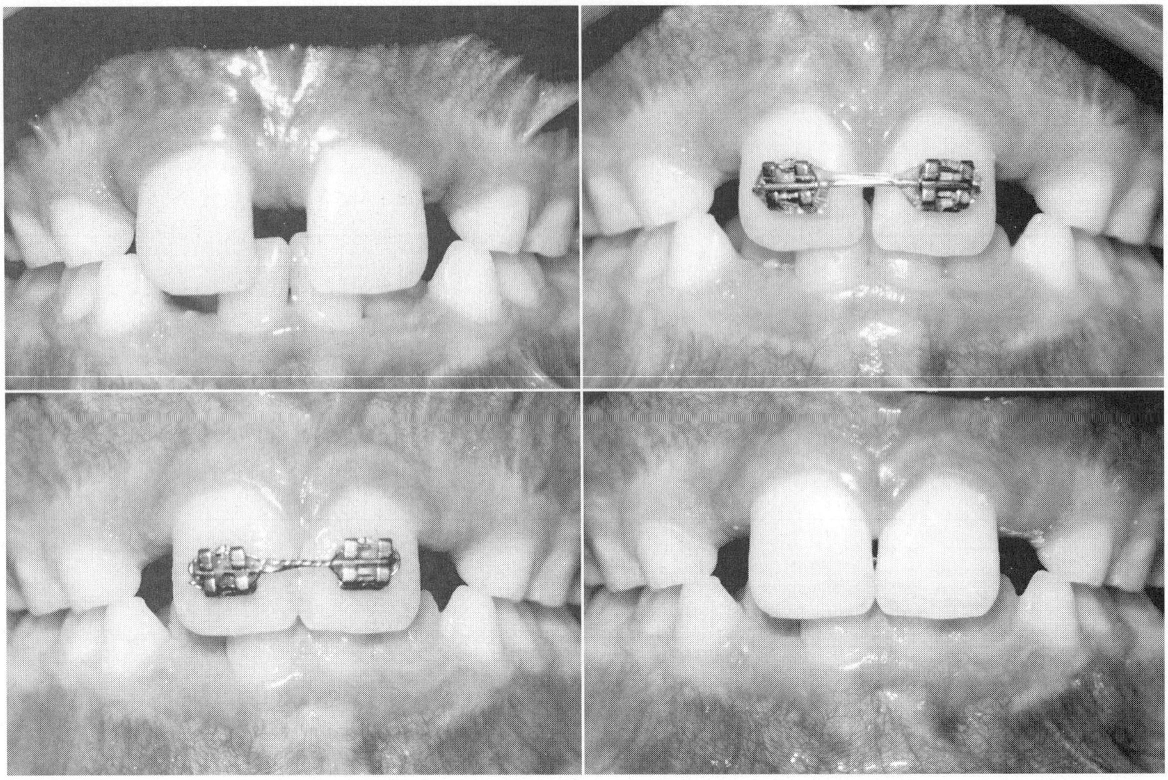

FIGURE 12-55 Closure of a diastema with a fixed appliance. **A,** This diastema requires closure by moving the crowns and roots of the central incisors. **B,** The bonded attachments and rectangular wire control the teeth in three planes of space while the elastomeric chain provides the force to slide the teeth along the wire. **C,** Immediately after space closure, the teeth are retained, preferably with **(D)** a fixed lingual retainer (see Figure 12-56 and 17-12), at least until the permanent canines erupt.

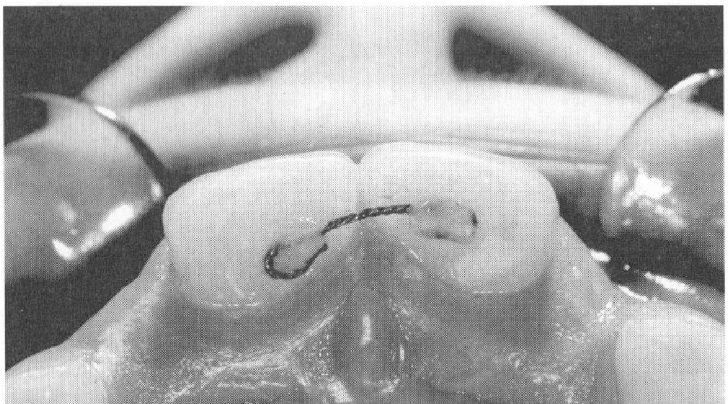

FIGURE 12-56 A fixed retainer to maintain diastema closure. A bonded 17.5 mil multistrand wire with loops bent into the ends is bonded to the lingual surfaces of anterior teeth to serve as a permanent retainer. This flexible wire allows physiologic mobility of the teeth and reduces bond failure but can be used only when the overbite is not excessive.

cause for maxillary incisor protrusion is a Class II malocclusion that often has a skeletal component, and in that case treatment must address the larger problem (see Chapter 13).

If there is adequate vertical clearance and space within the arch, maxillary incisors that have been displaced by a sucking habit can be tipped lingually with a removable or a fixed appliance. A Hawley-type removable appliance utilizing multiple clasps and a labial bow can be effective for this purpose (Figure 12-57). When the teeth require bodily movement or correction of rotations, a fixed appliance almost always is required (Figure 12-58). In these cases, an archwire should be used with bands on posterior teeth and bonded brackets on anterior teeth. This appliance must provide a retracting and space closing force, which can be obtained from closing loops incorporated into the archwire or from a section of elastomeric chain. Bodily incisor retraction places a large strain on the posterior teeth, which tends to pull them forward. Depending on the amount of incisor retraction and space closure, a headgear, chosen with consideration for vertical facial and dental characteristics, may be necessary for supplemental anchorage support.

If the overbite is enough to bring the upper and lower incisors into vertical contact, however, the upper incisors

A

B

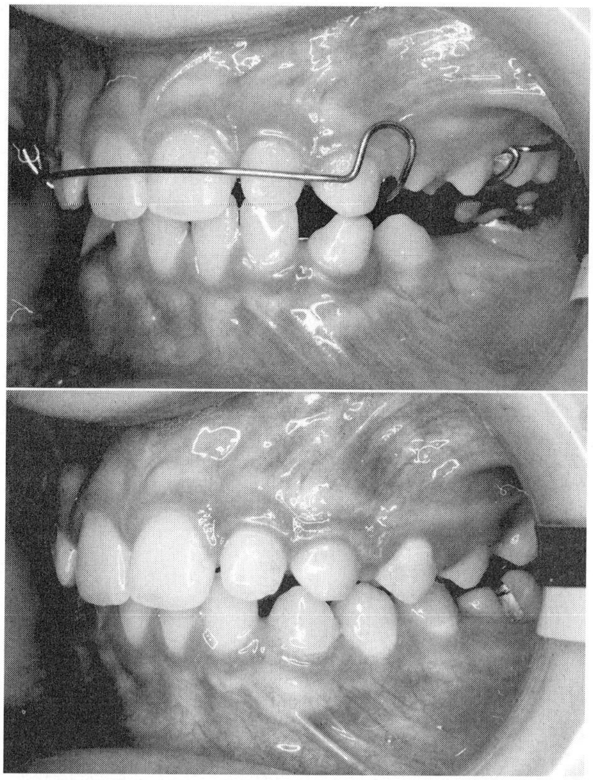

Figure 12-57 A removable appliance can be used in the mixed dentition to retract spaced and protruding anterior teeth. **A,** The labial bow is activated 1.5 to 2 mm and will achieve approximately 1 mm of retraction per month as the maxillary anterior teeth tip lingually. At each appointment, the labial bow should be adjusted and lingual acrylic removed to provide space for the tooth movement. **B,** A near normal occlusion in the late mixed dentition.

cannot be retracted to close spaces between them until the overbite is corrected. In some properly selected patients this can be addressed with a biteplate that allows eruption of posterior teeth and reduces the overbite, but it is rare that Class II malocclusion is not part of the total picture when excessive overjet and overbite both are present. This presents a much more complex treatment problem (see Chapter 13).

Missing Permanent Teeth

When permanent teeth are congenitally missing, the patient must have a thorough evaluation to determine the correct treatment because any of the diagnostic variables of profile, incisor position, tooth color and shape, skeletal and dental development, and space availability or deficiency can be crucial in treatment planning. The most commonly missing permanent teeth are second premolars (especially mandibular) and maxillary lateral incisors. These two conditions pose different problems.

Missing Second Premolars. If the patient has an ideal or an acceptable occlusion, maintaining the primary second molars is a reasonable plan, since many can be retained at least until the patient reaches the early twenties (Figure 12-59). Many reports exist of primary molars surviving until the patient is 40 to 60 years of age. Some reduction of their mesiodistal width often is necessary to improve the interdigitation of the posterior teeth. Most clinicians believe that when the size of primary molar is reduced, the mesiodistal diverging roots of the primary molar will resorb when they contact the adjacent permanent tooth roots. Even if eventual replacement of the primary molar with an implant or bridge is required, keeping the primary molar as long as possible is an excellent way to maintain alveolar bone in that area.

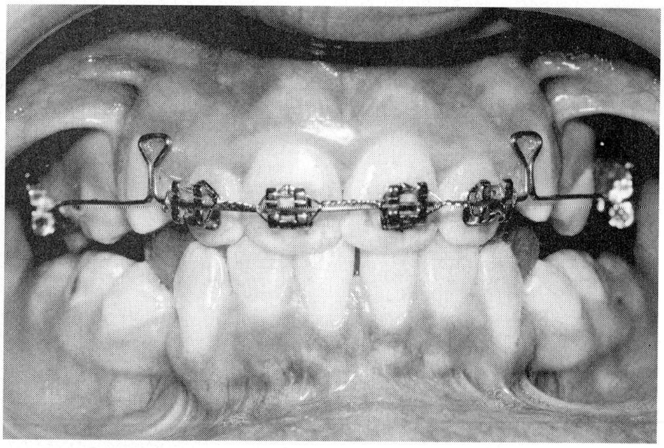

Figure 12-58 This closing loop archwire was used to retract protrusive maxillary incisors and close space. Each loop was activated approximately 1 mm per month, and the posterior anchorage was reinforced with headgear.

The second premolars have a tendency to form late and may be thought to be missing, only to be discovered to be forming at a subsequent visit. Good premolars seldom form after the child is 8 years of age. If the space, profile and jaw relationships are good or somewhat protrusive, it is possible to extract primary second molars that have no successor at age 7 to 9 and allow the first molars to drift mesially (Figure 12-60). This can produce partial or even complete space closure. Unfortunately, the amount and direction of mesial drift varies (Figure 12-61). Unless the second premolars are missing in all quadrants, it may be necessary to extract teeth in the opposing arch.

Early extraction can reduce the treatment time when the space of missing second premolars is to be closed, but later comprehensive orthodontic treatment usually is needed.[37] If only one primary molar is missing, unless there has been true unilateral space loss or there is considerable crowding on the contralateral side, restorative rather than orthodontic resolution of the problem is indicated. It is nearly impossible to close space unilaterally without affecting the midlines and other anterior interarch relationships.

Missing Maxillary Lateral Incisors. Long-term retention of primary laterals, in contrast to primary molars, is almost never an acceptable plan. When the lateral incisors

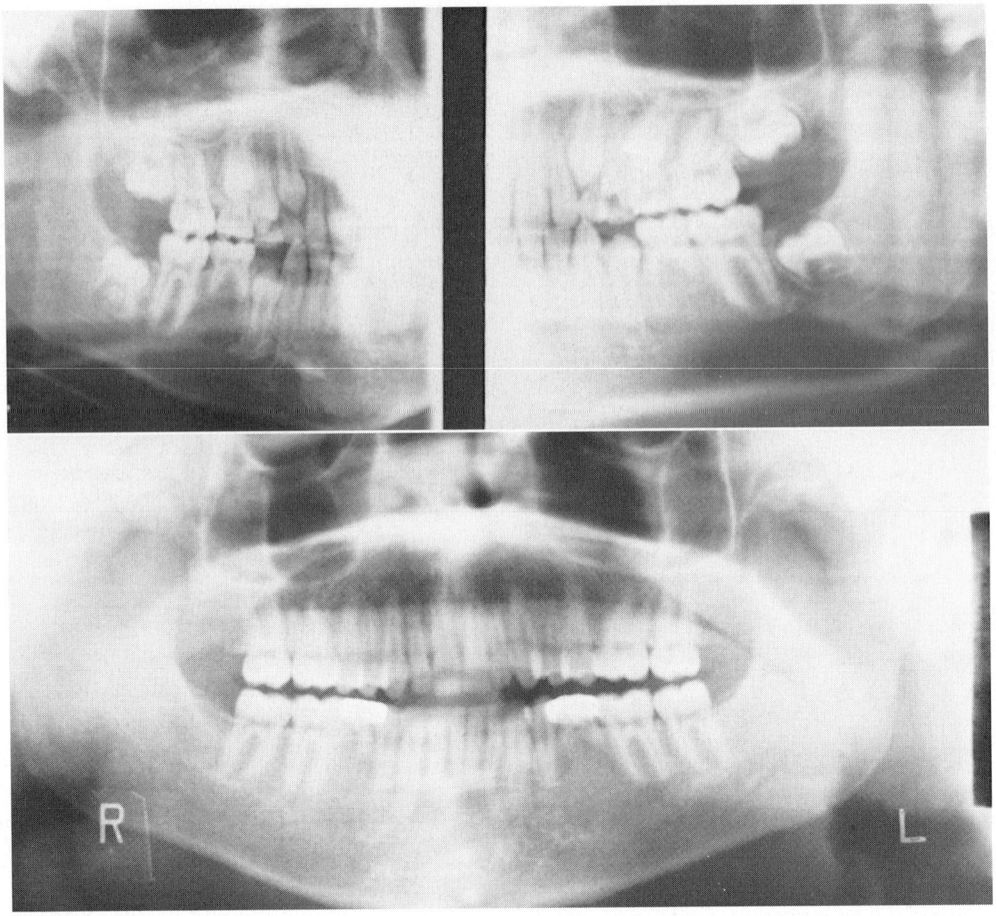

FIGURE 12-59 Primary mandibular second molars can be retained when the second premolars are missing. **A,** This patient was identified before orthodontic treatment as having missing mandibular second premolars. **B,** The decision was to retain the primary mandibular second molars because of the lack of crowding in the mandibular arch and their excellent root structure. These teeth were reduced mesiodistally and restored with stainless steel crowns during the finishing stages of orthodontic treatment to provide good occlusion.

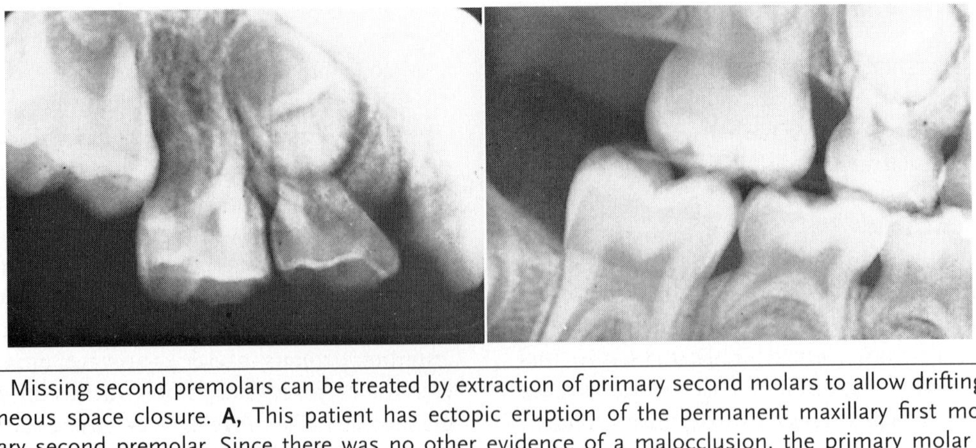

FIGURE 12-60 Missing second premolars can be treated by extraction of primary second molars to allow drifting of the permanent teeth and spontaneous space closure. **A,** This patient has ectopic eruption of the permanent maxillary first molar and a missing permanent maxillary second premolar. Since there was no other evidence of a malocclusion, the primary molar was extracted and **(B)** the permanent molar drifted anteriorly and closed the space during eruption. This eliminates the need for a prosthesis at a later date.

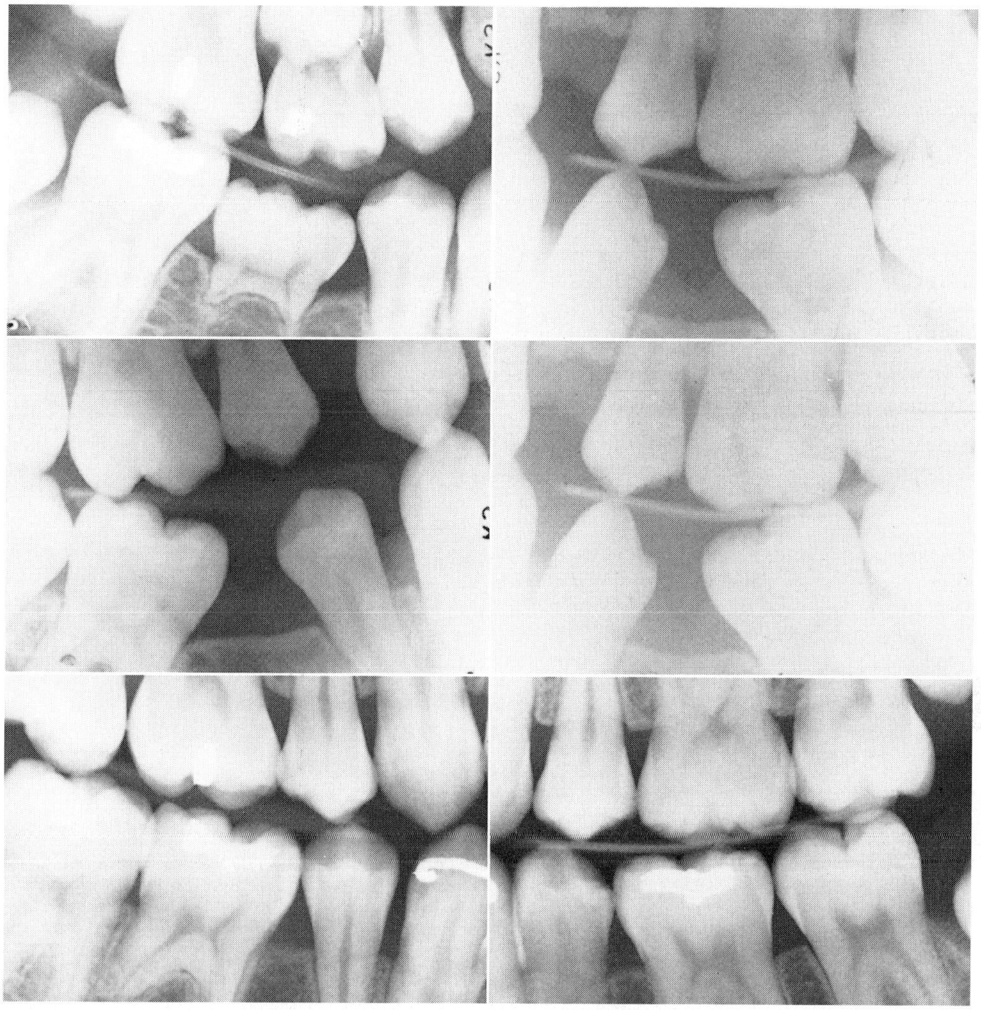

Figure 12-61 **A, B,** In this patient with bilaterally missing permanent mandibular second premolars, the decision was made to extract the retained primary molars to allow as much spontaneous drift and space closure as possible before full appliance therapy. **C, D,** Although posterior teeth did drift anteriorly and the anterior teeth distally, the space did not completely close. The pattern of drift to close the space of congenitally missing mandibular second premolars is highly variable and unpredictable. **E, F,** The residual space was closed and the roots paralleled with full appliances.

are missing, one of two sequelae usually is observed. In some patients, the erupting permanent canine resorbs the primary lateral incisor and spontaneously substitutes for the missing lateral incisor, which means that the primary canine has no successor and is sometimes retained (Figure 12-62). Some of these patients are seen as adults with primary canines in place, but most primary canines are lost by the end of adolescence even if their successors have erupted mesially. Less often, the primary lateral is retained when the permanent canine erupts in its normal position. Having the permanent canine erupt in the position of a congenitally missing lateral incisor is advantageous, whether or not the ultimate treatment is substitution of the canine for the lateral or opening space for a prosthetic replacement, because it generates alveolar bone in that area. Additionally, the canine shape and color can be determined which may have some influence on whether they are retracted or substituted for the lateral incisors and the space closed.

If space closure is the goal and the primary lateral incisors are replaced by the permanent canines, little immediate attention is necessary. Sometimes the absence of lateral incisors causes a large diastema to develop between the permanent central incisors. To maximize mesial drift of the erupting permanent canines, this diastema can be closed and retained (Figure 12-63). Later in the transition to the permanent dentition, the primary canines should be extracted if they are not resorbing, so the premolars can migrate into the canine positions and other posterior teeth can move mesially and close space (Figure 12-64).

Generally, unilateral orthodontic space closure in the anterior region of the mouth is not recommended. There is probably a better chance of matching the existing teeth with

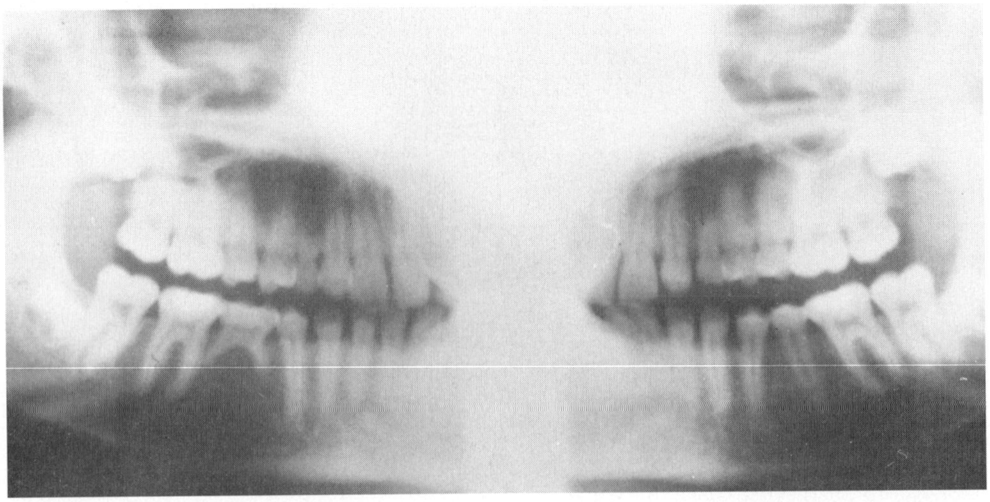

Figure 12-62 Missing permanent maxillary lateral incisors are often replaced spontaneously by permanent canines. This phenomenon occurs without intervention, but the resorption noted on the retained primary canines probably will continue to progress. If implants to eventually replace the missing laterals are planned, it is desirable for the canines to erupt mesially so that alveolar bone forms in the area of the future implant. The canines can be moved into their final position just prior to the implant surgery (see Chapter 18).

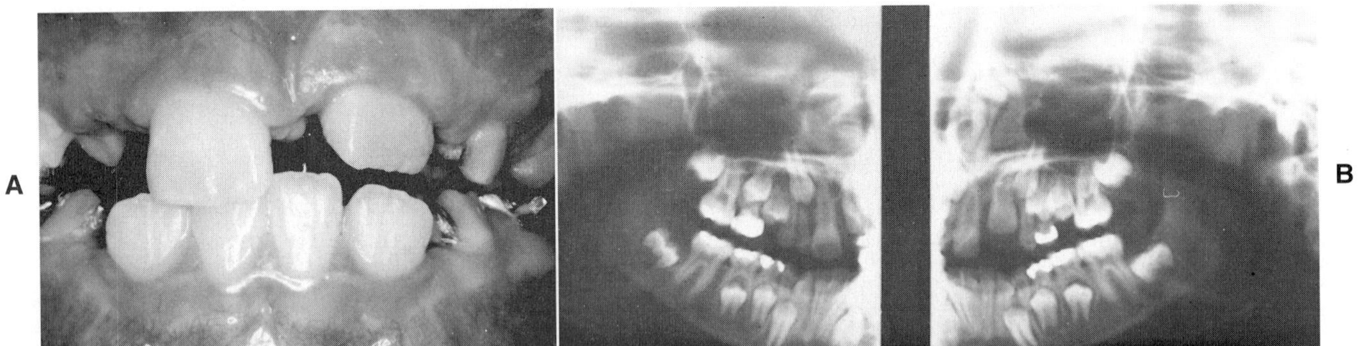

Figure 12-63 When permanent lateral incisors are congenitally missing, often a large diastema develops between the permanent central incisors. **A,** This patient has that type of diastema, and the unerupted permanent canines will be substituted for the missing lateral incisors. **B,** This radiograph shows the unerupted canines in an excellent position for substitution for the lateral incisors. **C,** The diastema has been closed to obtain maximum mesial drift of the canines. **D,** This technique enables the canines to erupt closer to their final position and eliminates unnecessary tooth movement during full appliance therapy.

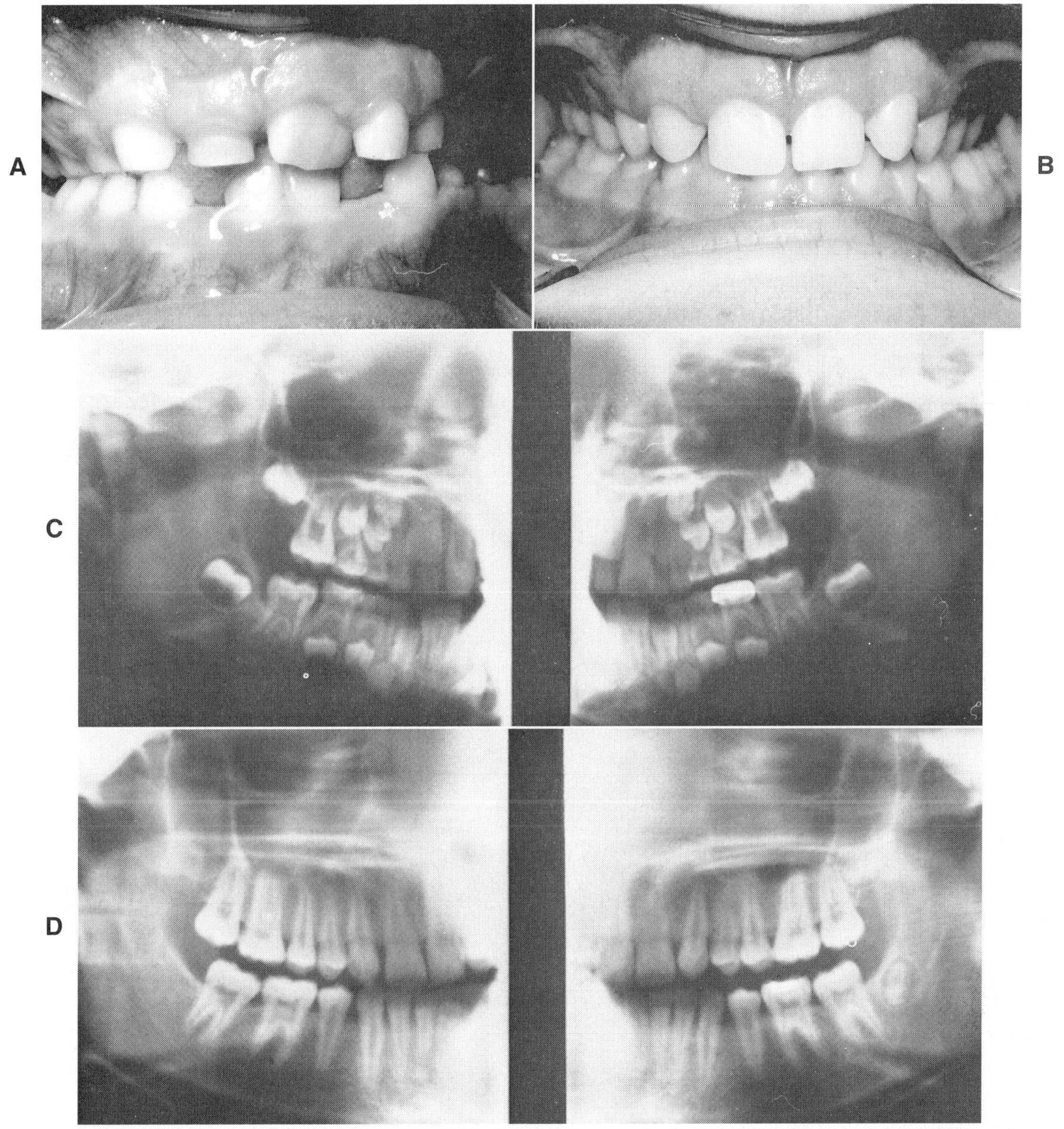

FIGURE 12-64 Selective removal of primary teeth when permanent maxillary lateral incisors are missing can lead to a shortened second phase of fully banded treatment. **A, B,** This patient had primary canines and primary first molars extracted to maximize the mesial drift of the permanent posterior teeth. **C, D,** This intervention resulted in good tooth position that will require little fixed appliance therapy to complete.

restorative solutions or substituting for both lateral incisors than with reshaping the existing teeth on only one side. A unilateral missing lateral incisor might require the extraction of the other lateral incisor prior to eruption of the canines to maximize the drift pattern for ultimate space closure and substitution (Figure 12-65), but generally the option to move the canines back into their proper position exists prior to premolar eruption. These same considerations generally apply for the lower anterior area, too, where one or two lateral incisors sometimes are missing. The details for completing comprehensive treatment and finishing for missing laterals are covered in Chapters 14 and 18.

Autotransplantation. In patients with a congenitally missing tooth or teeth in one area but crowding in another, autotransplantation also is a possible solution. Teeth can be transplanted from one position to another in the same mouth with a good prognosis for long-term success, if this is done when the transplanted tooth has approximately one-half of its root formed.[38] This means that the decision for autotransplantation must be made during the mixed dentition (Figure 12-66).

Transplantation is most commonly used to move premolars into the location of missing incisors. It can also be used to replace missing first molars with third molars, a decision

A

B

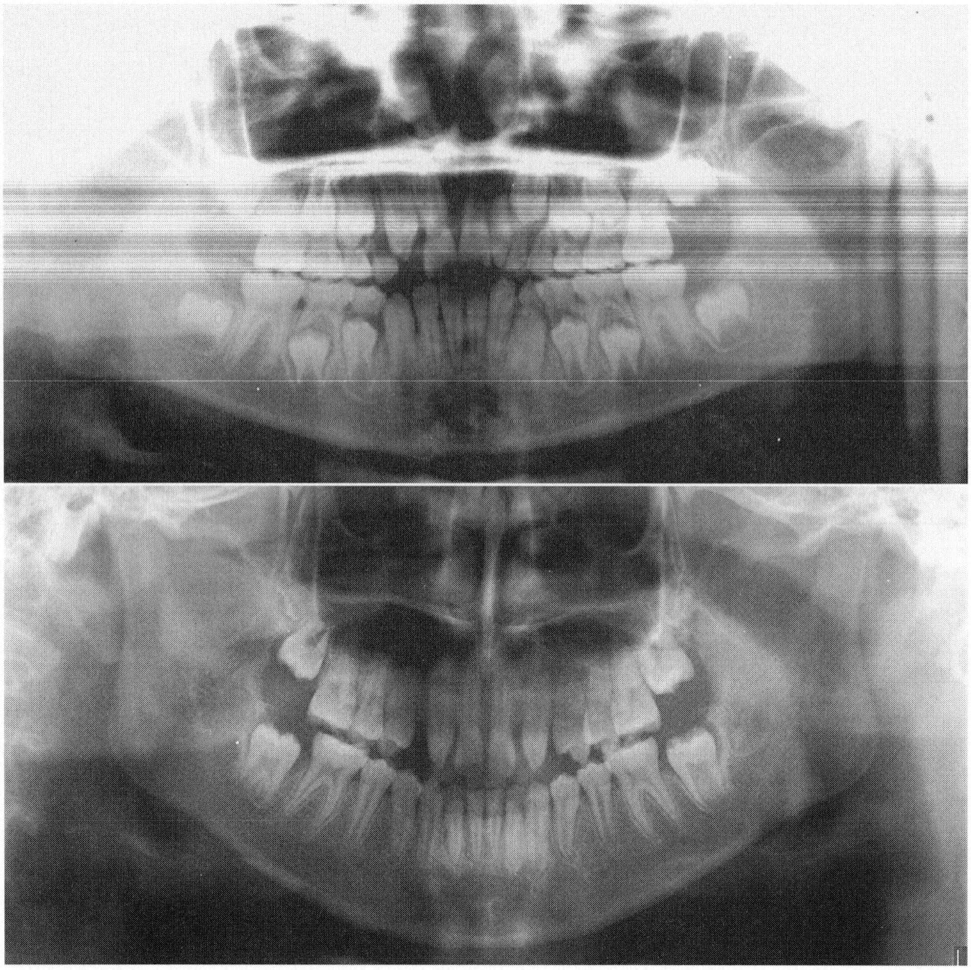

FIGURE 12-65 **A,** This patient's panoramic radiograph shows that one permanent maxillary lateral incisor is missing and the other peg-shaped. **B,** Instead of opening or closing space unilaterally the peg lateral was extracted and the teeth allowed to drift and erupt. The patient will now be treated with bilateral space closure or implants to improve symmetry and esthetics.

that can be made a little later (Figure 12-67).[39] A combination of careful surgical intervention and positioning of the transplant, followed by light orthodontic forces to achieve final tooth position and restorative treatment to recontour the crown of the transplanted tooth, can result in long-term functional and esthetic success.[40] The success rate with type of treatment is high and predictable.

Premature Tooth Loss With Adequate Space: Space Maintenance

Early loss of a primary tooth presents a potential alignment problem because drift of permanent or other primary teeth is likely unless it is prevented. Space maintenance is appropriate only when adequate space is available and all unerupted teeth are present and at the proper stage of development. If there is not enough space or if succedaneous teeth are missing, space maintenance alone is inadequate. The indications and contraindications for space maintenance are discussed in Chapter 7; the discussion here focuses on the treatment procedures.

Several treatment techniques can be used successfully for space maintenance, depending on the specific situation. Because these appliances are at risk for breakage and loss, they must be monitored carefully to be successful.

Band and Loop Space Maintainers

The band and loop is a unilateral fixed appliance indicated for space maintenance in the posterior segments. The simple cantilever design makes it ideal for isolated unilateral space maintenance (Figure 12-68). Because the loop has limited strength, this appliance must be restricted to holding the space of one tooth and is not expected to accept functional forces of chewing. Although bonding a rigid or flexible wire across the edentulous space has been advocated as an alternative, this has not proved satisfactory clinically. It also is no

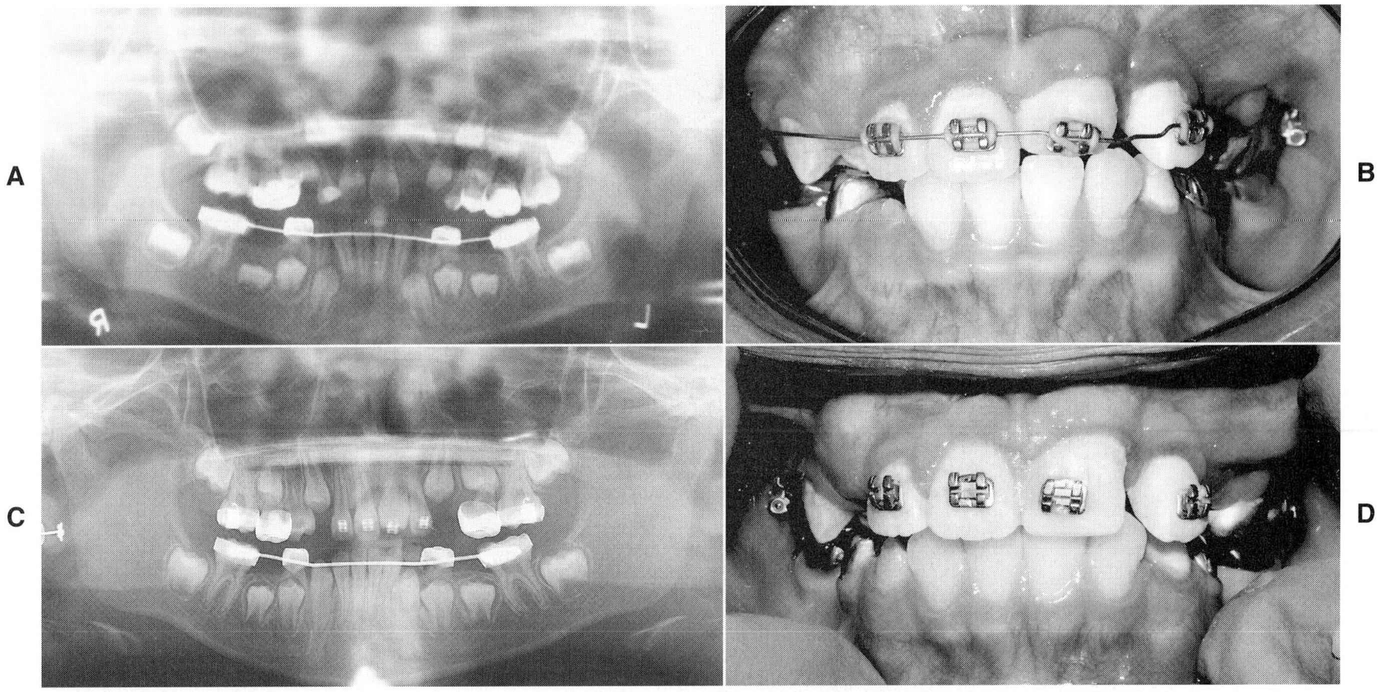

Figure 12-66 A, This patient has an unerupted permanent maxillary left central incisor due to a dilacerated root. It was determined that it could not be repositioned surgically or moved orthodontically. **B,** To relieve crowding, premolar extraction was indicated, and the maxillary left first premolar was transplanted to the maxillary left central incisor position and moved after a short healing period. **C,** Root development and healing have continued and indicate a vital tooth. **D,** The tooth will continue to be recontoured and restored with resin prior to definitive restorative treatment.

longer considered advisable to solder the loop portion to a stainless steel crown because this precludes simple appliance removal and replacement. Teeth with stainless steel crowns should be banded like natural teeth.

If a primary second molar has been lost, the band can be placed on either the primary first molar or the erupted permanent first molar. Some clinicians prefer to band the primary tooth in this situation because of the risk of decalcification around any band, but primary first molars are challenging to band because of their morphology, which converges occlusally and makes band retention difficult. A more important consideration is the eruption sequence of the succedaneous teeth. The primary first molar should not be banded if the first premolar is developing more rapidly than the second premolar, because loss of the banded abutment tooth would require replacement of the appliance.

Before eruption of the permanent incisors, if a single primary molar has been lost bilaterally, a pair of band and loop maintainers are recommended instead of the lingual arch that would be used if the patient were older. This is advisable because the permanent incisor tooth buds are lingual to the primary incisors and often erupt lingually. The bilateral band and loops enable the permanent incisors to erupt without interference from a lingual archwire. At a later time the two band-and-loop appliances can be replaced with a single lingual arch if necessary.

Partial Denture Space Maintainers

The partial denture is most useful for bilateral posterior space maintenance when more than one tooth has been lost per segment and the permanent incisors have not yet erupted. In these cases, because of the length of the edentulous space, band and loop space maintainers are contraindicated, and the lingual position of the unerupted permanent incisors and their likely lingual position at initial eruption make the lingual arch a poor choice. The partial denture also has the advantage of replacing occlusal function.

Another indication for this appliance is posterior space maintenance in conjunction with replacement of missing primary or delayed permanent incisors, for esthetics (Figure 12-69). Anterior space maintenance is unnecessary because arch circumference generally is not lost even if the teeth drift and redistribute the space, so replacement of missing anterior teeth is done solely to improve appearance. This has social advantages even for young children.

Distal Shoe Space Maintainers

The distal shoe is the appliance of choice when a primary second molar is lost before eruption of the permanent first

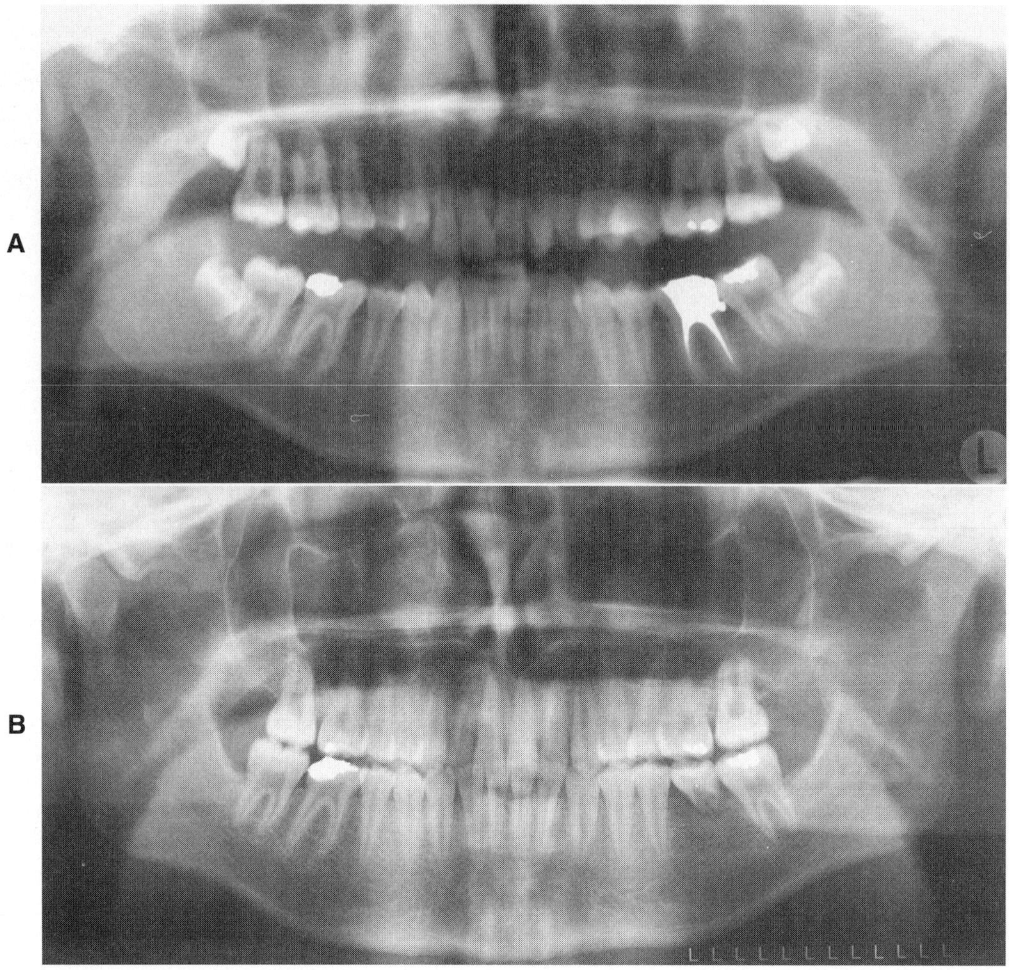

FIGURE 12-67 **A,** The mandibular permanent first molar was restoratively compromised. With the developing third molar in the same quadrant available **(B),** it was decided to transplant it into the first molar position when the root development was appropriate, rather than plan a restoration for the first molar. The transplanted third molar was subsequently repositioned during orthodontic treatment and served well as a replacement.

molar. This appliance consists of a metal or plastic guide plane along which the permanent molar erupts. The guide plane is attached to a fixed or removable retaining device (Figure 12-70). When fixed, the distal shoe is usually retained with a band instead of a stainless steel crown so that it can be replaced by another type of space maintainer after the permanent first molar erupts. Unfortunately, this design limits the strength of the appliance and provides no functional replacement for the missing tooth. If primary first and second molars are missing, the appliance must be removable and the guide plane is incorporated into a partial denture because of the length of the edentulous span. This type of appliance can provide some occlusal function.

To be effective, the guide plane must extend into the alveolar process so that it contacts the permanent first molar approximately 1 mm below the mesial marginal ridge, at or before its emergence from the bone. An appliance of this type is tolerated well by most children, but is contraindicated in patients who are at risk for subacute bacterial endocarditis or are immuno-compromised, because complete epithelialization around the intra-alveolar portion has not been demonstrated.[41] Careful measurement and positioning are necessary to ensure that the blade will ultimately guide the permanent molar. Faulty positioning is the most common problem with this appliance.

Lingual Arch Space Maintainers

A lingual arch is indicated for space maintenance when multiple primary posterior teeth are missing and the permanent incisors have erupted (Figure 12-71, *A, B*). A conventional lingual arch, attached to bands on the primary second or permanent first molars and contacting the maxillary or mandibular incisors, prevents anterior movement of the posterior teeth and posterior movement of the anterior teeth.

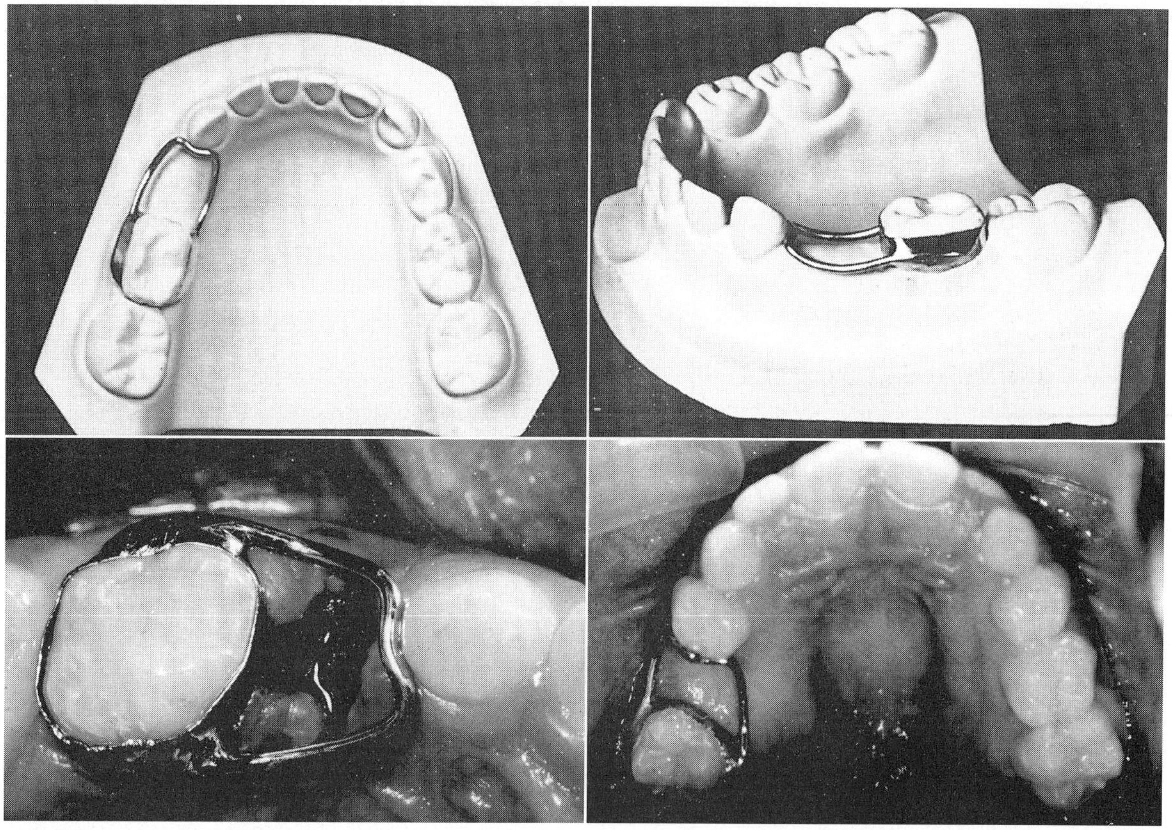

Figure 12-68 A band-and-loop space maintainer is generally used in the mixed dentition to save the space of a single prematurely lost primary molar. It consists of a band on either a primary or permanent molar and a wire loop to maintain space. **A,** The loop portion made from 36 mil wire is carefully contoured to the abutment tooth without restricting lateral movement of the primary canine and **(B)** the loop is also contoured to within 1.5 mm of the alveolar ridge. The solder joints should fill the angle between the band and wire to avoid food and debris accumulation. **C,** A completed band and loop maintainer in place after extraction of a primary first molar; **D,** an occlusal rest, shown here on the primary first molar, can be added to the loop portion to prevent the banded teeth from tipping mesially.

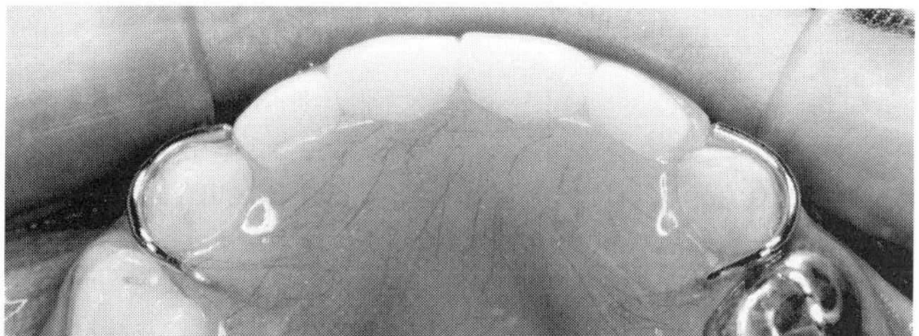

Figure 12-69 In a young child, a removable partial denture is used to replace anterior teeth for esthetics. At the same time, it can maintain the space of one or more prematurely lost primary molars. For this patient, the four incisors and the primary right first molar are replaced by the partial denture. Multiple clasps, preferably Adams' clasps, are necessary for good retention. Both the clasps and the acrylic need frequent adjustment to prevent interference with physiologic adjustment of primary teeth during eruption of permanent teeth. The C-clasps on the primary canines provide limited retention and are good examples of clasps that need continued careful attention.

A lingual arch space maintainer is usually soldered to the molar bands but can be removable, depending on the number of adjustments anticipated and the care of the appliance expected from the patient. Removable lingual arches (e.g., those that fit into attachments welded onto the bands) are more prone to breakage and loss. Regardless of whether it is removable, the lingual arch should be positioned to rest on the cingula of the incisors, approximately 1 to 1.5 mm off the soft tissue, and should be stepped to the lingual in the canine region to remain away from the primary molars and unerupted premolars (Figure 12-71, *C*). The most common problems with lingual arches are distortion, breakage and loss. Careful instructions to parents and patients can reduce these problems.

Maxillary lingual arches as space maintainers are not familiar to many clinicians but are contraindicated only in patients whose bite depth causes the lower incisors to contact the archwire on the lingual of the maxillary incisors (Figure 12-71, *D*). When bite depth does not allow use of a conventional design, either the Nance lingual arch (Figure 12-71, *E*) or a transpalatal arch (Figure 12-71, *F*) can be used. The Nance arch is an effective space maintainer, but soft tissue

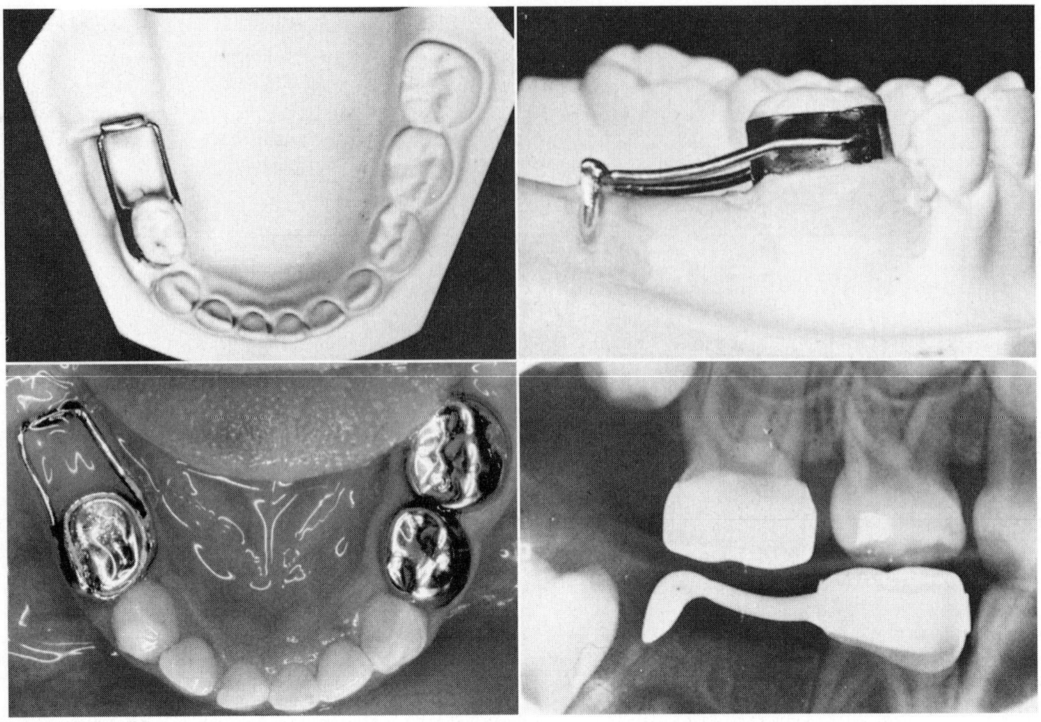

FIGURE 12-70 The distal-shoe space maintainer is indicated when a primary second molar is lost before eruption of the permanent first molar and is usually placed at or very soon after the extraction of the primary molar. **A,** The loop portion, made of 36 mil stainless steel wire, and the intra-alveolar blade are soldered to a band so the whole appliance can be removed and replaced with another space maintainer after the permanent molar erupts. **B,** The loop portion must be contoured closely to the ridge since the appliance cannot resist excessive occlusal forces from the opposing teeth. **C,** This distal shoe space maintainer was placed at the time of extraction of the primary second molar. **D,** The blade portion must be positioned so that it extends approximately 1 mm below the mesial marginal ridge of the erupting permanent tooth to guide its eruption. This position can be measured from pretreatment radiographs and verified by a radiograph taken at try-in or post-cementation. An additional occlusal radiograph can be obtained if the faciolingual position is in doubt.

irritation can be a problem. The best indication for a transpalatal arch is when one side of the arch is intact and several primary teeth are missing on the other side. In this situation, the rigid attachment to the intact side usually provides adequate stability for space maintenance. When primary molars have been lost bilaterally, however, both permanent molars may tip mesially despite the transpalatal arch, and a conventional lingual arch or Nance arch is preferred.

A flowchart is provided to help guide decision making for space maintenance (Figure 12-72).

Localized Space Loss (3 mm or less): Space Regaining

After premature loss of a primary tooth, space may be lost from drift of other teeth before a dentist is consulted. Then, repositioning the teeth to regain space rather than just space maintenance is required. Up to 3 mm of space can be reestablished in a localized area with relatively simple appliances and a good prognosis. Space loss greater than that constitutes a severe problem and usually requires comprehensive treatment to achieve acceptable results. Either space can be regained using complex appliance therapy or permanent teeth need to be extracted. The methods to regain the space are considered later under moderate or severe crowding. The treatment necessary to regain the space during the mixed dentition, especially if a second stage of treatment will be required in any event, may be more than is reasonable when one analyzes the cost/benefit ratio. Extraction with space closure often is a better choice. In that circumstance, often the crowding can be accepted during the mixed dentition so that the ultimate space closure occurs under control when the complete fixed appliances are present.

Maxillary Space Regaining

Generally, space is easier to regain in the maxillary than in the mandibular arch, because of the increased anchorage for removable appliances afforded by the palatal vault and the possibility for use of extraoral force (headgear). Permanent maxillary first molars can be tipped distally to regain space with either a fixed or removable appliance, but bodily

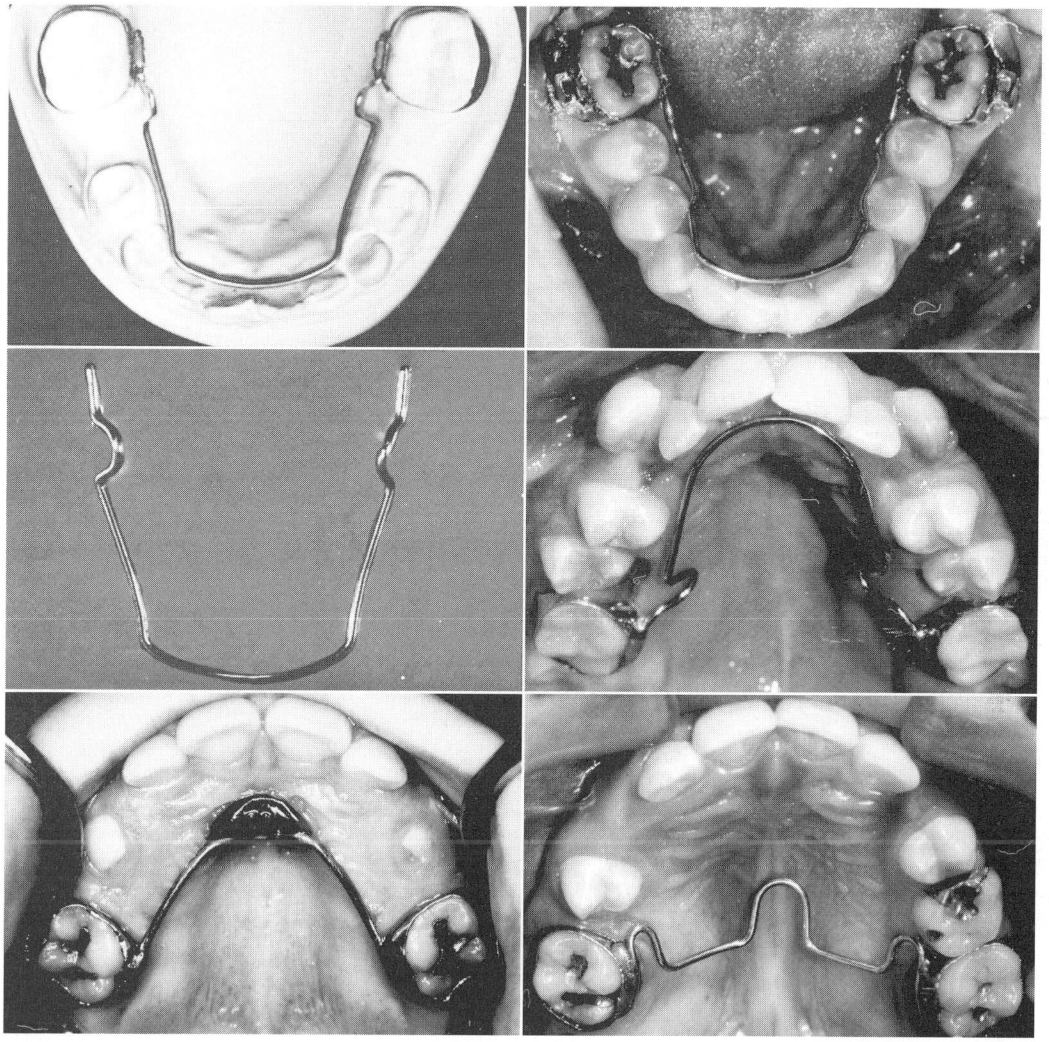

Figure 12-71 A lingual holding arch usually is the best choice to maintain space for premolars after premature loss of the primary molars when the permanent incisors have erupted. **A,** The lingual arch is made of 36 mil wire with adjustment loops mesial to the permanent first molars. **B,** This soldered lingual arch successfully maintained the space for the premolars. **C,** The lingual arch is stepped away from the premolars to allow their eruption without interference, which results in a keyhole design. The wire is also 1.5 mm away from the soft tissue at all points. **D,** A maxillary lingual arch is used when the overbite is not excessive, or **(E)** a Nance arch with an acrylic button in the palatal vault is indicated if the overbite is excessive. The palatal button must be monitored because it may cause soft tissue irritation. **F,** The transpalatal arch prevents a molar from rotating mesially into a primary molar extraction space, and this largely prevents its mesial migration. Several teeth should be present on at least one side of the arch when a transpalatal design is employed as a sole space maintainer.

movement requires a fixed appliance. Because the molars tend to tip forward and rotate mesiolingually, distal tipping to regain 2-3 mm often is satisfactory.

A removable appliance retained with Adams' clasps and incorporating a helical fingerspring adjacent to the tooth to be moved is very effective. This appliance is the ideal design for tipping one molar (Figure 12-73). One posterior tooth can be moved up to 3 mm distally during 3 to 4 months of full-time appliance wear. The spring is activated approximately 2 mm to produce 1 mm of movement per month. The molar generally will derotate spontaneously as it is tipped distally.

For unilateral bodily space regaining, a fixed intra-arch appliance is preferred. The excellent anchorage provided by the remaining teeth and palate can support the forces generated by a coil spring on a segmental archwire to produce distal movement of the molar on only one side, with good success (Figure 12-74).

If bodily movement of both permanent maxillary first molars is necessary in regaining space, this can be accomplished by using a banded and bonded fixed appliance or headgear. Sometimes both molars need to be moved distally, but one requires substantially more movement than the other. To accomplish this, an asymmetric facebow with a

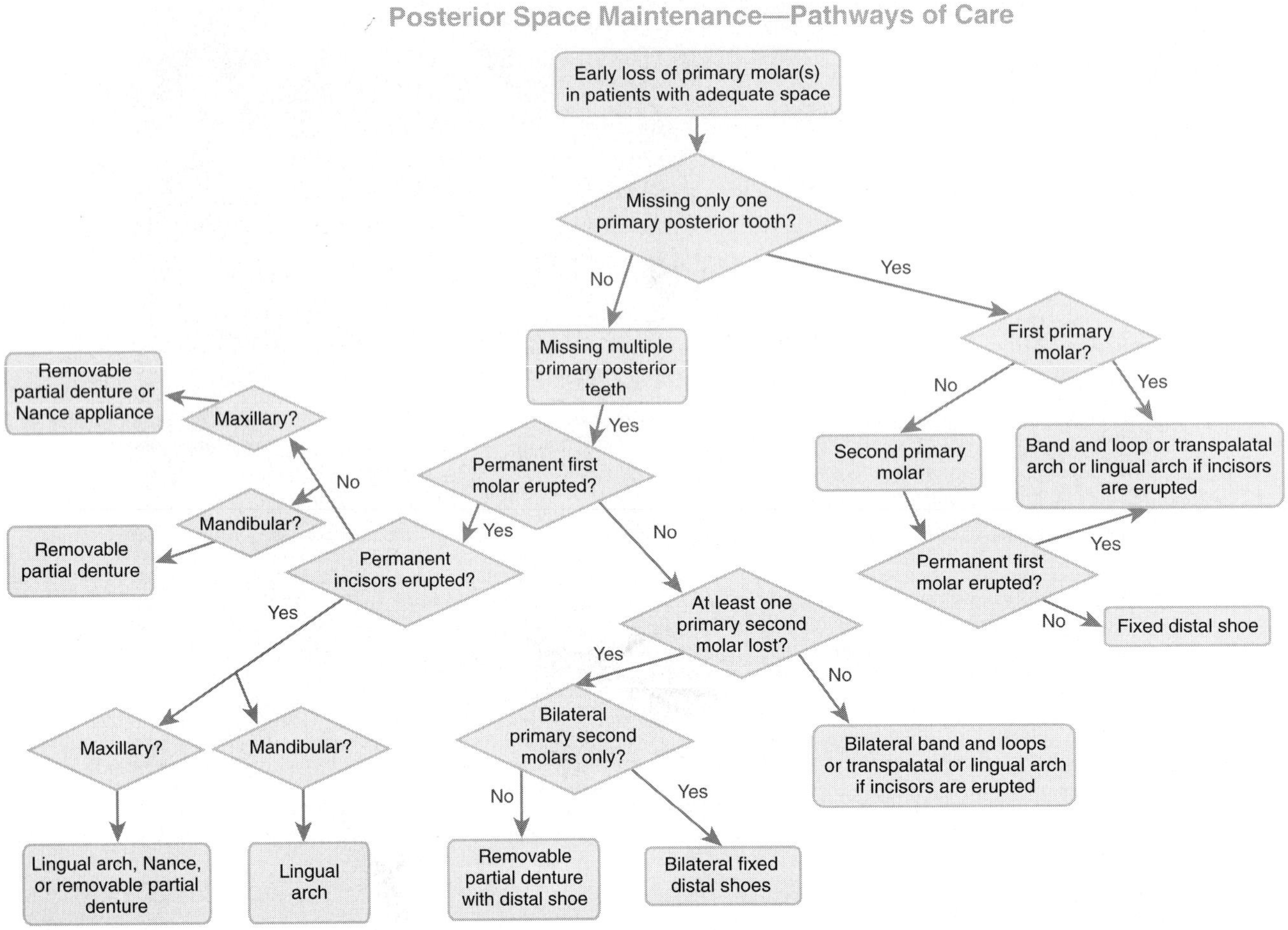

FIGURE 12-72 This flowchart can be used to aid decision making regarding possible options for space maintenance in the primary and mixed dentitions.

neckstrap attachment can be used (Figure 12-75).[42] This will result in more movement on the side with the longer outer bow but will also move that tooth toward lingual crossbite. Asymmetric cervical headgear is neither as easy to adjust nor as comfortable to wear as symmetric headgear, and it requires excellent patient compliance. For space regaining, it should be used only to deal with bilateral but asymmetric space loss—not true unilateral space loss, which is treated best with a removable or fixed appliances. A complete discussion of the clinical use of headgear is included in Chapter 13.

Regardless of the method used to regain these limited amounts of space, a space maintainer is required when adequate space has been restored. A fixed space maintainer is recommended, rather than trying to maintain the space with the removable appliance that was used for space regaining.

Mandibular Space Regaining

For moderate amounts of space regaining, removable appliances can be used in the mandibular arch just as they are in the maxillary arch, but as a rule they are less satisfactory because they are more fragile and prone to breakage. They do not fit as well and lack the palatal anchorage support. Problems with tissue irritation frequently are encountered, and patient acceptance tends to be poorer than with maxillary removable appliances.

For unilateral mandibular space regaining, the best choice is a fixed appliance and an archwire, which provides excellent anchorage. A lingual arch can be used to support the tooth movement and provide anchorage when used in conjunction with a segmental archwire and coil spring (Figure 12-76). If space has been lost bilaterally, there are two choices short of bands and brackets, an adjustable lingual arch and a lip bumper. When an active lingual arch pits posterior movement of both molars against the anchorage offered by the incisors, significant forward displacement of the incisors must be expected (Figure 12-77). With the lip bumper, a labial appliance fitted to tubes on the molar teeth (Figure 12-78), the idea is that the appliance presses against the lip, which creates a distal force to tip the molars posteriorly without affecting the incisors. Although some posterior movement of the molars can be observed when a

A 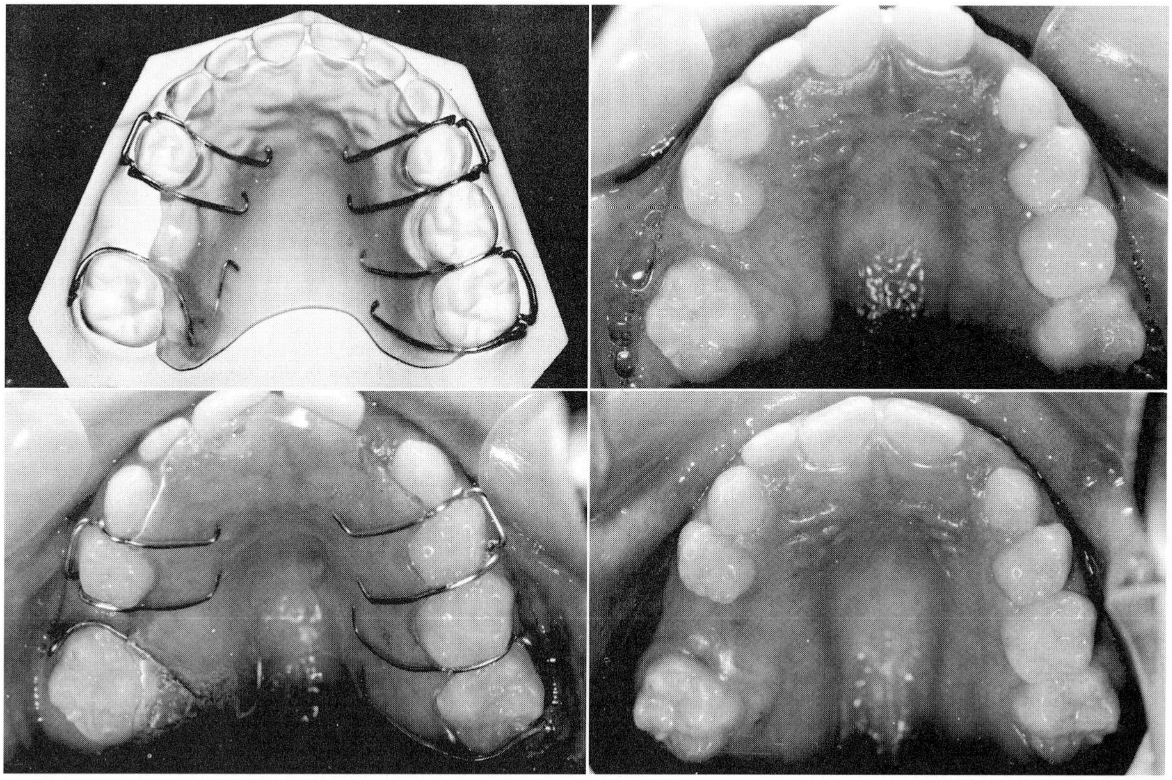 B

C D

Figure 12-73 A removable appliance with a fingerspring can be used to regain space by tipping a permanent first molar distally. **A,** The appliance incorporates multiple Adams' clasps and a 28 mil helical spring that is activated 1 to 2 mm per month. **B,** Premature loss of the primary second molar has led to mesial drift and rotation of the permanent first molar. **C,** This removable appliance can be used to regain up to 3 mm of space. **D,** After space regaining, the space should be maintained with a band and loop or lingual arch if the permanent incisors have erupted.

A 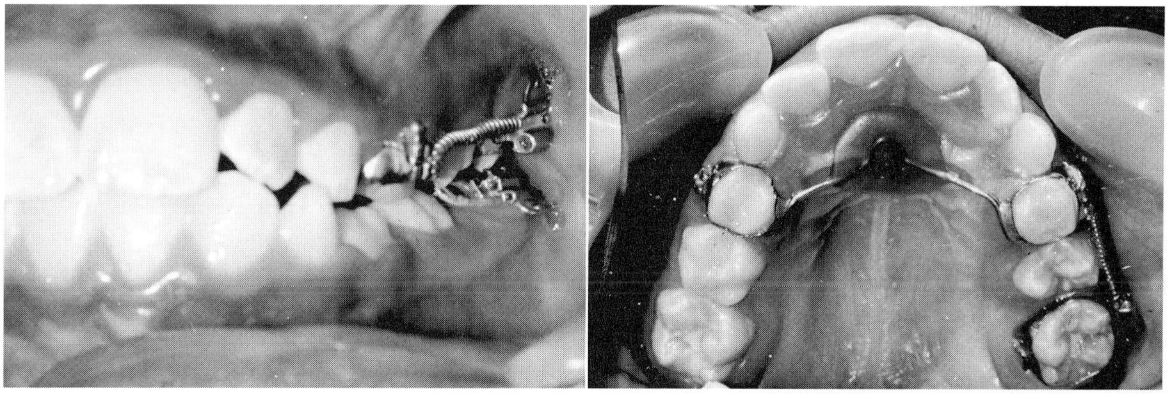 B

Figure 12-74 **A,** A fixed appliance also can be used to regain space in the maxillary posterior regions, with a coil spring generating the distalizing force. **B,** Palatal anchorage was gained using a Nance arch and the erupted teeth.

lip bumper is used, the appliance also alters the equilibrium of forces against the incisors, removing any restraint from the lip on these teeth. The result is forward movement of the incisors.[43] Depending on the type of lip bumper used and its clinical manipulation, transverse widening also may occur.[44]

On balance, the effects of the active lingual arch and the lip bumper are similar. A lingual arch can be left in place as a space maintainer after space has been regained. A lip bumper is not a good space maintainer and should be replaced with a lingual arch when long-term maintenance of the regained space is needed.

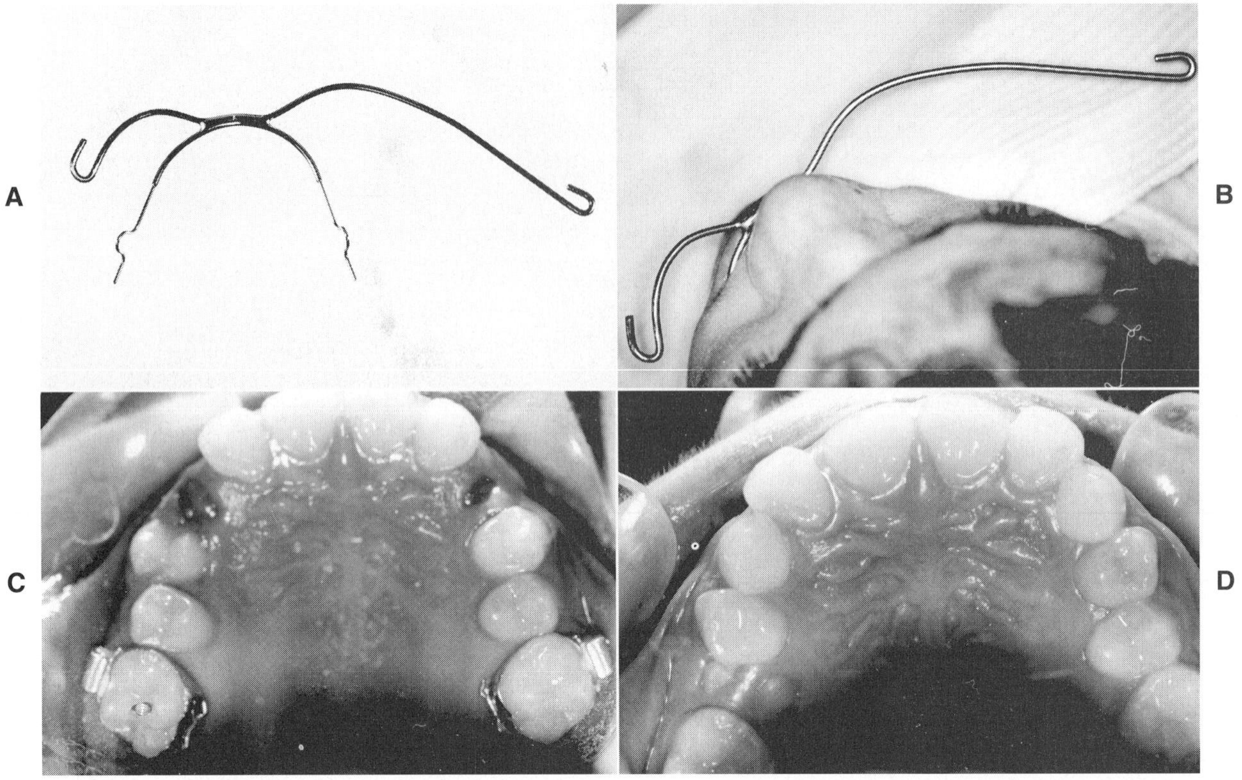

FIGURE 12-75 Asymmetric force, achieved with a headgear by using an asymmetric outer bow, can be useful in regaining bilateral but asymmetric lost space. **A,** The outer bow is cut short on the side that needs the smaller distal movement and is left long on the side requiring the greater distal correction. **B,** When the appliance is in place, before the neckstrap is attached, the side with the long outer bow should be approximately 4 to 5 cm from the cheek. The distance is reduced when force is applied by the strap and the outer bow rotates toward the face. **C,** Intraorally a bilateral space shortage is evident, more on the right side than the left, because of premature loss of a primary molar. **D,** Good asymmetric headgear wear resulted in space available for all succedaneous teeth.

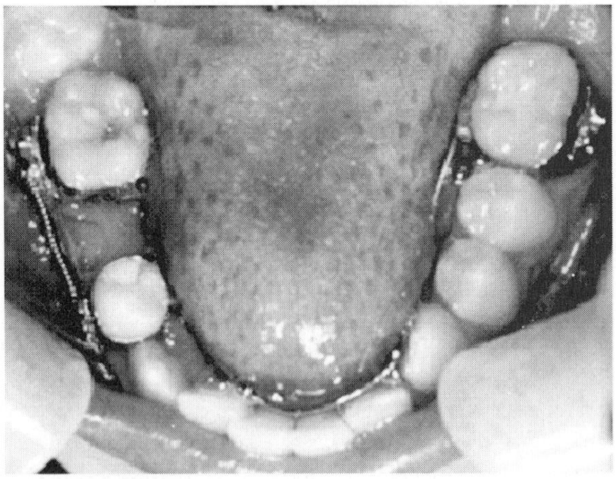

FIGURE 12-76 Moving molars distally in the mandibular arch is quite challenging and requires support from a number of teeth. Using a lingual arch, to incorporate anchorage from the permanent and primary molars as well as the incisors, and force from a coil spring can be effective.

Mild to Moderate Crowding of Incisors With Adequate Space

Irregular Incisors, Minimal Space Discrepancy

In some children space analysis shows that enough space for all the permanent teeth ultimately will be available, but relatively large permanent incisors and primary molars cause transient crowding of the permanent incisors. This crowding is usually expressed as mild faciolingual displacement or rotation of individual anterior teeth.

Studies of children with normal occlusion indicate that when they go through the transition from the primary to the mixed dentition, up to 2 mm of incisor crowding may resolve spontaneously without treatment (see Chapter 4). From this perspective, as a general rule there is no need for treatment when mild incisor crowding is observed during the mixed dentition. Not only is reduction of this small amount of crowding probably not warranted, there is no evidence that long-term stability will be greater if the child receives early treatment to improve alignment. The only reason for treatment is temporary esthetic improvement.

A

B

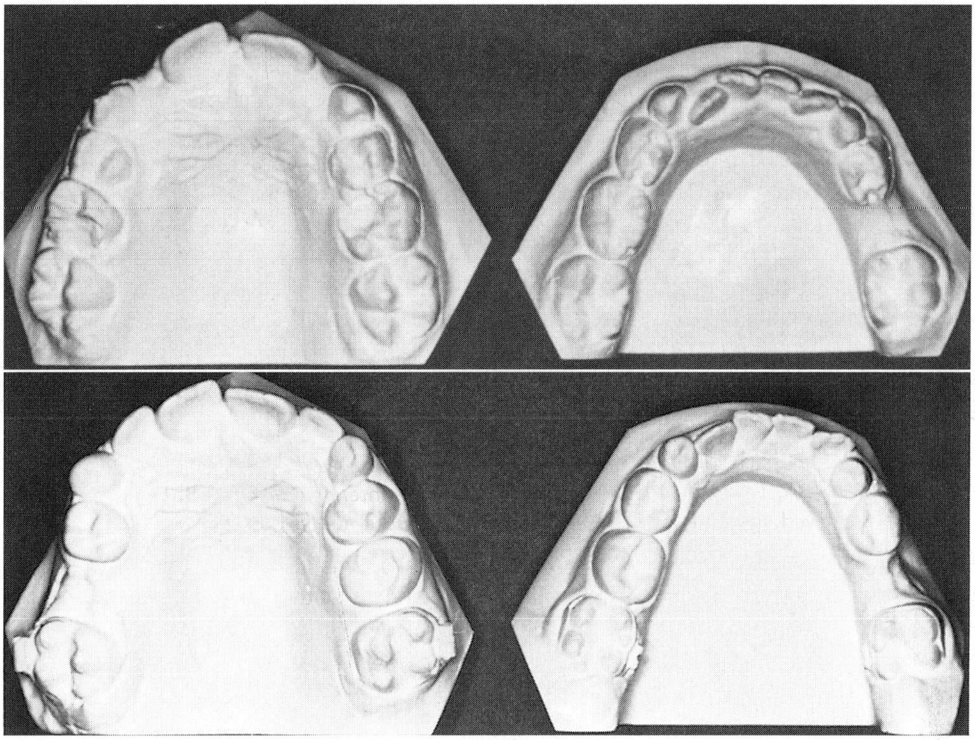

Figure 12-77 Space regaining in a child with space loss in the upper and lower arches. **A,** Casts demonstrating loss of space as a result of caries and early loss of a primary molar. **B,** Using an active lingual arch and headgear for the mandibular and maxillary arches, respectively, space regaining was achieved. At this point, space maintainers will be needed.

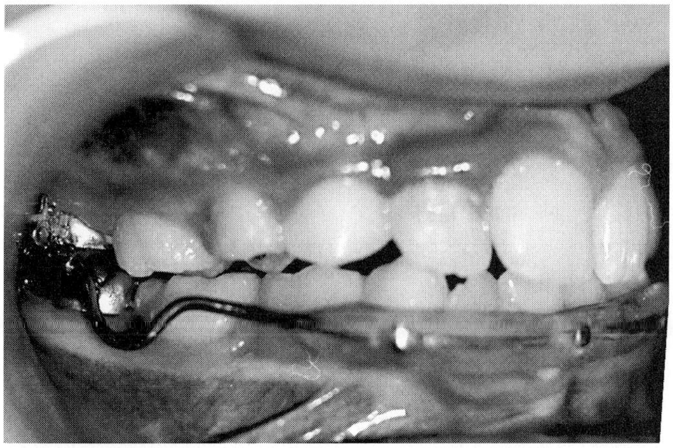

Figure 12-78 A lip bumper constructed of a 36 mil wire bow with an acrylic pad, which fits into tubes on the permanent first molars, is sometimes used to increase arch length. This occurs when the appliance stretches the lower lip and transmits force to move the molars back. The appliance also disrupts the equilibrium between the lip and tongue and allows the anterior teeth to move facially. The result is nearly equal molar and incisor change. (Courtesy Dr. M. Linebaugh.)

If exaggerated parental concern makes mild or moderate crowding a problem, one could consider disking the interproximal enamel surfaces of the remaining primary incisors or canines (Figure 12-79) as the anterior teeth erupt. It is possible to gain as much as 3 to 4 mm of anterior space through this procedure. Remember, at this point in the transitional dentition no disking or interproximal stripping should be attempted on permanent teeth. This could create a tooth-size discrepancy that later could not be resolved. Permanent tooth stripping should not be undertaken until all the permanent teeth have erupted and their interarch size relationship can be evaluated.

Correction of any incisor rotations caused by this transitional crowding requires space and controlled movement to align and derotate them, using an archwire and bonded attachments on the incisors. It is rare that a child who needs this type of treatment in the mixed dentition does not require further treatment after all permanent teeth have erupted, so extensive early treatment is not often indicated.

Mandibular Midline Shifts

When one primary canine is lost prematurely, treatment is needed to prevent or correct a midline shift. In mild or moderate crowding when no permanent teeth will be extracted to provide additional space in the arch, this problem needs

A

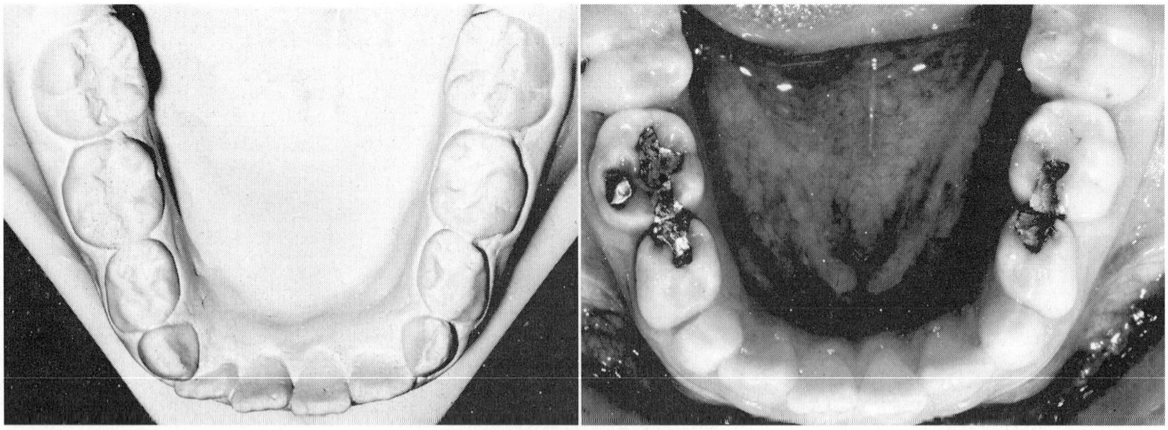

B

FIGURE 12-79 Disking can be used on multiple surfaces of primary teeth—especially the primary canines—when limited transitional crowding is apparent. **A,** This pretreatment cast shows minor anterior crowding. **B,** Disking of the mesial and distal surfaces of the primary canines allowed spontaneous alignment to occur without appliance therapy.

A

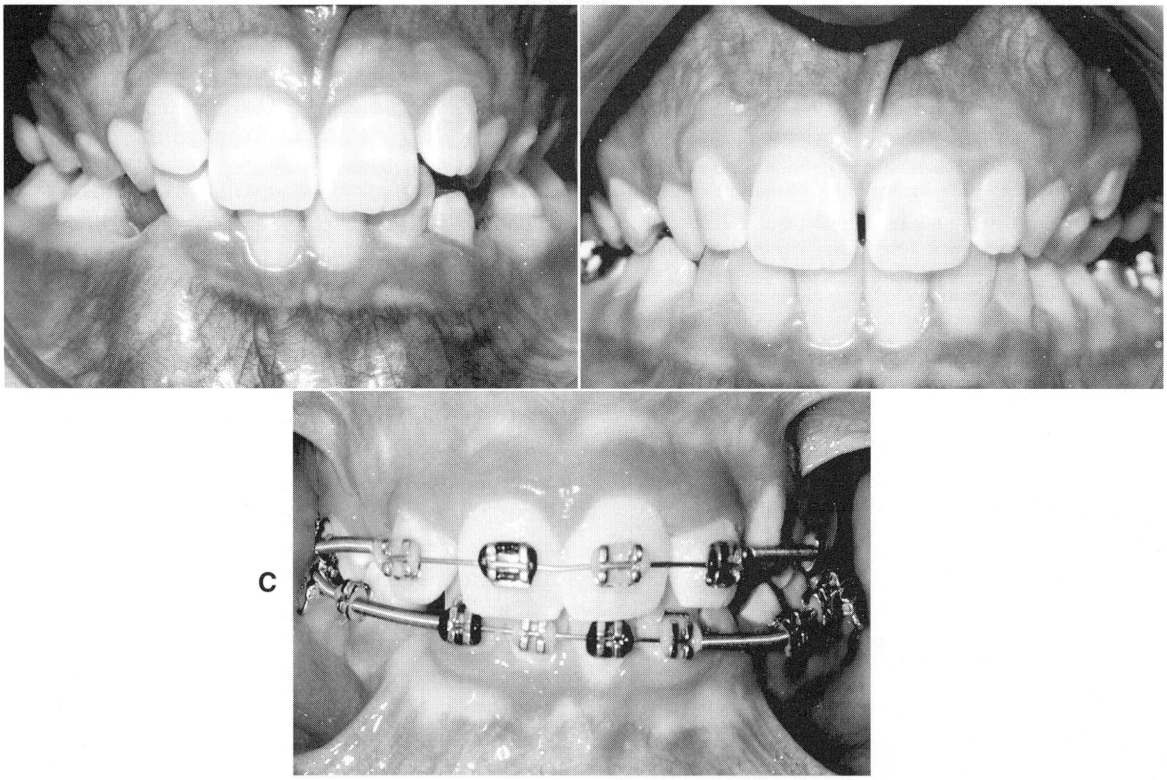

B

C

FIGURE 12-80 Some midline shifts require bodily tooth movement. **A,** The midline of the mandibular arch has bodily shifted to the patient's right because of premature loss of a primary canine. **B,** The teeth were moved back to their proper position using a fixed appliance and are supported until eruption of the canines with a lingual holding arch. **C,** The type of movement (illustrated in another patient) is best achieved with an archwire and coil springs to generate the tooth moving forces. Active coil springs can be replaced with passive coils to gain stability prior to retention.

to be addressed before the remaining permanent teeth erupt, because as more teeth erupt in asymmetric positions, overall arch perimeter will shorten and lead to a substantial space discrepancy with total arch asymmetry. If the midline has not changed, the contralateral canine can be removed and a lingual arch seated to prevent lingual tipping of the incisors. Another option is to maintain the position of the lateral incisor on the side of the canine loss using a lingual arch with a spur (see Figure 12-35).

If a midline shift has occurred (Figure 12-80, *A, B*) the incisors can be aligned and moved back to their optimum location using a bonded and banded appliance with an archwire. The force to move the teeth is usually generated by a coil spring placed on the archwire (Figure 12-80, *C*). Often the molar positions need to be supported with a lingual arch to maintain the arch form. Regardless of the type of tooth movement or the appliance used for correction, retention will be needed until the remaining permanent teeth erupt. In some cases, disking or extraction of a primary canine or molar will be required to provide the necessary room for this correction even if space in the arch is predicted to be adequate.

If both mandibular canines are lost, the permanent incisors tend to tip lingually, which reduces the arch circumference and increases the apparent crowding. In this situation, an active lingual arch for expansion and then a passive arch for maintenance will be required.

Some practitioners have advocated arch expansion in the primary[45] and early mixed dentitions[46] on the theory that this would assure more space at a later time. To date, there is no credible evidence that early intervention to "prepare," "develop," "balance," or expand arches by any other name has any efficacy in providing a less crowded permanent dentition later. Unfortunately, even in children who had mild crowding initially, incisor irregularity can recur soon after early treatment if retention is not managed carefully.[47] Parents and patients should know the issues and uncertainties associated with this type of treatment.

Space Deficiency Largely Due to Allowance for Molar Shift

In some children, more severe transitional crowding occurs when the incisors erupt. Space analysis often shows that a major component of the projected space deficiency is the allowance for mesial movement of the permanent first molars when the second primary molars are lost. For these patients, if the loss of leeway space could be prevented, there would be little or no space deficiency. Gianelly reported that in patients seeking treatment at Boston University, 70% would have enough space to align the teeth if molar drift were prevented.[48,49] One can look at these children from two perspectives: there is minimal benefit from early treatment unless there are major esthetic concerns, and therefore little or no reason to intervene; or alternatively, this group does not need much treatment, it should be relatively easy to provide, and there is always the possibility that if early treatment is done, later treatment might not be necessary.

Rather than begin treatment in the early mixed dentition, the current recommendation for the patients with moderate crowding is to begin comprehensive fixed appliance treatment in the late mixed dentition, just before the second primary molars exfoliate. The transitional incisor crowding would simply be tolerated up to that time, on the theory that it could be corrected most easily when the space became available. In these patients, beginning treatment earlier is not judged to be cost-effective—it takes longer for both patient and doctor, without producing a better long-term result.

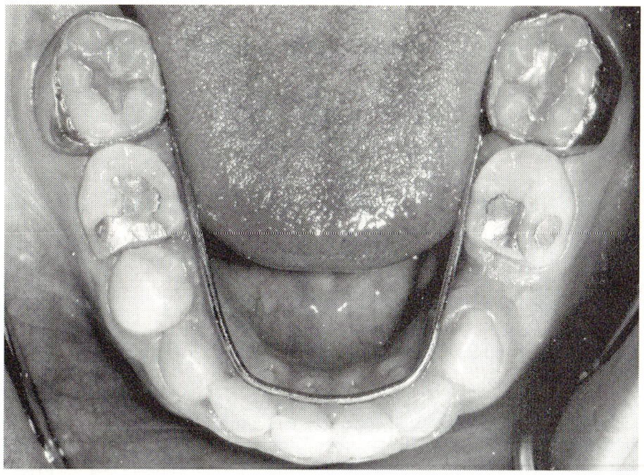

Figure 12-81 Disking primary posterior teeth in conjunction with space maintenance is an effective method to use the leeway space and all available arch length. Note that the disking must be completed perpendicular to the occlusal plane so that the height of contour of the tooth is reduced. Occlusally-convergent slices that do not reduce the mesiodistal width of the tooth are not helpful.

A primary indication does exist, however, for starting treatment earlier in some of these patients: early loss of a primary canine as the lateral incisors erupt (loss of both canines usually indicates more severe crowding that may indicate a different treatment approach—see below). This requires placement of a lingual arch to maintain symmetry and prevent distal movement of the incisors that shortens arch length. The lingual arch can be left in position until the second premolars erupt, so the start of comprehensive treatment can be delayed.

In the absence of early loss of primary teeth, the major reason for early intervention in a child who has a moderate space discrepancy is esthetic concern because of the obvious crowding. If the parents insist on doing something sooner rather than later, a combination of early extraction of primary canines and disking to reduce the width of primary molars can provide space to allow the permanent incisors, canines and premolars to erupt and align (Figure 12-81). The minimum orthodontic appliance therapy is a lingual arch that will support the incisor teeth and control the molar position and arch perimeter by preventing any mesial shift. The lingual arch can be activated slightly to tip molars distally and incisors facially to obtain a modest increase in arch length (Figure 12-82). A lip bumper also can be used in the lower arch to maintain the position of the molars or perhaps tip them slightly distally, while removing lip pressure and allowing the incisors to move facially. The effect of lingual arches and lip bumpers in the lower arch is remarkably similar; forward movement of the incisors is the major way in which additional space is gained.

When space is created in this way, the incisors often align spontaneously if the irregularity is from faciolingual tipping, but rotations are less likely to resolve. An exception is the

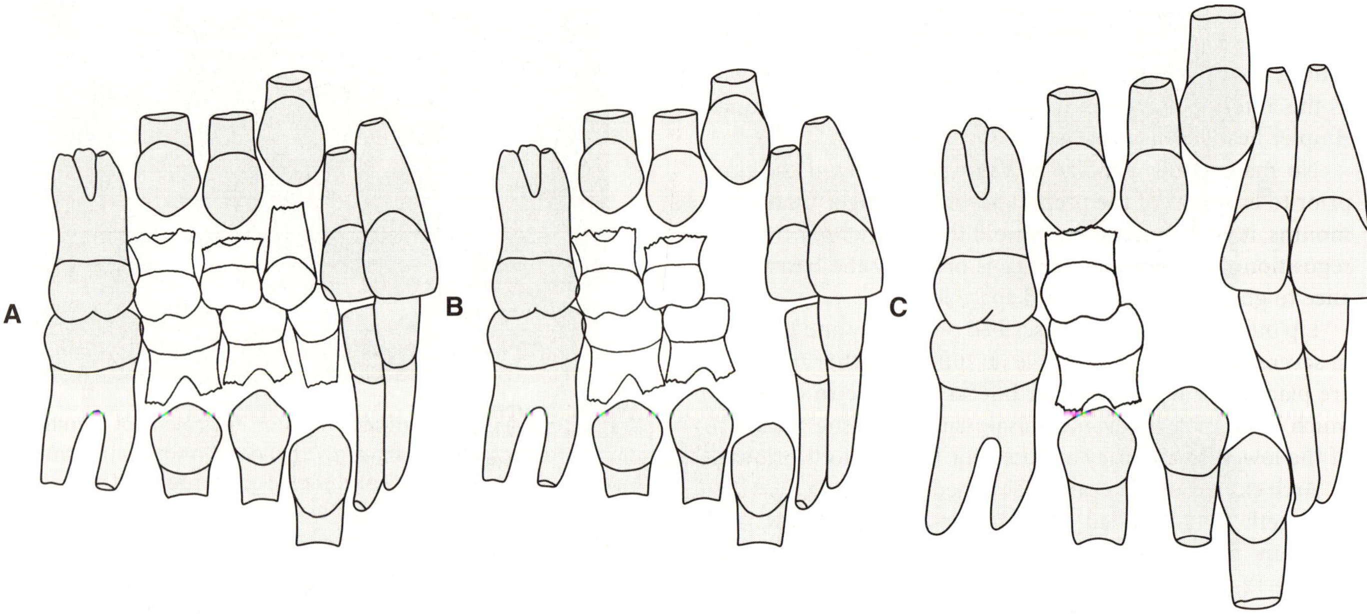

Figure 12-92 **Serial extraction is used to relieve severe arch length discrepancies. A,** The initial diagnosis is made when a severe space deficiency is documented and there is marked incisor crowding. **B,** The primary canines are extracted to provide space for alignment of the incisors. **C,** The primary first molars are extracted when one-half to two-thirds of the first premolar root is formed, to speed eruption of the first premolars.

therapy, but is now viewed as an adjunct to later comprehensive treatment instead of a substitute for it. Although serial extraction makes later comprehensive treatment easier and often quicker, by itself it usually does not result in ideal tooth position or closure of excess space.

Serial extraction is directed toward *severe* dental crowding. For this reason, it is best used when no skeletal problem exists and the space discrepancy is large—greater than 10 mm per arch. If the crowding is severe, little space will remain after the teeth are aligned, which means there will be little tipping and uncontrolled movement of the adjacent teeth into the extraction sites. If the initial discrepancy is smaller, more residual space must be anticipated. It is unwise to start serial extraction in a child who has a skeletal problem, because the closure of extraction spaces would be affected by how the skeletal problem was being addressed.

Serial extraction treatment begins in the early mixed dentition with extraction of primary incisors if necessary, followed by extraction of the primary canines to allow eruption and alignment of the permanent incisors (Figure 12-92). As the permanent teeth align without any appliances in place, there is usually some lingual tipping of the lower incisors, and overbite often increases during this stage. Labiolingual displacements resolve better than rotational irregularity. After extraction of the primary canines, crowding problems are usually under control for 1 to 2 years, but foresight is necessary. The goal is to influence the permanent first premolars to erupt ahead of the canines so that they can be extracted and the canines can move distally into this space. The maxillary premolars usually erupt before the canines, so the eruption sequence is rarely a problem in the upper arch. In the lower arch, however, the canines often erupt before the first premolars, which causes the canines to be displaced facially. To avoid this result, the lower primary first molar should be extracted when there is $^1/_2$ to $^2/_3$ root formation of the first premolar. This usually will speed up the premolar eruption and cause it to enter the arch before the canine (Figure 12-92, *C*). The result is easy access for extraction of the first premolar before the canine erupts (Figure 12-92, *D*).

A complication can occur if the primary first molar is extracted early and the first premolar still does not erupt before the canine. This can lead to impaction of the premolar that requires later surgical removal (Figure 12-93). At the time the primary first molar is removed, it may be obvious that the canine will erupt before the premolar. In this case the underlying premolar can also be extracted at the same time—a procedure termed *enucleation*. If possible, however, enucleation should be avoided because the erupting premolar brings alveolar bone with it. Early enucleation can leave a bone defect that persists.

The increase in overbite mentioned previously can become a problem during later treatment. A variation in the extraction sequence can be used to help in controlling this problem. The mandibular primary canines are retained and some space for anterior alignment is made available when the permanent laterals erupt by extracting the primary first molars instead. With this approach, eruption of the permanent first premolars is encouraged, and the incisors are less

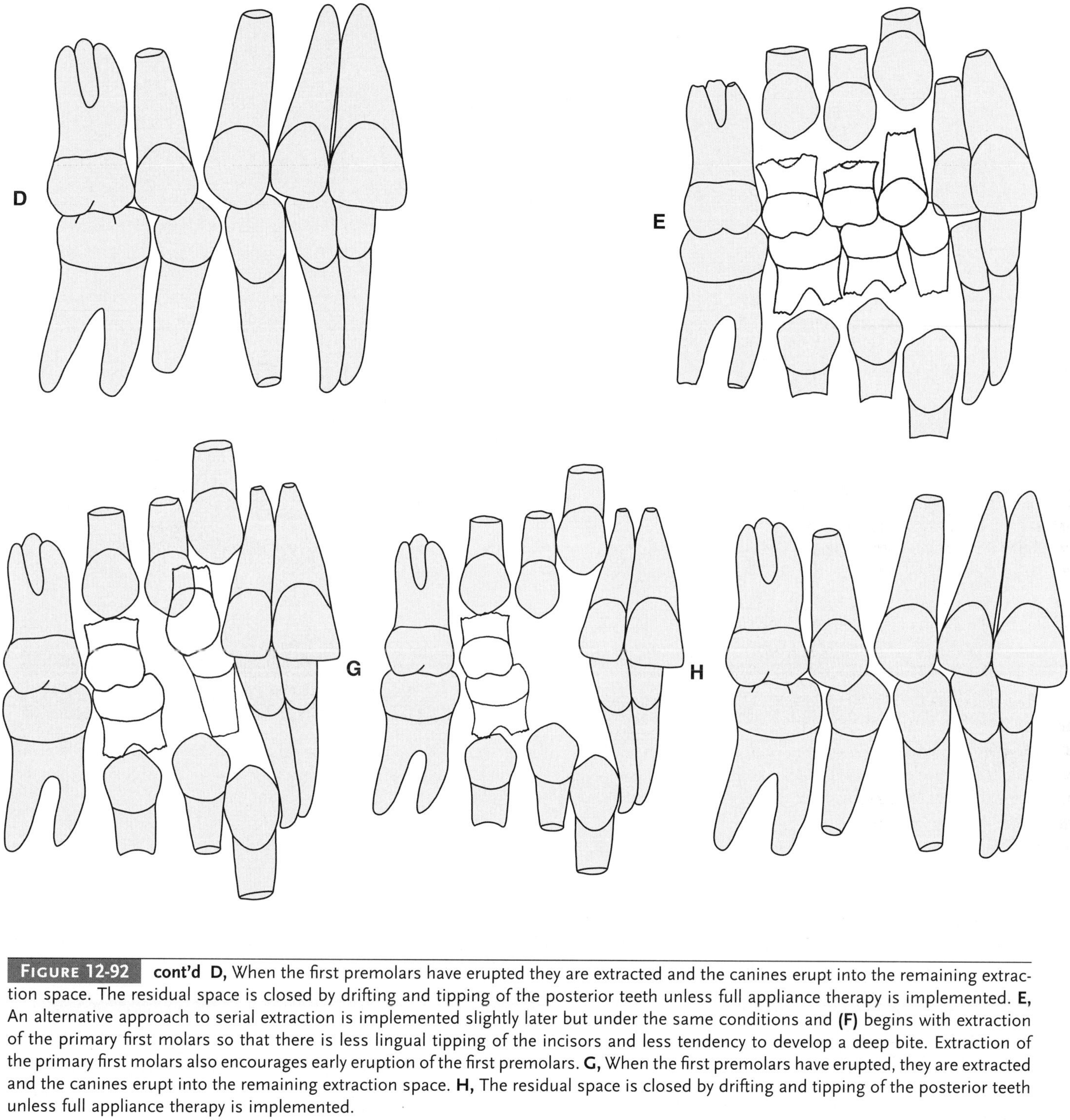

Figure 12-92 cont'd D, When the first premolars have erupted they are extracted and the canines erupt into the remaining extraction space. The residual space is closed by drifting and tipping of the posterior teeth unless full appliance therapy is implemented. **E,** An alternative approach to serial extraction is implemented slightly later but under the same conditions and **(F)** begins with extraction of the primary first molars so that there is less lingual tipping of the incisors and less tendency to develop a deep bite. Extraction of the primary first molars also encourages early eruption of the first premolars. **G,** When the first premolars have erupted, they are extracted and the canines erupt into the remaining extraction space. **H,** The residual space is closed by drifting and tipping of the posterior teeth unless full appliance therapy is implemented.

prone to tip lingually (Figure 12-92, *E* through *H*). The major goal of serial extraction is prevention of incisor crowding, however, and some crowding often persists if the primary canines are retained. In many patients with severe crowding, the primary canines are lost to ectopic eruption of the laterals and cannot be maintained.

After the first premolar has been extracted, the second primary molars should exfoliate normally. The premolar extraction spaces close partially by mesial drift of the second premolars and permanent first molars but largely by distal eruption of the canines. If serial extraction is not followed by mechanotherapy, ideal alignment, root positioning, correct rather than deep overbite, and space closure usually are not achieved (Figure 12-94).

Serial extraction was used much more frequently 20-30 years ago than now. It was overused then, and perhaps is

A

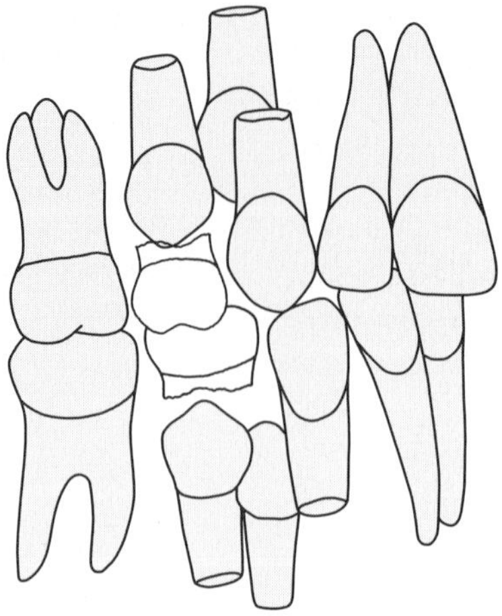

B

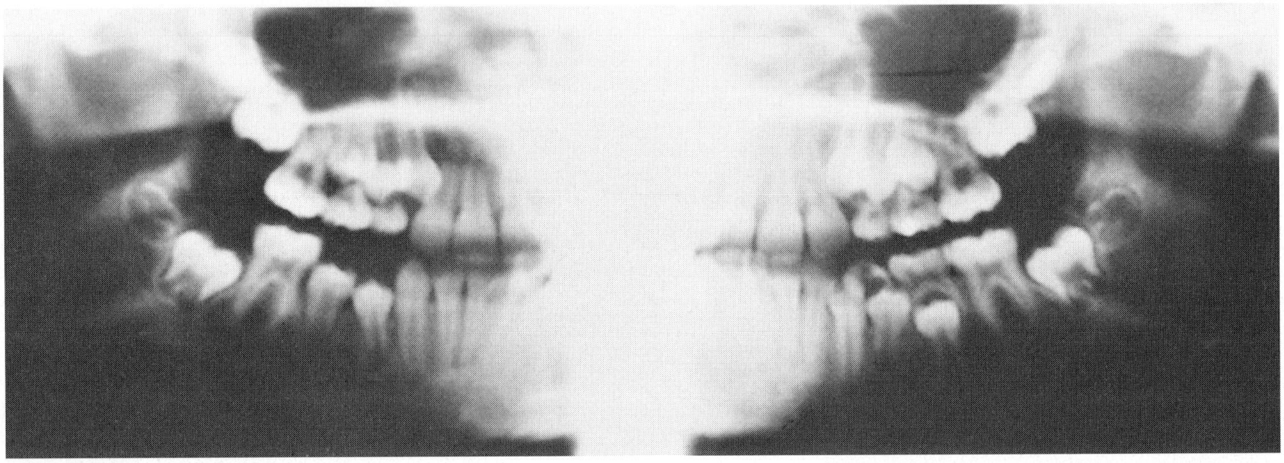

FIGURE 12-93 A complication of serial extraction is premature eruption of the permanent canines. **A,** When this occurs the first premolars are impacted between the canines and the second premolars. **B,** In this situation (note the lower right quadrant for this patient), the first premolars usually have to be surgically removed (a procedure often called enucleation).

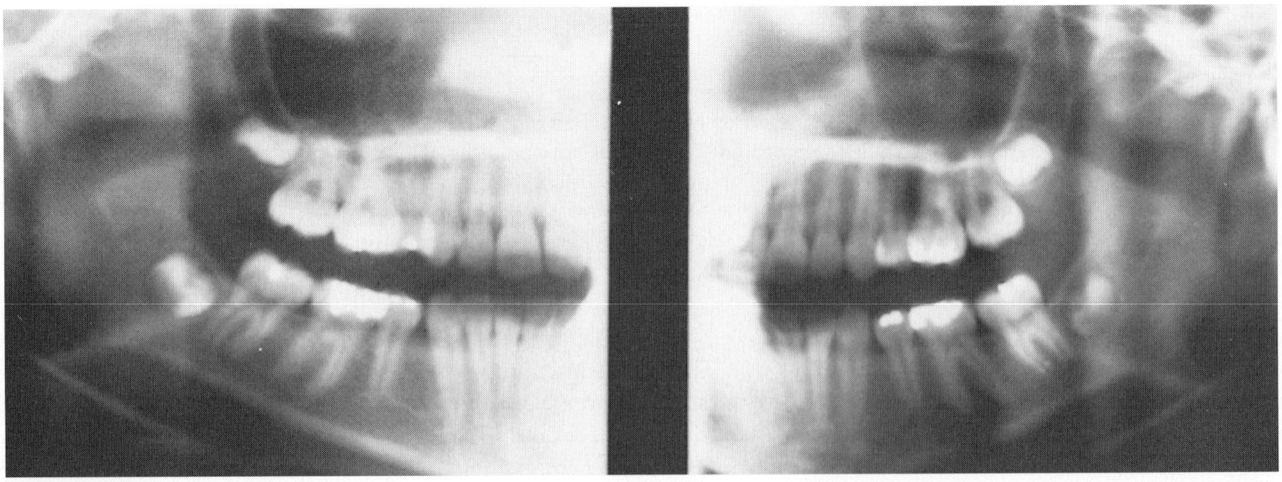

FIGURE 12-94 This patient had serial extraction that was not followed by fixed appliance treatment, with an excellent result. Properly-timed serial extraction usually results in incomplete space closure. Teeth drift together by tipping, which results in nonparallel roots between the canine and second premolar. Lack of root parallelism, residual space, and other irregularities can be addressed with subsequent fixed appliance therapy.

underused now. It can be a useful adjunct to treatment, shortening the time of comprehensive treatment if it is used correctly—but the patients must be chosen carefully and supervised carefully as they develop. It is far from a panacea for treatment of crowding.

The Borderline Crowding Case: What Do You Do?

If early extraction is only for the few patients with extremely severe crowding, and early expansion offers little advantage over expansion during later comprehensive treatment, what is the best approach to crowded and irregular teeth during the mixed dentition? The wisest course of action, in most cases, is simply to keep the options open for the later comprehensive treatment that these children will need. Unless crowding is very severe, maintaining leeway space during the last part of the transition to the permanent dentition increases the chance of successful nonextraction treatment. Early extraction of primary canines often can provide space for some spontaneous alignment of permanent incisors, and also can decrease the chance of canine impaction, but a lower lingual arch to maintain space is needed to keep the nonextraction open when this is done. Beyond that, the advantages of early appliance therapy are questionable, and must be viewed in the context of an increased burden of treatment versus little or no additional benefit.

REFERENCES

1. Langberg BJ, Arai K, Miner RM. Transverse skeletal and dental asymmetry in adults with unilateral lingual posterior crossbite. Am J Orthod Dento Orthop 127:6-15, 2005.
2. Adkins MD, Nanda RS, Currier GF. Arch perimeter changes on rapid palatal expansion. Am J Orthod 97:10-19, 1990.
3. Kutin G, Hawes R. Posterior cross-bite in the deciduous and mixed dentition. Am J Orthod 56:491-504, 1969.
4. Ranta R. Treatment of unilateral posterior crossbite: Comparison of the quad-helix and removable plate. J Dent Child 55:102-104, 1988.
5. Bell RA, LeCompte EJ. The effects of maxillary expansion using a quad-helix appliance during the deciduous and mixed dentitions. Am J Orthod 79:152-161, 1981.
6. Ngan P, Hu AM, Fields HW. Treatment of Class III problems begins with differential diagnosis of anterior crossbites. Pediatr Dent 19:386-395, 1997.
7. Ngan P, Fields H. Open bite: A review of etiology and management. Pediatr Dent 19:91-98, 1997.
8. Christensen JR, Fields HW, Adair SM. Oral habits. In: Pinkham JR, Casamassimo PS, Fields HW, McTigue DJ, Nowak AJ, eds. Pediatric Dentistry: Infancy to Adolescence. ed 4. Philadelphia: WB Saunders; 2005.
9. Paunio P, Rautava P, Sillanpa M. The Finnish family competence study: The effects of living conditions on sucking habits in 3-year-old Finnish children and the association between these habits and dental occlusion. Acta Odontol Scand 51:23-29, 1993.
10. Adair SM, Milano M, Dushku JC. Evaluation of the effects of orthodontic pacifiers on the primary dentitions of 24–59-month-old children: Preliminary study. Pediatr Dent 14:13-18, 1992.
11. Haryett R, Hansen R, Davidson P, et al. Chronic thumbsucking: The psychological effects and the relative effectiveness of the various methods of treatment. Am J Orthod 53:559-585, 1967.
12. Tyrologou S, Koch G, Kurol J. Location, complications and treatment of mesiodentes—a retrospective study in children. Swed Dent J 29:1-9, 2005.
13. Primosch R. Anterior supernumerary teeth assessment and surgical intervention in children. Pediatr Dent 3:204-215, 1981.
14. DiBase D. Mucous membrane and delayed eruption. Trans Br Soc Study Orthod 56:149-158, 1969-1970.
15. Kurol J, Thilander B. Infraocclusion of primary molars and the effect on occlusal development, a longitudinal study. Eur J Orthod 6:277-293, 1984.
16. Ekim SL, Hatibovic-Kofman S. A treatment decision-making model for infraoccluded primary molars. Int J Paediatr Dent 11:340-346, 2001.
17. Kurol J, Thilander B. Infraocclusion of primary molars with aplasia of the permanent successor: A longitudinal study. Angle Orthod 54:283-294, 1984.
18. Pulver F. The etiology and prevalence of ectopic eruption of the maxillary first permanent molar. J Dent Child 35:138-146, 1968.
19. Bjerklin K, Kurol J. Ectopic eruption of the maxillary first permanent molar: Etiologic factors. Am J Orthod 84:147-155, 1983.
20. Kennedy DB, Turley PK. The clinical management of ectopically erupting first permanent molars. Am J Orthod Dentofacial Orthop 92:336-345, 1987.
21. Bishara SE. Clinical management of impacted maxillary canines. Semin Orthod 4:87-98, 1998.
22. Ericson S, Kurol PJ. Resorption of incisors after ectopic eruption of maxillary canines: A CT study. Angle Orthod 70:415-423, 2000.
23. Baccetti T. A controlled study of associated dental anomalies. Angle Orthod 68:267-274, 1998.
24. Ericson S, Kurol J. Longitudinal study and analysis of clinical supervision of maxillary canine eruption. Community Dent Oral Epidemiol 14:172-176, 1986.
25. Ericson S, Kurol J. Early treatment of palatally erupting maxillary canines by extraction of the primary canines. Eur J Orthod 10:283-295, 1988.
26. Peck S, Peck L, Kataja M. Concomitant occurrence of canine malposition and tooth agenesis: Evidence of orofacial genetic fields. Am J Orthod Dent Orthop 122:657-660, 2002.
27. Shapira Y, Kuftinec MM. Intrabony migration of impacted teeth. Angle Orthod 73:738-743, 2003.
28. Peck S, Peck L. Classification of maxillary tooth transpositions. Am J Orthod Dent Orthop 107:505-517, 1995.
29. Shapira Y, Kuftinec MM. Tooth transposition—review of the literature and treatment considerations. Angle Orthod 59:271-276, 1989.
30. Proffit WR, Vig KW. Primary failure of eruption: A possible cause of posterior open-bite. Am J Orthod 80:173-190, 1981.
31. Bosker H, tenKate LP, Nijenhuis LE. Familial reinclusion of permanent molars. Clin Genet 13:314-320, 1978.
32. Andreasen JO, Andreasen FM. Textbook and Color Atlas of Traumatic Injuries to the Teeth. ed 3. Copenhagen: Munksgaard; 1994.
33. Turley PK, Crawford LB, Carrington KW. Traumatically intruded teeth. Angle Orthod 57:234-244, 1987.
34. Rodd HD, Davidson LE, Livesey S, Cooke ME. Survival of intentionally retained permanent incisor roots following crown root fractures in children. Dent Traumatol 18:92-97, 2002.
35. Little R, Riedel R. Postretention evaluation of stability and relapse—mandibular arches with generalized spacing. Am J Orthod 95:37-41, 1989.
36. Edwards J. The diastema, the frenum and the frenectomy: A clinical study. Am J Orthod 71:489-508, 1977.
37. Joondeph D, McNeill R. Congenitally absent second premolars: An interceptive approach. Am J Orthod 59:50-66, 1971.
38. Paulsen HU, Andreasen JO, Schwartz O. Pulp and periodontal healing, root development and root resorption subsequent to transplantation and orthodontic rotation: A long-term study of autotransplanted premolars. Am J Orthod 108:630-640, 1995.

39. Bauss O, Sadat-Khonsari R, Engelke W, Kahl-Nieke B. Results of transplanting developing third molars as part of orthodontics space management. Part 2: Results following the orthodontic treatment of transplanted developing third molars in cases of aplasia and premature loss of teeth with atrophy of the alveolar process. J Orofac Orthop 64:40-47, 2003.
40. Zachrisson BU, Stenvik A, Haanaes HR. Management of missing maxillary anterior teeth with emphasis on autotransplantation. Am J Orthod Dent Orthop 126:284-288, 2004.
41. Mayhew M, Dilley G, Dilley D, et al. Tissue response to intragingival appliances in monkeys. Pediatr Dent 6:148-152, 1984.
42. Hershey H, Houghton C, Burstone C. Unilateral face-bows: A theoretical and laboratory analysis. Am J Orthod 79:229-249, 1981.
43. O'Donnell S, Nanda RS, Ghosh J. Perioral forces and dental changes resulting from mandibular lip bumper treatment. Am J Orthod 113:247-255, 1998.
44. Nevant CT, Buschang PH, Alexander RG, Steffen JM. Lip bumper therapy for gaining arch length. Am J Orthod Dentofacial Orthop 100:330-336, 1991.
45. McInaney JB, Adams RM, Freeman M. A nonextraction approach to crowded dentitions in young children: Early recognition and treatment. J Am Dent Assoc 101:252-257, 1980.
46. Spillane LM, McNamara JA. Maxillary adaptation to expansion in the mixed dentition. Semin Orthod 1:176-187, 1995.
47. Little RM, Riedel RA, Stein A. Mandibular arch length increase during the mixed dentition: postretention evaluation of stability and relapse. Am J Orthod Dentofacial Orthop 97:393-404, 1990.
48. Gianelly AA. Crowding, timing of treatment. Angle Orthod 64:415-418, 1994.
49. Brennan M, Gianelly AA. The use of the lingual arch in the mixed dentition to resolve crowding. Am J Orthod Dent Orthop 117:81-85, 2000.
50. Lutz HD, Poulton D. Stability of dental arch expansion in the deciduous dentition. Angle Orthod 55:299-315, 1985.
51. McNamara JA, Brudon W. Orthodontic and Orthopedic Treatment in the Mixed Dentition. Ann Arbor, Mich: Needham Press; 1995.
52. Owen A. Morphologic changes in the sagittal dimension using the Frankel appliance. Am J Orthod 80:573-603, 1981.
53. Ten Hoeve A. Palatal bar and lip bumper in nonextraction treatment. J Clin Orthod 29:272-291, 1985.
54. Byloff FK, Darendeliler MA. Distal molar movement using the pendulum appliance, part 1: Clinical and radiographic indications. Angle Orthod 67:249-260, 1997.
55. Gianelly AA, Bednar J, Dietz VS. Japanese NiTi coils used to move molars distally. Am J Orthod 99:564-566; 1991.
56. Kurol J, Bjerklin K. Treatment of children with ectopic eruption of the maxillary first permanent molar by cervical traction. Am J Orthod 86:483-492, 1984.
57. Baumrind S, Korn EL, Isaacson RJ, et al. Quantitative analysis of orthodontic and orthopedic effects of maxillary traction. Am J Orthod 84:384-398, 1983.

CHAPTER

13

Treatment of Skeletal Problems in Children

CHAPTER OUTLINE

Whenever a jaw discrepancy exists, the ideal solution is to correct it by modifying the child's facial growth, so that the skeletal problem is corrected by more or less growth of one jaw than the other (Figure 13-1). Unfortunately, such an ideal solution is not always possible, but growth modification for skeletal problems can be successful.

Treatment planning for skeletal problems, and what has been learned about the optimum timing of treatment, have been discussed extensively in Chapter 8. The emphasis there is on new research that confirms the possibility of changing the way the jaws grow, emphasizes the variability of the treatment results, documents the relatively modest skeletal changes that often are produced, and notes the nearly inevitable dental changes that complement the skeletal changes to complete the treatment. These dentoalveolar changes are often overlooked, but are often the difference between successful and unsuccessful treatment.

This chapter briefly reviews the issues in treatment timing that were presented previously, but focuses on clinical treatment aimed at growth modification. Usually this is accomplished by applying forces directly to the teeth and secondarily and indirectly to the skeletal structures, instead of applying direct pressure to the bones. Tooth movement, in addition to any changes in skeletal relationships, is unavoidable. It is possible now to apply force directly against the bone by using temporary implants, bone anchors or bone screws (see Chapter 9). This approach is likely to be used more and more in the future because the dental changes that accompany growth modification often (but not always) are undesirable. Excessive tooth movement, whether it results from a weakness in the treatment plan, poor biomechanical control, or poor compliance, can cause growth modification to be incomplete and unsuccessful.

is almost impossible to control and often continues into the late teens. Excessive maxillary growth and deficient mandibular growth, which combine to produce skeletal Class II problems, fall into a middle ground. An acceleration of vertical and horizontal mandibular growth prior to adolescence usually can be generated. Even though this does not translate into a mandible that is significantly larger at the end of growth, it can benefit children who are having problems with jaw function and social acceptability. Excessive maxillary growth tends to be more vertical than horizontal, and treatment to control it has to be continued into adolescence even if it starts sooner.

Because of the rapid growth exhibited by children during the primary dentition years, it would seem that treatment of jaw discrepancies by growth modification should be successful at a very early age. The rationale for treatment at ages 4 to 6 would be that because of the rapid rate of growth and the relatively large forces on smaller and more plastic skeletal components, significant amounts of skeletal discrepancy could be overcome in a short time. This implies that once discrepancies in jaw relationships are corrected, proper function will cause harmonious growth thereafter without further treatment.

If this were the case, very early treatment (as in the primary dentition) would be advocated for many skeletal discrepancies. Unfortunately, although most anteroposterior and vertical jaw discrepancies can be corrected during the primary dentition years, relapse occurs because of continued growth in the original disproportionate pattern. If children are treated very early, they usually need further treatment during the mixed dentition and again in the early permanent dentition to maintain the correction. For all practical purposes, early orthodontic treatment for skeletal problems is mixed dentition treatment, and a second phase of treatment during adolescence will be required.

The opposite point of view would be that, since treatment in the permanent dentition will be required anyway, there is no point in starting treatment until then. Delaying treatment that long has two potential problems: (1) By the time the canines, premolars and second molars erupt there may not be enough growth remaining for effective modification, especially in girls; and (2) some children who need it would be denied the psychosocial benefits of treatment during an important period of development.

It now is clear that a child can benefit from treatment during the preadolescent years if esthetic and the resultant social problems are substantial, if he or she is trauma-prone, or if other specific indications exist—see Chapter 8. On the other hand, it seems to be neither necessary nor desirable to routinely begin treatment for many skeletal problems until the adolescent growth spurt. Beginning treatment too soon merely prolongs it unnecessarily. For each patient, the benefits of early treatment must be considered against the risk and cost of prolonging the total treatment period.

In the discussion of treatment techniques that follows, we assume that an appropriate treatment plan has been developed, based on the considerations discussed in the previous chapters.

Treatment of Transverse Maxillary Constriction

Skeletal maxillary constriction is distinguished by a narrow palatal vault (see Figure 6-66). It can be corrected by opening the midpalatal suture, which widens the roof of the mouth and the floor of the nose. This transverse expansion corrects the posterior crossbite, sometimes moves the maxilla forward, increases space in the arch, and repositions underlying permanent tooth buds. It can be done at any time prior to the end of the adolescent growth spurt. The major reasons for doing it sooner are to eliminate functional problems and mandibular shifts on closure, and to provide more space for the erupting maxillary teeth.[1,2]

Several methods of arch expansion are possible, but to obtain skeletal effects, it is necessary to place force directly across the suture. In preadolescent children, three methods can be used for palatal expansion: (1) a split removable plate with a jackscrew or heavy midline spring; (2) a lingual arch, often of the W-arch or quad-helix design; or (3) a fixed palatal expander with a jackscrew, which can be either attached to bands or incorporated into a bonded appliance. Removable plates and lingual arches produce slow expansion. The fixed expander can be activated for either rapid (0.5 mm or more per day), semi-rapid (0.25 mm/day), or slow (1 mm/week) expansion. For each of the possible methods, appropriate questions are: Does it achieve the expansion? Does it have iatrogenic side effects? and, Is the expansion stable?

Palatal Expansion in the Primary and Early Mixed Dentition

Because less force is needed to open the suture in younger children, it is relatively easy to obtain palatal expansion. In the early mixed dentition, all three types of expansion appliances produce both skeletal and dental changes.[3]

With a removable appliance, the rate of expansion must be quite slow, and the force employed during the process must be low, because faster expansion produces higher forces that create problems with retention of the appliance. Multiple clasps that are well adjusted are mandatory. Because of the instability of the teeth during the expansion process, failure to wear the appliance even for 1 day requires adjustment of the jackscrew, usually by the practitioner, to constrict the appliance until it again fits and expansion can be resumed. Compliance in activation and wear time are always issues with these appliances. Successful expansion with a removable appliance can take so much time that it is not cost-effective.

Lingual arches of the W-arch and quad helix designs (see Chapter 12) have been demonstrated to open the midpalatal

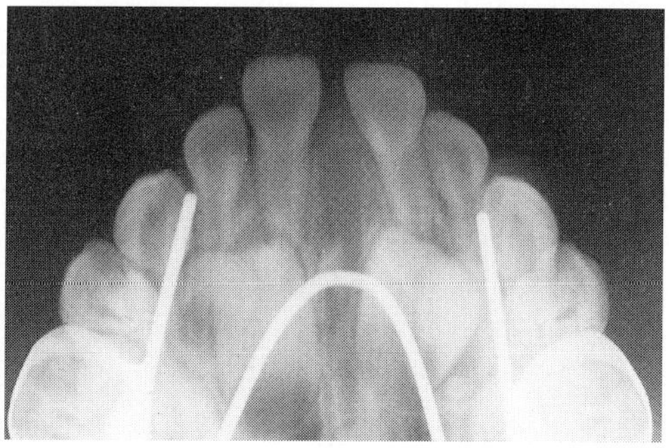

FIGURE 13-2 Prior to adolescence, the midpalatal suture can be opened during maxillary expansion using a number of methods. This occlusal radiograph taken during the primary dentition years illustrates sutural opening in response to the W-arch appliance.

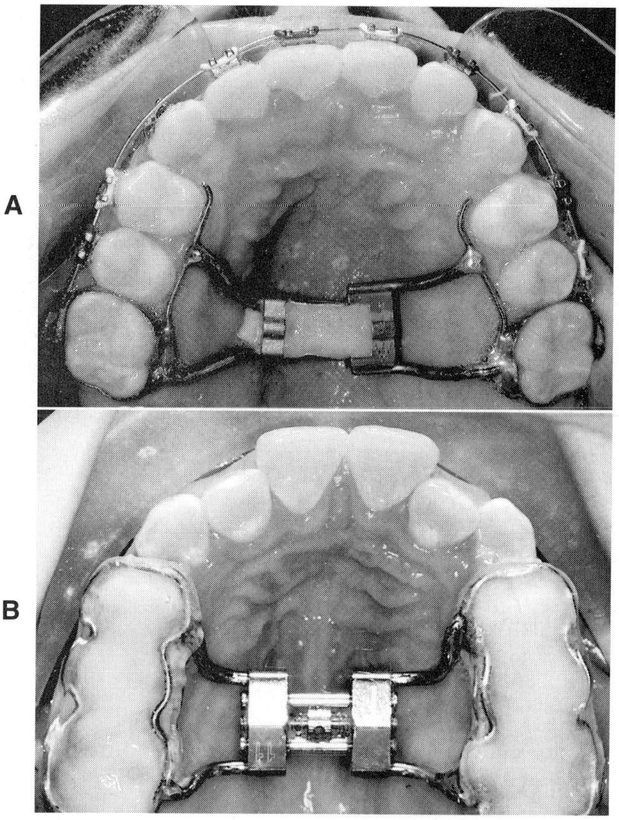

FIGURE 13-3 **A,** This banded palatal expander with a jack screw to supply the force has been stabilized using cold cure acrylic after rapid expansion to maintain the expansion while bone fills in at the suture. This will remain in place for 3 months. **B,** A bonded palatal expander in a mixed dentition child, with acrylic extending over the occlusal surfaces of the teeth to provide more surface for bonding. In effect, bite blocks have been placed between the posterior teeth, which decreases elongation of the teeth as expansion occurs and limits the amount of downward-backward rotation of the mandible.

suture in young patients (Figure 13-2). These appliances generally deliver a few hundred grams of force and provide slow expansion. They are relatively clean and reasonably effective, producing a mix of skeletal and dental change.

Fixed jackscrew appliances attached to bands or bonded splints also can be used in the early treatment of maxillary constriction. Banding permanent molars and primary second molars is relatively simple, but banding primary first molars can be challenging. Using a bonded appliance in the mixed dentition is relatively straightforward. This appliance can deliver a variety of forces and can extinguish habits by virtue of its bulk. In young children, in comparison with a lingual arch, there are two major disadvantages. First, the fixed jackscrew appliance is more bulky than an expansion lingual arch and more difficult to place and remove. The patient inevitably has problems in cleaning it, and either the patient or parent must activate the appliance. Second, a fixed appliance of this type can be activated rapidly, which in young children is a disadvantage, not an advantage. Rapid expansion should not be done in a young child. There is a risk of distortion of facial structures with rapid expansion (see Figure 8-14), and there is no evidence that rapid movement and high forces produce better or more stable expansion.

Many functional appliances incorporate some components to expand the maxillary arch either intrinsic force-generating mechanisms like springs and jackscrews or buccal shields to relieve buccal soft tissue pressure. When arch expansion occurs during functional appliance treatment, it is possible that some opening of the midpalatal suture contributes to it, but the precise mix of skeletal and dental change is not well-documented.

On balance, therefore, slow expansion with an active lingual arch is the preferred approach to maxillary constriction in young children in the primary and early mixed dentitions. A fixed jackscrew appliance is an acceptable alternative if activated carefully and slowly.

Palatal Expansion in the Late Mixed Dentition

With increasing age, the midpalatal suture becomes more and more tightly interdigitated, but in most individuals, it remains possible to obtain significant increments in maxillary width up to age 15 to 18. Expansion in adolescents is discussed in some detail in Chapter 14.

Even in the late mixed dentition, sutural expansion requires placing a relatively heavy force directed across the suture to move the halves of the maxilla apart. A fixed jackscrew appliance (either banded or bonded) is required (Figure 13-3). As many teeth as possible should be included in the anchorage unit. In the late mixed dentition, root resorption of primary molars may have reached the point that these teeth offer little resistance, and it may be wise to wait for eruption of the first premolars before beginning expansion.

Although some studies have reported increases in vertical facial height with maxillary expansion,[4] long-term

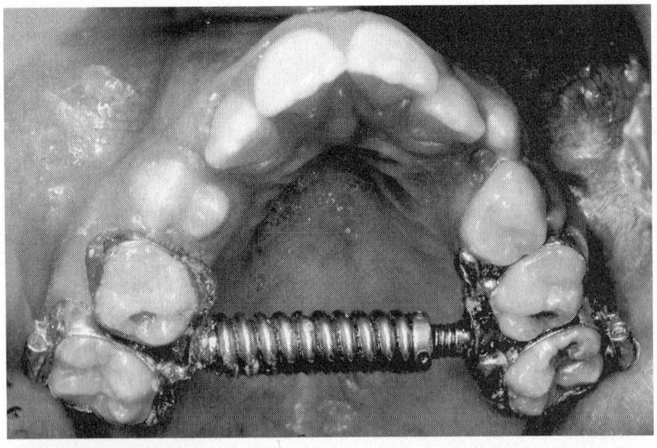

FIGURE 13-4 This expander uses a coil spring to provide the force as the stop on the threaded connector is turned. It takes more space in the palate, but can be calibrated to determine and monitor the amount of force that it delivers. This prevents either low or excessive forces when the expansion is moving faster or slower than expected, respectively. Note the attachment to banded second primary molars and permanent first molars.

evidence indicates this change is transitory.[5] A bonded appliance that covers the occlusal surface of the posterior teeth may be a better choice for a child with a long face tendency by producing less mandibular rotation than a banded appliance,[6] but this is not totally clear.[7] Perhaps the best summary is that the older the patient when maxillary expansion is done, the less likely it is that vertical changes will be recovered by subsequent growth.

Rapid or Slow Expansion?

In the late mixed dentition, either rapid or slow expansion is clinically acceptable. As we have reviewed in some detail in Chapter 8, it now appears that slower activation of the expansion appliance (i.e., at the rate of about 1 mm/week) provides approximately the same ultimate result over a 10- to 12-week period as rapid expansion, with less trauma to the teeth and bones (see Figure 8-15).

Rapid expansion typically is done with two turns daily of the jackscrew (0.5 mm activation). This creates 10 to 20 pounds of pressure across the suture—enough to create microfractures of interdigitating bone spicules. When a screw is the activating device, the force is transmitted immediately to the teeth and then to the suture. Sometimes a large coil spring is incorporated along with the screw, which modulates the amount of force, depending on the length and stiffness of the spring (Figure 13-4). The suture opens wider and faster anteriorly because closure begins in the posterior area of the midpalatal suture and there is a buttressing effect of the other maxillary structures in the posterior regions. With rapid or semi-rapid expansion, a diastema usually appears between the central incisors as the bones separate in this area (Figure 13-5). Expansion usually is continued until the maxillary lingual cusps occlude with the lingual inclines of the buccal cusps of the mandibular molars. When expansion has been completed, a 3-month period of retention with the appliance in place is recommended. After the 3-month retention period, the fixed appliance can be removed, but a removable retainer that covers the palate is often needed as further insurance against early relapse (Figure 13-6). A relatively heavy, expanded maxillary archwire provides retention if further treatment is being accomplished immediately.

The theory behind rapid activation was that force on the teeth would be transmitted to the bone, and the two halves of the maxilla would separate before significant tooth movement could occur. In other words, rapid activation was conceived as a way to maximize skeletal change and minimize dental change. It was not realized initially that during the time it takes for bone to fill in the space that was created between the left and right halves of the maxilla, skeletal relapse begins to occur almost immediately, even though the teeth are held in position. The central diastema closes from a combination of skeletal relapse and tooth movement created by stretched gingival fibers. The net treatment effect therefore is approximately equal skeletal and dental expansion.

Slow activation of the expansion appliance at the rate of 1 mm/week, which produces about 2 pounds of pressure in a mixed dentition child, opens the suture at a rate that is close to the maximum speed of bone formation.[8] The suture is not obviously pulled apart on radiographs, and no midline diastema appears, but both skeletal and dental changes occur. After 10 to 12 weeks, approximately the same roughly equal amounts of skeletal and dental expansion are present that were seen at the same time with rapid expansion. When bonded slow and rapid palatal expanders in early adolescents were compared, the major difference was greater expansion across the canines in the rapid expansion group. This translated into a predicted greater arch perimeter change but similar opening of the suture posteriorly.[9] So, by using slow palatal expansion (one turn every other day) in a typical fixed expansion appliance, or by using a spring to produce about 2 pounds of force, effective expansion with minimal disruption of the suture can be achieved for a late mixed dentition child.

Clinical Management of Palatal Expansion Devices

Most traditional palate expansion devices use bands for retention on first premolars and permanent first molars if possible. During the late mixed dentition years the first premolars often are not fully erupted and are difficult to band. If the primary second molars are firm, they can be banded along with the permanent first molars. Alternatively, only the permanent first molars can be banded. With this approach, the appliance is generally extended anteriorly, contacting the other posterior primary and erupting permanent teeth near their gingival margins.

The bands are stabilized in an impression while it is poured, so they are retained in the completed working model. A soldered wire framework and plastic palatal portions, if desired, are added during appliance fabrication.

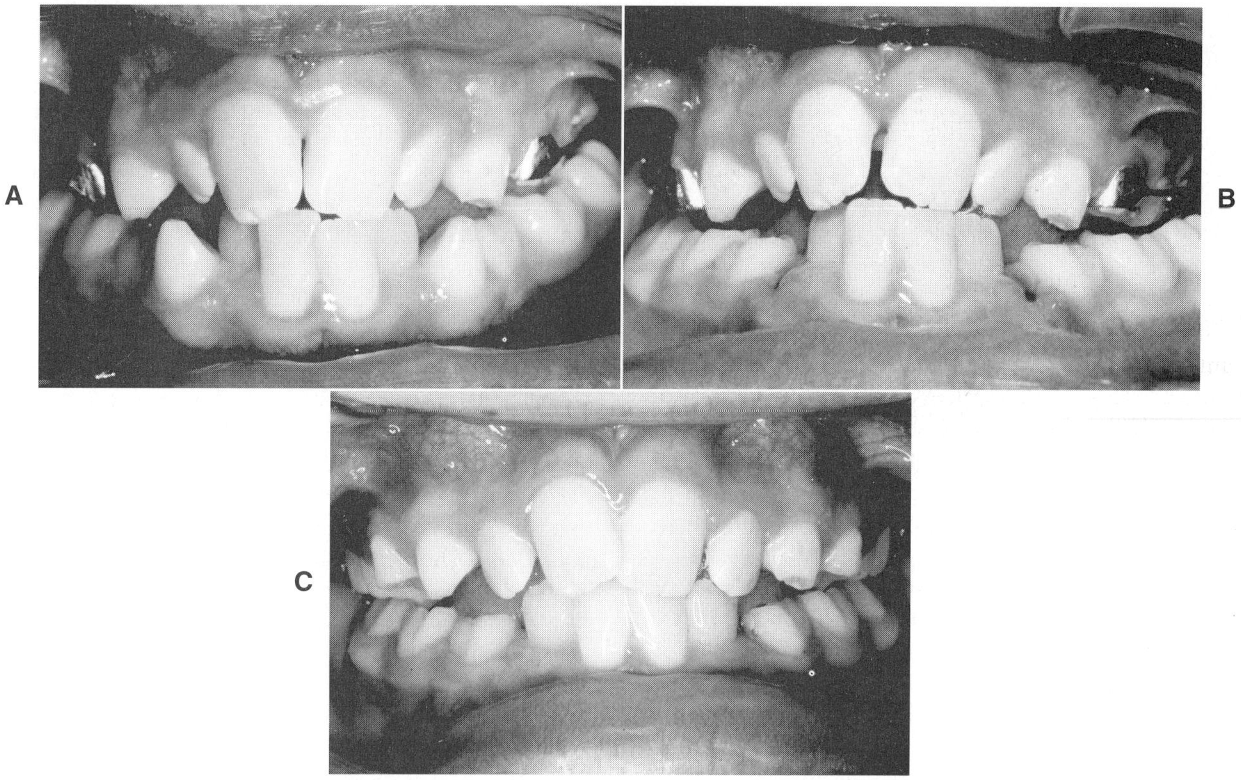

Figure 13-5 Spacing of the maxillary central incisors during rapid palatal expansion. **A,** When the appliance is placed and treatment begins, there is only a tiny diastema; **B,** After 1 week of expansion, the teeth have moved laterally with the skeletal structures. A larger diastema will be present as expansion continues; **C,** After retention, a combination of skeletal relapse and pull of the gingival fibers has brought the incisors together and closed the diastema.

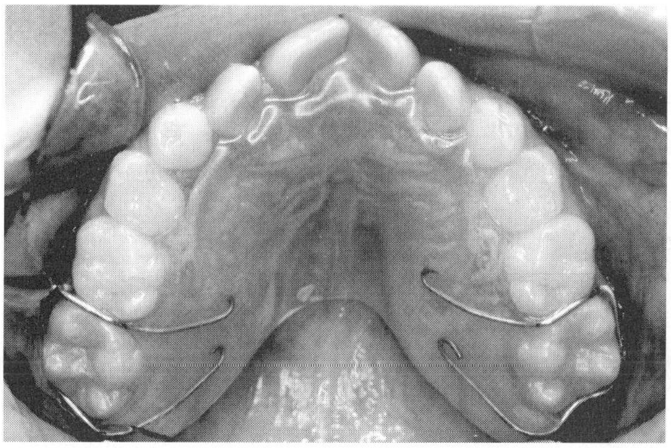

Figure 13-6 After the expander is removed, typically 3 months after palatal expansion is completed, an acrylic retainer that covers the palate still is needed to control relapse and stabilize the skeletal components.

After crossbite correction is completed, band removal can be difficult because the teeth are mobile and sensitive. In those cases, sectioning the bands is appropriate.

An alternative approach is to use a bonded palatal expander (see Figure 13-3, *B*). During fabrication of the working casts, plastic is generally extended over the occlusal and facial and lingual surfaces of the posterior teeth. When the appliance is returned from the laboratory, because of poor dimensional stability and distortion of the plastic portion, it may be necessary to relieve the acrylic where it seats on the maxillary teeth, reline this area with additional plastic, and refit the appliance in the mouth. By removing the appliance before final polymerization, it can be trimmed and further adjusted without complication. Generally, a composite resin is used to retain the appliance, with only the facial and lingual surfaces of the posterior teeth etched. Etching the occlusal surface is not recommended—bonding there is unnecessary for retention and can greatly complicate appliance removal.

Removal of the appliance is accomplished with a band remover engaged under a facial or lingual plastic margin, and is facilitated by including loops of wire extending from the facial surfaces (see Figure 14-12). The appliance can be sectioned, but this is time-consuming and usually unnecessary. Complete resin removal can be laborious, so using only an adequate amount of resin is crucial. There is a delicate balance. Inadequate resin will lead to excessive leakage onto the nonbonded surfaces, which can result in decalcification, or appliance loss. Too much resin, on the other hand, can make tooth and appliance cleaning, as well as appliance removal, difficult. For these reasons, some clinicians use glass ionomer cement for retention. The strength of the material usually is adequate but bonding failure may occur. Fluoride release from these cements may prove advantageous in the short term.

TREATMENT OF CLASS III PROBLEMS: MAXILLARY DEFICIENCY AND MANDIBULAR EXCESS

Anteroposterior and Vertical Maxillary Deficiency

Both anteroposterior and vertical maxillary deficiency can contribute to Class III malocclusion. If the maxilla is small or positioned posteriorly, the effect is direct. If it does not grow vertically, the mandible rotates upward and forward, producing an appearance of mandibular prognathism that may be due more to the position of the mandible than its size.

For children with a-p and vertical maxillary deficiency, the preferred treatment is to use a reverse-pull headgear (face mask) to move the maxilla into a more anterior and inferior position, which also increases its size as bone is added at the posterior and superior sutures. As with transverse expansion, it is easier and more effective to move the maxilla forward at younger ages, although recent reports indicate that some a-p changes can be produced up to the beginning of adolescence.[10,11] Probably a variety of ages are acceptable after the permanent incisors have erupted, up to the age of 10.[12] When force is applied to the teeth for transmission to the sutures, tooth movement in addition to skeletal change is inevitable. This type of treatment is best used in children who have true maxillary problems and not combinations of maxillary and mandibular problems. It is also most suited for those with modest to minor skeletal problems so that the teeth nearly touch in CR or are within several millimeters of each other.

Clinical Management of Facemask Treatment

Generally, it is better to defer maxillary protraction until the permanent first molars have erupted and can be incorporated into the anchorage unit. Many clinicians use protraction with a facemask following or simultaneously with palatal expansion, because some evidence suggests that the expansion makes antero-posterior skeletal change more likely.[12] There is other evidence that the expansion is optional and should be dictated by the maxillary arch width related to the lower arch width.[13]

The facemask obtains anchorage from the forehead and chin (Figure 13-7). The forward force on the maxilla is generated via elastics that attach to a maxillary appliance. To resist tooth movement as much as possible, the maxillary teeth should be splinted together as a single unit. The maxillary appliance can be banded, bonded, or removable (Figure 13-8). A removable plastic splint that covers the occlusal surfaces of the teeth often is satisfactory. Multiple clasps combined with plastic that extends over the incisal edges usually provide adequate retention. If necessary, the splint can be bonded in place, but this causes hygiene problems and should be avoided if possible for long-term use. It

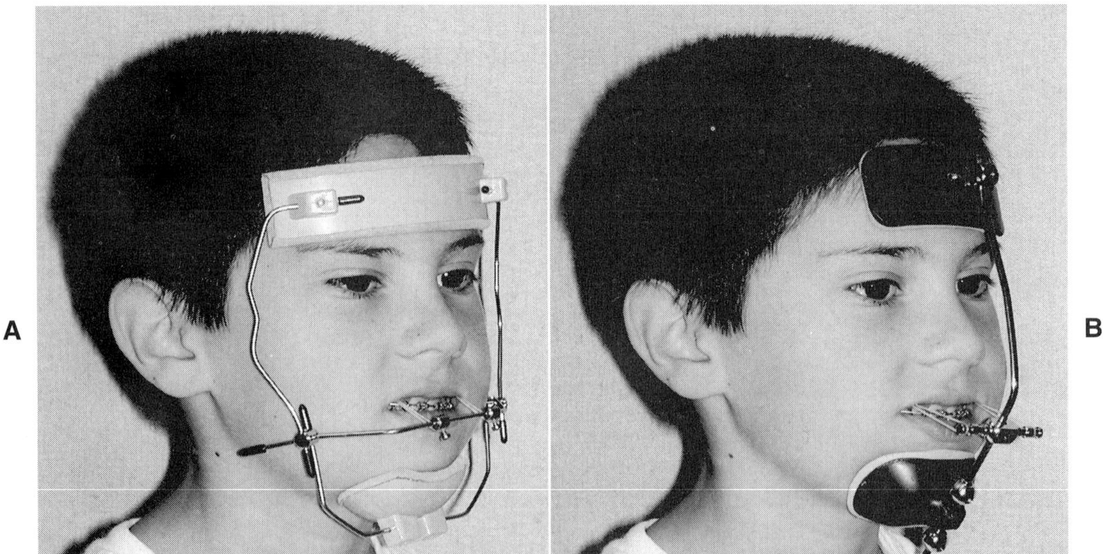

FIGURE 13-7 **A,** This Delaire-type face mask offers good stability when used for maxillary protraction. Note the direction of pull of the elastics is down and forward. **B,** This rail-style face mask provides more comfort during sleeping and is less difficult to adjust. It also can be adjusted to accommodate some vertical mandibular movement. Clinical experience indicates that some children will prefer one type over the other.

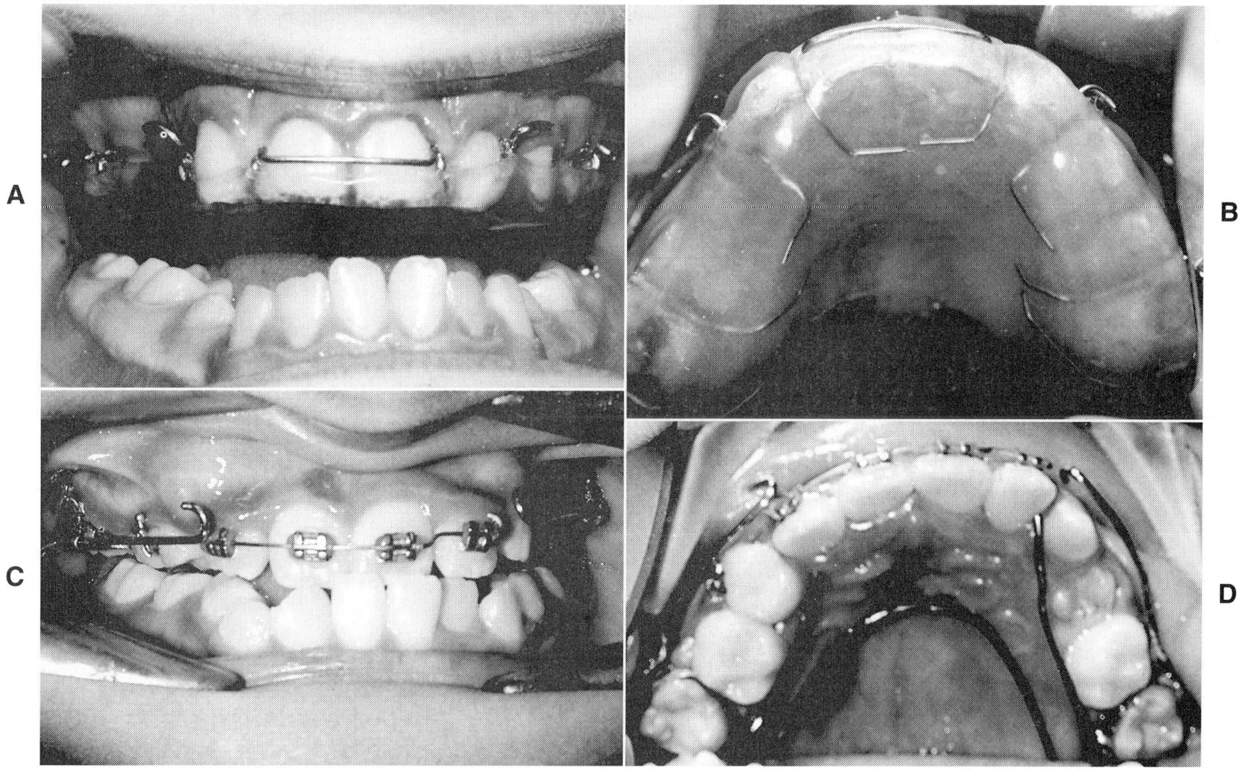

FIGURE 13-8 A maxillary removable splint is often used to make the upper arch a single unit for maxillary protraction. **A,** The splint incorporates hooks in the canine-premolar region for attachment of elastics and **(B)** should cover the anterior and posterior teeth and occlusal surfaces for best retention. Note that the hooks extend gingivally, so that the line of force comes closer to the center of resistance of the maxilla. Multiple clasps also aid in retention. **C-D,** A banded expander or wire splint also can be used. It consists of bands on primary and permanent molars (or just permanent molars) connected by a palatal wire for expansion and hooks on the facial for attachment of the face mask.

also is possible to use a heavy wire splint that incorporates a lingual arch (for arch expansion) cemented to the primary and molars and whatever permanent teeth are available (see Figure 13-8, *C*). Whatever the method of attachment, the appliance must have hooks for attachment to the face mask that are located in the canine-primary molar area above the occlusal plane. This places the force vector nearer the center of resistance of the maxilla and limits maxillary rotation (Figure 13-9).

For most young children, a facemask is as acceptable as conventional headgear. Contouring an adjustable facemask for a comfortable fit on the forehead is not difficult for most children. There are a variety of designs that accommodate mandibular movement and eyeglasses if necessary. The plastic forehead and chin pads occasionally require relining with an adhesive-backed protective pad for an ideal fit or to reduce soft tissue irritation.

Approximately 350-450 grams of force per side is applied for 12-14 hours per day. Most children with maxillary deficiency are deficient vertically as well as anteroposteriorly, which means that a slight downward direction of elastic traction between the intraoral attachment and the facemask frame often is desirable. Moving the maxilla down as well as forward rotates the mandible downward and backward,

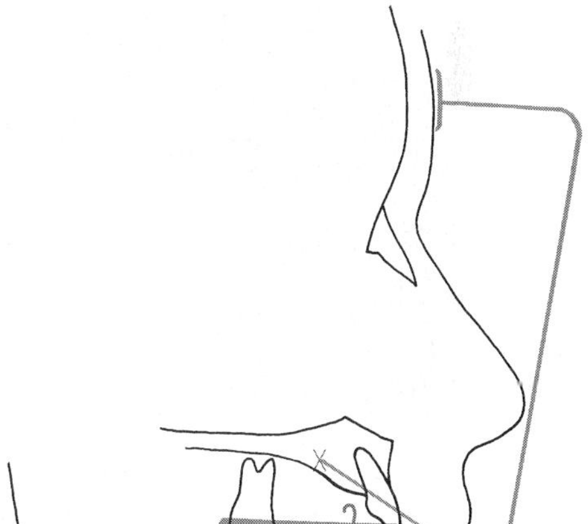

FIGURE 13-9 With the splint over the maxillary teeth and forward pull from the facemask, the hooks on the splint should be elevated. Even so, the line of force is likely to be below the center of resistance of the maxilla, so some downward rotation of the posterior maxilla and opening of the bite anteriorly can be anticipated.

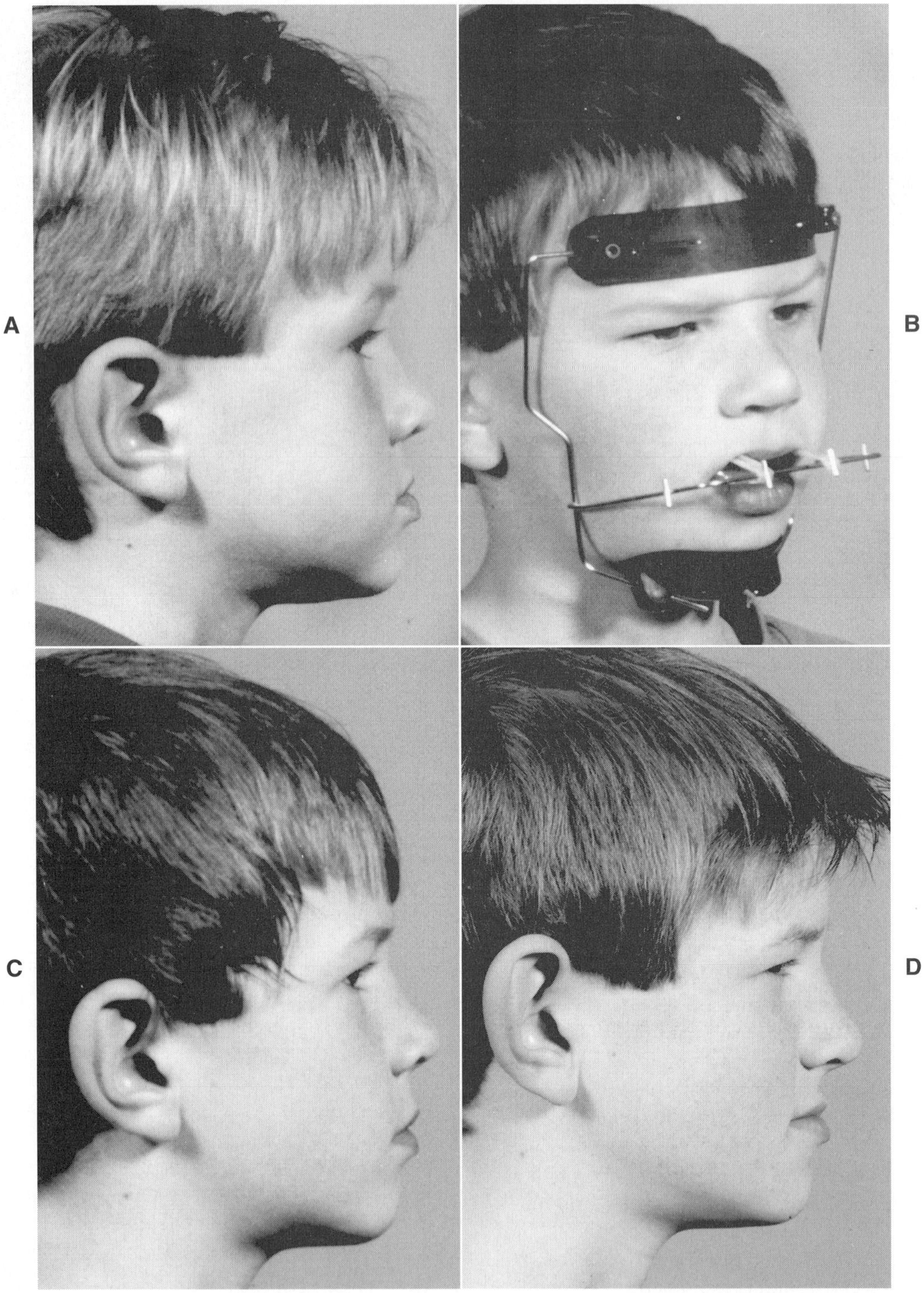

FIGURE 13-10 If forward traction is applied at an early age, it is possible to produce forward displacement of the jaw rather than just displacing teeth. **A,** Age 5 years 2 months, prior to treatment; **B,** Age 5-2, wearing a Delaire-style face mask; **C,** Age 7-10, at the time face mask treatment was discontinued. Note the increased fullness of the mid-face. **D,** Age 11-3, at the beginning of phase 2 treatment;

which contributes to correction of a skeletal Class III relationship. A downward pull would be contraindicated if lower face height were already large. Data for long-term outcomes of facemask treatment, however, suggest that when downward mandibular rotation occurs during the initial treatment, subsequent mandibular growth tends to have a greater horizontal component that increases the chance of eventual relapse into anterior crossbite.

Backward displacement of the mandibular teeth and forward displacement of the maxillary teeth also typically occur in response to this type of treatment (Figure 13-10).[14] As children come closer to adolescence, mandibular rotation

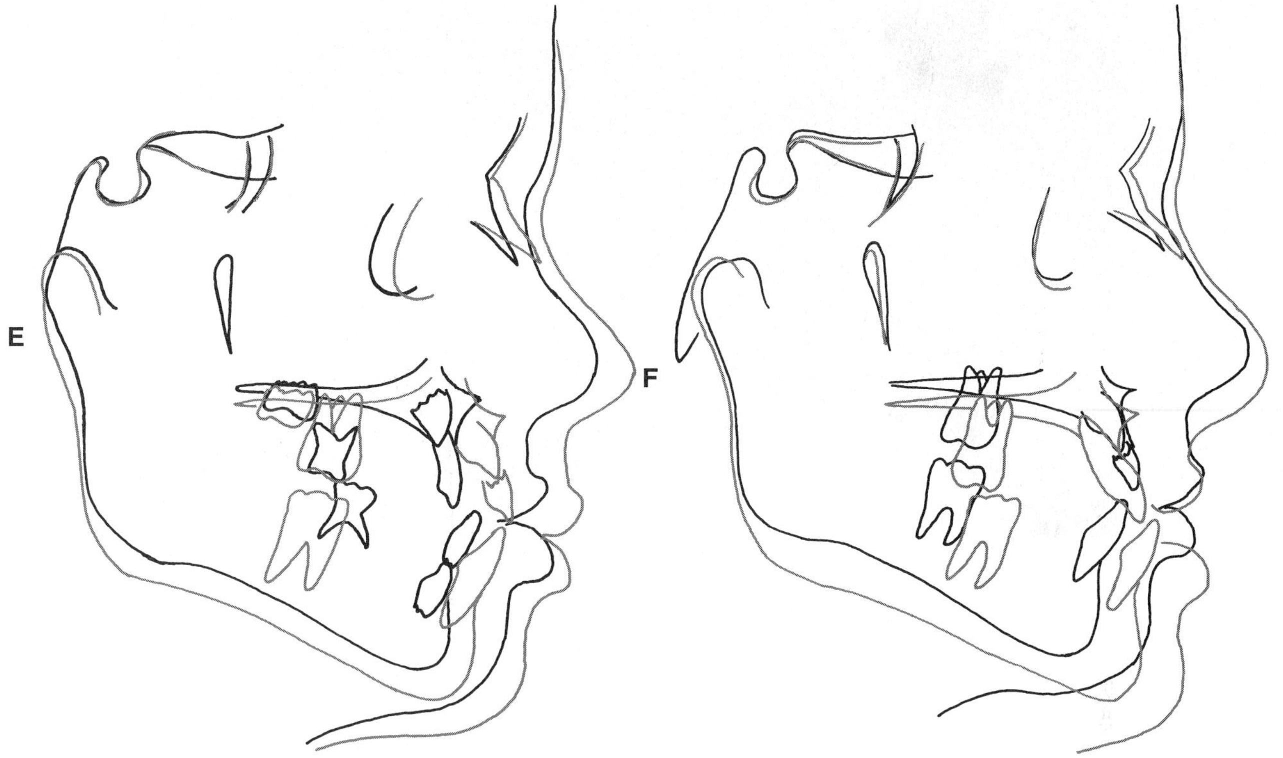

FIGURE 13-10 **cont'd E,** Cephalometric superimposition showing the changes during face mask treatment; **F,** Superimposition showing the changes ages 8-11 following treatment. When face mask treatment is discontinued, there usually is a rebound of mandibular growth similar to what occurred for this patient. Whether surgery eventually will be required will be determined by mandibular growth during and after adolescence. (From Proffit WR, White RP, Sarver DM. Contemporary Treatment of Dentofacial Deformity. St. Louis: Mosby; 2003.)

and displacement of maxillary teeth—not forward movement of the maxilla—are the major components of the treatment result.

Controlling Tooth Movement by Applying Force to Implants

Clearly, a major negative side effect of the maxillary protraction procedure is maxillary dental movement that detracts from the skeletal change. Shapiro and Kokich deliberately ankylosed primary canines so they could be used as "natural implants."[15] With traction against a maxillary arch stabilized by these teeth, they were able to demonstrate approximately 3 mm of maxillary protraction in 1 year, with minimal dental change. If a child with maxillary retrusion has spontaneous ankylosis of primary molars, a splint can be fabricated to use these teeth as implants and gain the same biomechanical advantage (Figure 13-11). It now is possible to use temporary bone anchors[16] (see Figure 19-16) as a point of attachment, avoiding pressure against the teeth and making protraction possible even if teeth are missing (see Figure 8-16), and it is likely that this method will come into regular clinical use in the near future. The lower density of the bone in preadolescents and avoiding damage to unerupted permanent teeth pose substantial problems to overcome, but the principle is sound.

Functional Appliances for Maxillary Protraction

Another possible treatment for correction of maxillary deficiency is a functional appliance made with the mandible positioned posteriorly and rotated open and with pads to stretch the upper lip forward. In theory, the lip pads used in Frankel's FR-III appliance (Figure 13-12), stretch the periosteum in a way that stimulates forward growth of the maxilla. The available data, however, indicate little true forward movement of the upper jaw.[17] Instead, most of the improvement is from dental changes. The appliance, which allows the maxillary molars to erupt and move mesially while holding the lower molars in place vertically and anteroposteriorly, tips the maxillary anterior teeth facially and retracts the mandibular anterior teeth (Figure 13-13). This tooth movement helps in the development of a normal overbite and overjet but has little effect on the skeletal malocclusion. Rotation of the occlusal plane also contributes to the change from a Class III to a Class I molar relationship (Figure 13-14). If the functional appliance rotates the chin down and back (see the following section), the Class III relationship will improve, but again with no effect on the maxilla. In short, functional appliance treatment, even with the use of upper lip pads, has little or no effect on maxillary retrusion and if considered should be used on extremely mild cases.

A,B

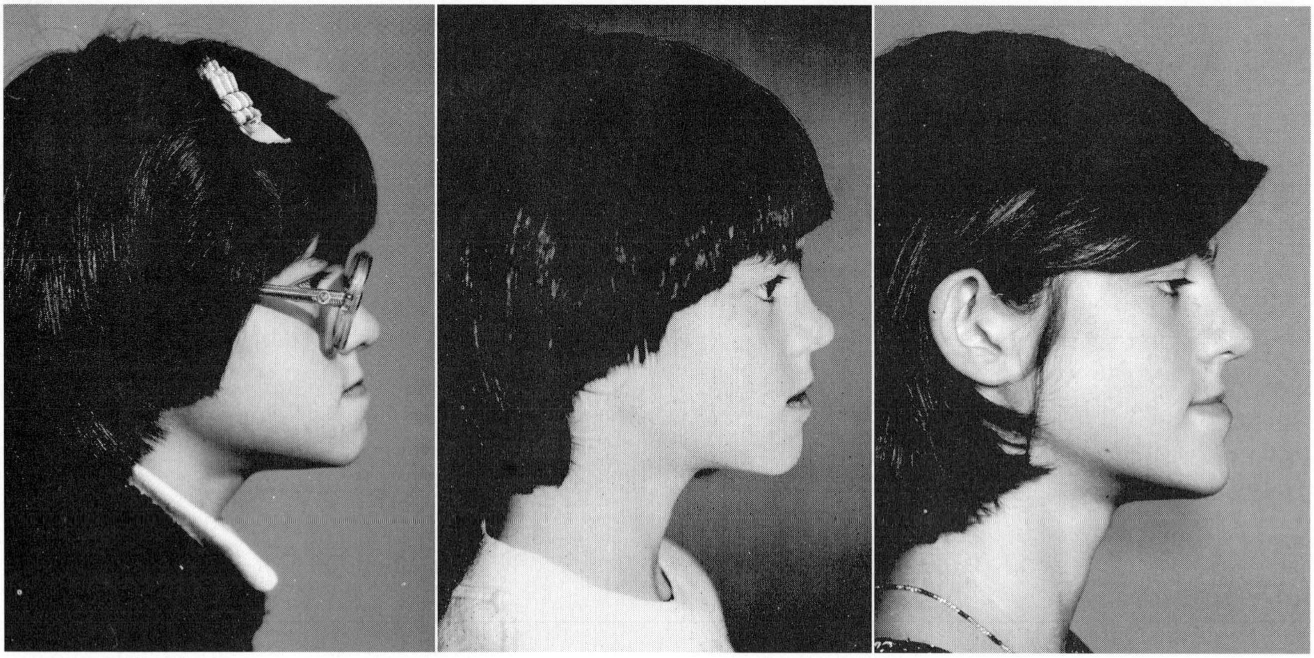

C

D

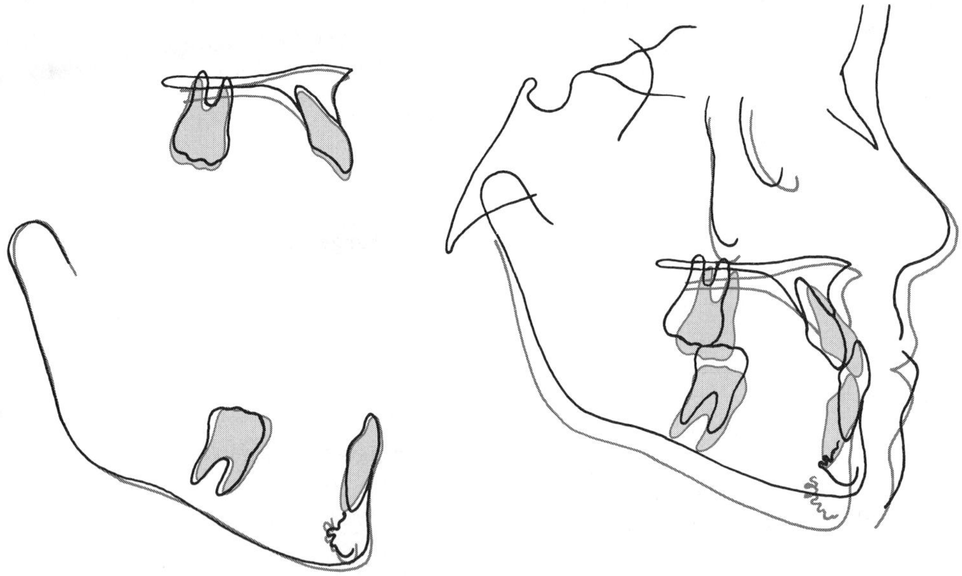

E

FIGURE 13-11 When ankylosed primary teeth are available for attachment of a facemask, an improved skeletal response can be obtained, as in this patient. **A,** Pre-treatment profile; **B,** Post-treatment profile; **C,** Profile 3 years later. Continued mandibular growth is always a risk, especially when a face mask is used for other than solely maxillary problems. **D,** Cephalometric superimpositions showing the changes during treatment. Note the improvement in the facial concavity and downward-backward rotation of the mandible, with almost totally skeletal and no dental change. The maxilla rotated down posteriorly, as would be predicted from the relationship of the line of force to its center of resistance. If sustained, this would have been an excellent result.

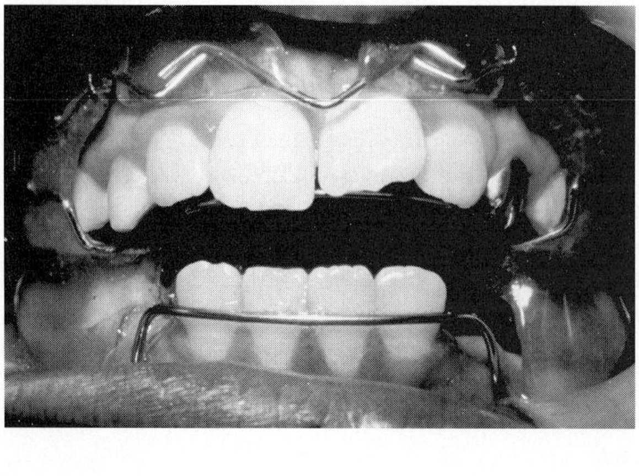

FIGURE 13-12 The Frankel-III appliance stretches the soft tissue adjacent to the maxilla, attempting to stimulate forward growth of the maxilla by stretching the periosteum, and does not advance the mandible. The vertical opening is used to enhance downward and forward eruption of maxillary posterior teeth.

A B

C

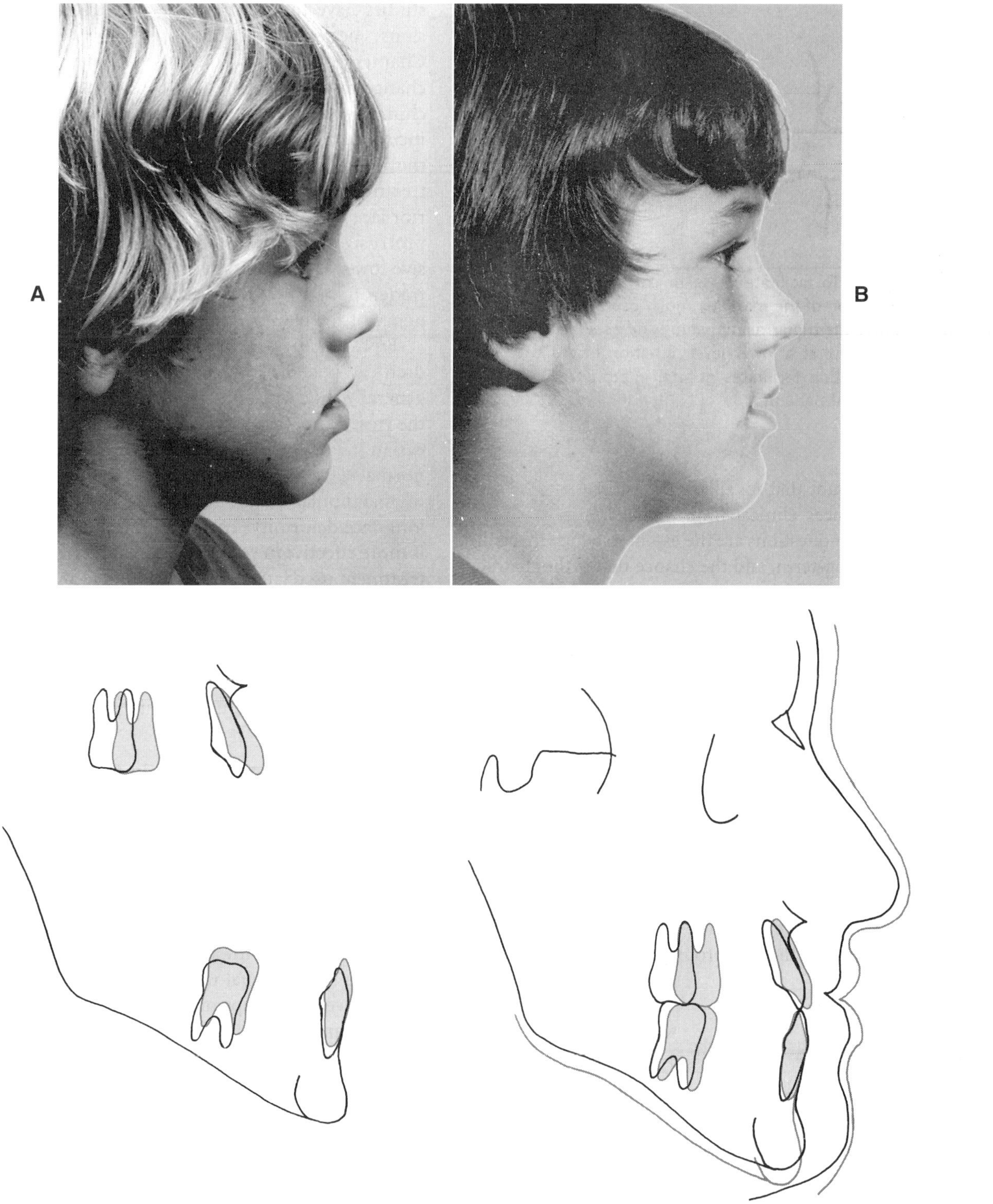

Figure 13-13 Response to a Class III functional appliance. **A,** Pre-treatment profile; **B,** Post-treatment profile; **C,** Cephalometric superimpositions. Note in the cranial base superimposition that the mandible rotated inferiorly and posteriorly to a less prominent position. The maxillary incisors moved facially and the mandibular teeth erupted so that occlusal contact was maintained. In essence, this method trades increased face height for decreased chin prominence.

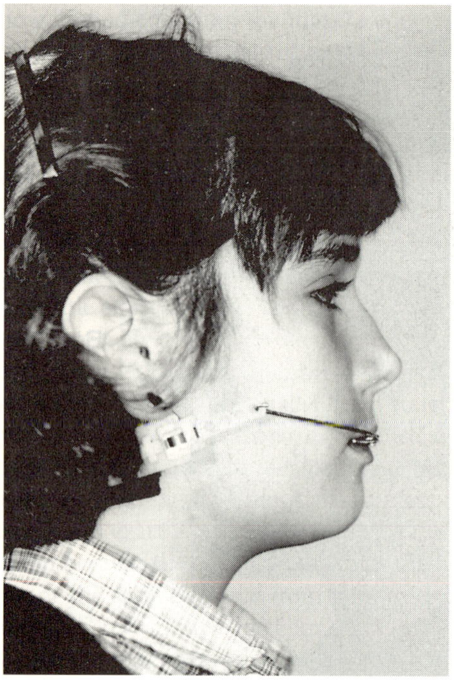

FIGURE 13-20 Kloehn-type cervical headgear. This appliance, which uses a cervical neckstrap and a facebow to produce distal force on the maxillary teeth and maxilla, is aimed at controlling maxillary size and position but is only effective if spontaneous mandibular growth also occurs.

appropriate working bite can be obtained with the mandible positioned anteriorly and inferiorly to correct the horizontal and vertical deficiency. To control their tendency to relapse lingually, the repositioned incisors should be held in place for several months before the active functional appliance therapy begins.

Impressions and Working Bite

The next step in the use of a removable functional appliance is to make impressions of the upper and lower arches and register the desired mandibular position, the "working bite." The impression technique depends on the appliance components that will be used. Good reproduction of the teeth and an accurate representation of the area where the lingual pads or flanges will be placed are mandatory. If buccal shields or lip pads are to be used, it is important not to overextend the impressions so that tissue is displaced, because this makes it difficult or impossible to accurately locate the appliance components in the vestibule. Improper location of the components leads to long-term soft tissue irritation, discomfort, difficulty in appliance adjustment, and poor patient compliance.

For the working bite, multiple layers of a wax hard enough to maintain its integrity after cooling to room temperature are needed. The patient's preliminary record casts can be used to trim the wax to a size that will register all posterior teeth, while not covering the anterior teeth or contacting the retromolar areas (Figure 13-23). With the anterior teeth exposed, the position of the mandible easily can be judged while the bite is being taken. Care must be exercised to avoid any soft tissue interference with the wax, which will deflect the mandible or interfere with closure. This is most likely to occur in the retromolar pad region. If such an interference is not detected, the finished appliance will not seat correctly. At best, this will require reduction of the posterior plastic stops if they were integrated into the design. At worst, a new bite registration and appliance will be necessary.

The working bite is obtained by advancing the mandible forward to move the condyles out of the fossa. Unless an asymmetry is to be corrected, the mandible should be advanced symmetrically so that the pretreatment midline relationships do not change appreciably. We recommend a 4 to 6 mm advancement, but always one that is comfortable for the patient and does not move the incisors past an edge-to-edge incisor relationship. From a scientific perspective it appears that quite large, modest or relatively small advancements all can produce growth modification, and that there is little difference between the results.[32]

The practical reason for recommending this modest advancement is better patient comfort, facial esthetics and patient compliance than with large advancements. Small advancements lead to the need for more appliance adjustments. The claim that small advancements are more effective because muscle adaptation is better have not been supported by evidence.

When the mandible is advanced, the bite also must be opened. There must be enough space for the laboratory technician to place wire and plastic between the teeth to connect major components of the appliance and construct occlusal and incisor stops. The minimal posterior opening to achieve the vertical space is about 3 to 4 mm. If dental changes from differential eruption are not a major part of the desired treatment response, wire occlusal stops (as in the Frankel appliance) can be used at this minimal opening. Interocclusal stops or facets to guide eruption, as in most activators and bionators, usually require 4 to 5 mm of posterior separation to be effective. If eruption of upper and lower posterior teeth is to be limited, as in a child with excessive vertical face height (see further discussion later in this chapter), the working bite should be taken with the patient open 2 to 3 mm past the resting vertical dimension (i.e., 5 to 6 mm total opening in the molar region), so that the soft tissue stretch against the bite blocks will produce a continuous force opposing eruption.

In preparation for obtaining the working bite, the wax is softened in hot water, while the child is directed to practice the working bite position. Some children can easily reproduce working bites after only a few practice tries, but others need more opportunities and perhaps some help. It is possible to aid these patients by constructing an index to guide them. This is most easily accomplished by using a stack of

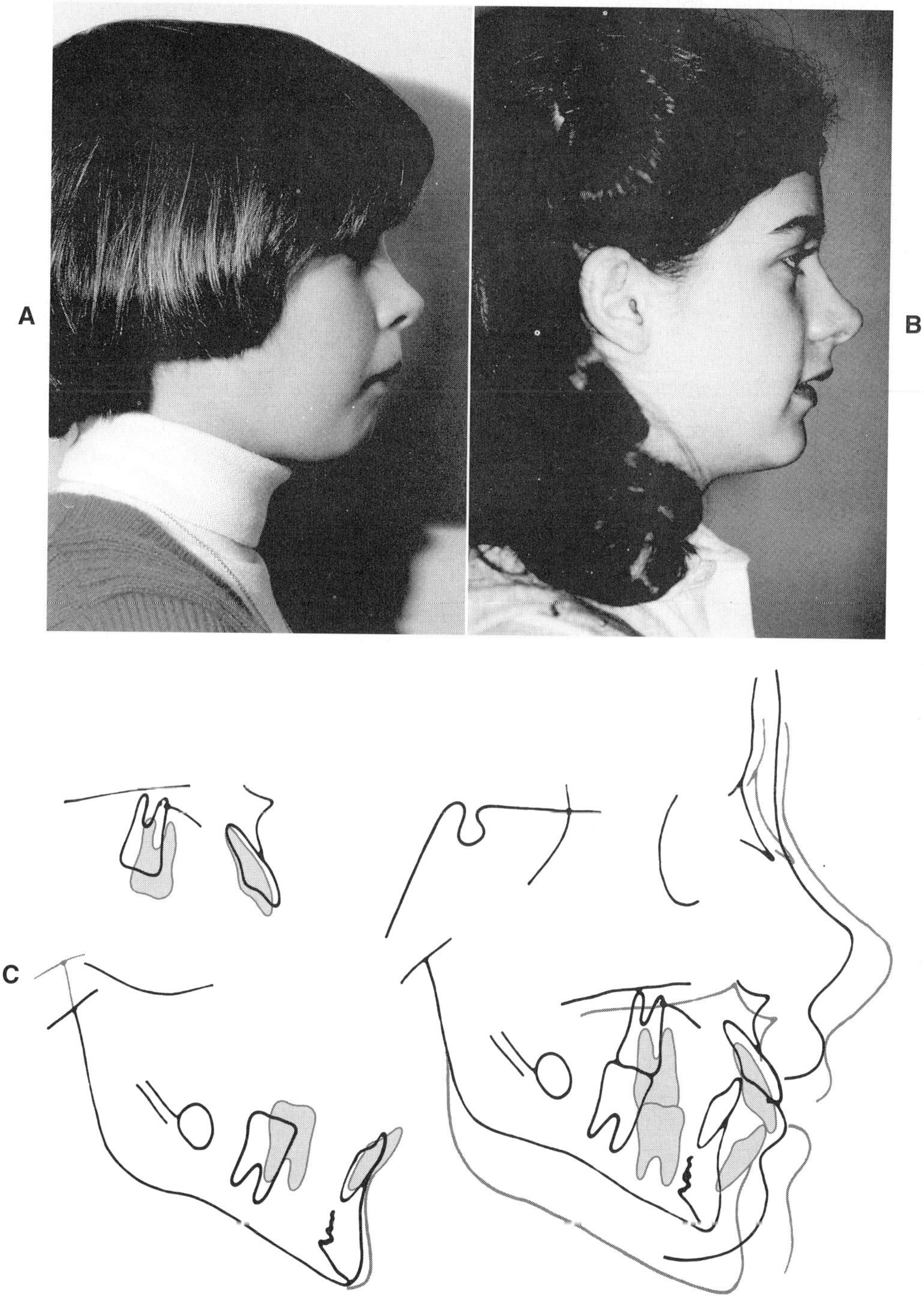

FIGURE 13-21 Headgear is sometimes used for patients with mandibular deficiencies. Facial appearance before **(A)** and after **(B)** treatment using headgear and Class II elastics; **C,** Cephalometric superimpositions of the treatment effects. This patient showed restriction of maxillary growth and some impressive mandibular growth, combined with distal movement of the upper teeth and mesial movement of the lower teeth, which were accompanied by posterior eruption.

tongue blades with notches carved into the top and bottom blade (see Figure 13-23, *D*). This guide will stop the bite closure at the predetermined jaw separation and determine the anteroposterior mandibular position at the same time. Other children can be directed very simply by estimating the closure and "coaching" (see Figure 13-23, *E*).

To produce the working bite, the technique follows the steps illustrated in Figure 13-23. First, firmly seat the softened wax on the maxillary arch so all teeth are indexed. Next, have the child position the mandible forward to the correct position and close to the desired position, paying careful attention to reproducing the previous midline

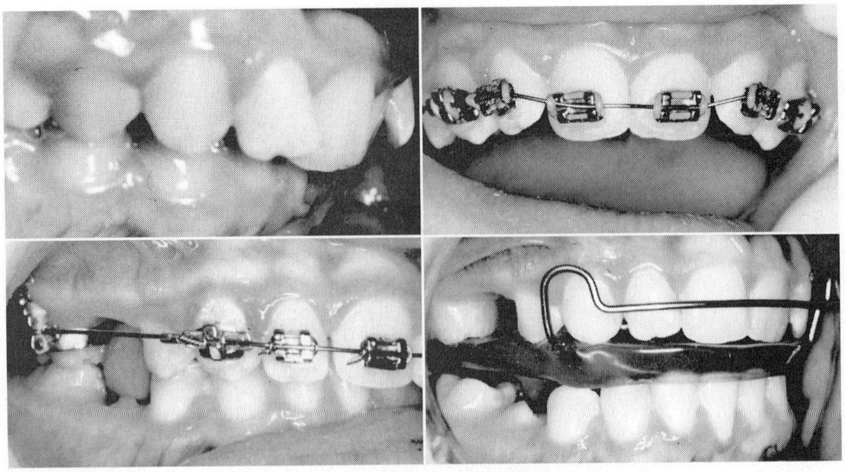

FIGURE 13-22 **A,** For this girl with a Class II division 2 malocclusion, it was impossible to take the bite registration for a functional appliance until the maxillary incisors were tipped facially; **B,** Although this change can be accomplished with a removable maxillary appliance with finger springs (and was done that way in traditional European removable appliance treatment), the pre-functional alignment now often can be accomplished more efficiently with a partial fixed appliance. In this case, the molars were banded, the canines and incisors bonded, and a superelastic NiTi wire was placed; **C,** Same patient two months later, with alignment accomplished and overjet established; **D,** Same patient four months later, with a deep bite bionator in place. (From Proffitt WR, White RP, Sarver DM. Contemporary Treatment of Dentofacial Deformity. St. Louis: Mosby; 2003.)

relationship. If a vertical stop made of tongue blades is used, it must remain in the proper orientation (parallel to the true horizontal). Otherwise, as the tongue blades incline either inferiorly or superiorly, the mandible will either be closed and retruded or opened, respectively to an incorrect position. When the correct bite has been obtained, the wax should be cooled and removed from the mouth. The bite should be examined for adequate dental registration and soft tissue interferences and rechecked for accuracy.

For a cemented, bonded, or partially fixed functional appliance, accurate impressions of the teeth are essential, but extension of the impressions into the vestibules is not important. If bands or steel crowns are used to retain a Herbst appliance (Figure 13-24), they can be fabricated indirectly by a laboratory on the cast by disking the teeth to create space, and many clinicians prefer this time saving method. Most clinicians have deserted bands for retention of fixed functional appliances because they have proved to be easily distorted and broken. Metal crowns, which are fit without reducing the teeth; cast splints that can be bonded; or bonded acrylic splints are more satisfactory. The bonded splints eliminate the need to separate teeth and therefore reduce both laboratory and clinical time. The working bite for a Herbst appliance is similar to the one for a removable functional appliance, typically with 4 to 6 mm advancement. Remember that pretreatment incisor positioning is just as important for these appliances.

Impressions for the twin block appliance (Figure 13-25) require little extensions past the teeth, because the appliance, again, is tooth-borne. The working bite is taken with advancement and opening in the same manner as for the bionator or activator.

Components for Functional Appliances

The design of a functional appliance generally follows the "components approach." An appropriate appliance prescription specifies the appliance components that would be most effective in solving the patient's specific problems. Most laboratories have incorporated the components into a checklist format that simplifies precise communication. It is important to have the appliance design in mind prior to the impressions, because the impression technique is affected by what appliance components are selected and where they will be placed. A bionator or an activator can include headgear tubes if a headgear is considered as an adjunct for treatment. If a vertical and/or distal extraoral force is desired, a facebow can be fitted into headgear tubes attached to almost any type of tooth-borne functional appliance (i.e., almost anything except a Frankel appliance) (Figure 13-26). This application of extraoral force may be useful for patients with a combination of mandibular deficiency and vertical maxillary excess who have a growth pattern in which the mandible tends to rotate downward and backward.

Components to Advance the Mandible. For most mandibular deficient patients, a bionator or activator-type appliance (Figure 13-27) is the simplest, most durable, and most readily accepted appliance. The flanges against the alveolar mucosa below the mandibular molars or lingual pads contacting the tissue behind the lower incisors provide the stimulus to posture the mandible to a new position (Figure

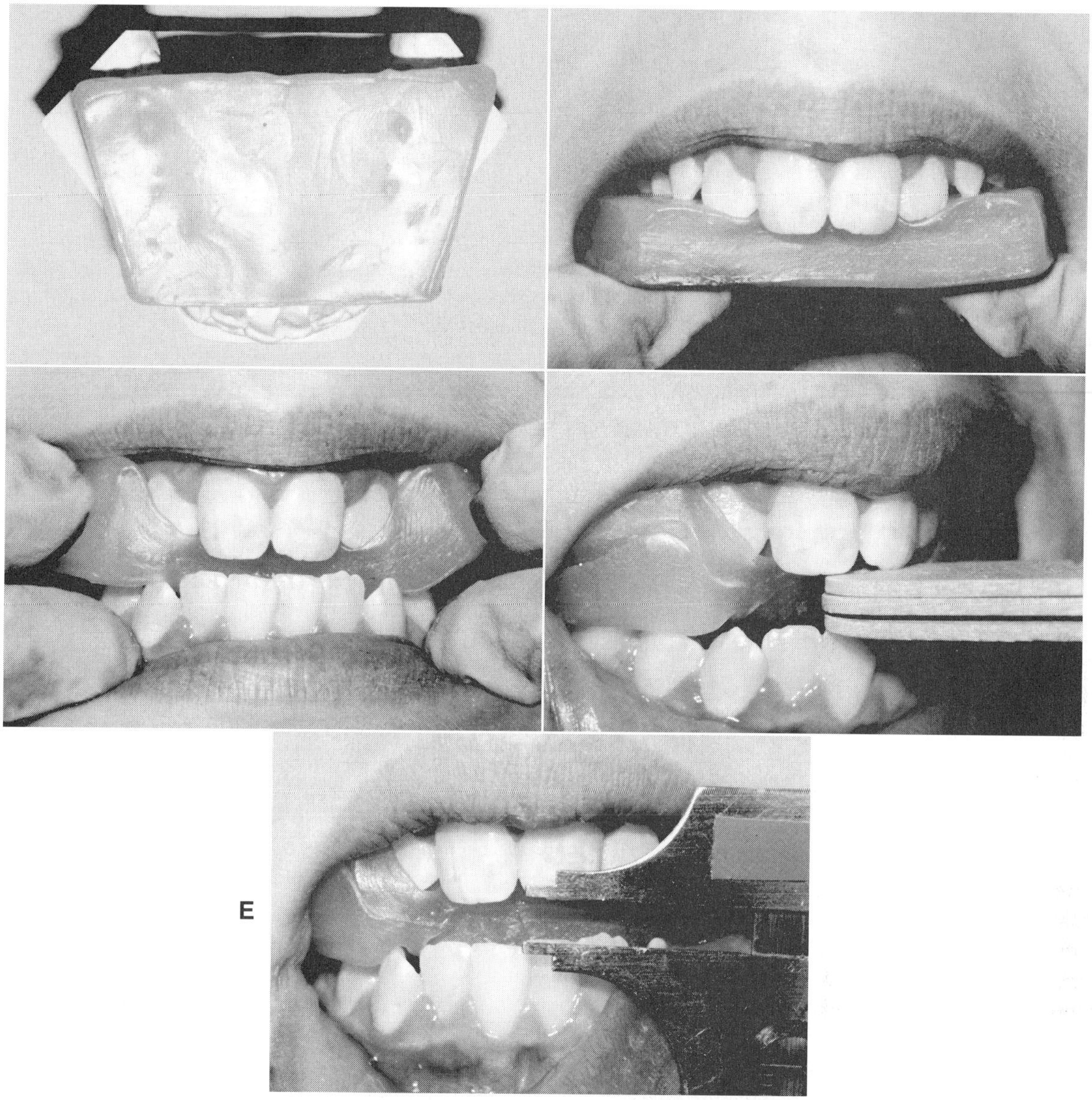

FIGURE 13-23 Steps for obtaining a "working bite" for functional appliance construction. **A,** Multiple layers of hard wax are luted together and cut to the size of the mandibular arch. Care must be taken not to cover the anterior teeth or extend the wax to areas of soft tissue interference. **B,** The softened wax is seated on the maxillary posterior teeth and pressed into place to ensure good indexing of the teeth. **C,** The mandible is guided to the correct anteroposterior and vertical position on observation of the midline relationships and the incisal separation. **D,** Either stacked tongue blades or **(E)** a Boley gauge can be used to control the amount of closure and help the patient reproduce the correct bite. The wax is then cooled with air and removed for inspection. Definite registration of both maxillary and mandibular teeth is required for proper appliance construction.

13-28). Growth modification is most effective if the patient uses his or her own musculature to posture the mandible forward, as opposed to the mandible being held forward by external pressure while the patient relaxes. Note that contact of the pad or flange with soft tissue, not the teeth, is the key to mandibular repositioning. If the lingual component of the appliance contacts the mandibular incisors, it also can produce a labially directed force against these teeth as the mandible attempts to return to normal resting posture. For this reason, activators and bionators usually are relieved behind the lower incisors.

Ramps supported by the teeth are another mechanism for posturing the mandible forward. It is much better to have two ramps in contact, as in the twin block appliance (see Figure 13-25), than to have the lower anterior teeth contact a ramp only on the upper appliance.

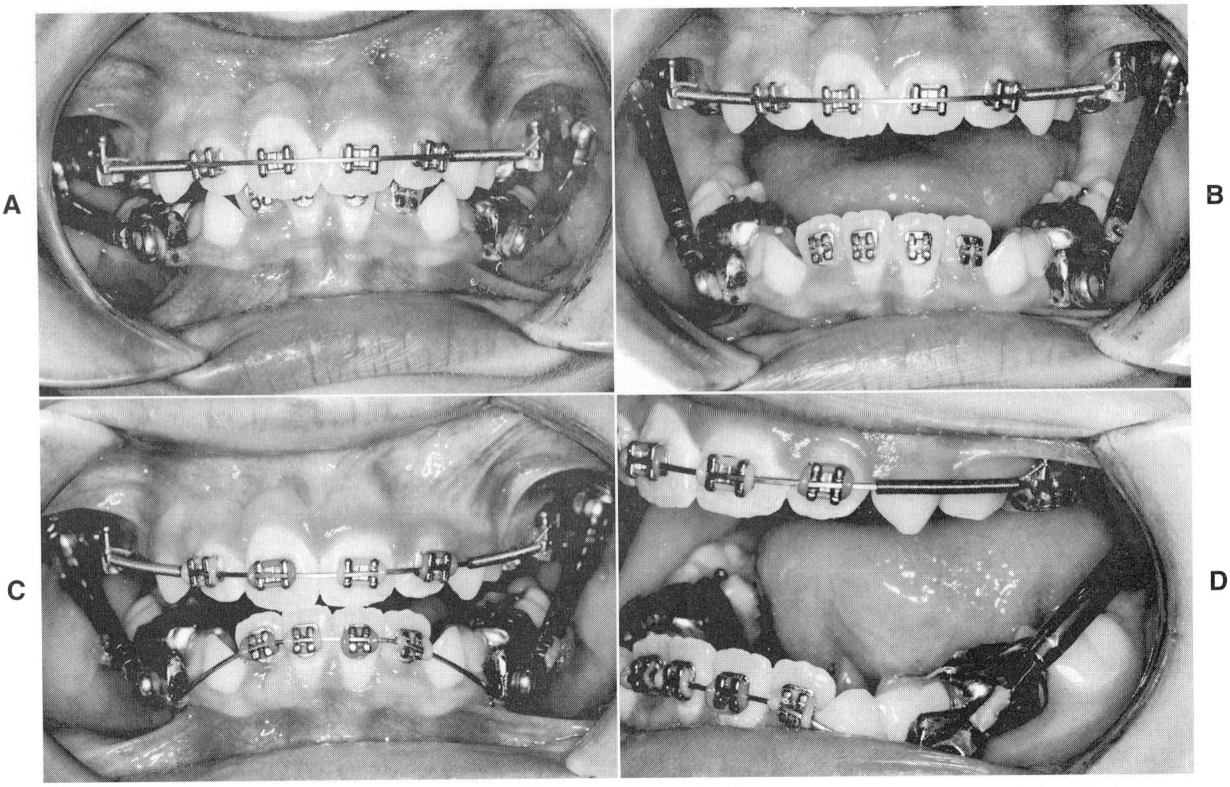

FIGURE 13-24 The Herbst appliance can be used in either the mixed or early permanent dentition. **A, B,** For this mixed dentition child, the arms of the Herbst appliance are attached to crowns on the maxillary first molars and mandibular second primary molars. Bonded brackets on the maxillary incisors and an arch wire with passive coil springs to maintain space are used to decrease retraction of the maxillary teeth. **C,** After initial alignment, the lower incisors have been added to the appliance, in this case to proceed toward leveling of the lower arch. **D,** As treatment continues, a spacer has been added to increase the amount of forward positioning of the mandible (see Figure 13-36 for details of this adjustment).

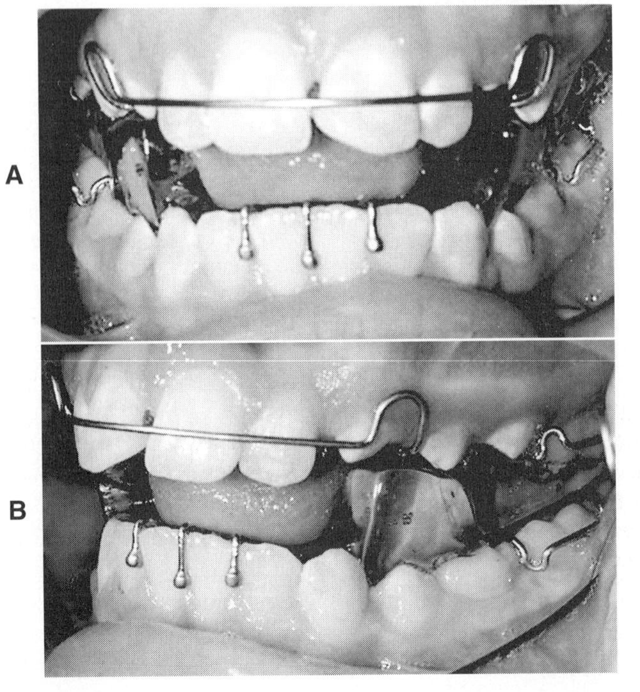

FIGURE 13-25 The twin block appliance can be used as a cemented (fixed) or removable appliance. This patient had a Class II deep bite malocclusion (A) treated with a twin block appliance that opened the bite and (B) advanced the mandible. The separate upper and lower units interdigitate via a ramp that can be seen extending forward from the maxillary primary canine area. This forces the mandible to a more protruded and vertically increased position. The appliance often is cemented at insertion and later made removable. Adjustments can be made to the occlusal coverage and the inclines to modify eruption and the amount of advancement. (Courtesy Dr. M. Mayhew.)

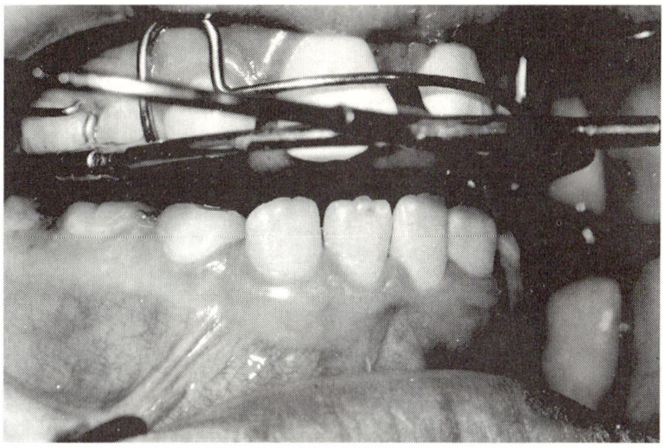

Figure 13-26 Headgear tubes can be incorporated into any tooth-borne functional appliance so that additional distal and vertical force can be applied with a facebow and headcap.

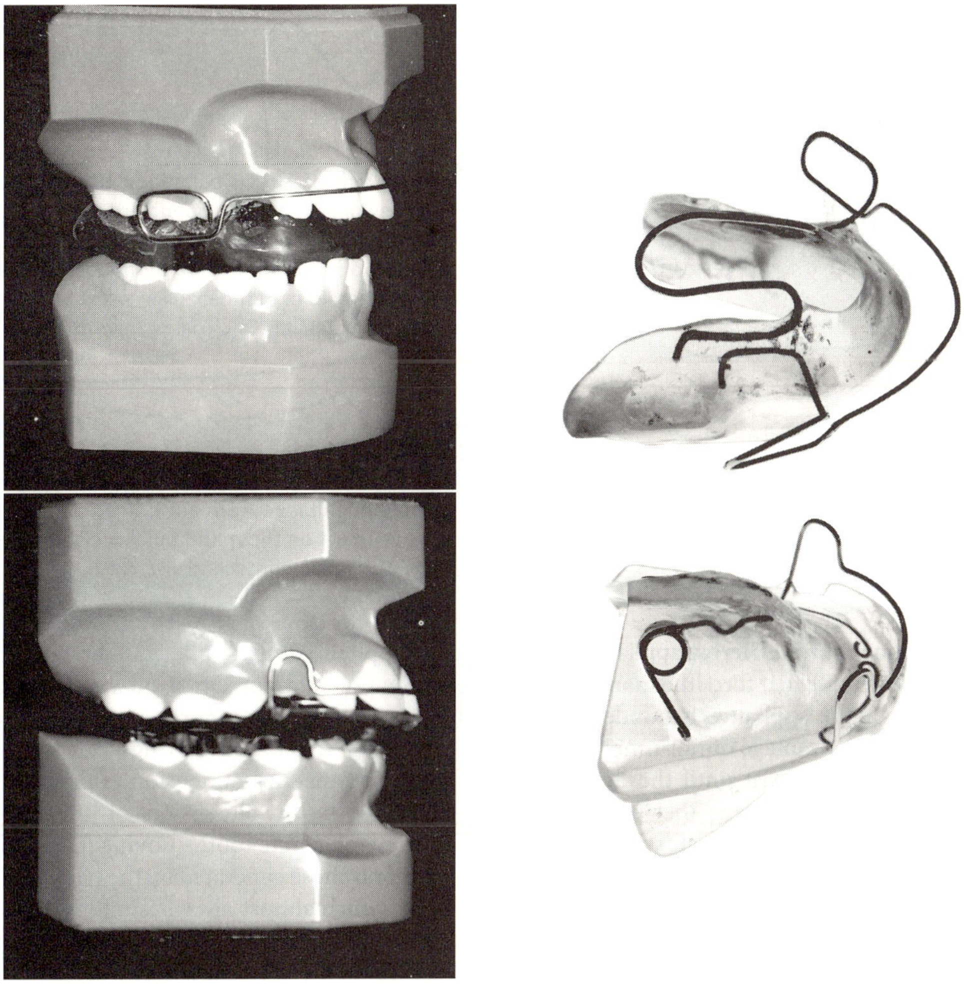

Figure 13-27 **A,** The bionator is borne on the teeth and advances the mandible. It usually has a buccal wire to maintain the lips off the teeth and can incorporate bite blocks between the posterior teeth and a tongue shield as this one does. **B,** The bionator also incorporates a major palatal connector to stabilize the posterior segments, but the appliance is limited in bulk and relatively easy for the patient to accommodate. **C,** The activator is also used to advance the mandible and can incorporate anterior and posterior bite blocks and a labial bow. **D,** The lingual shields usually extend deeper along the mandibular alveolus than other functional appliances, and sometimes the appliance incorporates a displacing spring that engages the maxillary first molar so that the appliance requires a closed and advanced mandibular posture to retain the appliance in place.

A

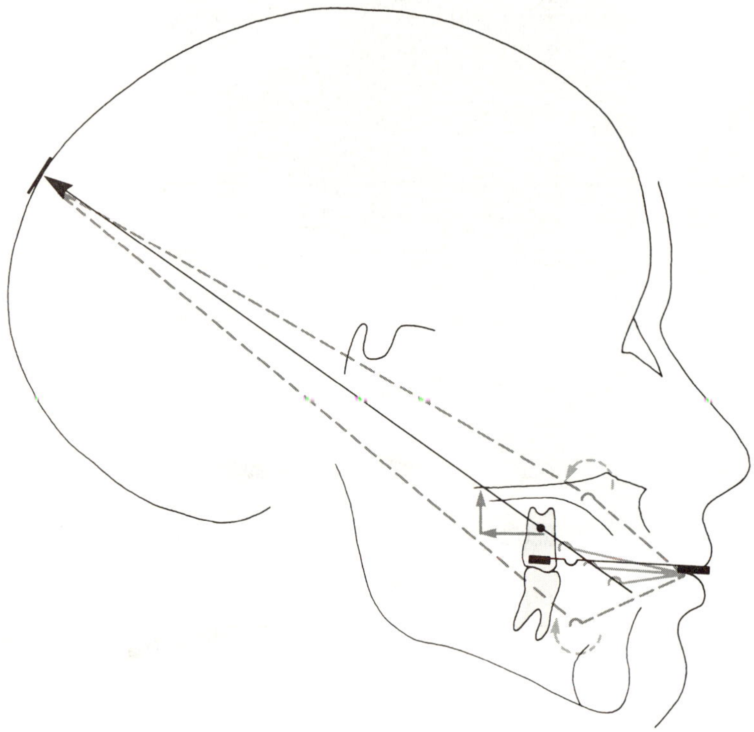

B

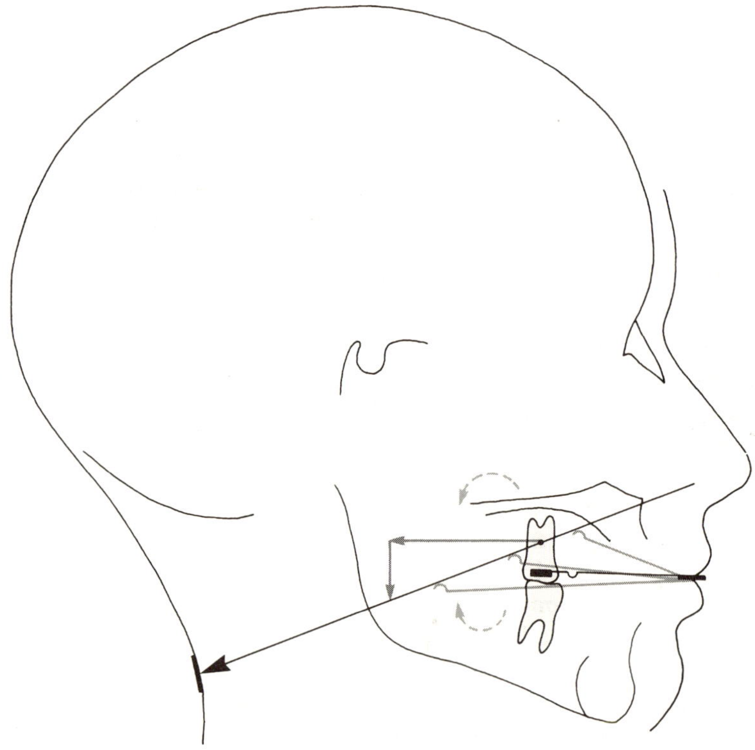

FIGURE 13-41 These diagrams illustrate effects of three commonly used types of facebow and extraoral anchorage attachments. In each diagram, the inner bow is shown in black, and the various outer bow possibilities in blue or dotted red. **A,** High-pull headgear (headcap) to the first molar. To produce bodily movement of the molar (no tipping), the line of force *(black arrow)* must pass through the center of resistance of the molar tooth. This will produce both backward and upward movement of the molar. Note that the line of force is affected by the length and position of the outer bow, so that a longer outer bow bent up or a shorter one bent down could produce the same line of force. If bow length or position produces a line of force above or below the center of resistance *(dotted red)*, the tooth will tip with the root or the crown, respectively, going distally because of the moment that is produced. **B,** Cervical headgear (neckstrap) to the first molar. Again, bodily movement is produced by an outer bow length and position that places the line of force through the center of resistance of the molar; but with a lower direction of pull, the tooth is extruded as well as moved backward. Note that the outer bow of a facebow used with cervical traction nearly always is longer than the outer bow used with a high-pull headcap. If the line of force is above or below its center of resistance, the tooth will tip with the root or crown, respectively, going distally as indicated by the dotted arrows.

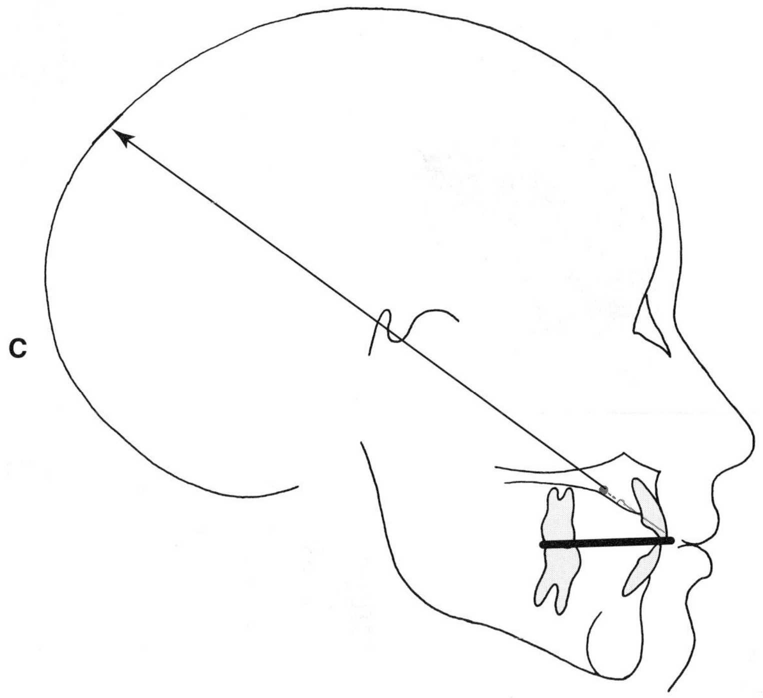

FIGURE 13-41 cont'd C, High-pull headgear to a short facebow inserted into a maxillary splint. With all the teeth splinted, it is possible to consider the maxilla as a unit and to relate the line of force to the center of resistance of the maxilla. As with headgear force against the first molar, the relationship of the line of force to the center of resistance of the maxilla determines the rotational effect on the maxilla.

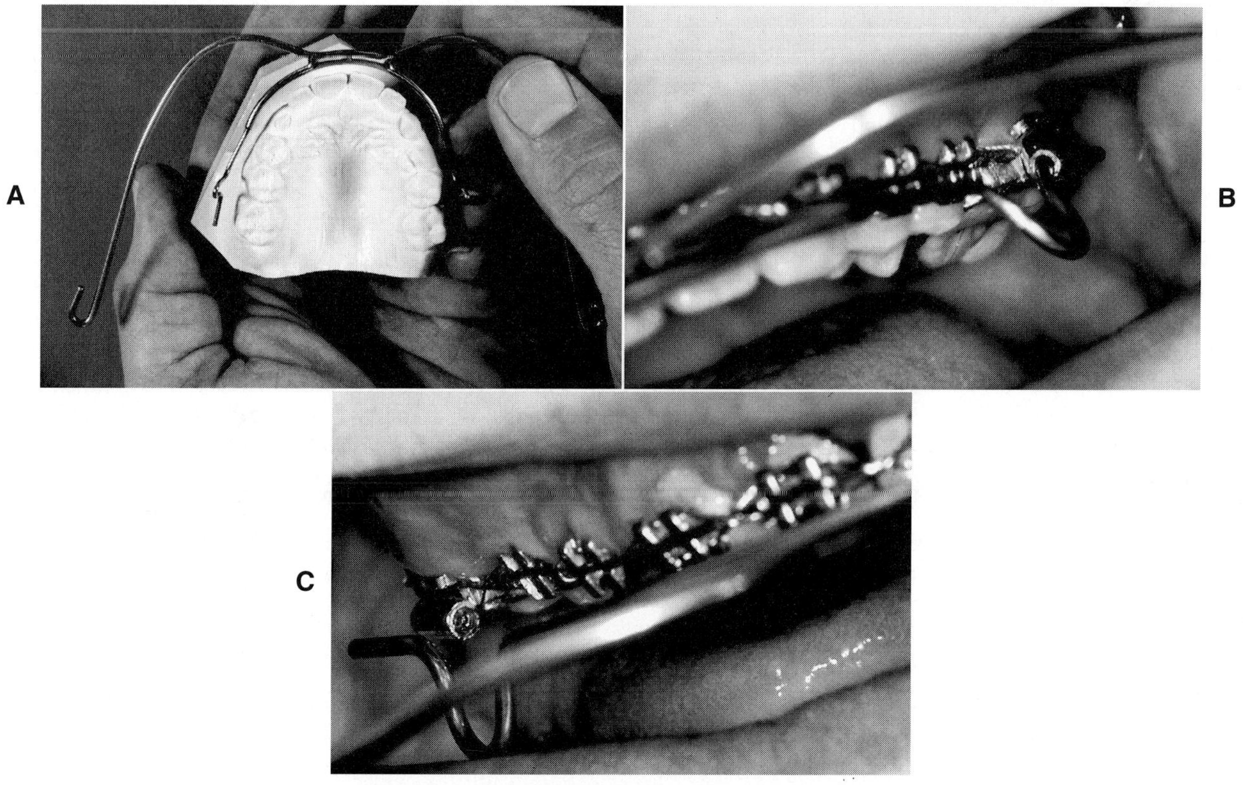

FIGURE 13-42 The steps for fitting a facebow for a headgear. **A,** Facebow inner bows come in graduated sizes. A simple method for selecting the appropriate size is to fit the bow to the pretreatment maxillary cast. **B,** After the bow is placed in one molar headgear tube, **(C)** it is adjusted to be passive and aligned with the tube on the other molar band. It should be easy to insert and remove at this point. Then the inner bow must be expanded by 1 to 2 mm to keep the posterior teeth out of crossbite as anterposterior changes are made. Often the adjustment loops mesial to the maxillary first molar need to be opened or closed to move the inner bow farther from or closer to the anterior teeth.

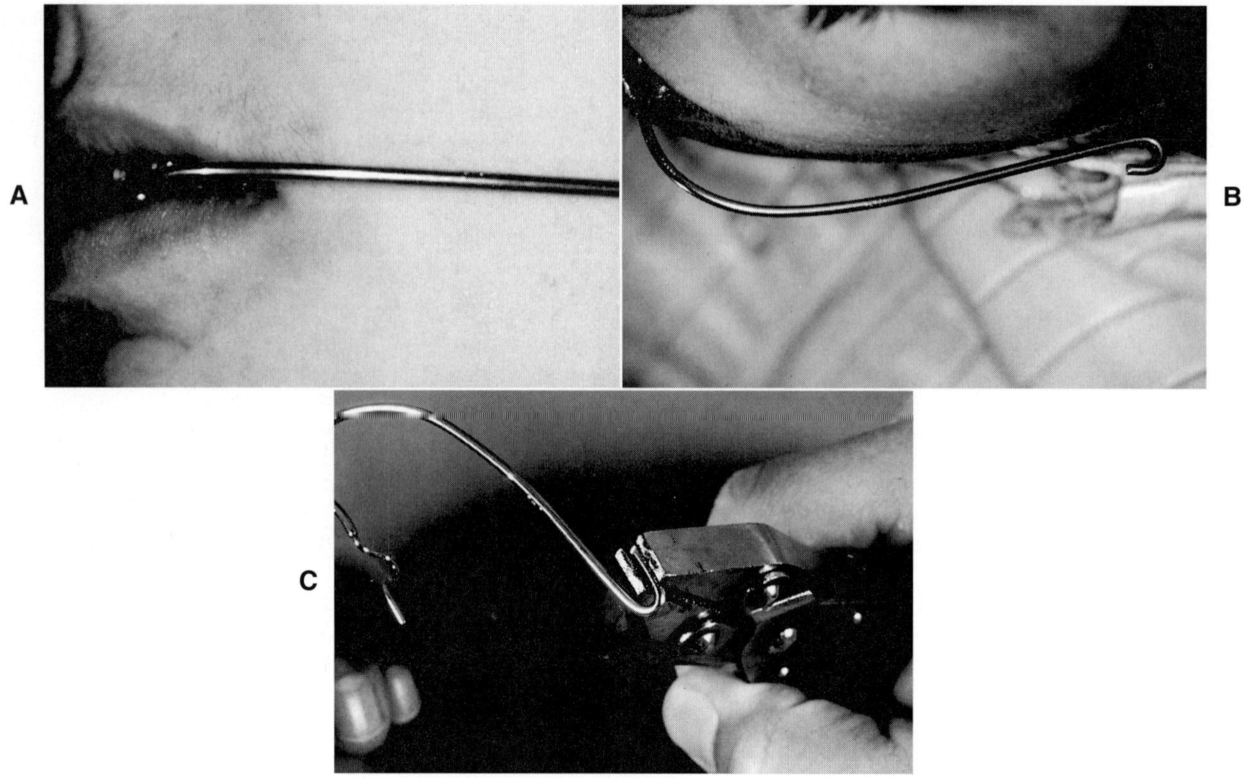

FIGURE 13-43 **A,** The facebow should be adjusted so that the junction of the inner and outer bows rests passively between the lips. **B,** The outer bow should rest several millimeters from the soft tissue of the cheek. This adjustment must be checked both before and after the straps for the headcap or neckstrap are attached. **C,** The length of the outer bow is critical to the desired dental changes. After the correct length is chosen and the outer bow cut with a pliers, a hook is bent at the end with a heavy pliers.

have a hook formed at the end (Figure 13-43, *C*). The length and the vertical position of the outer bow are selected to achieve the correct force direction relative to the center of resistance (see Figure 13-41).

This can actually be accomplished quite simply after the inner and outer bow relationships to the teeth and face have been adjusted. With the bow in place, by placing your fingers on the outer bow and simulating the direction of force application (e.g., up and back for highpull and down and back for cervical) at different points bilaterally (Figure 13-44), the reaction of the teeth can be determined. Force against the outer bow that lifts the junction of the inner and outer bows between the lips will move the roots distally. Conversely, if the force drops the bow between the lips, the molar crowns will tip distally. If neither occurs, the teeth will move bodily (Figure 13-45). Placing the terminal hook bend in the outer bow at the point where the type of movement you desire occurs will provide the correct direction of force.

The appropriate headcap or neckstrap is fitted by selecting the appropriate size. A spring mechanism—not elastic bands or straps—is strongly recommended to provide the force. The springs deliver consistent forces that can be documented and easily adjusted. The spring attachment is adjusted to provide the correct force with the patient sitting up or standing—not reclining in the dental chair (Figure 13-46, *A, B*). It is usually a good idea to start with a low force level to acclimate the patient to the headgear and then gradually increase the force at subsequent appointments. Even if the correct force level is set at the first appointment, the forces will drop when the strap stretches slightly and contours to the patient's neck. Once the forces are correct, the bow position must be rechecked since the pull of the straps and any adjustments to the inner or outer bow to improve fit and patient comfort can alter the previous bow position so that it needs adjustment.

The child should place and remove the headgear under supervision several times to be certain that he or she understands how to manipulate it and to ensure proper adjustment. Most headgear is worn after school, during relaxed evening hours and during sleep. It is definitely not indicated for vigorous activity, bicycle riding, or general roughhousing. Children should be instructed that if anyone grabs the outer bow, they should also grab the bow with their hands. This will prevent breakage and injury. The headgear straps must be equipped with a safety-release mechanism (Figure 13-46, *C, D*) to prevent the bow from springing back at the child and injuring him or her if it is grabbed and pulled by a playmate. Severe injuries, including loss of sight, have occurred from headgear accidents of this type.[45] In a review of commercially available headgear release mechanisms that

A

B

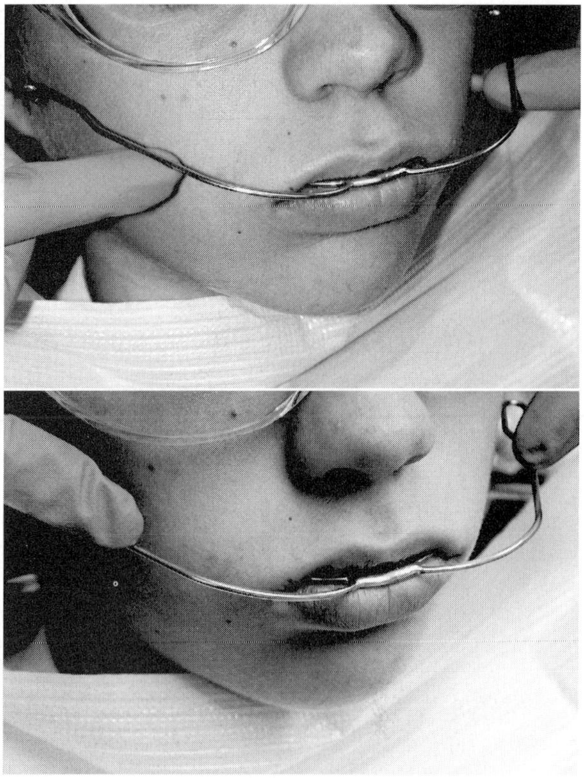

FIGURE 13-44 In order to determine the proper length needed for the outer bow, use the index fingers to apply pressure in the direction of the headgear selected. **A,** Pushing up and back in the direction of a high pull headgear and **(B)** pushing down and back in the direction of a cervical headgear. As the fingers are moved from the anterior portion of the outer bow to the posterior portion the position of the bow between the lips will change.

A

B

C

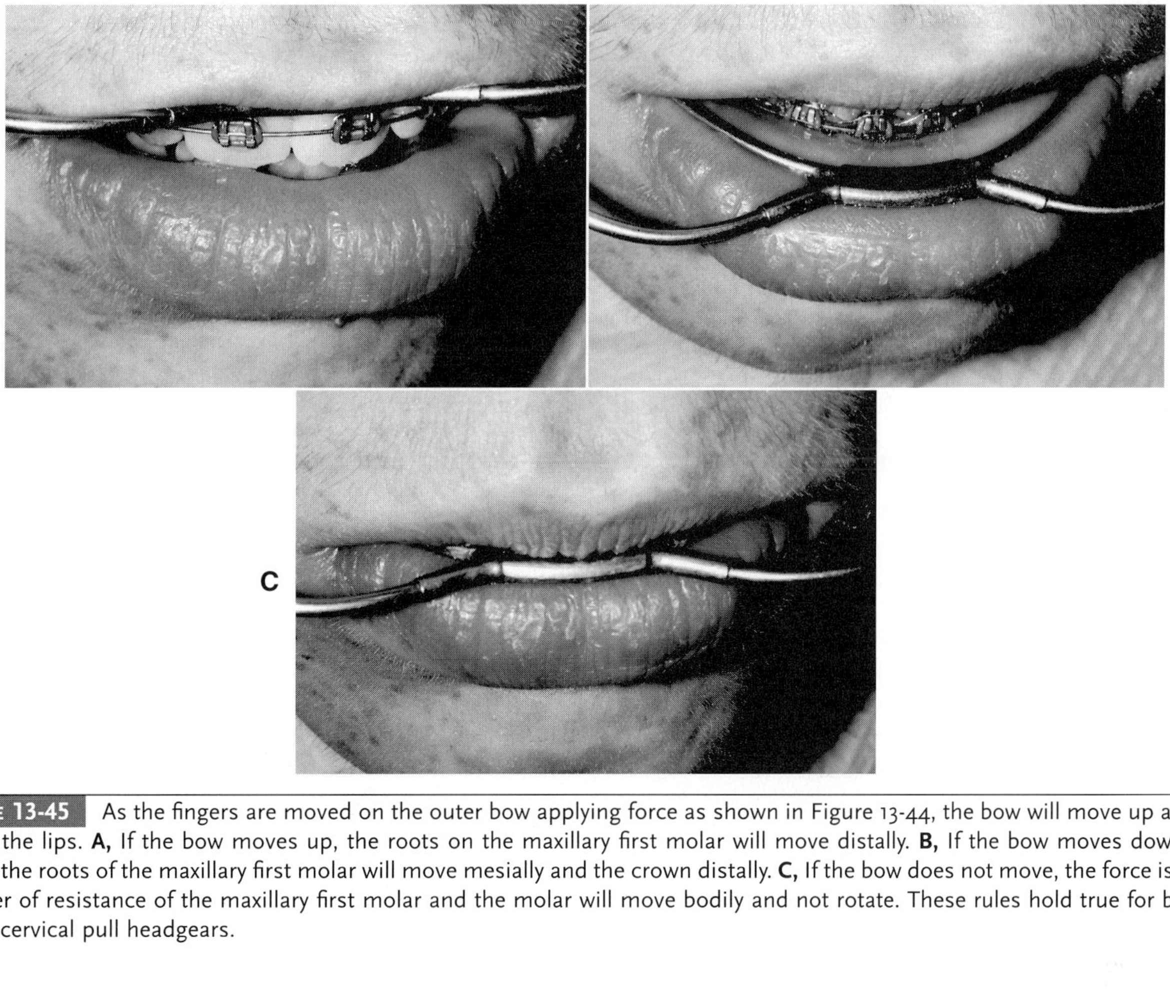

FIGURE 13-45 As the fingers are moved on the outer bow applying force as shown in Figure 13-44, the bow will move up and down between the lips. **A,** If the bow moves up, the roots on the maxillary first molar will move distally. **B,** If the bow moves down on the lower lip the roots of the maxillary first molar will move mesially and the crown distally. **C,** If the bow does not move, the force is through the center of resistance of the maxillary first molar and the molar will move bodily and not rotate. These rules hold true for both high pull and cervical pull headgears.

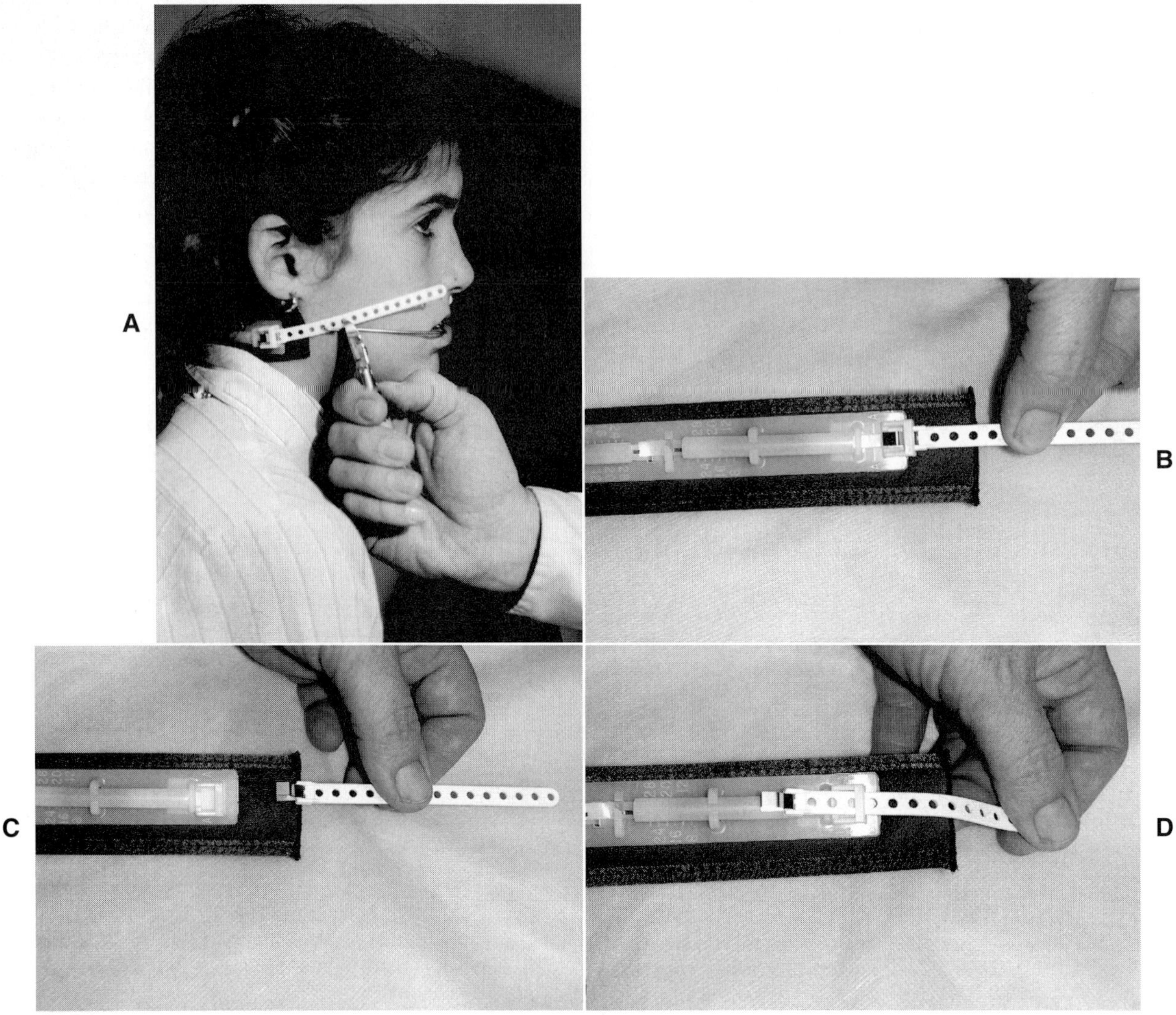

FIGURE 13-46 Adjustment of the neckstrap. **A,** The neckstrap is attached to the facebow and the proper force obtained from the spring mechanism by moving the hook to adjacent holes on the neckstrap. When the force is correct, the plastic connector is cut so that one extra hole is present in front of the correct hole. This provides a tab for the patient to grasp when placing the headgear. **B,** The spring mechanism delivers a predetermined force when the plastic connector is moved forward and aligned with a calibration mark. Here the rear of the tab is slightly anterior to the calibration mark. **C,** If the connector is stretched farther, such as it might be if someone grabbed the facebow and pulled on it, the plastic connector strap will release, preventing the bow from springing back into the patient's face and causing injury. **D,** The connector can be reassembled by threading it through the back of the safety release.

included 18 different designs, Stafford et al noted that almost all released at 10 to 20 pounds of force and concluded that the amount of extension before release occurred and the consistency of release were the most important variables from a safety perspective.[46]

COMBINED VERTICAL AND A-P PROBLEMS

Short Face/Deep Bite

Some children exhibit a skeletal vertical deficiency (short face), almost always in conjunction with an anterior deep bite and some degree of mandibular deficiency and often with a Class II, division 2 malocclusion. Skeletally, the condition often can be described as Class II rotated to Class I. The reduced face height is often accompanied by everted and prominent lips that would be appropriate if the face height were normal. Children with vertical deficiency can be identified at an early age.[47] They usually have a normal maxilla but have decreased eruption of maxillary and mandibular teeth. Many tend to have a low mandibular plane angle (skeletal deep bite) and a long mandibular ramus. Growth is expressed in an anterior direction, with a tendency toward upward and forward rotation of the mandible. The challenge in correcting these problems is to increase eruption of posterior teeth and influence the mandible to rotate downward without decreasing chin prominence too much.

In a patient with Class II malocclusion, one way to correct such problems is with cervical headgear, taking advantage of the extrusive tendency of extraoral force directed below the center of resistance of the teeth and the maxilla (Figure 13-47). This effect and eruption of the lower molar can be accomplished using a headgear and a biteplate to open the bite, a method used in the Florida prospective clinical trail.[24] With no posterior occlusion, both upper and lower teeth can erupt. The other way is to use a functional appliance (with or without mandibular advancement, depending on the anteroposterior jaw relationship) that allows free eruption of the posterior teeth.

Because most short face children also have a Class II malocclusion, it is important whether the eruption that occurs during treatment is primarily of the upper or the lower molars. Cervical headgear produces more eruption of the upper molars, while eruption can be manipulated with a functional appliance so that either the upper or lower molars erupt more. Class II correction, however, is easier if the lower molar erupts more than the upper, which means that—all other factors being equal—the functional appliance would be preferred (see Figure 8-22).

The ability of functional appliances to control eruption of posterior teeth can be used during treatment of children with a significant anteroposterior mandibular deficiency *and* reduced face height in an effort to take maximal advantage of mandibular growth by having it expressed in an anterior direction. First, all vertical eruption is blocked while an appliance with the mandible advanced is used. Then, after the anteroposterior correction is complete, a child treated in this manner may exhibit a posterior open bite when the appliance is not in place. At that point, the posterior bite block gradually is cut away while correct overbite is maintained anteriorly, so that slow eruption of posterior teeth back into occlusion can occur. This type of treatment places into sharp focus the interaction between the anteroposterior and vertical planes of space that must be addressed during growth modification treatment. The priority is placed on the most severe problem. It is remedied, and then the accompanying problems are addressed.

The fixed functional appliances tend not to be good choices in the mixed dentition treatment of short face problems. Certainly, the Herbst, with its propensity to intrude the upper molars, is not an attractive option for younger patients needing increased vertical dimensions, even though the mandibular plane angle usually does not change very much in Herbst treatment.[48] The twin block does offer some options to manage posterior eruption when the acrylic is modified during treatment.

It is appropriate to remember that eruption occurs more rapidly in some patients than others and probably is affected by resting mandibular posture and freeway space, as well as the amount of appliance wear. Some short face children show extremely rapid mandibular growth when the bite is opened and incisor overlap is removed, even with so simple an appliance as a bite plate. Unfortunately, this happens only occasionally, and except for the rare patients in whom there is no mandibular deficiency, posturing the mandible forward to allow the construction of a functional appliance is the better approach. Delivery and adjustment of a functional appliance for a vertically deficient patient is similar to that already discussed under mandibular deficiency.

Long Face/Open Bite

Excessive growth of the maxilla in children with Class II malocclusion often has more of a vertical than an anteroposterior component (i.e., there is more excessive growth downward than forward). Both components can contribute to skeletal Class II malocclusion, because if the maxilla moves downward, the mandible rotates downward and backward. The effect is to prevent mandibular growth from being expressed anteriorly. The goal of treatment is to restrict growth of the maxilla while the mandible grows into a more prominent and normal relationship with it (see Figure 13-37). Although the application of extraoral force is the obvious approach, functional appliance treatment also can be helpful.

Children with the long face pattern of growth generally have a maxilla that is rotated down posteriorly and/or a short mandibular ramus, which accounts for the steep mandibular plane and the large discrepancy between posterior and anterior face height. The ideal treatment for these patients would be to control all subsequent posterior vertical growth so that the mandible would rotate in an upward and forward direction (Figure 13-48). This could be accomplished by controlling all tooth eruption if there were adequate mandibular vertical ramus growth. Unfortunately, vertical facial growth continues through adolescence and into the postadolescent years, which means that even if growth can be modified successfully in the mixed dentition, active retention is likely to be necessary for a number of years. Although dramatic improvement can be demonstrated in selected patients, probably the most sensible use of any of the appliances to control vertical skeletal and dental development is to use them for the minor to moderate problems and intervene in adolescence toward the end of the growth period. That way, the problem is more manageable and treatment and retention are more circumscribed. Whatever the appliance and whenever the treatment started, retention would be critically important until growth was completed in the late teens or early 20s.

There are several possible approaches to the long face pattern of growth in preadolescent children. In the order of their clinical effectiveness, they are:

High-Pull Headgear to the Molars

One approach to vertical excess problems is to maintain the vertical position of the maxilla and inhibit eruption of the maxillary posterior teeth. This can be attempted with high-

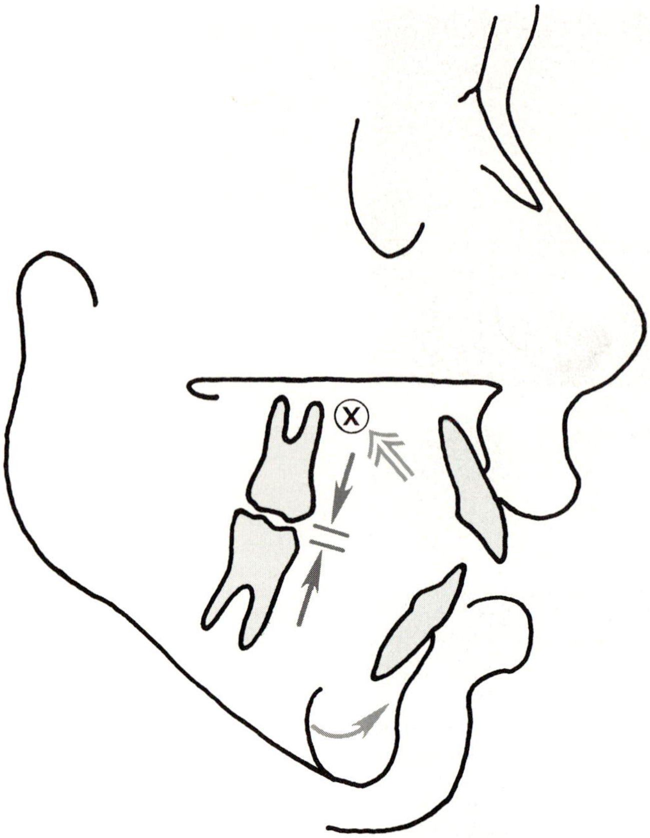

FIGURE 13-49 Mandibular-deficient children with excessive lower face height need treatment with an appliance that restricts posterior eruption and limits descent of the maxilla. This allows mandibular growth to be expressed anteriorly rather than vertically.

pull headgear to the posterior teeth, to be worn 14 hours a day with a force greater than 12 ounces per side (Figure 13-49). If this involves a conventional facebow to the first molar, delivery and adjustment of the headgear are identical to the high-pull headgear described previously for Class II problems. When comparisons are made using varied vertical and horizontal vectors of force, those with the greatest high-pull vector demonstrated the most vertical control of the upper molars.[49,50] This does not control eruption of the lower molars, which can be a problem in some patients. Lower molar eruption may contribute to the vertical facial change and outstrip changes made by controlling the upper molar with the headgear.

High-Pull Headgear to a Maxillary Splint

Another headgear approach for children with excessive vertical development is the use of a plastic occlusal splint (Figure 13-50) to which the facebow is attached.[51] This allows vertical force to be directed against all the maxillary teeth—not just the molars—and appears to have a substantial maxillary dental and skeletal effect with good vertical control. An appliance of this type would be most useful in a child with excessive vertical development of the entire maxillary arch and too much exposure of the maxillary incisors from beneath the lip (i.e., a long face child who does not have anterior open bite). To achieve both skeletal and dental correction, the patient must be compliant throughout what can be a very long treatment period.

Unfortunately, the maxillary splint allows mandibular posterior teeth to erupt freely, and if this occurs, there may be neither redirection of growth nor favorable upward and forward rotation of the mandible.

Functional Appliance with Bite Blocks

A more effective alternative is the use of a functional appliance that includes posterior bite blocks (Figure 13-51). The retraction force of the headgear is replaced by the somewhat lesser "headgear effect" of the functional appliance. The primary purpose of the appliance is to inhibit eruption of posterior teeth and vertical descent of the maxilla. The appliance can be designed with or without positioning the mandible anteriorly, depending on how much mandibular deficiency is present.

Regardless of whether the mandible is brought forward in the working bite, the bite must be opened past the normal resting vertical dimension if molar eruption is to be affected. When the mandible is held in this position by the appliance, the stretch of the soft tissues (including but not limited to the muscles) exerts a vertical intrusive force on the posterior teeth. In children with anterior open bites the anterior teeth are allowed to erupt, which reduces the open bite, while in the less common long face problems without open bite, all teeth are held by the bite blocks. Because there is no compensatory posterior eruption, all mandibular growth should be directed more anteriorly or at least to the extent that the overbite allows.

In the short term, this type of functional appliance treatment is effective in controlling maxillary vertical skeletal and dental growth.[52] This tends to project mandibular growth anteriorly and helps to close anterior open bites (Figure 13-52). Because of the long period of continued vertical growth, if a functional appliance is used for the first phase of treatment, posterior bite blocks or other components (such as bone screws for skeletal anchorage) will be needed to control vertical growth and eruption during fixed appliance therapy (Figure 13-53) and probably into retention. This is necessary because fixed appliances do not control eruption well and many biomechanical actions are extrusive.

High-Pull Headgear to a Functional Appliance with Bite Blocks

The most aggressive approach to maxillary vertical excess and a Class II jaw relationship is a combination of high-pull headgear and a functional appliance with posterior bite blocks to anteriorly reposition the mandible and control eruption.[53] The theory is that the extraoral force increases the control of maxillary growth and allows the force to be delivered to the whole maxilla rather than to simply the per-

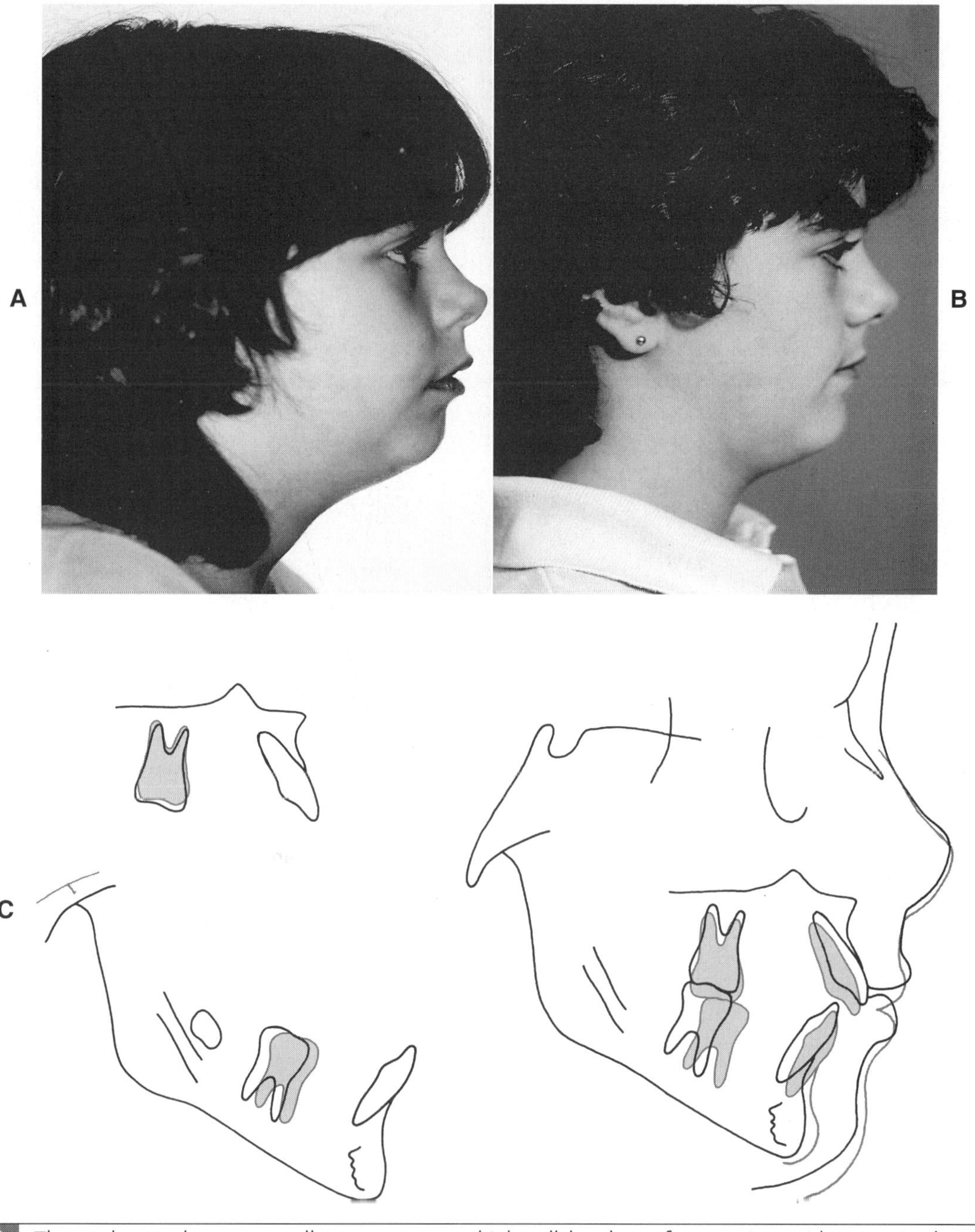

FIGURE 13-50 These photos show an excellent response to high-pull headgear for a patient with excessive lower face height. **A,** Pre-treatment profile; **B,** Post-treatment profile; **C,** Cephalometric superimposition. The cranial base superimposition shows that the maxilla and the maxillary teeth did not move inferiorly; as a result the mandible grew forward and not downward. The mandibular superimposition shows that the lower molar drifted forward into the leeway space. The incisor positions relative to the maxilla and mandible did not change.

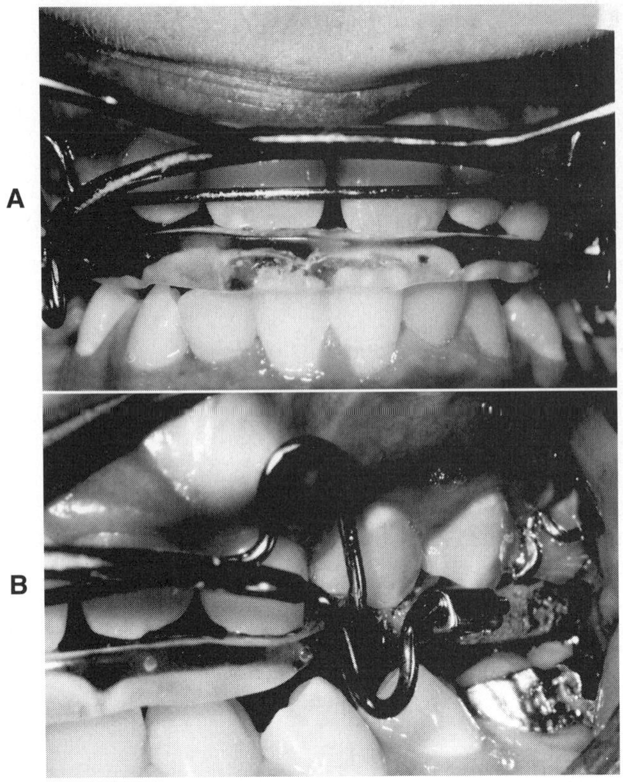

FIGURE 13-51 **A** and **B,** A plastic maxillary splint can be connected to a small conventional inner headgear bow and a high-pull headgear cap to deliver an upward and backward force to the entire maxilla. The splint limits dental eruption better than headgear just to the first molars.

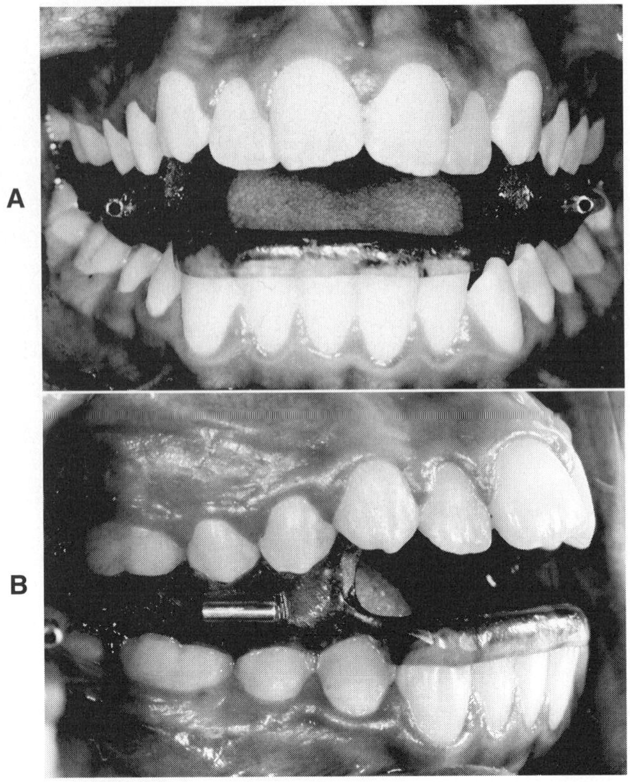

FIGURE 13-52 **A** and **B,** Bite blocks between the posterior teeth can be added to a functional appliance, as shown here, to provide more complete control of the eruption of posterior teeth. Highpull headgear can be worn with an appliance of this type if headgear tubes are included.

manent first molars (Figure 13-54). The high-pull headgear improves retention of the functional appliance and produces a force direction near the estimated center of resistance of the maxilla (see Figure 13-41, *C*). The functional appliance provides the possibility of enhancing mandibular growth while controlling the eruption of the posterior and anterior teeth. In reality, the addition of the headgear appears to provide little more than minimally more vertical control and probably insignificant maxillary skeletal impact.[54] This benefit should be weighed against the effects of the simpler open bite functional appliance without headgear.

When a headgear-activator combination is used, it is a good idea to add torquing springs to the activator (see Figure 13-34) to reduce the tipping effect on maxillary anterior teeth. In this case, which is a notable exception among the active functional appliances, the active components are designed to decrease dental and increase skeletal effects.[55]

Clinical management of the headgear-functional appliance is an amalgamation of techniques used for each of these appliances individually but with some interesting modifications. First, the impressions for the functional appliance are made and the working bite obtained as with any functional appliance. The headgear tubes are incorporated into the bite blocks in the premolar region (see Figure 13-26). At the time of functional appliance delivery, a headcap is made for the patient and a small, if not the smallest, facebow is adjusted to fit the headgear tubes. Usually the adjustment loops need to be closed so the bow is not placed too far anteriorly.

The facebow-functional appliance combination is taken to the mouth and adjusted (usually by shortening the outer bow) so the outer bow is consistent with a resultant force through the estimated center of resistance of the maxilla. With the inner bow resting passively between the lips as it should, the short outer bow must be bent upward. The headcap is connected to the facebow and the force adjusted to approximately 400 gm per side. After the facebow is attached, the headcap position may require additional adjustment.

As with any appliance, the patient should demonstrate competence in placement before leaving the initial appointment. The child is instructed to attach the facebow extraorally, place the facebow-functional appliance combination in the mouth, and then attach the headcap. If previous theory is correct, wearing this combination following the evening meal and during sleeping hours should be adequate. Of course, it is more demanding to wear both headgear and a functional appliance than either appliance alone, and this may be a stumbling block toward good compliance.

A

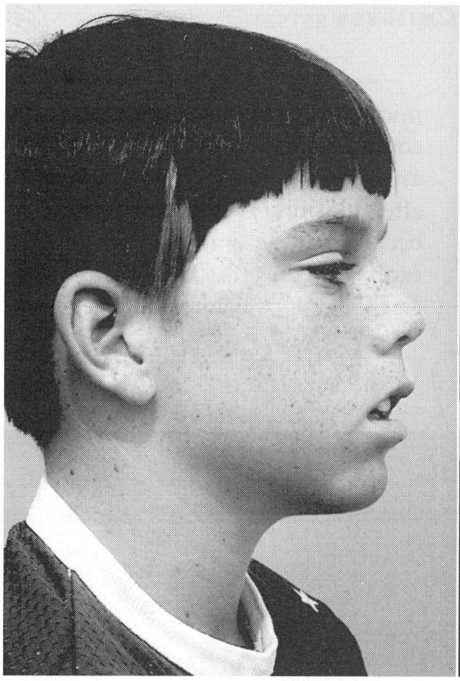

B

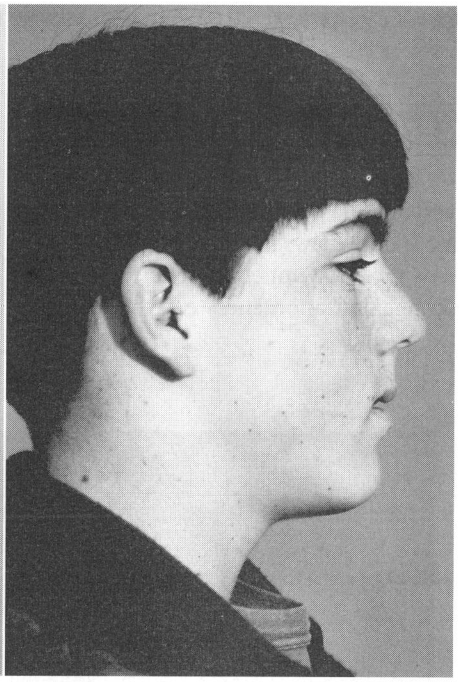

C

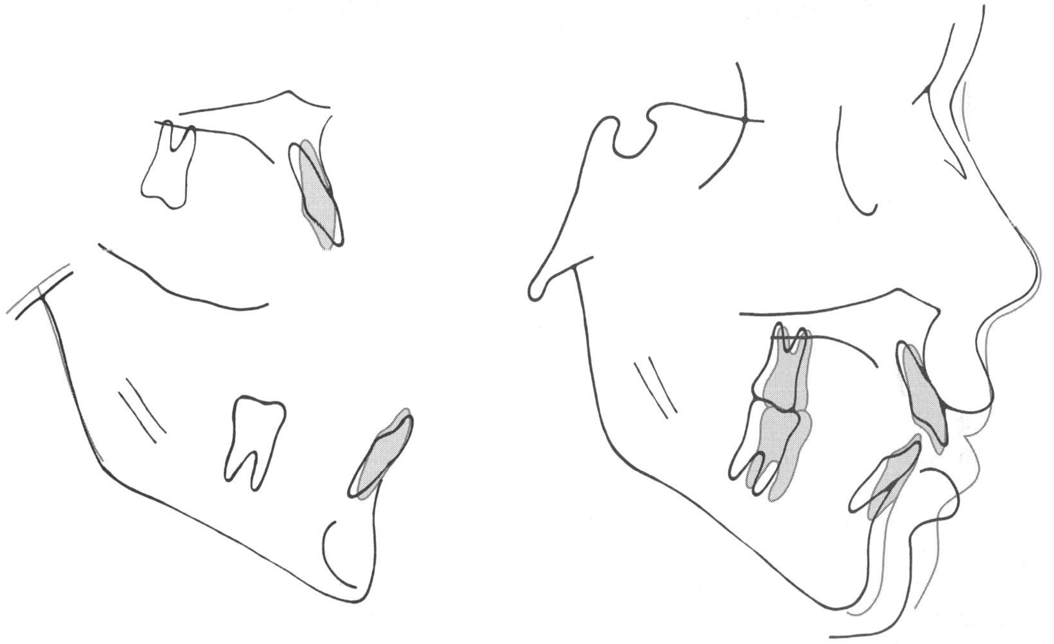

FIGURE 13-53 This patient demonstrates a good response to functional appliance treatment designed to control vertical development with posterior bite blocks in a child with excessive lower face height. **A,** Pre-treatment profile; **B,** Post-treatment profile. **C,** Cephalometric superimpositions indicate that no posterior eruption occurred, and all mandibular growth was directed anteriorly. Face height was maintained and anterior eruption closed the open bite. Maxillary and mandibular molar positions relative to their supporting bone were maintained.

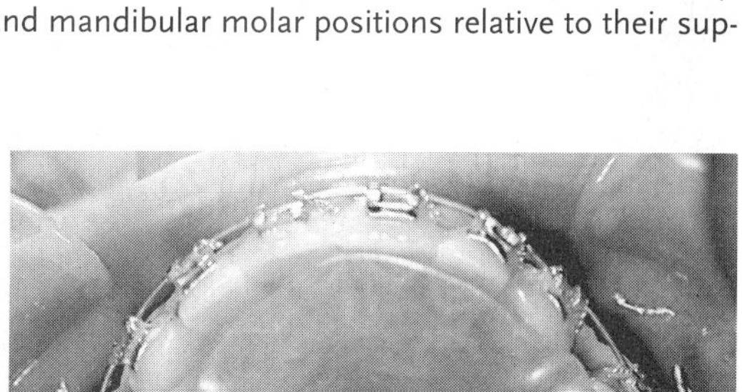

FIGURE 13-54 During fixed appliance treatment, posterior eruption can be controlled (after initial alignment and space closure are completed) by using removable posterior bite blocks to separate the posterior teeth beyond the resting vertical dimension. This creates an intrusive force on teeth in contact with the blocks, which is generated by the stretch of the facial soft tissues. The appliance is retained by clasps over the headgear tubes.

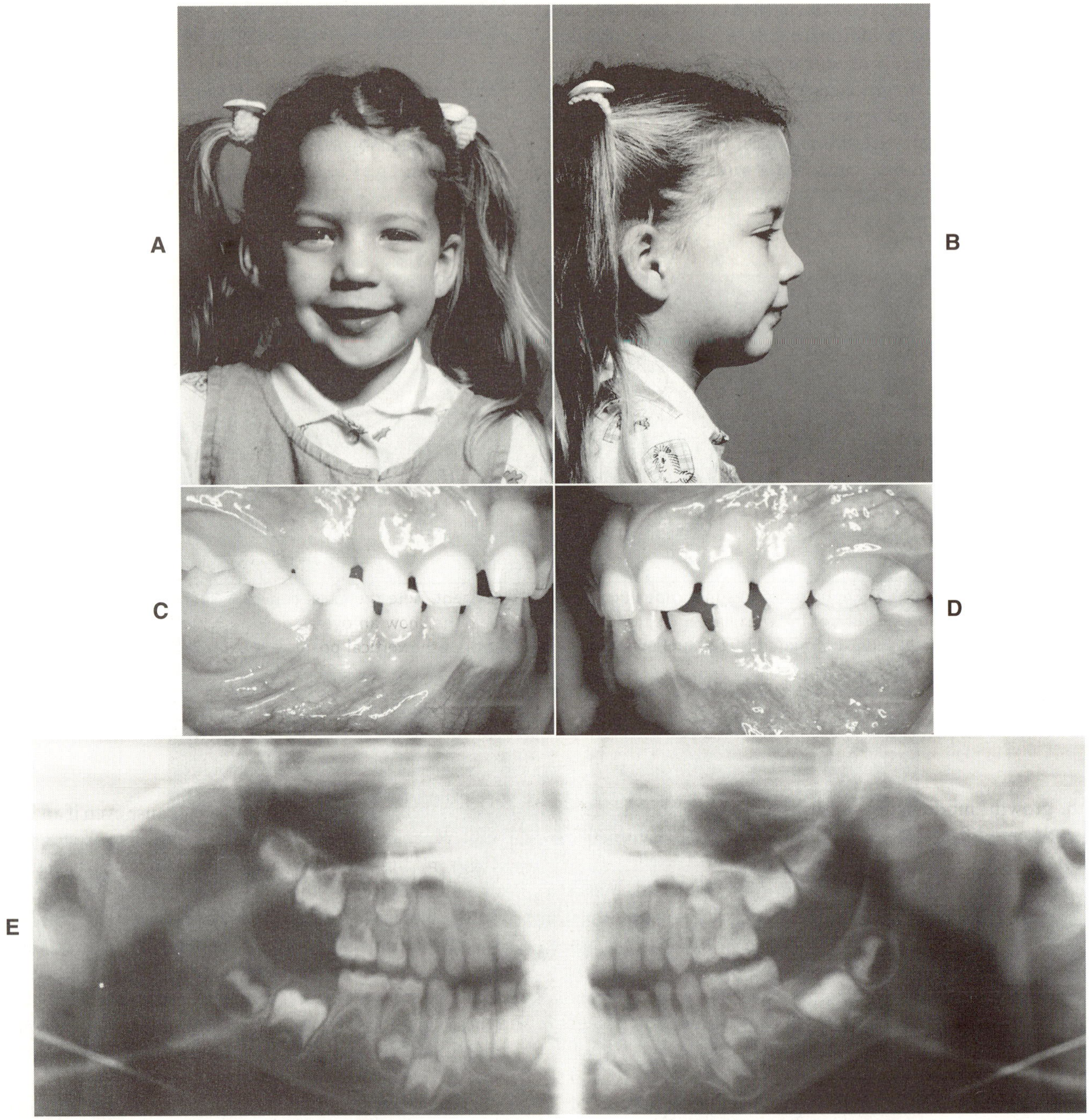

FIGURE 13-56 **A** and **B,** This 5-year-old girl's family dentist noted her facial asymmetry, with the chin off to the left (she deviated even more on opening) and referred her for further evaluation. **C** and **D,** Her buccal occlusion was normal (Class I) on the right and Class II on the left. **E,** The panoramic radiograph showed the classic appearance of a unilateral condylar fracture. Note the normal condyle on the right and only a condylar stub on the left. The injury almost surely occurred at age 2 when she fell but was not diagnosed at the time.

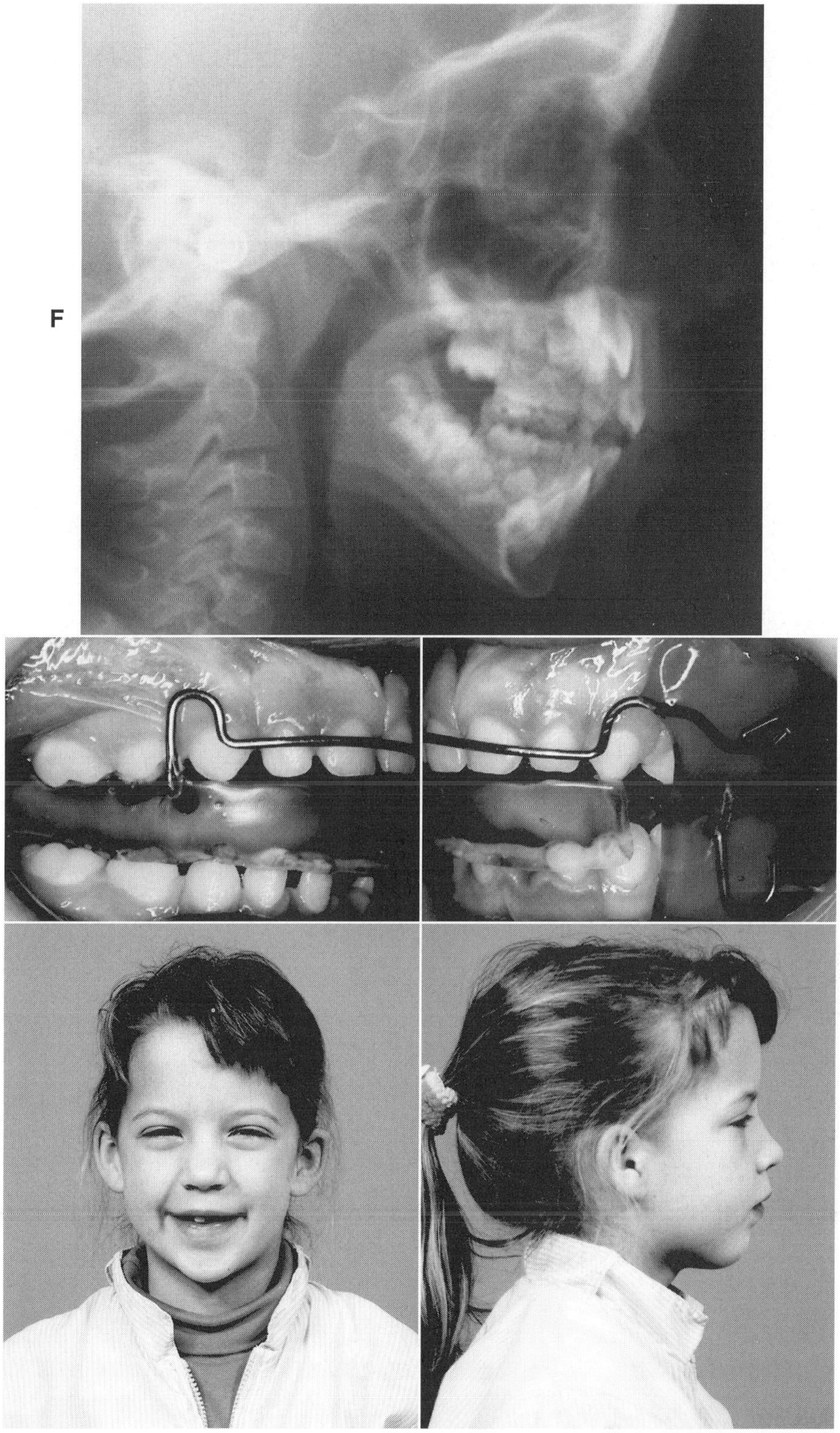

Figure 13-56 **cont'd F,** Note the two mandibular borders on the cephalometric radiograph due to the shorter ramus on the left. **G** and **H,** She was treated with a series of hybrid functional appliances, with buccal and lingual shields on the left, and a bite block anteriorly and on the right. The objective was to encourage mandibular growth and tooth eruption on the deficient left side and restrain eruption on the right. It is important to keep the tongue from between the teeth on the side where eruption is desired, thus the lingual shield on the left side (cannot be seen in the photos) was a critically important part of the appliance. **I** and **J,** Facial views 2 years later.

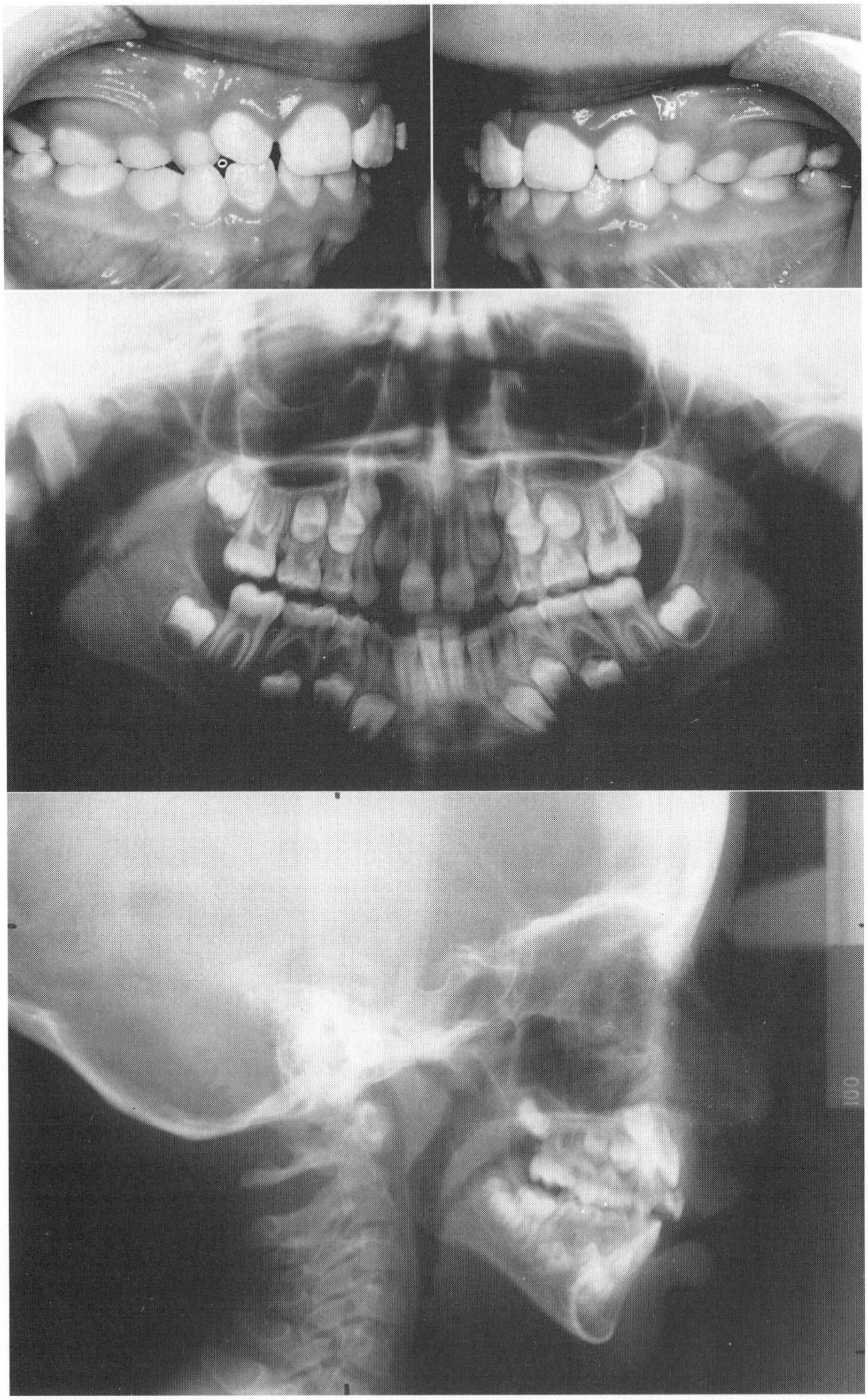

FIGURE 13-56 cont'd K and L, Intraoral views 2 years later. Note the improvement in both facial symmetry and occlusion. Treatment with hybrid functional appliances was continued. **M,** Panoramic and **(N)** cephalometric progress views. Note the regeneration of the left condyle and reduction in the difference in height of the two mandibular rami.

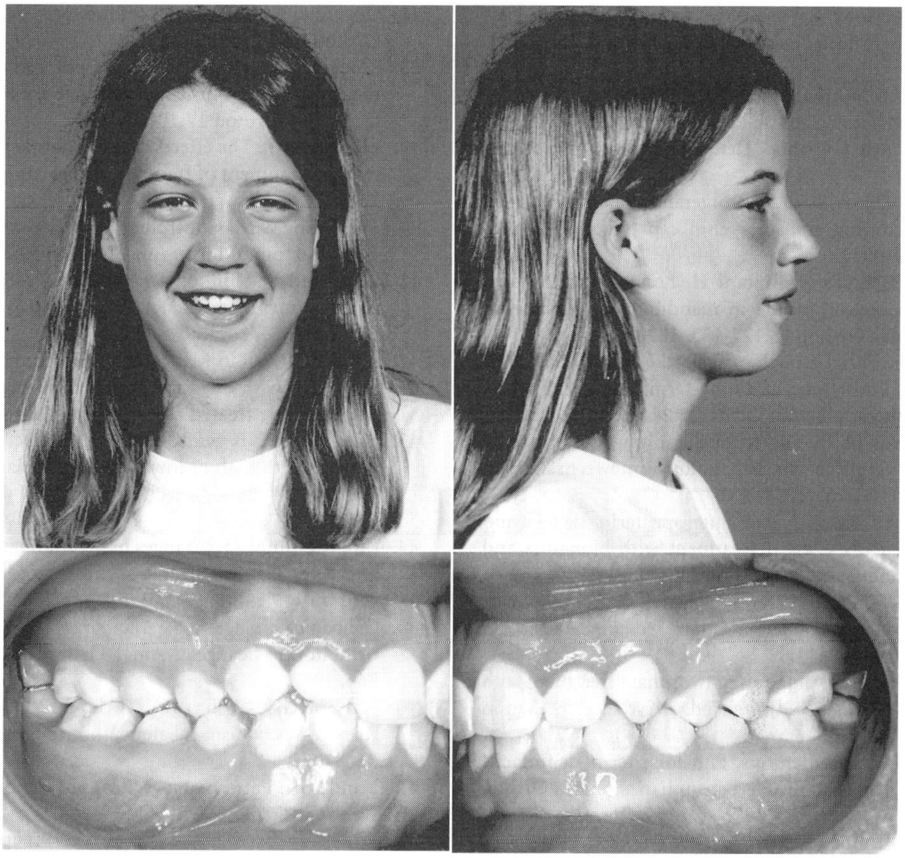

O P Q R

FIGURE 13-56 **cont'd** **O** and **P,** Facial, and **Q** and **R,** Intraoral views at age 13, with nearly complete resolution of the facial asymmetry although the mandible still deviates to the left on wide opening. Functional appliance treatment was discontinued at age 10, and there has been no further orthodontic therapy.

REFERENCES

1. Langberg BJ, Arai K, Miner RM. Transverse skeletal and dental asymmetry in adults with unilateral lingual posterior crossbite. Am J Orthod Dentofac Orthop 127:6-15, 2005.
2. Adkins MD, Nanda RS, Currier GF. Arch perimeter changes on rapid palatal expansion. Am J Orthod 97:10-19, 1990.
3. Sandikcioglu M, Hazar S. Skeletal and dental changes after maxillary expansion in the mixed dentition. Am J Orthod Dentofac Orthop 111:321-327, 1997.
4. daSilva Filho OG, Villas Boas M, Capelozza Filho L. Rapid palatal expansion in the deciduous and mixed dentitions: A cephalometric evaluation. Am J Orthod Dentofac Orthop 100:171-181, 1991.
5. Chang JY, McNamara JA Jr, Herberger TA. A longitudinal study of skeletal side effects induced by rapid maxillary expansion. Am J Orthod Dentofac Orthop 112:330-337, 1997.
6. Sarver DM, Johnston MW. Skeletal changes in vertical and anterior displacement of the maxilla with bonded rapid palatal expansion appliances. Am J Orthod Dentofac Orthop 95:462-466. 1989.
7. Reed N, Ghosh J, Nanda RS. Comparison of treatment outcomes with banded and bonded RPE appliances. Am J Orthod Dentofac Orthop 116:31-40, 1999.
8. Hicks E. Slow maxillary expansion: A clinical study of the skeletal versus the dental response to low magnitude force. Am J Orthod 73:121-141, 1978.
9. Akkaya S, Lorenzon S, Ucem TT. Comparison of dental arch and arch perimeter changes between bonded rapid and slow maxillary expansion procedures. Eur J Orthod 20:255-261, 1998.
10. Merwin D, Ngan P, Hagg U, et al. Timing for effective application of anteriorly directed orthopedic force to the maxilla. Am J Orthod Dentofac Orthop 112:292-299, 1997.
11. Franchi L, Baccetti T, McNamara JA. Postpubertal assessment of treatment timing for maxillary expansion and protraction therapy followed by fixed appliances. Am J Orthod Dentofac Orthop 126:555-568, 2004.
12. Kim JH, Viana MC, Graber TM, Omerza FF, BeGole EA. The effectiveness of protraction face mask therapy: A meta-analysis. Am J Orthod Dentofac Orthop 115:675-685, 1999.
13. Vaughn GA, Mason B, Moon HB, Turley PK. The effects of maxillary protraction therapy with or without rapid palatal expansion: A prospective, randomized clinical trial. Am J Orthod Dentofac Orthop 128:299-309, 2005.
14. da Silva Filho OG, Magro AC, Capelozza Filho L. Early treatment of the Class III malocclusion with rapid maxillary expansion and maxillary protraction. Am J Orthod Dentofac Orthop 113:196-203, 1998.
15. Shapiro PA, Kokich VG. Treatment alternatives for children with severe maxillary hypoplasia. Eur J Orthod 6:141-147, 1984.
16. Enacar A, Giray B, Pehlivanoglu M, Iplikcioglu H. Facemask therapy with rigid anchorage in a patient with maxillary hypoplasia and severe oligodontia. Am J Orthod Dentofac Orthop 123:571-577, 2003.
17. Ulgen M, Firatli S. The effects of the Frankel's function regulator on the Class III malocclusion. Am J Orthod Dentofac Orthop 105:561-567, 1994.

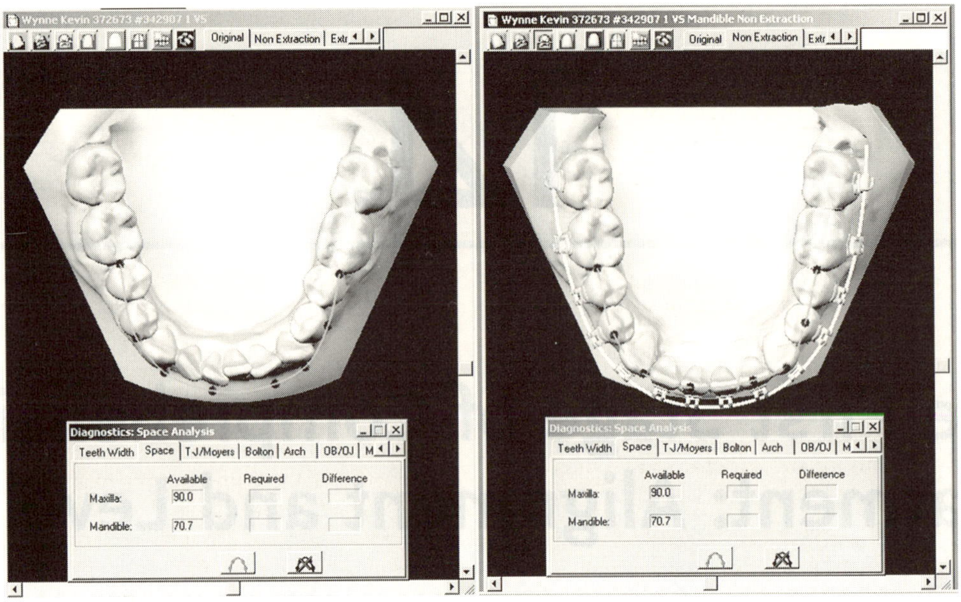

A

B

Figure 14-1 Digitized dental casts (here in the Ortho-CAD system) can be used quite effectively to calculate the amount of space needed to align the teeth, show the probable outcome of alignment and calculate the arch length needed. **A,** Pretreatment occlusal view of the lower arch, with a line showing the amount of space required for alignment; **B,** Virtual appliance in place.

In almost all patients with malocclusion, at least some teeth are initially malaligned. The great majority also have either excessive overbite, resulting from some combination of an excessive curve of Spee in the lower arch and an absent or reverse curve of Spee in the upper arch, or (less frequently) anterior open bite with excessive curve of Spee in the upper arch and little or none in the lower arch. The goals of the first phase of treatment are to bring the teeth into alignment and correct vertical discrepancies by leveling out the arches. In this form, however, neither goal is stated clearly enough. For proper alignment, it is necessary not only to bring malposed teeth into the arch, but also to specify and control the anteroposterior position of incisors, the width of the arches posteriorly, and the form of the dental arches. Similarly, in leveling the arch, it is necessary to determine and control whether the leveling occurs by elongation of posterior teeth, intrusion of incisors, or some specific combination of the two (see Chapter 7 for treatment planning details).

The form of the dental arches obviously varies between individuals. Although the orthodontist has some latitude in changing arch form, and indeed must do so in at least one arch if the upper and lower arch are not compatible initially, more stable results are achieved when the patient's original arch form is preserved during orthodontic treatment (see Chapter 12 for a discussion of arch form and archwire shape). The light resilient archwires used in the first stage of treatment need not be shaped to the patient's arch form as carefully as the heavier archwires used later in treatment, but from the beginning, the archwires should reflect each individual's arch form. If preformed archwires are used, from the beginning the appropriate large, medium or small arch form should be selected.

Because the orthodontic mechanotherapy will be different depending on exactly how alignment and leveling are to be accomplished, it is extremely important to clearly visualize the desired position of the teeth at the end of each stage of treatment before beginning that stage. Computer programs now exist to make this easier (Figure 14-1), but it is the thought process that counts. For instance, the best alignment procedures will result in incisors that are far too protrusive if the extractions necessary to prevent protrusion were not part of the plan. Similarly, unless leveling by intrusion is planned when it is needed, the appropriate mechanics are not likely to be selected.

In this and the subsequent chapters, it is expected that the appropriate goals for an individual patient have been clearly stated, and the discussion here concerns only the treatment techniques necessary to achieve those goals. Orthodontic treatment without specific goals can be an excellent illustration of the old adage, "If you don't know where you're going, it doesn't matter which road you take."

Alignment

Principles in the Choice of Alignment Arches

In nearly every patient with malaligned teeth, the root apices are closer to the normal position than the crowns, because malalignment almost always develops as the eruption paths of teeth are deflected. Putting it another way, a tooth bud occasionally develops in the wrong place, but (barring surgery that displaces all tissues in the area, as sometimes happens in cleft palate repairs, or the severe tipping from lip pressure that displaces maxillary central incisors in Class II, division 2 cases) the root apices are likely to be reasonably close to their correct positions even though the crowns have been displaced as the teeth erupted. To bring teeth into alignment, a combination of labiolingual and mesiodistal tipping guided by an archwire is needed, but root movement usually is not. Several important consequences for orthodontic mechanotherapy follow from this:

1. Initial archwires for alignment should provide light, continuous force of approximately 50 grams, to produce the most efficient tipping tooth movement. Heavy force, in contrast, is to be avoided.
2. The archwires should be able to move freely within the brackets. For mesiodistal sliding along an archwire, at least 2 mil clearance between the archwire and the bracket is needed, and 4 mil clearance is desirable. This means that the largest initial archwire that should be used with an 18-slot edgewise bracket is 16 mil, and 14 mil would be more satisfactory. With the 22-slot bracket, a 16 mil archwire would be satisfactory, and an 18 mil wire would not be too large from a bracket clearance point of view. Whatever the archwire, it should be ligated loosely in the bracket (indeed, this is probably the critical factor in determining frictional resistance to sliding). For that reason, more rapid alignment is a major advantage of self-ligating brackets that do not press the wire against the bottom of the bracket slot (see Chapter 11).
3. Rectangular archwires, particularly those with a tight fit within the bracket slot so that the position of the root apex could be affected, normally should be avoided. The principle is that it is better to tip crowns to position during initial alignment, rather than displacing the root apices; the corollary is that although a highly resilient rectangular archwire such as 17 × 25 A-NiTi could be used in the alignment stage, this is not advantageous because the rectangular archwire can create unnecessary and undesirable root movement during alignment (Figure 14-2). Superelastic NiTi wires have such low torsional strength that for all practical purposes they cannot torque roots,[2] so this complication is uncommon, but the larger wires nevertheless tend to slow the tipping movements needed for alignment. Round wires for alignment are preferred (Figure 14-3). There is no reason to pay extra for a high-performance rectangular wire for initial alignment, when alignment with it predictably will be slower and possibly more damaging to the roots than with a smaller round wire.
4. The springier the alignment archwire, the more important it is for the crowding to be at least reasonably symmetric. Otherwise, there is a danger that arch form will be lost as asymmetrically irregular teeth are brought into alignment. If only one tooth is crowded out of line, or if an impacted tooth has to be brought into alignment—a more severe version of the same thing—a rigid wire is needed so that arch form is maintained except where springiness is required, and an auxiliary wire should be used to reach the malaligned tooth. This important point is discussed in some detail below.

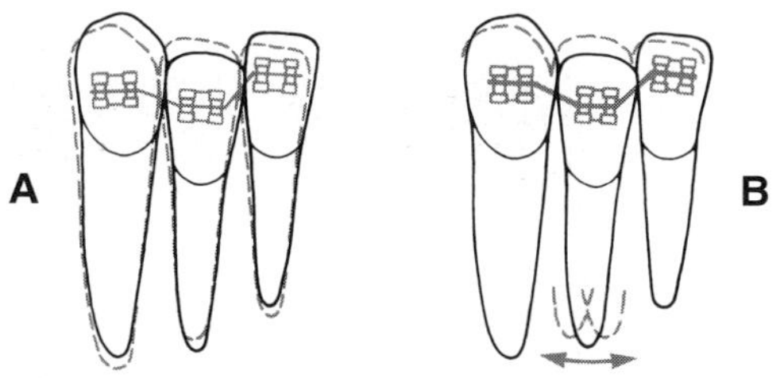

FIGURE 14-2 A tightly fitting resilient rectangular archwire for initial alignment is almost always undesirable because not only is frictional resistance to sliding likely to be problematic, the wire produces back-and-forth movement of the root apices as the teeth move into alignment. This occurs because the moments generated by the archwire change as the geometry of the system changes with alterations in tooth position. **A,** Diagrammatic representation of the alignment of a malposed lateral incisor with a round wire and clearance in the bracket slot. With minimal moments created within the bracket slot, there is little displacement of the root apex. **B,** With a rectangular archwire that has enough torsional stiffness to create root movement, back-and-forth movement of the apex occurs before the tooth ends up in essentially the same place as with a round wire. This has two disadvantages: it increases the possibility of root resorption, and it slows the alignment process.

Properties of Alignment Archwires

The wires for initial alignment require a combination of excellent strength, excellent springiness, and a long range of action. Ideally, there would be an almost flat load-deflection curve, with the wire delivering about 50 gm (the optimum force for tipping) at almost any degree of deflection. The variables in selecting appropriate archwires for alignment are the archwire material, its size (diameter or cross-section), and the distance between attachments (interbracket span). These factors have been discussed in Chapter 10 but are briefly reviewed here. Considering them in turn:

Archwire Material

The titanium-based archwires, both nickel-titanium (any of the NiTi wires) and beta-titanium (TMA), offer a better combination of strength and springiness than do steel wires (see Chapter 10). The NiTi wires, however, are both springier and stronger in small cross-section than beta-Ti. For this reason, NiTi wires are particularly useful in the first stage of treatment, and the remarkably flat load-deflection curve for

A

B

C

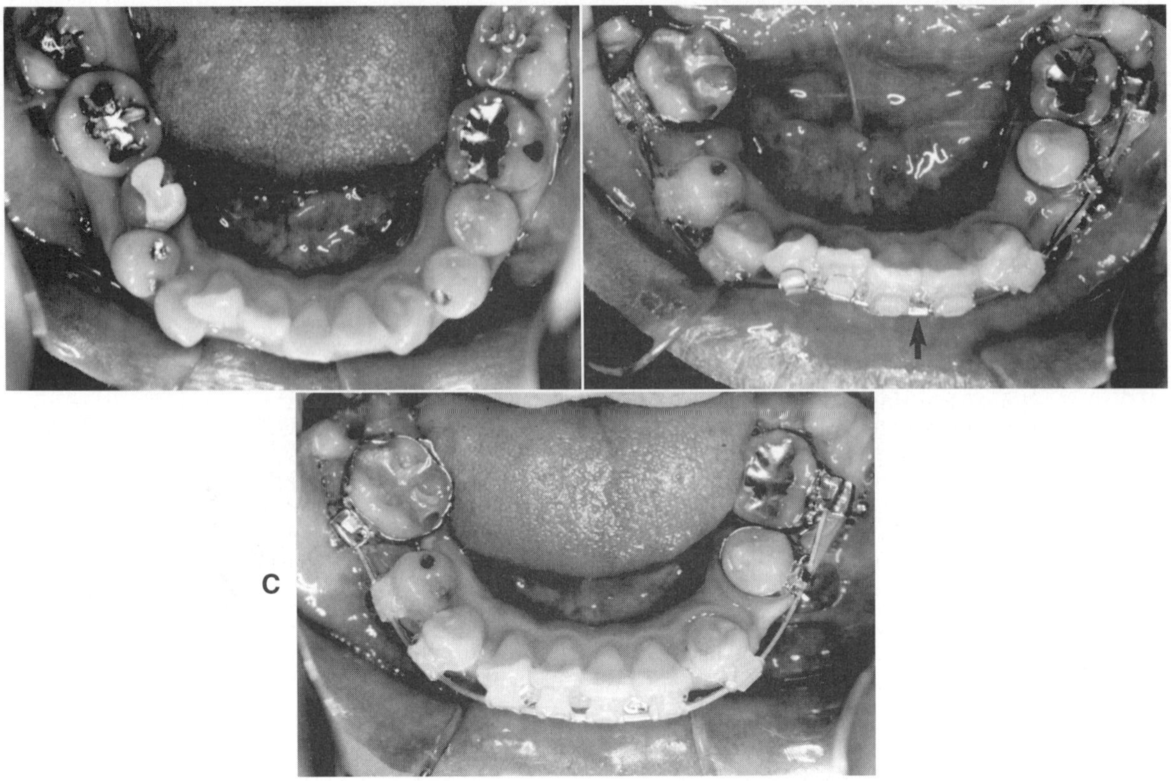

Figure 14-3 Alignment of severely crowded incisors with superelastic A-NiTi archwires in an adult. **A,** Pretreatment severe crowding; **B,** Progress with initial round A-NiTi archwire after premolar extraction to provide space. Note the split spacer crimped on the wire between the left central and lateral incisor brackets, to prevent archwire travel; **C,** Preliminary alignment completed, rectangular NiTi wire in place.

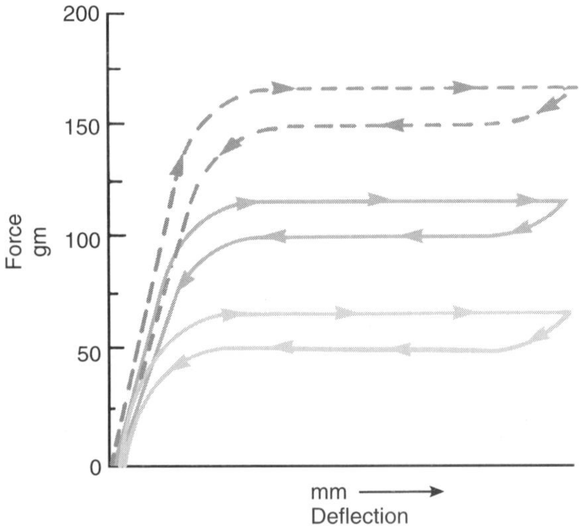

Figure 14-4 Force-deflection curves for 16 mil A-NiTi wires (Sentinol, GAC) prepared by the manufacturer to have different force delivery characteristics. For superelastic wires, the manufacturer's preparation, not the wire size, is the major factor in determining force delivery.

superelastic NiTi (austenitic NiTi, A-NiTi) makes it the preferred material (Figure 14-4). It is important to keep in mind that not all ostensibly superelastic wires offer the same performance, however. The choice of a superelastic wire should be based on performance data—and a product with advertising claims but no data should be regarded with considerable suspicion. If steel is used at this stage, either multistranded wires or loops to increase springiness (see following) are needed. Beta-Ti (TMA) rarely is the best choice for an initial archwire.

Size of Wire

For the superelastic A-NiTi wires, the manufacturer's preparation of the material determines the clinical performance, so wire size is a concern primarily with respect to clearance in the bracket slot. For the M-NiTi, beta-Ti or steel wires that now are used infrequently for initial alignment, wire size is an important criterion with respect to the wire properties. As wire size increases, strength increases rapidly, while springiness decreases even more rapidly, so the smallest diameter (and therefore the springiest) wire that has adequate strength would be preferred. When multiple strands of the same diameter wire are used, strength is added while springiness is relatively unaffected. This method of combining steel strands that individually would not be strong enough, makes steel wires without loops practical at the initial stage of treatment, but only if the irregularity is modest.

Distance Between Attachments

As the distance increases between the points of attachment of a beam, strength decreases rapidly while springiness increases even more rapidly. The width of brackets determines beam length when continuous archwires are used (unless brackets are bypassed): the wider the individual brackets, the smaller the interbracket span. For this reason, elastic archwires become very much stiffer when wide brackets reduce interbracket span. This is a particularly important consideration when non-superelastic wires are used initially.

As we have discussed in Chapter 10, it is logical to use narrow brackets with 18-slot edgewise, for two reasons: (1) In the latter stages of treatment the rectangular steel archwires that fill the slot are more effective with larger interbracket spans, and (2) sliding teeth along the archwire to close extraction spaces is relatively unimportant. With 22-slot edgewise, since the larger slot provides the clearance needed for sliding but makes it difficult to obtain close engagement of rectangular archwires with loops in closing extraction spaces, wider brackets are preferred. Prior to almost routine use of superelastic wires, bracket slot size and interbracket span were such strong influences on archwire choice that different initial wires often were used with the 18 and 22 slot appliances. This is no longer the case. But with superelastic wires it is necessary to pay more attention to maintaining arch form during alignment, to the point that now alignment when crowding is reasonably symmetric must be viewed differently from alignment in highly asymmetric situations.

Alignment of Symmetric Crowding

Archwire Choices

The flat load-deflection curve of superelastic NiTi (see Figure 14-4) makes it ideal for initial alignment when the degree of crowding is similar on the two sides of the arch. The superelastic wire provides remarkable range over which a tooth can be moved without generating excessive force. Under most circumstances initial alignment can be accomplished simply by tying 14 or 16 mil A-NiTi that delivers about 50 gm into the brackets of all the teeth, being careful not to tie too tightly, and observing the patient without the necessity of other changes (see Figure 14-3). The size of the superelastic wire is not a critical variable, except that 18 mil wires should not be used in the 18 slot appliance.

It is possible now to obtain superelastic wires that are almost totally passive when cold, but deliver the desired force when at mouth temperature. Placing a chilled wire is much easier than placing a springy one, and this can be significant advantage under some circumstances. On the other hand, once mouth temperature has been reached, there is no reason to expect such a thermally-sensitive wire to perform better than one without this feature.

When superelastic NiTi was first introduced, the major objection to it was that it is expensive. If a large range is not necessary, a triple-stranded 17.5 mil multistranded steel wire (3 × 8 mil) offers good properties at a fraction of the cost. In theory, this size would be too large for effective use in 18-slot brackets. Clinical research has shown, however, that in both the 18 and 22 appliance, if these wires are recontoured monthly and retied with elastomeric ligatures, the time to alignment is equivalent to A-NiTi.[3] Force levels certainly are more variable and patient discomfort probably is greater than with superelastic wires, but it is difficult to demonstrate this clinically.

The reason for this surprisingly good clinical performance probably is that flexible archwires allow the teeth to move relative to each other during chewing, as alveolar bone bends under masticatory loads (see Chapter 9). This releases frictional binding and allows the bracket to slide along the archwire to the next point at which friction stops it. But the lower cost of the steel archwire is quickly overbalanced by the additional clinical time necessary to retie it, especially if it must be taken out, adjusted to remove any areas of permanent distortion, and then re-ligated.

Laboratory data and clinical experience suggest that similar performance to the multistrand steel wire could be obtained with M-NiTi, a variety of more elaborate multi strand wires (coaxial wires, for instance, that have several smaller wires wound over a larger core wire), or with loops in small diameter steel wires. Both M-NiTi and coaxial multistrand wires are expensive, and the time to bend loops in 14 or 16 steel wires also is expensive. These wires, though they were the standard of treatment for initial alignment only a few years ago, have little or no place in current therapy.

As one might expect, the extreme springiness of superelastic wires is not a totally unmixed blessing. When these wires are tied into a malocclusion, they have a tendency to "travel" around the arch as the patient chews, especially if function is mostly on one side. Then the wire sticks out the back of the molar tube on one side, and may come out of the tube on the other side. Occasionally this can be extreme requires first opening enough space, then bringing the displaced tooth or teeth across the occlusion into proper position.

Occlusal interferences can make this difficult. The patient may tend to bite brackets off the displaced teeth, and as the teeth are moved "through the bite", occlusal force pushes them one way while the orthodontic appliance pulls them the other. It may be necessary to use a bite plate temporarily to separate the posterior teeth and create the vertical space needed to allow the teeth to move. The older the patient, the more likely it is that a bite plate will be needed. During rapid growth in early adolescence, often incisors that were locked in anterior crossbite can be corrected without a bite plate. After that, one probably will be required.

Transverse Maxillary Expansion by Opening the Midpalatal Suture

It is relatively easy to widen the maxilla by opening the midpalatal suture before and during adolescence, but this becomes progressively more difficult as patients become older. The chances of successful opening of the suture are nearly 100% before age 15, but decline thereafter because of the increased interdigitation of the sutures (see Figure 9-25).

Patients who are candidates for opening the midpalatal suture may have such severe crowding that even with this arch expansion, premolar extraction will be required. In these patients, however, separation of the suture should be the first step in treatment, before either extraction or alignment. The first premolar teeth are useful as anchorage for the lateral expansion and can serve for that purpose even if they are to be extracted later, and the additional space provided by the lateral expansion facilitates alignment.

Sometimes, transverse maxillary expansion can provide enough additional space to make extraction unnecessary, but rarely is it wise to use sutural expansion as a means of dealing with a crowding in an individual who already has normal maxillary width (see Chapter 8). Opening the midpalatal suture should be used primarily as a means of correcting a skeletal crossbite, making a narrow maxilla normal, not a normal maxilla abnormally wide.

In the early permanent dentition, the basic mechanism for separation of the midpalatal suture is a jackscrew built into a fixed appliance that is rigidly attached to as many posterior teeth as possible. The appliance can be made so that it has plastic palate-covering shelves or can consist solely of a metal or plastic framework against the teeth, not contacting the palatal tissue (Figure 14-11). In theory, the flanges extending into the palate could cause a more bodily repositioning of the alveolar processes, but in fact, there seems to be little or no difference in the skeletal or dental response to the two types of appliances.[4] Because the palate-covering appliance remains in contact with the soft tissue for an extended period, however, it can cause tissue irritation. For this reason, an appliance that does not contact the palate is preferred.

When the maxillary teeth move transversely, some extrusion may occur, and even if it does not, the tooth movement creates cuspal interferences that cause the mandible to rotate down and back. In deep bite patients who are still growing or in patients with a mild Class III tendency, this can be advantageous, but it is a problem in long face patients with a narrow maxilla. Adding bite blocks to a bonded expander is the best way to overcome this problem (Figure 14-12).[5]

Separation of the midpalatal suture can be produced by either rapid or slow expansion, and the same type of palate-separating appliance can be used for either approach (see Figure 8-16). Whether the expansion is done rapidly or slowly, the fixed appliance remains in place for approximately the same length of time, because a shorter period of post-expansion stabilization is sufficient with slow expansion. With rapid expansion, the expansion itself is carried out in approximately 2 weeks, but the screw should then be stabilized and the appliances maintained in place for 3 to 4 months of retention. With slow expansion, approximately $2\frac{1}{2}$ months are needed to obtain the expansion, and the appliance can be removed in another 2 months.

Some degree of relapse can be expected after palatal expansion because of the elasticity of the palatal soft tissue. Therefore it is wise to overcorrect the crossbite initially, bringing the maxillary lingual cusps into contact with the mandibular buccal cusps. Even if a period of stabilization with the palate-separating device has been provided, additional retention of the crossbite correction is needed when the fixed appliance is removed. A palate-covering removable retainer is satisfactory but may be somewhat awkward in combination with fixed appliances to align the teeth as the first stage of treatment proceeds. An alternative is a heavy labial archwire placed in the headgear tubes, which will maintain the lateral expansion while light resilient archwires are being used to align the teeth (Figure 14-13), or a lingual arch. The lingual arch gives better control of root position but the heavy labial arch can be fabricated much more quickly and easily. Unless a direct lingual arch can be placed as soon as the expansion appliance is removed, it is wise to use the heavy labial arch at least temporarily.

Correction of Dental Posterior Crossbites

Three approaches to correction of less severe dental crossbites are feasible: a heavy labial expansion arch, as shown in Figure 14-13, an expansion lingual arch, or cross-elastics. Removable appliances, although theoretically possible, are not compatible with comprehensive treatment and should be reserved for the mixed dentition or adjunctive treatment.

The inner bow of a facebow is also, of course, a heavy labial arch, and expansion of this inner bow is a convenient way to expand the upper molars. This expansion is nearly always needed for patients with a Class II molar relationship, whose upper arch usually is too narrow to accommodate the mandibular arch when it comes forward into the correct

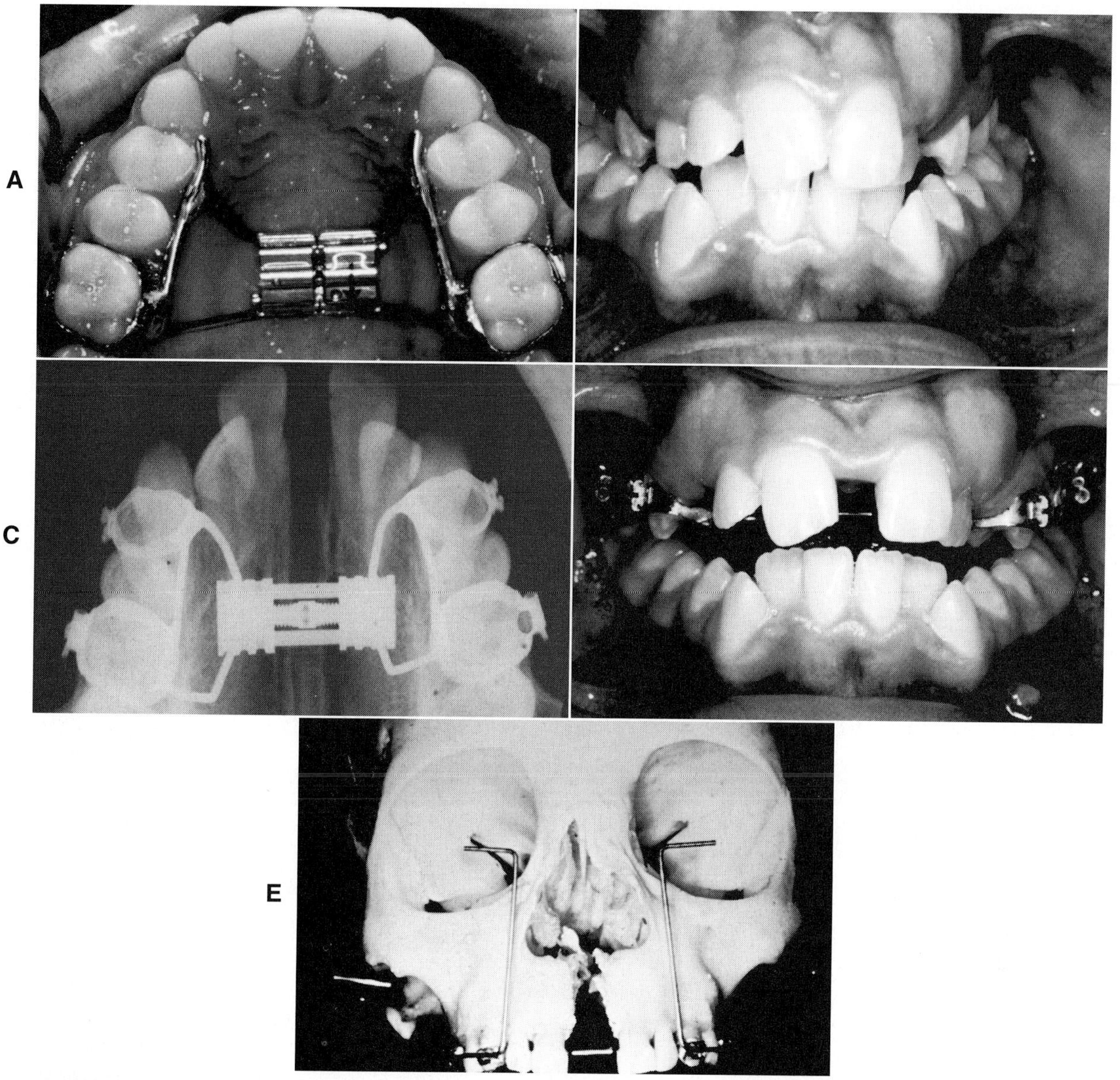

Figure 14-11 Palatal expansion in adolescents requires a rigid framework because of the heavy forces (2 to 4 pounds with slow expansion, 10 to 20 pounds with rapid expansion) that will be encountered. Although the various expansion appliances look quite different, they produce similar results. **A,** Hyrax expander with metal framework. Often an expander of this type is attached to bands on the first premolars as well as the molars. **B,** Severe maxillary constriction leading to bilateral crossbite; **C, D,** Progress with rapid expansion in this patient. Note the development of a space between the central incisors as the suture expands more anteriorly than posteriorly. **E,** Expansion on a skull, showing how the palate opens as if on a hinge at the base of the nose.

relationship because the upper molars are tipped lingually. The inner bow is simply adjusted at each appointment to be sure that it is slightly wider than the headgear tubes and must be compressed by the patient when inserting the facebow. If the distal force of a headgear is not desired, a heavy labial auxiliary can provide the expansion effect alone. The effect of the round wire in the headgear tubes, however, is to tip the crowns outward, and so this method should be reserved for patients whose molars are tipped lingually.

A transpalatal lingual arch for expansion must have some springiness and range of action. As a general principle, the more flexible a lingual arch is, the better it is for tooth movement but the less it adds to anchorage stability. This can be an important consideration in adolescent and adult patients. If anchorage is of no concern, a highly flexible lingual arch, like the quad helix design discussed in Chapter 12, is an excellent choice for correction of a dental crossbite. When the lingual arch is needed for both expansion and anchorage, however, the choices are 36 mil steel wire with an adjustment loop, or the newer system that allows the use of 32 × 32 TMA or steel wire (Figure 14-14).

The third possibility for dental expansion is the use of cross-elastics, typically running from the lingual of the upper molar to the buccal of the lower molar (Figure 14-15). These

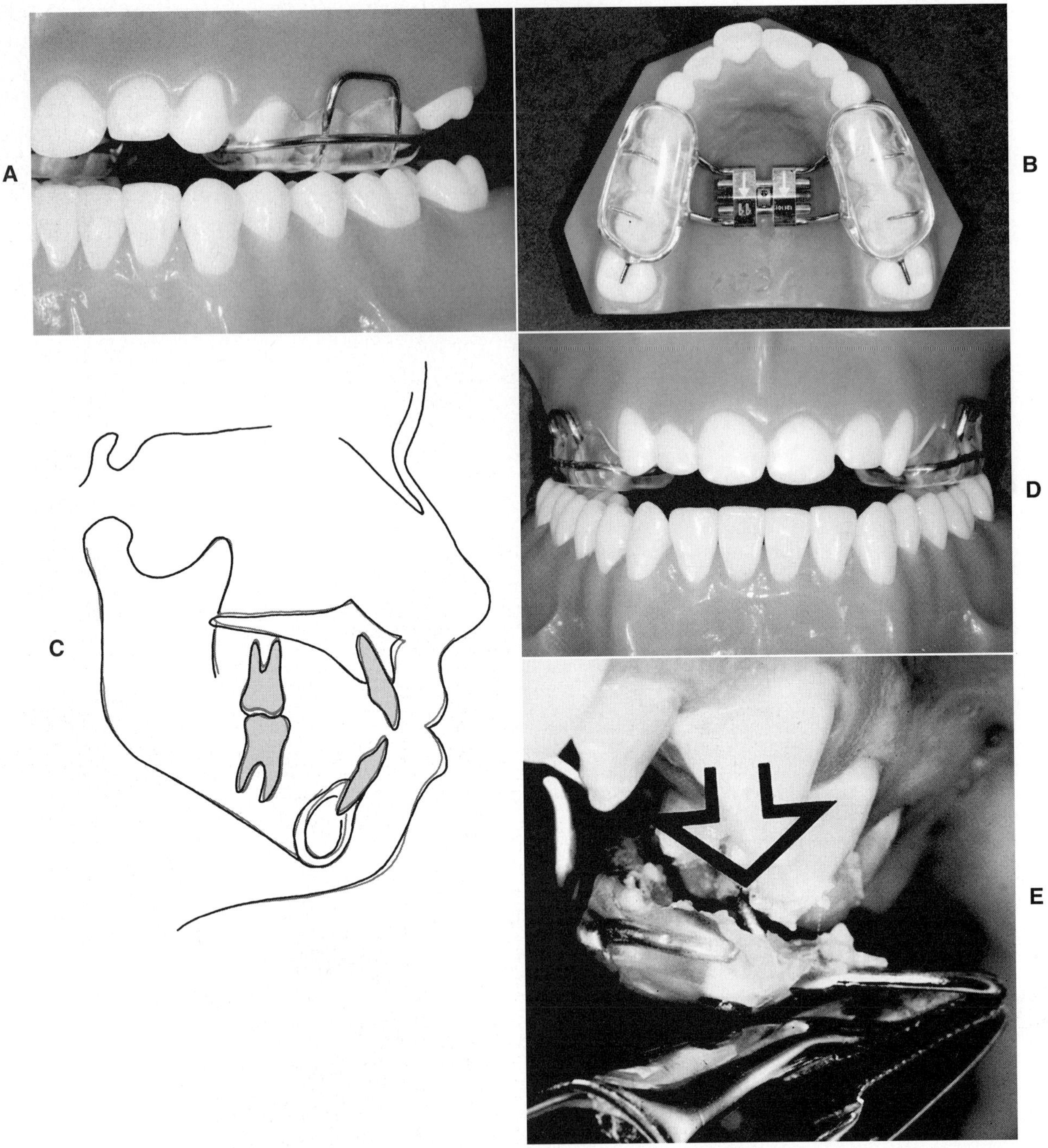

Figure 14-12 **A** and **B,** A bonded expander, shown here on a typodont, has two potential advantages over a banded type: occlusal force against the acrylic over the posterior teeth reduces the amount of extrusion and downward-backward rotation of the mandible that typically accompanies maxillary expansion, which is important in patients with a long face tendency; and the bonded type is easier to use in children in the mixed dentition. **C,** Cephalometric superimposition before and after expansion, showing the small amount of mandibular rotation when expansion was done with a device of this type, **D** and **E,** Removal of a bonded appliance of this type is facilitated by loops extending from the appliance that can be gripped and torqued.

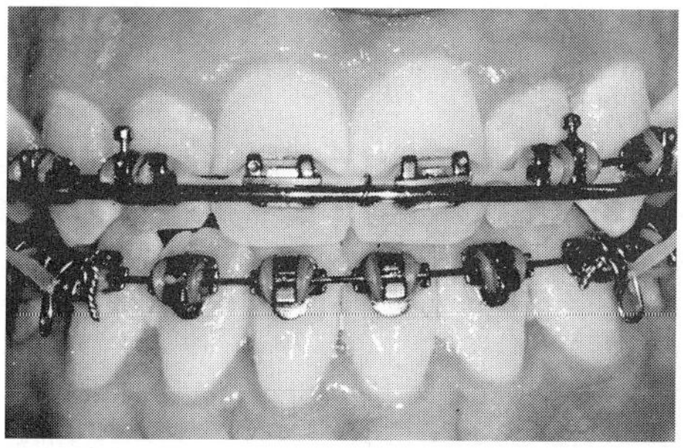

FIGURE 14-13 A heavy labial archwire (usually 36 or 40 mil steel) placed in the headgear tubes on first molars can be used to maintain arch width after palatal suture opening while the teeth are being aligned. This is more compatible with fixed-appliance treatment than a removable retainer and does not depend on patient cooperation. (From Proffit WR, White RP, Sarver DM. Contemporary Treatment of Dentofacial Deformity. St. Louis: Mosby; 2003.)

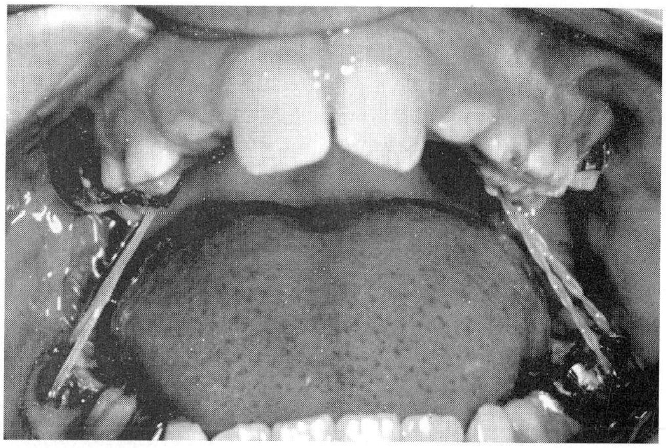

FIGURE 14-15 Cross-elastics from the lingual of the upper molars to the buccal of the lower molars. Cross-elastics are an effective way of correcting transverse dental relationships, but they also extrude teeth, and this must be kept in mind.

A

B

C

D

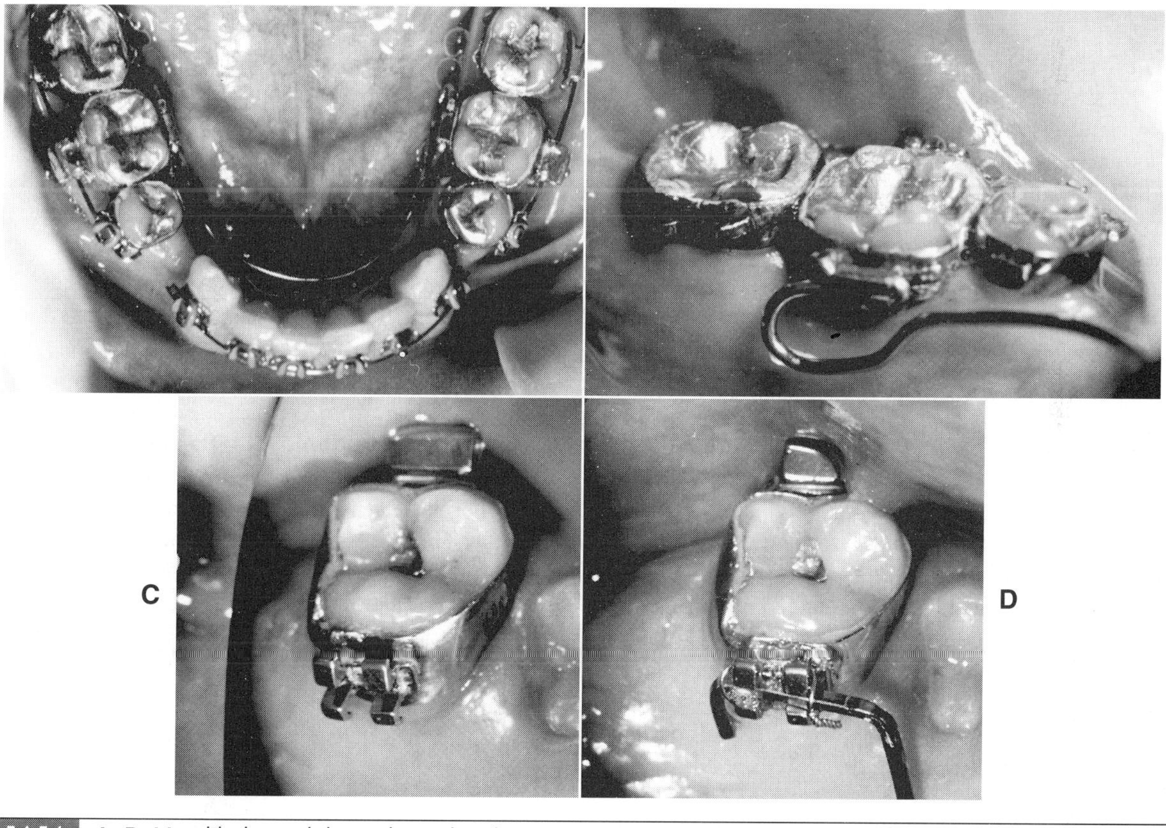

FIGURE 14-14 **A, B,** Mandibular stabilizing lingual arch. It is easier to insert a heavy lingual arch of this type from the distal of a horizontal tube on the first molar bands. Note that the lingual arch is contoured away from the incisors, so that it does not interfere with aligning and retracting them. **C, D,** A maxillary lingual arch can be active, typically to rotate the maxillary molars, or passive for stabilization. An active lingual arch can be placed in a horizontal tube or ligated into a special bracket on the molars. Ligation into a bracket makes it easier to remove and adjust the lingual arch, but over time gingival overgrowth can make re-ligation difficult.

elastics are effective, but their strong extrusive component must be kept in mind. As a general rule, adolescent patients can tolerate a short period of cross-elastic wear to correct a simple crossbite, because any extrusion is compensated by vertical growth of the ramus, but cross-elastics should be used with great caution, if at all, in adults. As any posterior crossbite is corrected, interference of the cusps increases posterior vertical dimension and thereby tends to rotate the mandible downward and backward, even if cross-elastics are avoided. The elastics accentuate this tendency.

If teeth are tightly locked into a posterior crossbite relationship, a bite plate to separate them vertically can make the correction easier and faster. In children and young adolescents, this is rarely needed. Use of a bite plate during transverse expansion indicates that elongation of the posterior teeth and downward-backward rotation of the mandible is an acceptable outcome.

IMPACTED OR UNERUPTED TEETH

Bringing an impacted or unerupted tooth into the arch creates a set of special problems during alignment. The most frequent impaction is a maxillary canine or canines, but it is occasionally necessary to bring other unerupted teeth into the arch, and the same techniques apply for incisors, canines and premolars. Impacted lower second molars pose a different problem and are discussed separately.

The problems in dealing with an unerupted tooth fall into three categories: (1) surgical exposure, (2) attachment to the tooth, and (3) orthodontic mechanics to bring the tooth into the arch.

Surgical Exposure

Before surgery to expose an unerupted tooth, it is obviously important to know with some precision where it is. A panoramic radiograph is the usual screening tool, but occlusal and periapical radiographs have proven more helpful in delineating the true position of the unerupted tooth and its possible overlap with the roots of erupted teeth.[6] The available options using the tube-shift method are a combination of the panoramic and an occlusal film (the vertical parallax method) or multiple periapical radiographs (the lateral cone shift method). The lateral cone shift method appears to do a better job of localizing maxillary canines.[7] With both methods, if the tooth in question is on the lingual of the reference object (an adjacent erupted tooth), it will move in the same direction as the tube is shifted. If it is on the buccal, it will move in the opposite direction as the tube shift.

It is important for a tooth to erupt through the attached gingiva, not through alveolar mucosa, and this must be considered when flaps to expose an unerupted tooth are planned. If the unerupted tooth is in the mandibular arch or on the labial side of the maxillary alveolar process, a flap should be reflected from the crest of the alveolus and sutured so that attached gingiva has been transferred to the region where the crown is exposed (see Figure 12-30). If this is not done, and the tooth is brought through alveolar mucosa, it is quite likely that tissue will strip away from the crown, leaving an unsightly and periodontally compromised gingival margin.[8] If the unerupted tooth is on the palatal side, similar problems with the heavy palatal mucosa are unlikely, and flap design is less critical.

Occasionally, a tooth will obligingly erupt into its correct position after obstacles to eruption have been removed by surgical exposure, but this is rarely the case after root formation is complete. At that stage, even a tooth that is aimed in the right direction usually requires orthodontic force to bring it into position.

Method of Attachment

The least desirable way to obtain attachment is for the surgeon to place a wire ligature around the crown of the impacted tooth. This inevitably results in loss of periodontal attachment, because bone destroyed when the wire is passed around the tooth does not regenerate when it is removed. Occasionally no alternative is practical, but wire ligatures should be avoided whenever possible.

Before the availability of direct bonding, a pin was sometimes placed in a hole prepared in the crown of an unerupted tooth, and in special circumstances, this remains a possible alternative. The best contemporary approach, however, is simply to expose an area on the crown of the tooth and directly bond an attachment of some type to that surface (Figure 14-16). In many instances, a button or hook is better than a standard bracket because it is smaller. Then, a piece of fine gold chain is tied to the attachment, and before the flap is repositioned and sutured into place, this is positioned so that it extends into the mouth. The chain is much easier to tie to than a wire ligature.

Mechanical Approaches for Aligning Unerupted Teeth

Orthodontic traction to pull an unerupted tooth toward the line of the arch should begin as soon as possible after surgery. Ideally, a fixed orthodontic appliance should already be in place before the unerupted tooth is exposed, so that orthodontic force can be applied immediately. If this is not practical, active orthodontic movement should begin no later than 2 or 3 weeks postsurgically.

This means that orthodontic treatment to open space for the unerupted tooth and allow stabilization of the rest of the

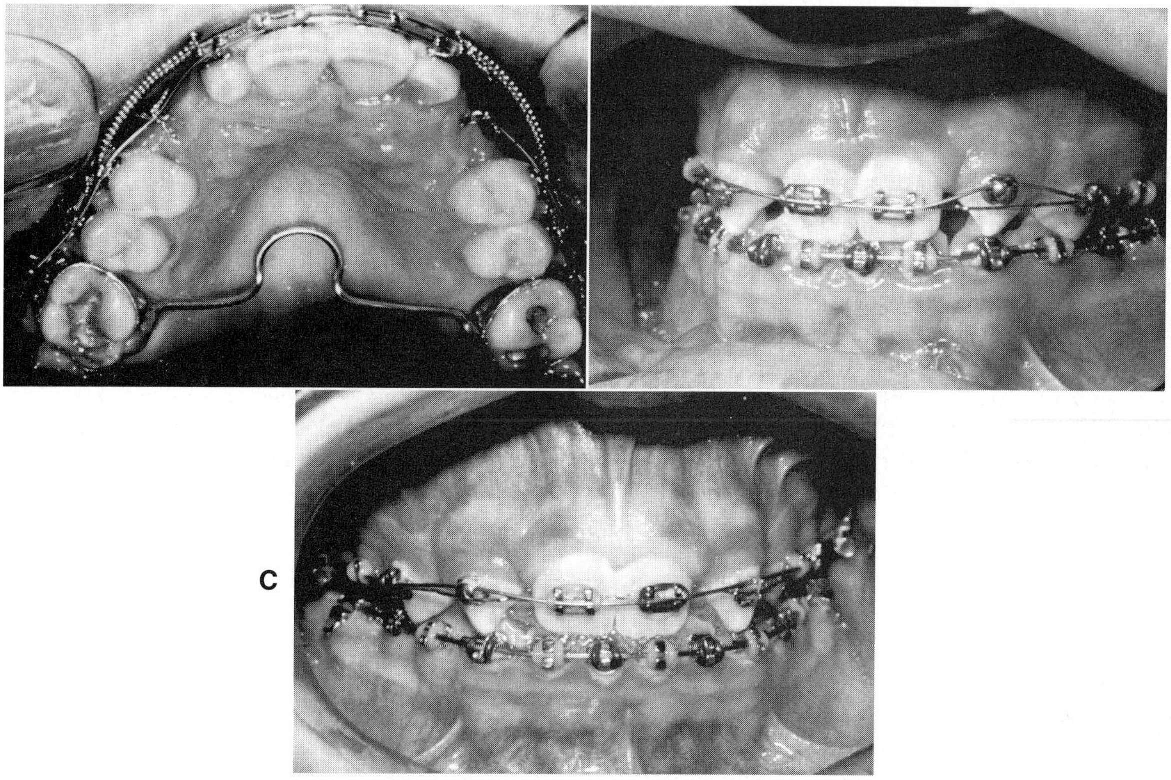

Figure 14-16 **A,** For this patient with bilateral impacted maxillary canines, a soldered lingual arch has been placed for better anchorage control; a heavy labial archwire is in place after space for the canines has been opened; and an auxiliary A-NiTi wire is tied to attachments (preferably, a segment of gold chain) that were bonded to the canines at the time they were exposed. **B,** Progress in the same patient, with the A-NiTi auxiliary now placed over a button that was bonded on the facial surface of the canine after it was brought down enough to allow this. **C,** When the tooth has elongated enough, the button is replaced with a standard canine bracket and alignment is complete.

dental arch must begin well before the surgical exposure. In this instance, the goals of presurgical orthodontic treatment are to create enough space if it does not exist, as often is the case; and to align the other teeth so that a heavy stabilizing archwire (at least 18 steel, preferably a rectangular steel wire) can be in position at the time of surgery. This allows postsurgical orthodontic treatment to start immediately.

As we have noted above, an unerupted tooth is an extreme example of an asymmetric alignment problem, with one tooth far from the line of occlusion. An auxiliary NiTi wire, overlaid on the stabilizing arch in the same way as recommended above for other asymmetric alignment situations (see Figure 14-16), now is the most efficient way to bring an impacted tooth into position. The numerous alternatives include a special alignment spring, either soldered to a heavy base archwire or bent into a light archwire, or a cantilever spring from the auxiliary tube on the first molar (Figure 14-17).

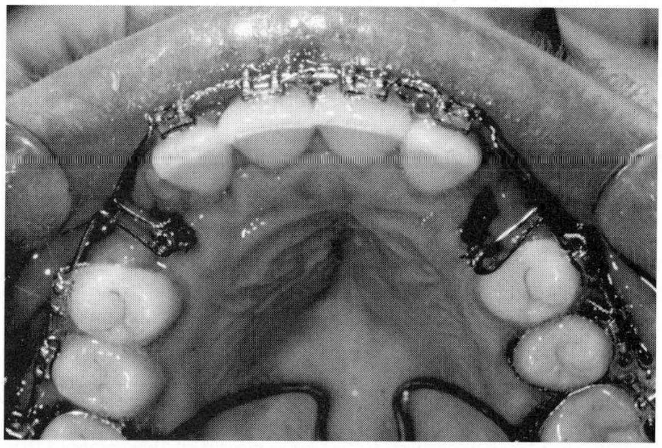

Figure 14-17 A vertical spring bent into a 14 mil steel archwire is an alternative approach to bring down an impacted canine. The spring is a loop of wire that faces downward before activation and is rotated 90° for attachment to the impacted tooth or teeth. This method is effective but less efficient than using a superelastic auxiliary wire.

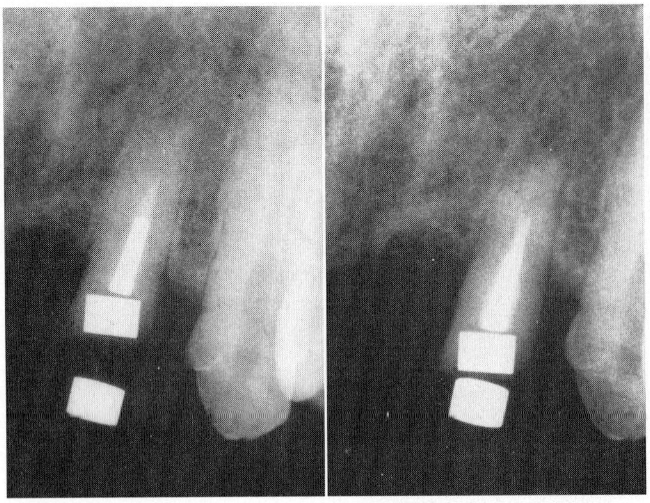

Figure 14-18 Use of magnets in attraction, one placed in the root of a fractured premolar and the other in a removable plate, to elongate a fractured tooth so that its crown can be restored.

Another possibility, magnetic force to initiate movement of an unerupted tooth, is especially attractive for a patient with other missing teeth in the maxillary arch because no mechanical connection is required. The technique involves bonding a small magnet to the unerupted maxillary tooth, and placing a larger magnet in attraction within a palate-covering removable appliance (Figure 14-18).[9,10] Unfortunately, success depends entirely on the patient's cooperation in wearing the removable appliance with the intraoral magnet all the time.

Ankylosis of an unerupted tooth is always a potential problem. If an area of fusion to the adjacent bone develops, orthodontic movement of the unerupted tooth becomes impossible, and displacement of the anchor teeth will occur. Occasionally, an unerupted tooth will start to move and then will become ankylosed, apparently held by only a small area of fusion. It can sometimes be freed to continue movement by anesthetizing the area and lightly luxating the tooth, breaking the area of ankylosis. If this procedure is done, it is critically important to apply orthodontic force immediately after the luxation, since it is only a matter of time until the tooth re-ankyloses. Nevertheless, this approach can sometimes allow a tooth to be brought into the arch that otherwise would have been impossible to move.

Unerupted/Impacted Lower Second Molars

Unlike impaction of most other teeth, which is an obvious problem from the beginning of treatment, impaction of lower second molars usually develops during orthodontic treatment (Figure 14-19). This occurs when the mesial marginal ridge of the second molar catches against the distal surface of the first molar or on the edge of a first molar band, so that the second molar progressively tips mesially instead of erupting. Moving the first molar posteriorly during the mixed dentition increases the chance that the second molar will become impacted. This possibility must be taken into account when procedures to increase mandibular arch length are employed.

Correction of an impacted second molar requires tipping the tooth posteriorly and uprighting it. In most cases, if the mesial marginal ridge can be unlocked, the tooth will erupt on its own. When the second molar is not severely tipped, the simplest solution is to place a separator between the two teeth. For more severe problems, an attachment must be bonded to the second molar as shown above. An auxiliary spring (Figure 14-20) often is useful to bring both upper and lower second molars into alignment when they erupt late in orthodontic treatment. The easiest way to do this is to use a segment of NiTi wire from the auxiliary tube on the first molar to the tube on the second molar. A rectangular wire, usually 16 × 22 M-NiTi, is preferred. This provides a light force to align the second molars while a heavier and more rigid wire remains in place anteriorly, which is much better than going back to a light round wire for the entire arch just to align the second molars.

Another possibility in adolescents is surgical uprighting of the impacted second molar, taking advantage of the space that is created when the third molar is extracted. In carefully selected cases, this can work quite nicely. Vitality of the second molar is retained because it essentially is rotated around the root apex, and the defect on the mesial of the uprighted tooth fills in with bone in the same way that it does when orthodontic uprighting is done (Figure 14-21).[11] The outcome is best when some vertical jaw growth remains so that the uprighted tooth does not remain elongated relative to the first molar.

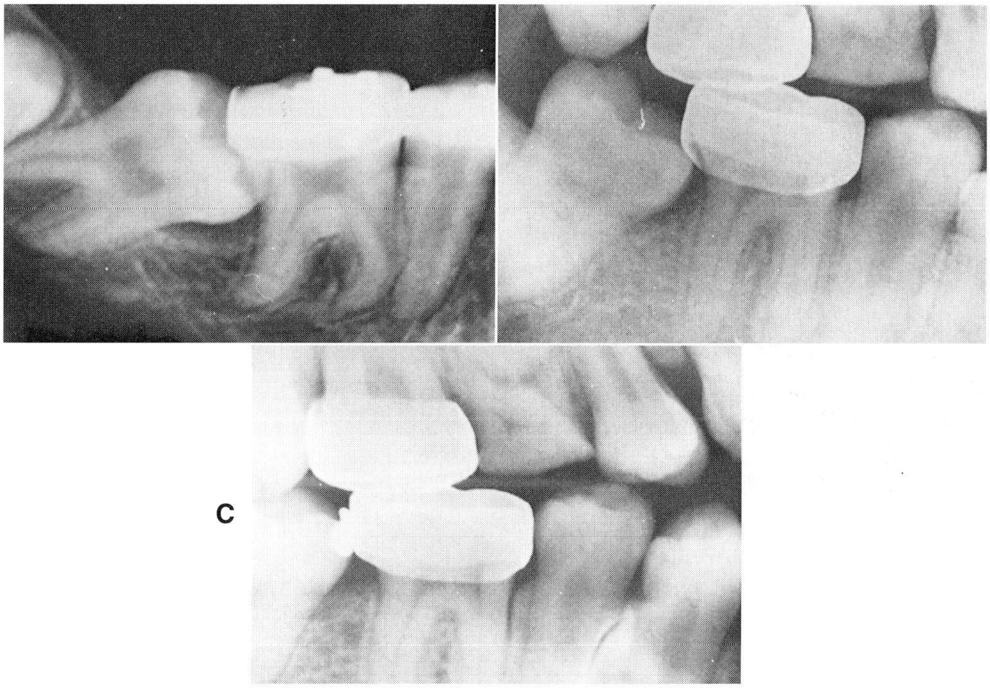

Figure 14-19 **A,** Radiographic view of an impacted mandibular second molar in a 16-year-old patient. Uprighting the tooth from this position requires surgical exposure of a portion of the facial surface of the crown and bonding an attachment (if possible, a tube) so that a spring can be used to tip it distally and bring it into the arch. **B,** For a second molar that is caught on the edge of a first molar band, a simpler approach is uprighting achieved with a 20 mil brass wire tightened around the contact. Usually it is necessary to anesthetize the area to place a separator on this type. **C,** Uprighting and distal movement obtained with the brass wire separator. A spring clip (one type is sold as the Arkansas de-impaction spring) can be used in the same way, but both brass wire and spring clips are effective only if the tooth is minimally tipped.

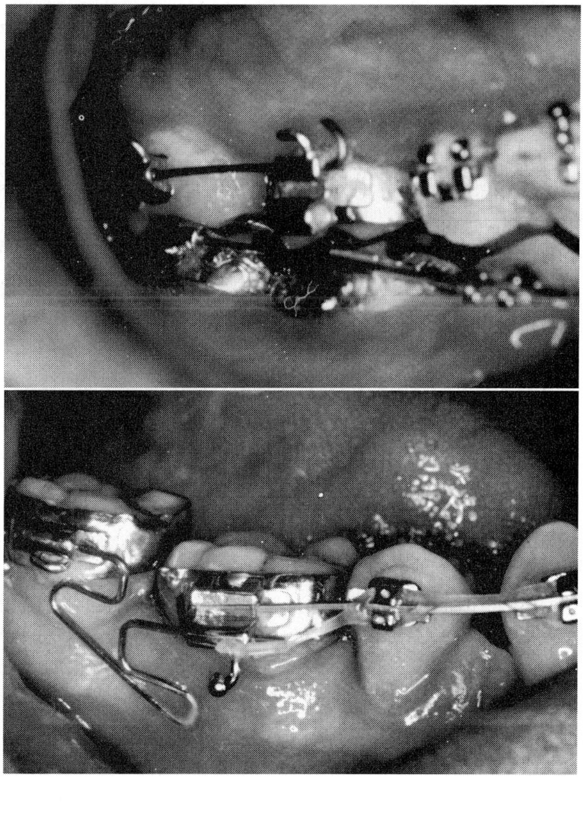

Figure 14-20 When a second molar is banded or bonded relatively late in treatment, often it is desirable to align it with a flexible wire while retaining a heavier archwire in the remainder of the arch. **A,** If the first molar carries an auxiliary tube, an auxiliary spring can be placed into the auxiliary tube, either a straight segment of rectangular A-NiTi wire, usually the most efficient procedure, or **(B)** a segment of steel wire with a loop as shown here.

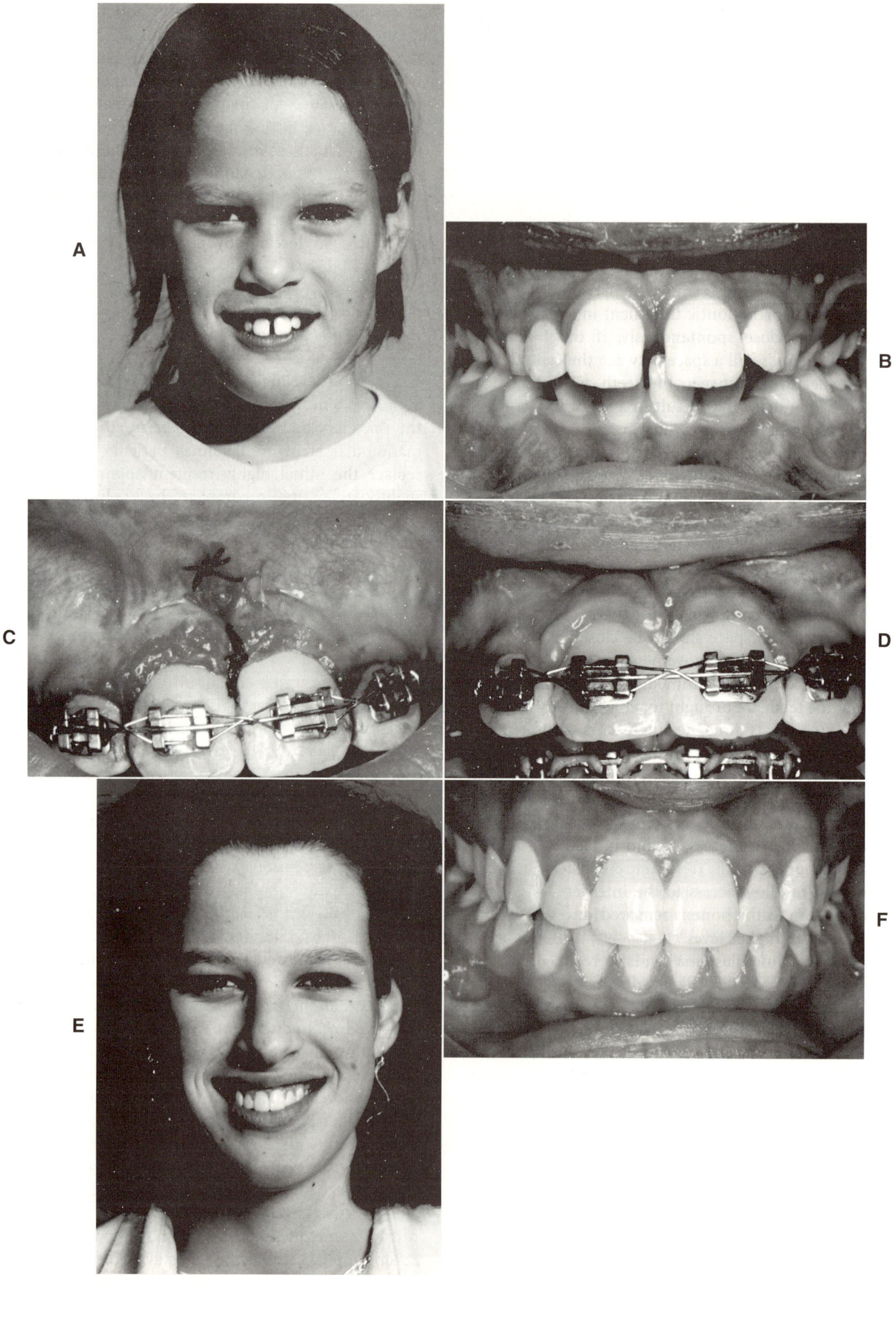
A
B
C
D
E
F

FIGURE 14-22 Management of a maxillary midline diastema. **A,** Facial appearance, showing the protruding maxillary incisors caught on the lower lip; **B,** Intraoral view before treatment; **C,** Teeth aligned and held tightly together with a figure-8 wire ligature, before frenectomy; **D,** Appearance immediately after frenectomy, using the conservative technique advocated by Edwards in which a simple incision is used to allow access to the interdental area, the fibrous connection to the bone is removed, and the frenal attachment is sutured at a higher level; **E,** Facial appearance 2 years after completion of treatment; **F,** Intraoral view 2 years after treatment.

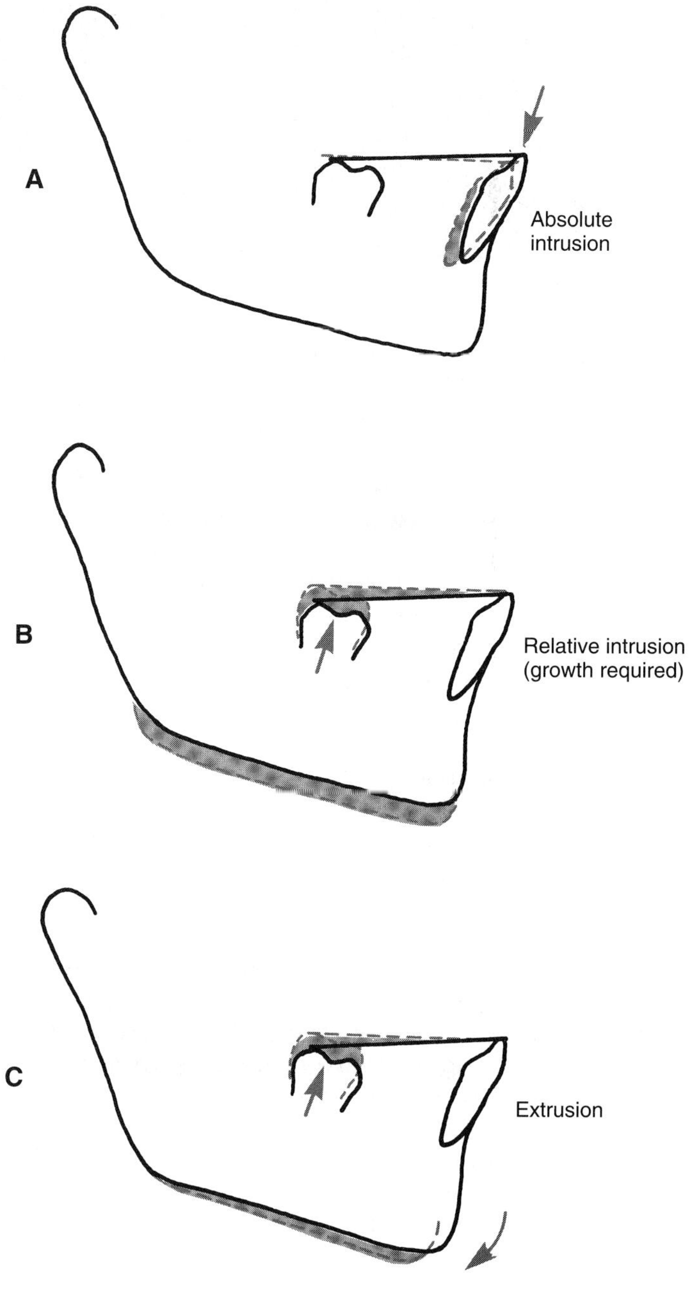

FIGURE 14-23 There are three possible ways to level a lower arch with an excessive curve of Spee: (1) absolute intrusion; (2) relative intrusion, achieved by preventing eruption of the incisors while growth provides vertical space into which the posterior teeth erupt; and (3) extrusion of posterior teeth, which causes the mandible to rotate down and back in the absence of growth. Note that the difference between (2) and (3) is whether the mandible rotates downward. This is determined by whether the ramus grows longer while the tooth movement is occurring.

Differential Growth in Adolescent Class II Treatment

The use of extraoral force or functional appliances to influence jaw growth is discussed in some detail in Chapter 13. The different timing of skeletal growth in males and females must be kept in mind when this approach is used. During adolescence, the mandible tends to grow forward more than the maxilla, providing an opportunity to improve a skeletal Class II jaw relationship. Girls mature considerably earlier than boys and are often beyond the peak of the adolescent growth spurt before the full permanent dentition is available and comprehensive orthodontic treatment can begin. Boys, who mature more slowly and have a more prolonged period of adolescent growth, are much more likely to have a clinically useful amount of anteroposterior growth during comprehensive treatment in the early permanent dentition.

Whether extraoral force (headgear) or a functional appliance is used to modify growth in Class II patients, a favorable response includes both restraint of maxillary growth and differential mandibular growth. Headgear is more compatible with the fixed appliances needed for comprehensive treatment, and functional appliance therapy alone is unlikely to provide a satisfactory result in the early permanent dentition. In skeletally immature patients with a permanent dentition, there is nothing wrong with a first phase of functional appliance treatment even though the permanent teeth have erupted, and then a fixed appliance to obtain detailed occlusal results, but it is likely that the functional appliance therapy will have to be modified or discontinued when the fixed appliance treatment begins. Many clinicians would like to believe that Class II elastics (or fixed springs that have the same effect) can influence growth as well as move teeth. Unfortunately, the evidence indicates that growth modification in adolescent patients is unlikely with elastics or flexible spring devices.[1] At this stage, headgear or a rigidly-coupled "fixed functional" like the Herbst appliance is preferred.

An ideal patient for headgear in the early permanent dentition is a 12- to 14-year-old boy with a Class II problem, whose skeletal maturity is somewhat behind his stage of dental development, and who has good growth potential (Figure 15-1). Boys at age 13, it must be remembered, are on the average at the same stage of maturation as girls at 11, and significant skeletal growth is almost always continuing. On the other hand, girls at age 13 are, on the average, at the same developmental stage as boys at 15, and by this time, clinically useful changes in jaw relationship from growth guidance are unlikely.

Although correction of molar relationship is a major goal of the second rather than the first stage of treatment, extraoral force should be applied against the first molars from the beginning in any patient for whom molar correction by differential growth is desired. There is no reason to wait for alignment and leveling to be completed, especially since every passing day decreases the probability of a favorable growth response. The extraoral force can also help control anchorage during alignment.

Although the main purpose of extraoral force is growth modification, some tooth movement in all three planes of space inevitably accompanies it. When there is good vertical growth and the maxillary molars are allowed to elongate, the maxillary teeth erupt downward and backward, and spaces may open up in the maxillary arch. Even though the extraoral force is applied against the first molar, it is unusual for space to develop between the first molar and second premolar. Instead, the second and, to a lesser degree, the first premolars follow the molars. The result is often a space distal to the canines, along with a partial reduction of overjet as the jaw relationship improves (Figure 15-2).

When this result occurs, the preferred approach is to consolidate space within the maxillary arch at a single location, using elastomeric chains to bring the canines and incisors into an anterior segment and the molar and premolars into a posterior segment. When the molar relationship has been corrected, the residual overjet is then reduced by retracting the incisors in this nonextraction patient in exactly the same way as in a patient who had a first premolar extraction space (see the following discussion). Extraoral force should be continued until an intact maxillary arch has been achieved. Discontinuing it when only the molar relationship has been corrected is unwise, both because the maximum skeletal effect probably has not been obtained at that point, and because the retraction of the incisor teeth requires posterior anchorage, which can be reinforced by the headgear.

Correction by Distal Movement of Upper Molars

The concept of "distal driving" of the maxillary posterior teeth has a long orthodontic history. After early cephalometric studies showed that little or no distal movement of upper molars was produced by the Class II elastic treatment of that era, headgear was re-introduced as a means of moving the upper molars back. Palatal anchorage also has been used to create distal movement of upper molars, to create a space into which the anterior teeth can be retracted, and skeletal anchorage (bone screws or bone anchors) now offers a more effective way to accomplish distal movement.

Although the modern methods discussed below have improved the situation, Class II correction by distal movement of upper molars has definite limits that it is important to understand and respect. With headgear, it is now clear that significant distal positioning of the upper posterior teeth relative to the maxilla occurs primarily in patients who have vertical growth and elongation of the maxillary teeth (see Figure 15-1). Without this, it is difficult to produce more than 2 to 3 mm of distal movement of the upper molars, unless the upper second molars are extracted (see below). Appliances based on palatal anchorage are somewhat more successful in moving upper molars back, but complete Class II correction by this mechanism is unlikely. Experience with skeletal anchorage still is rather limited, but moving first

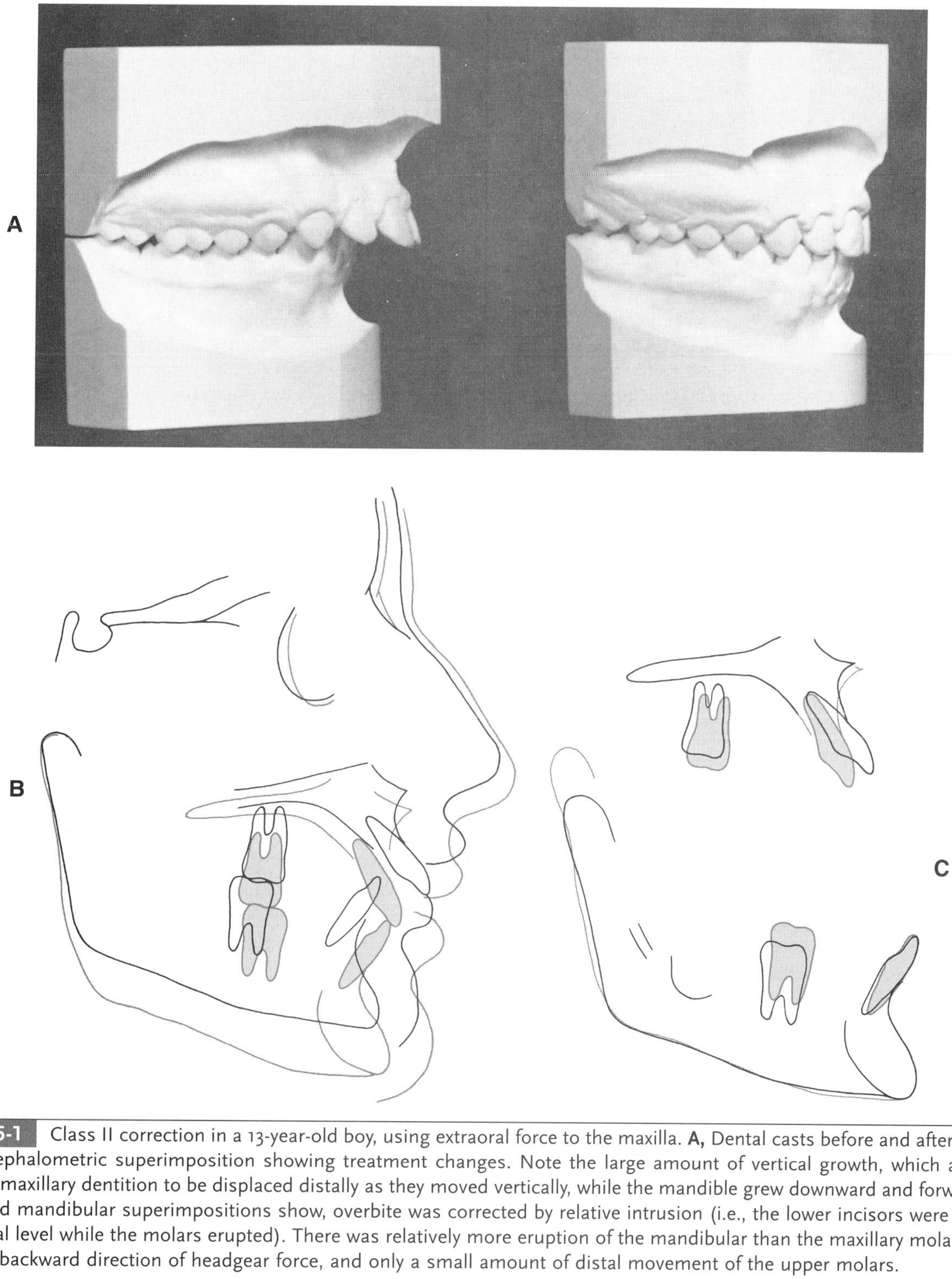

Figure 15-1 Class II correction in a 13-year-old boy, using extraoral force to the maxilla. **A,** Dental casts before and after treatment; **B** and **C,** Cephalometric superimposition showing treatment changes. Note the large amount of vertical growth, which allowed the maxilla and maxillary dentition to be displaced distally as they moved vertically, while the mandible grew downward and forward. As the maxillary and mandibular superimpositions show, overbite was corrected by relative intrusion (i.e., the lower incisors were held at the same vertical level while the molars erupted). There was relatively more eruption of the mandibular than the maxillary molar, reflecting the upward-backward direction of headgear force, and only a small amount of distal movement of the upper molars.

molars back requires space behind them, and second molar retraction may be required for major distalization.

Molar Rotation as a Factor in Distalization

In patients with mild to moderate skeletal Class II malocclusion, the upper molars are likely to have rotated mesially around the lingual root, and merely correcting the rotation changes the occlusal relationship in a Class I direction (see Figure 15-2). This can be done with a transpalatal lingual arch, an auxiliary labial arch or the inner bow of a facebow. Sometimes upper molars are so mesially rotated that it is difficult or impossible to insert a facebow until the rotation has been partially corrected with a more flexible appliance (such as a heavy labial arch, typically 36 mil steel, inserted into the

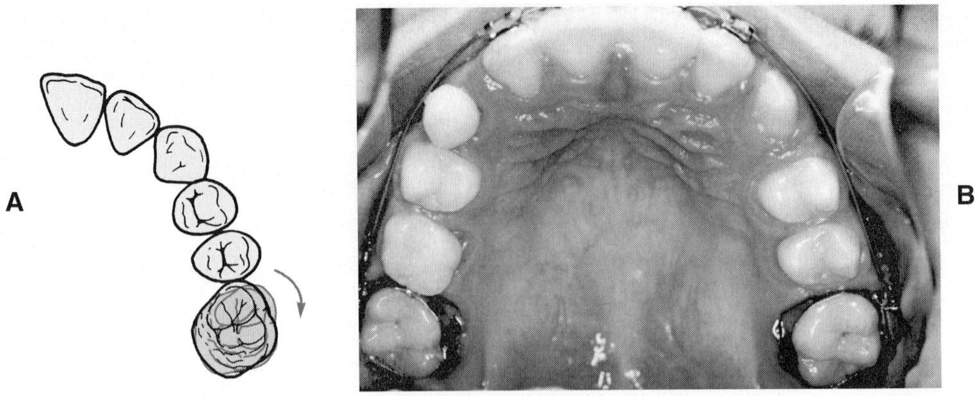

FIGURE 15-2 **A,** In patients with Class II malocclusion, the upper molars usually are rotated mesially, and part of the apparent backward movement of the first molar is a distal rotation of the buccal cusps as the tooth rotates around its lingual root. This type of rotation can be produced by a facebow or by a transpalatal lingual arch. **B,** Space tends to open within the maxillary arch when extraoral force to the upper first molars is used and the patient grows well, as in this patient after 12 months of headgear treatment during the adolescent growth spurt. Note the spacing in the premolar area, as gingival fibers produce distal rotation of these teeth also. When a complete fixed appliance is placed at this stage, one of the first steps is consolidation of the space distal to the canines.

headgear tubes and tied over an initial alignment archwire). Correction of rotated maxillary first molars is the first step in Class II treatment of almost every type.

Palatal Anchorage Systems for Distal Movement of Molars

Mesial movement of teeth is easier than distal movement, simply because there is much more resistance to distal movement. Successful distal movement of molars, therefore, requires more anchorage than can be supplied by just the other teeth. The relative stability of the anterior palate, both the soft tissue rugae and the cortical bone beneath them, is one possibility for obtaining this additional anchorage. Although removable appliances contact the palate, they are not effective in moving molars back, probably because they do not fit well enough. A fixed appliance that stabilizes the premolars and includes a plastic pad contacting the rugae is needed. Fortunately, most patients tolerate this with minimal problems, but contacting the palatal tissue has the potential to cause significant tissue irritation, to the point that the appliance has to be removed.

There are several possibilities for generating the molar distalizing force. A-NiTi coil springs compressed against the molars (from an anterior anchorage unit) produce an effective and nearly constant force system for the distal movement. Magnets in repulsion also can be used quite effectively (Figure 15-3), but the A-NiTi springs have the additional advantage of being less bulky and usually are a better choice. The pendulum appliance uses beta-Ti springs that extend from the palatal acrylic and fit into lingual sheaths on the molar tube (Figure 15-4). The effects of this appliance illustrate the potential of palatal anchorage for molar distalization.

In a small but well-characterized sample of patients who were treated to a super-Class I molar relationship with the pendulum appliance activated to produce 200 to 250 grams, Byloff et al found that molar movement averaged just over 1 mm/month (1.02 ± 0.68), with a considerable degree of distal tipping of the crown and an elevation of the molar (Figure 15-5).[2] As one would expect, despite the contact of the appliance with the palate, the premolars and incisors were tipped anteriorly, but the molar moved distally 2 to 3 times as far as the anchor teeth. When the appliance was modified to minimize distal tipping of the molar, the distal movement of the molar crown was similar, but greater distal movement of the roots was obtained at the cost of increased treatment time and some additional forward movement of the incisors (Figure 15-6).[3]

However the molars were moved distally, they must be held there while the other teeth are then retracted to correct the overjet (see Figure 15-4). It is one thing to move molars back, and something else to maintain them in that position. Simply leaving the distalization appliance in place for 2 to 3 months leads to distal movement of the premolars by stretched gingival fibers, but as soon as the original premolar-based lingual arch and palatal pad are removed, a new lingual arch and pad from the distalized molars must be placed. Even so, especially if the molar tipped distally, it will tip mesially again as the space closes. Placing a tip-back in the distalizing springs will keep the molar more upright and minimize relapse, but this increases the extrusive tendency, so as with headgear, the most successful molar distalization with the pendulum appliance occurs in patients who have vertical growth during their treatment. Even so, new data show that on the average, much of the original distalization is lost during the second phase of treatment with a complete fixed appliance.[4]

Force from Class II elastics also can be used to push the upper molars distally, but there are two problems. First, the elastics extrude the lower molars, which means that

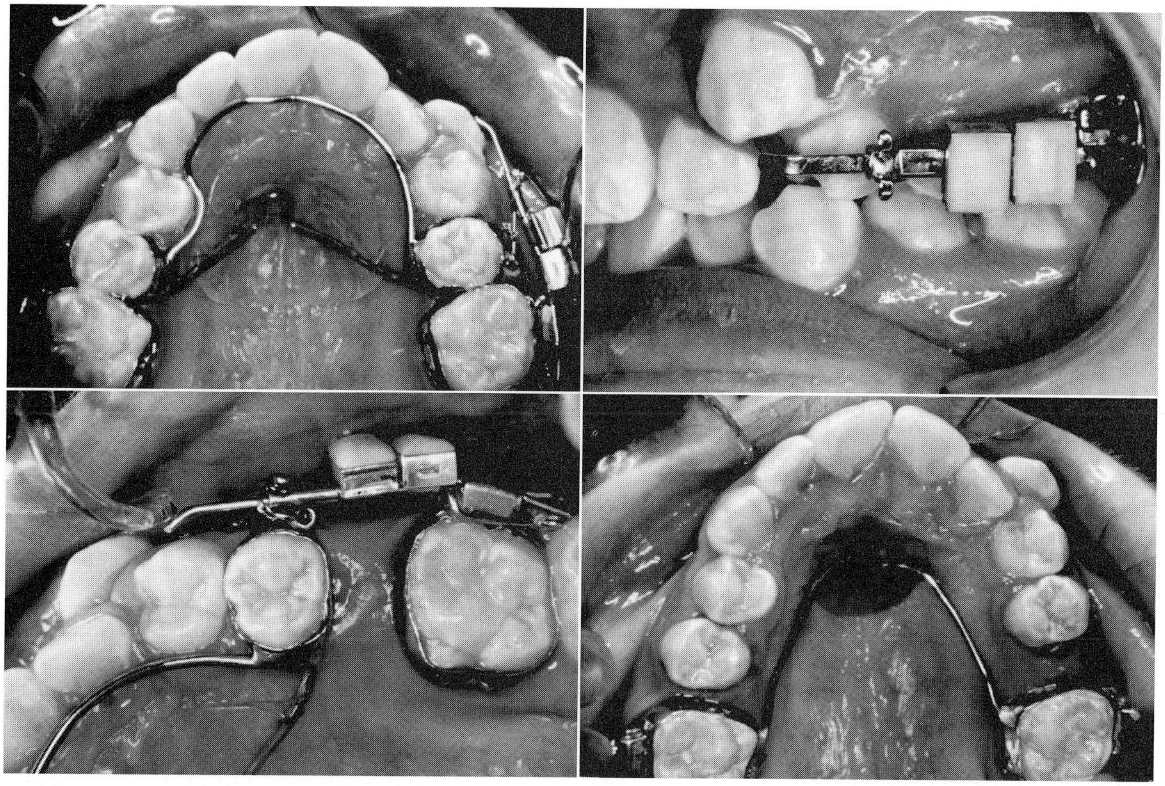

FIGURE 15-3 The use of magnets in repulsion to distalize maxillary first molars, initially only on the right side. **A,** Stabilizing lingual arch from second premolars, with one magnet attached to the premolar and the other to the first molar on the right side; **B,** Facial view of the magnet assembly. Note the arrangement for repositioning the premolar magnet as the molar moves back, to maintain the force; **C,** Progress: space opened at the rate of about 1 mm/month; **D,** Nance arch in place to maintain the molars (the left molar was distalized for 3 months, the right molar for 6 months) while distal drift of premolars occurs. A complete fixed appliance was placed a few months later to complete the treatment. (Courtesy Dr. Wick Alexander.)

downward-backward rotation of the mandible will occur unless the patient has some vertical growth during the period of treatment. Second, there is the risk of considerably more mesial movement of the lower teeth than distal movement of the upper teeth (Figure 15-7). In addition, Class II elastics tend to widen the lower molars to the point that they can produce a molar crossbite. A heavy rectangular archwire, slightly constricted across the molars, is needed to prevent this complication.

Distalization of First Molars After Second Molar Extraction

Moving upper first molars distally is much easier if space is created by extracting the upper second molars. Then vertical growth is not so critical in moving the first molars back, but even so, total Class II correction cannot be expected (Figure 15-8). For this reason, extraction of upper second molars to camouflage a skeletal Class II relationship should be considered only when specific indications are present (see Chapter 8). The key to success is a force system that moves the first molars and then the other teeth back without reciprocal protrusion of the anterior teeth. For this purpose, there are three possibilities: headgear, palatal anchorage, and skeletal anchorage.

The problem with headgear for tooth movement is that extraoral force of moderate intensity with long duration is needed. Skeletal effects in rapidly growing patients can be achieved with fewer hours per day of headgear wear than are necessary to successfully move teeth. To move the maxillary teeth posteriorly, the patient must wear the headgear full-time or nearly so. Molar extrusion should be avoided, so straight-pull or high-pull—but not cervical—headgear is indicated. The force magnitude should be large enough to simultaneously reposition all the maxillary teeth, which means that with an archwire tying the teeth together, the force should be approximately 300 gm on each side. Existing data show that with careful use of headgear to distalize first molars after second molar extraction, despite the potential problems, there is an excellent chance of clinical success and a 75% to 80% chance of maxillary third molars erupting into an acceptable position to replace the second molars.[5]

Occasionally unilateral molar distalization is indicated, typically when a unilateral Class II malocclusion is present and one side of the maxillary arch is crowded but the other

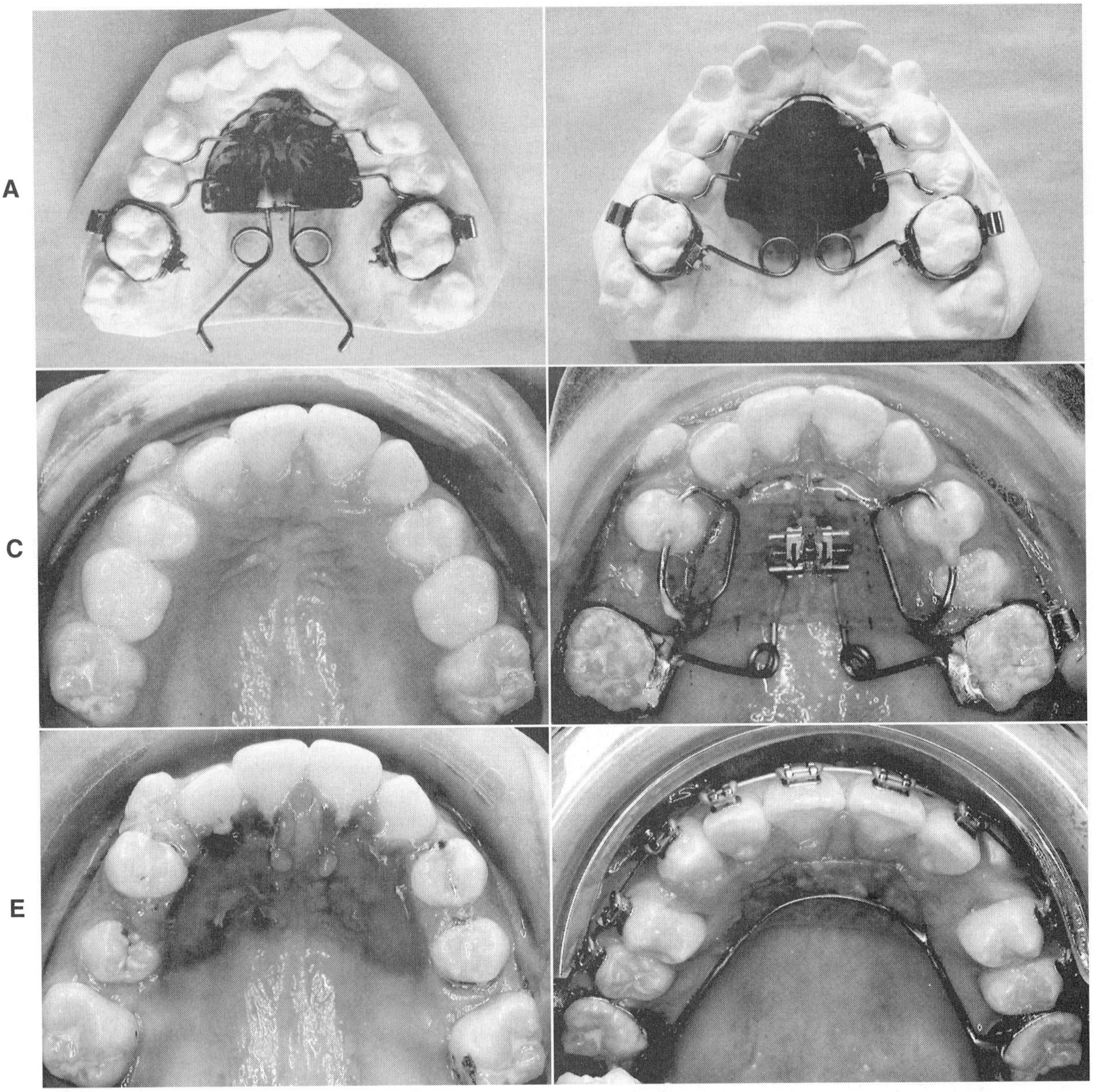

FIGURE 15-4 Pendulum appliance for molar distalization. **A, B,** Appliance on cast before and after activation of the springs. These are formed from beta-Ti wire and should deliver 200-250gm force (steel wire is too stiff, produces too much force). **C,** Occlusal view of a patient with the maxillary canines nearly blocked out of the arch (in an individual who can afford some increase in maxillary incisor prominence); **D,** Pendulum appliance with both a jackscrew for transverse expansion and molar distalizing springs (this modification is called the T-Rex appliance); **E,** Removal of the appliance. Note the increase in space in the arch, and the irritation of the palatal tissue beneath the appliance. Both are typical responses; **F,** A Nance lingual holding arch in place as fixed appliance treatment begins. It is easier to move maxillary molars distally than to keep them there as further treatment proceeds, and a lingual arch is necessary for stabilization before and during further treatment;

is not. In patients past the adolescent growth spurt who still have at least a little vertical growth remaining, extraction of one upper second molar and asymmetric cervical headgear can produce a satisfactory treatment outcome (Figure 15-9).

Palatal anchorage, as one would expect, is more successful in moving the first molar distally when the resistance of the second molar has been removed. Force levels against the first molar should be lower in second molar extraction cases. Bodily movement—not just tipping—is needed, and as with any technique that opens space mesial to the first molar, keeping the molar back while the other teeth are retracted is the key to success with this method (see Figure 15-7).

Skeletal anchorage is absolute or nearly so. Screws or anchors may become slightly loose, but even if they do, unwanted movement of anchor teeth is not a problem. If major retraction of the upper teeth to correct a Class II malocclusion is needed, it already is apparent that skeletal anchorage is a preferred way to accomplish it (Figure 15-10;

G
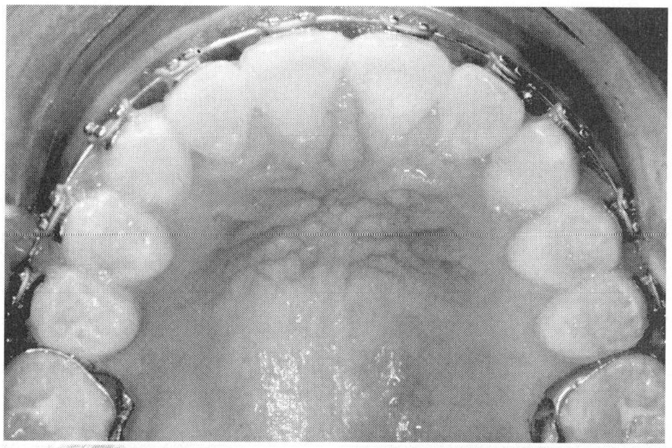

H
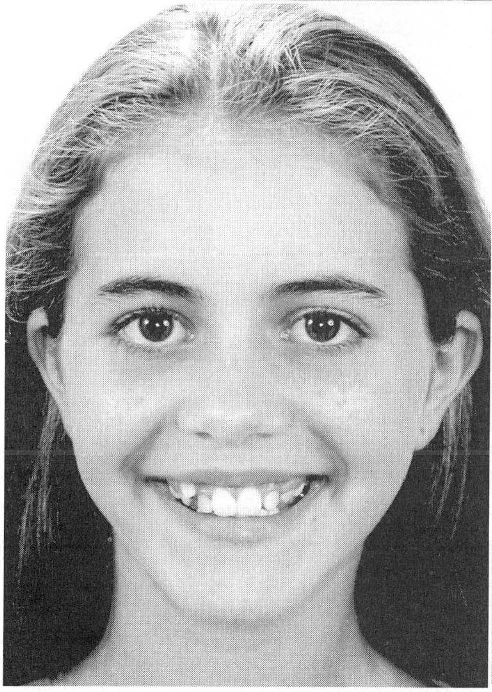

I
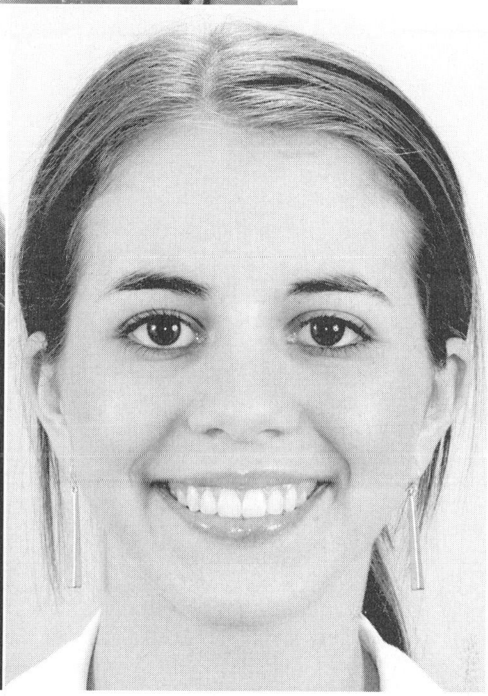

FIGURE 15-4 **cont'd G,** Alignment of the upper arch completed; **H,** Initial smile; **I,** Smile after treatment. (**A-B,** Courtesy Prof. A. Darendeliler.)

A
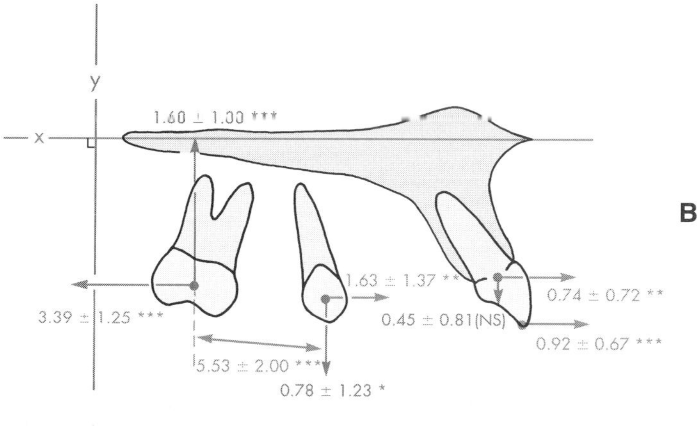

B
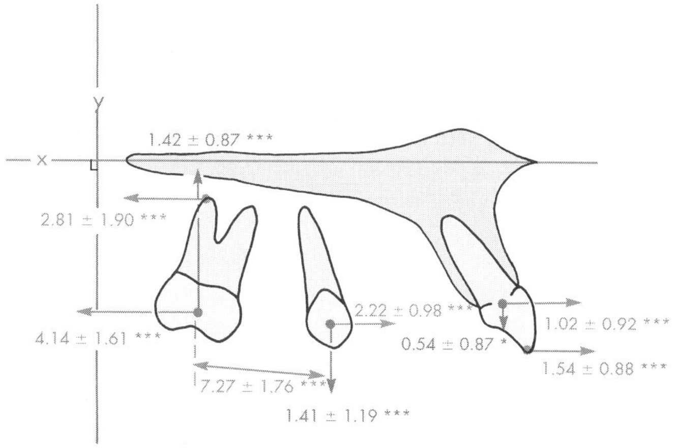

FIGURE 15-5 **A,** Mean changes in tooth position relative to the maxilla in a sample of 13 patients with activation of a pendulum appliance with 250 gm force and no tipback bends; **B,** Mean changes in 20 patients with a similar pendulum appliance incorporating tipback bends. The tipback bends reduced tipping of the molar as it moved distal and led to greater distal movement of the roots at the cost of increased displacement of the incisors and increased treatment time. (Redrawn from Byloff FK, Darendeliler MA, Clar E, Darendeliler A. Distal molar movement using the pendulum appliance. Part II, The effects of maxillary molar root uprighting bends. Angle Orthod 64:261-270, 1997.)

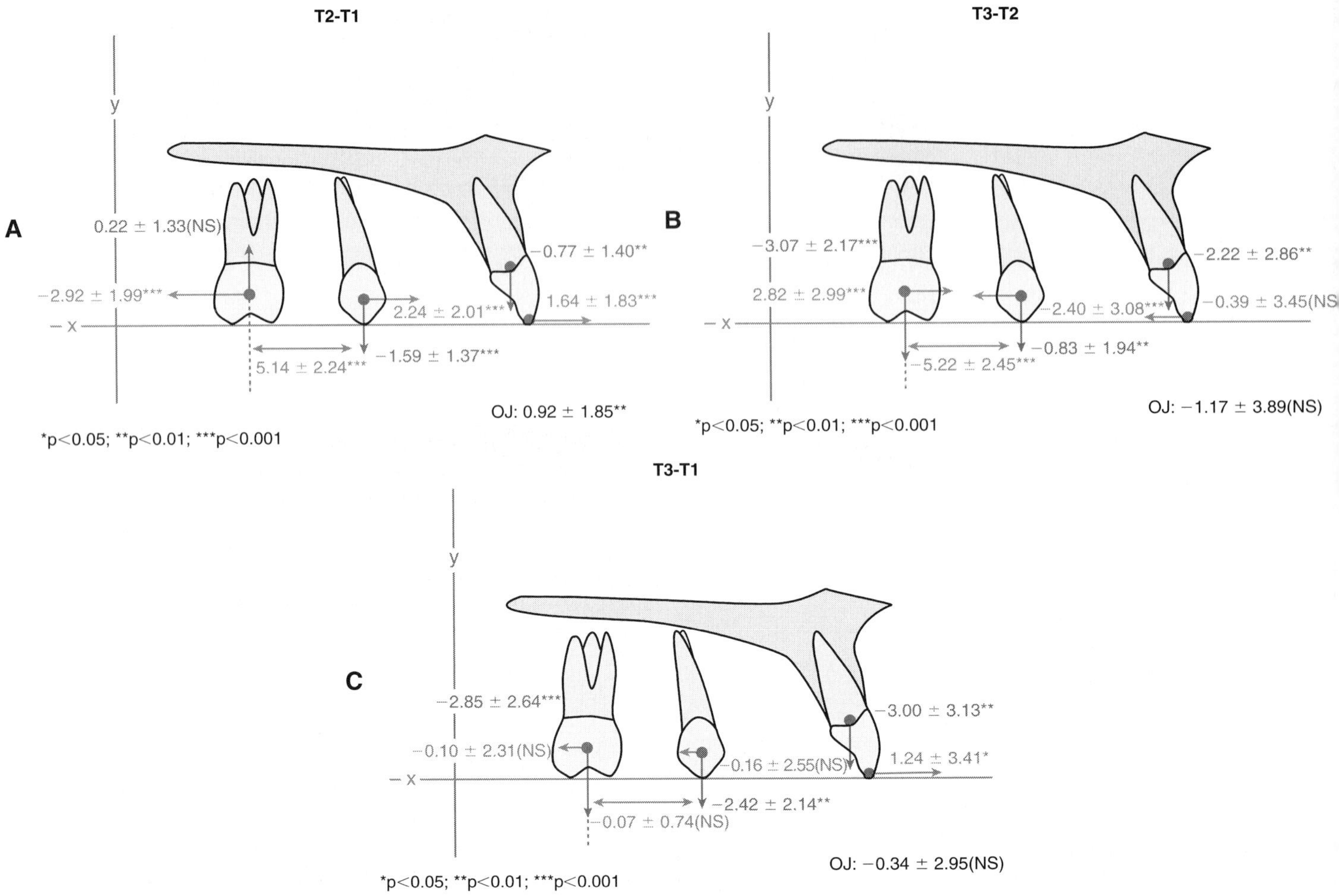

FIGURE 15-6 Mean changes in tooth position relative to the maxilla in a sample of 35 Class II patients treated with a first phase of molar distalization followed by comprehensive fixed appliance treatment. **A,** Changes during phase 1. The average age at the start of treatment was 12.3 years (S.D ± 1.5 years), and the treatment duration was 0.7 ± 0.2 years. Note that in phase 1, on the average the molar moved back about twice as far as the incisor moved forward, but the increase in space between the molar and premolar was due to nearly as much forward movement of the premolar as distal movement of the molar. The molar tended to intrude, while the premolar was extruded. The large standard deviations emphasize that, as usually is the case, changes in individual patients varied considerably. **B,** Changes during phase 2, duration 2.4 ± 0.6 years. During this time the changes in tooth positions relative to the maxilla that were created during pendulum treatment were recovered to a considerable extent. Note the vertical changes, consistent with vertical growth during adolescence. **C,** Changes from the beginning to completion of treatment, duration 3.1 ± 0.6 years, showing the small average net distalization of the molars relative to the maxilla. In the final analysis, successful correction of the malocclusion in many of these patients was due more to jaw growth, transverse expansion of the dental arches and forward movement of the incisors. Whether beginning treatment later with the pendulum appliance would have been as successful as the two-stage treatment used in this study has not yet been established. (From Poon Y, Byloff F, Petocz P, Darendeliler MA. Distal molar movement using the pendulum appliance. Part III, Outcome following phase 2 treatment with fixed appliances. Am J Orthod Dentofac Orthop, in press.)

see also Figure 18-46). Patients report that tolerating the presence of bone anchors or screws is less of a problem than wearing headgear, and probably is better accepted than palatal anchorage. It is difficult to distalize the upper teeth too much with headgear or palatal anchorage. Skeletal anchorage is so effective that over-retraction of the upper incisors is possible—which of course defeats the purpose of camouflage. Nevertheless, skeletal anchorage almost surely will displace the other ways to move molars distally in the near future.

Differential Anteroposterior Tooth Movement Using Extraction Spaces

There are two reasons for extracting teeth in orthodontics, as discussed in detail in Chapter 7: (1) to provide space to align crowded incisors without creating excessive protrusion, and (2) to allow camouflage of moderate Class II or Class III jaw relationships when correction by growth modification is not possible. A patient who is both Class II (or III) and crowded is a particular problem because the same space

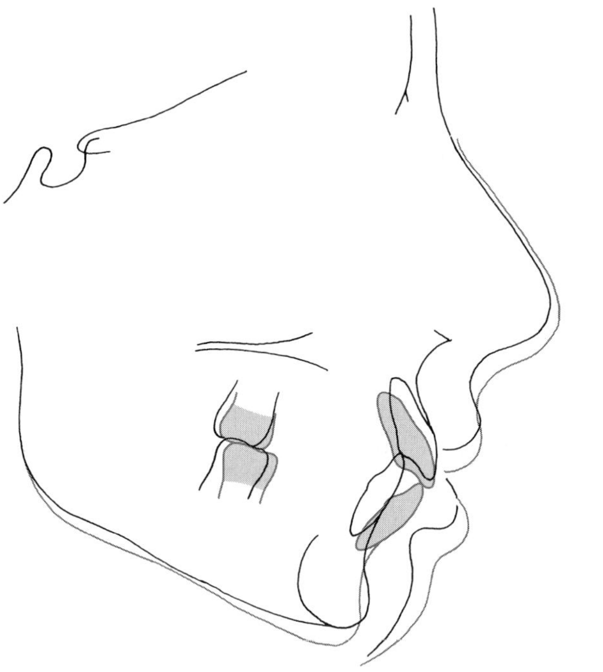

Figure 15-7 Cephalometric superimposition showing the response to Class II elastics in a girl in whom this was the major method for correcting a Class II malocclusion. Note that with rectangular archwires, some torque of the upper incisors was obtained. The rotational effects often associated with Class II elastics were less apparent for this patient than is sometimes the case (see also Figure 15-16), but the considerably greater forward displacement of the lower arch than retraction of the upper is typical.

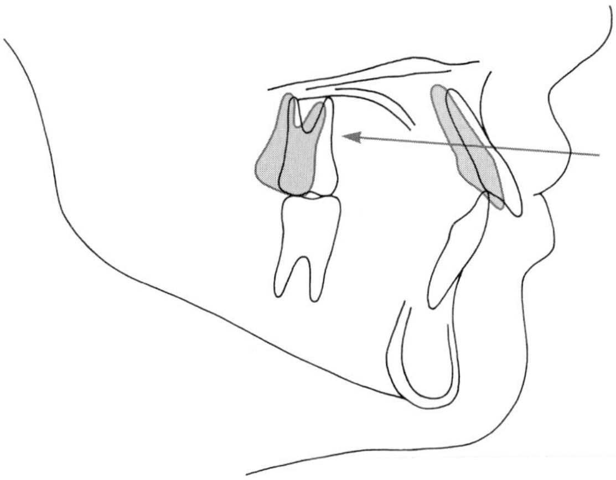

Figure 15-8 After extraction of maxillary second molars, extraoral force can successfully move the maxillary dentition posteriorly, as this cephalometric superimposition shows. To achieve this effect, extraoral force must be applied nearly full time, to promote efficient tooth movement. Until skeletal anchorage became available, the effective limit of movement of this type was 4 to 5 mm. (Retraced from Armstrong MM. Am J Orthod 59:215-243, 1971.)

cannot be used for both purposes. The more extraction space required for alignment, the less available for differential movement in camouflage, and vice versa.

An important part of treatment planning is deciding which teeth to extract and how the extraction spaces are to be closed (i.e., by retraction of incisor teeth, mesial movement of posterior teeth, or some combination). These decisions, reviewed in detail in Chapters 7 and 8, determine the orthodontic mechanics.

Class II Camouflage by Extraction of Upper First Premolars

Like upper second molar extraction, extraction of upper first premolars is a deceptively attractive solution to Class II problems and should be adopted only when its specific indications exist (see Chapter 8). With this approach, the objective during orthodontic treatment is to maintain the existing Class II molar relationship, closing the first premolar extraction space entirely by retracting the protruding incisor teeth (Figure 15-11). Anchorage must be reinforced, but one method, Class II elastics from the lower arch, is specifically contraindicated. The remaining possibilities are extraoral force to the first molars, a stabilizing lingual arch, retraction of the maxillary anterior segment with extraoral force directly against these teeth, or skeletal anchorage.

Excellent reinforcement of posterior anchorage can be obtained with extraoral force if it is applied consistently and for long durations. The more constant the headgear wear, the less a stabilizing lingual arch will be needed. Conversely, a stabilizing lingual arch augments the posterior anchorage full-time, while headgear is likely to be worn a good bit less.

It seems intuitively obvious that a lingual arch with a button against the palatal tissue should be more effective than a straight transpalatal lingual arch, but when first molars are being stabilized in a premolar extraction case, this is not necessarily true. The effect of the lingual arch is primarily to prevent the molars from rotating mesiolingually around their palatal root, and secondarily to prevent them from tipping mesially. A straight transpalatal lingual arch (see Figure 14-14) is as effective as one with a palatal button in preventing rotation, and for most patients, the marginally better stabilization with a palatal button is not worth the cost in tissue irritation. Note that this is true when a lingual arch is used to stabilize molars, but not true when the lingual arch is to stabilize premolars, as in the molar distalization technique discussed above. When pushed mesially, premolars tip more than they rotate, and a palatal button is needed on a lingual arch to stabilize them.

In addition to headgear and/or lingual arch stabilization, all the strategies described in Chapter 10 for reducing strain on anchorage (i.e., avoiding friction, retracting canines individually, skeletal anchorage) are appropriate with upper first premolar extraction and can be brought into use.

Retracting protruding maxillary anterior teeth with headgear attached to the archwire totally avoids strain on the

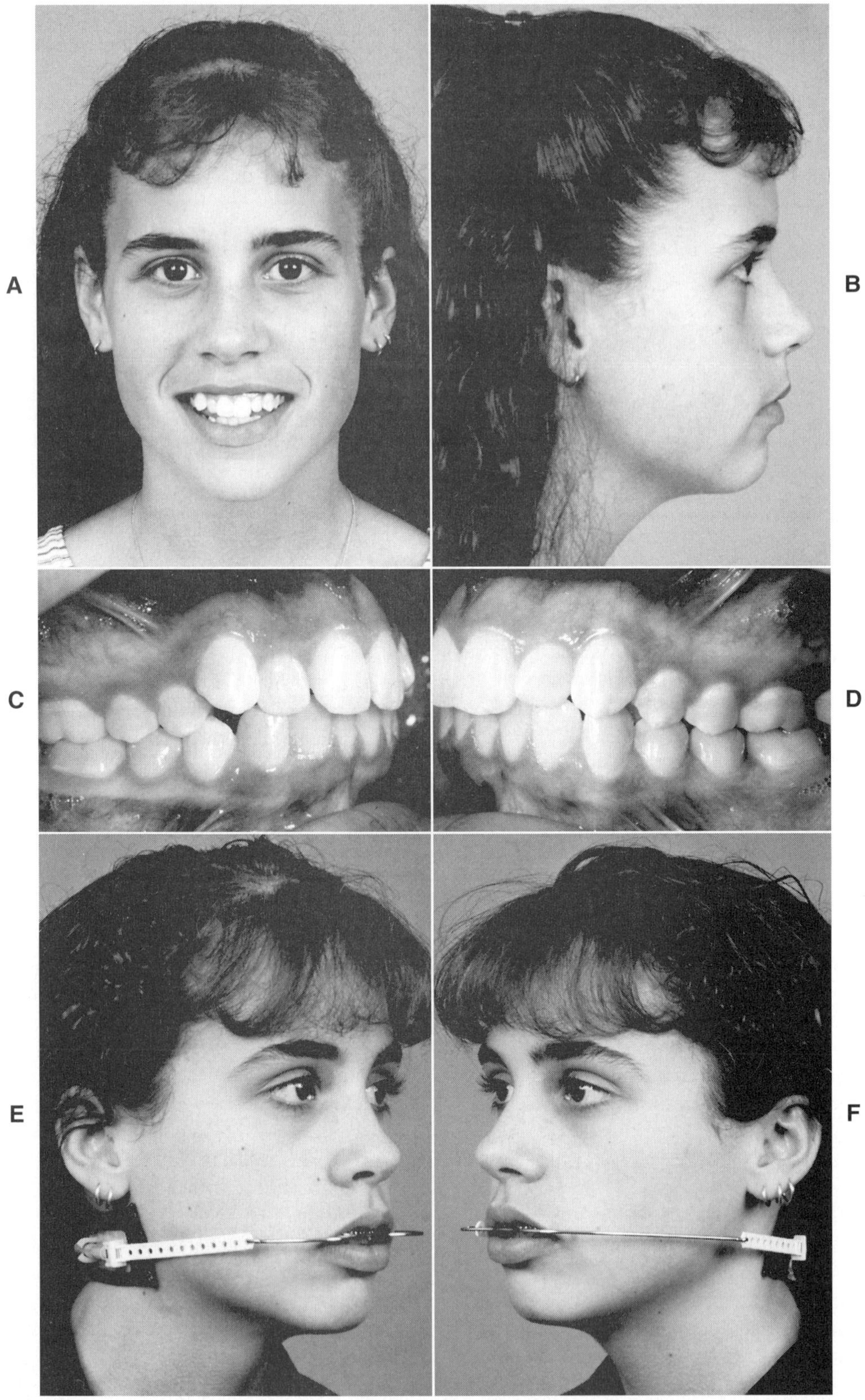

FIGURE 15-9 Unilateral Class II malocclusion in a teenage girl treated with extraction of one maxillary second molar and unilateral headgear. **A** to **D,** Prior to treatment. The maxillary midline was displaced to the right (with the right canine crowded out of the arch). There was only a moderate skeletal component of the malocclusion. **E** and **F,** Unilateral cervical headgear (for all practical purposes, unilateral headgear must be cervical). Note the longer outer bow on the side where greater tooth movement is desired.

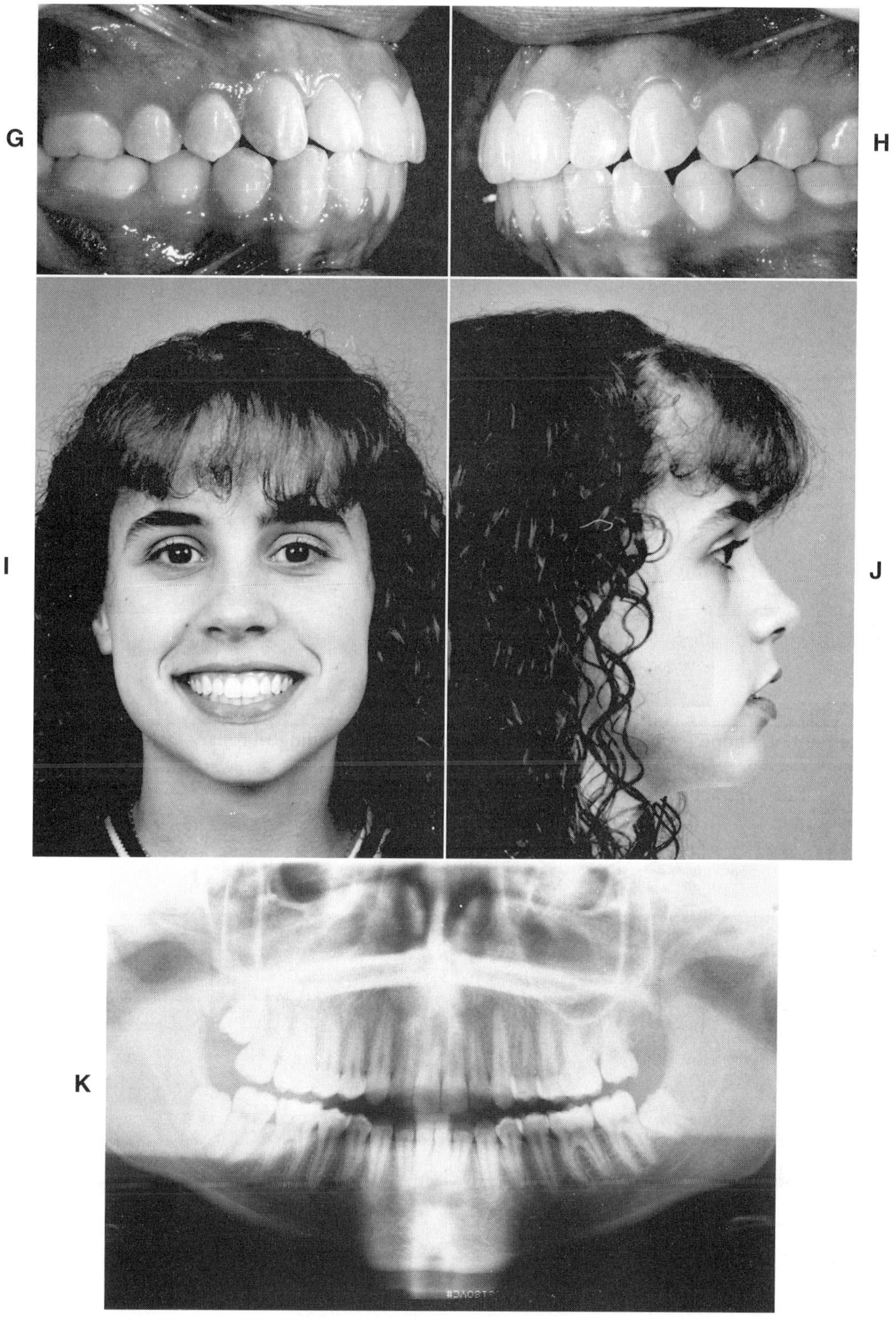

FIGURE 15-9 **cont'd G** to **J,** Post-treatment. Note the improvement of the dental midline as well as the correction of the molar relationship. **K,** Post-treatment panoramic radiograph, showing the upper left third molar well on the way to replacing the extracted second molar. There were minimal cephalometric changes, with no growth, as expected.

skeletal anchorage is an obvious and better tolerated replacement for headgear. The concern, of course, is that this might lead to excessive incisor retraction.

In the late 1980s, it was claimed by some dentists that extraction of upper first premolars would lead to later temporomandibular dysfunction (TMD) problems. The theory, to the extent that the proponents of this claim had one, was that retracting the upper incisors would inevitably lead to incisor interferences, and this would cause TMD. The claim was never supported by any evidence, and research data have refuted it.[6,7] It is important to limit first premolar extraction for camouflage of Class II malocclusion to the appropriate patients and not to extract the incisors too much, but if this is done, it can be an excellent treatment method.

Extraction of Maxillary and Mandibular Premolars

Correction of Class II buccal segment relationships with extraction of all four first premolars implies that the mandibular posterior segments will be moved anteriorly nearly the width of the extraction space. At the same time, the protruding maxillary anterior teeth will be retracted without forward movement of the maxillary buccal segments. This, in turn, implies (though it does not absolutely require) that Class II elastics will be used to assist in closing the extraction sites.

The Begg technique is a classic illustration of the use of Class II elastics to produce differential movement of the arch segments while correcting the molar relationship. In the Begg approach, at the beginning of the second stage of treatment, light interarch elastics are added to help close space, while Class II elastics are continued (Figure 15-12). An anchor bend is placed in the upper archwire so that the maxillary anterior teeth are tipped back in part by the force system associated with the archwire itself. In the lower arch, the anchor bend is used to control the amount of mesial tipping of the molars. The Class II elastics reinforce and accentuate the differential tooth movements along the archwires. It is extremely important to use only light forces, so that optimum force levels are reached where tipping is desired, while forces for bodily movement remain suboptimum.

A similar mechanical arrangement, of course, can be produced with the edgewise appliance. A round wire in an edgewise bracket allows tipping of the incisors in essentially the same way as with the Begg approach, but the mesiodistal width of the canine brackets tends to keep the canine teeth more upright, thereby increasing the strain on posterior anchorage. For this reason, when a Begg-like sliding space closure in both arches is used with the edgewise appliance, reinforcement of maxillary anchorage (with headgear or bone screws) is a good idea, and somewhat heavier Class II elastic force is needed.

It is also possible with the edgewise appliance to structure anchorage so that space closure by retraction of the maxillary anterior teeth and protraction of the mandibular posterior segments occurs without the use of Class II elastics. The best control is achieved with the segmented arch technique, using space-closing springs in each arch fabricated specifically for the type of space closure desired (see Closure of Extraction Spaces, this chapter).

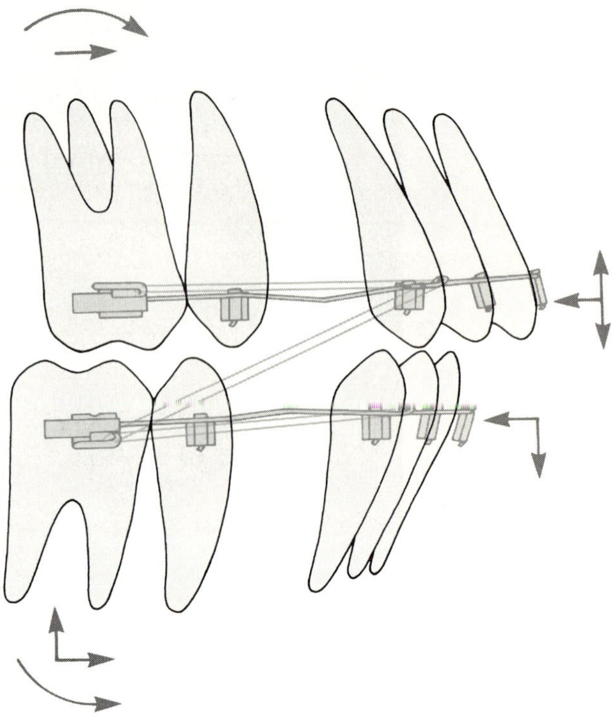

Figure 15-12 Diagrammatic representation of forces encountered in the second stage of Begg treatment, in which base archwires *(grey)* with anchor bends are combined with intra-arch and Class II elastics *(orange)*. The anchor bends produce bodily forward movement of the molars, but no couples are present on the incisors, so these teeth tip lingually. The anchor bends also depress the incisors and elongate the molars, which is counteracted by the Class II elastics for the upper arch but accentuated by the elastics for the lower.

When differential space closure without interarch elastics is desired, a more common approach with the edgewise appliance is to extract maxillary first and mandibular second premolars, thus altering the anchorage value of the two segments (Figure 15-13). With this approach, routine space-closing mechanics will move the lower molars forward more than the upper, particularly if maxillary posterior anchorage is reinforced with a stabilizing lingual arch or headgear. This upper first-lower second premolar extraction pattern greatly simplifies the mechanics needed for differential space closure with continuous-arch edgewise technique.

Occasionally, however, mesial movement of the lower first molar into a second premolar extraction space is difficult to produce. This is particularly likely when the second premolar was congenitally missing and a second primary molar was extracted, because bone resorption reduces the alveolar ridge dimensions before space closure can be completed. It can be

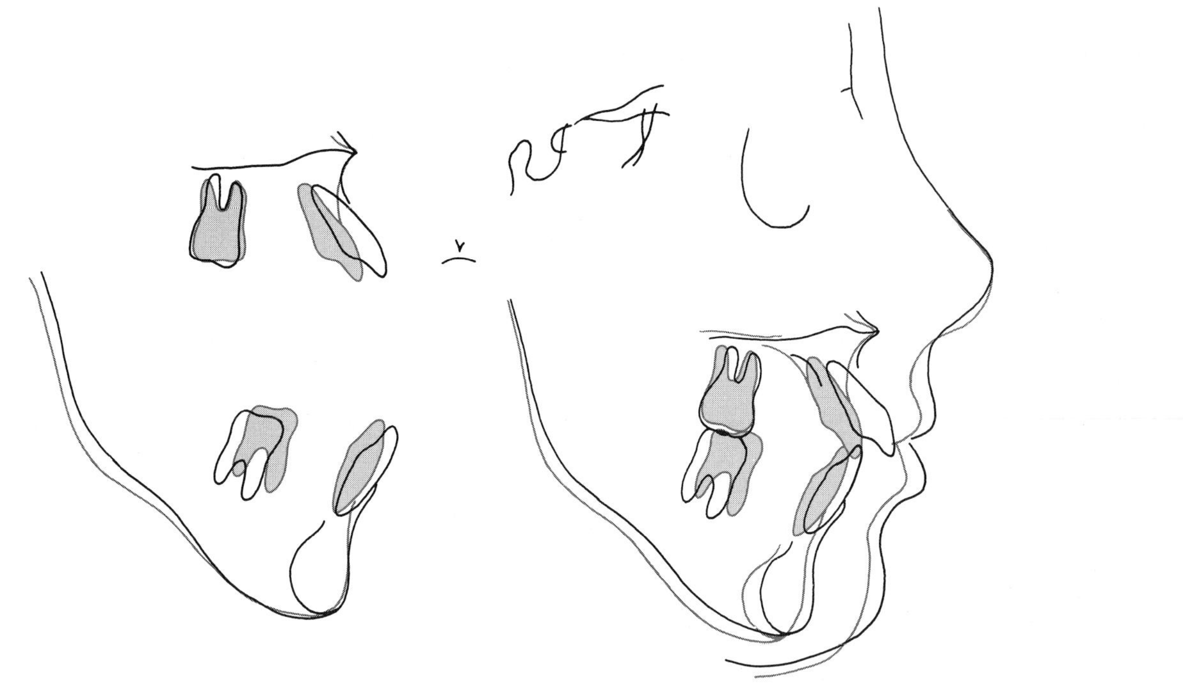

Figure 15-13 Cephalometric superimposition showing the result of treatment with extraction of upper first and lower second premolars. Even with second premolar extraction, some retraction of the mandibular incisors may occur, but most of the space closure will be by mesial movement of the lower molar. This adult patient experienced no growth, and a slight downward and backward rotation of the mandible occurred.

advantageous to remove only the distal root of the second primary molar, leaving the mesial part of the primary tooth in place (with a calcium hydroxide pulpotomy and temporary restoration) until the permanent tooth has been brought forward for that half of the total distance. Then the remaining half of the primary tooth is extracted, and space closure completed.[8]

Molar Correction With Inter-arch Elastics

Without extraction spaces, Class II elastics produce molar correction largely by mesial movement of the mandibular arch, with only a small amount of distal positioning of the maxillary arch (see Figure 15-7). When this pattern of tooth movement is desired, the amount of force varies with the amount of tipping allowed in the mandibular arch. With a well-fitting rectangular wire in the lower arch that is somewhat constricted posteriorly (to prevent rolling the lower molars facially and control the inclination of the lower incisors), approximately 250 gm per side is needed to displace one arch relative to the other. With a lighter round wire in the lower arch, not more than half that amount of force should be used. Incorporating the lower second molars in the appliance and attaching the elastics to a mesial hook on this tooth increase the anchorage and give a more horizontal direction of pull than hooking the elastic to the first molar.

It is important to keep in mind that with or without extraction, Class II elastics produce not only anteroposterior and transverse effects but also a vertical force (Figure 15-14). This force elongates the mandibular molars and the maxillary incisors, rotating the occlusal plane up posteriorly and down anteriorly. If the molars extrude more than the ramus grows vertically, the mandible itself will be rotated downward (Figure 15-15). Class II elastics, therefore, are contraindicated in nongrowing patients who cannot tolerate some downward and backward rotation of the mandible. The rotation of the occlusal plane, in and of itself, facilitates the desired correction of the posterior occlusion, but even if elongation of the lower molars can be tolerated because of good growth, the corresponding extrusion of the maxillary incisors can be unsightly.

Class II elastics, in short, may produce occlusal relationships that look good on dental casts but are less satisfactory when viewed from the perspective of skeletal relationships and facial esthetics. Because of this, prolonged use of Class II elastics, particularly with heavy forces, is rarely indicated. Using Class II elastics for 3 or 4 months at the completion of treatment of a Class II patient to obtain good posterior interdigitation is often acceptable. Applying heavy Class II force for 9 to 12 months as the major method for correcting a Class II malocclusion is rarely good treatment.

Class III elastics also have a significant extrusive component, tending to elongate the upper molars and the lower

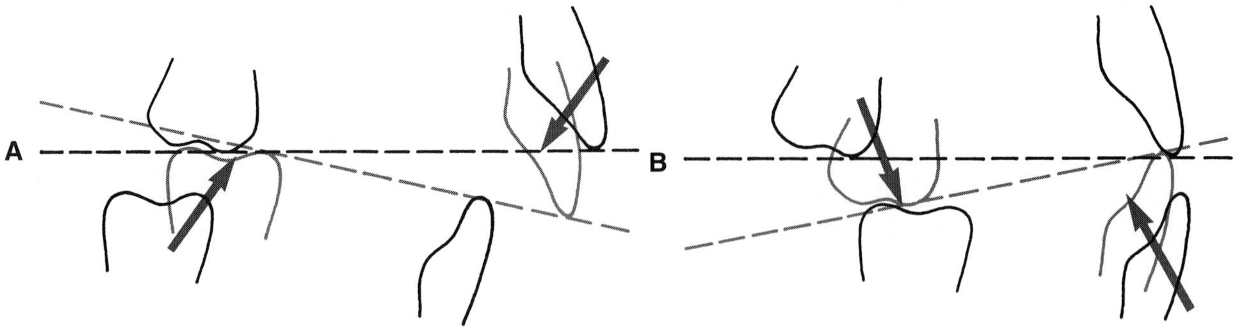

FIGURE 15-14 Rotation of the occlusal plane with **(A)** Class II and **(B)** Class III elastics. The rotation of the occlusal plane helps correct the molar relationship, and is helpful from that point of view, but it can be deleterious in some patients because elongation of the molars may cause undesirable rotation of the mandible or undesirable tooth-lip relationships.

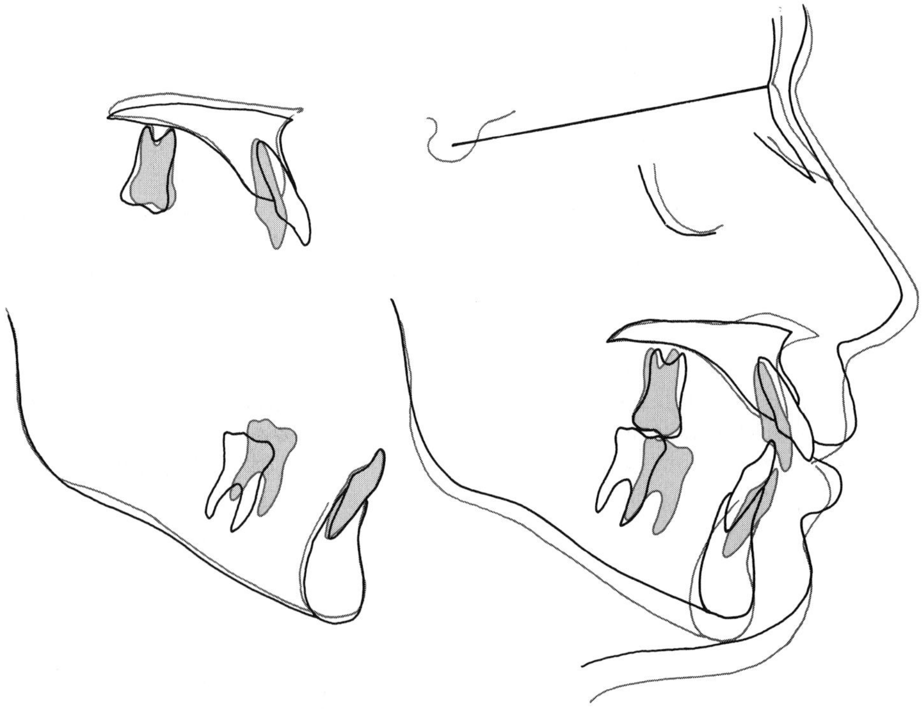

FIGURE 15-15 Cephalometric superimposition showing the vertical effects of Class II elastics in this patient, who had premolar extractions and did not have forward movement of the lower incisors despite the forward movement of the lower molars. Note the elevation of the lower molar, extrusion and distal tipping of the upper incisor, rotation of the occlusal plane, and downward and backward rotation of the mandible.

incisors. Elongating the molars enough to rotate the mandible downward and backward is disastrous in Class II treatment but, within limits, can help treatment of a Class III problem. If Class III elastics are used to assist in retracting mandibular incisors (see further discussion following), high-pull headgear to the upper molars worn simultaneously with the elastics can control the amount of elongation of the upper molars. Elongation of the lower incisors, however, still can be anticipated.

CLOSURE OF EXTRACTION SPACES

To obtain the desired result of closing spaces within the arch, it is essential to control the amount of incisor retraction vs. molar-premolar protraction. Indications for extraction have been discussed in Chapters 6 and 7, and the biomechanical concepts related to control of posterior anchorage and the amount of incisor retraction are described in Chapter 10. In this section, the focus is on contemporary mechanotherapy for space closure with the 18- and 22-slot edgewise appliances.

Moderate Anchorage Situations

Most patients fall into the moderate anchorage category, meaning that after alignment of the incisors has been completed, it is desired to close the remainder of the premolar extraction space with a 50:50 or 60:40 ratio of anterior retraction to posterior protraction. The different wire sizes in 18- and 22-slot edgewise appliances require a different approach to mechanotherapy.

Moderate Anchorage Treatment With 18-Slot Edgewise: Closing Loops

Although either sliding or loop mechanics can be used, the 18-slot appliance with single or narrow twin brackets on canines and premolars is ideally suited for use of closing loops in continuous archwires. Closing loop archwires should be fabricated from rectangular wire to prevent the wire from rolling in the bracket slots. Appropriate closing loops in a continuous archwire will produce approximately 60:40 closure of the extraction space if only the second premolar and first molar are included in the anchorage unit and some uprighting of the incisors is allowed. Greater retraction will be obtained if the second molar is part of the anchorage unit, less if incisor torque is required.

The performance of a closing loop, from the perspective of engineering theory, is determined by three major characteristics: its spring properties (i.e., the amount of force it delivers and the way the force changes as the teeth move); the moment it generates, so that root position can be controlled; and its location relative to the adjacent brackets, (i.e., the extent to which it serves as a symmetric or asymmetric V-bend in a continuous wire). In addition, clinical performance is affected by how well the loop conforms to additional design principles. Let us consider these in turn:

Spring Properties. The spring properties of a closing loop are determined almost totally by the wire material (at present, either steel or beta-titanium), the size of the wire, and the distance between points of attachment. This distance in turn is largely determined by the amount of wire incorporated into the loop but is affected also by the distance between brackets. Closing loops with equivalent properties can be produced from different types and sizes of wire by increasing the amount of wire incorporated into the loop as the size of the wire increases, and vice versa. Wires of greater inherent springiness or smaller cross-sectional area allow the use of simpler loop designs.

Figure 15-16, taken from the work of Booth,[9] illustrates the effects on the spring characteristics of a steel closing loop from changing wire size, the design of the loop, and the interbracket span (the combination of these latter two parameters, of course, determines the amount of wire in the loop). Note that, as expected, changing the size of the wire produces the largest changes in characteristics, but the amount of wire incorporated in the loop is also important. The same relative effect would be observed with beta-titanium wire. For any size of wire or design of loop, beta-Ti would produce a significantly smaller force than steel.

Root-Paralleling Moments. To close an extraction space while producing bodily tooth movement, a closing loop must generate not only a closing force but also appropriate

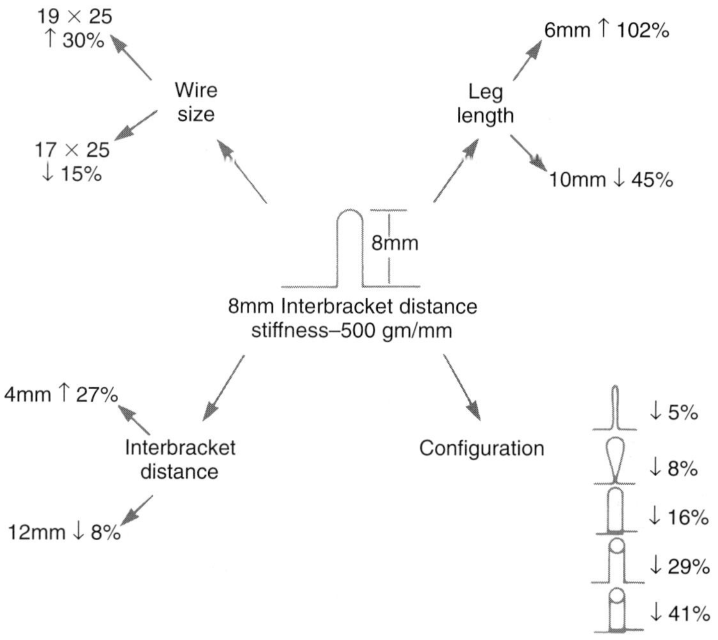

FIGURE 15-16 The effect of changing various aspects of a closing loop in an archwire. Note that an 8-mm vertical loop in 18×25 wire produces twice as much force as the desired 250 gm/mm. The major possibilities for producing clinically satisfactory loops are reducing wire size or incorporating additional wire by changing leg length, interbracket distance, and/or loop configuration. (Redrawn from Booth FA. MS Thesis, Optimum forces with orthodontic loops, Houston, University of Texas Dental Branch, 1971.)

moments to bring the root apices together at the extraction site. As discussed in Chapter 10, for bodily movement the moment of the force used to move the teeth must be balanced by the moment of a couple. If its center of resistance is 10-mm from the bracket, a canine tooth being retracted with a 100-gm force must also receive a 1000 gm-mm moment if it is to move bodily. If the bracket is 1 mm wide, a vertical force of 1000 gm must be produced by the archwire at each side of the bracket.

This requirement to generate a movement limits the amount of wire that can be incorporated to make a closing loop springier, because if the loop becomes too flexible, it will be unable to generate the necessary moments even though the retraction force characteristics are satisfactory. Loop design is also affected. Placing some of the wire within the closing loop in a horizontal rather than vertical direction improves its ability to deliver the moments needed to prevent tipping. Because of this and because a vertically tall loop can impinge on soft tissue, a closing loop that is only 7 to 8 mm tall while incorporating 10 to 12 mm or more of wire (e.g., a delta, L- or T-shaped loop) is preferred.

If the legs of a closing loop were parallel before activation, opening the loop would place them at an angle that in itself would generate a moment in the desired direction. Calculations show that unacceptably tall loops would be required to generate appropriate moments in this manner,[10] so additional moments must be generated by gable bends (or their equivalent) when the loop is placed in the mouth. An elegant solution to the design of a closing loop that would provide optimum and nearly constant moment-to-force ratios at variable activations was offered by Siatkowski in his Opus loop (Figure 15-17).[11]

Location of the Loop. A final engineering factor in the performance of a closing loop is its location along the span of wire between adjacent brackets. Because of its gable bends, the closing loop functions as a V-bend in the archwire, and the effect of a V-bend is quite sensitive to its position. Only if it is in the center of the span does a V-bend produce equal forces and couples on the adjacent teeth (see Figures 10-37 and 10-38). If it is one-third of the way between adjacent brackets, the tooth closer to the loop will be extruded and will feel a considerable moment to bring the root toward the V-bend, while the tooth farther away will receive an intrusive force but no moment.[12] If the V-bend or loop is closer to one bracket than one third of the distance, the more distant tooth will not be intruded but will receive a moment to move the root away from the V-bend (which almost never is desirable).

For routine use with fail-safe closing loops (as described later), the preferred location for a closing loop is at the spot that will be the center of the embrasure when the space is closed (Figure 15-18). This means that, in a first premolar extraction situation, the closing loop should be placed about 5 mm distal to the center of the canine tooth. The effect is to place the loop initially at the one-third position relative to the canine. The moment on the premolar increases as space closure proceeds. The design of the Opus loop calls for an off-center position with the loop 1.5 mm from the mesial (canine) bracket.

Additional Design Principles. An important principle in closing loop design is that, to the greatest extent possible, the loop should "fail safe." This means that, although a reasonable range of action is desired from each activation, tooth movement should stop after a prescribed range of movement even if the patient does not return for a scheduled adjustment. Too long a range of action with too much flexibility could produce disastrous effects if a distorted spring were combined with a series of broken appointments. The ideal loop design therefore would deliver a continuous, controlled force designed to produce tooth movement at a rate of approximately 1 mm per month but would not include more than 2 mm of range, so that movement would stop if the patient missed a second consecutive monthly appointment.

It also is important that the design be as simple as possible, because more complex configurations are less comfortable for patients, more difficult to fabricate clinically, and more prone to breakage or distortion. Engineering analysis, as the Opus loop demonstrates very nicely, shows that a relatively complex design is required to produce the best control of moment-force ratios. The possibilities of clinical

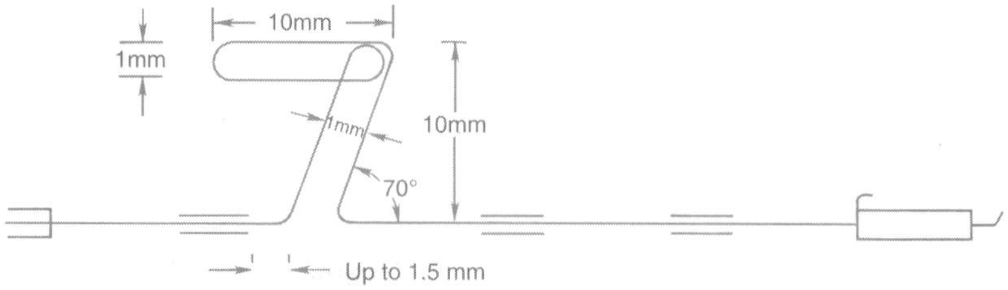

Figure 15-17 The Opus closing loop designed by Siatkowski offers excellent control of forces and moments, so that space can be closed under good control. The loop can be fabricated from 16 × 22 or 18 × 25 steel wire, or from 17 × 25 TMA wire. It is activated by tightening it distally behind the molar tube and can be adjusted to produce maximal, moderate, or minimal incisor retraction, but like all closing mechanisms with a long range of action, must be monitored carefully. (Redrawn from Siatkowski RE. Continuous archwire closing loop design, optimization and verification, Parts I and II. Am J Orthod Dentofac Orthop 112:393-402, 484-495, 1997.)

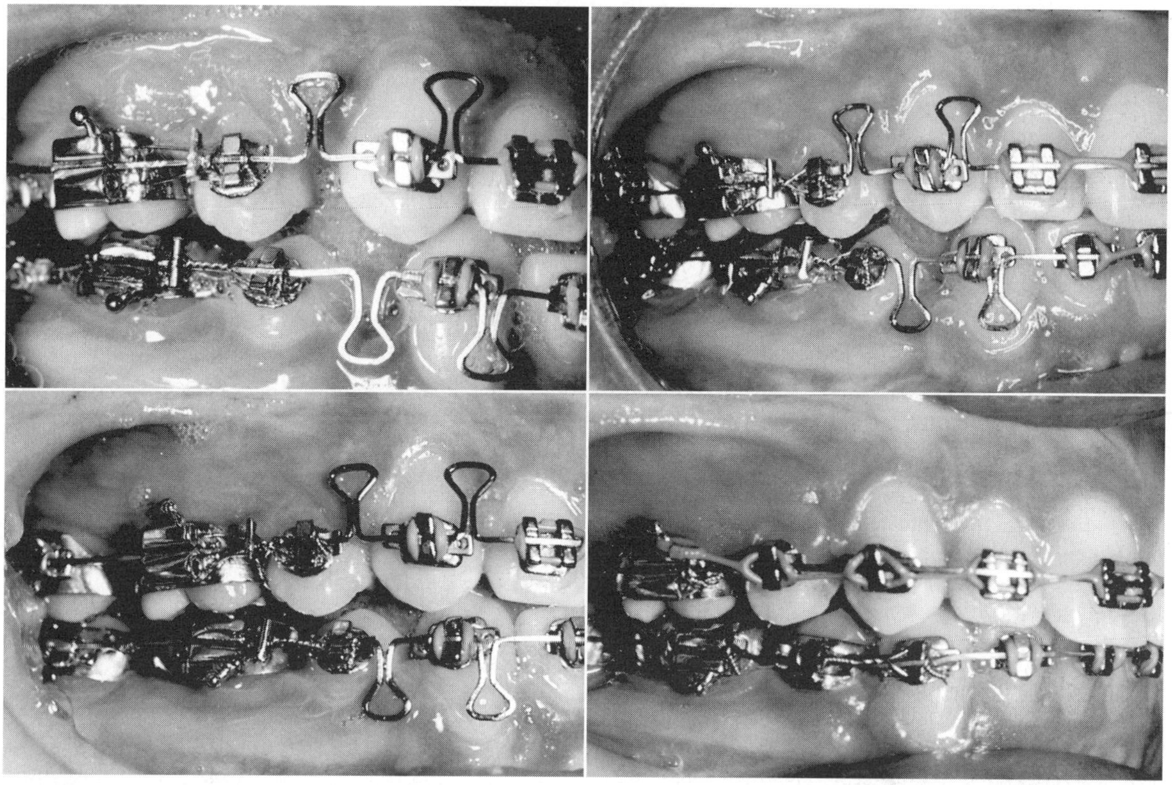

Figure 15-18 Space closure with preformed closing loops in the 18-slot appliance. **A,** 16 × 22 closing loops at initial activation, after the completion of stage 1 alignment and leveling. Note the location of the closing loops and the soldered tiebacks for activation. **B,** Three months later; **C,** Spaces closed at 4 months; **D,** 17 × 25 beta-Ti wire to begin the finishing phase of treatment.

problems from increased complexity always must be balanced against the potentially greater efficiency of the more complex design. The Opus loop has not been widely adopted because of concerns about its complexity and sturdiness. Clinical experience suggests that the average adolescent orthodontic patient can—and probably will—destroy almost any orthodontic device that is not remarkably resistant to being distorted.

A third design factor relates to whether a loop is activated by opening or closing. All else being equal, a loop is more effective when it is closed rather than opened during its activation. On the other hand, a loop designed to be opened can be made so that when it closes completely, the vertical legs come into contact, effectively preventing further movement and producing the desired fail-safe effect (Figure 15-19). A loop activated by closing, in contrast, must have its vertical legs overlap. This creates a transverse step, and the archwire does not develop the same rigidity when it is deactivated. The smaller and more flexible the wire from which a closing loop arch is made, the more important it is that the wire become rigid when the loop is deactivated.

Clinical Recommendations. These design considerations indicate that an excellent closing loop for 18-slot edgewise is a delta-shaped loop in 16 × 22 wire that is activated by opening, as shown in Figure 15-17. Such a wire fits tightly enough in an 18 × 25 mil bracket to give good control of root position. With 10 mm of wire in the loop, the force delivery is close to the optimum, and the mechanism fails safe because contact of the vertical legs when the loop is deactivated limits movement between adjustments and makes the archwire more rigid. It is important to activate the upper horizontal portion of a delta or T-loop so that the vertical legs are pressed lightly together when the loop is not activated (Figure 15-20). This also ensures that the loop will still be active until the legs come into contact.

With 16 × 22 wire and a loop of the delta design (so that the mechanism fails safe), with an activation of 1.0 to 1.5 mm, and with narrow 18-slot brackets, a gable bend of approximately 20 degrees on each side is needed to achieve an appropriate moment-force ratio (Figure 15-21). With wider brackets, a smaller gable bend would generate the same moment. With the same loop in stiffer wire like 17 × 25, a gable bend of any given magnitude would produce a larger moment than in 16 × 22 wire. Remember, however, that the moment-force ratio determines how teeth will move, so with a stiffer wire and the same activation a larger force would be generated and a larger moment would be needed. Optimum moment-force ratios can be achieved with several combinations of wire size, loop configuration and gable angle and, as Siatkowski has shown, can be

A

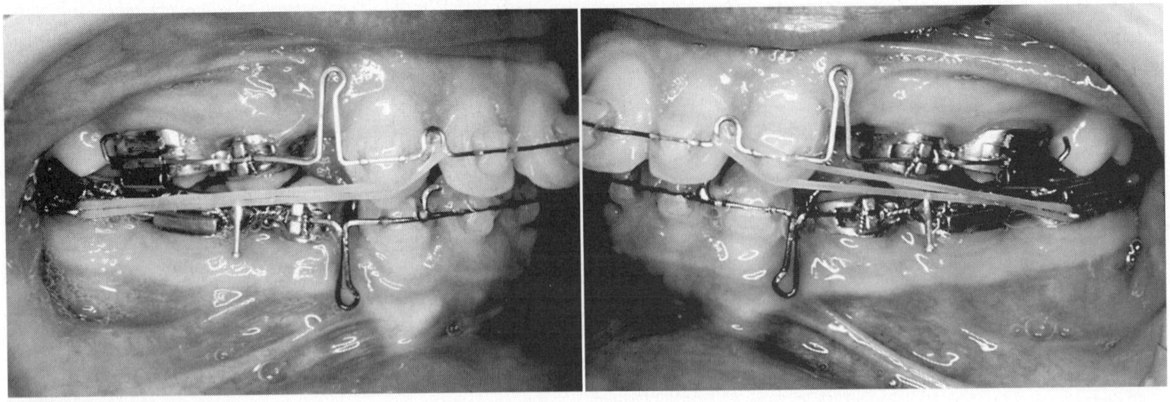

B

FIGURE 15-19 Closing loops in 16 × 22 wire of fail-safe design and 8-mm height used with Class II elastics in this patient. Note that the maxillary loop has been activated by pulling the wire through the molar tube and bending it up. In the mandibular arch, the loop is not active at this time, and the approximation of the legs to create a rigid archwire is apparent. The lower archwire has a tieback mesial to the first molar, so that this loop can be activated by tying a ligature from the posterior teeth to the wire rather than by bending over the end of the wire distal to the molar tube.

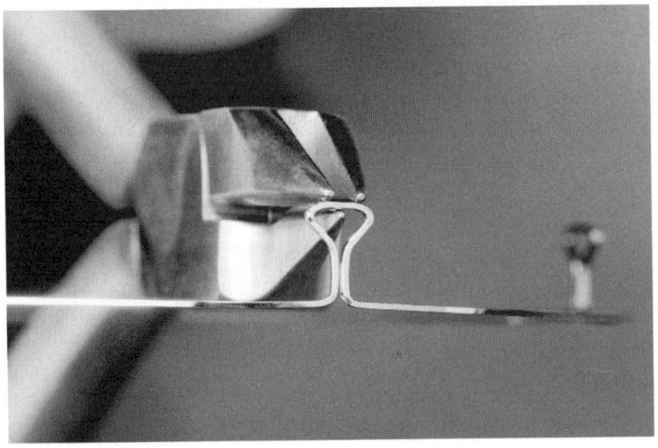

FIGURE 15-20 A three-prong pliers can be used to bring the vertical legs of a closing loop together if they are separated. The legs should touch lightly before activation of the loop by opening it.

A

B

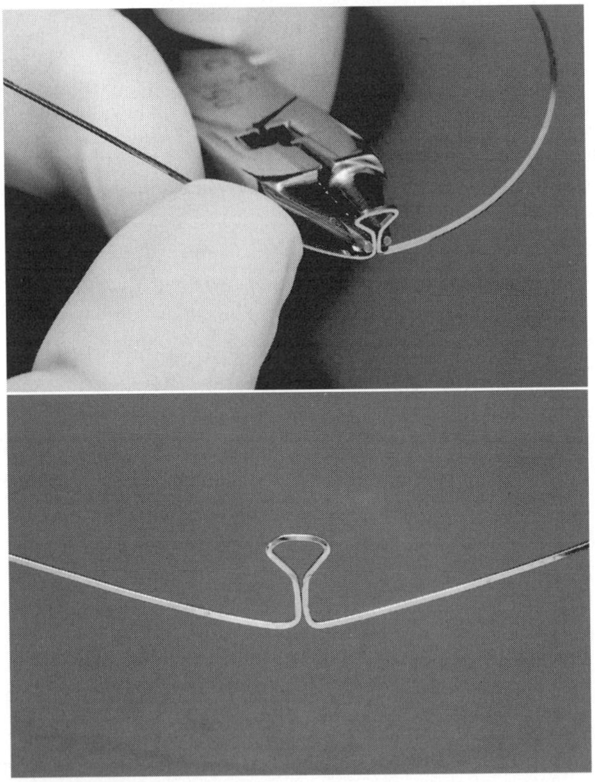

FIGURE 15-21 Gable bends for the closing loop archwire. **A,** Gable bends are placed by bending the wire at the base of the loop; **B,** Appropriate gable for a 16 × 22 closing loop (40 to 45 degrees total, half that on each side).

maintained over a variety of activations at the cost of design complexity.

A closing loop archwire is activated by pulling the posterior part of the archwire distally through the molar tubes, which activates the closing loop the desired amount (1 to 1.5 mm) and then fastening the wire in that position. The wire slides through the brackets and tubes only when it is being activated. After that, as the closing loop returns to its original configuration, the teeth move with the archwire, not along it. There are two ways to hold the archwire in its activated position. The simplest is by bending the end of the archwire gingivally behind the last molar tube. The alternative is to place an attachment—usually a soldered tieback (see Figure 15-18)—on the posterior part of the archwire, so that a ligature can be used to tie the wire in its activated position.

With a 16 × 22 closing loop, usually it is necessary to remove the archwire and reactivate the gable bends after 3 to 4 mm of space closure, but a quick reactivation is all that is needed at most appointments during space closure. As a general rule, if it is anticipated that a closing loop archwire will not have to be removed for adjustment (i.e., the distance to be closed is 4 mm or less), bending the posterior end of the wire is satisfactory. It can be quite difficult to remove an archwire that has been activated by bending over the end, however, and it saves time in the long run to use tiebacks for closing loop archwires that will have to be removed and readjusted.

Specific recommendations for closing loop archwires with the 18-slot appliance and narrow brackets are:

1. 16 × 22 wire, delta or T-shaped loops, 7 mm vertical height, and additional wire incorporated in the loop to make it equivalent to 10 mm of vertical height
2. Gable bends of 40 to 45 degrees total (half on each side of the loop)
3. Loop placement 4 to 5 mm distal to the center of the canine tooth at the center of the space between the canine and second premolar with the extraction site closed

These recommendations certainly are not the only clinically effective possibilities. The principle should be that if a heavier wire (e.g., 17 × 25 mil) is used, the loop design should be altered to incorporate additional wire for better force-deflection characteristics. Also, the gable angulations should be adjusted according to both the springiness of the loop and the width of the brackets. With wide brackets on the canines, for instance, the reduced interbracket span would make any loop somewhat stiffer, and both this and the longer moment arm across the bracket would dictate a smaller gable angle (but the range of the loop would be reduced, which is why wide brackets are not recommended).

Moderate Anchorage Space Closure With 22-Slot Edgewise

As a general rule, space closure in moderate anchorage situations with the 22-slot edgewise appliance is done in two steps: first retracting the canines, usually sliding them along the archwire, and second, retracting the four incisors, usually with a closing loop. This two-step space closure will produce an approximately 60 : 40 closure of the extraction space, varying somewhat depending on whether second molars are included in posterior anchorage and incisor torque requirement.

A 19 × 25 wire is the largest on which sliding retraction of a canine should be attempted (because clearance in the bracket slot is needed), and 18 × 25 wire also can be used. An archwire with a posterior stop, usually in front of the first molar tube, is needed. This stop has the effect of incorporating all the teeth except the canine into the anchorage unit. The canine retraction can then be carried out with a coil spring, a spring soldered to the base archwire, an intra-arch latex elastic, or an elastomeric material. As a general rule, A-NiTi coil springs are preferred because they produce an almost ideal light constant force (Figure 15-22). Elastics produce variable and intermittent forces, and both elastomeric chains and steel coil springs produce rapidly decaying interrupted forces.

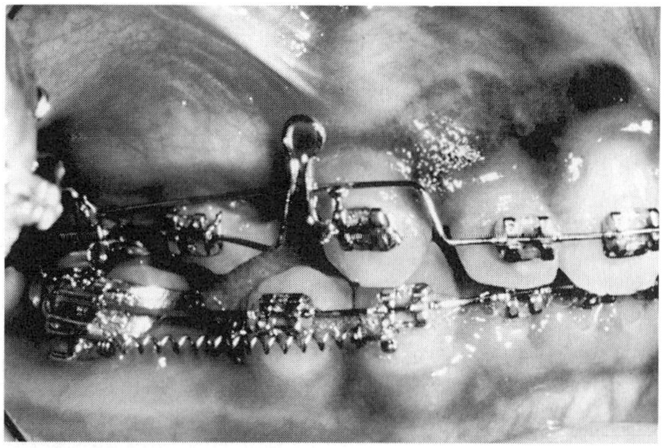

Figure 15-22 In this patient with a 22-slot appliance, sliding space closure in the lower arch is being carried out with a NiTi coil spring, while a segmental closing loop is being used in the upper arch for retraction of the canine.

In addition to its convenience and straightforward design, this type of sliding space closure has the important advantage that it fails safe in two ways: (1) The moments necessary for root paralleling are generated automatically by the twin brackets normally used with the 22-slot appliance. Unless the archwire itself bends, there is no danger that the teeth will tip excessively. (2) The rigid attachment of the canine to the continuous ideal archwire removes the danger that this tooth will be moved far outside its intended path if the patient does not return for scheduled adjustments. For this reason, a long range of action on the retraction springs is not dangerous, as long as the force is not excessive. The ideal force to slide a canine distally is 150-200 gm, since at least 50-100 gm will be used to overcome friction (see Chapter 10). A-NiTi springs can produce this level of force over a wide enough range to close an extraction space with a single activation.

The second stage in the two-stage retraction is usually accomplished with a closing loop, although it is possible to close the space now located mesial to the canines by again sliding the archwire through the posterior brackets. For this stage of incisor retraction, a rectangular wire with its smallest side at least 18 mil is needed—anything smaller rolls in the 22-slot and would allow the incisors to tip while being retracted. An 18 × 25 steel wire with a T-loop, though still too stiff, serves this purpose reasonably well while retaining the fail-safe design. Although loops in a 19 × 25 steel wire also can be used, the better force-deflection characteristics of 18 × 25 wire make it the preferred choice: the 19 × 25 loop either has to give up the fail-safe design or is much too stiff. A third alternative, in many ways now the preferred approach, is a closing loop in 19 × 25 beta-Ti wire. This provides better properties than 18 × 25 steel (quite close to 16 × 22 steel), at the cost of more difficulty in forming the archwire.

Although the two-step procedure is predictable and has excellent fail-safe characteristics, which explains why it remains commonly used, it takes longer to close space in two steps than one. It is possible to use a closing loop archwire for one-step (en masse) closure in the 22-slot appliance, as described previously for 18-slot edgewise. There are several possibilities, unfortunately none of them ideal. The Opus loop has excellent properties and can be used with 22-slot edgewise but is more effective in 18-slot because of the wire size. If a fail-safe design is preferred, a T-loop in 18 × 25 steel or 19 × 25 beta-Ti wire can be considered. All three of these possibilities provide less than ideal torque control of incisors during the retraction because the wire is so much smaller than the bracket slot. If en masse space closure is desired with the 22-slot appliance, a segmented arch technique offers advantages.

The segmented arch approach to space closure[13] is based on incorporating the anterior teeth into a single segment, and both the right and left posterior teeth also into a single segment, with the two sides connected by a stabilizing lingual arch. A retraction spring (Figure 15-23) is used to connect these stable bases, and the activation of the spring is varied to produce the desired pattern of space closure. Because the spring is separate from the wire sections that engage the bracket slots, a wire size and design that produce optimum properties can be used. An auxiliary rectangular tube, usually positioned vertically, is needed on the canine bracket or on the anterior wire segment to provide an attachment for the retraction springs (see Chapter 11). The posterior end of each spring fits into the auxiliary tube on the first molar tooth. With beta-Ti wire, the design of the retraction spring can be more simplified than the design necessary with steel wire. These springs are very effective, and with careful initial activation, an impressive range of movement can be produced before reactivation is necessary.

The greatest disadvantage of segmented arch space closure is not its increased complexity, but that it does not fail safe. Without a rigid connection between the anterior and posterior segments, there is nothing to maintain arch form and proper vertical relationships if a retraction spring is distorted or activated incorrectly. For this reason, despite the excellent results usually obtained with segmented arches and retraction springs, it is important to monitor these patients especially carefully and to avoid long intervals without observation.

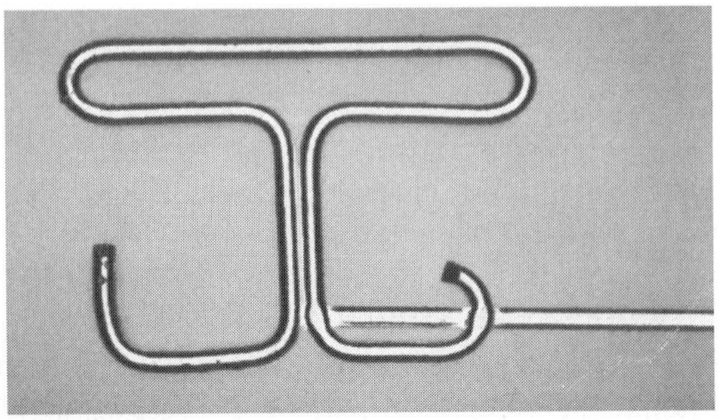

FIGURE 15-23 Composite retraction spring designed by Burstone for use with the segmented arch technique, consisting of 18 mil beta-Ti wire (the loop) welded to 17 × 25 beta-Ti. This spring can be used either for en masse retraction of incisors or canine retraction.

Maximum Incisor Retraction (Maximum Anchorage)

It is not always desirable to retract the anterior teeth as far as possible after premolars have been extracted. In fact, overretraction of incisors is as much of a potential problem as leaving them too prominent by not maintaining adequate posterior anchorage. When maximum retraction is needed, however, it is vital that the orthodontic mechanotherapy be structured to provide this. Techniques to produce maximum retraction combine two possible approaches. The first is reinforcement of posterior anchorage by appropriate means, including extraoral force, stabilizing lingual arches, interarch elastics and more recently, skeletal anchorage (indicated only if an extremely severe problem exists). The second approach involves reduction of strain on the posterior anchorage, which includes any combination of eliminating friction from the retraction system (as with closing loops), tipping the incisors before uprighting them (as in Begg technique), or retracting the canines separately (as in Tweed technique).

Maximum Retraction With the 18-Slot Appliance

With the 18-slot appliance, friction from sliding usually is avoided by employing closing loops, and tipping/uprighting is rarely part of the anchorage-control strategy. To obtain greater retraction of the anterior teeth, a sequence of steps to augment anchorage and reduce anchorage strain could be as follows:

1. Add stabilizing lingual arches and proceed with en masse space closure. The resulting increase in posterior anchorage, though modest, will change the ratio of anterior retraction to posterior protraction to approximately 2 : 1.
2. Reinforce maxillary posterior anchorage with extraoral force and (if needed) use Class III elastics from high-pull headgear to supplement retraction force in the lower arch, while continuing the basic en masse closure approach. Depending on how well the patient cooperates, additional improvement of retraction, perhaps to a 3 : 1 or 4 : 1 ratio, can be achieved.
3. Retract the canines independently, preferably using a segmental closing loop, and then retract the incisors with a second closing loop archwire. Used with stabilizing lingual arches (which are needed to control the posterior segments in most patients), this technique will produce a 3 : 1 retraction ratio. When this procedure is reinforced with headgear, even better ratios are possible.

A more detailed discussion of each of these approaches follows.

Reinforcement With Stabilizing Lingual Arches. Stabilizing lingual arches must be rigid and should be made from

36 mil or 32 × 32 steel wire. These can be soldered to the molar bands, but it is convenient to be able to remove them, and Burstone's designs (see Chapter 11) are preferred.

It is important for a lower stabilizing lingual arch to lie behind and below the lower incisors, so that it does not interfere with their retraction. If 36 mil round wire is used, the lower lingual arch is more conveniently inserted from the distal than from the mesial of the molar tube. The maxillary stabilizing lingual arch is a straight transpalatal design. Because maximum rigidity is desired for anchorage reinforcement, an expansion loop in the palatal section of this wire is not recommended unless a specific indication exists for including it.

If lingual arches are needed for anchorage control, they should be present during the first and second stages of treatment but can and should be removed after space closure is complete. Their presence during the finishing stage of treatment, after extraction spaces have been closed, is not helpful and may interfere with final settling of the occlusion.

Reinforcement With Headgear and Interarch Elastics. Extraoral force against the maxillary posterior segments is an obvious and direct method for anchorage reinforcement. It is also possible to place extraoral force against the mandibular posterior segments, but is usually more practical to use Class III elastics to transfer the extraoral force from the upper to the lower arch.

Inter-arch elastics for anchorage reinforcement were a prominent part of the original Tweed method for maximum retraction of protruding anterior teeth. In the Tweed approach to bimaxillary protrusion, "anchorage preparation," achieved by tipping the molars and premolars distally, was done before space closure. As anchorage was being prepared in the lower arch, Class III elastics were used to maintain lower incisor position while this is done. After the lower incisors were retracted, sliding the canine initially and then using a closing loop, the lower arch was stabilized and Class II elastics were used to prepare anchorage by tipping back the upper molars, before the upper incisors were retracted.

Although the original Tweed approach can be used with the contemporary 18-slot appliance, it is rarely indicated. Prolonged use of Class II and Class III elastics is extrusive and requires good vertical growth for acceptable results. Distally tipping the molars augments their anchorage value primarily by first moving these teeth distally, then mesially.

Segmented Retraction of the Canines. Segmented retraction of the canines with frictionless springs is an attractive method for reducing the strain on posterior anchorage and is a readily available approach with the modern 18-slot appliance. It is also possible to retract the canines by sliding them on the archwire, but the narrow brackets usually used with the 18-slot appliance and the tight clearance and relatively low strength of a 17 × 25 archwire produce less-than-optimum sliding.

For frictionless retraction of the canines, an auxiliary tube on the molar is needed. An auxiliary tube on the canine is unnecessary, because the retraction spring can fit directly into the canine bracket. The PG spring designed by Gjessing is an efficient current design (Figure 15-24).[14] Closing loops, either in a continuous archwire or with a segmented arch approach, are then used for the second stage of retraction of the incisors.

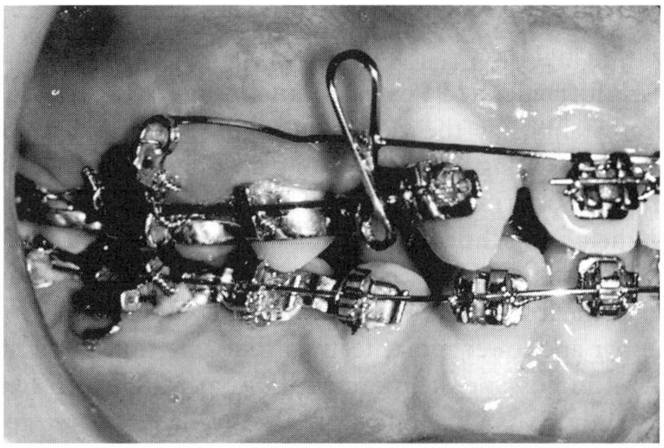

FIGURE 15-24 For canine retraction, the Gjessing retraction spring offers excellent control of forces and moments and probably is the most effective current design of a spring for this purpose.

Segmented canine retraction of this type presents two problems. The first is that it is difficult to control the position of the canine in all three planes of space as it is retracted. If the canine is pulled distally from an attachment on its buccal surface, the point of attachment is not only some distance occlusal but is also buccal to the center of resistance. This means that without appropriate moments, the tooth will tip distally and rotate mesiobuccally. Both a root-paralleling moment and an antirotation moment must be obtained by placing two different gable bends in the same spring. Control of the vertical position of the canine, particularly after the gable bends in two planes of space have been placed, can be a significant problem.

Second, much more than with en masse retraction using segmented mechanics, segmental retraction of canines does not fail safe. The canine is free to move in three-dimensional space, and there are no stops to prevent excessive movement in the wrong direction if a spring is improperly adjusted or becomes distorted. Loss of vertical control is particularly likely. A missed appointment and a distorted spring can lead to the development of a considerable problem, and patients must be monitored carefully.

Maximum Retraction With the 22-Slot Appliance

The same basic approaches are available with the 22- as with the 18-slot appliance: to increase the amount of incisor retraction, a combination of increased reinforcement of posterior anchorage and decreased strain on that anchorage is needed. All the possible strategies for anchorage control can be used. With a 22-slot appliance in which sliding retraction of canines is the approach to moderate anchorage, the

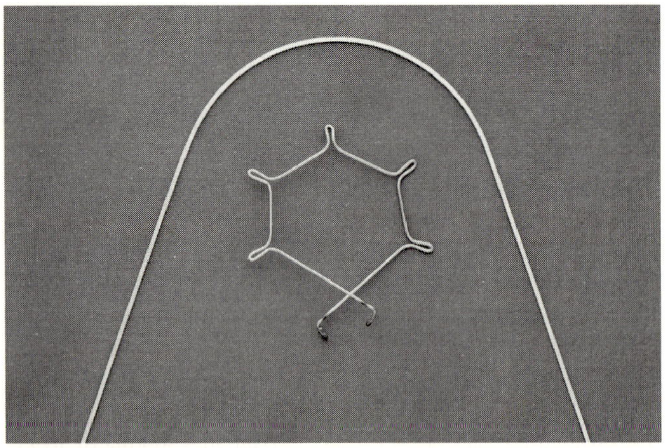

Figure 16-4 Torquing auxiliary archwires exert their effect when the auxiliary, originally bent in a tight circle as shown, is forced to assume the form of a base archwire over which it will be placed. This tends to distort the base archwire, which therefore should be relatively heavy—at least 18 mil steel.

A

B

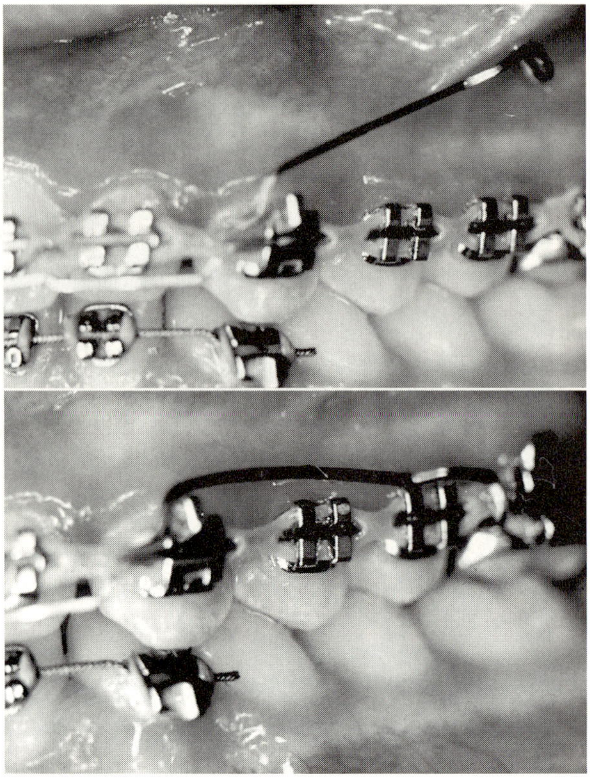

Figure 16-5 The Burstone torquing auxiliary (also see Figure 10-41) is particularly useful in Class II, division 2 cases where maxillary central incisors need a large amount of torque. The torquing auxiliary is full-dimension steel wire (21 × 25 or 17 × 25, in 22- or 18-slot brackets respectively) that fits in the brackets only on the incisors. It can be used only on the centrals or on the centrals and laterals, as shown here. The base arch (preferably also full-dimension rectangular wire) extends forward from the molars through the canine or lateral incisor brackets, then steps down and rests against the labial surface of the teeth to be torqued. When the torquing auxiliary is passive **(A),** its long posterior arms are up in the buccal vestibule. It is activated **(B)** by pulling the arms down and hooking them beneath the base archwire mesial to the first molar. The segment of the base arch that rests against the labial surface of the central incisors prevents the crowns from going forward, and the result is efficient lingual root torque.

anchorage is required to maintain overjet correction while upper incisor roots are torqued lingually. For that reason, Class II elastics are likely to be necessary when active torque is needed during the final stage of Class II treatment.

With a modern edgewise appliance, only moderate additional torque should be necessary during the finishing stage. With the 18-slot appliance, a 17 × 25 steel archwire has excellent properties in torsion, and torque with this archwire is entirely feasible. Building torque into the bracket slot initially means that it is unnecessary to place torquing bends in the archwire, making the accomplishment of torque as a finishing procedure relatively straightforward.

With the 22-slot appliance, full-dimension steel rectangular wires are far too stiff for effective torquing (see Figure 10-11). If incisors have been allowed to tip lingually too much, as can happen in the correction of maxillary incisor protrusion, correcting this merely by placing a rectangular steel archwire is not feasible. Prior to brackets with built-in torque and titanium archwires, torquing auxiliaries were commonly used with the 22-slot appliance. One of the great virtues of torque-slot brackets is that tipping of incisors, for the most part, can be prevented during retraction and space closure. In addition, full-dimension M-NiTi or beta-Ti archwires can be used to torque incisors with 22-slot brackets (provided the brackets have torque built in), further reducing any need for auxiliary arches. For these reasons, torquing auxiliaries for 22-slot edgewise have almost disappeared from contemporary use.

One torquing auxiliary deserves special mention: the Burstone torquing arch (Figure 16-5). It can be particularly helpful in patients with Class II, division 2 malocclusion whose maxillary central incisors are severely tipped lingually and require a long distance of torquing movement, while the lateral incisors need little if any torque. Because of the long lever arm, this is the most effective torquing auxiliary for use with the edgewise appliance. It is equally effective with the 18- or 22-slot appliance. If all four incisors need considerable torque, a wire spanning from the molar auxiliary tube to the incisors, with a V-bend so that the incisor segment receives the greater moment, is a highly efficient approach.[2]

Two factors determine the amount of torque that will be expressed by any rectangular archwire in a rectangular slot: the inclination of the bracket slot relative to the archwire, and the tightness of the fit between the archwire and the bracket. The variations in torque prescriptions in

TABLE 16-1

Effective Torque

Wire size	Play (degrees)	BRACKET TORQUE ANGLE (DEGREES) 10	22	30
		EFFECTIVE TORQUE		
18-Slot Bracket				
16 × 16	10.9	0.0	11.1	19.1
16 × 22	9.3	0.7	12.7	20.7
17 × 25	4.1	5.9	17.9	25.9
18 × 18	1.5	8.5	20.5	28.5
18 × 25	1.0	9.0	21.0	29.0
22-Slot Bracket				
16 × 22	21.9	0	0.1	8.1
17 × 25	15.5	0	6.5	13.5
19 × 25	9.6	0.4	12.4	20.4
21 × 25	4.1	5.9	17.9	25.9
21.5 × 28	1.8	8.2	20.2	28.2

Note based on nominal wire and/or slot sizes; actual play is likely to be greater. (From Semetz: *Kieferorthop Mitteil* 7:13-26, 1993.)

contemporary edgewise appliances are shown in Table 11-6. These variations largely reflect different determinations of the average contour of the labial and buccal surfaces of the teeth, but some differences are also related to the expected fit of archwires. With the 18-slot appliance, it is assumed that the rectangular archwires used for finishing will fit tightly in the bracket slot (i.e., that the finishing archwires will have a minimum dimension of 17 or 18 mil). With the 22-slot appliance, on the other hand, some prescriptions have extra built-in torque to compensate for rectangular finishing archwires that will have more clearance. Torque will not be expressed to the same extent with a 19 × 25 wire in a 22-slot bracket as with a 17 × 25 wire in an 18-slot bracket. The difference amounts to several degrees of difference in incisor inclination. The "effective torque" of various wire-bracket combinations is shown in Table 16-1. Obviously, when the torque prescription for a bracket is established, it is important to know what finishing wires are intended.

For full expression of the torque built into brackets in the 22-slot appliance, the best finishing wire usually is 21 × 25 beta-Ti. This wire's torsional stiffness is less than that of 17 × 25 steel (see Figure 10-11), but the shorter interbracket distances with 22-slot brackets bring its performance in torsion close to that of the smaller steel wire. Braided rectangular steel wires are available in a variety of stiffnesses, and the stiffest of these in 21 × 25 dimension also can be useful in 22-slot finishing. A solid 21 × 25 steel wire cannot be recommended because of its stiffness and the resulting extremely high forces and short range of action. If a solid steel wire of this size is used (the major reason would be surgical stabilization), it should be preceded by 21 × 25 beta-Ti.

CORRECTION OF VERTICAL INCISOR RELATIONSHIPS

If the first two stages of treatment have been accomplished perfectly, no change in the vertical relationship of incisors will be needed during the finishing stage of treatment. Minor adjustments often are needed, however, and major ones occasionally are required. At this stage, anterior open bite is more likely to be a problem than residual excessive overbite, but either may be encountered.

Excessive Overbite

Before attempting to correct excess overbite at the finishing stage of treatment, it is important to carefully assess why the problem exists, and particularly to assess two things: the vertical relationship between the maxillary lip and maxillary incisors, and anterior face height. If the display of the maxillary incisors on smile is appropriate, it is important to maintain this and make any overbite correction by repositioning the lower incisors. If display is excessive, intrusion of the upper incisors would be indicated. If face height is short, elongating the posterior teeth slightly (almost always, the lower posterior teeth) would be acceptable; if face height is long, intrusion of incisors would be needed.

If intrusion is indicated and a rectangular finishing archwire is already in place, the simplest approach is to cut this archwire distal to the lateral incisors and install an auxiliary intrusion arch (Figure 16-6). Remember that when a maxillary auxiliary intrusion arch is used, a stabilizing transpalatal lingual arch may be needed to maintain control of transverse relationships and prevent excessive distal tipping of the maxillary molars. The greater the desired vertical change in incisor position, the more important it will be to have a stabilizing lingual arch in place, and vice versa. Small corrections during finishing usually do not require placing a lingual arch.

Alternatively, if slight elongation of the posterior teeth is indicated, step bends in a flexible archwire would be satisfactory. The intermediate arch wire before the final torquing archwire is the one for implementation of these step bends (17 × 25 TMA with the 18-slot appliance, 17 × 25 M-NiTi with the 22-slot appliance). An auxiliary depressing arch for overbite correction can be effective, but only if the base archwire is a relatively small round wire (see Chapter 14), so this is not the preferred approach for a modest amount of final overbite correction.

Anterior Open Bite

As with deep bite, it is important to analyze the source of the difficulty if an anterior open bite persists at the finishing

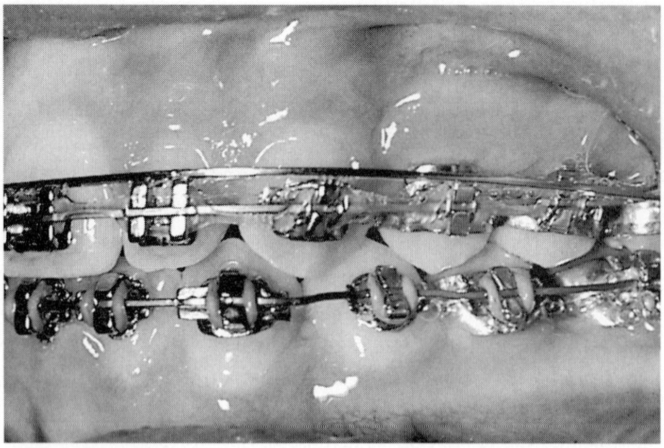

FIGURE 16-6 Use of an auxiliary leveling arch at the finishing stage to correct a mildly excessive overbite. If a continuous base archwire is in place, as in this patient, further leveling will occur by elongation of teeth in the premolar region—which is quite satisfactory in adolescents with some vertical growth remaining. If incisor intrusion is desired, the base arch must be segmented.

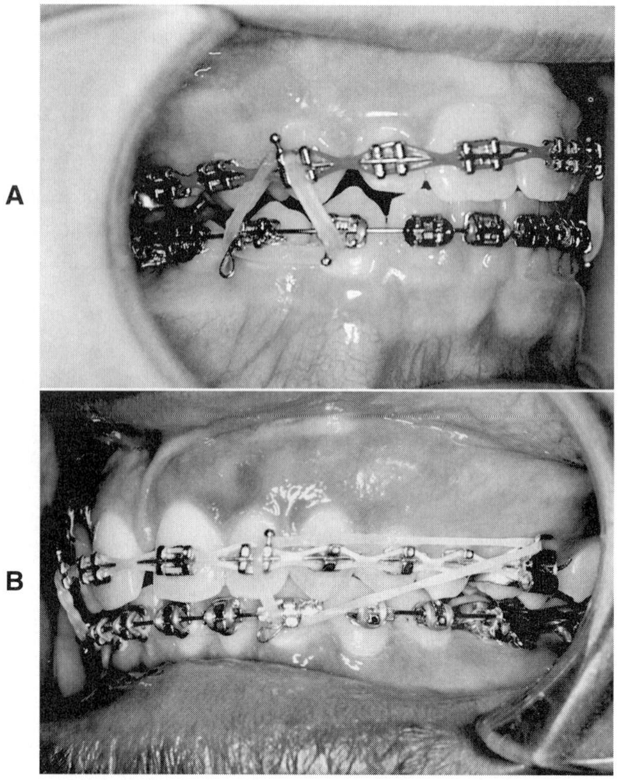

FIGURE 16-7 **A,** Anterior vertical elastics, either in the bilateral arrangement shown here or as a single anterior box, can be used to help close a mild anterior open bite at the end of treatment, but this is effective only if the archwires are contoured to allow the tooth movement. Elastics cannot overpower a stiff archwire that is maintaining the open bite. **B,** Class III (and Class II) elastics tend to extrude molars, and can lead to the development of anterior open bite. Using a triangular Class III elastic, as shown here, helps to control the open bite tendency. Use of these elastics, of course, presupposes that some elongation of the molars and incisors is acceptable.

stage of treatment, and as with deep bite, the relationship of the upper incisors to the lip and anterior face height are critical in determining what to do. If the open bite results from excessive eruption of posterior teeth, whether from a poor growth pattern or improper use of interarch elastics, correcting it at the finishing stage can be extremely difficult. The most effective approach to intrusion of posterior teeth is skeletal anchorage. Placing bone screws at the finishing stage to accomplish this implies that the earlier stages of treatment were not completed satisfactorily, but this might be necessary in some patients with a severe long face pattern of growth.

If no severe problems with the pattern of facial growth exist, however, a mild open bite at the finishing stage of treatment often is due to an excessively level lower arch. This condition is managed best by elongating the lower but not the upper incisors, thereby creating a slight curve of Spee in the lower arch. Because of the stiffness of the rectangular archwires used for finishing, even with 18-slot edgewise, it is futile to use vertical elastics to deepen the bite without altering the form of the archwires. Steps in an appropriately flexible lower archwire, while maintaining a stiffer upper wire, can be effective when supplemented with light vertical elastics (Figure 16-7). Obviously, if display of the upper incisors was inadequate, elongation of those teeth to close the bite would be indicated, and the same approach with the flexible/stabilizing archwires reversed would be indicated. Elongating the lower incisors to close a moderate anterior open bite is a quite stable procedure. Elongating the upper incisors is less stable, and this should be kept in mind when retention is planned.

MIDLINE DISCREPANCIES

A relatively common problem at the finishing stage of treatment is a discrepancy in the midlines of the dental arches. This can result either from a preexisting midline discrepancy that was not completely resolved at an earlier stage of treatment or an asymmetric closure of spaces within the arch. Minor midline discrepancies at the finishing stage are no great problem, but it is quite difficult to correct large discrepancies after extraction spaces have been closed and occlusal relationships have been nearly established.

As with any discrepancy at the finishing stage, it is important to establish as clearly as possible exactly where the discrepancy arises. Although coincident dental midlines are a component of functional occlusion—all other things being equal, a midline discrepancy will be reflected in how the posterior teeth fit together—it is undesirable esthetically to

A

B

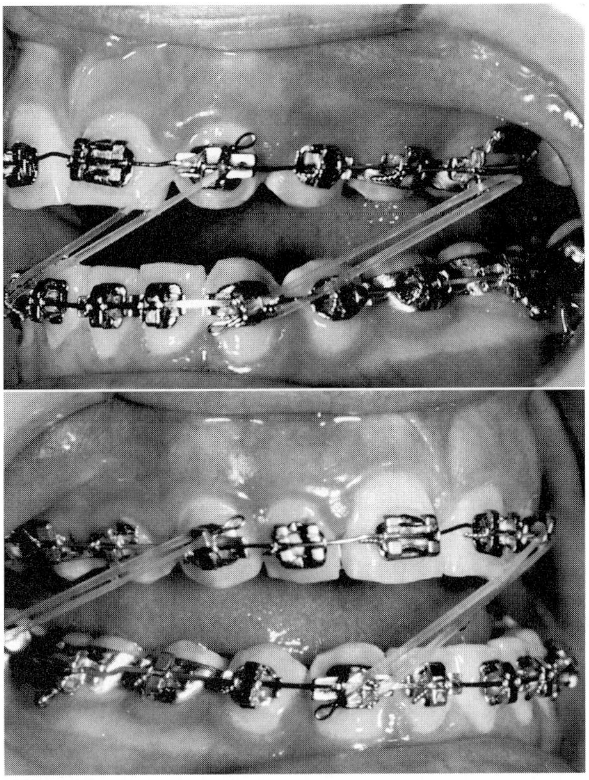

FIGURE 16-8 Midline correction can be approached with any combination of asymmetric posterior and anterior diagonal elastics. In this patient, a combination of Class II, Class III, and anterior diagonal elastics are being used, with a rectangular archwire in the lower arch and a round wire in the upper arch, attempting to shift the maxillary arch to the right.

displace the maxillary midline, bringing it around to meet a displaced mandibular midline. If a dental midline discrepancy results from a skeletal asymmetry, it may be impossible to correct it orthodontically, and treatment decisions will have to be made in the light of camouflage vs. surgical correction (see discussion in Chapter 8).

Fortunately, midline discrepancies in the finishing stage usually are not this severe and are caused only by lateral displacements of maxillary or mandibular teeth accompanied by a mild Class II or Class III relationship on one side. In this circumstance, the midline often can be corrected by using asymmetric Class II (or Class III) elastic force. As a general rule, it is more effective to use Class II or Class III elastics bilaterally with heavier force on one side than to place a unilateral elastic. However, if one side is totally corrected while the other is not, the patient usually tolerates a unilateral elastic reasonably well. It is also possible to combine a Class II or Class III elastic on one side with a diagonal elastic anteriorly, to bring the midlines together (Figure 16-8). This approach should be reserved for small discrepancies. Prolonged use of Class II or Class III elastics during the finishing stage of treatment should be avoided. Coordinated steps in the archwires also can be used to shift the teeth of one arch more than the other.[3]

An important consideration in dealing with midline discrepancies is the possibility of a mandibular shift contributing to the discrepancy. This can arise easily if a slight discrepancy in the transverse position of posterior teeth is present. For instance, a slightly narrow maxillary right posterior segment can lead to a shift of the mandible to the left on final closure, creating the midline discrepancy. The correction in this instance, obviously, must include some force system (usually careful coordination of the maxillary and mandibular archwires, perhaps reinforced by a posterior cross-elastic) to alter the transverse arch relationships. Occasionally, the entire maxillary arch is slightly displaced transversely relative to the mandibular arch so that with the teeth in occlusion, relationships are excellent, but there is a lateral shift to reach that position. Correction again would involve posterior cross-elastics, but in a parallel pattern as shown in Figure 16-8.

TOOTH SIZE DISCREPANCIES

Tooth size discrepancy problems must be taken into account when treatment is planned initially (see Chapter 7), but many of the steps to deal with these problems are taken in the finishing stage of treatment. Reduction of interproximal enamel (stripping) is the usual strategy to compensate for discrepancies caused by excess tooth size. When the problem is tooth size deficiency, it is necessary to leave space between some teeth, which may or may not ultimately be closed by restorations.

One of the advantages of a bonded appliance is that interproximal enamel can be removed at any time. When stripping of enamel is part of the original treatment plan, most of the enamel reduction should be done initially, but final stripping can be deferred until the finishing stage. This procedure allows direct observation of the occlusal relationships before the final tooth size adjustments are made. A topical fluoride treatment always is recommended immediately after stripping is done.

Tooth size deficiency problems often are caused by small maxillary lateral incisors. A small space distal to the lateral incisor can be esthetically and functionally acceptable, but a composite resin build-up of the small lateral incisor usually is the best plan for small incisors (Figure 16-9; see also [Steve Dickens series]). Precise finishing is easier if the build-up is done during the finishing stage of the orthodontic treatment. This can be accomplished simply by removing the bracket from the small tooth or teeth for a few hours while the restoration is done, then replacing the bracket and archwires. Alternatively, the composite build-ups should be done as soon possible after the patient is in retention. This requires an initial retainer to hold the space, and a new retainer immediately after the restoration is completed. The main reason for waiting until after the orthodontic appliance has

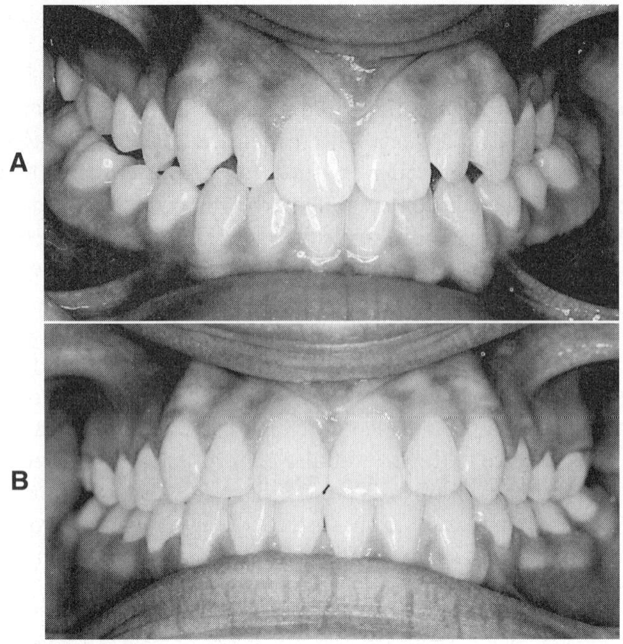

Figure 16-9 Small maxillary lateral incisors create tooth-size discrepancy problems that may become apparent only late in treatment. **A,** Small maxillary lateral incisors, one of which is distorted, prior to treatment. **B,** After treatment, in which space was created mesial and distal to the laterals so that laminates could be placed to bring the teeth to normal size and appearance.

been removed is to allow any gingival inflammation to resolve itself.[4]

More generalized small deficiencies can be masked by altering incisor position in any of several ways. To a limited extent, torque of the upper incisors can be used to compensate: leaving the incisors slightly more upright makes them take up less room relative to the lower arch and can be used to mask large upper incisors, while slightly excessive torque can partially compensate for small upper incisors. These adjustments require third-order bends in the finishing archwires. It is also possible to compensate by slightly tipping teeth, or by finishing the orthodontic treatment with mildly excessive overbite or overjet, depending on the individual circumstances.[5]

Final "Settling" of Teeth

At the conclusion of Class II or Class III correction, particularly if interarch elastics have been used, the teeth tend to rebound back toward their initial position despite the presence of rectangular archwires. In addition, it is not uncommon for a full-dimension rectangular archwire, no matter how carefully made, to hold some teeth slightly out of occlusion.

Because of the rebound after Class II or Class III treatment, it is important to slightly overcorrect the occlusal relationships. In a typical Class II anterior deep bite patient, the teeth should be taken to an end-to-end incisor relationship, with both overjet and overbite totally eliminated, before the headgear or elastic forces are discontinued. This provides some latitude for the teeth to rebound or settle into the proper relationship.

The more precisely a stiff finishing archwire fits the brackets and the more bends that it requires to compensate for bracket positioning, the more likely that some teeth will be almost but not quite in occlusion. This phenomenon was recognized by the pioneers with the edgewise appliance, who coined the term "arch-bound" to describe it. They found that with precisely fitting wires, it was almost impossible to get every tooth into solid occlusion, although one could come close.

These considerations lead to the formulation of two rules in finishing treatment:

1. Interarch elastics and headgear should be discontinued, and the rebound from their use allowed to express itself, 4 to 8 weeks before the orthodontic appliances are removed.
2. As a final step in treatment, the teeth should be brought into a solid occlusal relationship without heavy archwires present.

The final step of finishing therefore is appropriately called "settling," since its purpose is to bring all teeth into a solid occlusal relationship before the patient is placed in retention. There are three ways to settle the occlusion:

1. By replacing the rectangular archwires at the very end of treatment with light round arches that provide some freedom for movement of the teeth (16 mil in the 18-slot appliance, 16 or 18 mil in the 22-slot appliance) and allowing the teeth to find their own occlusal level;
2. With laced posterior vertical elastics after removing the posterior segments of the archwires; or
3. After the bands and brackets have been removed, with the use of a tooth positioner.

Replacing full-dimension rectangular wires with light round wires at the very end of treatment was the original method for settling, recommended by Tweed in the 1940s and perhaps by other edgewise pioneers earlier. These light final arches must include any first- or second-order bends used in the rectangular finishing arches. It is usually unnecessary for the patient to wear light posterior vertical elastics during this settling, but they can be used if needed. These light arches will quickly settle the teeth into final occlusion and should remain in place for only a few weeks at most.

The difficulty with undersized round wires at the end of treatment is that some freedom of movement for settling of posterior teeth is desired, but precise control of anterior teeth is lost as well. It was not until the 1980s that orthodontists realized the advantage of removing only the posterior part of the rectangular finishing wire, leaving the anterior segment (typically canine-to-canine) in place, and

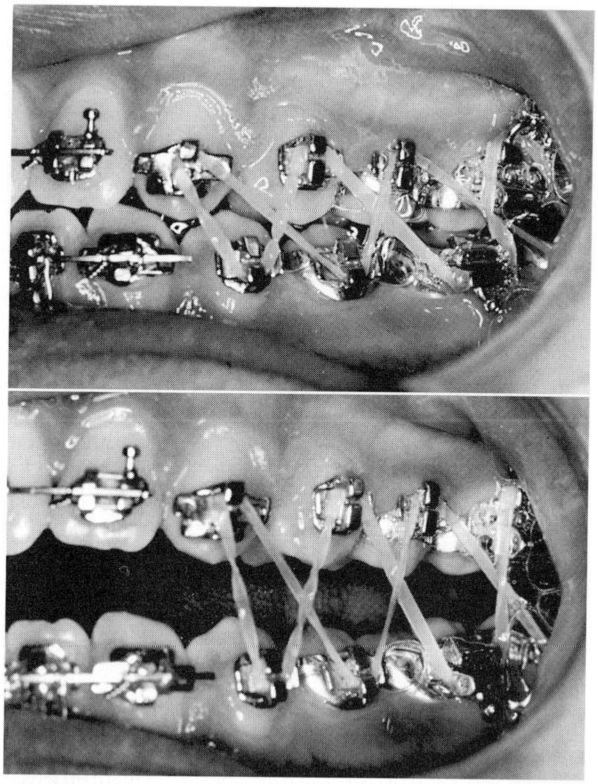

A

B

FIGURE 16-10 Use of laced elastics for settling the teeth into final occlusion at the end of treatment. The elastics can be used either with light round archwires, or (usually preferred) with rectangular segments in the anterior brackets and no wire at all posteriorly. The last step in treatment then becomes cutting the rectangular finishing archwires distal to the lateral incisors or canines, and removing the posterior segments.

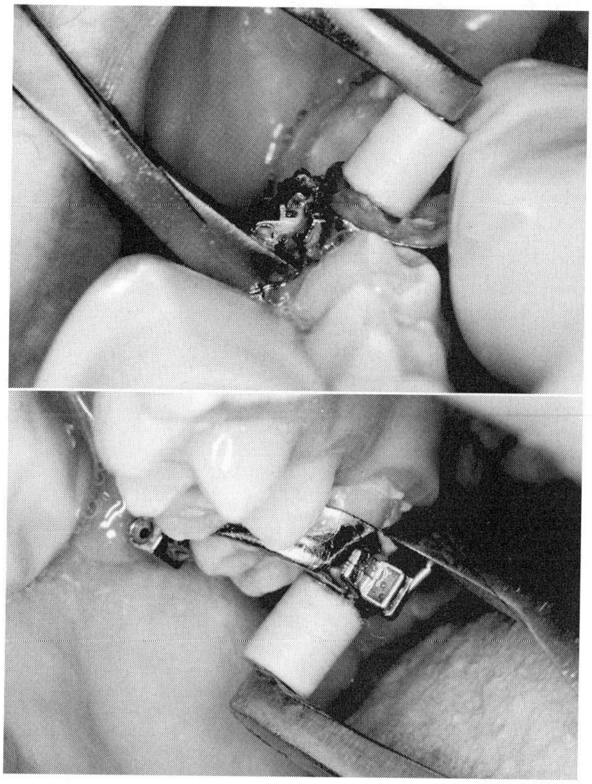

A

B

FIGURE 16-11 Removal of molar bands with band-removing pliers. **A,** Lower posterior bands are removed primarily with pressure from the buccal surface; **B,** Upper posterior bands are removed with pressure primarily against the lingual surface, which is easier when a lingual tube (as seen here), cleat or other attachment was welded to the band initially.

using laced elastics to bring the posterior teeth into tight occlusion (Figure 16-10).[6] This method sacrifices a large degree of control of the posterior teeth, and therefore should not be used in patients who had major rotations or posterior crossbite. For the majority of patients who had well-aligned posterior teeth from the beginning, however, this is a remarkably simple and effective way to settle the teeth into their final occlusion. It is the last step in active treatment for the majority of patients at present.

The elastics for this settling are laced around the tubes and brackets as shown in Figure 16-11. A typical arrangement is to use light $^{3}/_{4}$-inch elastics, with a Class II or Class III direction depending on whether slightly more correction is desired. An alternative is to use a pair of $^{5}/_{16}$ $^{3}/_{8}$ inch elastics on both sides in a vertical triangle. These elastics should not remain in place for more than 2 weeks, and 1 week usually is enough to accomplish the desired settling. At that point, the fixed appliances should be removed and the retainers placed.

REMOVAL OF BANDS AND BONDED ATTACHMENTS

Removal of bands is accomplished by breaking the cement attachment and then lifting the band off the tooth—which sounds simpler than it is in some instances. For upper molar and premolar teeth, a band-removing instrument is placed so that first the lingual, then the buccal surface is elevated (Figure 16-11). A welded lingual bar is needed on these bands to provide a point of attachment for the pliers if lingual hooks or cleats are not a part of the appliance. For the lower posterior teeth, the sequence of force is just the reverse: the band-remover is applied first on the buccal, then the lingual surface.

Bonded brackets must be removed, insofar as possible, without damaging the enamel surface. This is done by creating a fracture within the resin bonding material or between the bracket and the resin, and then removing the residual resin from the enamel surface. With metal brackets, applying a cutting pliers to the base of the bracket so that the bracket bends (Figure 16-12) has the disadvantage of

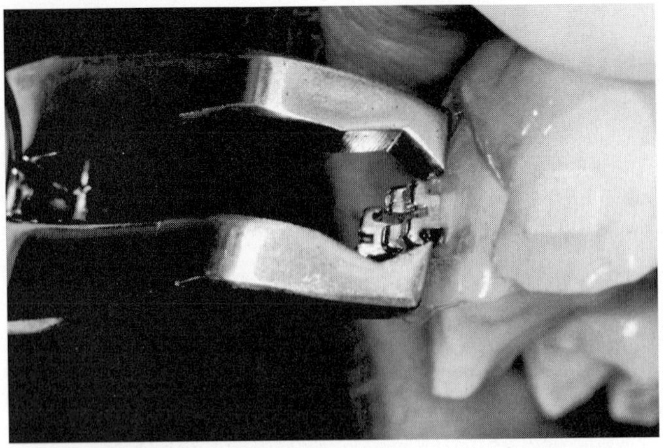

FIGURE 16-12 Removal of bonded brackets. A special plier can be used to fracture the bonding resin, which usually results in much of the resin left on the tooth surface. This works particularly well with twin brackets. The advantage of this method is that the bracket usually is undamaged; the disadvantage is heavy force that may cause enamel damage. The alternative is to use a cutter to distort the bracket base. The first approach is more compatible with recycling of brackets, but the second is safer and usually leaves less resin to remove from the tooth surface.

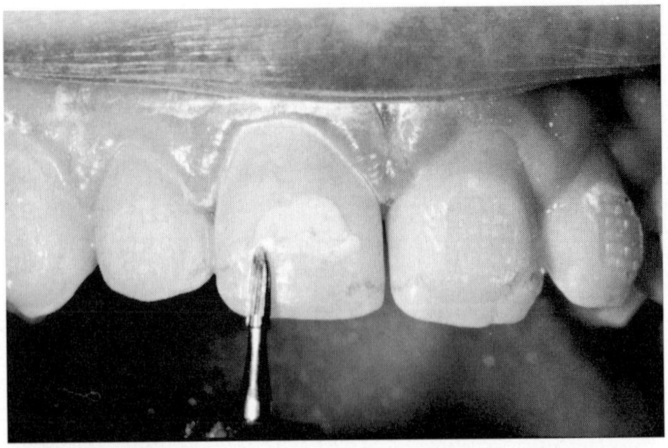

FIGURE 16-13 Upon debonding, the bond failure usually occurs between the base of the bracket and the resin, leaving excess resin on the tooth. Removing excess bonding resin is best accomplished with a smooth 12-fluted carbide bur, followed by pumicing. The carbide bur is used with a gentle wiping motion to remove the resin.

destroying the bracket, which otherwise could be reused, but this is the safest method.

Enamel damage from debonding metal brackets is rare, but there have been a number of reports of enamel fractures and removal of chunks of enamel when ceramic brackets are debonded (see Chapter 11 for a more detailed discussion). It also is easy to fracture a ceramic bracket while attempting to remove it, and if that happens, large pieces of the bracket must be ground away with a diamond stone in a handpiece. These problems arise because ceramic brackets have little or no ability to deform—they are either intact or broken. Shearing stresses are applied to the bracket to remove it, and the necessary force can become alarmingly large.

There are three approaches to these problems in debonding ceramic brackets:

1. Modify the interface between the bracket and the bonding resin to increase the chance that when force is applied, the failure will occur between the bracket and the bonding material. Chemical bonds between the bonding resin and the bracket can be too good, and most manufacturers now have weakened them or abandoned chemical bonding altogether;
2. Use heat to soften the bonding resin, so that the bracket can be removed with lower force[7]; or
3. Modify the bracket so that it breaks predictably when debonding force is applied. One advantage of a metal slot in a ceramic bracket is that then the bracket can be engineered to fracture in the slot area, which makes it much easier to remove.

Electrothermal and laser instruments to heat ceramic brackets for removal now are available. There is no doubt that less force is needed when the bracket is heated, and research findings indicate that there is little patient discomfort and minimal risk of pulpal damage. Nevertheless, the ideal solution would be to perfect the third approach so that ceramic brackets can be debonded without heating as readily as metal ones.

Cement left on the teeth after debanding can be removed easily by scaling, but residual bonding resin is more difficult to remove. The best results are obtained with a 12-fluted carbide bur at moderate speeds in a dental handpiece (Figure 16-13).[8] This bur cuts resin readily but has little effect on enamel. Topical fluoride should be applied when the cleanup procedure has been completed, however, since some of the fluoride-rich outer enamel layer may be lost with even the most careful approach.

POSITIONERS FOR FINISHING

An alternative to segmental elastics or light round archwires for final settling is a rubber or plastic tooth positioner. A positioner is most effective if it is placed immediately on removal of the fixed orthodontic appliance. Normally, it is fabricated by removing the archwires 4 to 6 weeks before the planned removal of the appliance, taking impressions of the teeth and a registration of occlusal relationships, and then resetting the teeth in the laboratory, incorporating the minor changes in position of each tooth necessary to produce appropriate settling (Figure 16-14). All erupted teeth should be included in the positioner, to prevent supereruption. As part of the laboratory procedure, bands and brackets are trimmed away, and any band space is closed.

This indirect approach allows individual tooth positions to be adjusted with considerable precision, bringing each

A

B

C

D

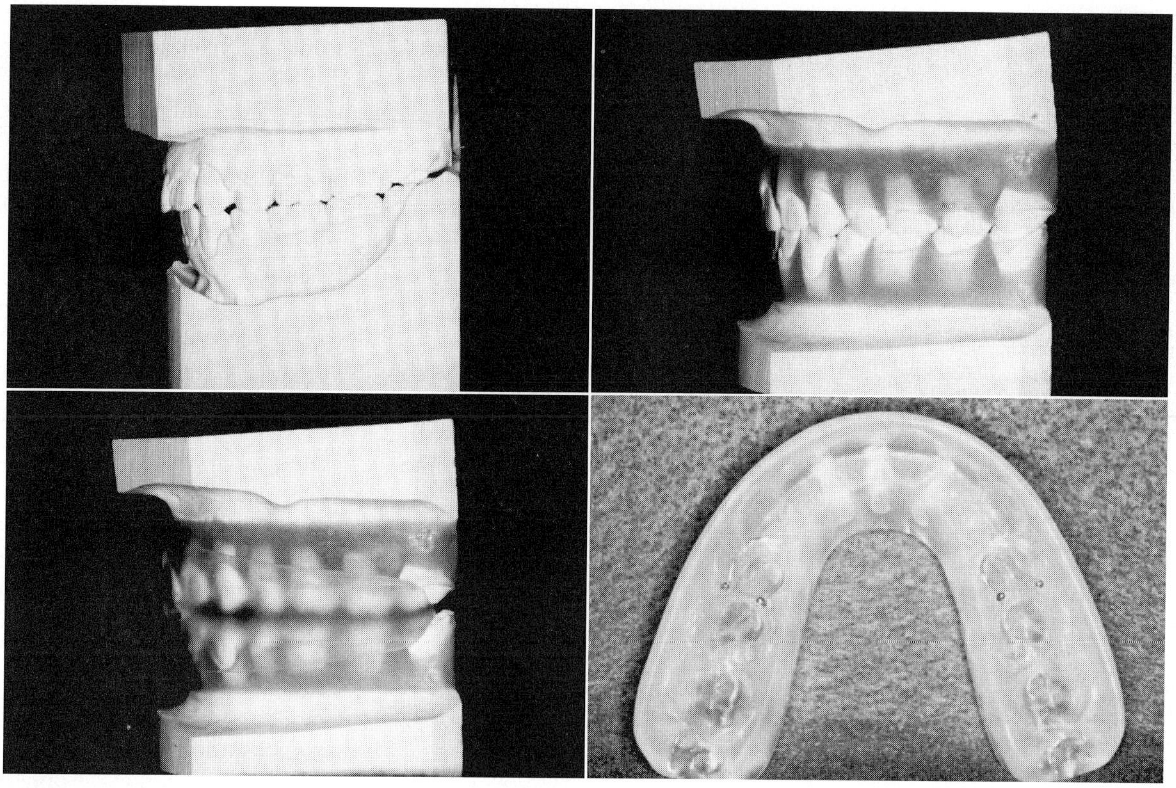

Figure 16-14 Use of a positioner for finishing. **A,** Dental casts after appliance removal; **B,** The positioner setup. Often the positioner impression is taken one month before debanding, with bands and brackets carved off the teeth in the laboratory, so the positioner can be delivered immediately after the appliance is removed; **C,** Transparent positioner on setup; **D,** Maxillary occlusal view of the positioner. Note the clasps in the premolar region that help to prevent space from opening. Their use is particularly important when a positioner is used in a maxillary premolar extraction case.

tooth into the desired final relationship. The positioning device is then fabricated by forming either a plastic material (now usually polyurethane) around the repositioned and articulated casts, producing a device with the inherent elasticity to move the teeth slightly to their final position as the patient bites into it.

The use of a tooth positioner rather than final settling archwires has two advantages: (1) it allows the fixed appliance to be removed somewhat more quickly than otherwise would have been the case (i.e., some finishing that could have been done with the final archwires can be left to the positioner), and (2) it serves not only to reposition the teeth but also to massage the gingiva, which is almost always at least slightly inflamed and swollen after comprehensive orthodontic treatment. The gingival stimulation provided by a positioner is an excellent way to promote a rapid return to normal gingival contours (Figure 16-15).

The use of positioners for finishing also has disadvantages. First of all, these appliances require a considerable amount of laboratory fabrication time, and therefore are expensive. Second, settling with a positioner tends to increase overbite more than the equivalent settling with light elastics. This is a disadvantage in patients who had a deep overbite initially but can be advantageous if the initial problem was an anterior open bite. Third, a positioner does not maintain the correction of rotated teeth well, which means that minor rotations may recur while a positioner is being worn. Finally, good cooperation is essential.

With modern edgewise appliances, the first advantage is not nearly so compelling as it was previously. It is an error to remove a fixed appliance early and depend on a positioner to accomplish more than minimal settling of the occlusion. At present, therefore, there are two main indications for use of a positioner: (1) a gingival condition with more than the usual degree of inflammation and swelling at the end of active orthodontics, or (2) an open bite tendency, so that settling by mild depression rather than elongation of posterior teeth is needed. Severe malalignment and rotated teeth, a deep bite tendency, and an uncooperative patient are contraindications for positioner use.

A positioner should be worn by the patient at least 4 hours during the day and during sleep. Since the amount of tooth movement tends to decline rapidly after a few days of use, an excellent schedule is to remove the orthodontic appliances, clean the teeth and apply a fluoride treatment, and place the positioner immediately, asking the patient to wear it as nearly full time as possible for the first 2 days. After that, it can be worn on the usual night-plus-4 hours schedule.

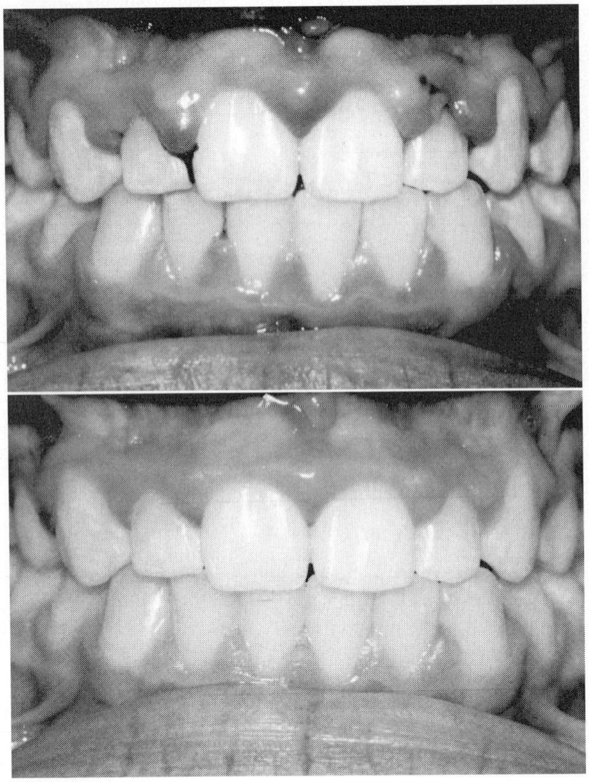

FIGURE 16-15 Gingival improvement with positioner wear. **A,** Swollen maxillary papillae immediately after band removal, just before placement of an immediate positioner; **B,** 2 weeks later. This degree of gingival swelling and puffiness occurs only rarely during fixed appliance treatment, but when it does, a positioner is one of the best means to resolve it.

As a general rule, a tooth positioner in a cooperative patient will produce any changes it is capable of within 2-3 weeks. Final (posttreatment) records and retainer impressions can be taken 2 or 3 weeks after the positioner is placed. Beyond that time, if the positioner is continued, it is serving as a retainer rather than a finishing device—and positioners, as a rule, are not good retainers.

SPECIAL FINISHING PROCEDURES TO AVOID RELAPSE

Relapse after orthodontic treatment has two major causes: (1) continued growth by the patient in an unfavorable pattern, and (2) tissue rebound after the release of orthodontic force.

Control of Unfavorable Growth

Changes resulting from continued growth in a Class II, Class III, deep bite or open bite pattern contribute to a return of the original malocclusion, and so are relapse in that sense. These changes are due to the pattern of skeletal growth, not just to tooth movement. Controlling this type of relapse requires a continuation of active treatment after the fixed appliances have been removed, rather than specific finishing procedures to prevent relapse.

For patients with skeletal problems who have undergone orthodontic treatment, this "active retention" takes one of two forms. One possibility is to continue extraoral force in conjunction with orthodontic retainers (high-pull headgear at night, for instance, in a patient with a Class II open bite growth pattern). The other appropriate option, which often is more acceptable to the patient, is to use a functional appliance rather than a conventional retainer after the completion of fixed appliance therapy. This important subject is discussed in more detail in Chapter 17.

Control of Soft Tissue Rebound

A major reason for retention is to hold the teeth until soft tissue remodeling can take place. Even with the best remodeling, however, some rebound from the application of orthodontic forces occurs, and indeed the tendency for rebound after interarch elastics are discontinued has already been discussed. There are two ways to deal with this phenomenon: (1) overtreatment, so that any rebound will only bring the teeth back to their proper position, and (2) adjunctive periodontal surgery to reduce rebound from elastic fibers in the gingiva. In some cases, permanent retention is required to maintain the desired relationships, but this need not be planned if either of the two approaches described here would make it unnecessary.

Overtreatment

Since it can be anticipated that teeth will rebound slightly toward their previous position after orthodontic correction, it is logical to position them at the end of treatment in a somewhat overtreated position. Only a small degree of overtreatment is compatible with precise finishing of orthodontic cases as described previously, but it is nevertheless possible to apply this principle during the finishing phase of treatment. Consider three specific situations:

Correction of Class II or Class III Malocclusion. The rebound or settling after Class II or Class III correction has already been discussed. After headgear or elastics have been discontinued, it can be expected that the teeth will rebound 1 to 2 mm relatively quickly. Especially when elastics are used, the patient should be taken to a slightly overcorrected position, and elastics discontinued for 3-4 weeks to allow rebound to occur, before appliances are removed.

Particularly when a patient has been wearing Class II elastics, he or she may begin to posture the mandible forward, so that the malocclusion looks more corrected than it really is. For this reason also, it is important to allow a period of time without elastics before ending active treatment, to be sure that the patient really has been corrected and is not just posturing. This is different from rebound, which occurs independently of mandibular posturing, but obviously it is important to detect. Rebound is a 1-2 mm phenomenon; posturing can produce an apparent 4-5 mm relapse. The best plan is to reduce the force on Class II elastics when the apparently correct degree of overcorrection has been achieved but maintain them full-time for 3-4 weeks, then wear them just at night for another appointment period, and finally discontinue them completely for at least 4 weeks before removing the appliances.

Crossbite Correction. Whatever the mechanism used to correct crossbite, it should be overcorrected by at least 1 to 2 mm before the force system is released. If the crossbite is corrected during the first stage of treatment, as should be the case, the overcorrection will gradually be lost during succeeding phases of treatment, but this should improve stability when transverse relationships are established precisely during the finishing phase.

Irregular and Rotated Teeth. Just as with crossbites, irregularities and rotations can be overcorrected during the first phase of treatment, carrying a tooth that has been lingually positioned slightly too far labial, for instance, and vice versa. It is wise to hold the teeth in a slightly overcorrected position for at least a few months, during the end of the first stage of treatment and the second stage. As a general rule, however, it is not wise to build this overcorrection into rectangular finishing archwires.

Similarly, a tooth being rotated into position in the arch can be overrotated. Maintaining an overrotated position can be done by adjusting the wings of single brackets, or by pinching shut one of a pair of twin brackets. Maintaining overcorrected labiolingual positions of incisors is done readily with first-order bends in working archwires. Rotated teeth should be maintained in an overcorrected position as long as possible, but even then, these teeth are often candidates for the periodontal procedures described following.

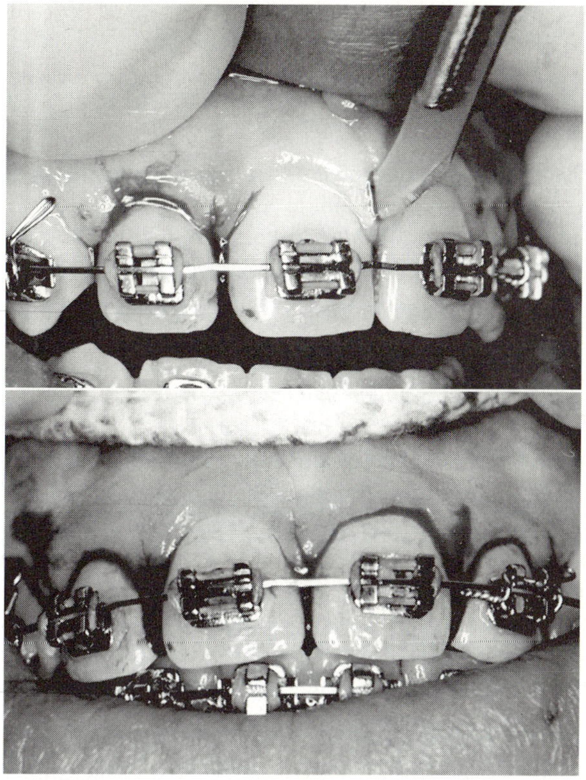

FIGURE 16-16 The "papilla split" procedure is an alternative to the "around the tooth" CSF approach for sectioning gingival circumferential fibers to improve post-treatment stability. It is particularly indicated for esthetically sensitive areas like the maxillary anterior region. Vertical cuts are made in the gingival papillae without separating the gingival margin at the papilla tip. **A,** The blade inserted to make the vertical cut; **B,** View at completion of the papilla splits before sutures are placed. Another advantage of this procedure is that it is easier to perform with an orthodontic appliance and archwire in place.

Adjunctive Periodontal Surgery

A major cause of rebound after orthodontic treatment is the network of elastic supracrestal gingival fibers. As teeth are moved to a new position, these fibers tend to stretch, and they remodel very slowly. If the pull of these elastic fibers could be eliminated, a major cause of relapse of previously irregular and rotated teeth should be eliminated. In fact, if the supracrestal fibers are sectioned and allowed to heal while the teeth are held in the proper position, relapse caused by gingival elasticity is greatly reduced.

Surgery to section the supracrestal elastic fibers is a simple procedure that does not require referral to a periodontist unless possible gingival recession is an esthetic concern. It can be carried out by either of two approaches. The first method, originally developed by Edwards,[9] is called *circumferential supracrestal fibrotomy* (CSF). After infiltration with a local anesthetic, the procedure consists of inserting the sharp point of a fine blade into the gingival sulcus down to the crest of alveolar bone (Figure 16-16). Cuts are made interproximally on each side of a rotated tooth and along the labial and lingual gingival margins unless, as is often the case, the labial or lingual gingiva is quite thin, in which case this part of the circumferential cut is omitted. No periodontal pack is necessary, and there is only minor discomfort after the procedure.

An alternative method is to make an incision in the center of each gingival papilla, sparing the margin but separating the papilla from just below the margin to 1 to 2 mm below the height of the bone buccally and lingually (see Figure 18-23).[10] This modification is said to reduce the possibility that the height of the gingival attachment will be reduced after the surgery, and it is particularly indicated for esthetically sensitive areas (i.e., the maxillary incisor region). Nevertheless, there is little if any risk of gingival recession with the original CSF procedure unless cuts are made across thin labial or lingual tissues. From the point of view of improved stability after orthodontic treatment, the surgical procedures appear to be equivalent.

Neither the CSF nor the papilla-dividing procedure should be done until malaligned teeth have been corrected and held in their new position for several months, so this surgery is always done toward the end of the finishing phase of treatment. It is important to hold the teeth in good alignment while gingival healing occurs. This means that either the surgery should be done a few weeks before removal of the orthodontic appliance or, if it is performed at the same time the appliance is removed, a retainer must be inserted almost immediately. It is easier to do the CSF procedure after the orthodontic appliances have been removed, although it can be carried out with appliances in place. An advantage of the papilla-dividing procedure may be that it is easier to perform with the orthodontic appliance still in place. The only problem with placing a retainer immediately after the surgery is that it may be difficult to keep the retainer from contacting soft tissue in a sore area.

Experience has demonstrated that sectioning the gingival fibers is an effective method to control rotational relapse but does not control the tendency for crowded incisors to again become irregular. The primary indication for gingival surgery therefore is a tooth or teeth that were severely rotated. This surgery is not indicated for patients with crowding without rotations.

REFERENCES

1. Burstone CJ, Koenig HA. Creative wire bending—the force system from step and V bends. Am J Orthod Dentofac Orthop 93:59-67, 1988.
2. Isaacson RJ, Rebellato J. Two-couple orthodontic appliance systems: Torquing arches. Semin Orthod 1:31-36, 1995.
3. Gianelly AA. Asymmetric space closure. Am J Orthod Dentofac Orthop 90:335-341, 1986.
4. Kokich VG, Kokich VO. Interrelationship of orthodontics with periodontics and restorative dentistry. In: Nanda R, ed. Biomechanics and Esthetic Strategies in Clinical Orthodontics. Philadelphia: Elsevier/Saunders; 2005.
5. Fields HW. Orthodontic-restorative treatment for relative mandibular anterior excess tooth size problems. Am J Orthod 79:176-183, 1981.
6. Steffen JM, Haltom FT. The five-cent tooth positioner. J Clin Orthod 21:528-529, 1987.
7. Azzeh E, Feldon PJ. Laser debonding of ceramic brackets: A comprehensive review. Am J Orthod Dentofac Orthop 123:79-83, 2003.
8. Eliades T, Gioka C, Eliades G, Makou M. Enamel surface roughness following debonding using two resin grinding methods. Eur J Orthod 26:333-338, 2004.
9. Edwards JG. A long-term prospective evaluation of the circumferential supracrestal fiberotomy in alleviating orthodontic relapse. Am J Orthod Dentofac Orthop 93:380-387, 1988.
10. Edwards JG. Soft-tissue surgery to alleviate orthodontic relapse. Dent Clin North Am 37:205-225, 1993.

CHAPTER

17

Retention

CHAPTER OUTLINE

At sporting events, no matter how good things look for one team late in the game, the saying is "It's not over till it's over." In orthodontics, although the patient may feel that treatment is complete when the appliances are removed, an important stage lies ahead. Orthodontic control of tooth position and occlusal relationships must be withdrawn gradually, not abruptly, if excellent long-term results are to be obtained. The type of retention should be included in the original treatment plan.

WHY IS RETENTION NECESSARY?

There is extensive literature on retention and post-treatment stability, which has been reviewed in some depth recently.[1,2] Although a number of factors can be cited as influencing long-term results, orthodontic treatment results are potentially unstable, and therefore retention is necessary, for three major reasons: (1) the gingival and periodontal tissues are affected by orthodontic tooth movement and require time for reorganization when the appliances are removed; (2) the teeth may be in an inherently unstable position after the treatment, so that soft tissue pressures constantly produce a relapse tendency; and (3) changes produced by growth may alter the orthodontic treatment result. If the teeth are not in an inherently unstable position, and if there is no further growth, retention still is vitally important until gingival and periodontal reorganization is completed. If the teeth are unstable, as often is the case following significant arch expansion, gradual withdrawal of orthodontic appliances is of no value. The only possibilities are accepting relapse or using permanent retention. Finally, whatever the situation, retention cannot be abandoned until growth is essentially completed.

Reorganization of the Periodontal and Gingival Tissues

Widening of the periodontal ligament space and disruption of the collagen fiber bundles that support each tooth are normal responses to orthodontic treatment (see Chapter 9). In fact, these changes are necessary to allow orthodontic tooth movement to occur. Even if tooth movement stops before the orthodontic appliance is removed, restoration of the normal periodontal architecture will not occur as long as a tooth is strongly splinted to its neighbors, as when it is attached to a rigid orthodontic archwire (so holding the teeth with passive archwires cannot be considered the beginning of retention). Once the teeth can respond individually to the forces of mastication (i.e., once each tooth can be displaced slightly relative to its neighbor as the patient chews), reorganization of the periodontal ligament (PDL) occurs over a 3- to 4-month period, and the slight mobility present at appliance removal disappears.

This PDL reorganization is important for stability because of the periodontal contribution to the equilibrium that normally controls tooth position. To briefly review our current understanding of the pressure equilibrium (see Chapter 5 for a detailed discussion), the teeth normally withstand occlusal forces because of the shock-absorbing properties of the periodontal system. More importantly for orthodontics, small but prolonged imbalances in tongue-lip-cheek pressures or pressures from gingival fibers that otherwise would produce tooth movement are resisted by "active stabilization" due to PDL metabolism. It appears that this stabilization is caused by the same force-generating mechanism that produces eruption. The disruption of the PDL produced by orthodontic tooth movement probably has little effect on the stabilization against occlusal forces, but it reduces or eliminates the active stabilization, which means that immediately after orthodontic appliances are removed, teeth will be unstable in the face of occlusal and soft tissue pressures that can be resisted later. This is the reason that every patient needs retainers for at least a few months.

The gingival fiber networks are also disturbed by orthodontic tooth movement and must remodel to accommodate the new tooth positions. Both collagenous and elastic fibers occur in the gingiva, and the reorganization of both occurs more slowly than that of the PDL itself.[3] Within 4 to 6 months, the collagenous fiber networks within the gingiva have normally completed their reorganization, but the elastic supracrestal fibers remodel extremely slowly and can still exert forces capable of displacing a tooth at one year after removal of an orthodontic appliance. In patients with severe rotations, sectioning the supracrestal fibers around severely malposed or rotated teeth, at or just before the time of appliance removal, is a recommended procedure because it reduces relapse tendencies resulting from this fiber elasticity[4] (see Chapter 16).

This timetable for soft tissue recovery from orthodontic treatment outlines the principles of retention against intra-arch instability. These are:

1. The direction of potential relapse can be identified by comparing the position of the teeth at the conclusion of treatment with their original positions. Teeth will tend to move back in the direction from which they came, primarily because of elastic recoil of gingival fibers but also because of unbalanced tongue-lip forces (Figure 17-1).

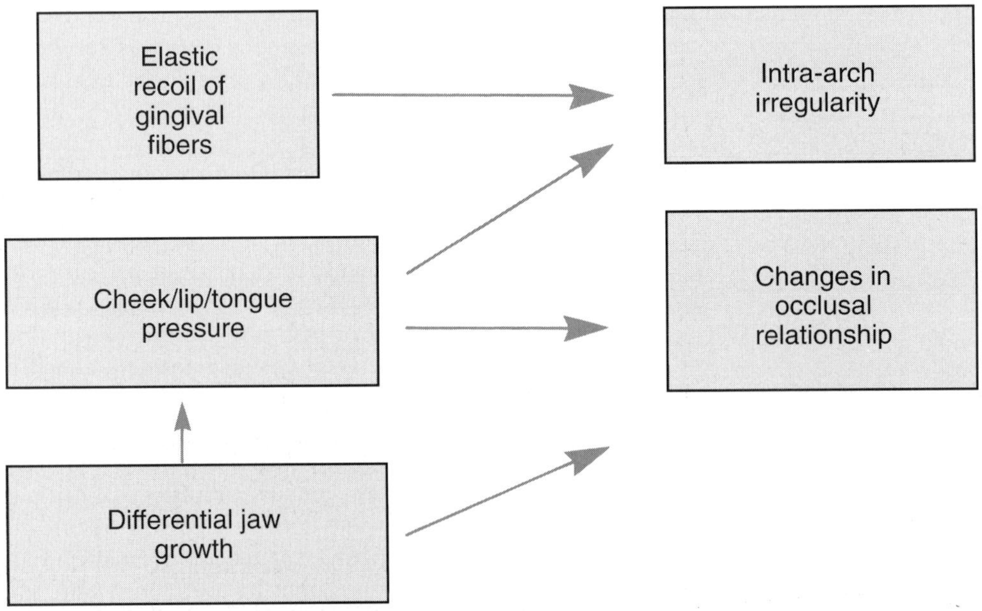

FIGURE 17-1 The major causes of relapse after orthodontic treatment include the elasticity of gingival fibers, cheek/lip/tongue pressures, and jaw growth. Gingival fibers and soft tissue pressures are especially potent in the first few months after treatment ends, before PDL reorganization has been completed.

2. Teeth require essentially full-time retention after comprehensive orthodontic treatment for the first 3 to 4 months after a fixed orthodontic appliance is removed. To promote reorganization of the PDL, however, the teeth should be free to flex individually during mastication, as the alveolar bone bends in response to heavy occlusal loads during mastication (see Chapter 9). This requirement can be met by a removable appliance worn full-time except during meals or by a fixed retainer that is not too rigid.
3. Because of the slow response of the gingival fibers, retention should be continued for at least 12 months if the teeth were quite irregular initially but can be reduced to part-time after 3 to 4 months. After approximately 12 months, it should be possible to discontinue retention in non-growing patients. More precisely, the teeth should be stable by that time if they ever will be. Some patients who are not growing will require permanent retention to maintain the teeth in what would otherwise be unstable positions because of lip, cheek, and tongue pressures that are too large for active stabilization to balance out. Patients who will continue to grow, however, usually need retention until growth has reduced to the low levels that characterize adult life.

Occlusal Changes Related to Growth

A continuation of growth is particularly troublesome in patients whose initial malocclusion resulted, largely or in part, from the pattern of skeletal growth. Skeletal problems in all three planes of space tend to recur if growth continues (Figure 17-2), because most patients continue in their original growth pattern as long as they are growing. Transverse growth is completed first, which means that long-term transverse changes are less of a problem clinically than changes from late anteroposterior and vertical growth.

Comprehensive orthodontic treatment is usually carried out in the early permanent dentition, and the duration is typically between 18 and 30 months. This means that active orthodontic treatment is likely to conclude at age 14 to 15, while anteroposterior and particularly vertical growth often do not subside even to the adult level until several years later. Long-term studies of adults have shown that very slow growth typically continues throughout adult life, and the same pattern that led to malocclusion in the first place can contribute to a deterioration in occlusal relationships many years after orthodontic treatment is completed.[5] In late adolescence, continued growth in the pattern that caused a Class II, Class III, deep bite or open bite problem in the first place is a major cause of relapse after orthodontic treatment and requires careful management during retention.[6]

Retention After Class II Correction

Relapse toward a Class II relationship must result from some combination of tooth movement (forward in the upper arch, backward in the lower arch, or both) and differential growth of the maxilla relative to the mandible (Figure 17-3). As might be expected, tooth movement caused by local periodontal and gingival factors can be an important short-term problem, whereas differential jaw growth is a more important long-term problem because it directly alters jaw position and this contributes to repositioning of teeth.

Overcorrection of the occlusal relationships as a finishing procedure is an important step in controlling tooth movement that would lead to Class II relapse. Even with good retention, 1 to 2 mm of anteroposterior change caused by adjustments in tooth position is likely to occur after treatment, particularly if Class II elastics were employed. This change occurs relatively quickly after active treatment stops.

In Class II treatment, it is important not to move the lower incisors too far forward, but this can happen easily with Class II elastics. In this situation, lip pressure will tend to upright the protruding incisors, leading relatively quickly (often in only a few months after full-time retainer wear is discontinued) to crowding and return of both overbite and overjet. As a general guideline, if more than 2 mm of forward repositioning of the lower incisors occurred during treatment, permanent retention will be required.

The slower long-term relapse that occurs in some patients who did not have inappropriate tooth movement results primarily from differential jaw growth. The amount of growth remaining after orthodontic treatment will obviously depend on the age, sex and relative maturity of the patient, but after treatment that involved growth modification, further growth almost surely will result in some loss of the previous correction as the original growth pattern persists.

In Class II patients, this relapse tendency can be controlled in one of two ways. The first, the traditional fixed appliance approach of the 1970s and earlier, is to continue headgear to the upper molars on a reduced basis (at night, for instance) in conjunction with a retainer to hold the teeth in alignment. This requires leaving the first molar bands on when everything is removed at the end of active treatment. It is quite satisfactory in well-motivated patients who have been wearing headgear and are willing to continue it during treatment, and is compatible with traditional retainers that are worn full-time initially—but compliance with headgear becomes a problem with all but the most cooperative patients .

The other method is to use a functional appliance of the activator-bionator type to hold both tooth position and the occlusal relationship (Figure 17-4). To the patient, this intraoral device is just another variety of retainer, and compliance is less of a problem. If the patient does not have excessive overjet, as should be the case at the end of active treatment, the construction bite for the functional appliance is taken without any mandibular advancement—the idea is to prevent a Class II malocclusion from recurring, not to actively treat one that already exists.

A potential difficulty is that the functional appliance will be worn only part-time, typically just at night, and daytime retainers of conventional design also will be needed to

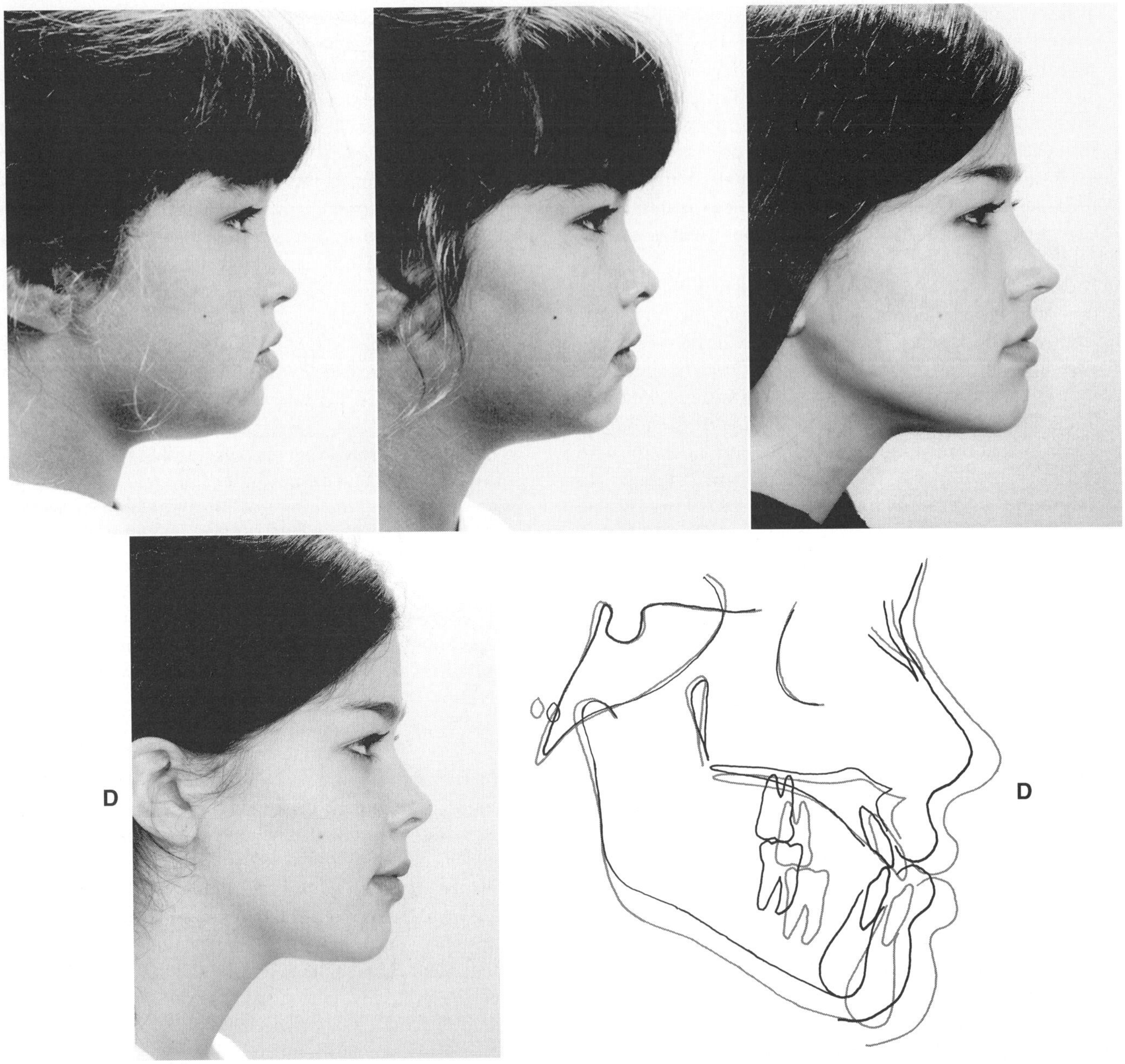

Figure 17-2 Growth after early rreatment of a Class III problem is likely to cause the problem to reappear, as in this girl. **A**, Profile at age 7, prior to treatment; **B**, Age 8, after treatment with reverse-pull headgear (face mask); **C**, 5 years later, after the adolescent growth spurt; **D**, After orthognathic surgery; **E**, Cephalometric superimposition showing the pattern of growth from the end of the face mask treatment *(black)* through adolescence to just prior to surgery *(red)*.

control tooth position during the first few months. The extra retainer from the beginning makes sense for a patient with a severe growth problem. For patients with less severe problems, in whom continued growth may or may not cause relapse, it may be more rational to use only conventional maxillary and mandibular retainers initially, and replace them with a functional appliance to be worn at night if relapse is beginning to occur after a few months.

This type of retention is often needed for 12 to 24 months or more in a patient who had a skeletal problem initially. The guideline is: the more severe the initial Class II problem and the younger the patient at the end of active treatment, the more likely that either headgear or a functional appliance will be needed during post-treatment retention. It is better, and much easier, to prevent relapse from differential growth than to try to correct it later.

Retention After Class III Correction

Retaining a patient after correcting a Class III malocclusion early in the permanent dentition can be frustrating, because

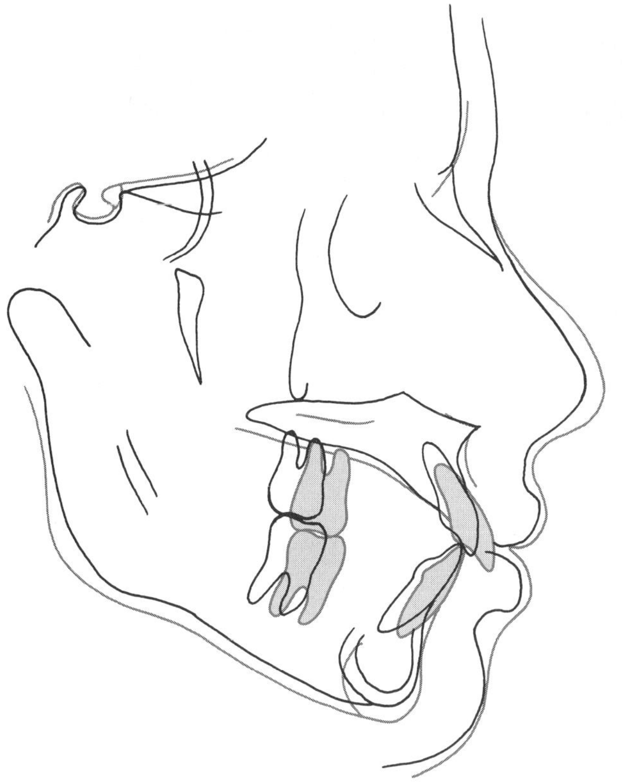

FIGURE 17-3 Cephalometric superimposition demonstrating growth-related relapse in a patient treated to correct Class II malocclusion. *Black,* Immediate posttreatment, age 13; *red,* Recall, age 17. After treatment, both jaws grew downward and forward, but mandibular growth did not match maxillary growth, and the maxillary dentition moved forward relative to the maxilla. As in Class III patients, early treatment has little or no effect on the underlying growth pattern.

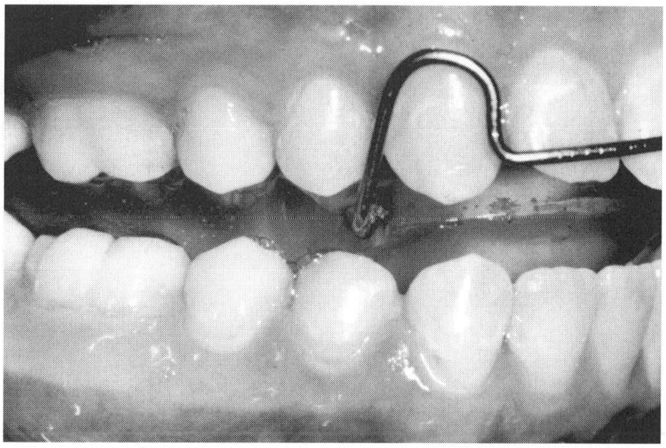

FIGURE 17-4 In patients in whom further growth in the original Class II pattern is expected after active treatment is completed, a functional appliance worn at night can be used to maintain occlusal relationships. In a typical Class II deep bite patient, the lower posterior teeth are allowed to erupt slightly, while other teeth are tightly controlled.

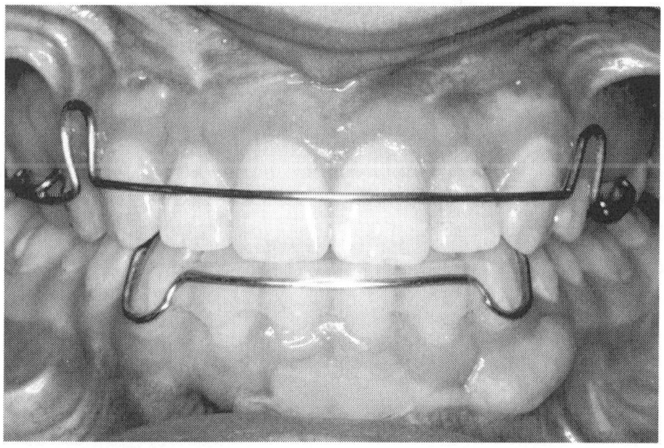

FIGURE 17-5 Control of the vertical position of teeth in retention is as important as controlling alignment, especially in patients who had a deep bite or open bite initially. For this deep bite patient, note that the lower incisors contact the palatal acrylic of the upper retainer, while the upper incisors contact the facial surface of the lower retainer. This prevents incisor eruption that would lead to return of excessive overbite.

relapse from continuing mandibular growth is very likely to occur and such growth is extremely difficult to control. Applying a restraining force to the mandible, as from a chincup, is not nearly as effective in controlling growth in a Class III patient as applying a restraining force to the maxilla is in Class II problems. As we have noted in previous chapters, a chincup tends to rotate the mandible downward, causing growth to be expressed more vertically and less horizontally, and Class III functional appliances have the same effect. If face height is normal or excessive after orthodontic treatment and relapse occurs from mandibular growth, surgical correction after the growth has expressed itself may be the only answer. In mild Class III problems, a functional appliance or a positioner may be enough to maintain the occlusal relationships during posttreatment growth.

Retention After Deep Bite Correction

Correcting excess overbite is an almost routine part of orthodontic treatment, and therefore the majority of patients require control of the vertical overlap of incisors during retention. This is accomplished most readily by using a removable upper retainer made so that the lower incisors will encounter the baseplate of the retainer if they begin to slip vertically behind the upper incisors (Figure 17-5). The procedure, in other words, is to build a potential bite plate into the retainer, which the lower incisors will contact if the bite begins to deepen. The retainer does not separate the posterior teeth.

Because vertical growth continues into the late teens, a maxillary removable retainer with a bite plane often is needed for several years after fixed appliance orthodontics is completed. Bite depth can be maintained by wearing the retainer only at night, after stability in other regards has been achieved.

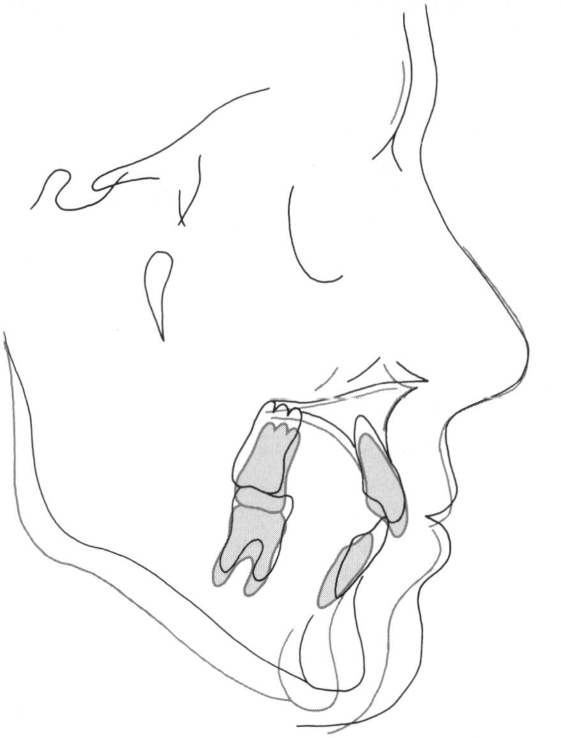

Figure 17-6 Four years after removal of the orthodontic appliances, this 17-year-old has an anterior open bite, 5 mm of overjet with an end-on molar relationship, and severe crowding of the mandibular incisors. Relapse of this type is associated with a downward and backward mandibular rotation and eruption of the upper posterior teeth during post-treatment growth, as shown in the cephalometric superimposition from the end of treatment to 4 year recall. The incisor crowding is due to uprighting and lingual repositioning of the incisors as the mandibular rotation thrusts them into the lower lip.

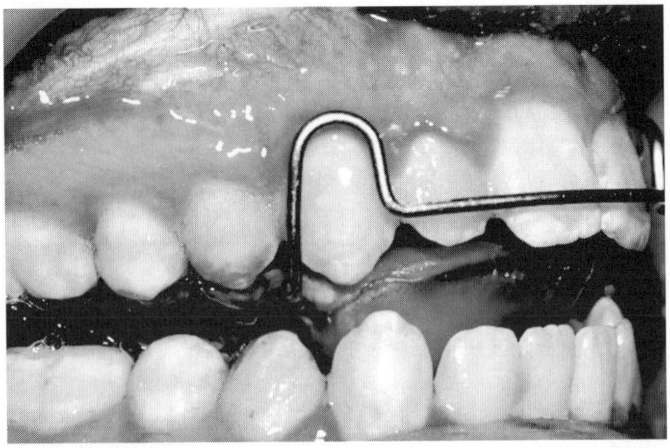

Figure 17-7 Controlling the eruption of posterior teeth during late vertical growth is the key to preventing open-bite relapse. There are two major approaches to accomplishing this: a functional appliance with bite blocks to impede eruption, as shown here in a patient soon after his severe open bite was corrected, or high-pull headgear. Both must be continued as a nighttime retainer through the late teens. Although the high-pull headgear can be quite effective in a cooperative patient, the functional appliance is a better choice for most patients for two reasons: it controls eruption of both the upper and lower molars, and usually it is better accepted because it is easier for the patient to wear.

Retention After Anterior Open Bite Correction

Relapse into anterior open bite can occur by any combination of depression of the incisors and elongation of the molars. Active habits (of which thumbsucking is the best example) can produce intrusive forces on the incisors, while at the same time leading to an altered posture of the jaw that allows posterior teeth to erupt. If thumbsucking continues after orthodontic treatment, relapse is all but guaranteed. Tongue habits, particularly tongue-thrust swallowing, are often blamed for relapse into open bite, but the evidence to support this contention is not convincing (see discussion in Chapter 5). In patients who do not place some object between the front teeth, return of open bite is almost always the result of elongation of the posterior teeth, particularly the upper molars, without any evidence of intrusion of incisors (Figure 17-6). Controlling eruption of the upper molars therefore is the key to retention in open bite patients.

High-pull headgear to the upper molars, in conjunction with a standard removable retainer to maintain tooth position, is one effective way to control open bite relapse. A better tolerated alternative is an appliance with bite blocks between the posterior teeth that creates several millimeters of jaw separation (an open bite activator or bionator) (Figure 17-7). This stretches the patient's soft tissues to provide a force opposing eruption. Excessive vertical growth and eruption of the posterior teeth often continue until late in the teens or early twenties, making a persistent open bite tendency difficult to control, but this can be accomplished with good patient cooperation over a long enough period.

A patient with a severe open bite problem is particularly likely to benefit from having conventional maxillary and mandibular retainers for daytime wear, and an open bite bionator as a nighttime retainer, from the beginning of the retention period.

Retention of Lower Incisor Alignment

Not only can continued skeletal growth affect occlusal relationships, it has the potential to alter the position of teeth. If the mandible grows forward or rotates downward, the effect is to carry the lower incisors into the lip, which creates a force tipping them distally. For this reason, continued mandibular growth in normal or Class III patients is strongly associated with crowding of the lower incisors (see Figure 17-1). Incisor crowding also accompanies the downward and backward rotation of the mandible seen in skeletal open bite problems (see Figure 17-6). A retainer in the lower incisor region is needed to prevent crowding from developing, until growth has declined to adult levels.

It often has been suggested that orthodontic retention should be continued, at least on a part-time basis, until the third molars have either erupted into normal occlusion or have been removed. The implication of this guideline, that pressure from the developing third molars causes late incisor crowding, is almost surely incorrect (see Chapter 5). On the other hand, because eruption of third molars or their extraction usually does not take place until the late teen years, the guideline is not a bad one in its emphasis on prolonged retention in patients who are continuing to grow.

Most adults, including those who had orthodontic treatment and once had perfectly aligned teeth, end up with some crowding of lower incisors. In a group of patients who had first premolar extraction and treatment with the edgewise appliance, only about 30% had perfect alignment 10 years after retainers were removed and nearly 20% had marked crowding.[7] Which individuals would have post-treatment crowding could not be predicted from the characteristics of the original malocclusion or variables associated with treatment. It seems likely that late mandibular growth is the major contributor to this crowding tendency. It makes sense, therefore, to routinely retain lower incisor alignment until mandibular growth has declined to adult levels (i.e., until the late teens in girls and into the early 20s in boys).

Timing of Retention: Summary

In summary, retention is needed for all patients who had fixed orthodontic appliances to correct intra-arch irregularities. It should be:

- Essentially full-time for the first 3 to 4 months, except that the retainers not only can but should be removed while eating (unless periodontal bone loss or other special circumstances require permanent splinting)
- Continued on a part-time basis for at least 12 months, to allow time for remodeling of gingival tissues
- If significant growth remains, continued part-time until completion of growth.

For practical purposes, this means that nearly all patients treated in the early permanent dentition will require retention of incisor alignment at least until their late teens, and in those with skeletal disproportions initially, part-time use of a functional appliance or extraoral force probably will be needed.

REMOVABLE APPLIANCES AS RETAINERS

Removable appliances can serve effectively for retention against intra-arch instability and are also useful as retainers (in the form of modified functional appliances or part-time headgear) in patients with growth problems. If permanent retention is needed, a fixed retainer should be used in most instances, and fixed retainers (see p. 626) are also indicated for intra-arch retention when irregularity in a specific area is likely to be a problem.

Hawley Retainers

By far the most common removable retainer is the Hawley retainer, designed in the 1920s as an active removable appliance. It incorporates clasps on molar teeth and a characteristic outer bow with adjustment loops, spanning from canine to canine (Figure 17-8). Because it covers the palate, it automatically provides a potential bite plane to control overbite.

The ability of this retainer to provide some tooth movement was a particular asset with fully banded fixed appliances, since one function of the retainer was to close band spaces between the incisors. With bonded appliances on the anterior teeth or after using a tooth positioner for finishing, there is no longer any need to close spaces with a retainer. However, the outer bow provides excellent control of the incisors even if it is not adjusted to retract them.

When first premolars have been extracted, one function of a retainer is to keep the extraction space closed, which the standard design of the Hawley retainer cannot do. Even worse, the standard Hawley labial bow extends across a first premolar extraction space, tending to wedge it open. A common modification of the Hawley retainer for use in extraction cases is a bow soldered to the buccal section of Adams clasps on the first molars, so that the action of the bow helps hold the extraction site closed (see Figure 17-8). Alternative designs for extraction cases are to wrap the labial bow around the entire arch, using circumferential clasps on second molars for retention; or to bring the labial wire from the baseplate between the lateral incisor and canine and to bend or solder a wire extension distally to control the canines (Figure 17-9). The latter alternative does not provide an active force to keep an extraction space closed, but avoids having the wire cross through the extraction site, and gives positive control of canines that were labially positioned initially (which the loop of the traditional Hawley design may not provide).

The clasp locations for a Hawley retainer must be selected carefully, since clasp wires crossing the occlusal table can disrupt rather than retain the tooth relationships established during treatment. Circumferential clasps on the terminal molar may be preferred over the more effective Adams clasp if the occlusion is tight.

The palatal coverage of a removable plate like the maxillary Hawley retainer makes it possible to incorporate a bite plane lingual to the upper incisors, to control bite depth. For any patient who once had an excessive overbite, light contact of the lower incisors against the baseplate of the retainer is desired.

Removable Wraparound Retainers

A second major type of removable orthodontic retainer is the wraparound or clip-on retainer, which consists of a plastic bar (usually wire-reinforced) along the labial and

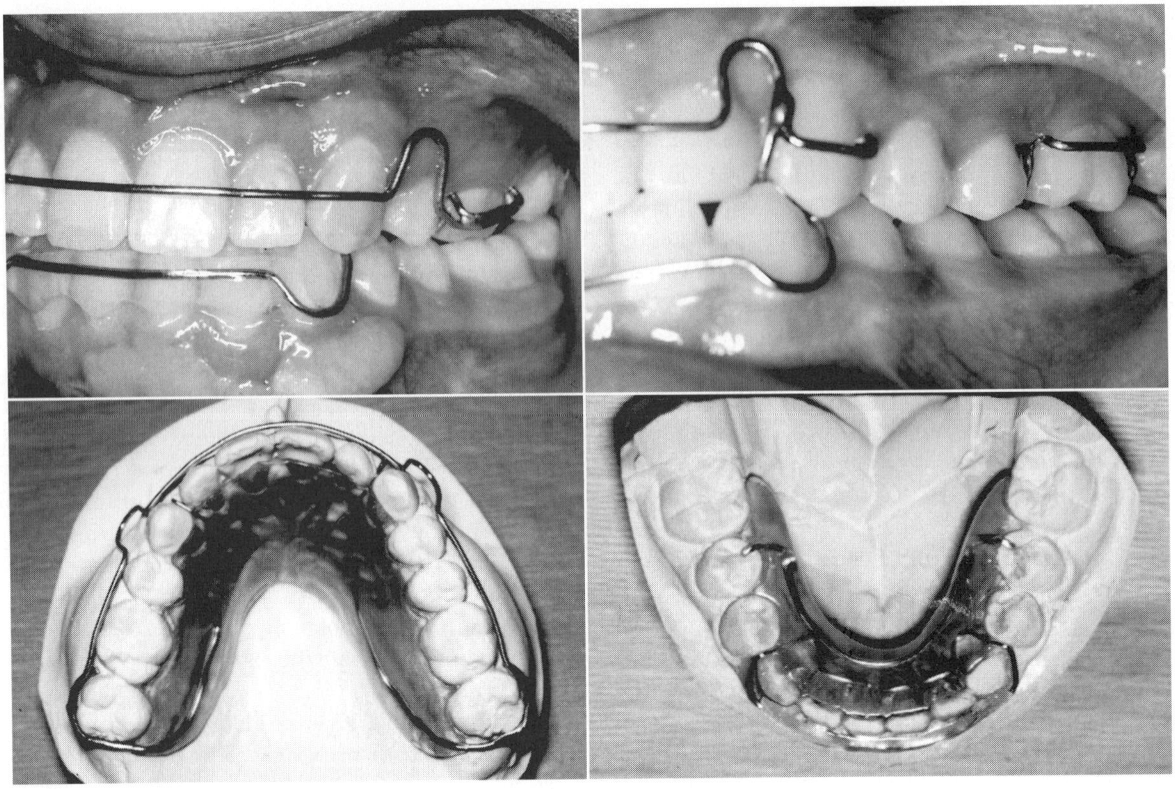

Figure 17-8 A canine-to-canine anterior bow and clasps on molars are the characteristic features of the Hawley retainer design. **A,** A Hawley retainer for a patient with maxillary premolar extractions, with the anterior bow soldered to Adams clasps on the first molars so that the extraction site is held closed. **B,** The adjustment loop of the Hawley anterior bow keeps the wire from having full contact with the canines. If this is needed, as in this patient whose canines were facially positioned before treatment, a wire that extends across the canines can be soldered to the anterior bow. **C,** In a patient whose second molars have erupted, a wraparound outer bow soldered to C-clasps on the second molars provides a way to avoid interference as the retainer wire crosses the occlusion. **D,** For a mandibular retainer, the wire Hawley bow is less effective than a wire-reinforced acrylic bar that tightly contacts the lower incisors. This Moore design has almost completely replaced the Hawley design for lower removable retainers that extend to the posterior teeth.

lingual surfaces of the teeth (see Figure 17-9). A full-arch wraparound retainer firmly holds each tooth in position. This is not necessarily an advantage, since one object of a retainer should be to allow each tooth to move individually, stimulating reorganization of the PDL. In addition, a wraparound retainer, though quite esthetic, is often less comfortable than a Hawley retainer and may not be effective in maintaining overbite correction. A full-arch wraparound retainer is indicated primarily when periodontal breakdown requires splinting the teeth together.

A variant of the wraparound retainer, the canine-to-canine clip-on retainer, is widely used in the lower anterior region. This appliance has the great advantage that it can be used to realign irregular incisors, if mild crowding has developed after treatment (see Active Retainers, on p. 628), but it is well tolerated as a retainer alone. An upper canine-to-canine wraparound occasionally is useful in adults with long clinical crowns but rarely is indicated and usually would not be tolerated in younger patients because of occlusal interferences.

In a lower extraction case, usually it is a good idea to extend a canine-to-canine wraparound distally on the lingual only to the central groove of the first molar (see Figure 17-9). This is called a Moore retainer. It provides control of the second premolar and the extraction site, but the retainer must be made carefully to avoid lingual undercuts in the premolar and molar region. Posterior extension of the lower retainer, of course, also is indicated when the posterior teeth were irregular before treatment.

Positioners as Retainers

A tooth positioner also can be used as a removable retainer, either fabricated for this purpose alone, or more commonly, continued as a retainer after serving initially as a finishing device. Positioners are excellent finishing devices and under special circumstances can be used to an advantage as retainers. For routine use, however, a positioner does not make a good retainer. The major problems are:

1. The pattern of wear of a positioner does not match the pattern usually desired for retainers. Because of its

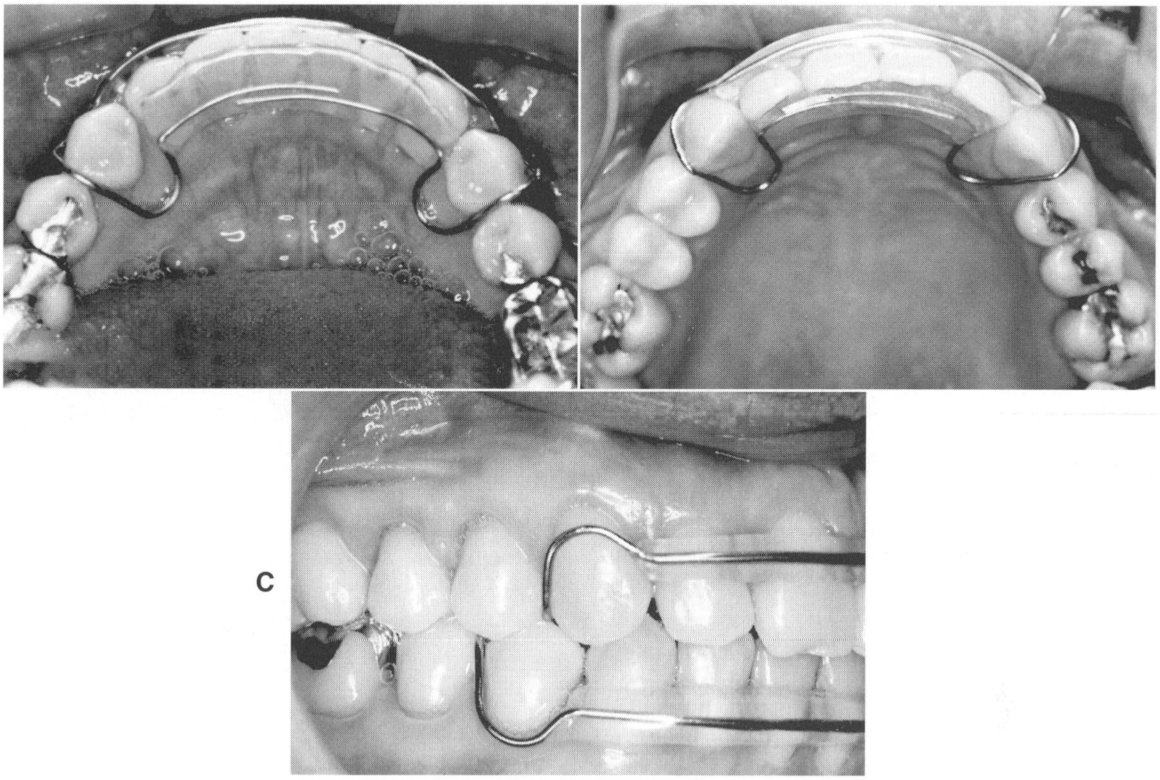

FIGURE 17-9 **A,** a removable clip-type retainer that controls alignment of only the anterior teeth (3-3 clip or, as shown here, 4-4 clip) often is preferred as a removable lower retainer, because if the lower posterior teeth were well aligned prior to treatment, retention of these teeth usually is unnecessary, and undercuts lingual to the lower molars make it difficult to place a lower retainer that extends further posteriorly. **B,** An anterior clip retainer in the maxillary arch is particularly useful when it is necessary to keep spaces from reopening. It also can be used to prevent re-rotation of maxillary incisors, but the wider upper incisors allow a broad contact with just a retainer wire, and contact of the lower incisors with a maxillary clip retainer often becomes a problem. **C,** Anterior clip retainers in both arches for this patient, who had maxillary and mandibular anterior spacing prior to treatment.

bulk, patients often have difficulty wearing a positioner full-time or nearly so. In fact, positioners tend to be worn less than the recommended 4 hours per day after the first few weeks, although they are reasonably well tolerated by most patients during sleep.

2. Positioners do not retain incisor irregularities and rotations as well as standard retainers. This problem follows directly from the first one: a retainer is needed nearly full-time initially to control intra-arch alignment. Also, overbite tends to increase while a positioner is being worn, and this effect as well probably relates in large part to the fact that it is worn only a small percentage of the time.

A positioner does have one major advantage over a standard removable or wraparound retainer, however—it maintains the occlusal relationships as well as intra-arch tooth positions. For a patient with a tendency toward Class III relapse, a positioner made with the jaws rotated somewhat downward and backward may be useful. Although a positioner with the teeth set in a slightly exaggerated "supernormal" from the original malocclusion can be used for patients with a skeletal Class II or open bite growth pattern, it is less effective in controlling growth than part-time headgear or a functional appliance.

In fabricating a positioner, it is necessary to separate the teeth by 2 to 4 mm. This means that an articulator mounting that records the patient's hinge axis allows more accurate fabrication. As a general guideline, the more the patient deviates from the average normal, and the longer the positioner will be worn, the more important it is to make it on articulator-mounted casts. If a positioner is to be used for only 2 to 4 weeks as a finishing device in a patient who will have some vertical growth during later retention, and if the patient has an approximately normal hinge axis, an individualized articulator mounting makes little or no practical difference.

The usual sign of a positioner made to an incorrect hinge axis is some separation of the posterior teeth when the incisors are in contact. Patients wearing a positioner as a retainer should be checked carefully to see that this effect is not occurring.

FIXED RETAINERS

Fixed orthodontic retainers are normally used in situations where intra-arch instability is anticipated and prolonged retention is planned, especially the mandibular incisor area. There are four major indications:

1. Maintenance of lower incisor position during late growth. As has been discussed previously, the major cause of lower incisor crowding in the late teen years, in both patients who have had orthodontic treatment and those who have not, is late growth of the mandible in the normal growth pattern. Especially if the lower incisors have previously been irregular, even a small amount of differential mandibular growth between ages 16 and 20 can cause recrowding of these teeth. Relapse into crowding is almost always accompanied by lingual tipping of the central and lateral incisors in response to the pattern of growth. An excellent retainer to hold these teeth in alignment is a fixed lingual bar, attached only to the canines (or to canines and first premolars) and resting against the flat lingual surface of the lower incisors above the cingulum (Figure 17-10). This prevents the incisors from moving lingually and is also reasonably effective in maintaining correction of rotations in the incisor segment.

   Fixed canine-to-canine retainers must be made from a wire heavy enough to resist distortion over the rather long span between these teeth. Usually 28 or 30 mil steel is used for this purpose (see Figure 17-1), with a loop bent in the end of the wire to improve retention. With this design, a bonded retainer can remain in place for many years. Although there has been concern about a long-term effect on periodontal health, long-term recall of patients who have worn a bonded lower retainer for more than 20 years has shown no periodontal problems.[8]

   It is also possible to bond a fixed lingual retainer to one or more of the incisor teeth. The major indication for this variation is a tooth or teeth that had been severely rotated. Whatever the type of retainer, however, it is desirable not to hold the teeth rigidly during retention. For this reason, if the span of the retainer wire is reduced by bonding an intermediate tooth or teeth, a more flexible wire should be used. A good choice for a fixed retainer with adjacent teeth bonded is a braided steel archwire of 17.5 mil diameter (Figure 17-11).

2. Diastema maintenance. A second indication for a fixed retainer is a situation where teeth must be permanently or semi-permanently bonded together to maintain the closure of a space between them. This is encountered most commonly when a diastema between maxillary central incisors has been closed. Even if a frenectomy has been carried out (see Chapters 7 and 15), there is a tendency for a small space to open up between the upper central incisors. The best retainer for this purpose is a bonded section of flexible wire, as shown in Figure 17-12. The wire should be contoured so that it lies near the cingulum to keep it out of occlusal contact. The object of the retainer is to hold the teeth together while allowing them some ability to move independently during function, hence the importance of a flexible wire. An alternative (Figure 17-13) is a solid wire configured to avoid the tooth contacts to facilitate flossing, which also can incorporate stops to prevent deepening of the bite.

   A removable retainer is not a good choice for prolonged retention of a central diastema. In troublesome cases, the diastema is closed when the retainer is removed but opens up quickly. The tooth movement

A
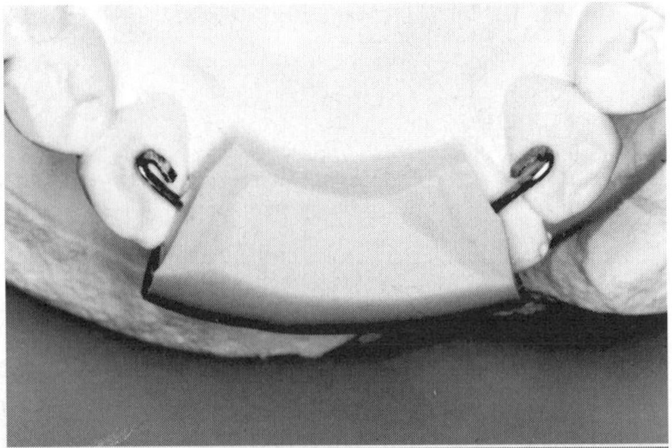
B
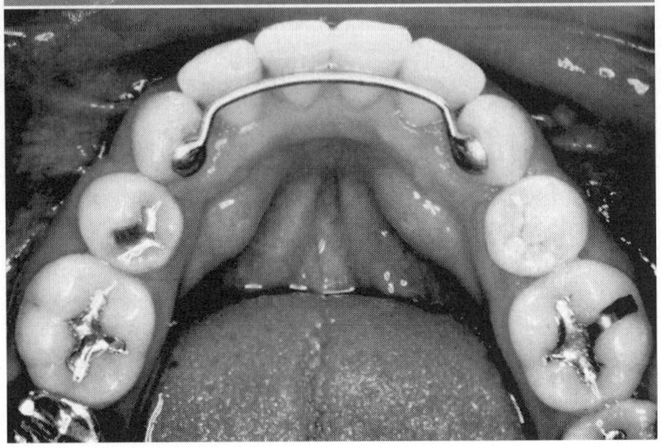

FIGURE 17-10 **A,** A bonded canine-to-canine retainer in the lower arch is an excellent way to maintain alignment. It is fabricated on a lower cast, often with a carrier to hold it in position while being bonded. Note the design with wire loops on the canines to provide retention when the retainer is bonded. **B,** A bonded canine-to-canine retainer, with retention pads, in place. Data now show that wire retention loops decrease the chance that the retainer will break loose.

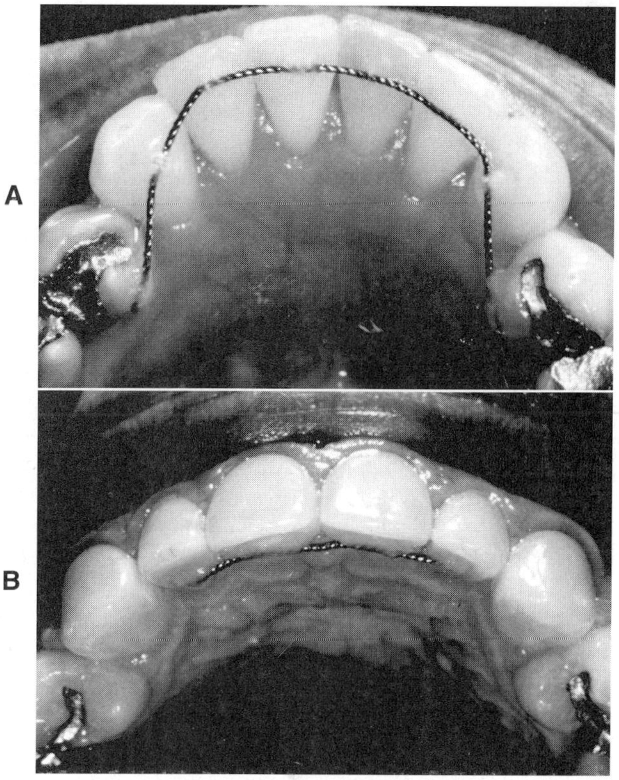

FIGURE 17-11 **A,** Bonding a wire to all the mandibular anterior teeth (canine-to-canine or premolar-to-premolar) is indicated if spaces existed in the lower anterior segment prior to treatment, or if severe rotations were corrected. A lighter wire (17.5 or 19.5 mil twist) should be used. A retainer of this type must be kept under observation, because a bond failure on one tooth is unlikely to be noticed by the patient and severe decalcification can occur in that area. **B,** A bonded section of twist wire also can be used to maintain alignment of maxillary teeth that were severely displaced initially (as in Class II, division 2), or keep a maxillary diastema closed. Multiple bonded attachments on the lingual of the upper incisors also can serve to prevent deepening of the bite as lower incisors erupt.

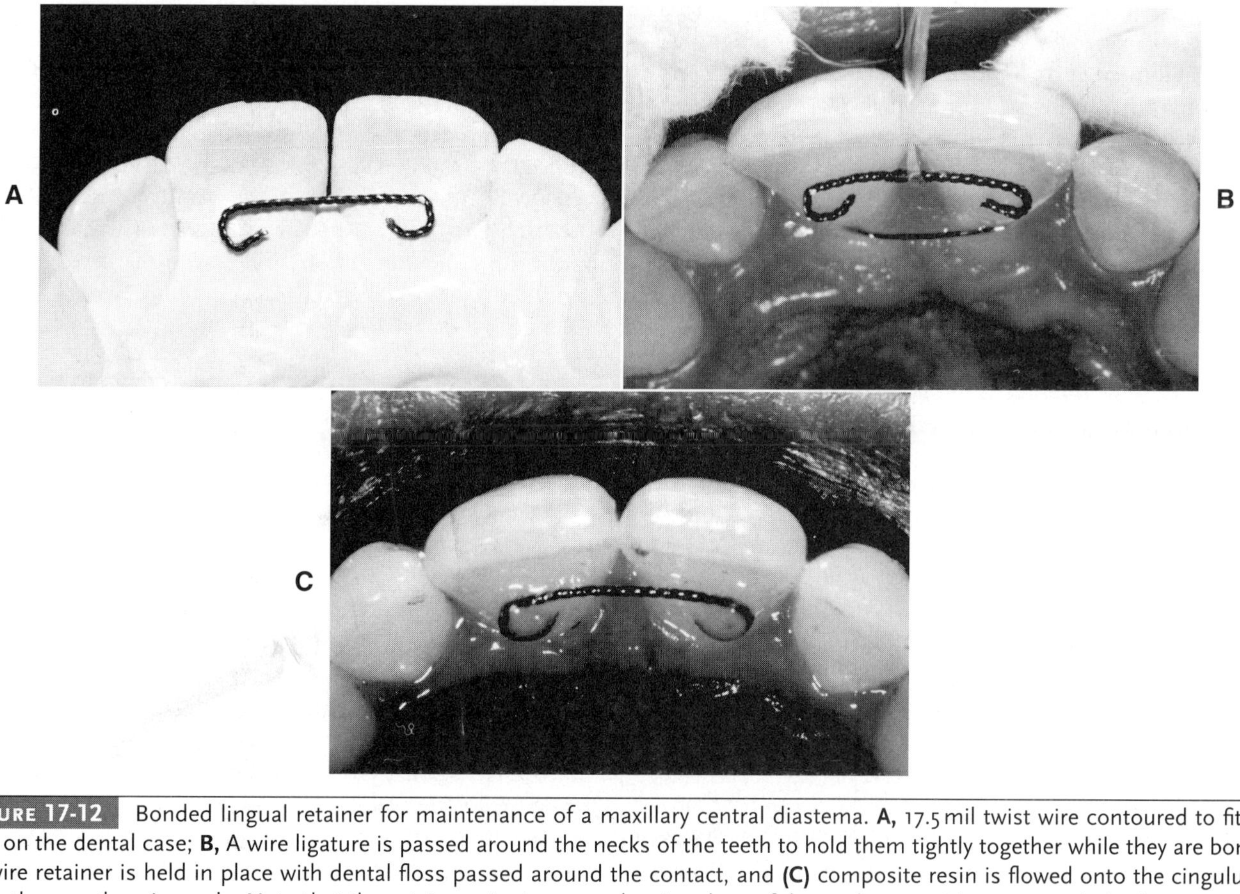

FIGURE 17-12 Bonded lingual retainer for maintenance of a maxillary central diastema. **A,** 17.5 mil twist wire contoured to fit passively on the dental case; **B,** A wire ligature is passed around the necks of the teeth to hold them tightly together while they are bonded. The wire retainer is held in place with dental floss passed around the contact, and **(C)** composite resin is flowed onto the cingulum of the teeth, over the wire ends. Note that the retainer wire is up on the cingulum of the teeth, to avoid contact with the lower incisors.

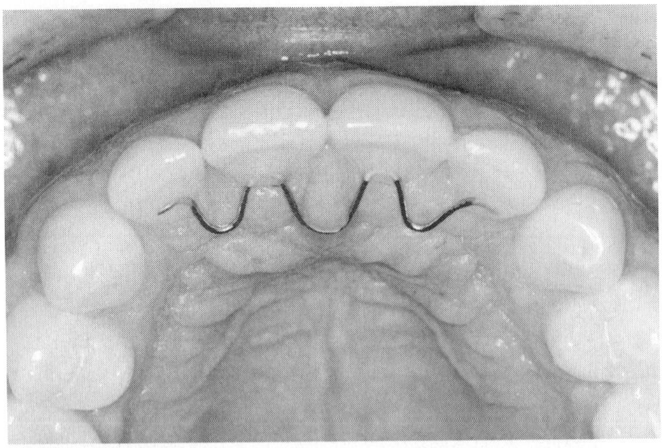

FIGURE 17-13 An alternative design for a bonded retainer for the maxillary incisors. The wire is contoured so that flossing is not impeded, and the bonded attachment areas also serve to keep the bite from deepening.

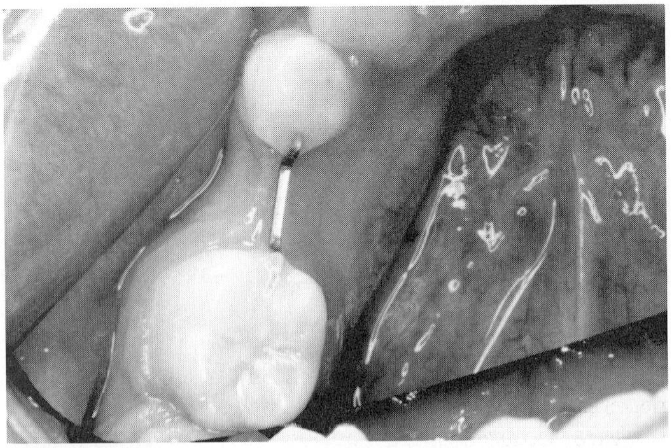

FIGURE 17-14 Fixed retainer (sometimes called an A-splint retainer) to maintain space for eventual replacement of a missing second premolar. A shallow preparation has been made in the enamel of the marginal ridges adjacent to the extraction site, and a section of 21 × 25 wire, stepped down away from the occlusion, is bonded as a retainer.

that accompanies this back-and-forth closure is potentially damaging over a long period.

3. Maintenance of pontic or implant space. A fixed retainer is also the best choice to maintain a space where a bridge pontic or implant eventually will be placed. Using a fixed retainer for a few months reduces mobility of the teeth and often makes it easier to place the fixed bridge that will serve, among other functions, as a permanent orthodontic retainer. If further periodontal therapy is needed after the teeth have been positioned, several months or even years can pass before a bridge is placed, and a fixed retainer is definitely required. Implants should be placed as soon as possible after the orthodontics is completed, so that integration of the implant can occur simultaneously with the initial stages of retention.

   The preferred orthodontic retainer for maintaining space for posterior restorations is a heavy intracoronal wire, bonded to the adjacent teeth (in shallow preparations if these are future abutment teeth for a bridge) (Figure 17-14). Obviously, the longer the span, the heavier the wire should be. Bringing the wire down out of occlusion decreases the chance that it will be displaced by occlusal forces.

   Anterior spaces need a replacement tooth, which can be attached to a removable retainer. This approach guarantees nearly full-time wear and is satisfactory for short periods. After a few months, especially if an implant or permanent bridge will be delayed for a long time while adolescent vertical growth is completed, it is better to place a fixed retainer in the form of a bonded bridge.

4. Keeping extraction spaces closed in adults (see Figure 17-11, *A*). A fixed retainer is both more reliable and better tolerated than a full-time removable retainer, and spaces reopen unless a retainer is worn consistently. It may be better in adults to bond a fixed retainer on the facial surface of posterior teeth when spaces have been closed.

The major objection to any fixed retainer is that it makes interproximal hygiene procedures more difficult. As Figure 17-13 demonstrates, a maxillary fixed retainer wire can be contoured to allow access to the interproximal area. It is possible to floss between teeth that have a fixed retainer across the interdental contact area by using a floss-threading device. With proper flossing, there is no reason that fixed retainers, if needed, cannot be left in place indefinitely.

ACTIVE RETAINERS

"Active retainer" is a contradiction in terms, since a device cannot be actively moving teeth and serving as a retainer at the same time. It does happen, however, that relapse or growth changes after orthodontic treatment lead to a need for some tooth movement during retention. This usually is accomplished with a removable appliance that continues as a retainer after it has repositioned the teeth, hence the name. A typical Hawley retainer, if used initially to close a small amount of band space, can be considered an active retainer, but the term usually is reserved for two specific situations: realignment of irregular incisors with spring retainers, and management of Class II or Class III relapse tendencies with modified functional appliances.

Realignment of Irregular Incisors: Spring Retainers

Re-crowding of lower incisors is the major indication for an active retainer to correct incisor position. The shape of the incisor crowns can contribute to re-crowding,[9] but the cause of the problem in these cases usually is late mandibular growth that uprighted the incisors. If late crowding has developed, it often is necessary to reduce the interproximal width of lower incisors before realigning them, so that the crowns do not tip labially into an obviously unstable position. Not only does stripping of contacts reduce the mesiodistal width of the incisors, decreasing the amount of space required for their alignment, it also flattens the contact areas, increasing the inherent stability of the arch in this region. As with any procedure involving the modification of teeth, however, stripping must be done cautiously and judiciously.[10,11] It is not indicated as a routine procedure.

Interproximal enamel can be removed with either abrasive strips (Figure 17-15), thin discs in a handpiece or thin flame-shaped diamond stones. Obviously, enamel reduction should not be overdone, but if necessary, the width of each lower incisor can be reduced up to 0.5 mm on each side without going through the interproximal enamel. If an additional 2 mm of space can be gained, reducing each incisor 0.25 mm per side, it is usually possible to realign typically crowded incisors.

If the irregularity is modest, a canine-to-canine clip-on is usually the active retainer used to realign crowded incisors. The steps in making such an active retainer are: (1) reduce the interproximal width of the incisors and apply topical fluoride to the newly exposed enamel surfaces; (2) prepare a laboratory model, on which the teeth can be reset into alignment; and (3) fabricate a canine-to-canine clip-on appliance (Figure 17-16).

If there is more than a modest degree of relapse, however, a fixed appliance for retreatment must be considered. With bonded brackets on the lower arch from premolar to premolar, space can be opened and superelastic NiTi wires can be used to bring the incisors back into alignment quite efficiently (Figure 17-17). If the incisors are advanced toward the lip when this is done, a bonded lingual retainer should be placed before the brackets are removed. Permanent retention obviously will be required after the realignment.

A

B

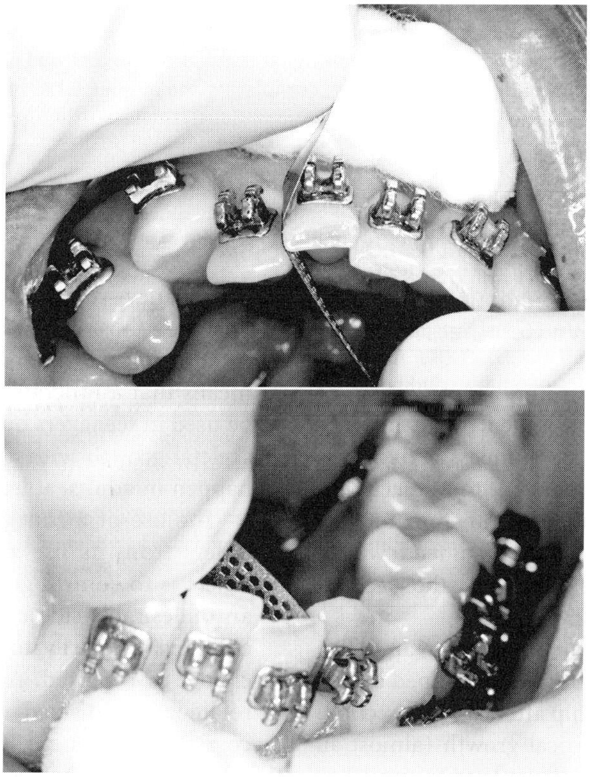

Figure 17-15 Removal of interproximal enamel to facilitate alignment of crowded lower incisors. **A, B,** Use of a carbide-coated strip to remove enamel. The surfaces are polished after the stripping is completed. Topical fluoride should be applied immediately after stripping procedures, because the fluoride-rich outer layer of enamel has been removed.

CHAPTER

18

Special Considerations in Treatment for Adults

CHAPTER OUTLINE

ADJUNCTIVE VERSUS COMPREHENSIVE TREATMENT

Adjunctive orthodontic treatment for adults is, by definition, tooth movement carried out to facilitate other dental procedures necessary to control disease, restore function and/or enhance appearance. Almost always, it involves only a part of the dentition, and the primary goal usually is to make it easier or more effective to replace missing or damaged teeth. Making it easier for the patient to control periodontal problems is a frequent secondary goal, and sometimes is the primary goal. The treatment duration tends to be a few months, rarely more than a year, and long-term retention usually is supplied by the restorations. With the distinction made in this way, most of the adjunctive treatment discussed in this chapter can be carried out within the context of general dental practice. Whether one or several practitioners are involved, adjunctive orthodontics must be coordinated carefully with the periodontal and restorative treatment.

In contrast, the goal of comprehensive orthodontics for adults is the same as for adolescents: to produce the best combination of dental occlusion, dental and facial appearance, and stability of the result to maximize benefit to the patient. Typically, comprehensive orthodontics requires a complete fixed orthodontic appliance, intrusion of some teeth is likely to required, orthognathic surgery may be considered to improve jaw relationships, and the duration of treatment from braces on to braces off exceeds 1 year. Adults receiving comprehensive treatment are the main candidates for esthetically-enhanced appliances, the prime examples being clear aligners, lingual appliances, and ceramic facial brackets. The complexity of the treatment procedures means that an orthodontic specialist is likely to be significantly more efficient in delivering the care.

The first part of this chapter is devoted to adjunctive treatment, carried out in large part with fixed appliances that involve only selected areas of the dental arches. The second part covers non-surgical comprehensive adult treatment. The integration of orthodontics and orthognathic surgery is discussed in Chapter 19.

GOALS OF ADJUNCTIVE TREATMENT

Typically, adjunctive orthodontic treatment will involve any or all of several procedures: (1) repositioning teeth that have drifted after extractions or bone loss so that more ideal fixed or removable partial dentures can be fabricated, or so that implants can be placed; (2) alignment of anterior teeth to allow more esthetic restorations or successful splinting, while maintaining good interproximal bone contour and embrasure form; (3) correction of crossbite if this compromises jaw function (not all do); and (4) forced eruption of badly broken down teeth to expose sound root structure on which to place crowns.

Whatever the occlusal status originally, the goals of adjunctive treatment should be to:

Improve periodontal health by eliminating plaque-harboring areas and improving the alveolar ridge contour adjacent to the teeth

Establish favorable crown-to-root ratios and position the teeth so that occlusal forces are transmitted along the long axes of the teeth

Facilitate restorative treatment by positioning the teeth so that

- More ideal and conservative techniques (including implants) can be used
- Optimal esthetics can be obtained with bonding, laminates or full coverage porcelain restorations

An old rule says that to make it clear what something is, it helps to point out what it isn't but might be mistaken for. So, some important corollaries:

- Orthodontic treatment for temporomandibular dysfunction should not be considered adjunctive treatment
- Although intrusion of teeth can be an important part of comprehensive treatment for adults, it should be avoided as an adjunctive procedure because of the technical difficulties involved and the possibility of periodontal complications. As a general guideline for adjunctive treatment, lower incisor teeth that are excessively extruded are best treated by reduction of crown height, which has the added advantage of improving the ultimate crown-to-root ratio of the teeth. For other teeth, tooth-lip relationships must be kept in mind when crown height reduction is considered.
- Crowding of more than 3-4 mm should not be attempted by stripping enamel from the contact surfaces of the teeth. It may be advantageous to strip posterior teeth to provide space for alignment of the incisors, but this requires a complete orthodontic appliance and cannot be considered adjunctive treatment.

PRINCIPLES OF ADJUNCTIVE TREATMENT

Diagnostic and Treatment Planning Considerations

Planning for adjunctive treatment requires two steps: (1) collecting an adequate diagnostic data base and (2) developing a comprehensive but clearly stated list of the patient's problems, taking care not to focus unduly on any one aspect of a complex situation. The importance of this planning stage in adjunctive orthodontic treatment cannot be overemphasized, since the solution to the patient's specific problems may involve the synthesis of many branches of dentistry. In adjunctive treatment, the restorative dentist usually is the principal architect of the treatment plan, and the orthodontics (whether or not an orthodontist is part of the treatment team) is to allow better restorative treatment.

Nevertheless, the steps outlined in Chapter 6 should be followed when developing the problem list. The interview and clinical examination are the same, whatever the type of orthodontic treatment. Diagnostic records for adjunctive orthodontic patients, however, differ in several important ways from those for adolescents and children.

For this adult and dentally compromised population, the records usually should include individual intraoral radiographs to supplement the panoramic film that often suffices for younger and healthier patients (Figure 18-1). When active dental disease is present, the panoramic radiograph does not give sufficient detail. The revised guidelines promulgated by the U.S. Food and Drug Administration in late 2004 (see Chapter 6) should be followed in determining exactly what radiographs are required in evaluating the patient's oral health status.

For adjunctive orthodontics, pretreatment cephalometric radiographs usually are not required, but it is important to anticipate the impact of various tooth movements on facial esthetics. In some instances, the computer prediction methods used in comprehensive treatment (see Chapter 7) can be quite useful in planning adjunctive treatment.

Articulator-mounted casts are likely to be needed, because they facilitate the planning of associated restorative procedures.

Once all the problems have been identified and categorized, the key treatment planning question is: Can the occlusion be restored within the existing tooth positions, or must some teeth be moved to achieve a satisfactory, stable, healthy and esthetic result? The goal of adjunctive treatment, to provide a physiologic occlusion and facilitate other dental treatment, has little to do with Angle's concept of an ideal occlusion.

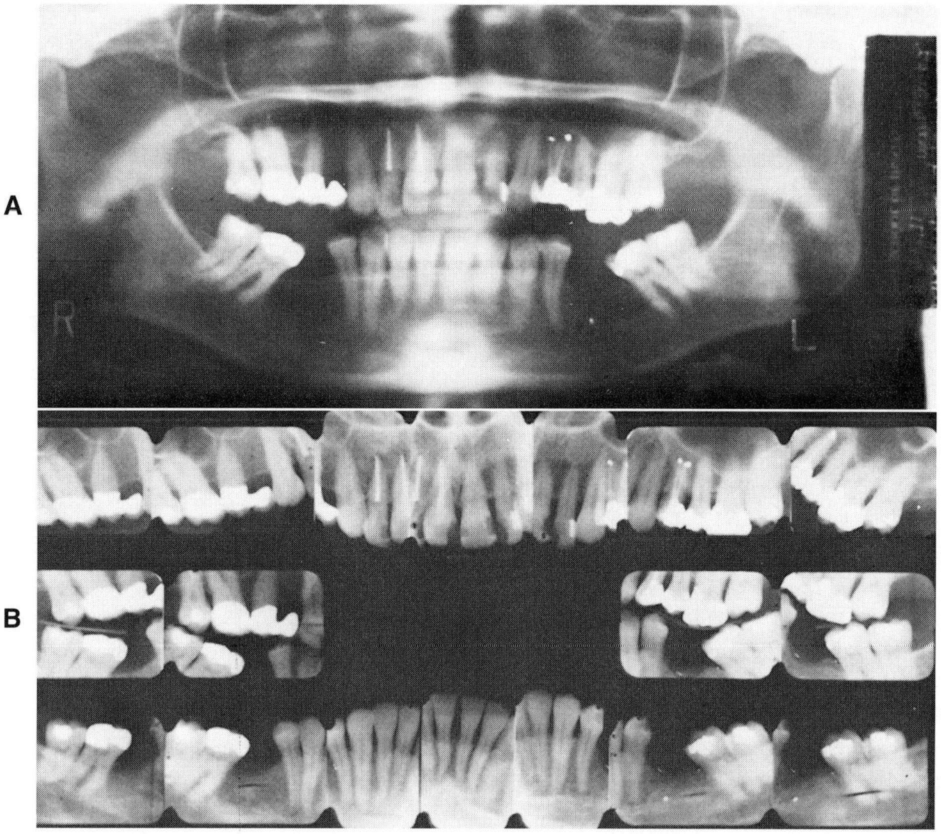

Figure 18-1 For the periodontically compromised adults who are the usual candidates for adjunctive orthodontics, periapical radiographs of the areas that will be treated, as well as a panoramic radiograph, usually are needed. Periodontal disease now is the major indication for periapical radiographs. For this patient who is a candidate for adjunctive orthodontic treatment, adequate detail of root morphology, dental disease, and periodontal breakdown is obtained only from carefully taken periapical radiographs.

Obviously, the time needed for any orthodontic treatment depends on the severity of the problem and the amount of tooth movement desired, but with efficient use of orthodontic appliances, it should be possible to reach the objectives of adjunctive treatment within 6 months. As a practical matter, this means that like comprehensive orthodontics, most adjunctive orthodontics cannot be managed well with traditional removable appliances. It requires either fixed appliances or a sequence of clear aligners to get the job done in a reasonable period of time. In addition, it is becoming increasingly apparent that skeletal anchorage makes adjunctive tooth movement more effective and efficient. For adjunctive treatment, this is almost always in the form of bone screws.

Biomechanical Considerations

Characteristics of the Orthodontic Appliance

For adjunctive treatment, with the possible exception of alignment of anterior teeth, we recommend the 22-slot edgewise appliance with twin brackets (one-half the width of the crown). The rectangular (edgewise) bracket slot permits control of buccolingual axial inclinations, the relatively wide bracket helps control undesirable rotations and tipping, and the larger slot size allows the use of stabilizing wires that are somewhat stiffer than ordinarily might be used in comprehensive treatment.

Recently, the development of clear aligner therapy (CAT—see Chapter 11) has provided an effective type of removable appliance that can be well-suited to alignment of anterior teeth. Removable appliances of the traditional plastic-and-wire type are rarely satisfactory for adjunctive (or comprehensive) treatment. They often are uncomfortable, and are likely to be worn for too few hours per day to be effective. With CAT, both discomfort and interference with speech and mastication are minimized, and patient cooperation improves. A fixed appliance on posterior teeth only is all but invisible, but it is quite apparent on anterior teeth, and the better appearance of a clear aligner also is a factor in choosing it to align anterior teeth. Despite this esthetic advantage, there are biomechanical limitations. Clear aligners make control of root position extremely difficult, and it also is difficult to correct rotations and to extrude teeth. If these limitations are not important in a particular adjunctive case, CAT can be considered. If they are, in nearly all cases adults who are candidates for adjunctive treatment will accept a visible fixed appliance.

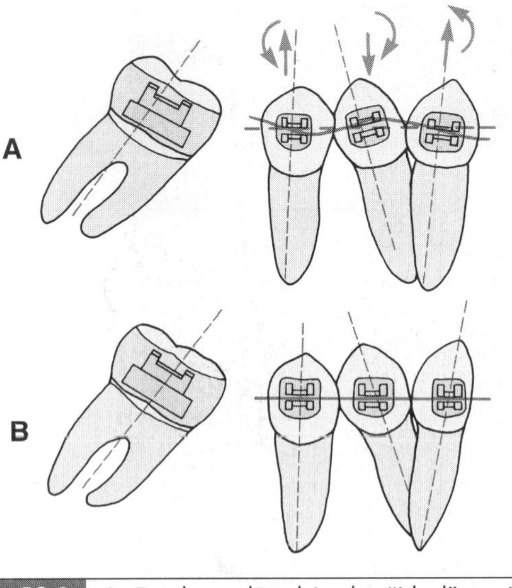

FIGURE 18-2 **A,** Brackets placed in the "ideal" position on moderately irregular anchor teeth for molar uprighting. For adjunctive orthodontic treatment, movement of the anchor teeth usually is undesirable, but a straight length of wire will move them as the brackets are repositioned. **B,** Brackets placed in the position of maximum convenience, lined up so that a straight length of wire can be placed without moving the anchor teeth. This makes things easier if no movement of the anchor teeth is desired. For adjunctive orthodontic procedures like molar uprighting, we recommend the use of fully adjusted "straight wire" brackets and working archwires that are somewhat smaller than the bracket slot, to reduce unwanted buccolingual movement of anchor teeth even though the brackets are lined up in the other planes of space.

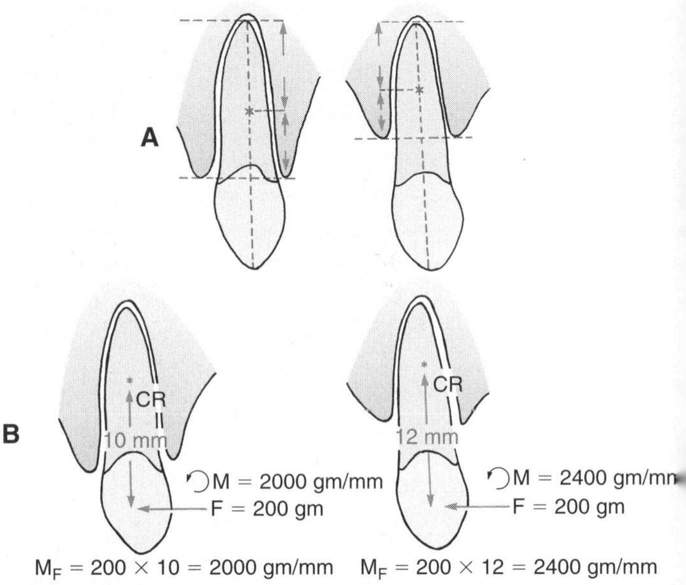

FIGURE 18-3 **A,** The center of resistance of a single rooted tooth lies approximately six-tenths of the distance between the apex of the tooth and the crest of the alveolar bone. Loss of alveolar bone height, as for the tooth on the right, moves the center of resistance closer to the root apex. **B,** The magnitude of the tipping moment produced by a force is equal to the force times the distance from the point of force application to the center of resistance. If the center of resistance moves apically, the tipping moment produced by the force (M_F) increases, and a larger countervailing moment produced by a couple applied to the tooth (M_C) would be necessary to affect bodily movement. This is almost impossible for traditional removable appliances and very difficult with clear aligners even when bonded attachments are added. For all practical purposes, a fixed appliance is required (see Chapter 10 for more detail).

Modern edgewise brackets of the straight wire type (see Chapter 11) are designed for a specific location on an individual tooth. Placing the bracket in its ideal position on each tooth implies that every tooth will be repositioned if necessary to achieve ideal occlusion (Figure 18-2, *A*). Since adjunctive treatment is concerned with only limited tooth movements, usually it is neither necessary nor desirable to alter the position of every tooth in the arch. For this reason, in a partial fixed appliance for adjunctive treatment, the brackets are placed in an ideal position only on teeth to be moved, and the remaining teeth to be incorporated in the anchor system are bracketed so that the archwire slots are closely aligned (Figure 18-2, *B*). This allows the anchorage segments of the wire to be engaged passively in the brackets with little bending. Passive engagement of wires to anchor teeth produces minimal disturbance of teeth that are in a physiologically satisfactory position. This important point is illustrated in more detail in the sections on specific treatment procedures that follow.

Effects of Reduced Periodontal Support

Since patients who need adjunctive orthodontic treatment often have lost alveolar bone to periodontal disease before it was brought under control, the amount of bone support of each tooth is an important special consideration. When bone is lost, the periodontal ligament (PDL) area decreases, and the same force against the crown produces greater pressure in the PDL of a periodontally compromised tooth than a normally supported one. The absolute magnitude of force used to move teeth must be reduced when periodontal support has been lost (see Figure 18-13, p. 645). In addition, the greater the loss of attachment, the smaller the area of supported root and the further apical the center of resistance will become (Figure 18-3). This affects the moments created by forces applied to the crown and the moments needed to control root movement (see Chapter 10). In general terms, tooth movement is quite possible despite bone loss, but lighter forces and relatively larger moments are needed.

Timing and Sequence of Treatment

In the development of any orthodontic treatment plan, the first step is the control of any active dental disease (Figure 18-4). Before any tooth movement, active caries and pulpal pathology must be eliminated, using extractions, restorative procedures, and pulpal or apical treatment as necessary. Endodontically treated teeth respond normally to orthodontic force, providing all residual chronic inflammation has been eliminated.[1] Prior to orthodontics, teeth should be restored with well-placed amalgams or composite resins. Restorations requiring detailed occlusal anatomy should not be placed until any adjunctive orthodontic treatment has been completed, because the occlusion inevitably will be changed. That could necessitate remaking crowns, bridges, or removable partial dentures.

Periodontal disease also must be controlled before any orthodontics begins, because orthodontic tooth movement superimposed on poorly controlled periodontal health can lead to rapid and irreversible breakdown of the periodontal support apparatus.[2] Scaling, curettage (by open flap procedures, if necessary), and gingival grafts should be undertaken as appropriate. Surgical pocket elimination and osseous surgery should be delayed until completion of the orthodontic phase of treatment, because significant soft tissue and bony recontouring occurs during orthodontic tooth movement. Clinical studies have shown that orthodontic treatment of adults with both normal and compromised periodontal tissues can be completed without loss of attachment, providing there is good periodontal therapy both initially and during tooth movement.[3,4]

During this preparatory phase, the patient's enthusiasm for treatment and ability to maintain good overall oral hygiene should be carefully monitored. Adjunctive orthodontics has the potential to do more harm than good in patients who cannot or will not maintain good oral hygiene. If disease can be controlled, however, adjunctive orthodontics can significantly improve the final restorative and periodontal procedures.

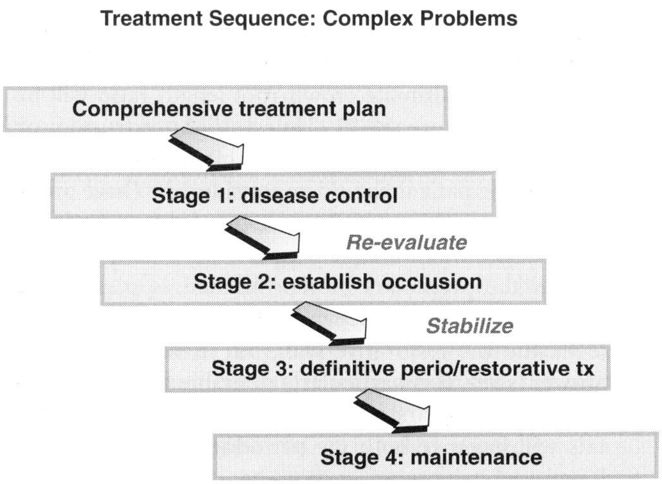

FIGURE 18-4 The sequence of steps in the treatment of patients requiring adjunctive orthodontics. Orthodontics is used to establish occlusion, but only after disease control has been accomplished, and the occlusion should be stabilized before definitive restorative treatment is carried out.

ADJUNCTIVE TREATMENT PROCEDURES

Uprighting Posterior Teeth

Treatment Planning Considerations

When a first permanent molar is lost during childhood or adolescence and not replaced, the second molar drifts mesially and the premolars often tip distally and rotate as space opens between them. As the teeth move, the adjacent gingival tissue becomes folded and distorted, forming a plaque-harboring pseudopocket that may be virtually impossible for the patient to clean (Figure 18-5). Repositioning the teeth eliminates this potentially pathologic condition and has the added advantage of simplifying the ultimate restorative procedures.

A

B

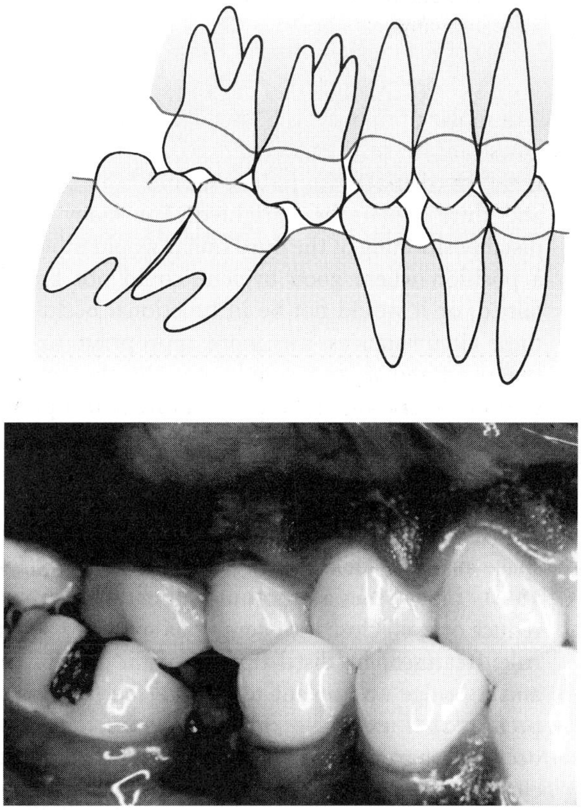

FIGURE 18-5 **A,** Loss of a lower molar can lead to tipping and drifting of adjacent teeth, poor interproximal contacts, poor gingival contour, reduced interradicular bone, and supra-eruption of unopposed teeth. Since the bone contour follows the cementoenamel junction, pseudopockets form adjacent to the tipped teeth. **B,** Note the loss of alveolar bone in the area where a mandibular first molar was extracted many years previously. Mesial drift and tipping of the second molar has closed half the space. The patient's posterior crossbite, however, is unrelated to early loss of the molar.

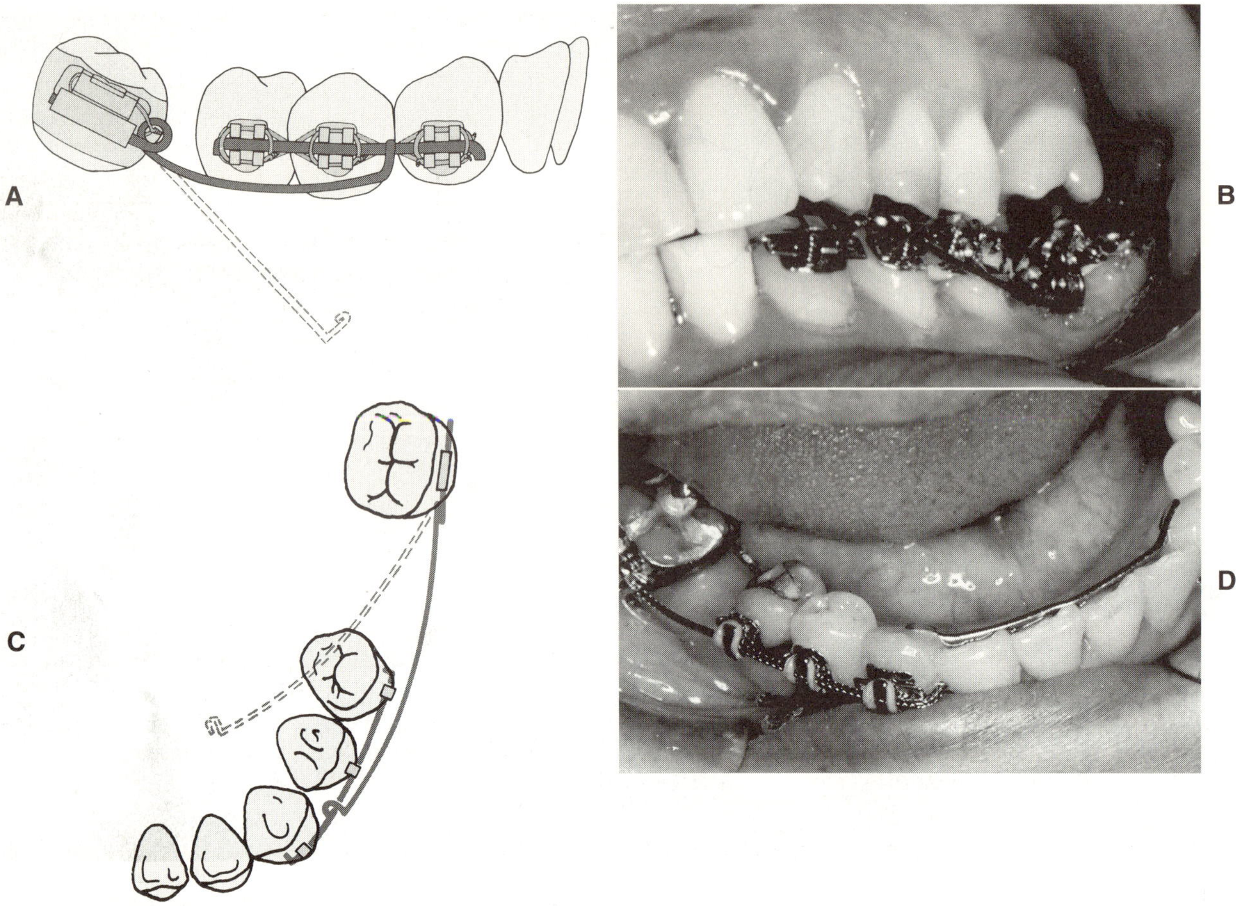

FIGURE 18-9 Uprighting with an auxiliary spring. **A,** If the relative alignment of the molar precludes extending the stabilizing segment into the molar bracket, then a rigid stabilizing wire, 19 × 25 stainless steel, is placed in the premolars and canine only (often with the brackets positioned so this wire is passive—see Figure 18-3). The mesial arm of the uprighting spring lies in the vestibule before engagement, and the spring is activated by lifting the mesial arm and hooking it over a stabilizing wire in the canine and premolar brackets. **B,** Auxiliary uprighting spring to molar just after initial placement. Note the helix bent into the steel wire that forms the spring, to provide better spring qualities. **C,** Because the force is applied to the facial surface of the teeth, an auxiliary uprighting spring tends not only to extrude the molar but also to roll it lingually, while intruding the premolars and flaring them buccally. To counteract this side effect, the uprighting spring should be curved buccolingually so that when it is placed into the molar tube, the hook would lie lingually to the archwire prior to activation *(dotted line)*. **D,** Better control of anchorage, with either a continuous wire or an auxiliary spring, is obtained when a canine-to-canine stabilizing wire is bonded on the lingual surface of these teeth.

without a helical loop, or 17 × 25 steel wire with a loop added to provide more springiness. The mesial arm of the helical spring should be adjusted to lie passively in the vestibule and upon activation should hook over the archwire in the stabilizing segment. It is important to position the hook so that it is free to slide distally as the molar uprights. In addition, a slight lingual bend placed in the uprighting spring is needed to counteract the forces that tend to tip the anchor teeth buccally and the molar lingually (Figure 18-9, *C*).

Mesial Root Movement. If mesial root movement is desired, an alternative treatment approach is indicated (Figure 18-10). After initial alignment of the anchor teeth with a light flexible wire, a single "T-loop" sectional archwire 17 × 25 stainless steel or 19 × 25 beta-Ti wire is adapted to fit passively into the brackets on the anchor teeth and gabled at the T to exert an uprighting force on the molar. Insertion into the molar can be from the mesial or distal. If the treatment plan calls for maintaining or closing rather than increasing the pontic space, the distal end of the archwire should be pulled distally through the molar tube, opening the T-loop by 1 to 2 mm, and then bent sharply gingivally to maintain this opening. This activation provides a mesial force on the molar that counteracts distal crown tipping while the tooth uprights (Figure 18-10, *D*). If opening the space is desired, the end of the wire is not bent over so the tooth can slide distally along it.

The T-loop appliance also is indicated if the molar to be uprighted is severely tipped but has no occlusal antagonist.

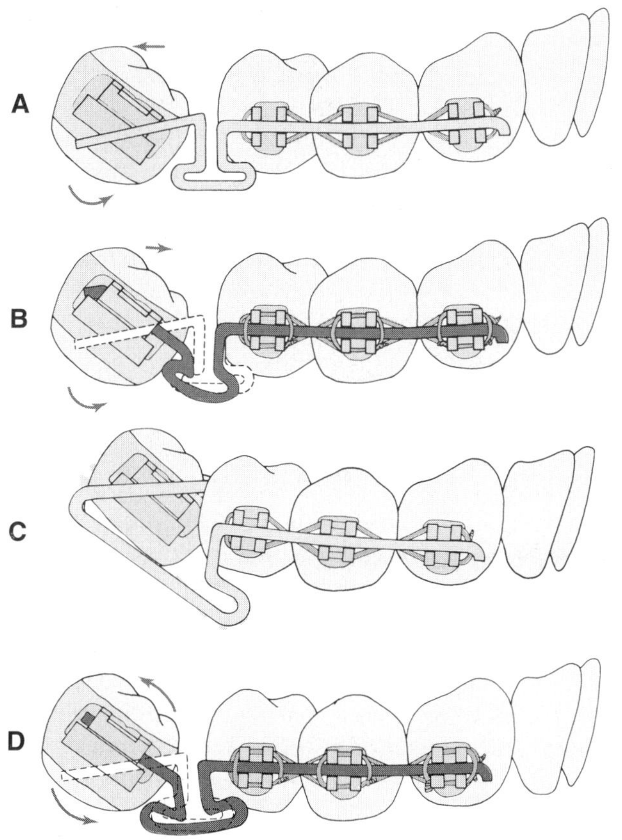

FIGURE 18-10 **A,** T-loop spring in 17 × 25 steel wire, showing the degree of angulation of the wire before inserting it into the molar tube that is necessary to upright a single tipped molar. **B,** If a T-loop is activated by pulling the distal of the wire through the molar tube and bending it, the tooth cannot move distally. This generates a moment that results in molar uprighting by mesial root movement with space closure. **C,** A T-loop for uprighting by distal tipping. Note that the tooth can move back by sliding along the wire. **D,** Modification of a T-loop that can be used to upright a severely tipped or rotated molar by distal tipping. The wire is inserted into the distal end of the tube on the molar spring active to upright the tooth by distal crown tipping.

In that circumstance, a T-loop minimizes the extrusion that accompanies uprighting, which can be excessive with the other methods when there is no antagonist.

Final Positioning of Molar and Premolars. Once molar uprighting has been almost accomplished, often it is desirable to increase the available pontic space and close open contacts in the anterior segment. This is done best using a relatively stiff base wire, with a compressed coil spring threaded over the wire to produce the required force system. With 22-slot brackets, the base wire should be 18 mil round or 17 × 25 rectangular steel wire, which should engage the anchor teeth and the uprighted molar more or less passively. The wire should extend through the molar tube, projecting about 1 mm beyond the distal. An open coil steel spring (.009 wire, .030 lumen) is cut so that it is 1-2 mm longer than the space, slipped over the base wire (Figure 18-11), and compressed between the molar and distal premolar. It should exert a force of approximately 150 gm to move the premolars mesially while continuing to tip the molar distally. The coil spring can be reactivated without removing it by compressing the spring and adding a split spacer to maintain the compression (Figure 18-11, *B*).

Uprighting Two Molars in the Same Quadrant

Because the resistance offered when uprighting two molars is considerable, only small amounts of space closure should be attempted. The goal should be a combination of modest lingual crown movement and distal crown tipping, which typically would leave space for a premolar-sized implant or pontic. In the lower arch, a bonded canine-to-canine lingual stabilizing wire (which is similar to a bonded retainer—see Chapter 17) is needed to control the position of the anterior teeth (see Figure 18-9). Trying to upright both the second and third molars bilaterally at the same time is not a good idea—significant movement of the anchor teeth is inevitable.

When both the second and third molars are to be uprighted, the third molar should carry a single rectangular tube and the second molar a bracket. Since the second molar is usually more severely tipped than the third molar, increased flexibility of the wire mesial and distal to the

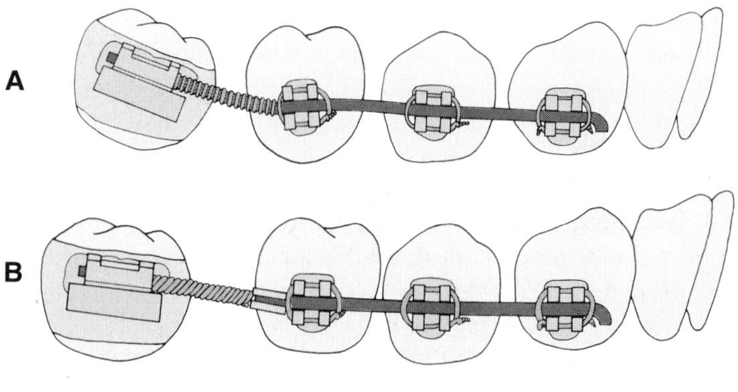

FIGURE 18-11 **A,** Compressed coil spring on a round wire (usually 18 mil steel) may be used to complete molar uprighting while closing remaining spaces in the premolar region. **B,** The coil spring may be reactivated by compressing it against a split spacer crimped over the archwire.

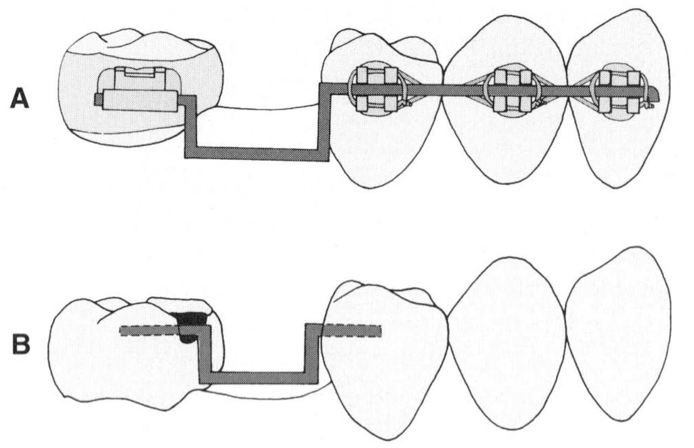

FIGURE 18-12 A molar that has been uprighted is unstable and must be maintained in its new position until a fixed bridge or implant is placed to stabilize it. There are two ways to provide temporary stabilization: **A,** An extracoronal splint using 19 × 25 steel wire engaging the brackets passively; **B,** An intracoronal splint (often called an A-splint) that is bonded in shallow preparations in the proximal enamel with composite resin (also see Figure 17-14). This causes minimal tissue disturbance. The intracoronal splint is preferred, particularly if retention is to be continued for more than a few weeks.

second molar is required. The best approach is to use a modern highly flexible wire initially, and 17 × 25 A-NiTi usually is a good choice. Excessive mobility of the teeth can result from failure to reduce occlusal interferences.

Retention

After molar uprighting, the teeth are in an unstable position until the prosthesis that provides the long-term retention is placed. Long delays in making the final prosthesis should be avoided if possible. As a general guideline, a fixed bridge can and should be placed within 6 weeks after uprighting is completed. Especially if an implant is planned, there may be a considerable delay while a bone graft heals and the implant becomes integrated. If retention is needed for more than a few weeks, the preferred approach is an intracoronal wire splint (19 × 25 or heavier steel wire), bonded into shallow preparations in the abutment teeth (Figure 18-12). This type of splint causes little gingival irritation and can be left in place for a considerable period, but it would have to be removed and rebonded to allow bone grafting and implant surgery.

Crossbite Correction

Posterior crossbites frequently are corrected using "through the bite" elastics from a conveniently placed tooth in the opposing arch, which moves both the upper and lower tooth (Figure 18-13, *A*). This tips the teeth into the correct occlusion but also tends to extrude them. For this reason, elastics must be used with caution to correct posterior crossbites in adults, because the extrusion can change occlusal relationships throughout the mouth. One way to obtain more movement of a maxillary tooth than its antagonist in the lower arch is to have several teeth in the lower arch stabilized by a heavy archwire segment (Figure 18-13, *B-E*). Of course, the same approach could be used in reverse to produce more movement of a mandibular tooth. If a mesially tipped lower molar also is in buccal crossbite, an auxiliary uprighting spring can be contoured to help move it lingually (see Figure 18-36).

If a deep overbite exists on the teeth in crossbite, correction will be much easier if a temporary bite plane that frees the occlusion is added. This bite plane should be carefully constructed to contact the occlusal surfaces of all teeth to prevent any supereruption during treatment.

Establishing a good overbite relationship is the key to maintaining crossbite correction. Crown reconstruction can be used to provide positive occlusal indexing, while eliminating any balancing interferences from the lingual cusps of posterior teeth.

If an anterior crossbite is due only to a displaced tooth and if correcting it requires only tipping (as perhaps in the case of a maxillary incisor that was tipped lingually into crossbite), then a removable appliance or clear aligner may be used to tip the tooth into a normal position. However, when using either type of removable appliance, tipping a tooth facially or lingually also produces a vertical change in occlusal level (Figure 18-14). Tipping maxillary incisors labially to correct anterior crossbite nearly always produces an apparent intrusion and a reduction in overbite. This can present a problem during retention, since a positive overbite serves to retain the crossbite correction. A fixed appliance generally is necessary for vertical control in correction of anterior crossbites.

Forced Eruption

Treatment Planning

For teeth with defects in or adjacent to the cervical third of the root, controlled extrusion can be an excellent alternative to extensive crown-lengthening surgery.[6] Extruding the tooth can allow isolation under rubber dam for endodontic therapy when it would not be possible otherwise. Forced eruption also allows crown margins to be placed on sound tooth structure while maintaining a uniform gingival contour that provides improved esthetics (Figure 18-15). In addition, the alveolar bone height is not compromised, the apparent crown length is maintained, and the bony support of adjacent teeth is not compromised. As the tooth is extruded, the attached gingiva should follow the cementoenamel junction. This returns the width of the attached gingiva to its original level. However, it usually is necessary to perform some limited recontouring of the gingiva, and perhaps of the bone, to produce a contour even with the adjacent teeth and a proper biologic width between bone and depth of sulcus.

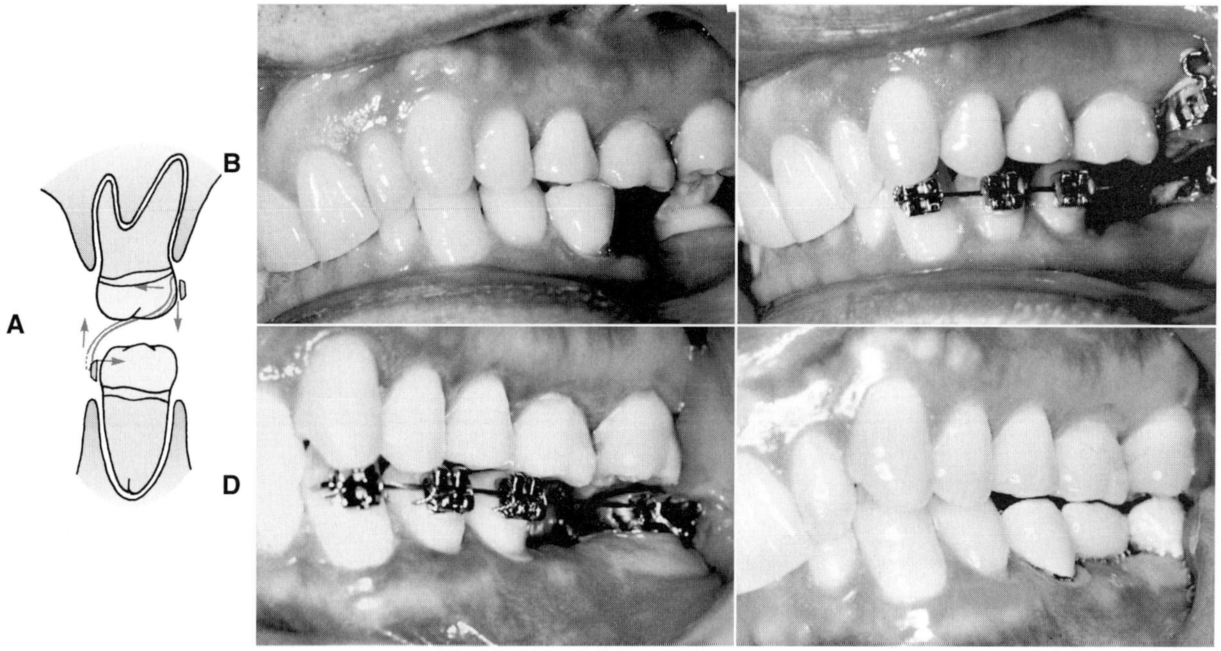

FIGURE 18-13 **A,** "Through the bite" or cross elastics produce both horizontal and vertical forces and will extrude the teeth while moving them buccolingually. If these elastics are used to correct posterior crossbite in adults, care must be taken not to open the bite anteriorly too much. Cross elastics are rarely indicated for an anterior crossbite. **B,** Buccal crossbite of the second molars in a patient at age 50 who had lost the mandibular first molar years previously. The lower second molar had tipped mesially and lingually. **C,** The standard orthodontic appliance for uprighting a lower molar was used, consisting of a band on the mandibular second molar, a bonded canine-to-canine mandibular lingual wire to augment anchorage, and bonded brackets on the facial of the premolars and canine. In addition, a lingual cleat was placed on the lower band, and a band with a facial hook was placed on the maxillary second molar, so that cross elastics could be worn. **D,** The molar uprighting was completed after the crossbite was corrected. **E,** The completed bridge in place. This is classic adjunctive orthodontics. The anterior deep bite and incisor alignment were not problems for this patient and were not corrected.

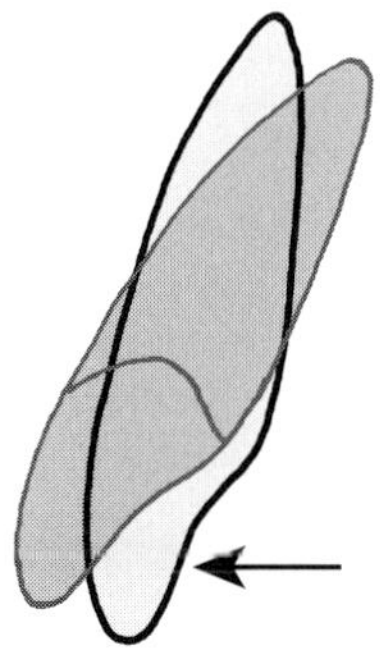

FIGURE 18-14 A labially directed force against a maxillary incisor from a removable appliance will tip the tooth and cause an apparent intrusion of the crown, which reduces the open bite.

As a general rule, endodontic therapy should be completed before extrusion of the root begins. For some patients, however, the orthodontic movement must be completed before definitive endodontic procedures, because one purpose of extrusion may be to provide better access for endodontic and restorative procedures. If so, preliminary endodontic treatment to relieve symptoms is done initially, and the tooth is maintained with a temporary root filling or other palliative treatment until it has been moved to a better position.

The distance the tooth should be extruded is determined by three things: (1) the location of the defect (fracture line, root perforation, etc.); (2) space to place the margin of the restoration so that it is not at the base of the gingival sulcus (typically, 1 mm is needed); and (3) an allowance for the biological width of the gingival attachment (about 2 mm). Thus if a fracture is at the height of the alveolar crest, the tooth should be extruded about 3 mm; if it is 2 mm below the crest, 5 mm of extrusion ideally would be needed. The crown-to-root ratio at the end of treatment should be 1 : 1 or better. A tooth with a poorer ratio can be maintained only by splinting it to adjacent teeth.

Isolated one- or two-wall vertical pockets pose a particular esthetic problem if they occur in the anterior region of the mouth. Surgical correction may be contraindicated simply on esthetic grounds. Forced eruption of such teeth, with concomitant crown reduction, can improve the periodontal condition while maintaining excellent esthetics.

In general, extrusion can be as rapid as 1 mm per week without damage to the PDL, so 3 to 6 weeks is sufficient for almost any patient. Too much force, and too rapid a rate of movement, runs the risk of tissue damage and ankylosis.

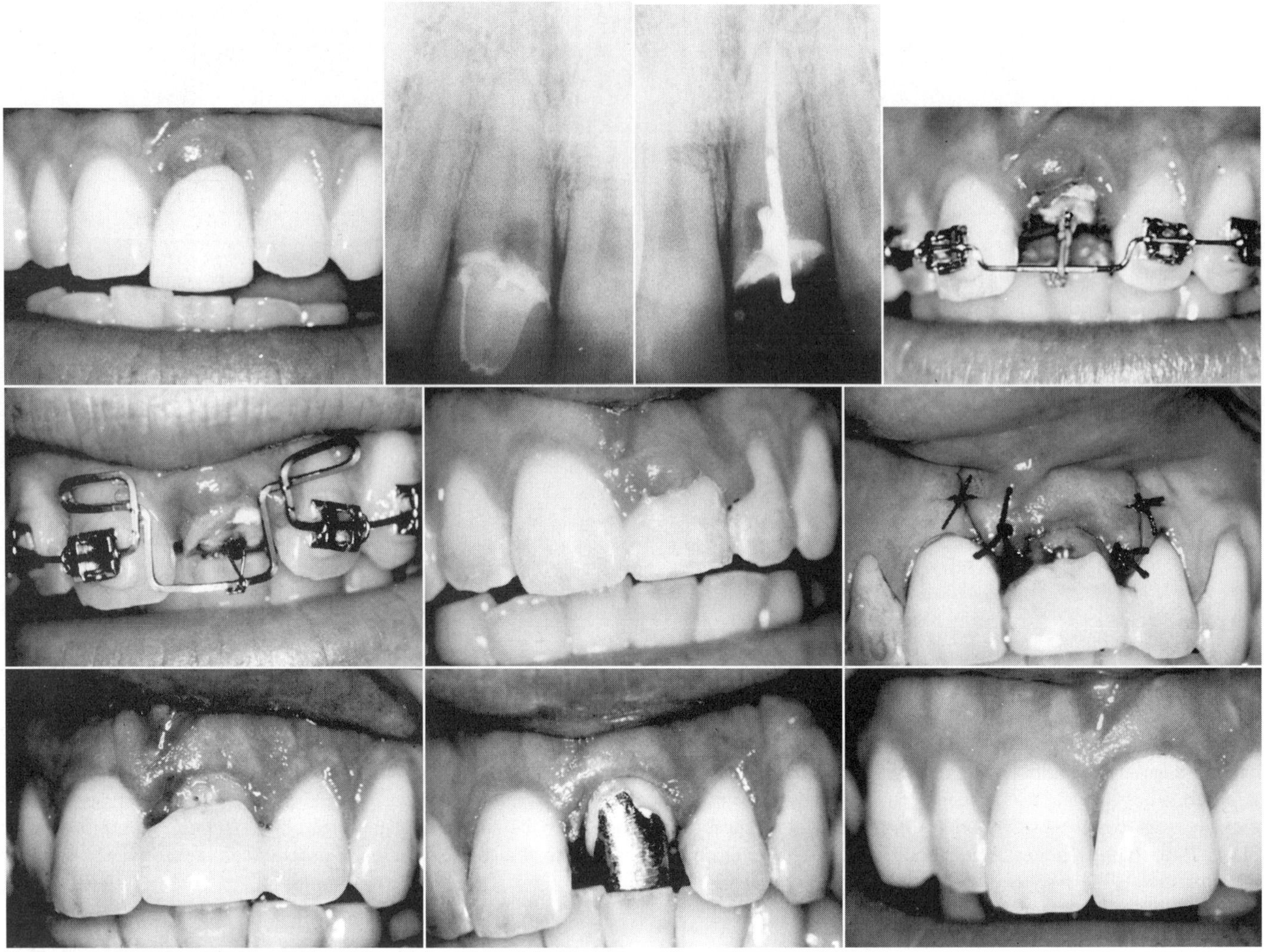

A,B C,
E,F G
H,I J

FIGURE 18-15 Forced eruption can move a tooth that is unrestorable because of subgingival pathology into a position that allows treatment. **A,** This central incisor had a crown placed after being chipped previously, but now showed gingival inflammation and elongation. **B,** A periapical radiograph revealed internal root resorption below the crown margin. The treatment plan was **C,** Endodontic treatment to arrest the internal resorption, then elongation of the root so that a new crown margin could be placed on sound root structure. **D,** Initially, an elastomeric tie was used from an archwire segment to an attachment on the post that was cemented in the root canal; then **E,** Loops in a flexible rectangular wire (17 × 25 beta-Ti) were employed for quicker and more efficient tooth movement. **F,** 4 mm elongation occurred in as many weeks, and a temporary restoration was placed. **G, H,** An apically repositioned flap was used to create the correct gingival contour, then **I** to **J,** A coping and final ceramic crown were prepared. Extraction of the tooth was avoided and a highly esthetic restoration was possible.

Orthodontic Technique

Since extrusion is the tooth movement that occurs most readily and intrusion the movement that occurs least readily, ample anchorage is usually available from adjacent teeth. The appliance needs to be quite rigid over the anchor teeth, and flexible where it attaches to the tooth that is being extruded. A continuous flexible archwire (see Figure 18-15) produces the desired extrusion but must be managed carefully because it also tends to tip the adjacent teeth toward the tooth being extruded, reducing the space for subsequent restorations and disturbing the interproximal contacts within the arch (Figure 18-16, *A*). A flexible cantilever spring to extrude a tooth (Figure 18-16, *B*), or a rigid stabilizing wire and an auxiliary elastomeric module or spring for extrusion (Figure 18-16, *C*) provide better control.

Two methods are suggested for extrusion in uncomplicated cases. The first employs a stabilizing wire, 19 × 25 or 21 × 25 stainless steel, bonded directly to the facial surface of the adjacent teeth (Figure 18-17).[7] A post and core with temporary crown and pin is placed on the tooth to be extruded, and an elastomeric module is used to extrude the tooth. This appliance is simple and provides excellent control of anchor teeth, but better control can be obtained when orthodontic brackets are used.

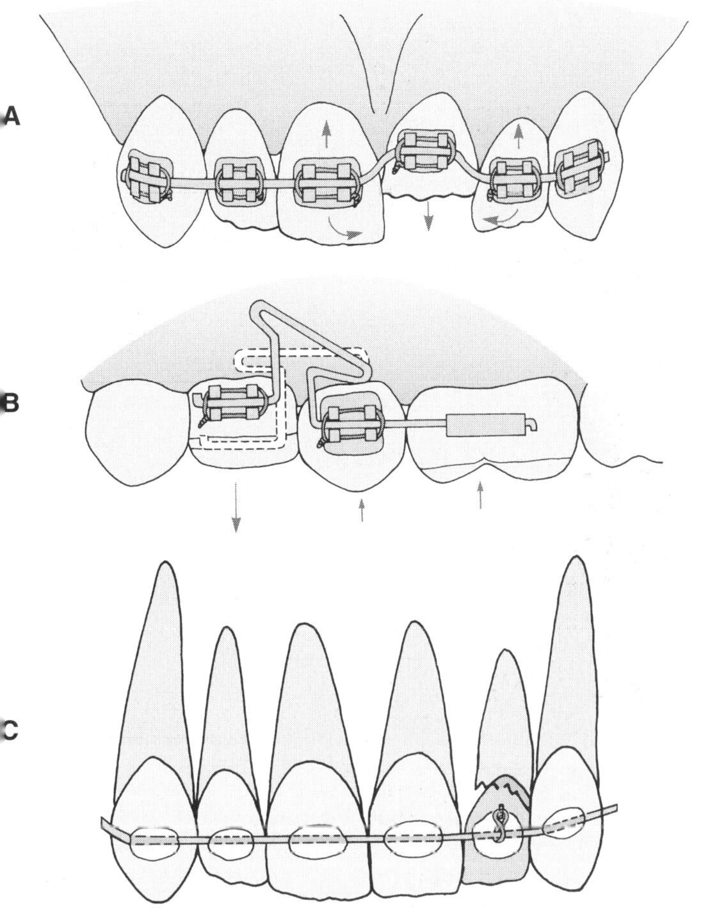

FIGURE 18-16 **A,** Although a straight orthodontic wire activated apically will produce an extrusive force on a tooth, it will also cause the teeth on either side to tip toward each other, reducing the space available for the extruding tooth. **B,** A modified T-loop in a rectangular wire (17 × 25 steel in 18 slot brackets, 19 × 25 beta-Ti in 22 slot) will extrude a tooth while controlling mesio-distal tipping. **C,** Extrusion also can be done without conventional orthodontic attachments, by bonding a 19 × 25 steel stabilizing wire directly to the facial surface of adjacent teeth. An elastomeric module is stretched between the stabilizing wire and a pin placed directly into the crown of the tooth to be extruded. If a temporary crown is used for better esthetics while the extrusion is being done, it must be progressively cut away to make the tooth movement possible. (**C,** courtesy Dr. L. Osterle.)

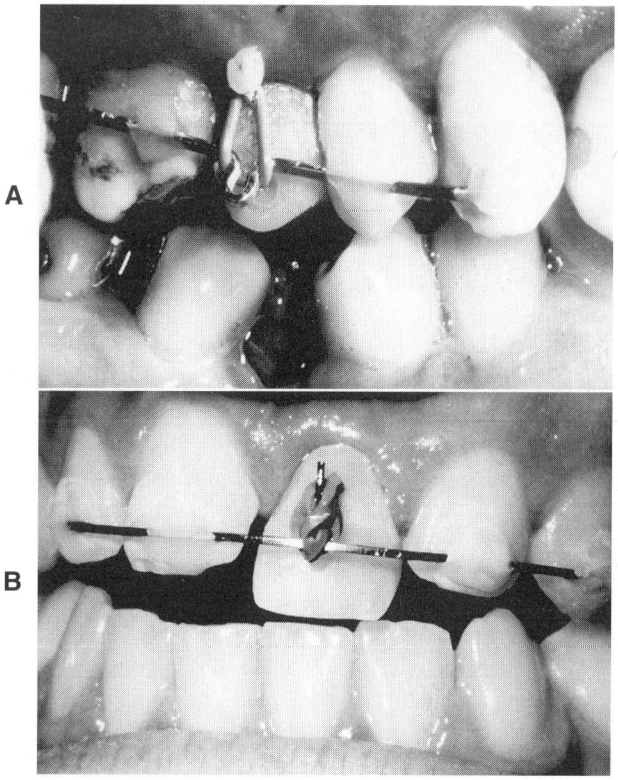

FIGURE 18-17 Possible approaches to Extrusion of a single tooth can be done without conventional orthodontic attachments, by bonding a 19 × 25 steel stabilizing wire directly to the facial surface of adjacent teeth. **A,** An elastomeric module is stretched between the stabilizing wire and a pin placed directly into the crown of the tooth to be extruded, in this case a fractured maxillary premolar. **B,** The same technique can be used to extrude an incisor. A temporary restoration placed on the tooth while it is being extruded needs to be reduced at frequent intervals. (Courtesy Dr. L. Osterle.)

The alternative is to bond brackets to the anchor teeth, bond an attachment (often a button rather than a bracket) to the tooth to be extruded, and use interarch elastics (Figure 18-18) or a flexible archwire (Figure 18-19). If the buccal surface of the tooth to be extruded is intact, a bracket should be bonded as far gingivally as possible.

If the crown of a posterior tooth is hopelessly destroyed, an orthodontic band with a bracket usually can be placed over the remaining root surface. An orthodontic band has the benefit of helping isolation procedures during emergency endodontic treatment. Once endodontic treatment is completed, a pin in the tooth can be used for the attachment, and a temporary crown can be placed if needed for esthetics. Adjacent teeth are bonded to serve as the anchor unit.

With any technique for forced eruption, the patient must be seen every 1 to 2 weeks to reduce the occlusal surface of the tooth being extruded if this is needed (see Figure 18-17), control inflammation and monitor progress. After active tooth movement has been completed, at least 3 but not more than 6 weeks of stabilization is needed to allow reorganization of the periodontal ligament. If periodontal surgery is needed to recontour the alveolar bone and/or reposition the gingiva, this can be done 1 month after completion of the extrusion. As with molar uprighting, it is better to complete the definitive prosthetic treatment without extensive delay.

A

B

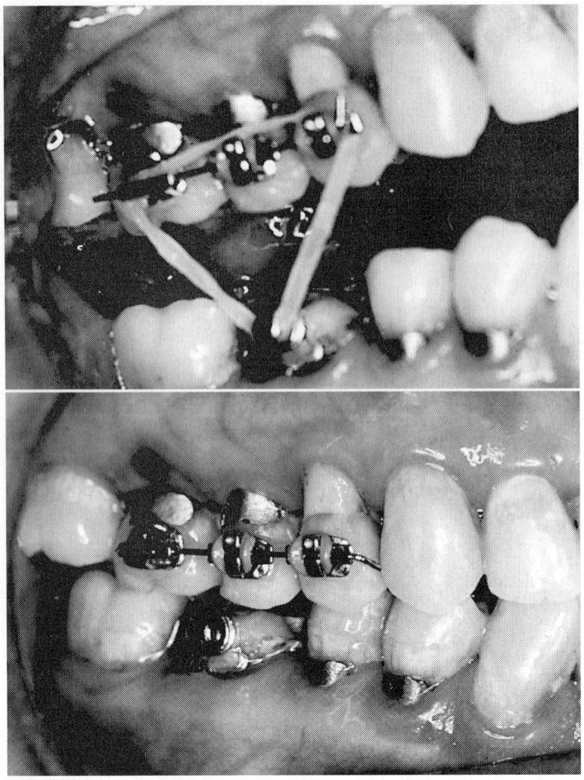

Figure 18-18 For this lady in her 60s, the facial surface of a lower first molar fractured to below the gingival margin. **A,** The maxillary premolars and first molar were bonded and stabilized, and an elastic to a button bonded on the lower molar was used to elongate it to the point, **B,** The fracture line was exposed and a satisfactory crown preparation was possible.

A

B

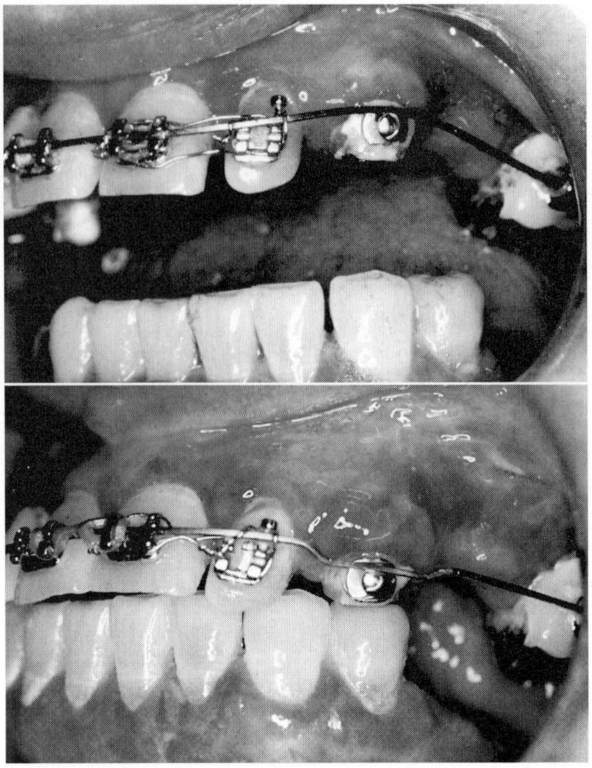

Figure 18-19 A bridge attached to the maxillary left canine failed because of caries beneath the crown on the canine tooth. After it was treated endodontically, a button was bonded to an amalgam temporary build-up on the root, and **A,** a continuous arch wire (17 × 25 beta-Ti) was used to extrude the tooth to the point that a permanent restoration could be placed. **B,** At that point all the amalgam build-up had been removed, and the tooth had been elongated 5 mm.

Alignment of Anterior Teeth

Anterior Diastema Closure and Space Redistribution

The major indication for adjunctive orthodontic treatment to correct malaligned anterior teeth is preparation for build-ups, veneers or implants to improve the appearance of the maxillary incisor teeth. The most frequent problem is a maxillary central diastema, often further complicated by irregular spacing related to small or missing lateral incisors.

A "diagnostic setup" is very helpful in planning the correction of such problems. For this procedure, the study casts are duplicated and the malaligned teeth are carefully cut from the model, repositioned and the teeth are then waxed back onto the cast in a new position. If digital casts are available, a modern alternative is to do this on a computer screen (see Figure 14-1), and this is part of routine treatment planning when a sequence of clear aligners will be used in comprehensive treatment (see below). This allows evaluation of the feasibility of the orthodontic treatment in light of the crown and root movements required, the anchorage available, the periodontal support for each tooth, and the possible occlusal interferences.

There are two possible orthodontic techniques: a partial fixed appliance, typically with bonded brackets on the maxillary incisors and a bonded tube on the first molars for additional anchorage control; or a sequence of clear aligners. With a fixed appliance, initial alignment is carried out using a light wire such as 16 mil A-NiTi or 17.5 mil braided steel. This wire is replaced, after the teeth are aligned, with a 16 or 18 mil round steel wire along which the teeth are repositioned using elastomeric modules or coil springs (Figure 18-20). There is always a tendency for the space to reopen after any degree of diastema closure. Bonding a flexible wire on the lingual of the incisors as a semi-permanent retainer is recommended (see Figure 17-12).

An alternative is the use of a sequence of clear aligners. These are available commercially in two ways: (1) for modest amounts of tooth movement, aligners made by re-setting the teeth on dental casts that can be reshaped by the doctor (see Figure 11-12) and (2) for more extensive tooth movement, a set of 15-50 aligners fabricated on stereolithographic models created from computer models of the projected tooth movement (Invisalign, OrthoClear). In adjunctive treatment, the first method is potentially quite useful. The second method, discussed in more detail in the latter part of this chapter, is almost prohibitively expensive unless comprehensive treatment is planned.

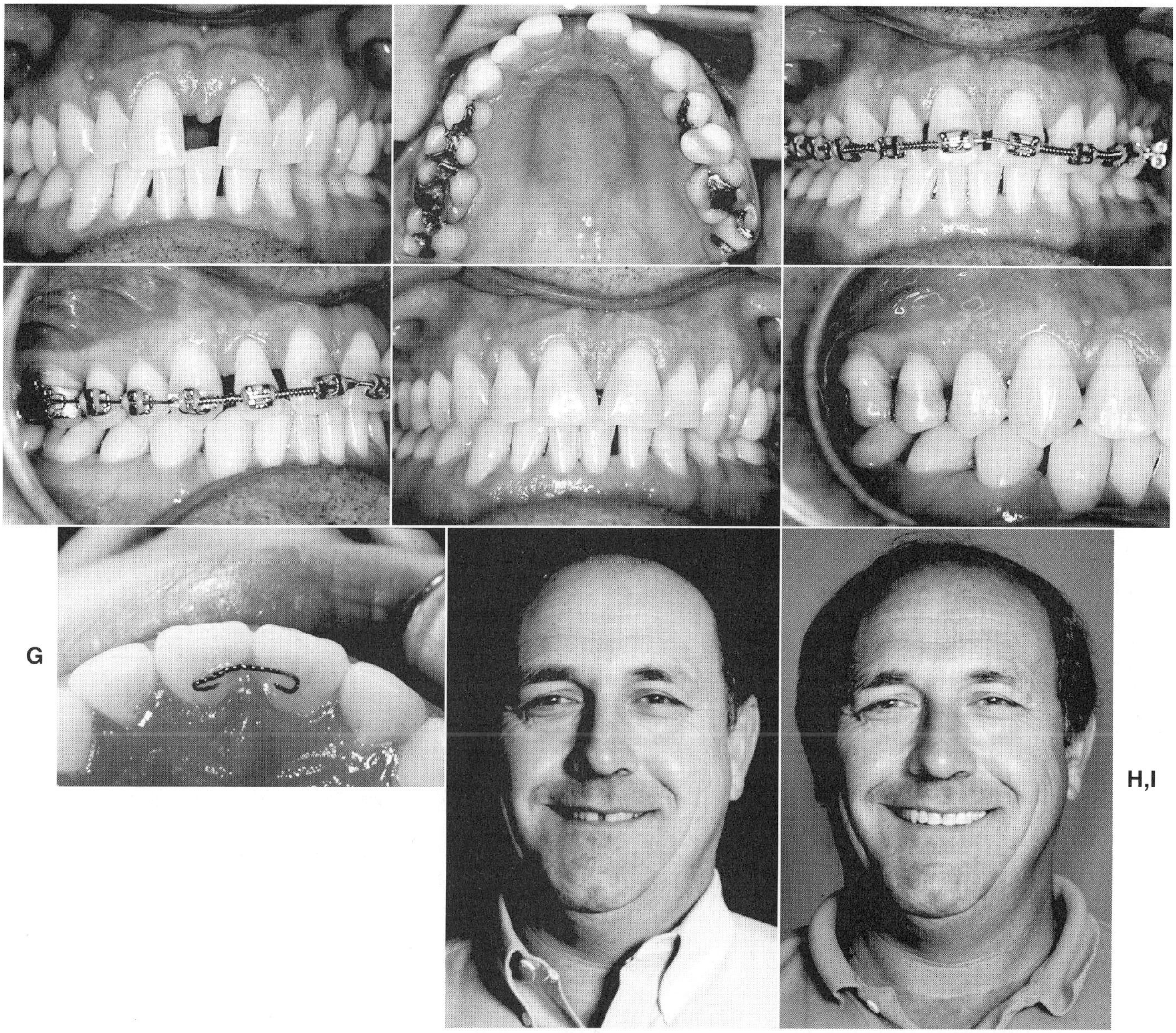

Figure 18-20 If spacing of maxillary incisors is related to small teeth and a tooth-size discrepancy, composite build-ups are an excellent solution, but satisfactory esthetics may require redistribution of the space before the restorations are placed, as in this patient who was concerned about his large central diastema. **A** and **B,** Before treatment, age 48; **C** and **D,** Redistribution of the space using a fixed appliance with coil springs on a 16 mil steel archwire, immediately before removal of the orthodontic appliance and placement of the restorations (to be done the same day). For this patient, a 17.5 mil multistrand wire was used for initial alignment, before the coil springs were placed; **E** and **F,** Completed restorations (composite build-ups). **G,** Note the retainer of bonded 21.5 mil multistrand wire on the lingual of the central incisors to prevent partial reopening of the midline space. Surgical revision of the frenum was not performed, partially in deference to the patient's age. **H,** Appearance on smile before and **I,** after treatment.

Alignment of Crowded, Rotated, and Displaced Incisors

As a rule, spacing is the problem when maxillary incisors need realignment to facilitate other treatment. Crowding usually is the problem when alignment of lower incisors is considered, to provide access for restorations, achieve better occlusion, or enable the patient to maintain the teeth. In some cases, alignment of incisors in both arches must be considered. The key question is whether the crowding should be resolved by expanding the arch, removing some interproximal enamel from each tooth to provide space,[8] or removing one lower incisor.

Expansion of a crowded incisor segment can be done with clear aligners, but if only the lower arch is to be treated, the esthetics of the appliance is not a consideration, and a partial fixed appliance is more efficient and cost-effective (Figure 18-21). A segment of A-NiTi wire, with stops to make it slightly advanced, usually is the best way to bring the teeth

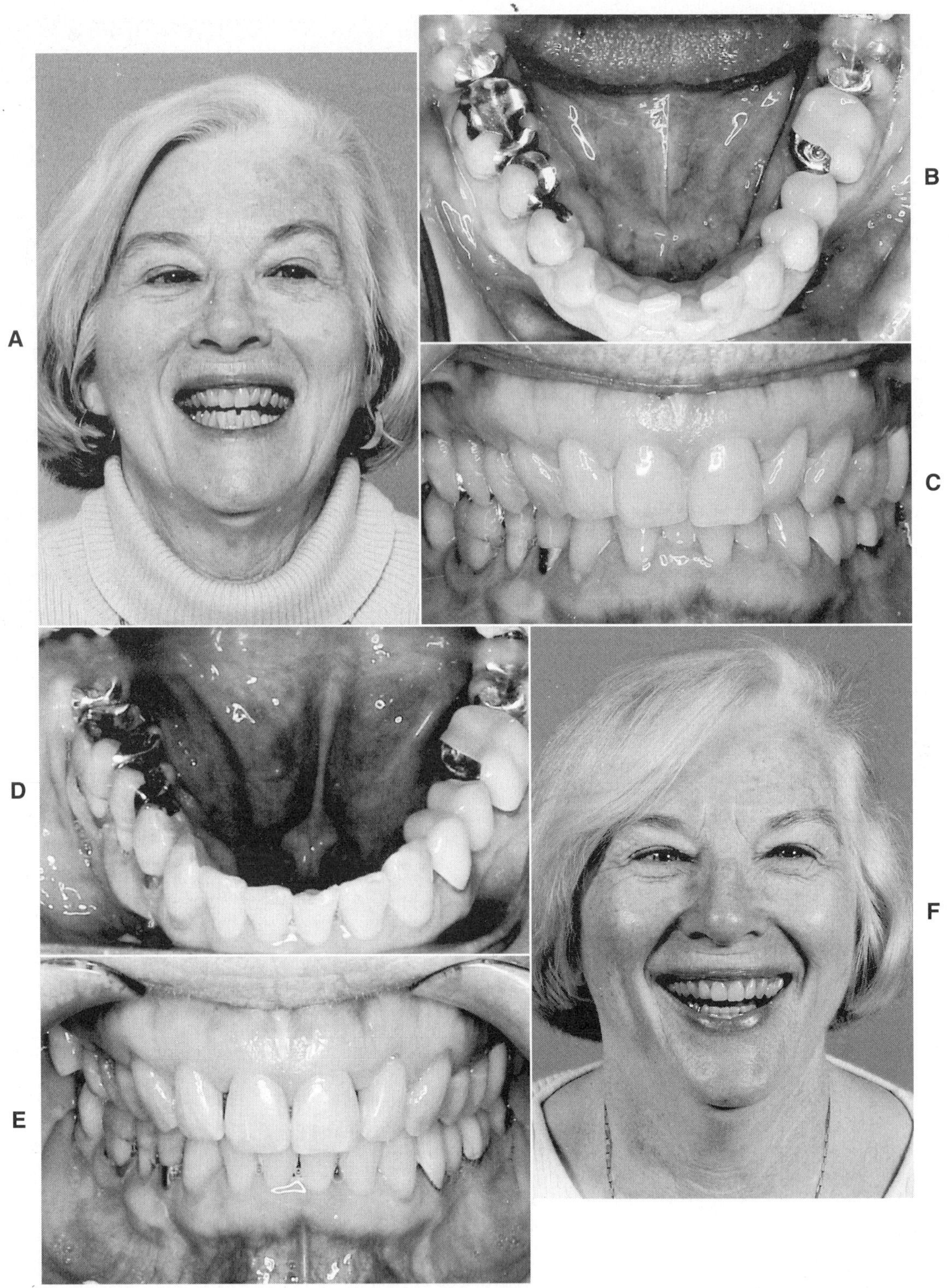

FIGURE 18-21 The decision to extract a damaged lower incisor in an adult with crowding and use the space to align the remaining teeth, or to align the teeth and restore the damaged one, has an esthetic component because the lower incisors are visible on smile in older individuals. In this patient, aligning the lower incisors without extraction would also require aligning the upper incisors—but this expansion would increase lip support and improve the overall facial appearance as well as the dental appearance. **A,** Smile before treatment, after loss of one corner of the lower right central incisor; **B,** Mandibular occlusal view; **C,** Frontal view. Note the moderately deep bite and lack of overjet. The restorative dentist sought orthodontic consultation, thinking that extraction of the damaged tooth might be the best plan. The patient wanted the best esthetic result, and accepted a period of treatment with a fixed appliance on both arches, after which the incisor would be restored. The orthodontic alignment required 5 months. **D,** Mandibular occlusal view after alignment; **E,** Frontal view; **F,** Smile after restoration was completed.

into alignment. For root positioning, this should be succeeded by a segment of rectangular NiTi wire.

Stripping the contact points of the teeth to remove enamel can provide space for alignment of mildly irregular lower incisors, and either a fixed appliance or a clear aligner sequence can provide the tooth movement. This should be undertaken with caution, however, because it may have an undesirable effect on overjet, overbite, posterior intercuspation, and esthetics. In severe crowding, removing one lower incisor and using the space to align the other three incisors can produce a satisfactory result (Figure 18-22). The treatment time and difficulty, whatever the type of appliance, put this at or across the border of comprehensive treatment. Neither stripping nor incisor extraction should be undertaken without a diagnostic set-up to verify feasibility.

Remember that stretched gingival fibers are a potent force for relapse after rotations have been corrected, and that good long-term stability may require a fiberotomy (see Chapter 16). Whether clear aligners or a fixed appliance was used, retention is necessary until restorative or other treatment is completed. This can be the final aligner in a sequence, a molded thermoplastic retainer after a fixed appliance is removed, a canine-to-canine clip retainer or a bonded fixed retainer (see Chapter 17).

Comprehensive Treatment in Adults: Why Do They Seek It?

For our purposes in this chapter, comprehensive orthodontic treatment is defined as treatment that involves all the teeth rather than selected areas (i.e., a complete rather than a partial orthodontic appliance is needed), and will require more than a few months for completion. That does not mean other dental treatment is not part of the overall plan. The major distinction between adjunctive and comprehensive orthodontics is how extensive the orthodontic treatment will be, not the extent to which other dental treatment also will be required.

Adults who seek comprehensive orthodontics can be divided into two major groups, which overlap to some extent:

1. A younger group (age 20 to early 40s) whose goal is to improve their quality of life. This usually means improving their dental and facial appearance to overcome perceived social handicaps. Often they wanted orthodontic treatment at an earlier age but didn't get it. A typical comment is that "I always wanted treatment, and now that I have a good job and can afford it, I really want to get these teeth fixed". Because appearance is important, these patients are the ones most likely to request an esthetic or invisible appliance.
2. An older group (30s to 60s) whose goal is to keep what they have. Typically, they have experienced periodontal disease that would be easier to keep under control if their teeth were not so malaligned, have lost some teeth that are proving difficult to replace because of malocclusion, or both. Integration of extensive orthodontics into a larger treatment plan, therefore, usually is required. The appearance of the teeth and face may not be the primary concern, but it is not unimportant. These patients usually are quite willing to tolerate a visible orthodontic appliance if the appearance of their teeth will be improved at the end of treatment.

Psychological Considerations

A major motivation for orthodontic treatment of younger patients is the parents' desire to do the best they can for their children. The typical child or adolescent accepts orthodontics in about the same rather passive way that he or she accepts going to school, summer camp, and the inevitable junior high school dance—as just another in the series of events that one must endure while growing up. Occasionally, of course, an adolescent actively resists orthodontic treatment, and the result can be unfortunate for all concerned if the treatment becomes the focus of an adolescent rebellion. In most instances, however, children tend not to become emotionally involved in their treatment.

Adults in both the younger and older groups, in contrast, seek comprehensive orthodontic treatment because they themselves want something. For the younger group who are trying to improve their lot in life, that something is not always clearly expressed, and in fact some young adults have a remarkably elaborate hidden set of motivations. It is important to explore why an individual wants treatment, and why now as opposed to some other time, to avoid setting up a situation in which the patient's expectations from treatment cannot possibly be met. Sometimes orthodontic treatment is sought as a last-ditch effort to improve personal appearance to deal with a series of complicated social problems. Orthodontic treatment obviously cannot be relied on to repair personal relationships, save jobs or overcome a series of financial disasters. If the prospective patient has unrealistic expectations of that sort, it is much better to deal with them sooner rather than later.

Most adults in both the younger and older groups, fortunately, understand why they want orthodontics and are realistic about what they can obtain from it. One might expect those who seek treatment to be less secure and less well adjusted than the average adult, but for the most part, they have a more positive self-image than average.[9] It apparently takes a good deal of ego strength to seek orthodontic treatment as an adult, and ego strength rather than weakness characterizes most potential adult patients. A patient who seeks treatment primarily because he or she wants it (internal motivation) is more likely to respond well psychologically than a patient whose motivation is the urging of others or the expected impact of treatment on others (external motivation). External motivation is often accompanied by an increasing impact of the orthodontic problem on per-eating and chewing. To produce myofascial pain, the patient must be clenching or grinding the teeth for many hours per day, presumably as a response to stress. Great variations are seen in the way different individuals respond to stress, both in the organ system that feels the strain (those who develop an ulcerated colon rarely have TMD also) and in the amount of stress that can be tolerated before symptoms appear (tense individuals develop stress-related symptoms before their relaxed colleagues do). For this reason, it is impossible to say that occlusal discrepancies of any given degree will lead to TMD symptoms.

It is possible to demonstrate that some types of occlusal discrepancies predispose patients who clench or grind their teeth to the development of TMD symptoms. It must be kept in mind, however, that it takes two factors to produce myofascial pain: an occlusal discrepancy *and* a patient who clenches or grinds the teeth. Perhaps the most compelling argument against malocclusion as a primary cause of TMD is the observation that TMD is no more prevalent in patients with severe malocclusion than in the general population.[11] The dictum "let your teeth alone" would solve myofascial pain problems if it could be followed by the patient.

Treatment Indications

From this perspective, three broad approaches to myofascial pain symptoms can be considered: reducing the amount of stress; reducing the patient's reaction to the stress; or improving the occlusion, thereby making it harder for the patient to hurt himself or herself. Drastic alteration of the occlusion, by either restorative dental procedures or orthodontics, is logical only if the less invasive stress-control and stress-adaptation approaches have failed. In that circumstance, orthodontic treatment to alter the occlusion so that the patient can better tolerate parafunctional activity may be worth attempting. In some instances, that may involve orthognathic surgery to reposition the jaws.

The extent to which TMD symptoms in many adults disappear when comprehensive orthodontic treatment begins can be surprising and overly gratifying to those who do not understand the etiology of myofascial pain. Orthodontic intervention can appear almost magical in the way that TMD symptoms disappear long before the occlusal relationships have been corrected. The explanation is simple—orthodontic treatment makes the teeth sore, grinding or clenching sensitive teeth as a means of handling stress does not produce the same subconscious gratification as previously, the parafunctional activity stops, and the symptoms vanish. The changing occlusal relationships also contribute to breaking up the habit patterns that contributed to the muscle fatigue and pain. No matter what the type of orthodontic treatment, symptoms are unlikely to be present while movement of a significant number of teeth is occurring, as long as treatment that produces strongly deflective contacts is avoided. Prolonged use of Class II or Class III elastics may not be well tolerated in adults who have had TMD problems and should be avoided (for that matter, prolonged use of elastics should be avoided in most other adult patients as well).

A

B

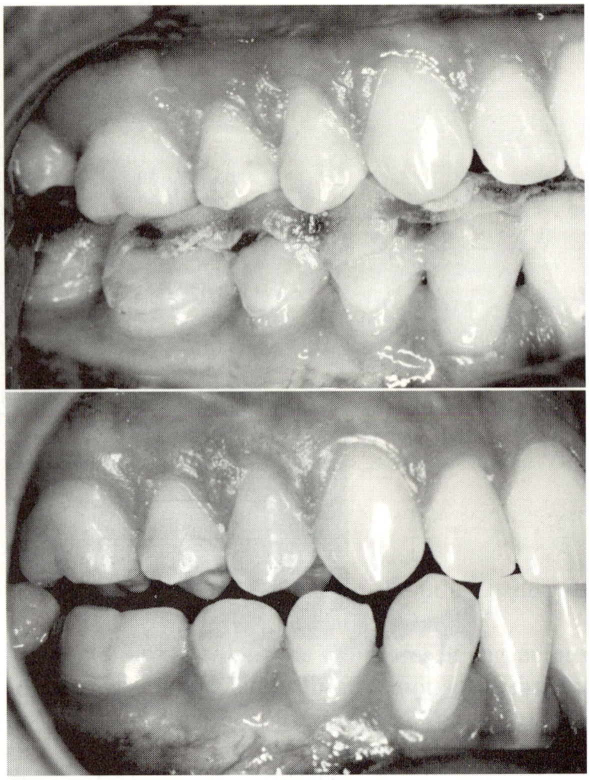

FIGURE 18-27 Occlusal relationships in a 24-year-old woman who had worn a splint covering only her posterior teeth for the previous 18 months. Note the posterior open bite when the splint was taken out. This was created by a combination of intrusion of the posterior teeth and further eruption of the anterior teeth. Discarding the splint had become impossible.

The moment of truth for TMD patients who have had orthodontic treatment comes some time after the orthodontics is completed, when the clenching and grinding that originally caused the problem tend to recur. At that point, even if the occlusal relationships have been significantly improved, it may be impossible to keep the patient from moving into extreme jaw positions and engaging in parafunctional activity that produces pain. The use of interocclusal splints in this situation may be the only way to keep symptoms from recurring. In short, the miraculous cure that orthodontic treatment often provides for myofascial pain tends to disappear with the appliance. Those who have had symptoms in the past are always at risk of having them recur.

Occasionally, orthodontic treatment is made more complicated by previous splint therapy for TMD problems. If an occlusal splint for TMD symptoms covers the posterior but not the anterior teeth, the anterior teeth that have been taken out of occlusion begin to erupt again and may come back into occlusion even though the posterior teeth are still separated (Figure 18-27). Clinically, it may appear that the posterior teeth are being intruded, but incisor eruption usually

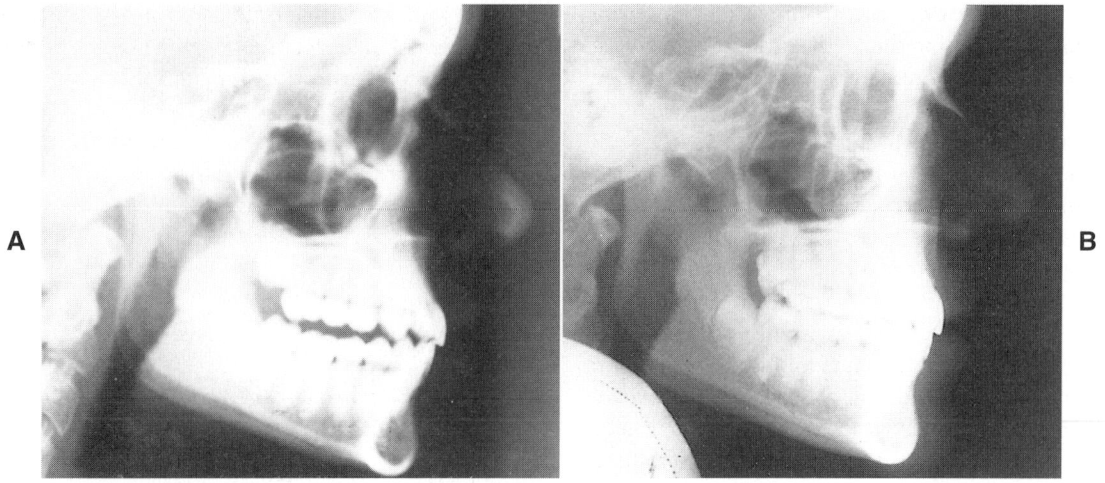

Figure 18-28 Cephalometric films for the patient shown in Figure 18-26. **A,** Before and **(B)** after orthodontic treatment to extrude the posterior teeth back into occlusion.

is a greater contributor to the development of posterior open bite. In only a few months, the patient may end up in a situation in which discarding the splint has become impossible. Then the only treatment possibilities are elongation of the posterior teeth, either with crowns or orthodontic extrusion, or intrusion of the anterior teeth.

Orthodontic intervention at this stage is difficult, because TMD symptoms are likely to develop immediately if the splint is removed, and it is not possible to elongate the posterior teeth orthodontically without discarding or cutting down the splint. Placing orthodontic attachments on the posterior teeth and using light vertical elastics to the posterior segments (Figure 18-28) can be used to bring the posterior teeth back into occlusion, if the patient can tolerate this treatment. Some reintrusion of the elongated anterior teeth is likely to occur, but a significant increase in face height is often maintained. Although permanently increasing the vertical dimension to control disk displacement can be accomplished in this way, this treatment plan should be used with extreme caution.

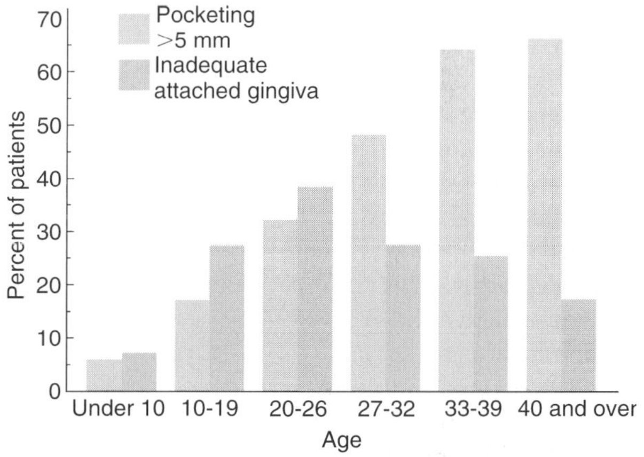

Figure 18-29 The prevalence of periodontal pockets greater than 5 mm and inadequate attached gingiva as a function of age in 1,000 consecutive patients with severe orthodontic problems who were referred to the university of north carolina dentofacial clinic for possible surgical-orthodontic treatment. (Redrawn from Morarity JD, Simpson DM. J Dent Res 63:[Special Issue A, #1249], 1984.)

Periodontal Considerations

Periodontal problems are rarely a major concern during orthodontic treatment of children and adolescents, because periodontal disease usually does not arise at an early age and tissue resistance is higher in younger patients. For the same reasons, periodontal considerations are increasingly important as patients become older, regardless of whether periodontal problems were a motivating factor for orthodontic treatment.

The prevalence of periodontal disease as a function of age in a large group of potential orthodontic patients with severe malocclusion is shown in Figure 18-29. Note that up to the late thirties, there is nearly a straight-line relationship between age and periodontal pocketing (defined here as the presence of pockets greater than 5 mm). In contrast, the prevalence of mucogingival problems peaks in the twenties. The odds are that any patient over the age of 35 has some periodontal problems that could affect orthodontic treatment, and mucogingival considerations are important in treatment of the younger adult group.

Periodontal disease is not a continuous and steadily progressive degenerative process.[12] Instead, it is characterized by episodes of acute attack on some but usually not all areas of the mouth, followed by quiescent periods. It is obviously important to identify high-risk patients and high-risk sites. At present, persistent bleeding on probing is the best indicator of active and presumably progressive disease. New diagnostic procedures to evaluate subgingival plaque and crevicular fluids for the presence of indicator bacteria, enzymes, or other chemical mediators show promise and are likely to be clinically useful in the near future. There appear to be at least three risk groups in the population: those with rapid progression (about 10%), those with moderate progression (the great majority, about 80%), and those with no progression despite the presence of gingival inflammation (about 10%).[13]

There is no contraindication to treating adults who have had periodontal disease and bone loss, as long as the disease has been brought under control (Figure 18-30). Progression of untreated periodontal breakdown must be anticipated, however, and the periodontal situation must receive major attention in planning and executing orthodontic treatment for all adults.

Treatment of Patients With Minimal Periodontal Involvement

Any patient undergoing orthodontic treatment must take extra care to clean the teeth, but this is even more important in adult orthodontics. Bacterial plaque is the main etiologic factor in periodontal breakdown, and plaque-induced gingivitis is the first step in the disease process. Orthodontic appliances simultaneously make maintenance of oral hygiene more difficult and more important. In children and adolescents, even if gingivitis develops in response to the presence of orthodontic appliances, it almost never extends into periodontitis. This cannot be taken for granted in adults, no matter how good their initial periodontal condition.[14]

The periodontal evaluation of a potential adult orthodontic patient must include not only the response to periodontal probing but also the level and condition of the attached gingiva. Labial movement of incisors in some patients can be followed by gingival recession and loss of attachment. The risk is greatest when irregular teeth are aligned by expanding the dental arch.

The present concept is that gingival recession occurs secondarily to an alveolar bone dehiscence, if overlying tissues are stressed. The stress can be due to any of several causes. Major possibilities are toothbrush trauma, plaque-induced inflammation, or the stretching and thinning of the gingiva that might be created by labial tooth movement. Once recession begins, it can progress rapidly, especially if there is little or no keratinized attached gingiva and the attachment is only alveolar mucosa.

It was once thought that the width of the gingival attachment determined whether recession occurred. The concept now is that two characteristics are important: the width of the attached gingiva (not all keratinized gingiva is attached), and the thickness of the gingival tissue. The width of the attached gingiva can be observed most readily by inserting a periodontal probe and observing the distance between the point at which the gingival attachment is encountered and the point at which the alveolar mucosa begins. Lower incisors in patients with a prominent chin and compensation in the form of lingual tipping of these teeth (Figure 18-31) are at particular risk of recession, and thin gingival tissue probably is the reason.

For adult orthodontic patients, it is much better to prevent gingival recession than to try to correct it later. For this reason, a gingival graft (Figure 18-32) must be considered in adults with minimal attached gingiva or thin tissue, particularly those for whom arch expansion will be used to align incisors and those who will have surgical mandibular advancement or genioplasty (see Chapter 19).

Moderate Periodontal Involvement

Before orthodontic treatment is attempted for patients who have preexisting periodontal problems, dental and periodontal disease must be brought under control. Preliminary periodontal therapy can include all aspects of periodontal treatment except osseous surgery. It is important to remove all calculus and other irritants from periodontal pockets before any tooth movement is attempted, and it is often wise to use surgical flaps to expose these areas to ensure the best possible scaling. Treatment procedures to facilitate the patient's long-term maintenance, like osseous recontouring or repositioned flaps to compensate for areas of gingival recession, are best deferred until the final occlusal relationships have been established. A period of observation following preliminary periodontal treatment, to make sure that the patient is adequately controlled and to allow healing after the periodontal therapy, should precede comprehensive orthodontics.

Disease control also requires endodontic treatment of any pulpally involved teeth. There is no contraindication to the orthodontic movement of an endodontically treated tooth, so root canal therapy before orthodontics will cause no problems. Attempting to move a pulpally involved tooth, however, is likely to cause a flare-up of the periapical condition.

The general guideline for preliminary restorative treatment is that temporary restorations should be placed to control caries, with the definitive restorative dentistry delayed until after the orthodontic phase of treatment. Temporary restoration, however, should not be taken to mean the use of a short-lived material that will last only a few months. Composite resin is now the preferred temporary restorative material while orthodontics is being carried out. Cast restorations should be delayed until after the final occlusal relationships have been established by orthodontic treatment.

Because the margins of bands can make periodontal maintenance more difficult, it usually is better to use a fully bonded orthodontic appliance for periodontally involved adults. Self-ligating brackets or steel ligatures also are preferred for periodontally involved patients rather than elastomeric rings to retain orthodontic archwires, because patients with elastomeric rings have higher levels of microorganisms in gingival plaque.[15]

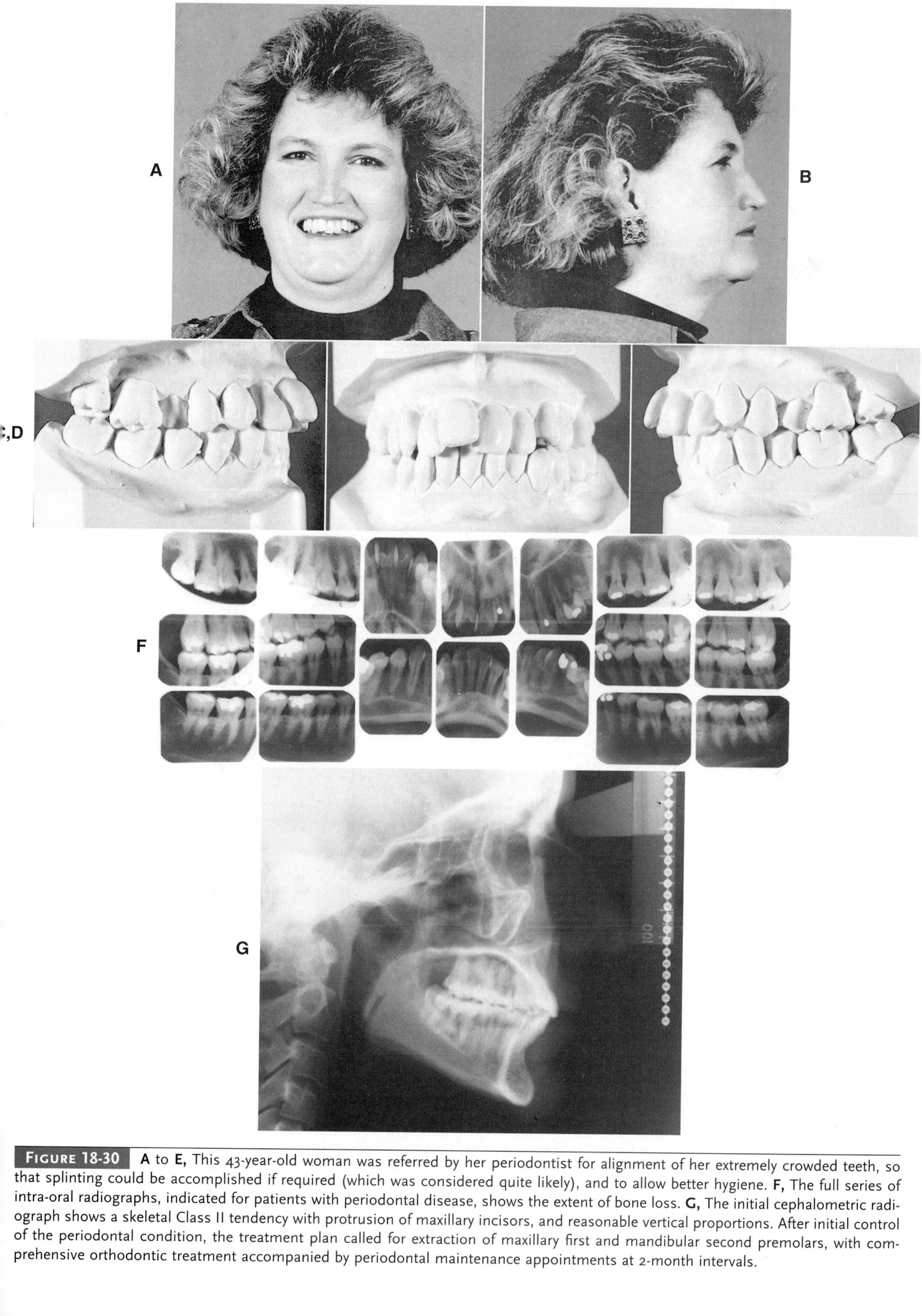

FIGURE 18-30 **A** to **E,** This 43-year-old woman was referred by her periodontist for alignment of her extremely crowded teeth, so that splinting could be accomplished if required (which was considered quite likely), and to allow better hygiene. **F,** The full series of intra-oral radiographs, indicated for patients with periodontal disease, shows the extent of bone loss. **G,** The initial cephalometric radiograph shows a skeletal Class II tendency with protrusion of maxillary incisors, and reasonable vertical proportions. After initial control of the periodontal condition, the treatment plan called for extraction of maxillary first and mandibular second premolars, with comprehensive orthodontic treatment accompanied by periodontal maintenance appointments at 2-month intervals.

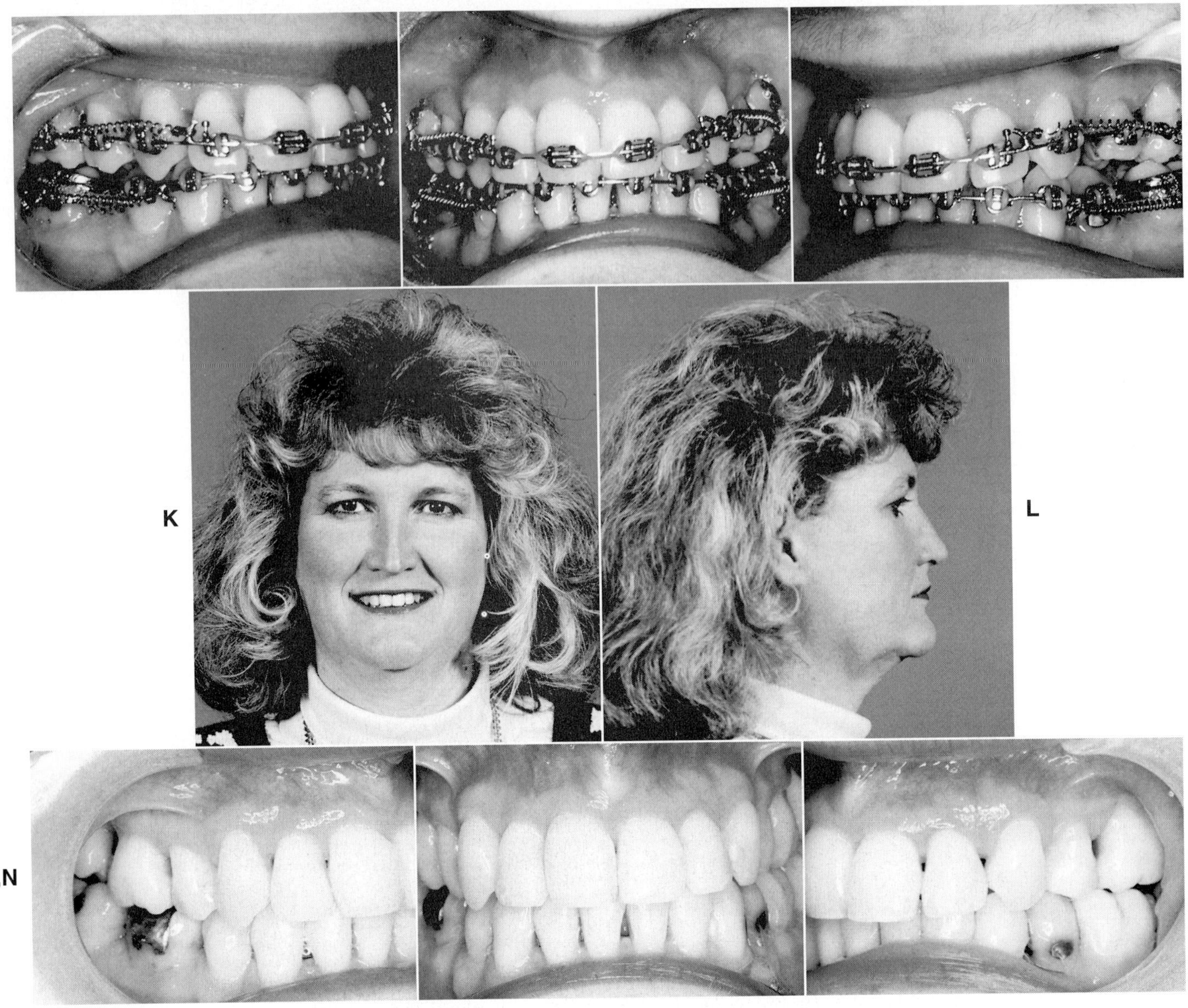

Figure 18-30 **cont'd H** to **J,** To keep orthodontic forces as light as possible, space closure was carried out using 150-gm super-elastic coil springs; after the spaces were closed, light Class II elastics also were employed for 3 months. **K** to **O,** After 21 months of orthodontic treatment, both occlusion and alignment were greatly improved, and the patient was pleased with the change in dental and facial appearance.

During comprehensive orthodontics, a patient with moderate periodontal problems must be on a maintenance schedule, with the frequency of cleaning and scaling depending on the severity of the periodontal disease. Periodontal maintenance therapy at 2- to 4-month intervals is the usual plan. Adjunctive chemical agents between appointments (including chlorhexidine if needed) also should be considered.

Severe Periodontal Involvement

The general approach to treatment for patients with severe periodontal involvement is the same as that outlined earlier, but the treatment itself must be modified in two ways: (1) periodontal maintenance should be scheduled at more frequent intervals, perhaps with the patient being seen as frequently for periodontal maintenance as for orthodontic appliance adjustments (i.e., every 4 to 6 weeks); and (2) orthodontic treatment goals and mechanics must be modified to keep orthodontic forces to an absolute minimum, because the reduced area of the periodontal ligament (PDL) after significant bone loss means higher pressure in the PDL from any force (Figure 18-33). Sometimes it is helpful to temporarily retain a tooth that is hopelessly involved periodontally, using it to help support an orthodontic appliance that will contribute to saving other teeth.

P

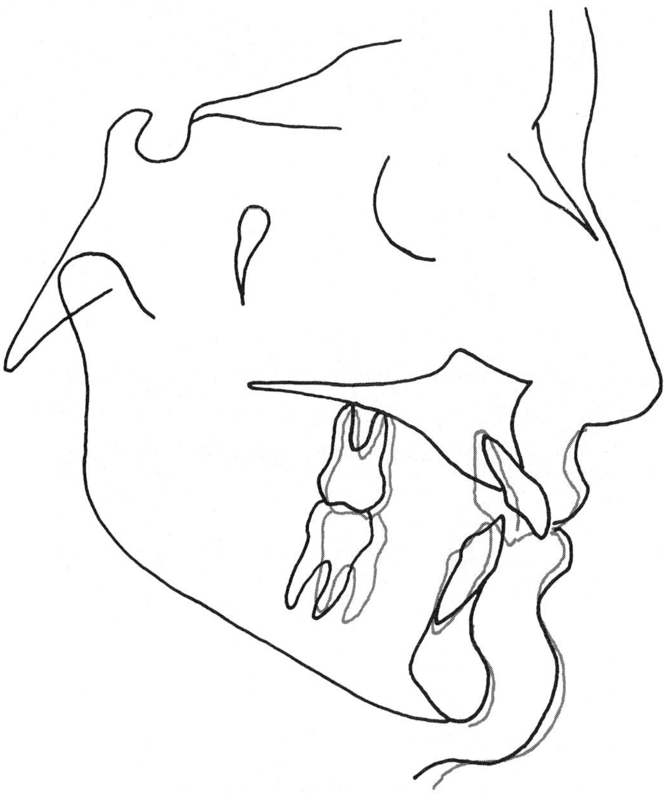

Q

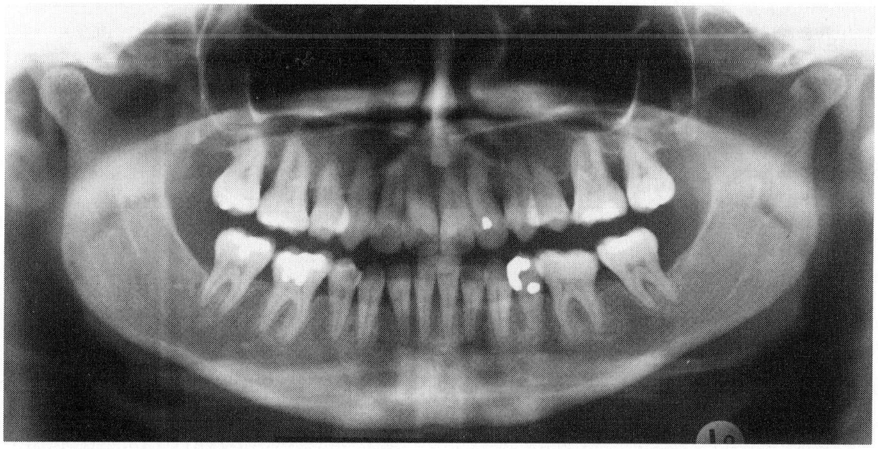

FIGURE 18-30 cont'd P, Cephalometric superimposition shows the changes that occurred, with some retraction of the upper but not the lower incisors. Because of the extreme bone loss, suckdown retainers, which splint the teeth, were used full-time for the first 6 months, then just at night. **Q,** Panoramic radiograph 1 year after the completion of treatment. Note that the periodontal condition remained stable. Some root resorption had already occurred before the orthodontic treatment began, especially on premolars and molars (see the initial periapical radiographs). These teeth were relatively unchanged, but some shortening of maxillary incisor roots did occur during the orthodontic treatment. It remains unclear whether patients who have experienced severe periodontal disease are more susceptible to root resorption during subsequent orthodontic treatment.

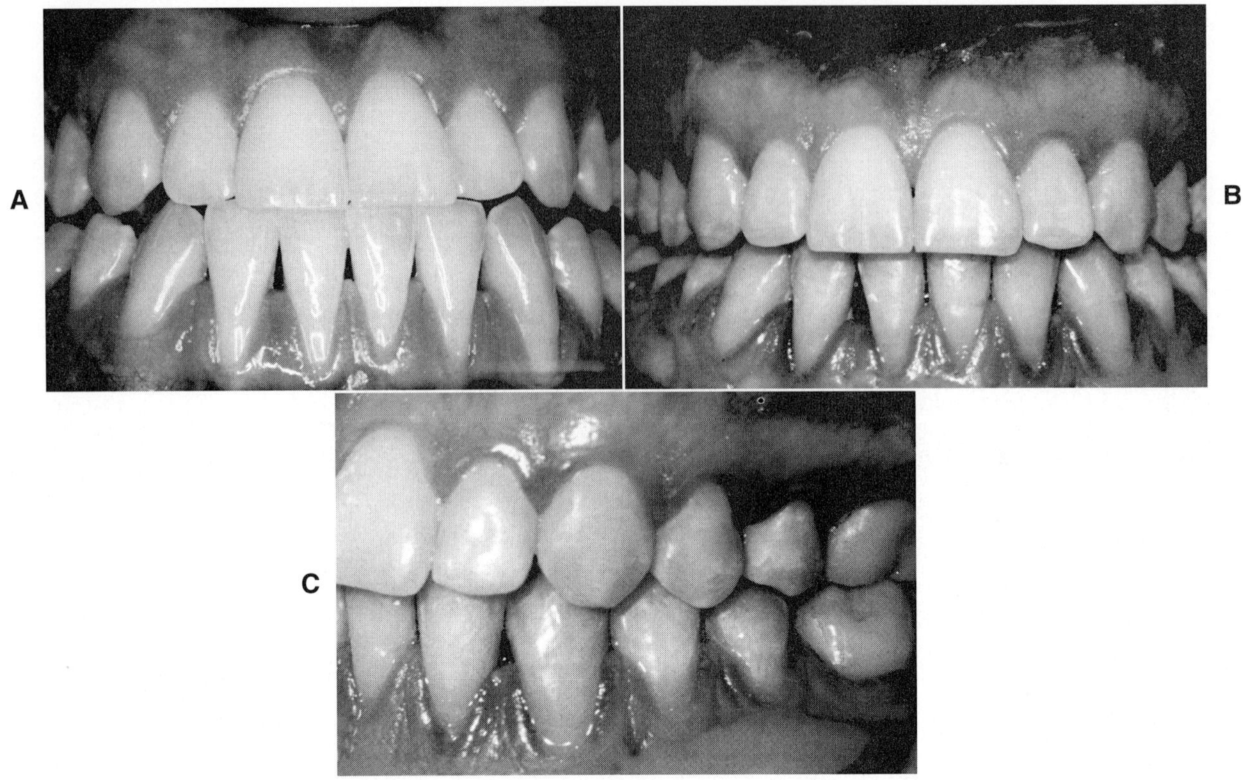

FIGURE 18-31 **A,** This young adult had been treated orthodontically with expansion of a crowded lower arch that led to gingival recession; **B, C,** After extensive gingival grafting and orthodontic-surgical re-treatment. It is much better to place a gingival graft before recession occurs, if there is a risk of recession.

It is interesting that even after severe periodontal problems have developed, orthodontic treatment can be carried out with further loss of alveolar bone *if* good control of the periodontal condition is maintained. Space closure in areas of major bone loss sometimes leads to an improvement in bone height (Figure 18-34), but this is unpredictable. Patients can be told that they can have comprehensive orthodontic treatment without undue risk of making their periodontal situation worse, but should not be promised an improvement.

Modifications in treatment mechanics are discussed at the end of this chapter.

Prosthodontic–Implant Interactions

Adults presenting for comprehensive orthodontic treatment often also have dental problems that require restorations. Such problems include loss of tooth structure from wear and abrasion or trauma, gingival esthetic problems, and missing teeth that require replacement with either conventional prosthodontics or implants.

Problems Related to Loss of Tooth Structure

The positioning of damaged, worn or abraded teeth during comprehensive orthodontics must be done with the eventual restorative plan in mind. Early consultation with the restorative dentist obviously becomes important. There are three particularly important considerations in deciding where the orthodontist should position teeth that are to be restored: the total amount of space that should be created, the mesiodistal positioning of the tooth within the space, and the buccolingual positioning (Figure 18-35).

When tooth structure has been lost all the way to beyond the normal contact point, the tooth becomes abnormally narrow, and restoration of the lost crown width as well as height is important. The orthodontic positioning obviously should provide adequate space for the appropriate addition of the restorative material. The ideal position may or may not be in the center of the space mesio-distally—this would depend on whether the most esthetic restoration would be produced by symmetric addition on each side of the tooth, or whether a larger build-up on one side would be better. Similarly, the ideal bucco-lingual position of a worn or damaged tooth would be influenced by how the restoration was planned. If a crown or composite build-ups are planned, the tooth should be in the center of the dental arch. But if a facial veneer is to be used (see Figure 18-35 and Figure 1-6), the orthodontist should place the tooth more lingually than otherwise would be the case, to allow for the thickness of the veneer on the facial surface. Finally, better restorations can be done if the orthodontist provides slightly more space than is required, so there is room for the restorative dentist to

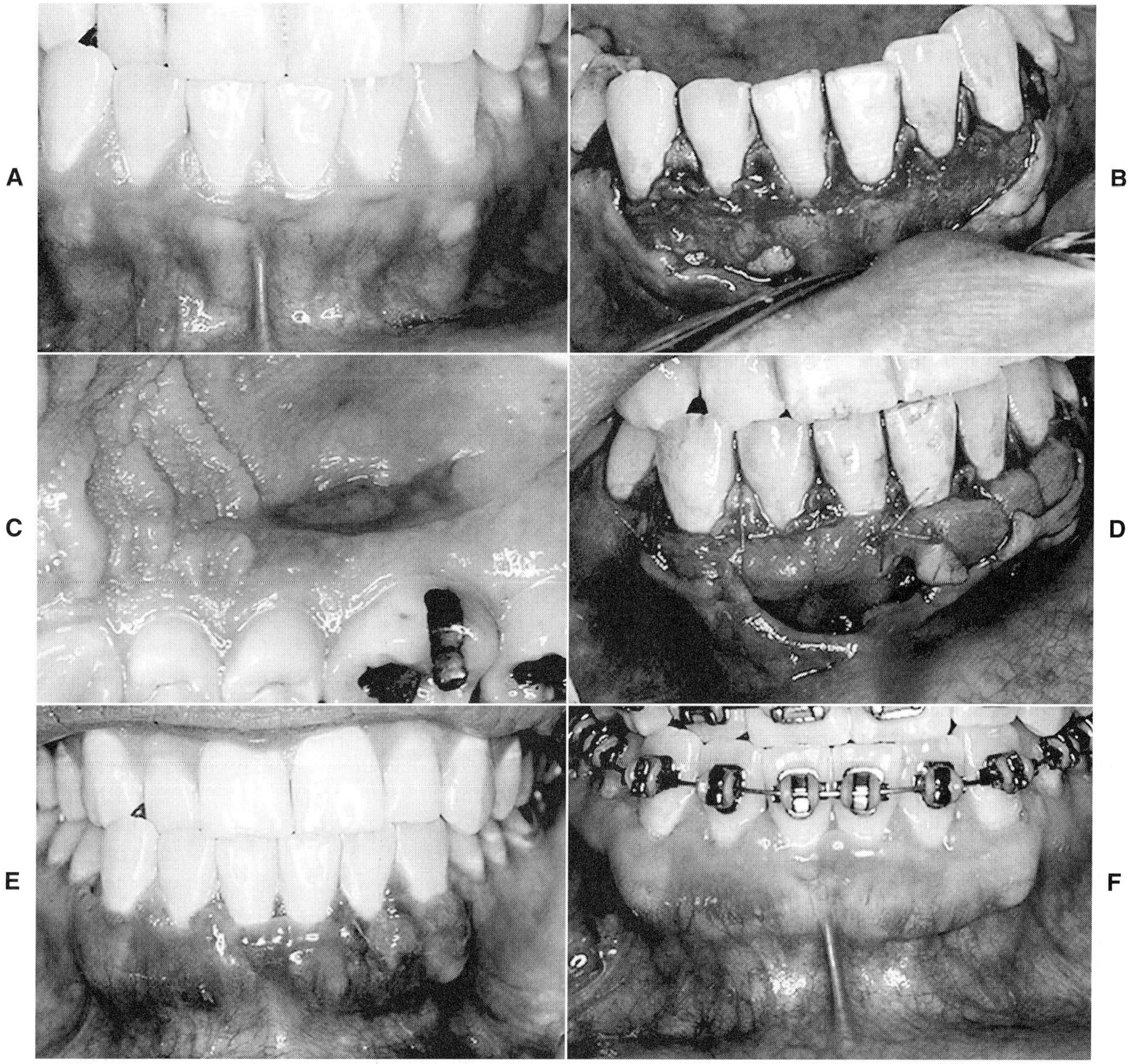

FIGURE 18-32 In adults who will have comprehensive orthodontic treatment, gingival grafting to create adequate quantity and thickness of attached gingiva is important before beginning orthodontic tooth movement. **A,** Lack of attached gingiva and thin gingival tissue in the mandibular anterior region in a patient whose lower incisors must be advanced to align them. Note the alveolar mucosa extending almost to the gingival margin on all anterior teeth; **B,** surgical preparation of a bed for grafting; **C,** the palatal donor site for tissue for the gingival graft; **D,** the graft sutured in place; **E,** healing 1 week later, showing incorporation of the grafts; **F,** initial alignment archwire in place 3 months later, with the gingival grafts creating both a thicker contour of the gingival tissue and a generous band of attachment. (Courtesy Dr. J. Morarity.)

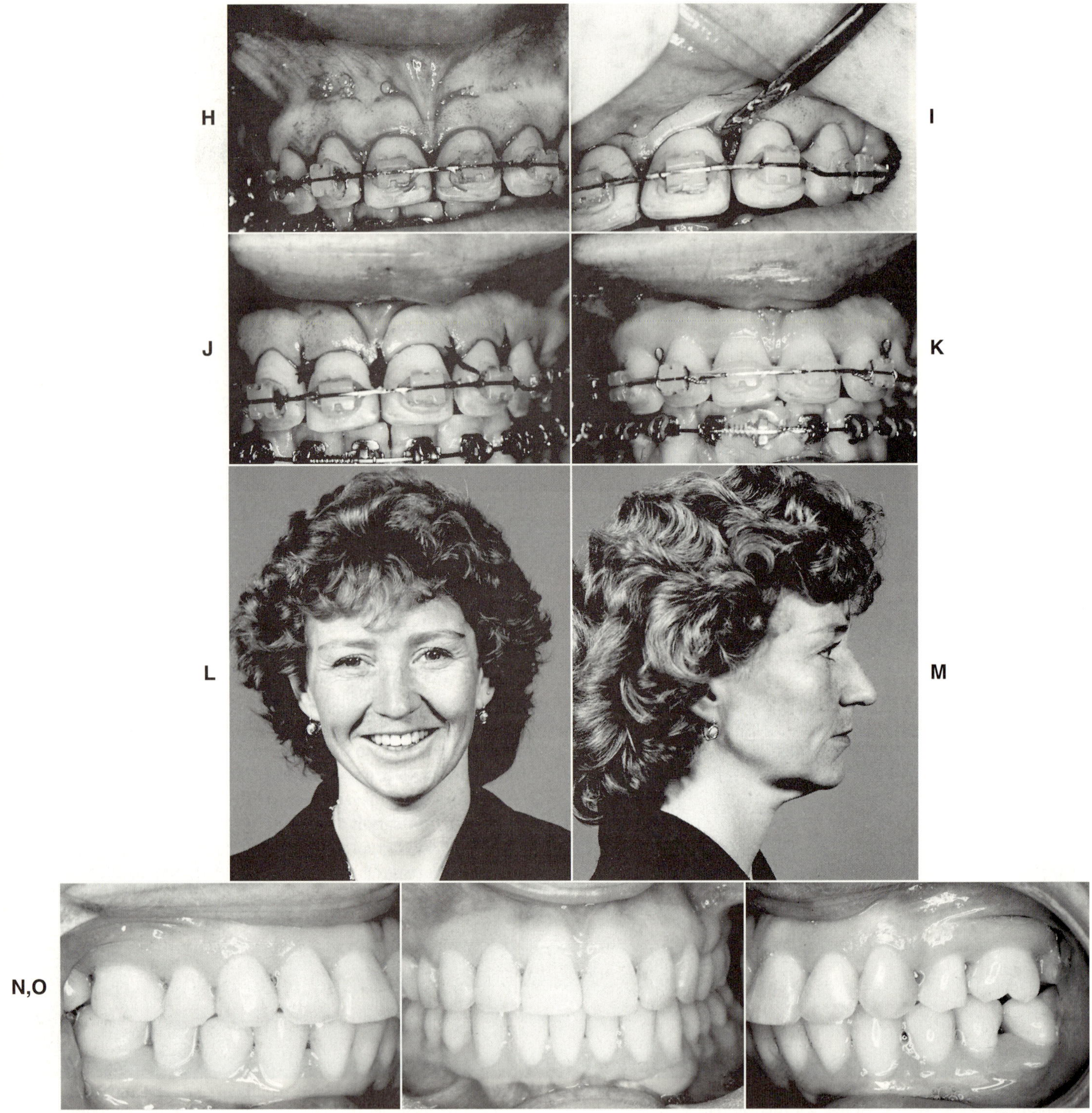

FIGURE 18-34 cont'd H to **J,** Because of the severe rotations of the irregular maxillary incisors, after alignment was completed but with the orthodontic appliance still in place, repositioning of the maxillary frenum and sectioning of the elastic gingival fibers were carried out; **K,** Three weeks later. **L** to **P,** After 18 months of treatment, both the occlusion and appearance of the teeth were greatly improved.

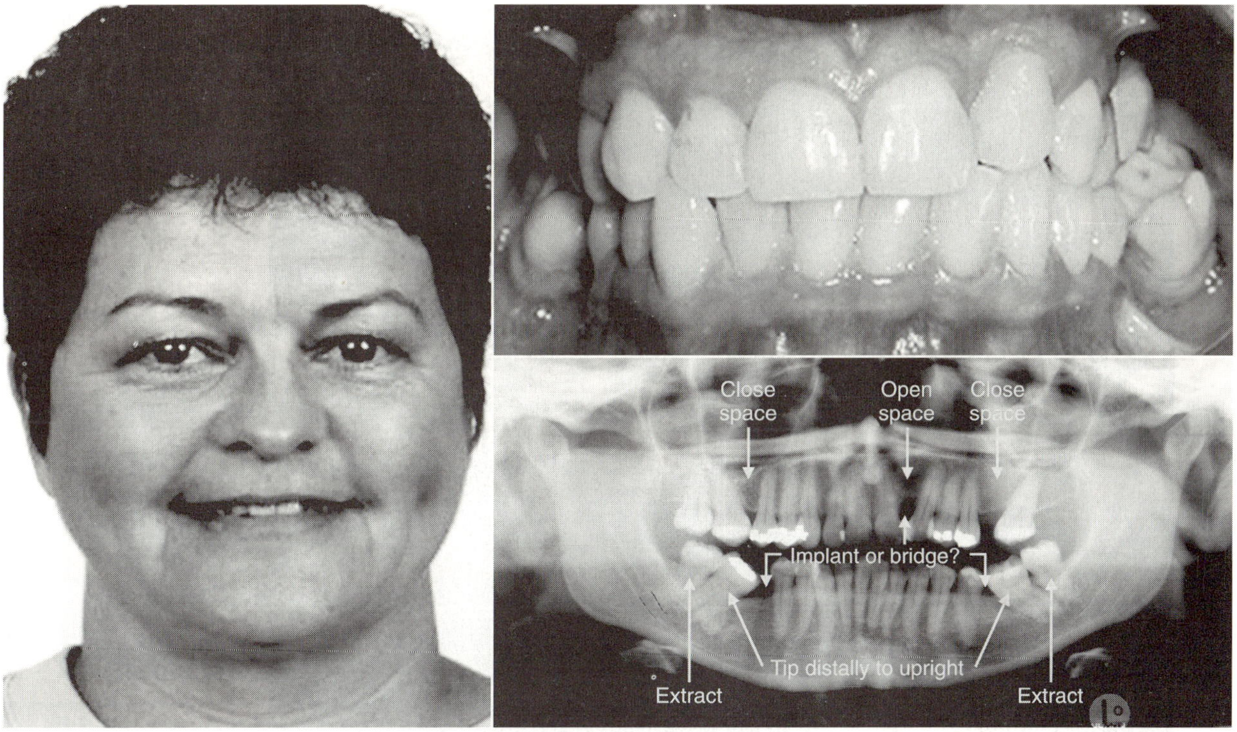

FIGURE 18-36 **A,** At age 48, this woman sought treatment to replace missing teeth and improve her appearance, especially her "crooked smile." She commented that she had provided orthodontic treatment for her two children and sent both through college, and "Now it's my turn". **B,** The maxillary left lateral incisor and all four first molars were missing. The left canine had had a composite buildup to close the remaining lateral incisor space. The maxillary posterior teeth were in a crossbite relationship, especially on the left side. **C,** Areas of periodontal bone loss were present, but at this point, active periodontal disease had been brought under control. The key questions in planning treatment revolved around whether to close old extraction spaces or open them for prosthetic replacements. To improve symmetry in the maxillary arch and obtain better smile esthetics, opening space for replacement of the missing lateral incisor was needed, and space closure in the maxillary left molar area would facilitate opening the anterior space. The mandibular third molars would be extracted so the second molars could be uprighted and rolled lingually to improve the crossbite.

by tipping it distally, and then a bridge is placed. If comprehensive treatment is planned, should the space be closed by bringing the first molar mesially? That depends very much on the specific problems of an individual patient (Figures 18-36, 18-37). Often it is better judgment to open a partially closed old extraction site and replace the missing tooth with a bridge or implant. This decision should be considered carefully in consultation between the orthodontist and prosthodontist.

If it is desired to move lower molars forward into an old first molar or second premolar extraction site, a temporary implant in the ramus can be used to provide the necessary anchorage and avoid retracting the lower anterior teeth. This technique, pioneered by Roberts,[16] offers a level of control that cannot be obtained in any other way (Figure 18-38). Mesial root movement is technically much more difficult than distal tipping, but the larger problem is that cortical bone remodeling usually is required to close the space because of atrophy after the old extraction. With only other teeth as anchorage, the anterior teeth are likely to be retracted more than desirable. Even with skeletal anchorage, the space closure is likely to be quite slow.

Tooth Loss Due to Periodontal Disease. A space closure problem is also posed by the loss of a tooth to periodontal disease. Sometimes closure of the space where a hopelessly involved tooth was extracted results in an improvement of the periodontal situation (see Figure 18-34). As a general rule, however, it is better to move teeth away from such an area, in preparation for a prosthetic replacement, because of the risk that normal bone formation will not occur as the tooth moves into the defect.

However, there is an exception. First molars and incisors are lost in some adolescents and young adults to aggressive periodontitis, which differentially attacks these teeth and is characterized by the presence of a specific microbe, *Actinobacillus actinomycetemcomitans.* Once the disease process has been brought under control, which now typically involves antibiotic therapy, the causative agent seems to disappear.[17] Although bone around the first molars is often totally destroyed, neither the second molar nor the second

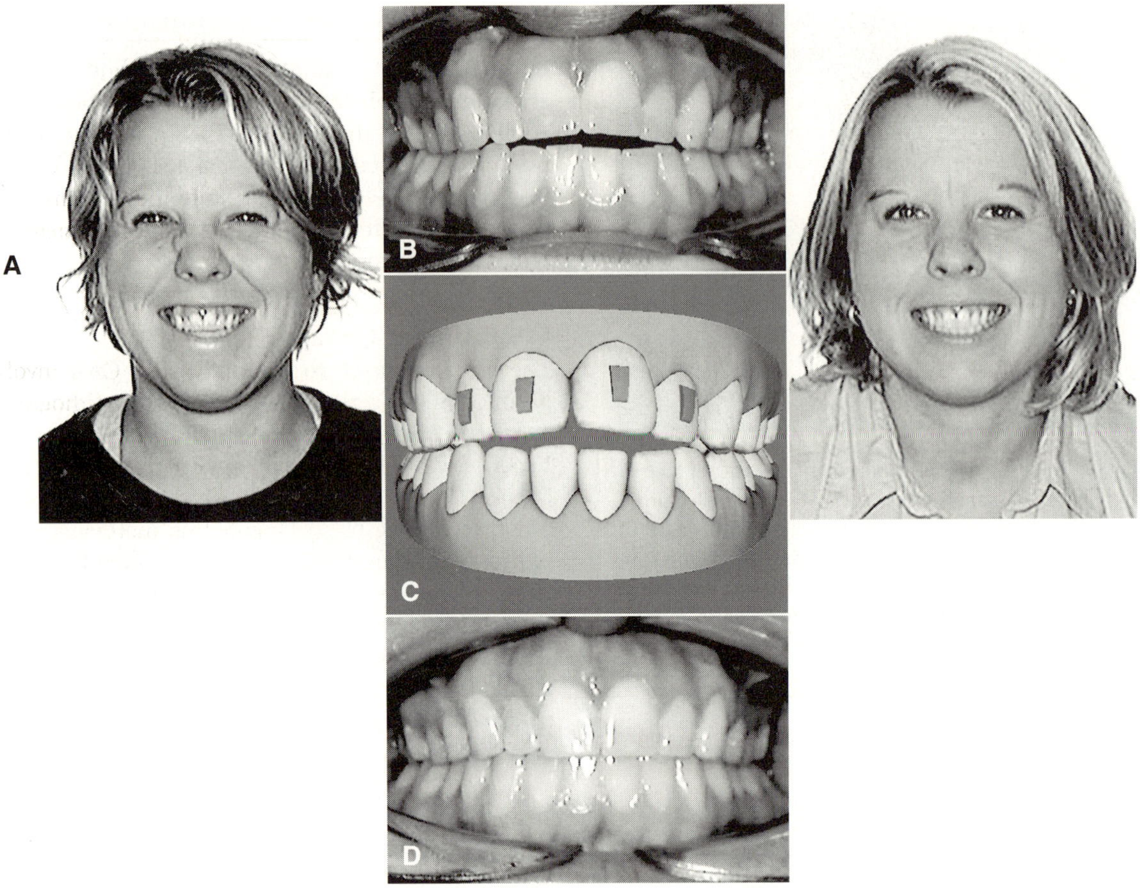

FIGURE 18-41 Extrusion of teeth, as in this patient to close an anterior open bite, is difficult with invisalign, but can be accomplished with the use of bonded attachments on the teeth so the aligners have a better grip. **A, B,** Age 24, prior to treatment. She reported previous orthodontic treatment at age 12; the open bite developed during subsequent adolescent growth. **C,** The ClinCheck form, showing the attachments to be placed on the teeth (see Figure 18-22 for the clinical appearance of clear plastic bonded attachments). Air-rotor stripping was performed in the upper arch to provide space to retract the incisors and reduce overbite (see Figure 11-16 for the reproximation form that accompanies the ClinCheck form when this is part of the treatment plan). She had 19 upper and 10 lower aligners. Treatment required $9^1/_2$ months. **D, E,** Age 25, after treatment. A lower bonded retainer and a maxillary suckdown retainer were placed. The occlusion was stable on 2-year recall. (Courtesy Dr. W. Gierie.)

do this that did not exist when lingual orthodontics was tried, and largely abandoned in the United States, in the late 1980s and early 1990s. Because the lingual surfaces of the incisors, canines, and posterior teeth do not line up nearly as well as the facial surfaces, there is no way to avoid considerable shaping of lingual archwires. Laser scans to obtain the information, and remotely forming the wires on a wire-bending robot, make archwire formation a much more precise and less time-consuming procedure now. One way to look at it is that although modern lingual orthodontics is quite different from clear aligner therapy, it is based on computer technology to a similar extent. With lingually-bonded brackets and archwires, any type of tooth movement now can be produced quite efficiently and root positioning at extraction sites is not a particular problem (Figures 18-42 to 18-44).

Intrusion and Skeletal Anchorage

Considerations for Intrusion

In adolescents and young adults (up to about age 18 in females and 20 in males), the choice between intrusion or extrusion to correct a deep overbite and level an excessive curve of Spee often can be resolved in favor of extrusion, because vertical growth will compensate for it. In adults, the choice often must be intrusion, which is much more effective when skeletal anchorage in the form of miniplates or screws is available, and when segmented rather than continuous archwires are used. The practical effect is to make both skeletal anchorage and segmented arch treatment more important in adults than in younger patients.

One potential problem with intrusion in periodontally involved adults is the prospect that a deepening of peri-

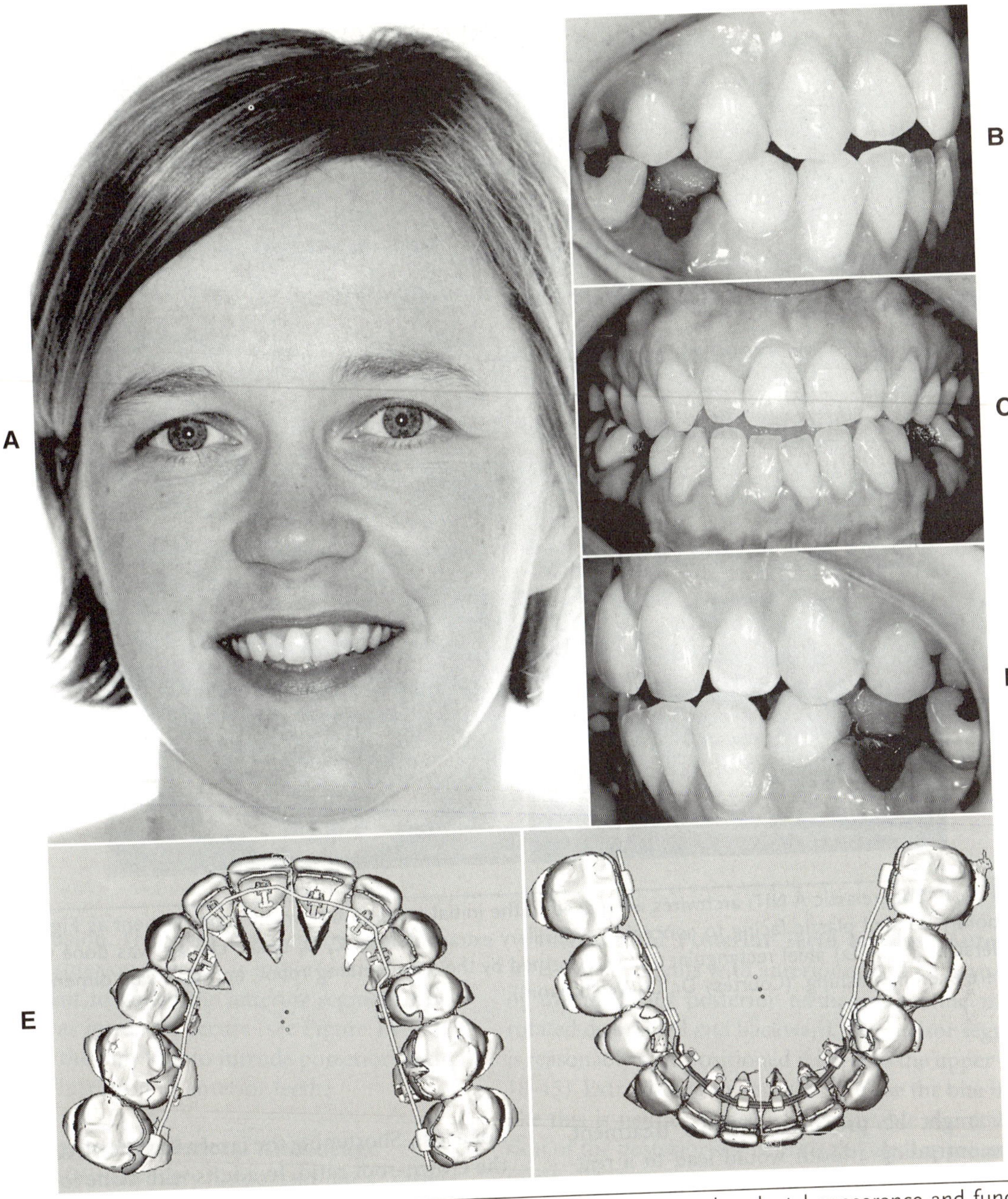

FIGURE 18-42 This 31-year-old woman sought orthodontic treatment to improve her dental appearance and function, and chose lingual orthodontics to avoid the outward appearance of braces on her teeth. **A,** Smile before treatment; **B** to **D,** Pretreatment intraoral views. She had moderately severe crowding of her lower incisors, posterior crossbite, and an anterior open bite that would have placed her in anterior crossbite if corrected without retraction of the lower incisors. Her maxillary right first premolar had been extracted when she was a child, and the dental midline was deviated to the right. The treatment plan called for extraction of the mandibular second premolars and maxillary left second premolar to provide space for alignment and repositioning of the anterior teeth. **E, F,** Laser scans of her dental casts were used in the Incognito software to plan both the contour of the custom lingual bonding pads for each tooth and the shape of the archwires that would be produced by a wire-bending robot. (Courtesy Dr. D. Weichmann.)

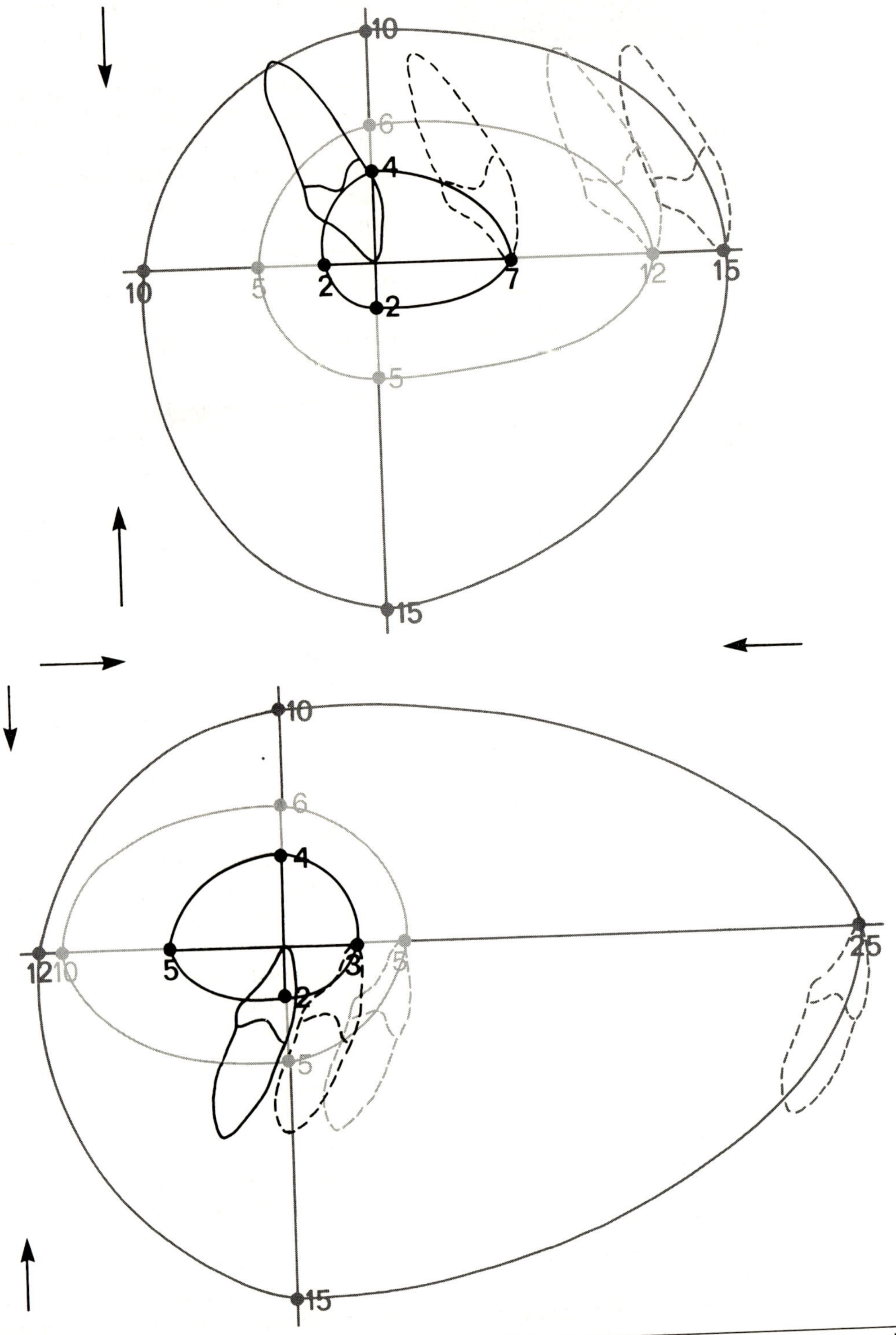

FIGURE 19-4 With the ideal position of the upper and lower incisors shown by the origin of the *x* and *y* axes, the envelope of discrepancy shows the amount of change that could be produced by orthodontic tooth movement alone (the inner envelope of each diagram); orthodontic tooth movement combined with growth modification (the middle envelope); and orthognathic surgery (the outer envelope). Note that the possibilities for each treatment are not symmetric with regard to the planes of space. There is more potential to retract than procline teeth and more potential for extrusion than intrusion. Since growth of the maxilla cannot be modified independently of the mandible, the growth modification envelope for the two jaws is the same. Surgery to move the lower jaw back has more potential than surgery to advance it.

G

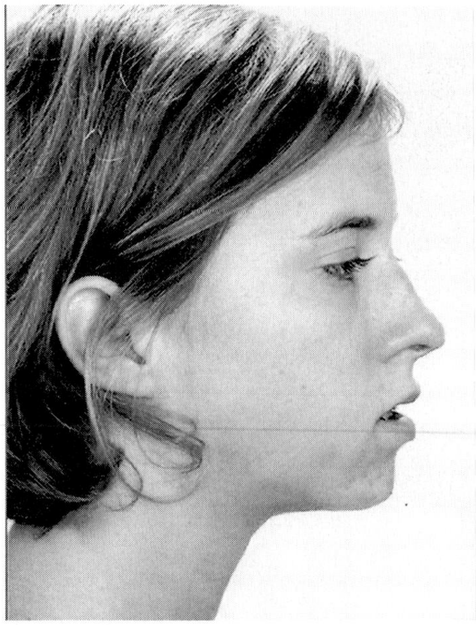

FIGURE 19-6 A, Pretreatment profile im
Class II malocclusion; **B,** The first step in c
position of a digitized cephalometric tracing
retraction of the protruding upper incisors.
bly would be more negative than positive; D
are protrusive relative to the chin, chin defic
augment the chin; **F,** Simulation of adding
and recontour the drooping nasal tip; **G,** C
outcome of treatment with this surgical pla
malocclusion.

alone, or lower first and upper second
general rule, Class III problems are less ar
flage than Class II, because retracting the
make the chin appear even more promin
site of effective camouflage (see Figure 8-3
ration of a Class III patient often requ
upper first premolars so that upper inciso
correcting their axial inclination and inc
overjet (Figure 19-7). If space were needed
second rather than first premolar extra
I logical choice so that the lower incisors w

It obviously is important for the pati
treated either way to understand all these
the decision between camouflage and sur
patient can and must make the decision, i
some conditions can be treated better
alone than others, simply because the
esthetics is likely to be better. Some chara
make the difference between satisfactory
as ment and failure are summarized in Box
ar covered in considerable detail in recent te

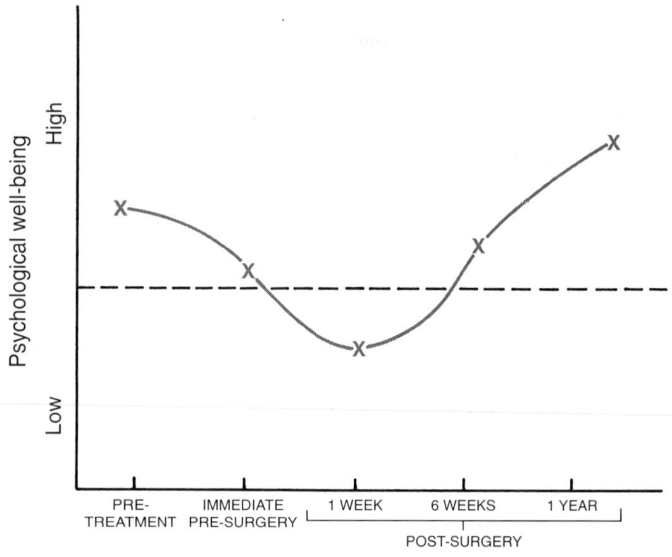

FIGURE 19-5 A generalized representation of the typical psychological response to orthognathic surgery, based on the work of Kiyak.[9] Prior to treatment, patients who seek orthognathic surgery tend to be above the mean on most psychologic parameters. Immediately before surgery, they are not quite so positive, as anxiety and other concerns increase. In the days immediately after surgery, a period of negativism typically occurs (depression, dissatisfaction, etc.). This is related in part to steroid use at surgery and withdrawal afterward, but is not totally explained by this. By six weeks post-surgery, the patients usually are well on the positive side of normal again, and at one year typically rate quite high for satisfaction with treatment and general psychological well-being.

Computer Simulation of Alternative Treatment Outcomes

It always has been a moral and ethical imperative to allow the patient to make important decisions about what treatment he or she will accept, and now it is a legal obligation as well.[5] Involving the patient as decisions are made about the choice of alternative treatments is an essential element of informed consent (see Chapter 7).

Computer image predictions are particularly valuable in helping patients decide between camouflage and surgery, and in planning surgical treatment. The patient can view the impact on the soft tissue profile of orthodontic camouflage versus surgery when these are realistic treatment alternatives (Figure 19-6), and also view the effect of varying amounts of surgical change—more or less mandibular advancement, for example, or the effect of genioplasty or rhinoplasty in addition to change in jaw position. Predictions of changes in the frontal view still are art work rather than scientifically based, but current computer prediction programs do a good job of predicting profile changes,[7] and steady improvements continue to occur. It is one thing to describe in words what the different outcomes of camouflage and surgery would be, and something else to help the patient visualize it by seeing image predictions.

At one point, there was great concern that showing predictions to patients might lead to unrealistic expectations and disappointment with the actual result, but patient responses show that this risk is minimal or non-existent. In a randomized trial, those who saw the prediction images before surgery were more, not less likely to be satisfied with their result.[8] Only the patient can decide whether the difference between surgical correction of jaw relationships and orthodontic camouflage would be worth it in terms of the additional risk and cost of surgery. Computer simulations help them do that.

Extraction of Teeth and the Camouflage/Surgery Decision

The decision for camouflage or surgery must be made before treatment begins, because the orthodontic treatment to prepare for surgery often is just the opposite of orthodontic treatment for camouflage. It is a serious error to attempt camouflage on the theory that if it fails, the patient can then be referred for surgical correction. At that point, another phase of "reverse orthodontics" to eliminate the effects of the original treatment will be required before surgery can provide both normal jaw relationships and normal occlusion.

The critical importance of deciding on camouflage or surgery at the beginning of treatment is illustrated by the difference in extractions needed with the two approaches. In camouflage, extraction spaces are used to produce dental compensations for the jaw discrepancy and the extractions are planned accordingly. For example, with orthodontic treatment alone, a patient with mandibular deficiency and a Class II malocclusion might have upper first premolars removed to allow the retraction of the maxillary anterior teeth. Extraction in the lower arch would be avoided and the lower incisors probably would be proclined to help reduce the overjet (Figure 19-6, *C*).

The extraction pattern for this same patient would be quite different if mandibular advancement were planned. Instead of creating dental compensation for the jaw deformity, the orthodontic treatment now would be planned to remove it. In the upper arch the position of the incisors relative to the maxilla often is normal or retrusive; if so, upper premolar extraction would be undesirable. Often in mandibular deficiency the lower incisors are protrusive relative to the chin. Then there are two possibilities: extraction in the lower arch to retract them and temporarily increase the overjet so the chin will be brought further forward when the mandible is advanced, or a lower border osteotomy to move the chin forward (Figure 19-6, *D*).

A similar but reversed situation would be seen in a patient with a skeletal Class III problem. If camouflage were planned, typical extractions might be lower first premolars

A

C

E

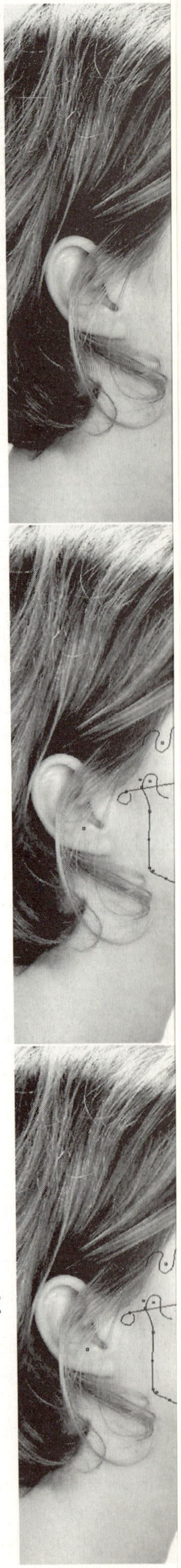

U